Blackwell's Five-Minute Veterinary Consult

Clinical Companion

Small Animal Dermatology

Third Edition

Blackwell's Five-Minute Veterinary Consult
Clinical Companion

Small Animal Dermatology

Third Edition

Karen Helton Rhodes
Ceffyl Consulting, LLC
Edisto Island, South Carolina, USA

Alexander H. Werner
Animal Dermatology Center
Studio City and Westlake Village, California and Reno, Nevada, U.S.A

WILEY Blackwell

This third edition first published 2018

Edition History
Lippincott, Williams, and Wilkins (1e, 2002), Wiley-Blackwell (2e, 2011)

Registered Office
John Wiley & Sons, Inc., 111 River Street, Hoboken, NJ 07030, USA

Editorial Office
The Atrium, Southern Gate, Chichester, West Sussex, PO19 8SQ, UK

For details of our global editorial offices, customer services, and more information about Wiley products visit us at www.wiley.com.

Wiley also publishes its books in a variety of electronic formats and by print-on-demand. Some content that appears in standard print versions of this book may not be available in other formats.

Library of Congress Cataloging-in-Publication Data

Names: Rhodes, Karen Helton, author. | Werner, Alexander H., author.
Title: Blackwell's five-minute veterinary consult clinical companion. Small animal dermatology / by Karen Helton Rhodes, Alexander H. Werner.
Other titles: Five-minute veterinary consult clinical companion. Small animal dermatology | Small animal dermatology
Description: Third edition. | Hoboken, NJ : Wiley, 2018. | Series: Blackwell's five-minute veterinary consult | Includes bibliographical references and index. |
Identifiers: LCCN 2017050000 (print) | LCCN 2017051137 (ebook) | ISBN 9781119337225 (pdf) | ISBN 9781119337294 (epub) | ISBN 9781119337249 (pbk.)
Subjects: LCSH: Dogs–Diseases–Handbooks, manuals, etc. | Cats–Diseases–Handbooks, manuals, etc. | Veterinary dermatology–Handbooks, manuals, etc. | Exotic animals–Diseases–Handbooks, manuals, etc. | MESH: Dog Diseases | Skin Diseases–veterinary | Cat Diseases | Handbooks
Classification: LCC SF992.S55 (ebook) | LCC SF992.S55 R46 2018 (print) | NLM SF 992.S55 | DDC 636.089/65–dc23
LC record available at https://lccn.loc.gov/2017050000

Cover image: Courtesy of Alexander Werner
Cover design by Wiley

Set in 10.5/13pt BerkeleyStd by Aptara Inc., New Delhi, India
Printed and bound in Singapore by Markono Print Media Pte Ltd

1 2018

This text is dedicated to:

To the eternal student
Karen Helton Rhodes

Mike
Alexander H. Werner

Contents

Preface ix
About the Companion Website xi

section 1 Basics 1

chapter **1** Epidermis in Clinical Dermatology 3
chapter **2** Lesion Description/Terminology 11
chapter **3** Diagnostic Culture and Identification (Bacterial and Fungal) 28
chapter **4** Obtaining a Diagnostic Biopsy 36
chapter **5** Practical Cytology 43
chapter **6** Symptom Checker (Lesional and Regional Dermatoses) 59
chapter **7** Antibiotic Stewardship and Emerging Resistant Bacterial Infections . . . 142

section 2 Diseases/Disorders 155

chapter **8** Acne (Canine and Feline) 157
chapter **9** Anal Furunculosis/Perianal Fistula 161
chapter **10** Anal Sac Disorders 169
chapter **11** Atopic Disease 173
chapter **12** Autoimmune Blistering Diseases 187
chapter **13** Bacterial Pyoderma 211
chapter **14** Behavioral or Self-Injurious Dermatoses 227
chapter **15** Biting and Stinging Insects 239
chapter **16** Contact Dermatitis 265
chapter **17** Cutaneous Adverse Drug Reaction, Erythema Multiforme, Stevens–Johnson Syndrome, and Toxic Epidermal Necrolysis 272
chapter **18** Cutaneous Adverse Food Reactions 286
chapter **19** Demodicosis (Canine and Feline) 296
chapter **20** Dermatomyositis, Canine Familial 312
chapter **21** Dermatophytosis 320
chapter **22** Endocrinopathies, Atypical 337
chapter **23** Eosinophilic Disease (Granuloma) Complex 351

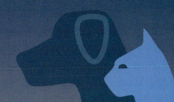

chapter **24** Epitheliotropic (Cutaneous) Lymphoma . . . 365
chapter **25** Histiocytic Proliferative Disorders . . . 380
chapter **26** Hyperadrenocorticism, Canine . . . 394
chapter **27** Hyperadrenocorticism, Feline Skin Fragility Syndrome . . . 409
chapter **28** Hypothyroidism . . . 416
chapter **29** Keratinization (Cornification) Disorders . . . 430
chapter **30** Leishmaniasis: Protozoan Dermatitis . . . 458
chapter **31** Lupus Erythematosus . . . 467
chapter **32** *Malassezia* Dermatitis . . . 480
chapter **33** Mast Cell Tumors . . . 494
chapter **34** Mycobacterial Infections . . . 510
chapter **35** Mycoses, Deep . . . 521
chapter **36** Nocardiosis and Actinomycosis . . . 535
chapter **37** Otitis Externa, Media, and Interna . . . 541
chapter **38** Panniculitis . . . 563
chapter **39** Photodermatoses . . . 574
chapter **40** Pododermatitis and Claw Disorders . . . 588
chapter **41** Pre- and Paraneoplastic Syndromes . . . 615
chapter **42** Sarcoptid Mites . . . 634
chapter **43** Sebaceous Adenitis, Granulomatous . . . 648
chapter **44** Sporotrichosis . . . 658
chapter **45** Superficial Necrolytic Dermatitis . . . 665
chapter **46** Tumors, Common Skin and Hair Follicle . . . 672
chapter **47** Uveodermatologic Syndrome . . . 692
chapter **48** Vasculitis . . . 698
chapter **49** Viral Dermatoses . . . 711
chapter **50** Zoonosis . . . 727
appendix **A** Canine Genodermatoses . . . 731
appendix **B** Drug Formulary . . . 747

Index . . . 821

Preface

This third edition of *Blackwell's Five-Minute Veterinary Consult Clinical Companion: Small Animal Dermatology* has been revised in both content and format.

The content is a compilation of current scientific literature and "state of the art" clinical specialty medicine in a compact handbook. This third edition presents a new body of work intended to complement but not duplicate the information found in *Blackwell's Five-Minute Veterinary Consult: Canine and Feline*. The *living epidermis* is briefly explored in relationship to clinical disorders. An introductory *lesional and regional differentials* chapter is formatted to act as a "symptom checker" to help direct the clinician. Diagnostic plans and therapeutic options are specifically outlined for each disorder. When appropriate, clinical and therapeutic myths are countered with scientific information to aid in daily clinician/client conversations.

We have retained the "easy to scan" bullet layout and included even more clinical color photographs to illustrate the text. The majority of photographs have been replaced or updated from previous editions. The chapters have been arranged in an alphabetical format for quick reference. An appendix of common canine genodermatoses is included with a listing of genetic reference labs for diagnostic purposes. A formulary of common dermatologic therapeutics is provided.

This dermatology *Clinical Companion* was written for both the veterinary clinician and the student of veterinary medicine. It is intended as a quick informative reference and vital clinical resource. The large number of clinical photographs and simplistic style also make this text a valuable addition to your client library in the examination room or reception area.

Karen Helton Rhodes and Alexander H. Werner

About the Companion Website

This book is accompanied by a companion website:

www.fiveminutevet.com/dermatology

The website includes:

- Client education handouts

section 1

BASICS

chapter 1

Epidermis in Clinical Dermatology

DEFINITION/OVERVIEW

- The skin is the largest organ in the body.
- Functions of the skin include (among others):
    - Physical barrier
    - Thermoregulation
    - Environmental protection
    - Immunoregulation
    - Sensory perception
    - Antimicrobial activity.
- The skin can renew itself and thus respond to a variety of hostile factors.
- The process of cell migration within the epidermis from the stratum basale to the stratum corneum (epidermal renewal) takes approximately 22 days.
- Epidermal renewal time line can be useful when discussing duration necessary for clinical improvement.
- A helpful correlation for the client may be to compare epidermal renewal to the short length of time that a suntan will last.
- The process of renewing the epidermis is a series of complex organized steps of:
    - Controlled cell renewal
    - Cell death
    - Cell removal.
- The epidermis – more specifically, the stratum corneum or "skin barrier" – has recently been the focus of research regarding the pathobiomechanisms of disease as well as for therapeutic advances.

Blackwell's Five-Minute Veterinary Consult Clinical Companion: Small Animal Dermatology, Third Edition.
Karen Helton Rhodes and Alexander H. Werner.

STRATUM CORNEUM BARRIER

- The outer portion of the epidermis, the stratum corneum, is composed of approximately 20 overlapping layers and is considered the skin's barrier. The stratum corneum layer (Figures 1.1, 1.2):
- Controls hydration by restricting water movement into and out of the skin. (i.e., 0.5 mL water vapor is lost through the normal stratum corneum per day in human skin)
- Is the primary defense against environmental hazards such as allergens, pollutants, and irritants by continuous desquamation (renewal and removal)
- Maintains homeostasis with commensal organisms via the production of antimicrobial peptides
- Absorbs UV light to protect sensitive underlying tissue.

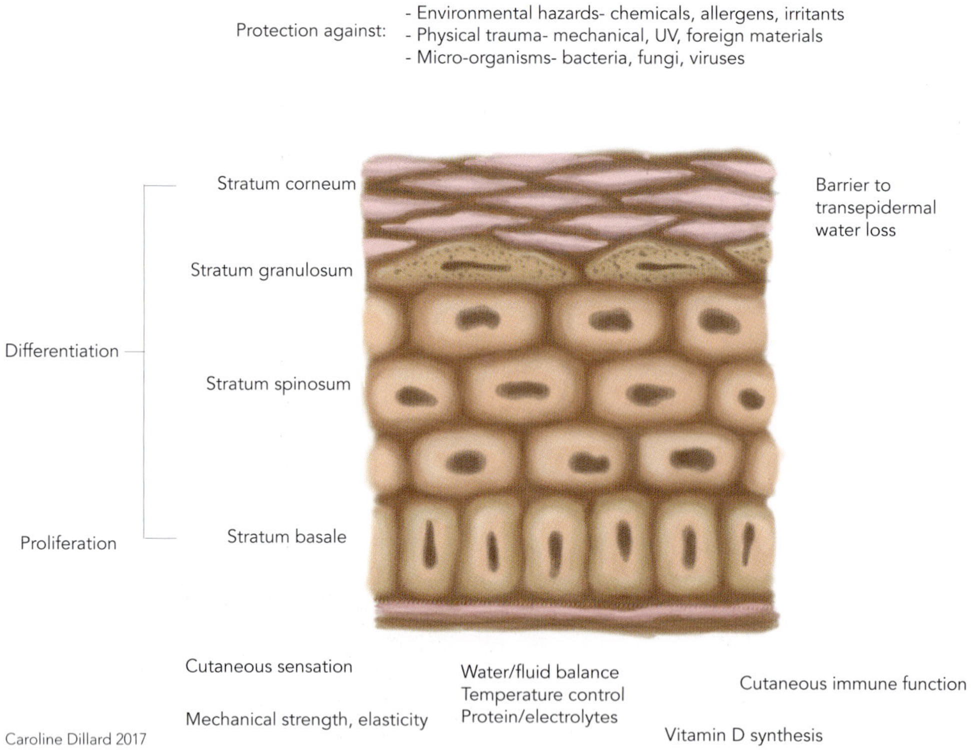

Fig. 1.1. Epidermal influence on homeostasis. Courtesy of Caroline Dillard.

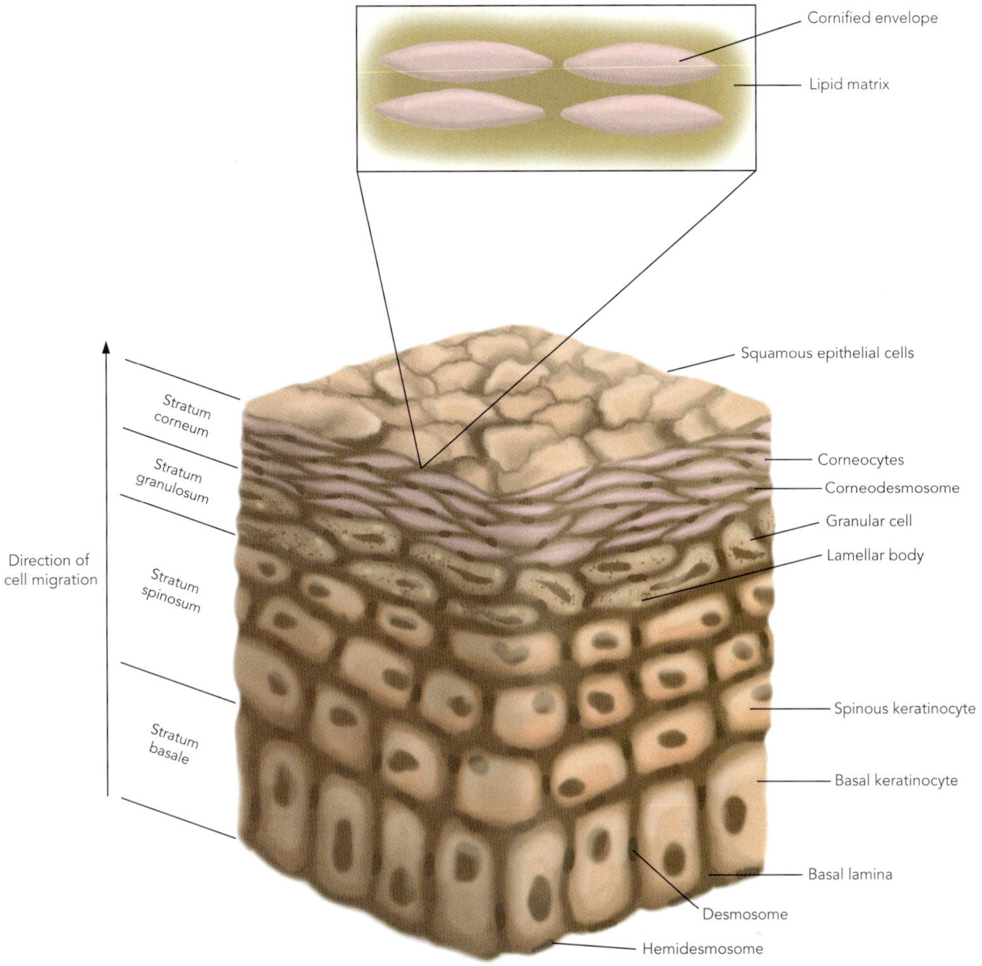

Fig. 1.2. Layers of the epidermis. Courtesy of Caroline Dillard.

PROCESS OF CORNIFICATION/KERATINIZATION

- Outline of basic steps in the cornification process to form the skin barrier (Figure 1.3).
    - Step 1: bundling of keratin within the corneocyte (keratinocyte) (Figure 1.4).
    - Step 2: replacement of the cell membrane with a thick cornified envelope (Figure 1.5).
    - Step 3: formation of lamellar lipid bilayers (Figure 1.6).
    - Step 4: desquamation (Figure 1.7).

- The final product of cornification is a tough hydrophobic "bricks and mortar" layer (Figure 1.8).
- The entire process of cell migration from the stratum basale to stratum corneum during normal cornification takes approximately 22 days in the dog.
- Understanding the specific steps of cornification is vital to the understanding of various clinical disorders.
- Defects in one small step of the cornification process can influence the entire process.

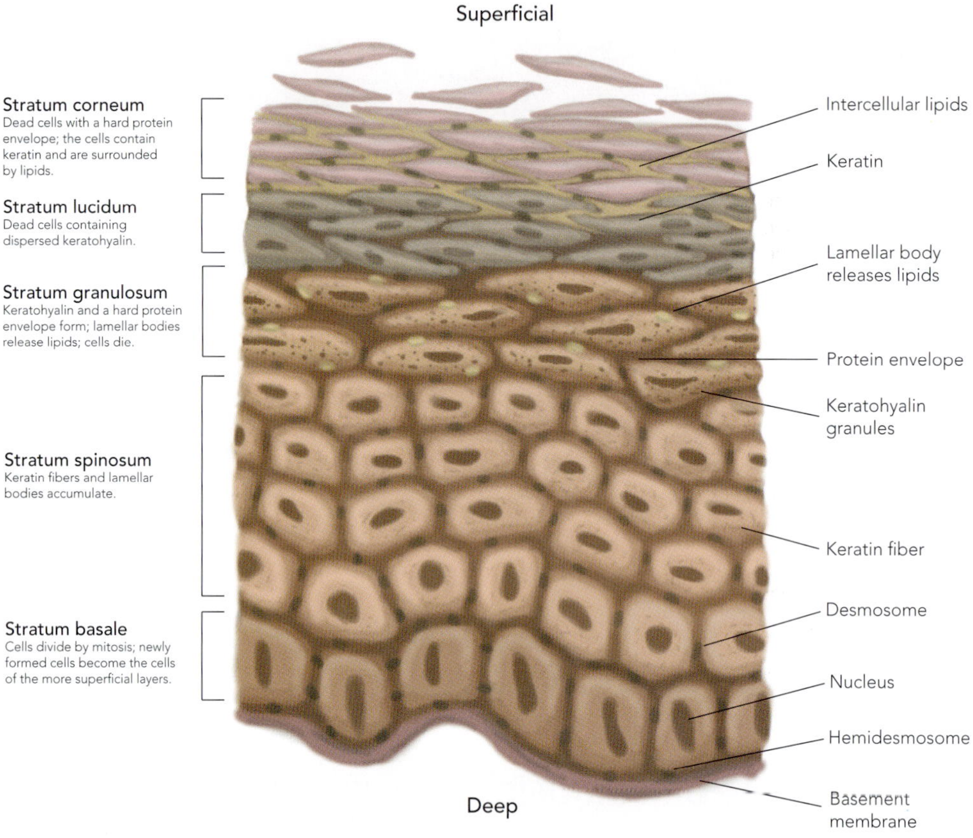

Fig. 1.3. Simplified process of cornification/keratinization. Courtesy of Caroline Dillard.

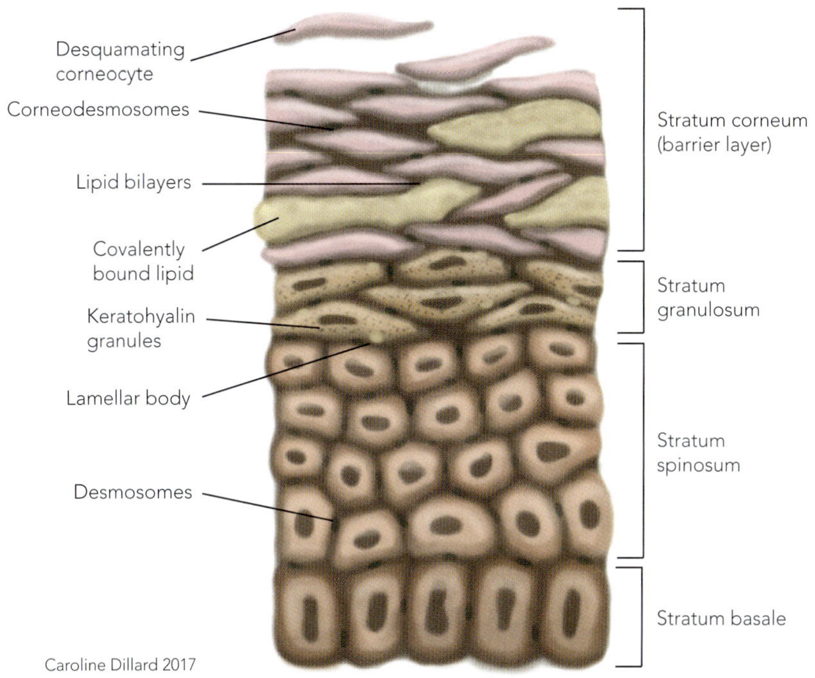

■ **Fig. 1.4.** Cornification step 1, bundling of keratin. Cell nuclei and organelles undergo proteolysis. Profillagrin in keratohyalin granules of the stratum granulosum layer dephosphorylates to fillagrin. Fillagrin bundles loose keratin filaments in the cell into a core unit. Courtesy of Caroline Dillard.

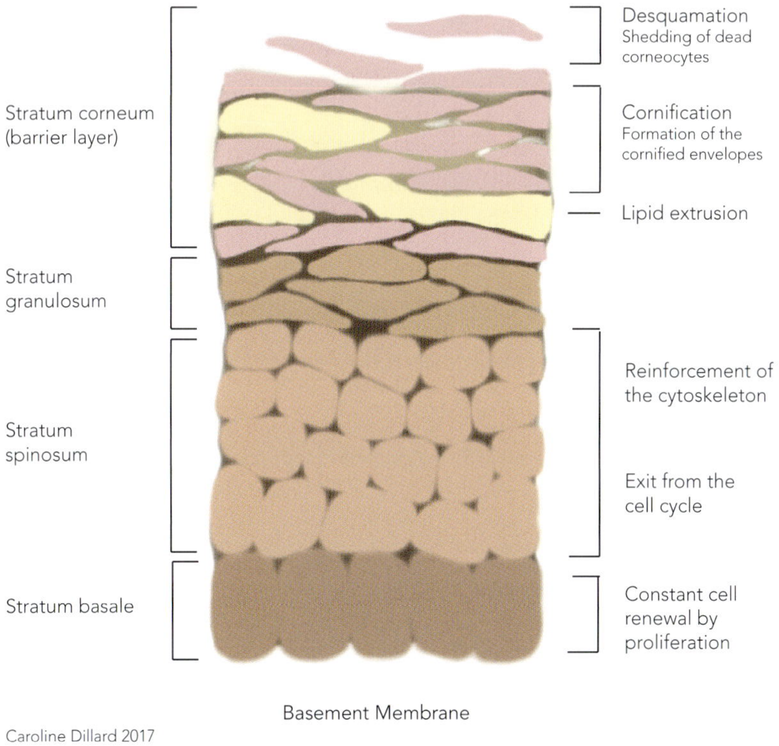

■ **Fig. 1.5.** Cornification step 2, transformation of the cell membrane into a cell envelope. Transglutaminases mediate calcium-dependent cross-linking of small peptides. Plasma membrane of the keratinocyte becomes a tough protein layer called the corneocyte envelope. Courtesy of Caroline Dillard.

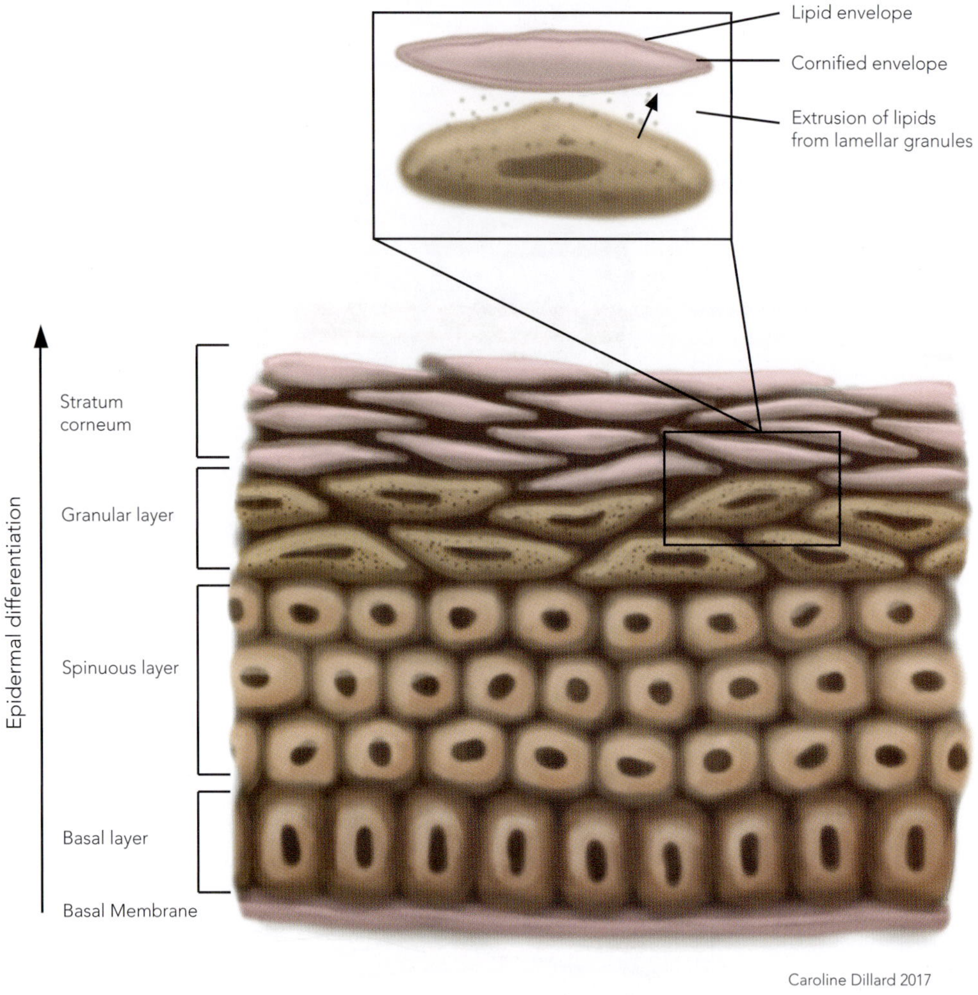

■ **Fig. 1.6.** Cornification step 3, formation of lipid bilayers. Lamellar bodies (small organelles containing lipid) are formed in the stratum spinosum. Lipid is secreted into the intercellular spaces at the level of the stratum granulosum and stratum corneum and forms into lamellar bilayers. Intercellular lipids include cholesterol, long-chain fatty acids, and ceramides. Courtesy of Caroline Dillard.

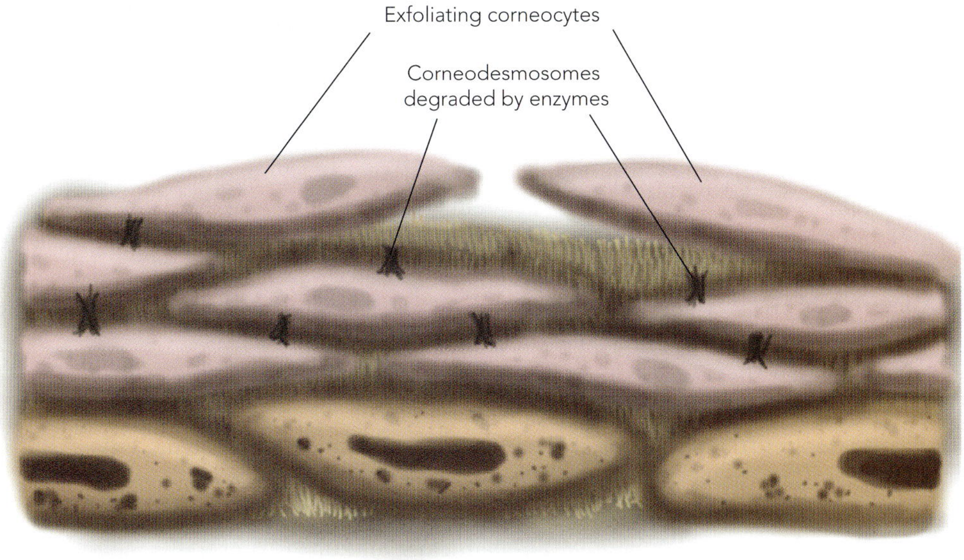

■ **Fig. 1.7.** Cornification step 4, desquamation. Proteases cleave intercorneocyte adhesions (desmosomes). Squames (exfoliating corneocytes), seen as scales or flakes, are released into the environment. Courtesy of Caroline Dillard.

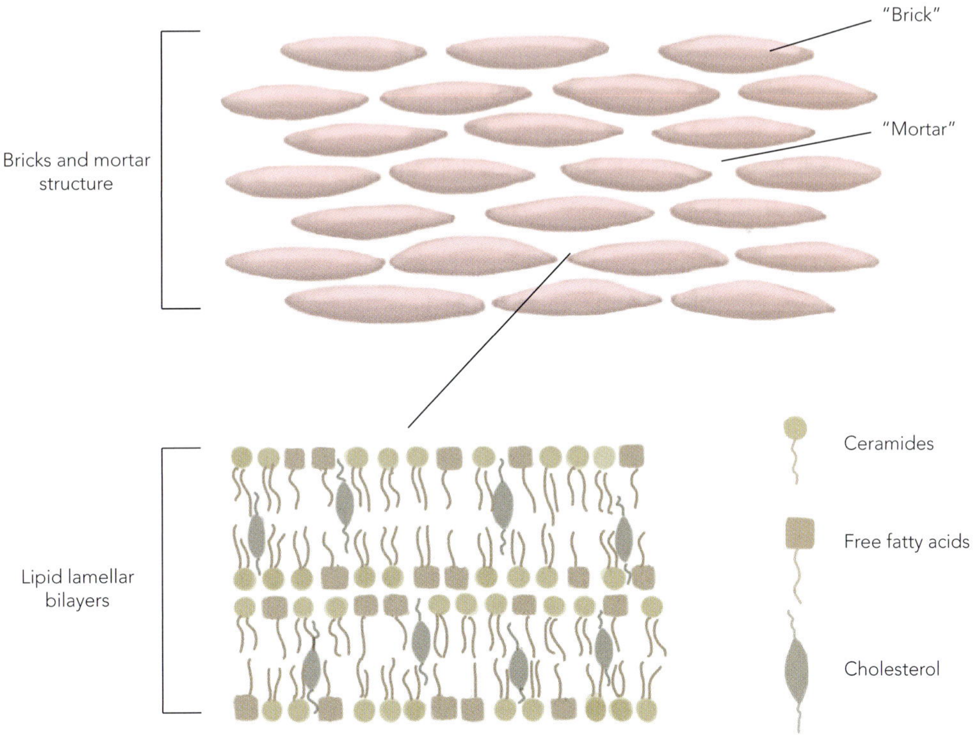

■ **Fig. 1.8.** Final product of cornification is a tough hydrophobic "bricks and mortar" layer that is a biochemically active barrier; bricks (corneocytes) and mortar (lipid). Courtesy of Caroline Dillard.

CATEGORIES OF SKIN BARRIER IMPAIRMENT

- Disorders can be divided into primary and secondary issues.
- Primary: defects in proteins or enzymes necessary for normal cornification.
- Secondary: inflammatory disorders that may have a negative effect on skin barrier function.
- An extensive list of factors (enzymes, proteins, etc.) can influence and regulate the process.
- Alteration in any step can lead to barrier dysfunction and abnormalities in permeability leading to clinical disorders (e.g., canine ichthyosis).
- There is much discussion regarding the relationship of atopic dermatitis and skin barrier function.
    - It is not currently known if there is a primary defect in these patients or if the alterations in the skin barrier are secondary to inflammation.
    - Most studies have shown some level of skin barrier abnormality in dogs with atopic dermatitis – functionally, chemically, and ultrastructurally.
    - The concept of skin barrier "repair" has also become important therapeutically (oral and topical).
    - Measurement of transepidermal water loss (TEWL) is a common tool to assess skin barrier function.

COMMENTS

- The skin is the only anatomic and physiologic barrier between the animal and the surrounding environment.
- It is not a simplistic cover but a living, vital, responsive organ.
- The skin has certain predictable reaction patterns (erythema, lichenification, etc.) that can aid the clinician in the establishment of a list of differential diagnoses.
- The skin may also relay information and clues regarding systemic processes (cutaneous manifestations of systemic disease).
- The skin is the most visible organ of the body, making it of vital concern for pet owners.

chapter 2

Lesion Description/ Terminology

DEFINITION/OVERVIEW

- The skin is the largest organ of the body; evaluating it in health and in disease can be overwhelming.
- An organized approach to the definition and recording of dermatologic lesions is helpful for the diagnosis and the monitoring of patients.
- From the macroscopic pattern to the specific lesion type, with an accurate description, an overall picture should emerge.
- Dermatologic diseases are often recurrent conditions: concise documentation in the record of the history and physical findings permits formulation of the differential list leading to a final diagnosis.
- Most electronic medical records limit record keeping to word descriptions of lesions; concise and accurate depictions require understanding of lesions and their causes.
- Practitioners should familiarize themselves with common dermatologic terminology to “paint a picture” with words.
- Example of a typical case description of flea allergic dermatitis might read: dorsal lumbosacral patch of alopecia with papules, crusts, excoriations, and lichenification.

DERMATOLOGIC TERMINOLOGY

- Terms to describe the overall hair coat:
  - Shiny
  - Dull
  - Oily
  - Dry
  - Brittle
  - Thick
  - Thin/hypotrichosis (partial alopecia)
  - Absent (alopecia)
  - Color:
    - Generalized changes from normal
    - Associated with specific colored hair.

Blackwell's Five-Minute Veterinary Consult Clinical Companion: Small Animal Dermatology, Third Edition.
Karen Helton Rhodes and Alexander H. Werner.

- Distribution of lesions:
  - Symmetrical or asymmetrical
  - Regional (examples):
    - Face/muzzle/head
    - Pinnae
    - Eyelid/periocular
    - Dorsal muzzle
    - Lipfold
    - Chin
    - Neck
    - Nasal planum
    - Mucous membrane (all or a specific region)
    - Mucocutaneous junction
    - Dorsal
    - Ventral
    - Truncal
    - Abdominal
    - Flank
    - Tail
    - Extremity
    - Paws/palmar/plantar
    - Claw/claw fold
    - Footpad.
- Pattern:
  - Diffuse
  - Generalized
  - Focal
  - Multifocal
  - Localized
  - Patchy
  - Regional.

CLINICAL FEATURES: PRIMARY LESIONS VERSUS SECONDARY LESIONS

- Primary lesions develop directly from the disease process:
  - Scale: a thin accumulation of keratinocytes; further defined as fine, coarse, greasy, dry, adherent, or loose (Figure 2.1); the normal skin sheds imperceptible individual cells; abnormal adhesion/dysadhesion of cells results in clumping of cells visible as scale, +/- admixed with crust; may be a result of an accelerated epidermal turnover rate (e.g., normal 22 days decreasing to 3–7 days in idiopathic seborrhea)
  - Crust: a thick accumulation of cells with dried exudate of serum, blood, purulent debris, or medications (Figure 2.2)

- Follicular cast: accumulation of keratinaceous or sebaceous material above the level of the follicular ostia; may be adherent to hair shaft (Figure 2.3)
- Milia: keratin filled cyst within the epidermis (Figure 2.4)
- Comedo: dilated hair follicle blocked by sebaceous and epidermal debris; when the follicular ostia is open to the air, debris will darken to form a "blackhead" (Figure 2.5)
- Lesions under 1 cm in diameter:
  - Macule: nonpalpable change in skin color; increased or decreased pigmentation, hemorrhage (nonblanching), or erythema (Figure 2.6)
  - Papule: solid elevation of the skin (Figure 2.7)
  - Vesicle: acellular fluid-filled lesion, within or just below the epidermis (Figure 2.8)
  - Pustule: cellular fluid-filled lesion, within or just below the epidermis; fluid most often contains neutrophils, but may also contain eosinophils (Figure 2.9)
  - Nodule: solid elevation of the skin that extends into deeper layers (Figure 2.10)
- Lesions over 1 cm in diameter:
  - Patch: nonpalpable change in skin color; large macule (Figure 2.11)
  - Plaque: flat, palpable and solid elevation; large or coalescing papules (Figure 2.12)
  - Wheal: temporary accumulation of fluid in the dermis; often creates a sharply demarcated (steep-walled) raised area; flattens with digital pressure (Figure 2.13)
  - Bulla: large accumulation of fluid, often extending into the dermis (Figure 2.14)
  - Abscess: very large accumulation of cellular fluid that extends deep into the dermis and subcutaneous tissues
  - Cyst: epithelium-lined cavity with fluid or semi-solid matter, often just beneath the epidermis (Figure 2.15)
  - Tumor: large mass that may involve the skin and deeper tissues (Figure 2.16)
- Pigmentation change:
  - Hyperpigmentation: increase in cutaneous pigmentation
  - Hypopigmentation: decrease in cutaneous pigmentation
  - Leukoderma: white skin (Figure 2.17)
  - Leukotrichia: white hair (Figure 2.18).

- Secondary lesions develop from primary lesions, most often induced by the patient or by the environment:
  - Epidermal collarette: circular accumulation of scale, resulting from the enlargement of a ruptured vesicle or pustule (Figure 2.19)
  - Excoriation: linear erosion with erythema and crusting as a result of self-trauma (Figure 2.20)
  - Lichenification: thickening of the skin with accentuation of the normal skin pattern caused by chronic inflammation and self-trauma (Figure 2.21)

- Erosion: defect in the skin that does not penetrate the dermal-epidermal junction (Figure 2.22)
- Ulcer: defect in the skin that penetrates the dermal-epidermal junction (Figure 2.23)
- Fissure: linear defect penetrating the epidermis to the dermis (Figure 2.24)
- Fistula: deep lesion with a draining site (Figure 2.25)
- Scar: area of fibrous tissue that has replaced normal skin; often palpates as a thinned or depressed defect (Figure 2.26).

COMMENTS

- Examination findings should be recorded in an organized and consistent manner; descriptions should provide a clear "picture" of the previous dermatologic condition during subsequent examinations.
- Findings should be organized from the "larger" to the "smaller" picture.
- Identifying specific lesions correctly and understanding how they develop provide invaluable pathophysiologic information.
- Many dermatoses have pathognomonic appearances that, when correlated with signalment and history, can provide an appropriate and limited differential diagnosis list.
- Alternatively, many dermatoses share similar physical findings; an accurate record of descriptions may permit the clinician to develop a concise plan for the diagnosis and treatment of patients with dermatologic disease.

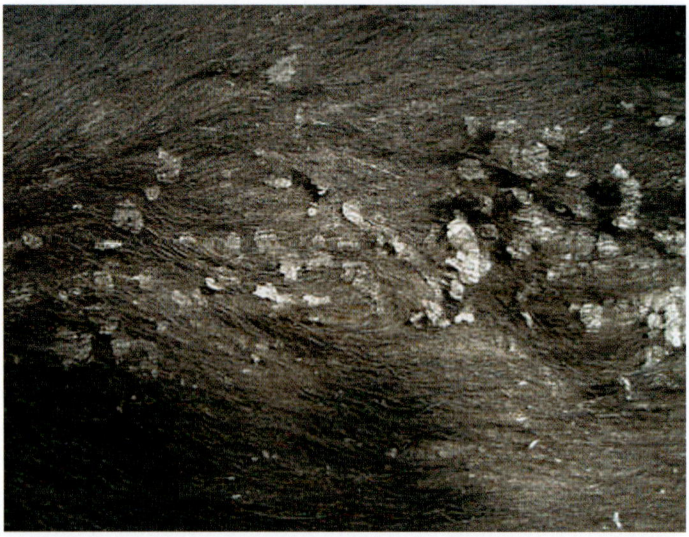

Fig. 2.1. Scale – coarse accumulation of keratinocytes.

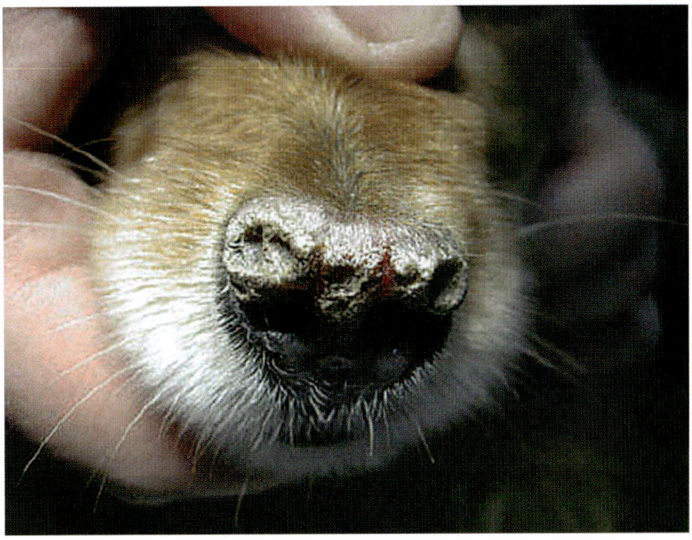

Fig. 2.2. Crust – thick accumulation of dried exudate on the nasal planum.

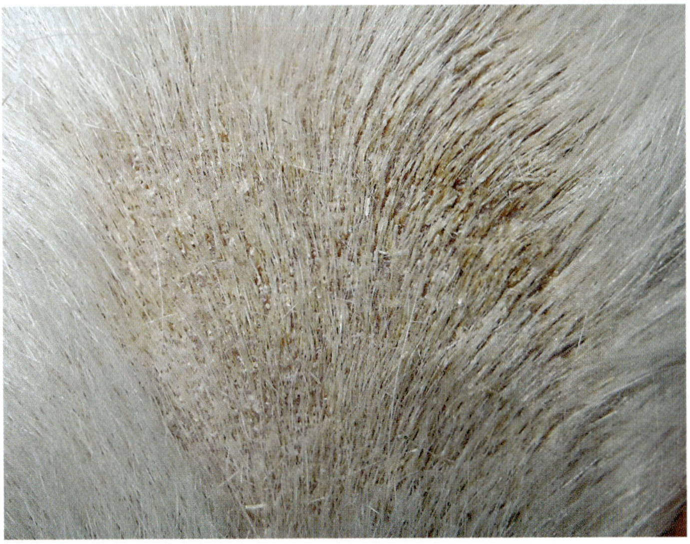

Fig. 2.3. Follicular cast – accumulation of keratin adherent to hair shaft (sebaceous adenitis).

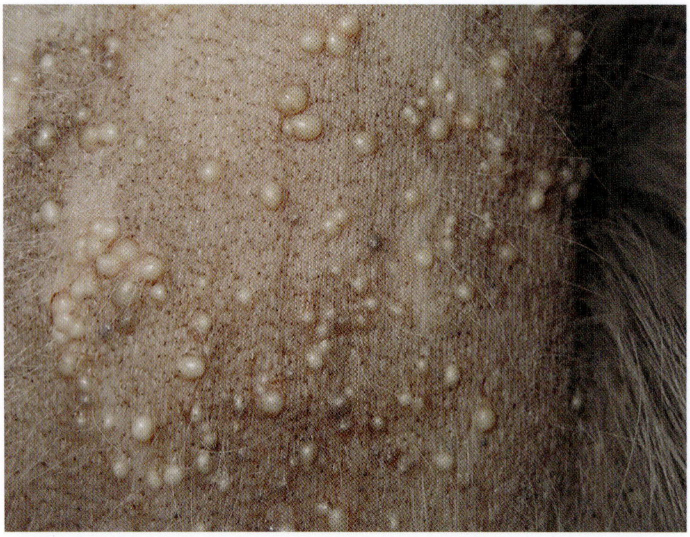

■ **Fig. 2.4.** Milia – keratin-filled cyst on the ventral neck.

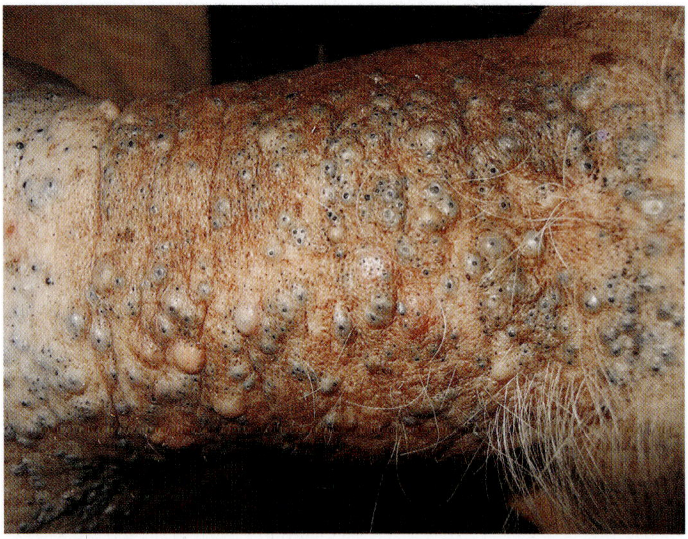

■ **Fig. 2.5.** Comedo – dilated hair follicle blocked by epidermal debris.

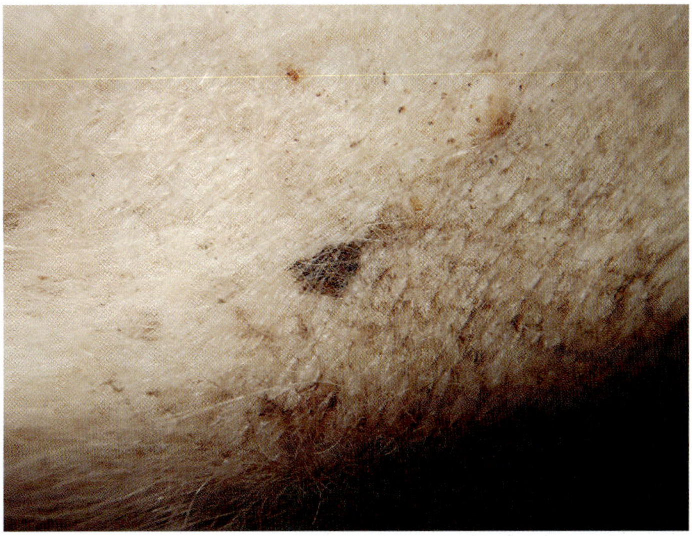

Fig. 2.6. Macule – nonpalpable change in skin color (hyperpigmented in this image).

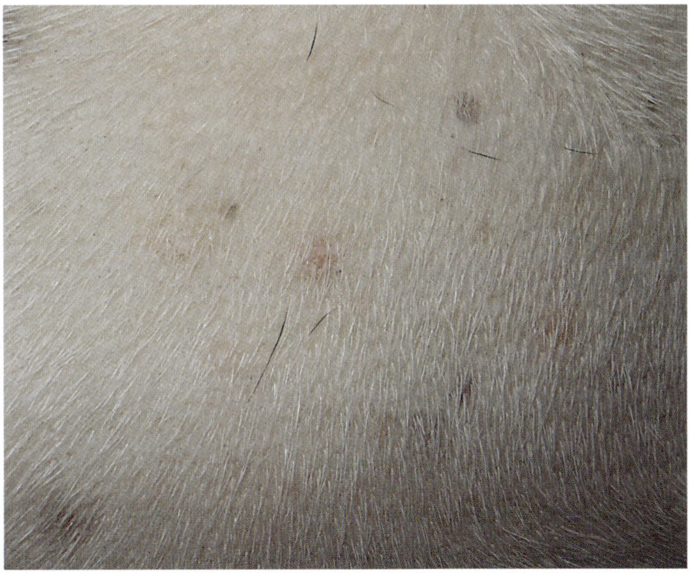

Fig. 2.7. Papule – solid elevation of the skin (i.e., flea bite).

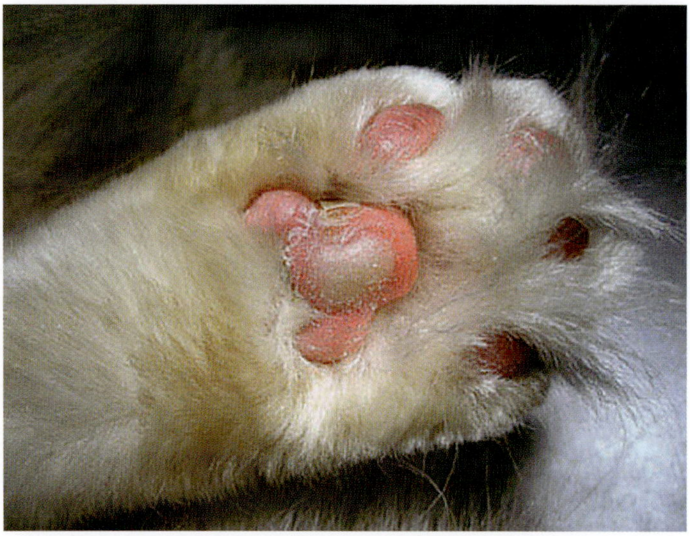

■ **Fig. 2.8.** Vesicle – acellular fluid-filled lesion (pemphigus foliaceus).

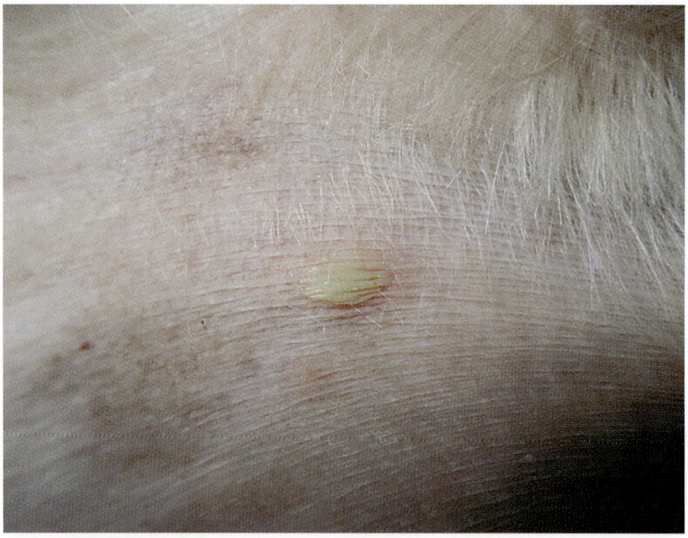

■ **Fig. 2.9.** Pustule – cellular fluid-filled lesion.

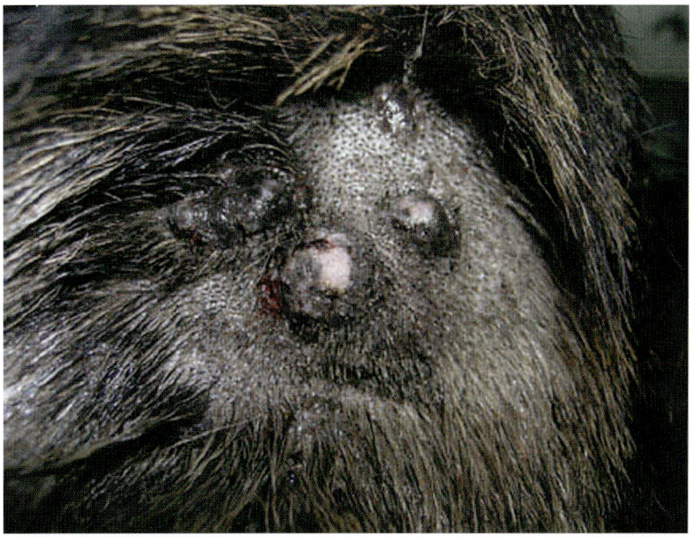

■ **Fig. 2.10.** Nodule – solid elevation of the skin that extends into deeper layers (fibropruritic nodules).

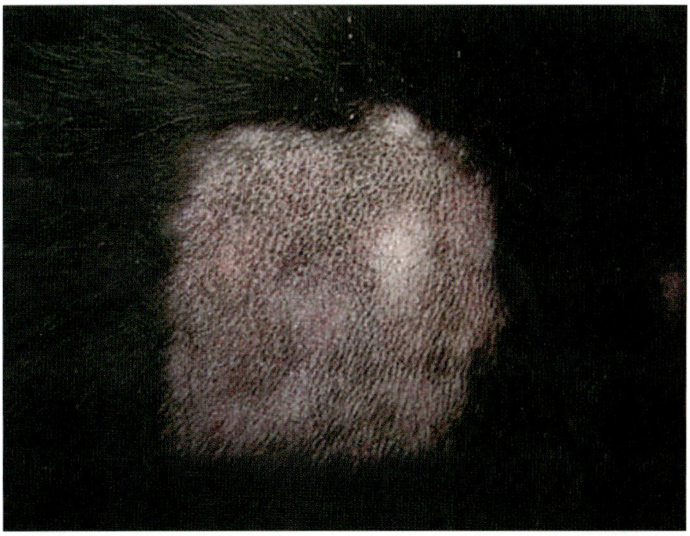

■ **Fig. 2.11.** Patch – large lesion of nonpalpable change in skin color (epitheliotropic lymphoma – hair clipped from lateral thorax).

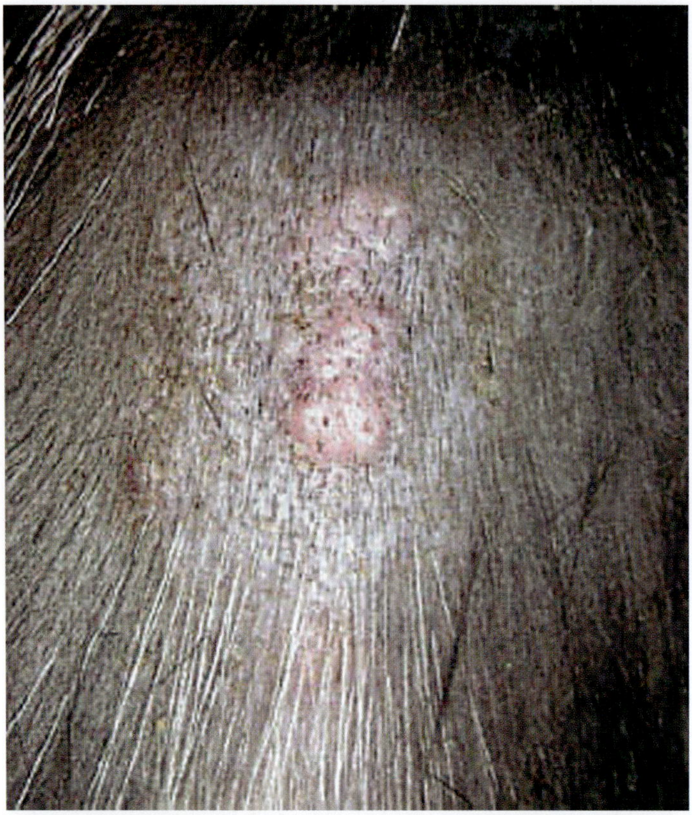

■ **Fig. 2.12.** Plaque – flat palpable and solid elevation (lipid).

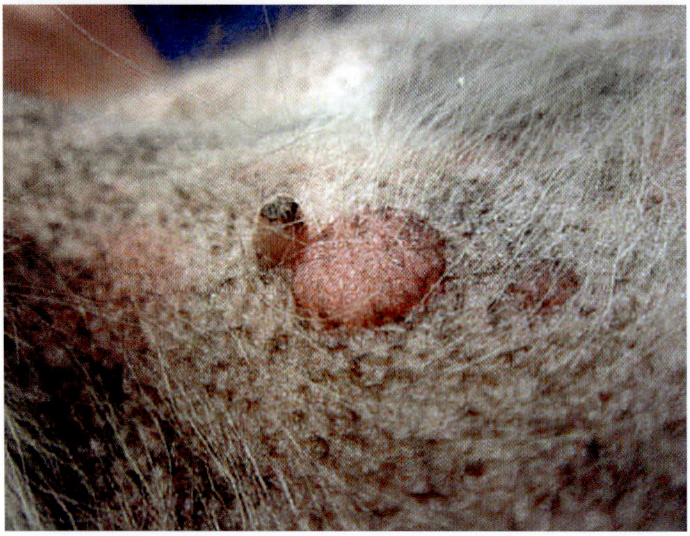

■ **Fig. 2.13.** Wheal – temporary accumulation of fluid that flattens with digital pressure.

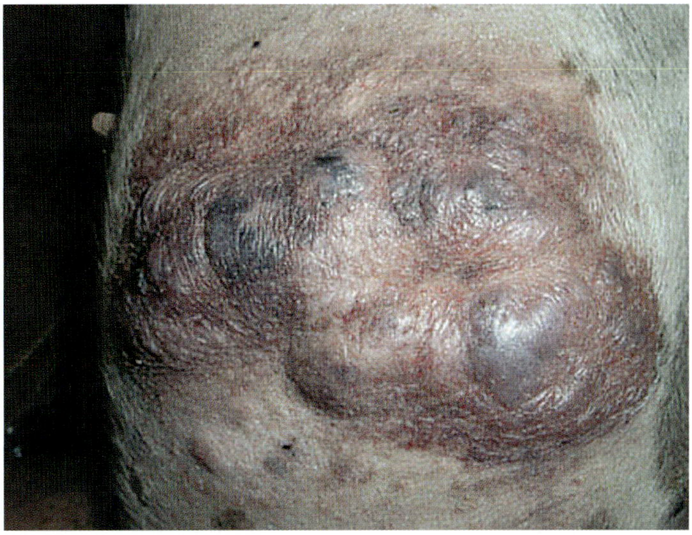

Fig. 2.14. Bulla – large accumulation of fluid, often extending into the dermis.

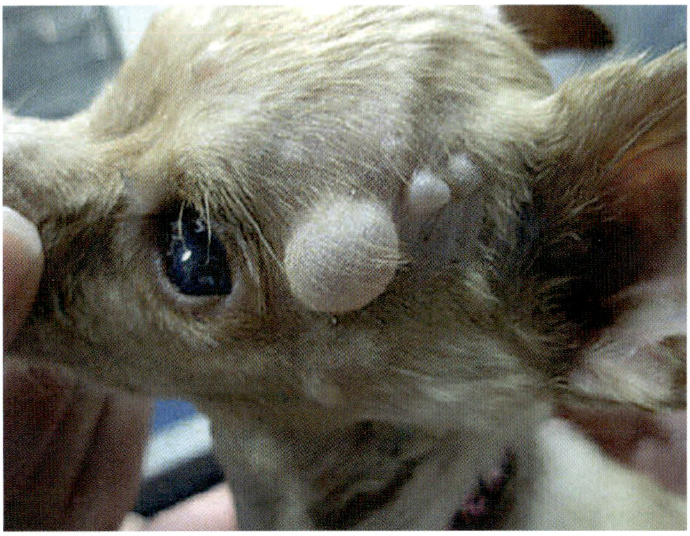

Fig. 2.15. Cyst – epithelium-lined cavity with fluid (apocrine cyst).

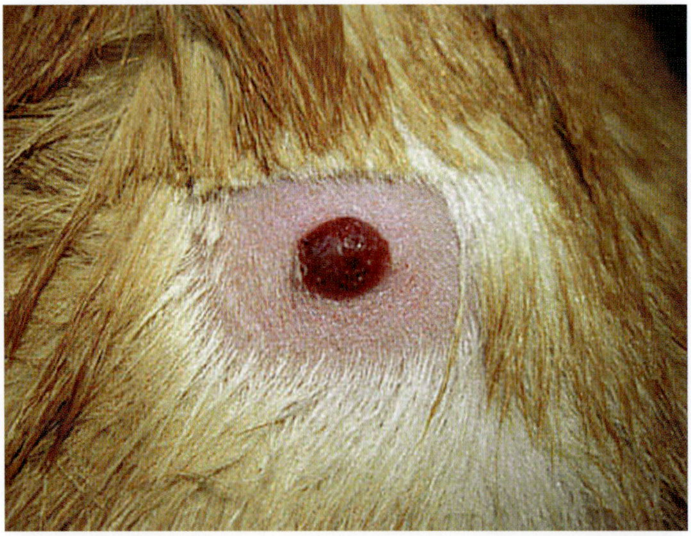

■ **Fig. 2.16.** Tumor – large mass that may involve the skin and deeper tissues (plasma cell tumor).

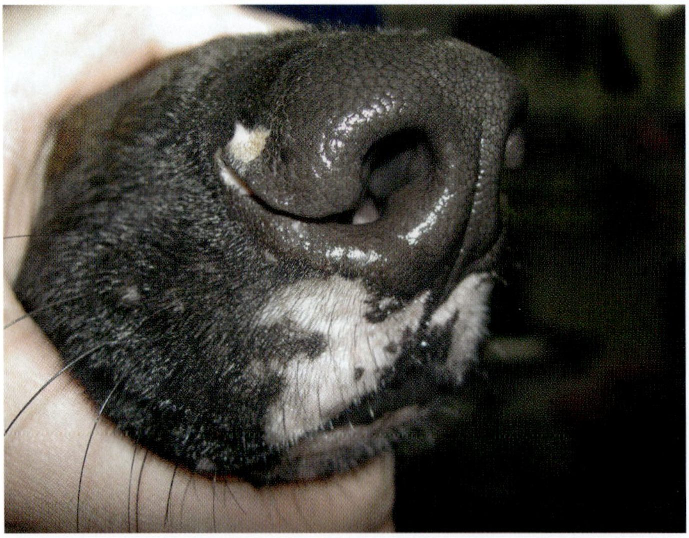

■ **Fig. 2.17.** Leukoderma – well-demarcated patch with loss of pigmentation of skin.

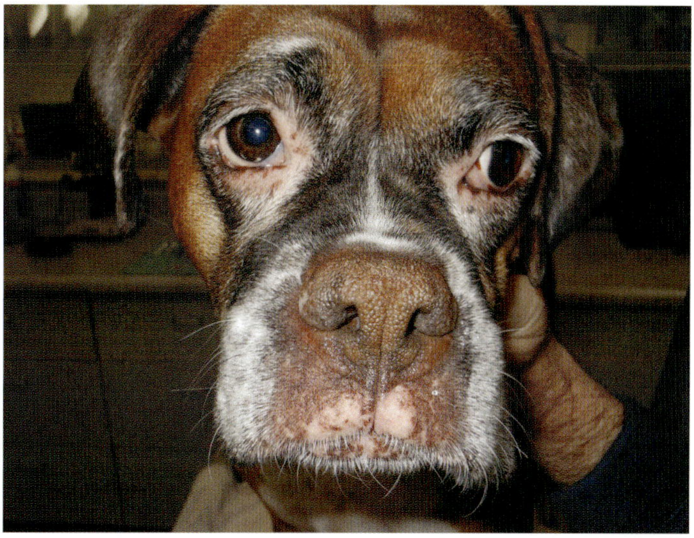

■ **Fig. 2.18.** Leukotrichia – loss of pigmentation of hair (vitiligo).

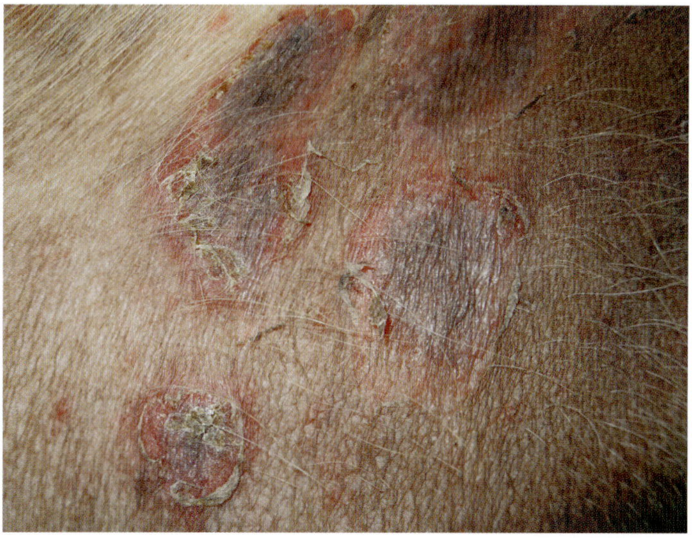

■ **Fig. 2.19.** Epidermal collarettes – multifocal circular accumulations of scale (often with central hyperpigmentation with chronicity).

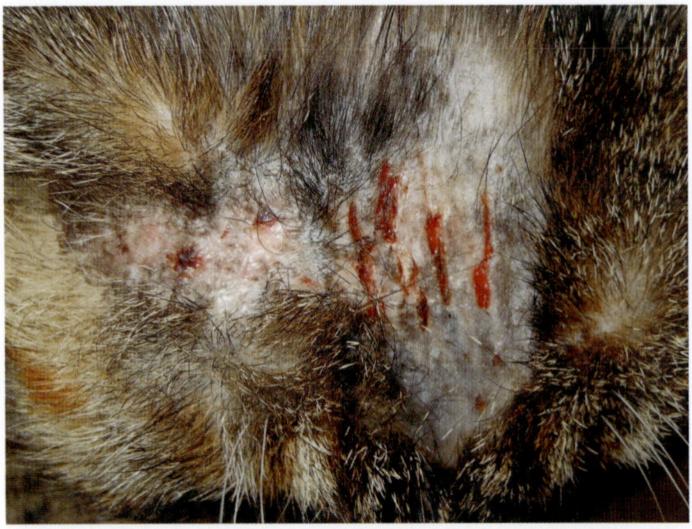

■ **Fig. 2.20.** Excoriation – linear erosions as a result of self-trauma on the neck of a DSH with allergic dermatitis.

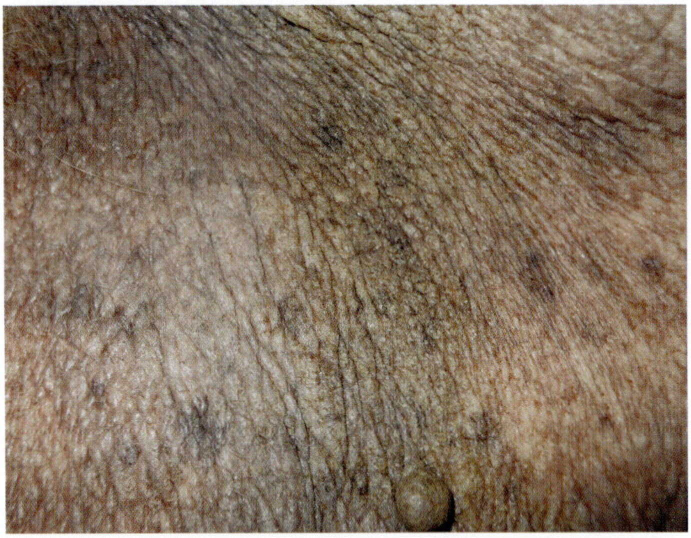

■ **Fig. 2.21.** Lichenification – thickening of the skin with accentuation of normal pattern from self-trauma.

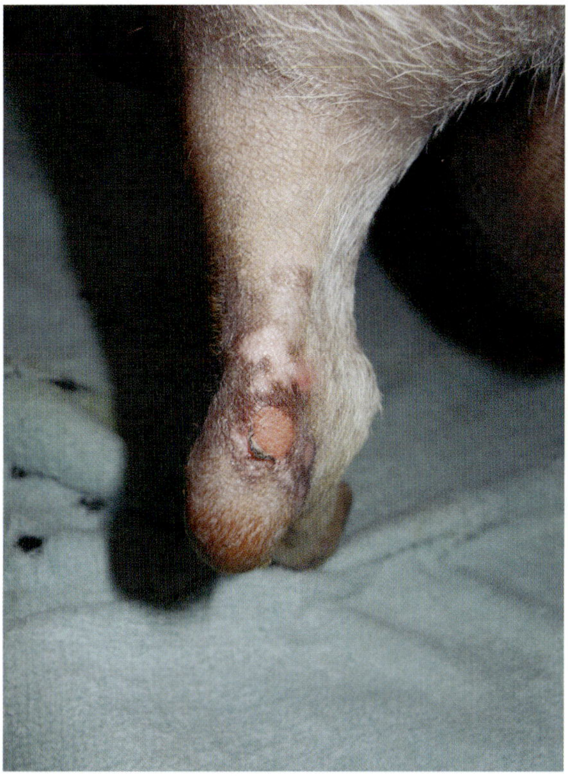

Fig. 2.22. Erosion – defect in the skin that does not penetrate the dermal-epidermal junction. The upper layers of the epidermis have peeled away from lower layers in this case of epidermolysis bullosa acquisita.

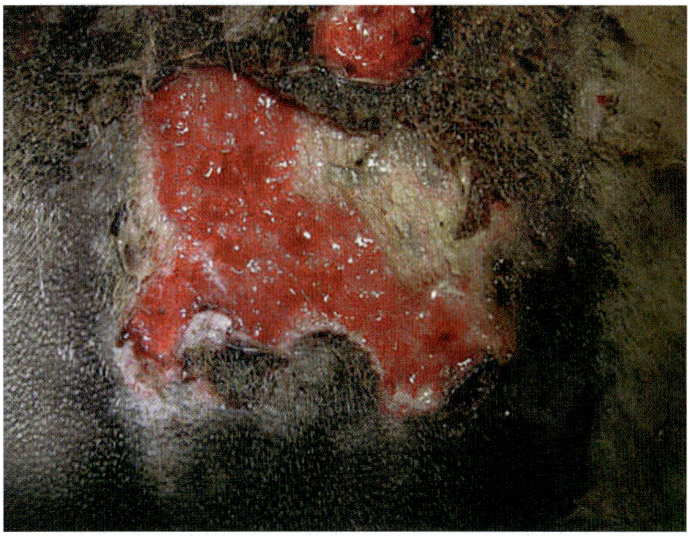

Fig. 2.23. Ulcer – defect in the skin that penetrates the dermal-epidermal junction.

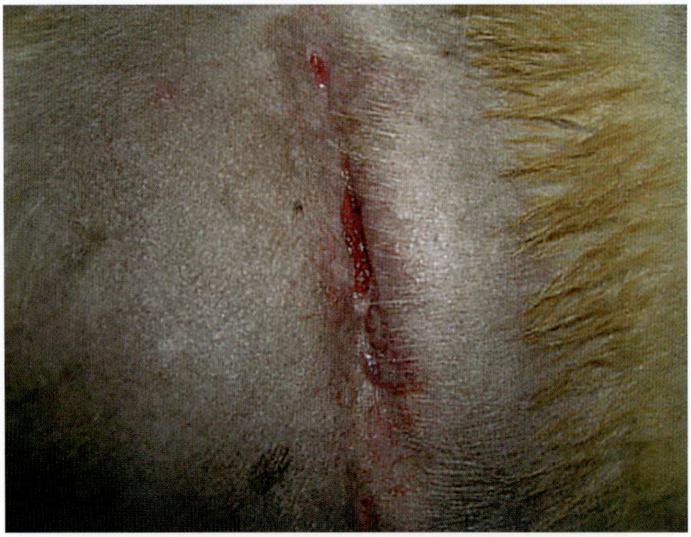

■ **Fig. 2.24.** Fissure – linear defect penetrating the epidermis on the lateral abdomen of a dog with panniculitis.

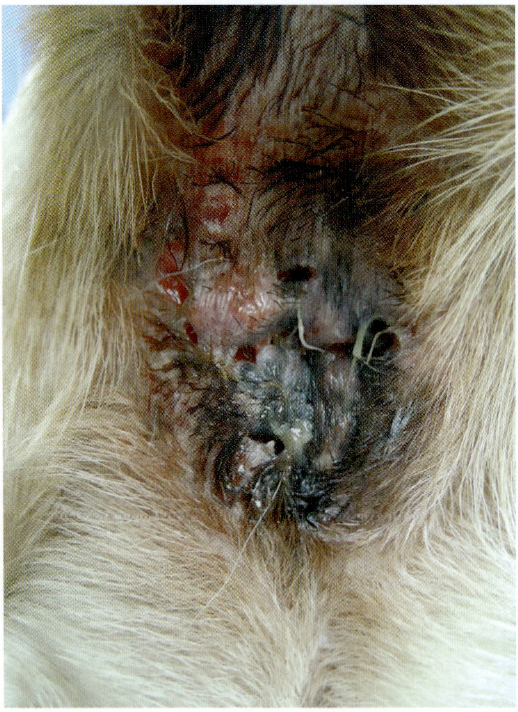

■ **Fig. 2.25.** Fistula – deep, often draining lesion or tract (perianal fistulae).

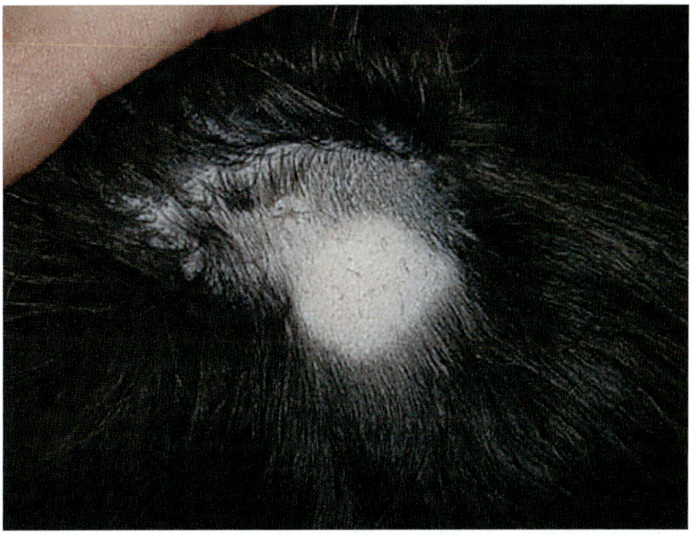

■ **Fig. 2.26.** Scar – area of fibrous tissue that has replaced normal skin (vaccination reaction).

chapter 3

Diagnostic Culture and Identification (Bacterial and Fungal)

DEFINITION/OVERVIEW

- Culturing dermatologic lesions for dermatophytes is always appropriate.
- Samples for culture should be submitted if fungal organisms (non-*Malassezia* spp.) are identified in epidermal or aural exudates.
- Bacterial culture and sensitivity testing is often not required for the treatment of routine bacterial folliculitis in the dog.
- Bacterial culture and sensitivity is indicated when cases fail to respond to an appropriate antibiotic choice.
- Bacterial culture and sensitivity is appropriate if rod bacteria are identified in epidermal or aural exudates.

DERMATOPHYTE CULTURE AND IDENTIFICATION

Culture Media

- Dermatophyte test medium (DTM): Sabouraud's dextrose agar modified by the addition of antimicrobials to discourage the growth of nondermatophytes, and phenol red as a pH indicator.
- Sabouraud's dextrose agar or rapid sporulating medium (RSM): agars used to encourage development of conidia for dermatophyte identification.
- DTM delays the development of conidia; products with a combination of agars are recommended.
- Media plates allow better access for inoculation of samples than small glass bottles.
- Incubate cultures at room temperature (75–80 °F), kept away from ultraviolet light, and prevented from desiccation by placing a small cup of water in the incubator. A small food storage container can act as an informal incubator.

Sample Collection

- Hair pluck (Figures 3.1, 3.2):
  - Remove hairs at the periphery of lesions with sterile forceps
  - Selection of hairs by Wood's lamp may increase success

Blackwell's Five-Minute Veterinary Consult Clinical Companion: Small Animal Dermatology, Third Edition.
Karen Helton Rhodes and Alexander H. Werner.

  - Examine directly under the microscope and/or gently press samples onto test medium.
- Toothbrush (Figure 3.3):
  - Samples from large or poorly demarcated lesions may be collected with a sterile (or new "in package") toothbrush
  - Brush hair against the direction of growth to encourage removal of fragile (infected) hair shafts
  - Gently stab the bristles into the test media – a large amount of debris does not need to be transferred.

Colony Growth and Identification

- Monitor culture plates for color change and colony growth daily.
- Observe for growth up to 28 days.
- DTM color changes from yellow to red *prior to* or *at the same time as* macroscopic colony growth.
- Dermatophytes preferentially metabolize proteins in the medium, creating an alkaline pH turning the yellow color of the DTM to red at the same time that the dermatophyte colony appears; most other fungi metabolize carbohydrates in the media first, creating an acidic environment with no color change *but over time,* they will consume the proteins and cause a red color change,
- Dermatophyte colonies are white, creamy, or lightly tan but not pigmented (Figure 3.4).
- Colonies may be cottony, wool-like, or powdery.

Fungal Identification

- Transfer colonies to a glass slide using clear acetate tape or a sterile loop.
- Lactophenol cotton blue stain is most often recommended to enhance the appearance of hyphae and conidia, but any dark stain will suffice (Figure 3.5).
- Examine slides for hyphae, macroconidia, and/or microconidia for identification (Figure 3.6).
- *Microsporum canis*, *Microsporum gypseum*, and *Trichophyton mentagrophytes* are the most common dermatophytes isolated from lesions of dogs; *Microsporum canis* is most commonly isolated from cats.
- Colonies that cannot be identified should be submitted to a reference laboratory for identification; consult with your laboratory prior to submitting samples.
- A multicenter study compared the interpretation skills of " in-house" cultures by clinicians (dermatologists and general practitioners) with reference mycology laboratory results: specialists (dermatologists) demonstrated a 3% error rate while general practitioners misdiagnosed 20% of the cases. This discrepancy may be due to a lack of microscopic identification or erroneous medium color change notation.

PCR for Dermatophytes (Polymerase Chain Reaction Test)

- Rapid test.
- Requires very little DNA to be present in the sample.
- Not reliable for diagnosing dermatophytosis: very small amount of contaminant DNA can yield a false-positive result.
- Dermatophyte DNA is ubiquitous; it can be found in the soil.
- An animal with a positive PCR may have contaminant DNA on the hair coat and not be a true transient carrier.
- Dermatophyte PCR is sensitive but not specific.

BACTERIAL CULTURE

- Submit samples to a reference laboratory experienced in the culture, identification, and sensitivity testing of bacterial organisms of veterinary significance.
- Inform the laboratory if you suspect an unusual or a zoonotic organism; obtain information regarding laboratory preferences for submission of samples suspected of being methicillin-resistant *Staphylococcus* spp.
- Obtain samples from superficial lesions using sterile swabs.
- Excessive debris that may contaminate results should be gently removed with alcohol-soaked gauze; do not scrub lesions with antiseptic solutions prior to sample collection.
- Samples for bacterial culture, identification, and sensitivity testing from the external and middle ear canals are discussed below and in the relevant chapter.

Samples from Superficial Lesions

- Most often used for culture and sensitivity in superficial and deep folliculitis.
- Apply sterile submission swab directly to a lesion (Figure 3.7).
- Collect sample from within a lesion by needle aspiration and apply to a sterile swab (Figure 3.8).
- Samples may be collected from:
    - Superficial exudates
    - Beneath crusts and scabs
    - Periphery of epidermal collarettes
    - Pricked pustules.

Samples Obtained from Tissue

- Most often used for culture and sensitivity in deep folliculitis and atypical bacterial infections.
- Use sterile biopsy technique.
- Place tissue sample on a sterile gauze and remove the epidermis by scalpel (the epidermis may be submitted with additional tissue for histopathologic examination).

- Submit remaining dermis and subcutaneous tissue in a sterile container; if an extended transport time is anticipated, a small amount of sterile saline should be added to the container to prevent tissue desiccation.

Samples Obtained from the Ear Canal

- Indicated with persistent infection.
- Indicated when rod bacteria are identified in cytology samples.
- Samples obtained from the proximal and distal external ear canal, from the middle ear, as well as from individual ears, may be different; submission of samples from each location may be necessary for accurate assessment of otitis externa and otitis media, especially if cytology results demonstrate disparate populations of organisms.
- Samples from the horizontal canal may be obtained by protecting a sterile swab with the cover of an intravenous or spinal catheter during insertion through the vertical canal.
- A spinal needle or sterile catheter may be inserted through the tympanic membrane to sample fluid within the bulla (Figure 3.9); sample contamination from the external ear canal is common.

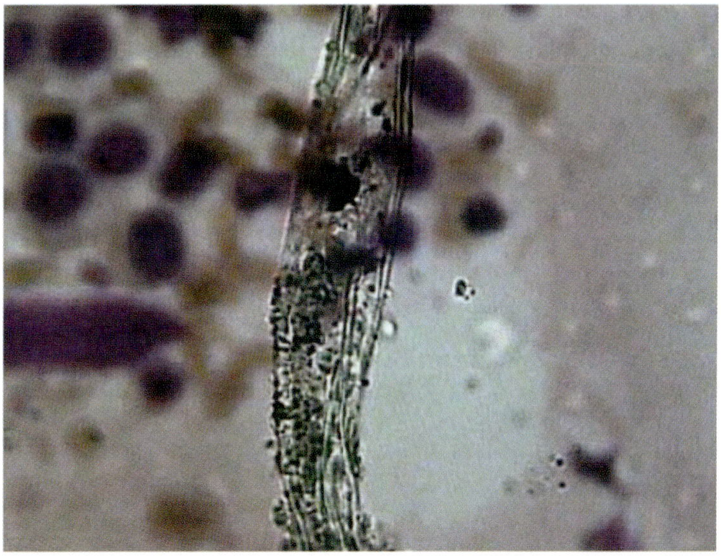

Fig. 3.1. Hair shaft infected with *Microsporum gypseum* hyphae.

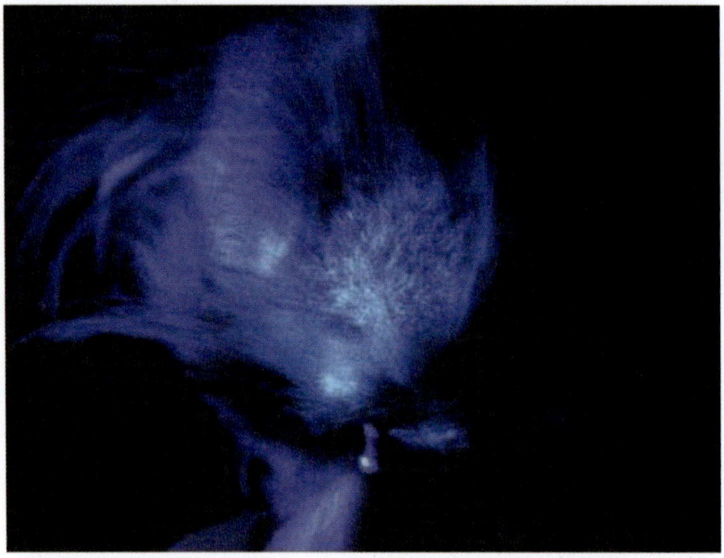

■ **Fig. 3.2.** Positive Wood's lamp fluorescence. Note bright staining of hair shafts on head.

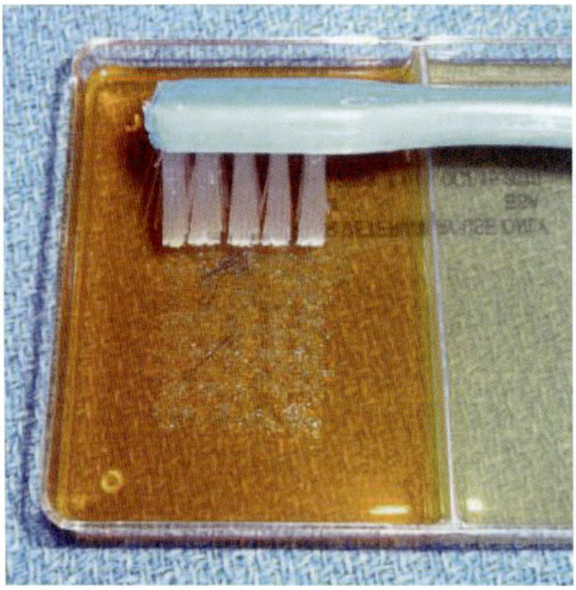

■ **Fig. 3.3.** Toothbrush technique for inoculating media. Tracks are produced by light pressing of brush onto the media.

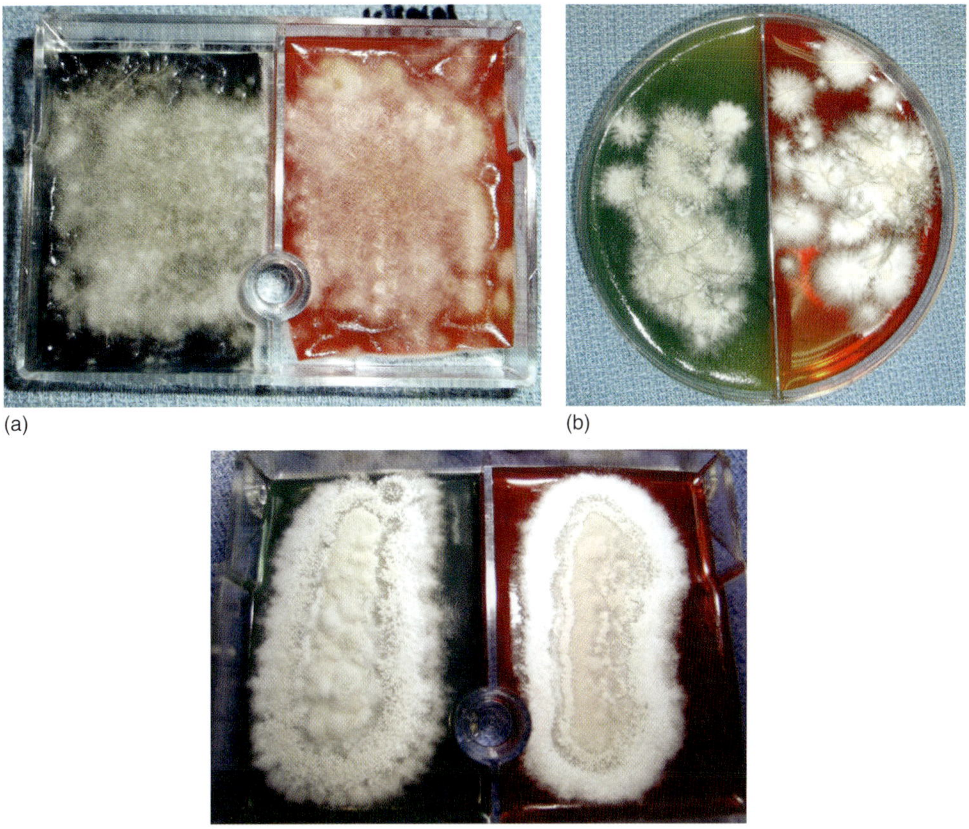

(a) (b) (c)

■ **Fig. 3.4.** (a) *Microsporum canis* colonies appear white/cottony. (b) *Microsporum gypseum* colonies appear ivory/granular. (c) *Trichophyton mentagrophytes* colonies appear white/powdery.

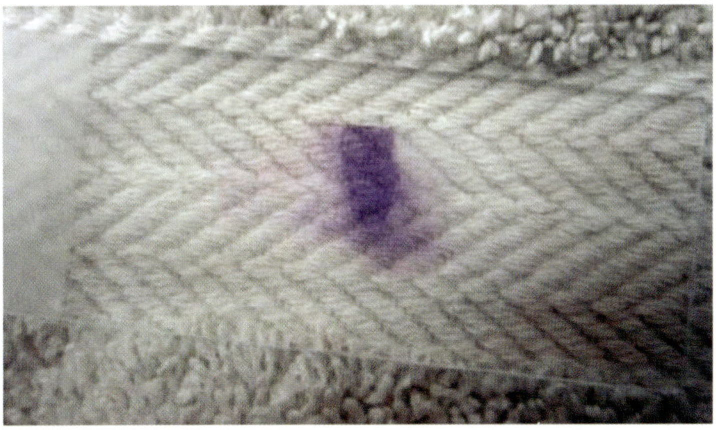

■ **Fig. 3.5.** Clear tape sampling of colony for identification with lactophenol cotton blue stain.

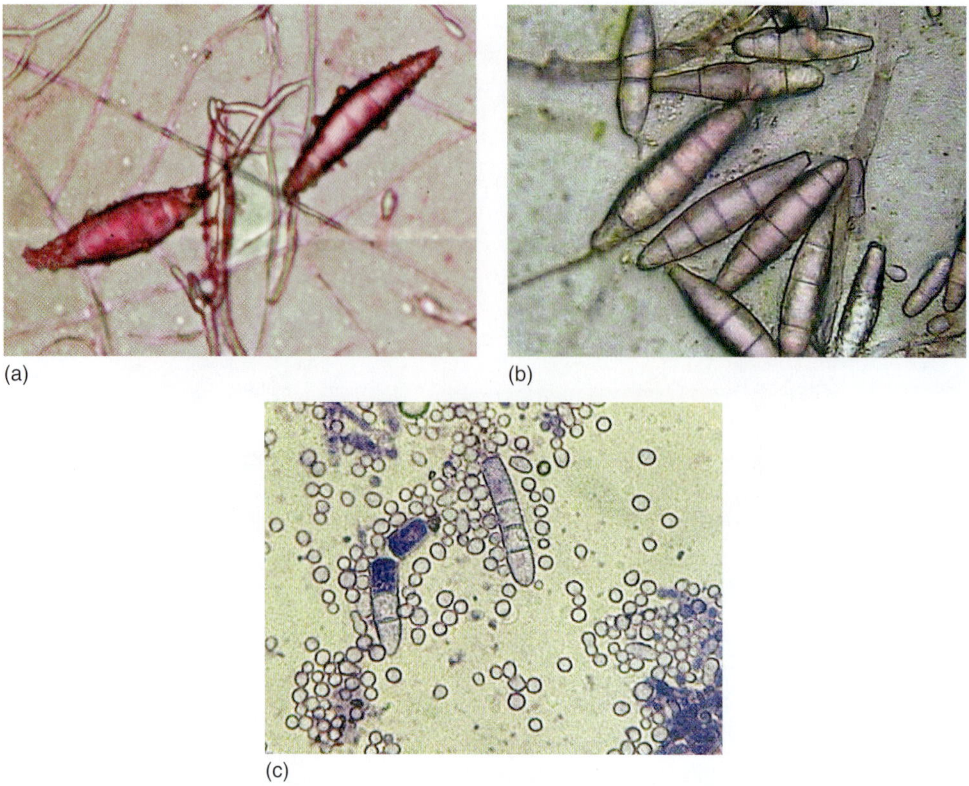

■ **Fig. 3.6.** (a) *Microsporum canis* macroconidia are spindle-shaped and thick-walled with a terminal knob. (b) *Microsporum gypseum* macroconidia are spindle to cigar-shaped and thin-walled. (c) *Trichophyton mentagrophytes* abundant microconidia common; cigar-shaped macroconidia uncommon.

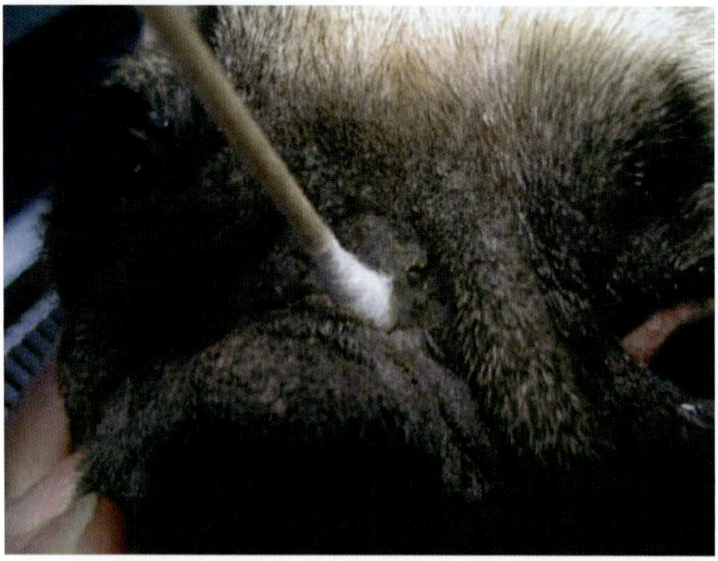

■ **Fig. 3.7.** Sampling for bacterial culture directly from skinfold.

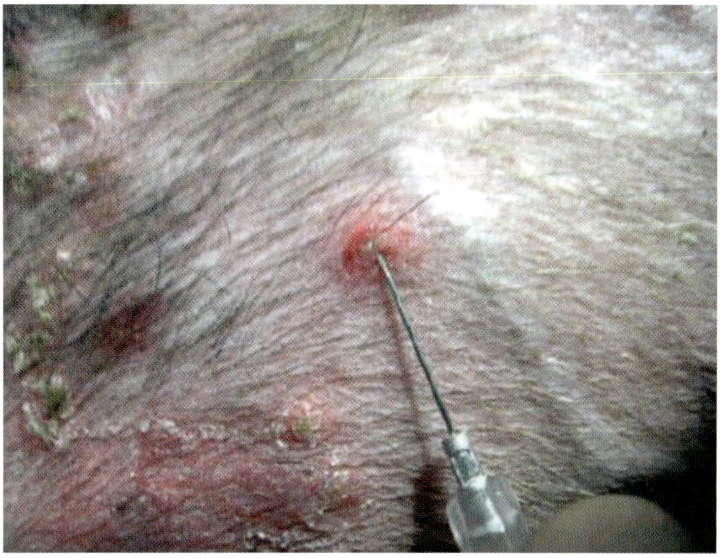

■ **Fig. 3.8.** Sampling for bacterial culture and cytology from pustule.

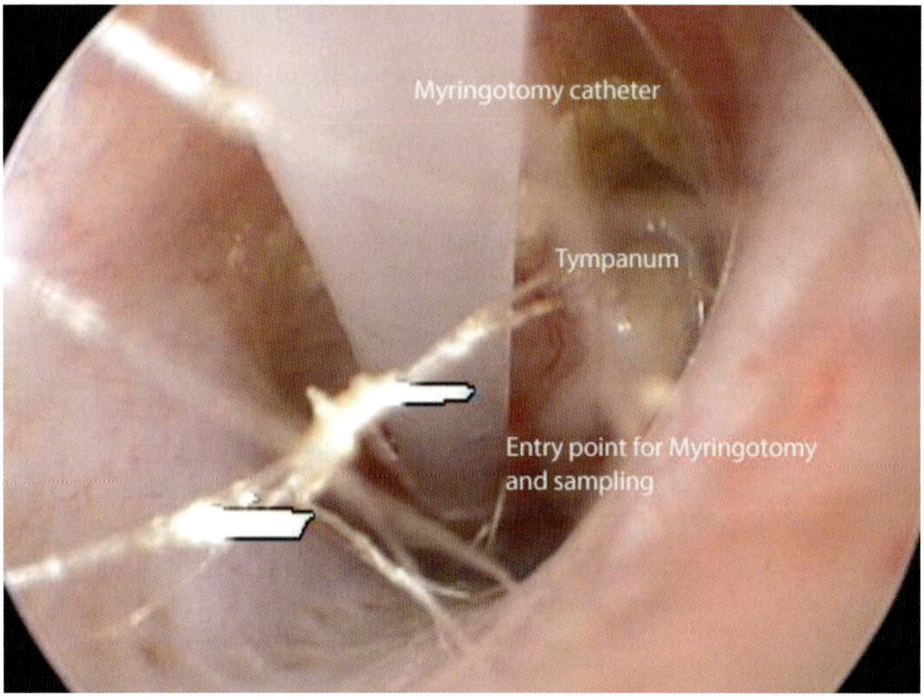

■ **Fig. 3.9.** Insertion of a sterile catheter through the tympanum (myringotomy) to collect sample for culture and cytology. Note catheter tube penetrating tympanic membrane in the lower quadrant.

chapter 4

Obtaining a Diagnostic Biopsy

DEFINITION/OVERVIEW

- The skin biopsy is one of the most important diagnostic tools available.
- Three factors are key to obtaining a diagnostic biopsy: site selection, tissue handling, and a qualified dermatopathologist.
- There are a number of recognized dermatopathologists available through a variety of commercial and private laboratories.
- Your local board certified veterinary dermatologist(s) may be helpful in providing names and locations of laboratories.
- The art of site selection and tissue handling are the responsibility of the submitting veterinarian.

THE DECISION TO BIOPSY

- There are a number of cutaneous disorders for which the biopsy is the only helpful diagnostic tool.
- The biopsy is equally important for what appears to be a "classic case" that continues to fail conventional therapy.

When to Biopsy

- Persistent lesions
- Neoplastic or suspected neoplastic disorders
- Persistent scaling dermatoses
- Vesicular dermatoses
- Undiagnosed alopecias
- Unusual dermatoses

SITE SELECTION

- Proper site and lesion selection is crucial to obtain accurate information from a tissue sample.

Blackwell's Five-Minute Veterinary Consult Clinical Companion: Small Animal Dermatology, Third Edition.
Karen Helton Rhodes and Alexander H. Werner.

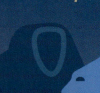

- Sampling only from the periphery of a lesion may cause pathology to be missed if the active section of dermatitis is small and not within the sectioned tissue.
- Choose representative lesions from multiple areas of skin; most laboratories permit submission of 3–5 samples for dermatopathologic examination.
- Submit samples from the tissue affected even if less amenable to biopsy (e.g., from the planum nasale – this area heals well after biopsy).

Where to Biopsy

- Choose several representative lesions because they may represent various stages of the same disorder or multiple problems.
- Include lesions characterized by scale, crust, erythema, erosion, ulceration, etc.; it is not always necessary to biopsy the edge of a lesion, although a sample taken within the center of an ulcer is rarely diagnostic.
- Pustules and vesicles should not be biopsied with a punch technique (unless smaller than 4 mm); the twisting motion of the punch will rupture or remove the roof of the lesion and disrupt the architecture of the sample; these lesions should be excised *in toto*.
- Ulcers or deep draining lesions are best taken by excision, rather than by punch technique, because the twisting motion may separate the pathologic tissue from the more normal tissue (e.g., vasculitis, panniculitis).
- If affected, biopsy footpads or the planum nasale; wedge samples are easier to close than circular punched samples – these areas heal well.
- Crusted lesions are excellent areas for biopsy; if the crust separates from the lesion during sampling, include the crust in the formalin jar and *make a notation for the technician to "please cut in the crust."*
- Heavily scaled areas are often good diagnostic sites.

BIOPSY TECHNIQUE

- Skin biopsy sites should be gently clipped (if needed) and should not be scrubbed or cleaned.
- Excessive cleaning will remove or alter potentially significant pathologic changes.
- Most skin biopsies can be obtained with local anesthesia; sedation may be necessary with fractious animals.
- When possible, use 6 mm or larger biopsy punches to avoid sampling error.

How to Biopsy

- Never scrub or cleanse the area before excision – the surface crust may contain the pathologic changes necessary to make a diagnosis.
- Use a surgical blade to obtain a wedge-shaped or elliptic biopsy specimen when sectioning the nose, footpad, vesicles, bullae, or deep lesions (e.g., vasculitis, panniculitis).

- A 6 mm biopsy punch is the preferred size to obtain skin tissue samples.
- When using a punch biopsy, tense the skin around the lesion to be biopsied and position the punch perpendicular to the skin and rotate smoothly in one direction only; do not twist back and forth to avoid artifactual damage of tissue (Figure 4.1).
- Biopsy punches are single-use: blades easily become dulled, causing the tissue to tear during the procedure.
- When using lidocaine, place the anesthesia in the subcutaneous compartment below the tissue to be sampled; do not inject intradermally.
- Use a small-gauge needle to manipulate the tissue, or grasp the tissue sample below the epidermis with a forceps to avoid crush artifacts.
- Separate the biopsy sample from underlying tissue by curved scissors placed beneath the lifted sample (Figure 4.2).
- Gently blot blood off the biopsy sample.
- Place the sample immediately in the formalin.
- Small or thin specimens may be placed on a small piece of a tongue depressor with the haired portion to the outside to prevent curling and then floated upside down in the formalin.
- Avoid freezing.

PATHOLOGY REPORT (TABLES 4.1, 4.2, BOX 4.1)

- All skin biopsy samples must be accompanied by a complete biopsy request.
- Some laboratories permit submission of clinical images with tissues or a copy of the written records (such as a summary or referral letter).
- Histopathology requests should include a thorough history (including drugs administered and responses), accurate and complete lesion description, clinical symptoms, and differential diagnoses.

TABLE 4.1. Dermatohistopathology Report

Report item	Remarks
Description	Summarizes the histologic changes noted in the tissue
History	Provides the pathologist's summary of the case as presented by the clinician (errors should be corrected with the pathologist if noted)
Morphologic diagnosis	Reports the overall histologic pattern recognized
Etiologic diagnosis	Identifies a causative disease or agent if recognized (e.g., bacteria, parasites, fungal, etc.)
Comments	The pathologist draws a correlation between the clinical features of the case (provided by the clinician) and the histopathologic features of the biopsy. The information provided by the clinician is vital for a valid conclusion to be given

TABLE 4.2. Common Histopathologic Terminology

Term	Meaning
Acanthosis	Increased thickness of epidermis (epidermal hyperplasia); often noted with chronic inflammation
Acantholysis	Loss of adhesion of keratinocytes (acantholytic keratinocytes); often due to autoimmune diseases such as pemphigus foliaceus; may also be seen in inflammatory disease
Amyloid	Hyaline, amorphous, eosinophilic material
Apoptosis	Individual premature keratinocyte death
Atrophy, epidermal	Thin epidermis; often associated with corticosteroid use
Ballooning degeneration	Koilocytosis, swollen cytoplasm without vacuolization; characteristic of viral infection
Bullae	Fluid-filled acellular spaces within or below the epidermis (vesicles are smaller bulla)
Cholesterol clefts	Appear as clear spicule-shaped spaces; often seen with xanthomatosis, panniculitis, and ruptured follicular cysts
Civatte bodies	Apoptotic cells in the stratum basale of the epidermis
Clefts	Slit-like spaces within the epidermis or dermoepidermal junction; caused by acantholysis, hydropic degeneration of basal cells, or processing artifacts
Collagenolysis	Denatured collagen, homogeneous, eosinophilic, often attracts mineralization
Crust	Surface accumulation of epidermal cells, serum proteins, RBCs, WBCs
Dermoepidermal junction	Interface between epidermis and dermis
Dell	Small depression on the surface of the epidermis
Desmoplasia	Fibroplasia induced by neoplasia
Diapedesis	RBCs within the intercellular spaces of the epidermis; implies loss of vascular integrity
Dyskeratosis	Premature faulty keratinization; may be seen with neoplasia or keratinization disorders
Dystrophic mineralization	Deposits of calcium along collagen fibers
Exocytosis	Migration of inflammatory cells, RBCs, or both into intercellular spaces
Fibroplasia	Increased amounts of fibrous tissue
Fibrosis	Advanced fibroplasia, thick parallel strands of collagen; characteristic of acral lick dermatitis
Flame figures	Areas of altered collagen surrounded by eosinophilic material, see collagenolysis; often noted with eosinophilic granulomas, also called excessive trichilemmal keratinization
Grenz zone	Marginal zone of collagen that separates the epidermis from an underlying dermal alteration; often seen in neoplastic and granulomatous disorders

(*Cont.*)

TABLE 4.2. (Continued)	
Hydropic degeneration	Vacuolar damage to the stratum basale; frequently seen with discoid lupus erythematosus
Hyper- and hypogranulosis	Denotes thickness of stratum granulosum (e.g., areas of lichenification reveal hypergranulosis)
Hyperkeratosis	Increased thickness of stratum corneum layer of epidermis; divided into orthokeratosis (nuclei lost) and parakeratosis (nuclei retained); assists in identifying an etiology (e.g., zinc-responsive dermatosis is characterized by parakeratosis)
Hypomelanosis	Decrease in pigment; as seen in vitiligo
Melanosis	Hyperpigmentation; seen in chronic inflammation
Microabscess, eosinophilic	Seen in EGC, allergy, pemphigus complex, Malassezia, eosinophilic folliculitis
Microabscess, Munro's	Accumulation of neutrophils within or below the stratum corneum; often seen in psoriasiform lichenoid dermatosis of springers
Microabscess, Pautrier's	Accumulation of abnormal lymphoid cells; often seen in epitheliotropic lymphoma
Microabscess, spongiform	Accumulation of neutrophils within stratum spinosum often seen with superficial suppurative necrolytic dermatitis of schnauzers
Mucinosis	Increased amounts of amorphous basophilic material in the dermis; characteristic of normal skin in the shar-pei dog and in hypothyroidism
Necrolysis	Epidermal coagulative necrosis with no dermal involvement and minimal inflammation; often seen with TEN and thermal burns
Papillomatosis	Epidermal proliferation due to papilloma virus infection, often exophytic; may be endophytic
Pigmentary incontinence	Melanin pigment dropped from the epidermis into the dermis and phagocytized by macrophages; often seen with DLE
Reticular degeneration	Multilocular intraepidermal edema with keratinocyte swelling; often seen with superficial necrolytic dermatitis/hepatocutaneous syndrome
Satellitosis	Cytotoxic lymphocytes surrounding an apoptotic cell; indicates cell-mediated immune response
Spongiosis	Epidermal intercellular edema
Sclerosis	Scar formation
Vacuolar degeneration	Intracellular edema

DLE, discoid lupus erythematosus; EGC, eosinophilic granuloma complex; RBC, red blood cell; TEN, toxic epidermal necrolysis; WBC, white blood cell.

Box 4.1 Histopathologic Patterns in Dermatology*

Perivascular
Interface
Vasculitis
Interstitial dermatitis
Nodular/diffuse
Intraepidermal vesicular/pustular
Subepidermal vesicular/pustular
Folliculitis/perifolliculitis/furunculosis
Panniculitis
Fibrosing dermatitis
Atrophic dermatopathy

*Used in the morphologic description in the report.

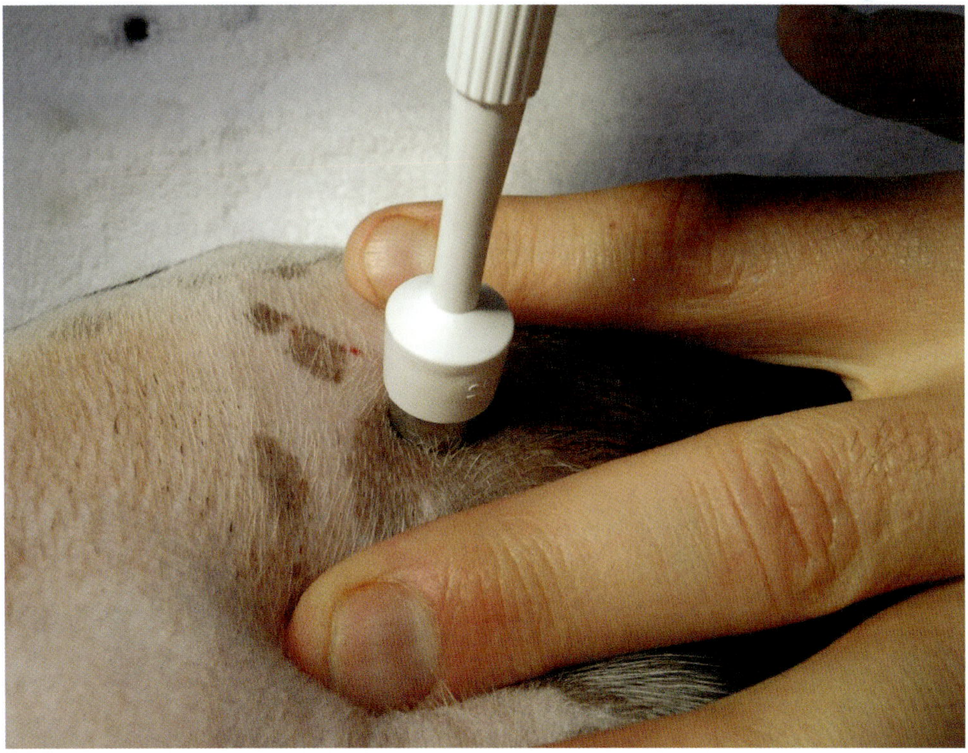

■ **Fig. 4.1.** The skin is tensed on either side of the lesion to be biopsied; the biopsy punch is positioned perpendicular to the skin and rotated smoothly in one direction.

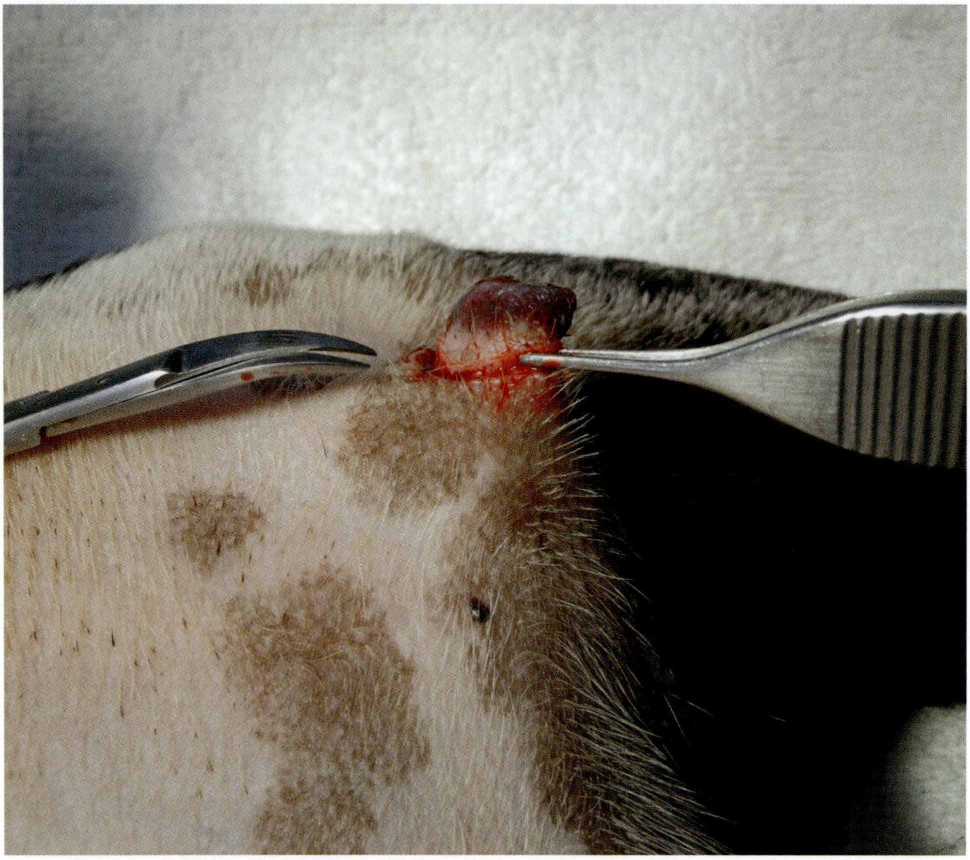

Fig. 4.2. To avoid crush artifacts, the sample is grasped from beneath and lifted to allow the curved ends of a scissors to separate the sample from underlying tissue.

chapter 5

Practical Cytology

DEFINITION/OVERVIEW

- Cutaneous cytology is an essential diagnostic tool.
- Samples should be obtained in almost every dermatologic case.
- The technical aspects of sample collection and slide preparation are critical for interpretive value.
- Skin scrapings and trichograms, otic swabs/smears, direct impression smears, fine-needle aspiration, and acetate tape preparation samples are the most frequently employed cytologic techniques in dermatology.

SKIN SCRAPINGS: SUPERFICIAL SAMPLE

To diagnose infestations of sarcoptes, notoedres, cheyletiella, *Demodex gatoi*, *Demodex cornei*, *Otodectes*.

- Select lesional skin.
- Place a small amount of mineral oil on a glass slide.
- Use a scalpel blade #10 or spatula.
- Apply a small amount of mineral oil either to the blade or directly onto the selected lesional skin (most helpful for sarcoptes).
- Scrape the area in the direction of hair growth and transfer accumulated material to the glass slide (Figure 5.1).
- Select several sites for sampling and, in cases of a suspect sarcoptes infestation, sample a large surface area.
- Certain sampling sites may be preferable depending on the suspect clinical diagnosis, i.e., sarcoptes – pinnal margins and elbows, demodex – dorsal midline or focal alopecic sites.
- Scan the slide using the 10× objective; adjust the microscope diaphragm and/or condenser to provide greater contrast.
- Note the proportion of live/dead mites and egg/young/adult forms present (Figure 5.2a).

Blackwell's Five-Minute Veterinary Consult Clinical Companion: Small Animal Dermatology, Third Edition.
Karen Helton Rhodes and Alexander H. Werner.

SKIN SCRAPINGS: DEEP SAMPLE

To diagnose infestations of *Demodex canis*, *Demodex injai*, *Demodex cati*, the technique is the same as that for a superficial scrape except that an extra step is added.

- After the initial material is placed on the slide, squeeze the site between the thumb and the forefinger, which initiates capillary oozing.
- Scrape the area again to collect additional material and place on the prepared slide.
- Pressure theoretically forces the mites toward the surface of the hair follicles.
- Scan the slide using the 10× objective; adjust the microscope diaphragm and/or condenser to provide greater contrast.
- Note the proportion of live/dead mites and egg/young/adult forms present (Figure 5.2b).
- *Caution*: edema and swelling, often seen with pododemodicosis, may make finding the mites more difficult; sample at the margins of lesions.

TRICHOGRAMS: HAIR PLUCKS

An adjunct to other types of sampling or when obtaining periocular samples.

- Place a small amount of mineral oil on a glass slide.
- Pluck a small sampling of hairs from lesional and/or perilesional skin with a hemostat and place directly in the mineral oil; *Demodex* mites may be seen clustered around the hair bulb of extracted hairs (Figure 5.3).
- Place the hairs on the slide in a unidirectional pattern so that all the hair bulbs line up, making the slide easier to read.
- Scan the slide using the 10× objective; adjust the microscope diaphragm and/or condenser to provide greater contrast.
- Note the number of anagen (growing) versus telogen (resting) hairs (a predominance of telogen hairs may indicate an endocrinopathy; as an exception, many Nordic breeds have telogen-dominated hair cycles) (Figure 5.4).
- Clumping of melanin (macromelanosomes) within the hair shafts may indicate a color dilution alopecia (Figure 5.5).
- Dermatophyte-infected hairs will demonstrate an invasion of the keratin of the hair shaft by arthroconidia and hyphae, resulting in a pale irregular appearance (Figure 5.6).

SQUEEZE TAPE IMPRESSIONS

An additional technique for identification of *Demodex* mites.

- Adhesive tape is placed onto the lesional skin and the underlying skin is squeezed for 2–3 seconds and repeated 3–4 times.
- Tape is placed onto a glass slide, sticky side down.

- This technique appears to have good sensitivity and specificity for the diagnosis of canine demodicosis (not evaluated in feline patients).
- Squeeze tape impressions are typically less invasive and may be more easily performed on multiple body sites or when dealing with a fractious animal.

OTIC SWABS/SMEARS

Used to diagnose bacterial and yeast overgrowth as well as to support the diagnosis of other differentials (neoplasia, keratinization disorders, mites, fungal infections); otic cytology should be performed on otitis cases at every examination (Table 5.1).

- Obtain the sample for cytology by positioning a cotton swab at the juncture of the vertical canal and the horizontal canal (approx. 75° angle; use caution straightening the canal to avoid puncturing tympanum).
- Roll the sample onto a glass slide; if desired, form letters R and L (or use the right and then left side of the slide) to identify which ear the sample represents so both samples can be placed on the same slide (Figure 5.7).
- Heat-fix the slide by passing a flame under the slide for 2–3 seconds (optional).
- Use Diff-Quik® stain (modified Wright's stain) and gently rinse the slide, being careful not to dislodge the sample.
- Initially examine the slide under 10× objective to identify the best field for observation; then use 40×, 100×, or oil immersion to identify the organisms and/or cellular population.

TABLE 5.1. Arbitrary scale for quantifying bacteria and yeast (external canal)

	Per high power (400×) field
Scale bacteria	
0	None
1	Fewer than 1–2 organisms
2	2–5 organisms
3	5–20 organisms
4	More than 20
Scale yeast	
0	None
1	Fewer than 1
2	1–5
3	5–10
4	More than 10

- Special considerations:
  - Inflammatory cells degenerate with infection but often remain intact with immune-mediated skin disease
  - Acantholytic cells may be present in large numbers and lend diagnostic information (e.g., pemphigus foliaceus)
  - Large number of epithelial cells with few bacteria may indicate a keratinization disorder or hypothyroidism
  - Keratinocytes may have melanin granules (may be mistaken for bacteria)
  - Normal cerumen does not take up stain
  - Neutrophils without bacteria may indicate a hypersensitivity reaction to medications being placed in the ear canal (e.g., neomycin, propylene glycol).

DIRECT IMPRESSION SMEARS: TOUCH IMPRINTS/TZANCK PREPARATION

Used to diagnose *Malassezia* overgrowth or to evaluate ulcers and plaques.

- Press a glass slide directly onto the surface of the skin several times in the same site – often used if the surface of the skin is greasy (Figure 5.8), *or*
- Press the slide onto a cut surface of a biopsy specimen or directly onto a plaque/ulcer/erosion (Figure 5.9).
- If obtaining samples from the cut surface of a biopsy specimen, gently blot excess blood from the surface using a dry gauze sponge prior to making the imprint and air dry the slide prior to staining.
- Heat-fix samples obtained from a greasy surface prior to staining unless adhesive slides are used (optional).
- Collect samples for yeast identification by cotton swab or spatula rolled onto the slide (especially sensitive areas such as the perivulvar and perianal regions), or by superficial skin scraping spread onto the slide.
- For interdigital lesions, samples may be collected by impression of the interdigital web directly onto the slide.
- For paronychia, nail bed debris may be obtained by using a tongue depressor or spatula scraping of the region and then spread onto the glass slide.
- Sample crusted lesions and epidermal collarettes by gently removing the surface or margins of the lesion with a sterile needle and imprinting the subjacent surface on a glass slide.
- Use the same arbitrary scale for quantification of yeast as used with otic swab.

FINE-NEEDLE ASPIRATION

Used to examine pustules, nodules, and tumors.

- Use a 22 gauge needle with attached 6 cc syringe for nodules/tumors.
- Use a 23 gauge needle with attached 3 cc syringe for smaller lesions (such as pustules).

- For solid nodules/tumors: carefully insert the needle into the center of the lesion, with the plunger pulled back to provide negative pressure; then release the negative pressure and repeat the process several times (sometimes while redirecting the needle).
- Always release the negative pressure prior to removing the needle from the lesion so that the sample collected remains in the needle or needle hub.
- Alternative method for solid nodules/tumors: draw 2 cc of air into the 6 cc syringe; using a stabbing motion, insert the needle into several areas of the nodule/tumor (Figure 5.10).
- Remove the needle from the syringe, fill the syringe with air, replace the needle onto the syringe, and expel the sample onto a clean microscope slide.
- Prior to staining, the sample should be gently distributed in a thin layer using a second slide.
- For smaller lesions (such as pustules): gently wipe alcohol onto the surface of the lesion, air dry, lance the roof of the lesion with a sterile needle, and "scoop up" the contents with the needle to place on a glass slide (Figure 5.11).

ACETATE TAPE PREPARATION

Used for identification of mites (*Cheyletiella* spp.) and yeast.

- Use "clear" acetate tape.
- For *Malassezia* identification:
  - Press the suspect area multiple times with the sticky side of the tape (Figure 5.12a)
  - Stain the tape with a modified Romanowsky stain (i.e., Diff-Quik®)
  - Do not put tape into the "fixative" to prevent dissolving of the adhesive and sample loss (Figure 5.12b)
  - Press the tape (sticky side down) onto a glass slide.
- For *Cheyletiella* identification:
  - Apply the tape to multiple sites (collecting as much scale as possible)
  - Directly press tape (sticky side down) onto a glass slide.

COMMENTS

- With direct impression, forcefully press the sample onto the surface of the slide for greater adherence.
- If heat fixing, heat fixation should be brief – do not "cook" the slide.
- The staining process should be gentle to avoid dislodging the material from the slide (immerse the slide in each fixative/stain and hold for the allotted time rather than repeated dippings).
- Use caution when rinsing the slide (low pressure).
- Change stain pots on a routine basis (weekly or when contaminated).

- Organisms will be clearer when using oil immersion (e.g., 1000×) or when a drop of immersion oil is placed on the slide with a cover slip applied when using high dry objective (e.g., 400×).
- Permanently save the slide by applying a small amount of mounting medium (e.g., Permount) with a cover slip.
- Tips for evaluating cytology samples:
  - Melanin granules can mimic bacteria in cytologic samples; they are typically round to oblong and have a green/brown coloration
  - Keratohyalin granules are pink to purple and irregular in shape and are typically seen within epidermal cells
  - Stain precipitate is amorphous and granular and often dark purple or black in color.

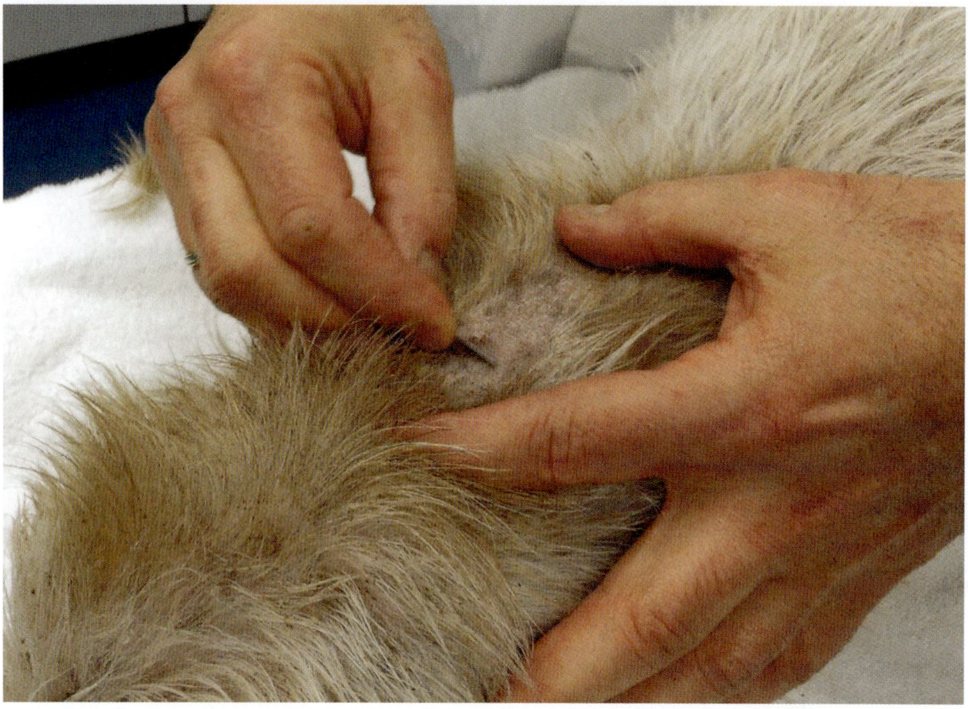

Fig. 5.1. Skin scraping technique: scrape in the direction of the hair growth, "scoop" up debris accumulated on blade, and transfer onto a glass slide.

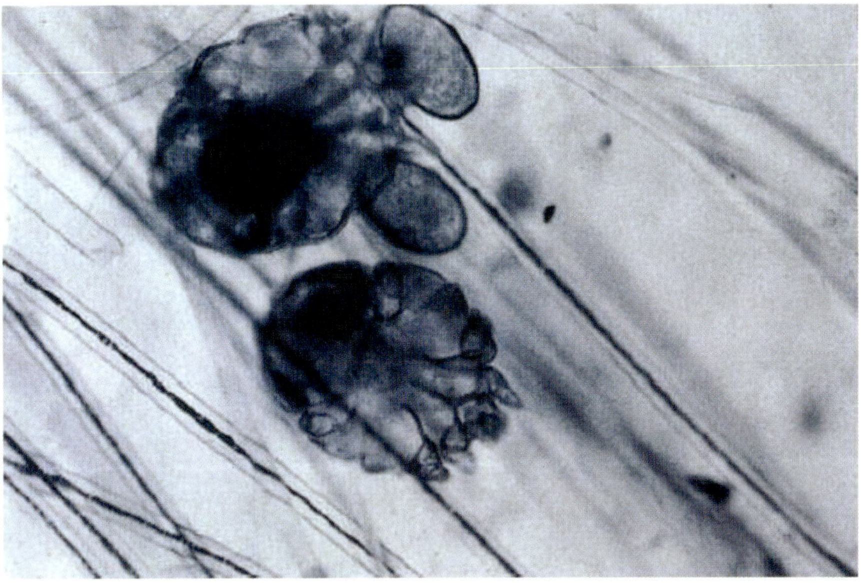

(a)

(b)

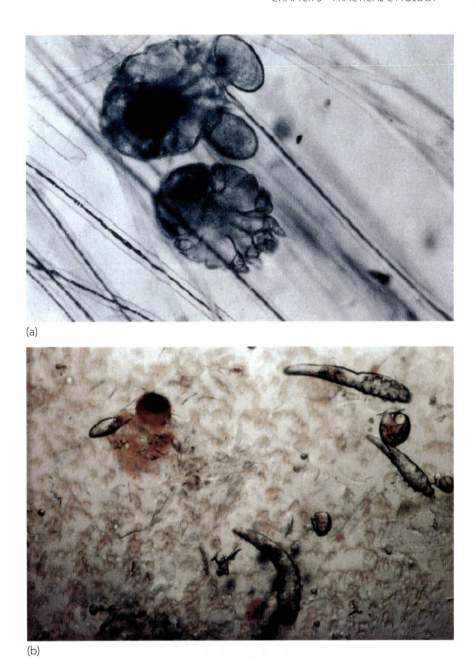

■ **Fig. 5.2.** (s) *Sarcoptes scabiei* mite and ova found on a superficial skin scraping of the ear margin. (b) *Demodex canis* mites: records should note the different stages of the mite found (adult, larva, and egg in the above sample). The presence of red blood cells indicates a sufficiently deep scraping.

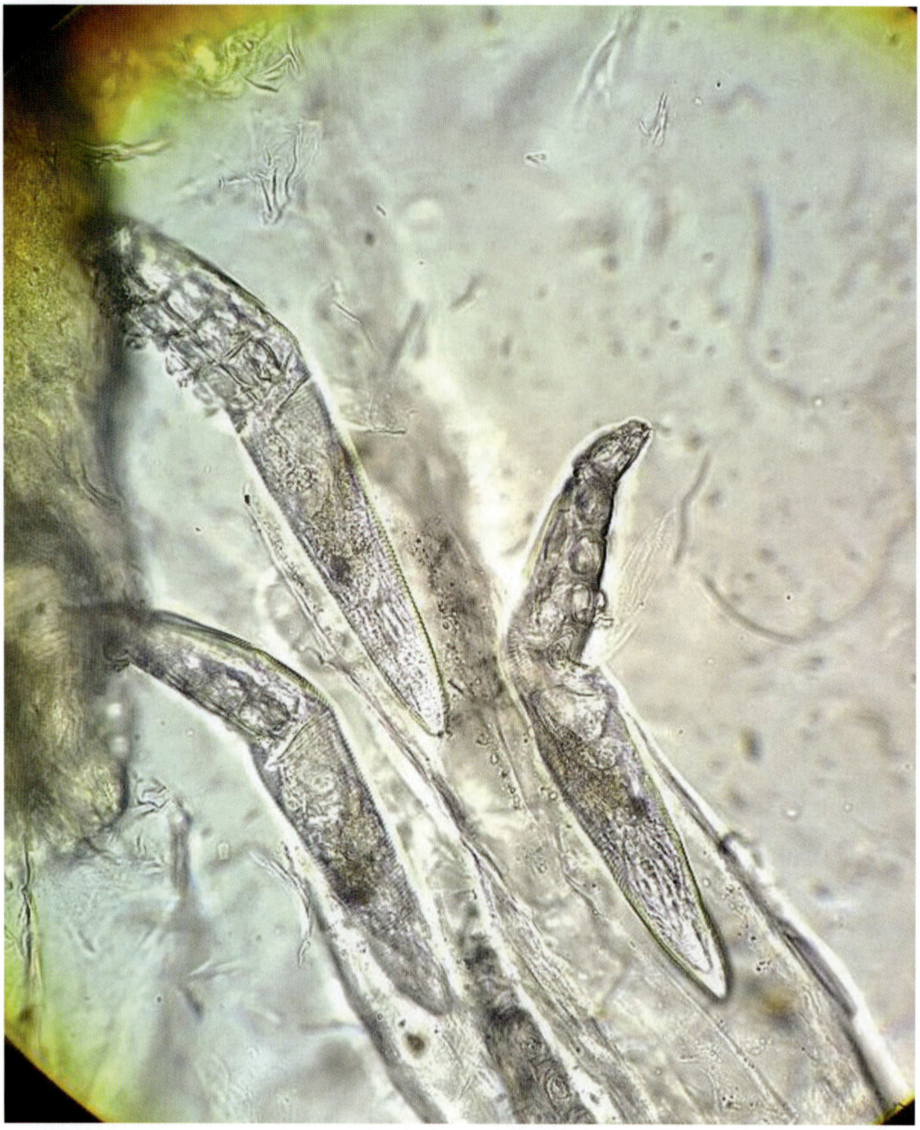

■ **Fig. 5.3.** *Demodex canis* mites at the hair bulb within follicle root sheath from a trichogram.

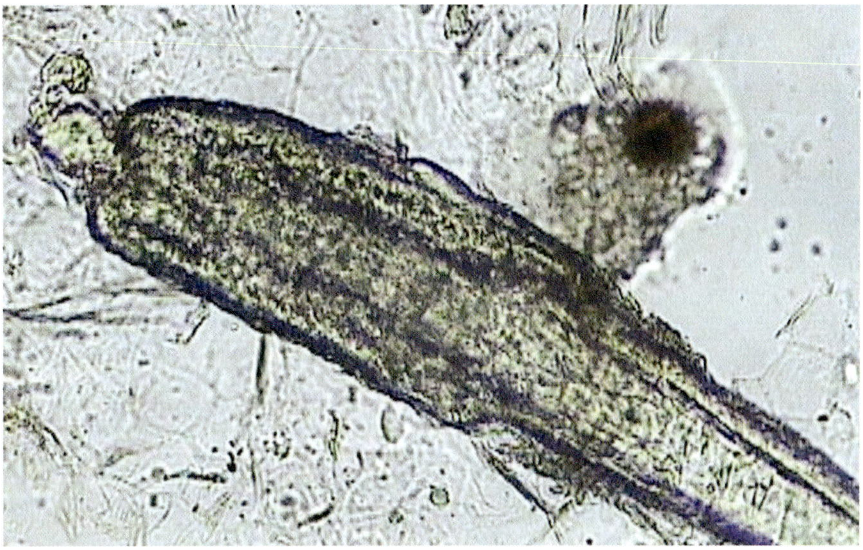

(a)

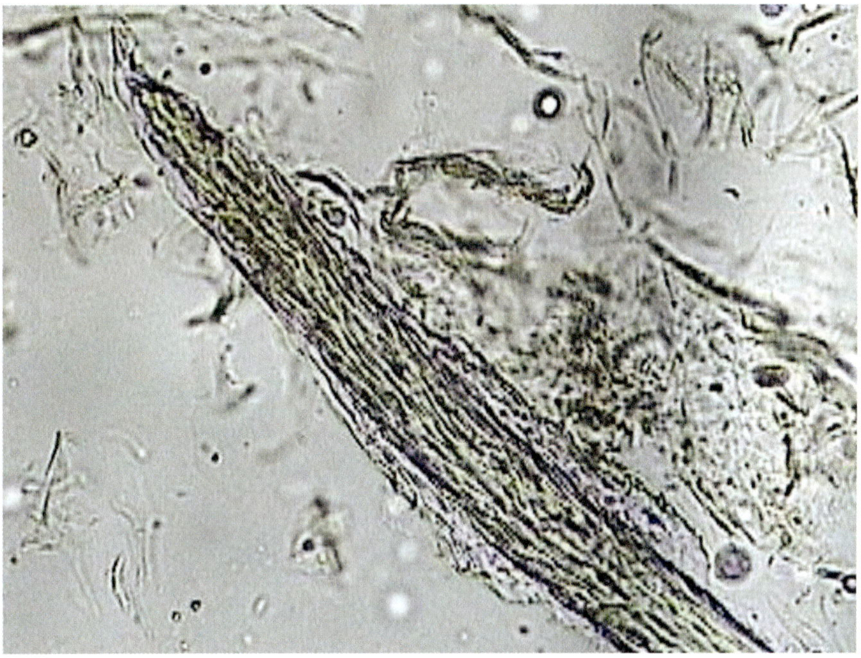

(b)

■ **Fig. 5.4.** Trichogram. (a) Anagen hair bulbs have rounded ends and may curl or bend. (b) Telogen hairs have a pointed or tapered end.

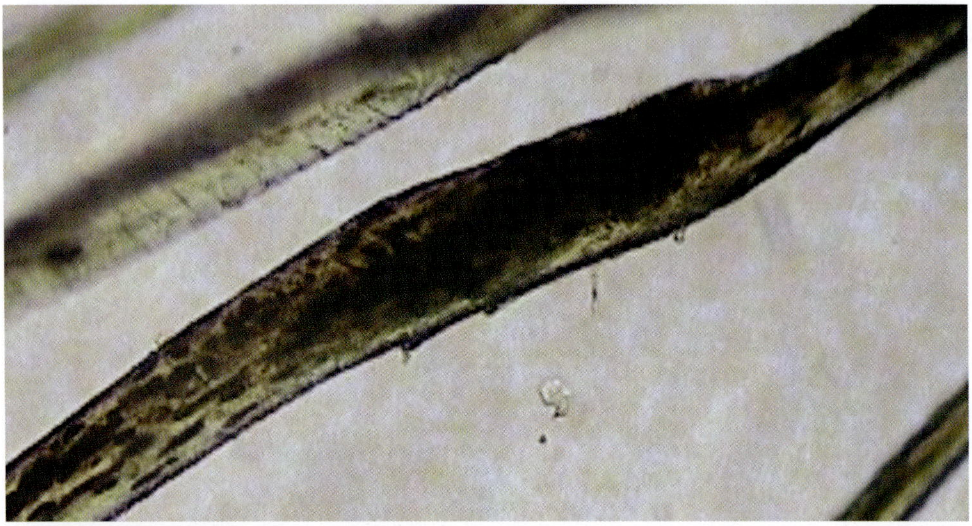

■ **Fig. 5.5.** Macromelanosome interrupting hair shaft in dog with color dilution alopecia.

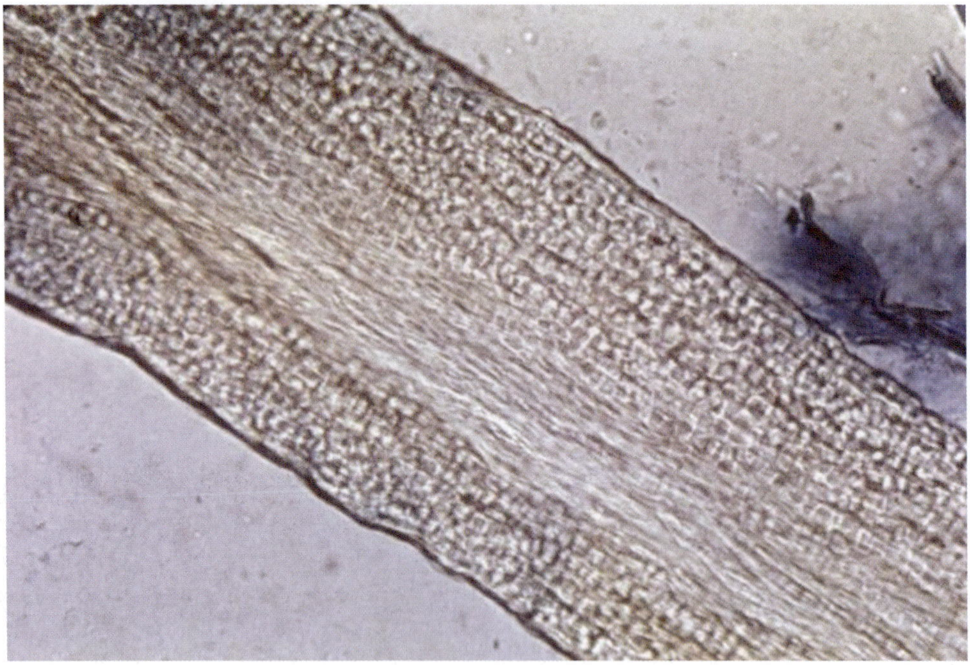

■ **Fig. 5.6.** Fungal hyphae invading hair shaft causing an irregular surface of the cuticle.

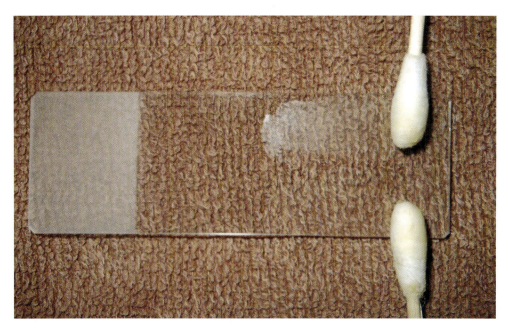

■ **Fig. 5.7.** Cytology slides from the ear, interdigital space, etc., are made by rolling the cotton-tipped applicator across the glass slide – samples from ears separated onto right (*lower*) and left (*upper*) sides of one slide.

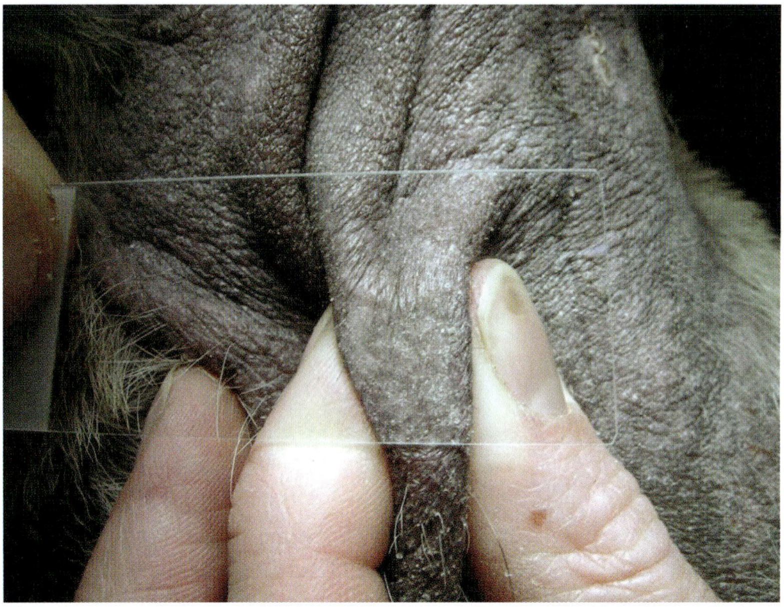

(a)

■ **Fig. 5.8.** (a) Impression smear for yeast; press a glass slide directly onto the surface of the skin several times in the same site. (b) Cytologic specimen (oil emersion, 1000×) from a patient with *Malassezia* pododermatitis.

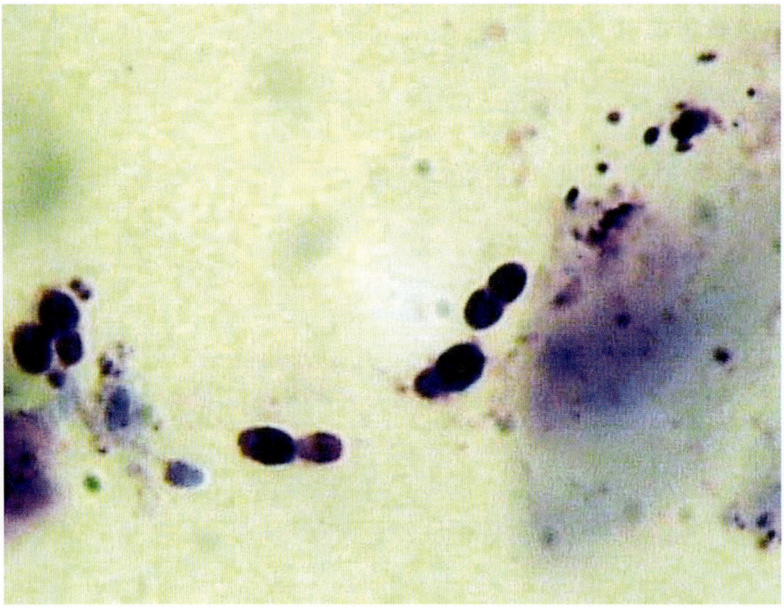

(b)

■ **Fig. 5.8.** (*Continued*)

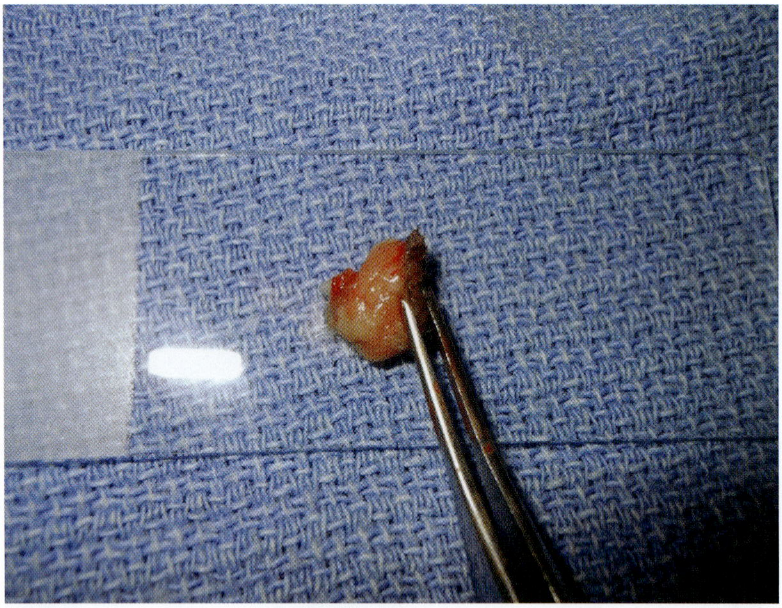

(a)

■ **Fig. 5.9.** Touch prep from biopsy sample. (a) Punch biopsy sample is transected; the flat portion is blotted on gauze to remove blood and pressed multiple times onto the glass slide. (b) Slide is dried and routinely stained. (c) Cytology from this biopsy demonstrating atypical lymphocytes in a patient with epitheliotropic lymphoma (oil immersion, 1000×).

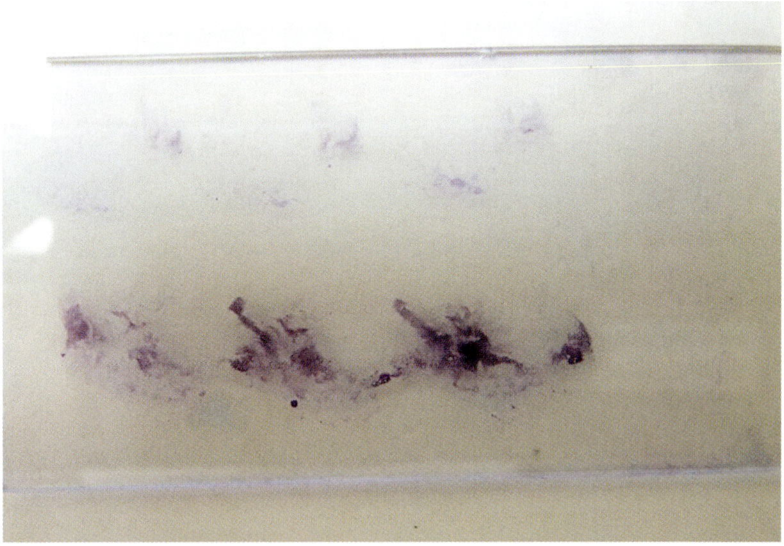

(b)

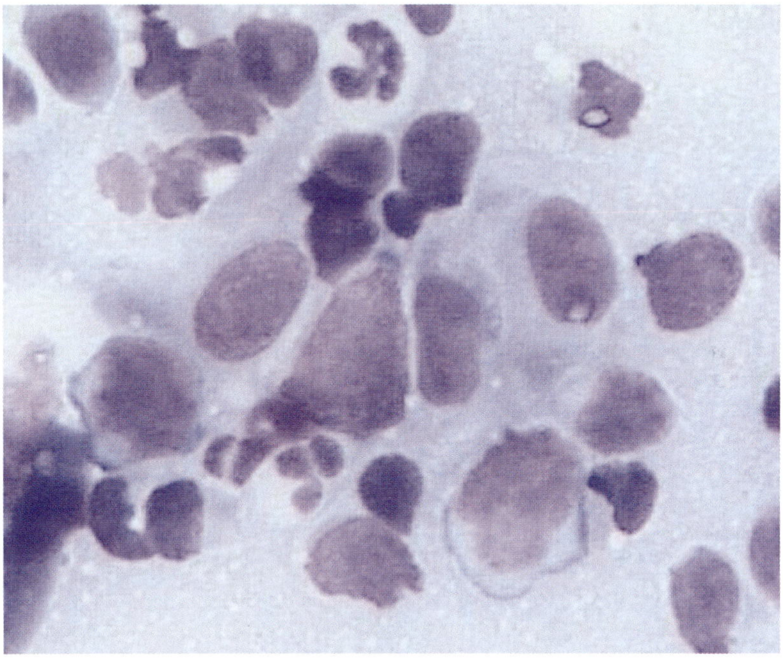

(c)

■ **Fig. 5.9.** *(Continued)*

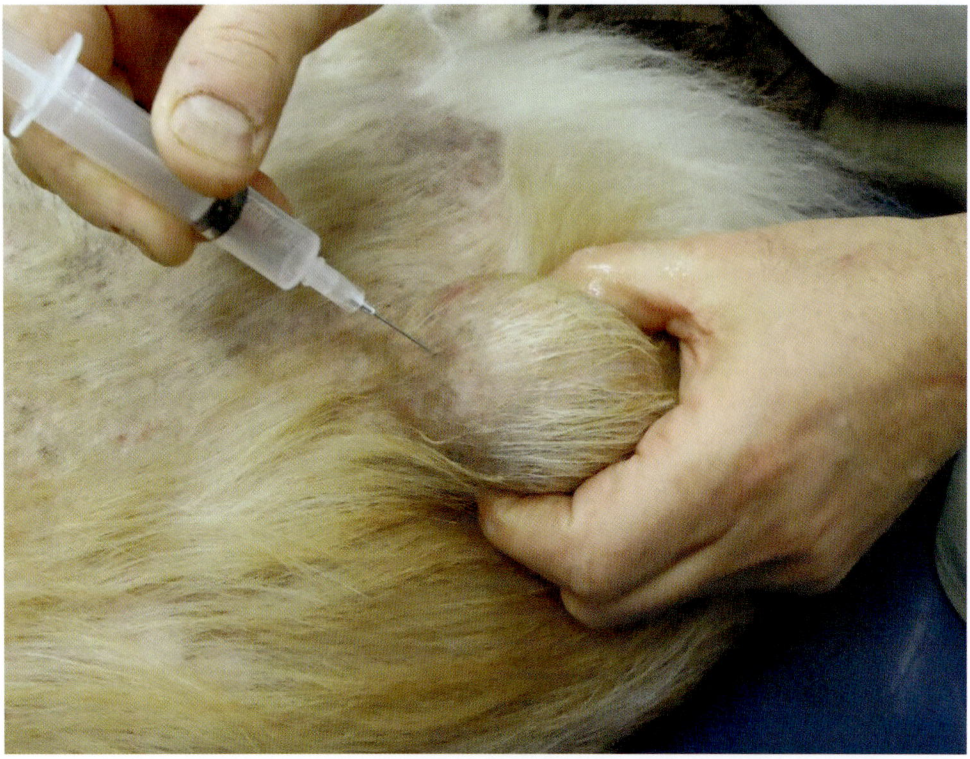

■ **Fig. 5.10.** A 22 gauge needle on a 6 cc syringe (with 2 mL air) is "stabbed" into a mass multiple times to obtain the sample. The contents are ejected onto a glass slide using a second slide to gently distribute the sample prior to staining.

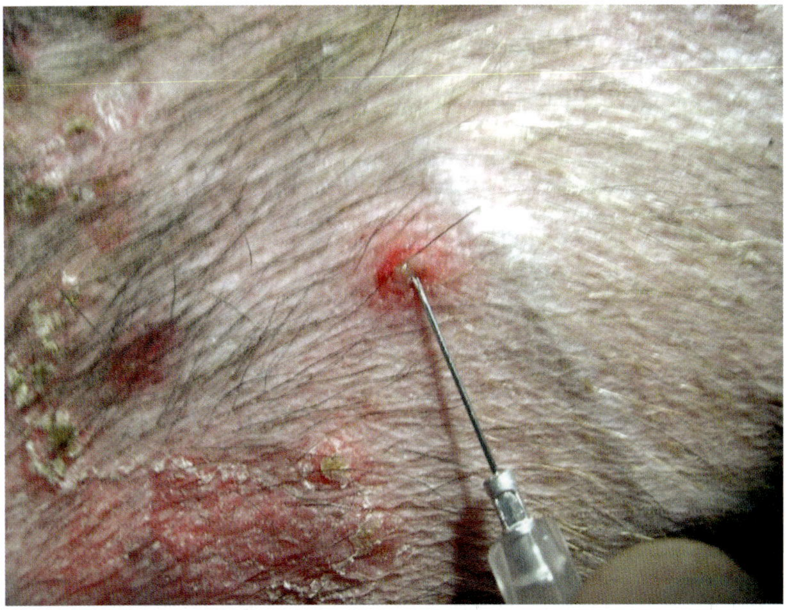

(a)

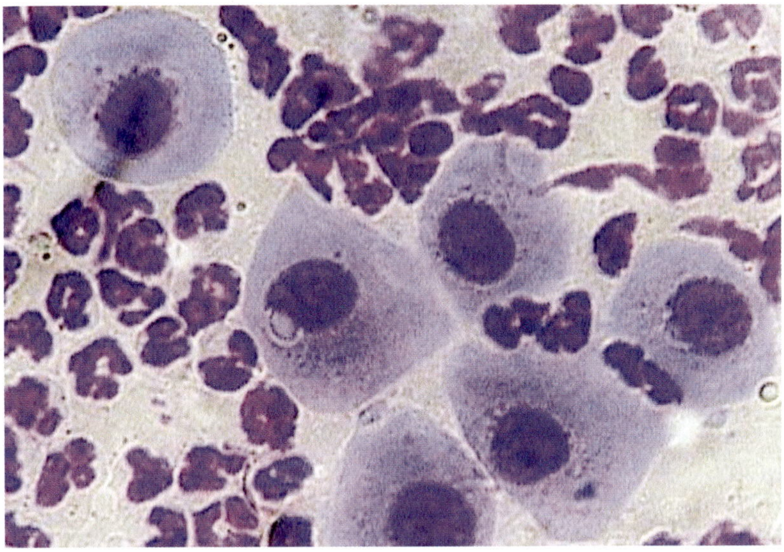

(b)

■ **Fig. 5.11.** (a) The roof of the lesion is lanced with a sterile needle, and the contents picked up by the needle to place on a glass slide. (b) Cytology from the same patient showing acantholytic keratinocytes and intact neutrophils seen with pemphigus foliaceus.

(a)

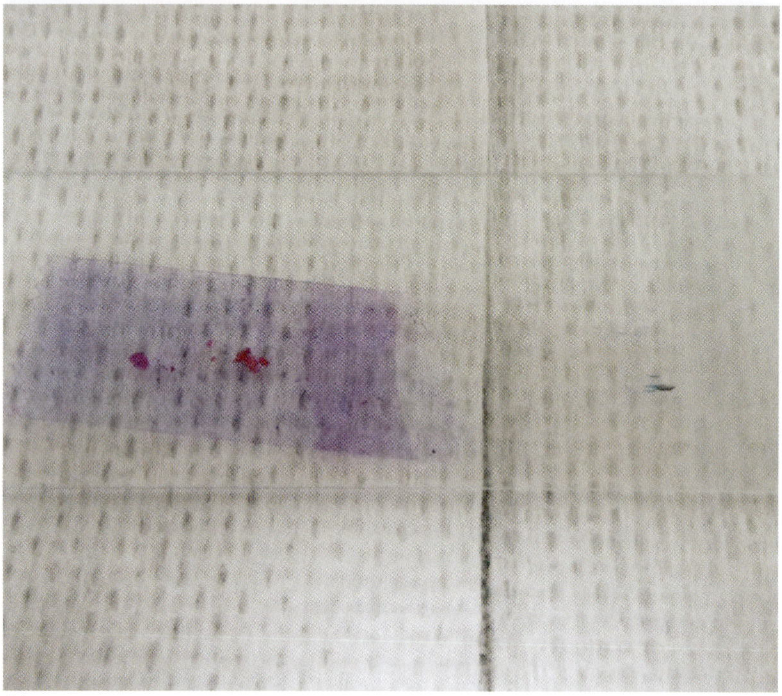

(b)

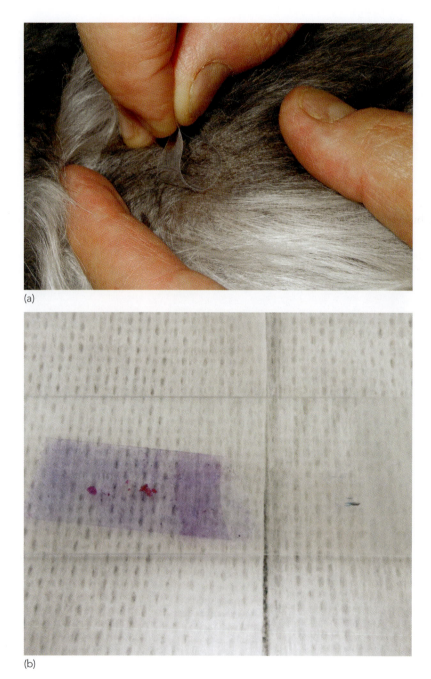

Fig. 5.12. (a) Sticky side of acetate tape is pressed repeatedly onto the skin to obtain sample. (b) Tape is stained and placed on a glass slide for examination.

chapter 6

Symptom Checker (Lesional and Regional Dermatoses)

DEFINITION/OVERVIEW

- Characteristics and patterns of lesions can often help narrow the differential list when examining a patient.
- The bulleted lists below are included as a tool to aid in formulating a differential list.
- It is impossible to make such a list all inclusive and completely accurate: many diseases/conditions have overlapping clinical signs.
- This chapter is intended to function as a preliminary guideline, a "symptom checker," for some of the more common dermatoses.

PATCHY ALOPECIA

- Demodicosis: often accompanied with hyperpigmentation, comedones, erythema, and secondary folliculitis (Figures 6.1, 6.2).
- Dermatophytosis: associated with scaling and folliculitis.
- Staphylococcal folliculitis: papules, pustules, crusts, epidermal collarettes, hyperpigmented macules, individual or large coalescing and "spreading" (Figure 6.3).
- Injection reaction: may be induration and/or atrophy at the site, often associated with repositol corticosteroid injection or routine vaccinations (Figure 6.4).
- Vaccine-induced vasculitis: lesion may or may not be associated with erythema, often rabies vaccine induced, may be observed 2–3 months after injection (Figure 6.5).
- Alopecia areata: noninflammatory complete focal alopecia, immune mediated, lymphocyte attack on hair bulb (Figure 6.6).
- Localized scleroderma: rare, shiny, smooth sclerotic patch (Figure 6.7).
- Sebaceous adenitis (short-coated breeds): annular to polycyclic areas, often associated with scaling (Figure 6.8).
- Anagen defluxion: sudden onset, stressful event or medication reaction, noninflammatory.
- Bowenoid *in situ* carcinoma (BISC): primarily seen in cats, possibly secondary to papillomavirus infection – pigmented scaling patches, often the head and pinnae (Figure 6.9).

Blackwell's Five-Minute Veterinary Consult Clinical Companion: Small Animal Dermatology, Third Edition.
Karen Helton Rhodes and Alexander H. Werner.

SPECIFIC LOCATION ALOPECIA

- Traction alopecia: associated with hairclips or rubber bands, dorsum of head (Figure 6.10).
- Postclipping alopecia: failure to regrow hair after clipping (often in Nordic breeds).
- Melanoderma/alopecia of Yorkshire terriers: alopecia and hyperpigmentation of pinnae, bridge of nose, sometimes tail and feet, puppies and young adults.
- Canine flank alopecia: localized cyclic serpiginous, follicular dysplasia on the flank associated with hyperpigmentation and comedones (Figure 6.11).
- Black hair follicular dysplasia: black hair only (Figure 6.12).
- Dermatomyositis: symmetric alopecia on the face, tip of tail, digits, carpi, tarsi, and pinnae; often associated with erythema and scarring; primarily in shelties and collies (Figure 6.13).
- Pinnal alopecia: miniaturization of hair, periodic or progressive, common in Siamese cats and dachshunds.
- Pattern baldness in dogs: Portuguese water dogs, American water spaniels, greyhounds, whippets, Boston terriers, Manchester terriers, Chihuahuas, Italian greyhounds, miniature pinscher (Figures 6.14, 6.15).
- Tail gland (supracaudal gland) alopecia: a patch of noninflamed alopecia located approximately 2 inches from the base of the tail along the dorsal surface (Figure 6.16).

GENERALIZED/DIFFUSE ALOPECIA

- Demodicosis: severe cases (Figure 6.17).
- Dermatophytosis: severe, chronic cases (Figure 6.18).
- Sebaceous adenitis: associated with phrynoderma (keratin casts), diffuse scaling, dorsum is always more affected than ventrum, dorsum of head involved (Figure 6.19).
- Cushing's syndrome (typical and atypical): truncal alopecia, comedones, rat tail, atrophic skin, phlebectasia, potbelly, pyoderma, hyperpigmentation (dog and cat); curling of tips of pinnae and skin fragility are characteristic in the cat (Figures 6.20–6.22).
- Hypopituitarism: failure to grow primary hair coat (Figure 6.23).
- Alopecia X: adrenal hyperplasia-like syndrome, symmetric truncal alopecia (Figure 6.24).
- Hypothyroidism: "tragic face"/myxedema in the dog, bilateral and symmetrical truncal and cervical alopecia (Figures 6.25, 6.26).
- Hyperthyroidism: cat, unkempt hair coat with partial alopecia, barbering along forelimbs, may mimic OCD (Figures 6.27, 6.28).
- Hyperestrogenism: rare symmetric alopecia of perineum, inguinal, flank regions; mammary glands and vulvar hyperplasia, cystic ovaries.
- Estrous related: intact female dogs, perineal and flank alopecia that may progress to generalized, cyclic.

- Testosterone-responsive dermatoses: progressive truncal alopecia of castrated male dogs.
- Sertoli cell tumor: male feminization, gynecomastia, alopecia of perineum and genital region (Figure 6.29).
- Castration-responsive dermatosis: hair loss in collar area, perineum, caudomedial thighs, flanks.
- Topical hormone replacement therapy exposure: more recently recognized cause of "endocrinopathy" appearance (Figures 6.30, 6.31).
- Diabetes mellitus: partial diffuse alopecia, may be associated with miliary dermatitis in the cat (Figure 6.32).
- Color dilution alopecia: thinning of haircoat, associated with folliculitis, progressive, often associated with blue coat color; common in Yorkshire terriers, dobermans, labradors (Figure 6.33).
- Follicular dysplasia: slow progressive alopecia (Irish water spaniels, Italian spinones).
- Follicular lipidosis: red points, young dogs, rottweilers.
- Congenital alopecia: bichon frise, beagle, basset hound, French bulldog, rottweiler; some breeds selected for this disorder – Chinese crested, Mexican dogs, American hairless terrier, Abyssinian cat, sphinx cat.
- Telogen defluxion: associated with stressful event (e.g., pregnancy).
- Keratinization disorder: associated with hyperkeratosis and excessive greasiness, most common in the cocker spaniel (Figure 6.34).
- Pemphigus: hair loss accompanied by scale, crust, pustules, erythema.
- Cutaneous epitheliotropic lymphoma: scale and alopecia initial stage; progresses to plaques, nodules, and ulceration, associated with depigmentation of mucous membranes (Figures 6.35–6.37).
- Feline hereditary hypotrichosis: autosomal recessive, Siamese, Devon rex, Burmese, birman; thin sparse haircoat.
- Feline alopecia universalis: hereditary defect, complete absence of primary hairs, decreased secondary hairs, thickened epidermis, oily skin, no whiskers, downy fur at tip of tail, paws, scrotum (sphinx, Canadian hairless).
- Feline symmetrical alopecia: psychogenic or allergic dermatitis most common etiology.
- Feline thymoma; exfoliative dermatitis, erythematous, nonpruritic, starts on the head and neck, becomes generalized, older cats.
- Feline paraneoplastic alopecia: acute onset, rapidly progressing, ventrally (may also affect eyes, nose, footpads) complete alopecia, smooth and glistening skin, pancreatic exocrine adenocarcinomas and bile duct carcinomas (Figure 6.38).
- Feline lymphocytic mural folliculitis: alopecia, scale, hyperpigmentation, ± pruritus may be a reaction pattern or paraneoplastic syndrome.
- Pseudopelade: lymphocytic attack on hair follicle isthmus with resultant alopecia, nonpruritic, noninflammatory (Figure 6.39).
- Alopecia mucinosa: mucinosis of hair follicle outer root sheath and epidermis.
- Trichorrhexis nodosa: excessive trauma to the hair, focal hair shaft swelling associated with cuticular damage.

EXFOLIATIVE DERMATOSES

- Dermatophytosis: can manifest as any clinical presentation, commonly exfoliative (Figure 6.40).
- Ectoparasites: cheyletiellosis, demodicosis, sarcoptid mite infestation (Figure 6.41).
- Feline thymoma: erythema, face, neck; older cats, nonpruritic, exfoliative.
- Keratinization disorders: keratin casts, secondary *Malassezia* overgrowth.
- Vitamin A-responsive dermatosis: nutritionally responsive; cocker spaniels, westies, dalmatians, labradors, shar-pei, fox terriers (Figure 6.42).
- Zinc-responsive dermatosis: alopecia, scale, crust, erythema; periocular, pinnal, lips, Alaskan breeds predisposed (Figure 6.43).
- Follicular dysplasias: alopecia associated with hyperkeratosis and abnormal hair morphology (structure/melanization) (Figure 6.44).
- Idiopathic canine nasodigital hyperkeratosis: accumulation of scale of the planum nasale and digital pad margins, generally asymptomatic (Figure 6.45).
- Sebaceous adenitis: diffuse keratin casts that mat the hair to the surface of the skin, dorsum of the body most affected including head (Figures 6.46, 6.47).
- Ichthyosis: severe congenital disorder of keratinization, golden retrievers, West Highland white terriers, cavalier King Charles spaniels, Jack Russell, Norfolk terrier, Yorkshire terriers; tightly adhered scale secondary pyoderma, poor prognosis (Figure 6.48).
- Epitheliotropic lymphoma (cutaneous T cell lymhoma – CTCL): static patches of scaling are often the first clinical signs of CTCL followed by plaques, nodules, and tumors; also associated with depigmentation and oral lesions (Figures 6.49–6.52).
- Actinic keratosis: crusted erythematous patches to plaques on sun-exposed skin (Figure 6.53).
- Lichenoid psoriasiform dermatosis: springer spaniels and German shepherds predisposed, medial aspect of pinnae and groin (Figure 6.54).
- Schnauzer comedone syndrome: scaling and comedones along the dorsal trunk.
- Ear margin dermatosis: dachshunds, idiopathic, ± vasculitis/vasculopathy, alopecia, fissures, keratin casts, notching (Figure 6.55).
- Hereditary nasal parakeratosis of labradors: may fissure and cause some discomfort, often nonsymptomatic, 6–12 months of age (Figure 6.56).
- Superficial necrolytic dermatosis: "hepatocutaneous syndrome"; hyperkeratosis, crusting, ulceration; pinnae, face, MCJ, joints, footpads (Figure 6.57).
- Dirty face syndrome of Persian cats: erythematous and exfoliative, pruritic, red/brown sebaceous accumulation, often *Malassezia* overgrowth, also recognized in Himalayan cats. (Figure 6.58).
- Acne: feline and canine; pyoderma variant in dogs; keratinization defect in cats (Figure 6.59).
- Exfoliative cutaneous lupus erythematosus: exfoliative, crusting, and scaling; facial distribution of German short-haired pointers; young dogs, wax and wane (Figure 6.60).

CRUSTING AND EROSIVE/ULCERATIVE DERMATOSES

- Pemphigus foliaceus: often more crusted than ulcerative; bridge of nose, footpads, pinnal initial presentation, IMSD, drug induced (Promeris), dermatophyte induced (Figures 6.61–6.64).
- Pemphigus vulgaris: ulcerative with adherent crust; may have oral lesions (Figure 6.65).
- Bullous pemphigoid: autoantibody directed against the basement membrane zone, ulcerative, mucocutaneous junctions often affected.
- Discoid lupus erythematosus: immune complex deposition; nasal planum, pinnae, footpads; depigmentation (Figure 6.66).
- Systemic lupus erythematosus: multisystemic disease, immune complex deposition targeting basement membrane zones (Figure 6.67).
- Exfoliative cutaneous lupus erythematosus: exfoliative, crusting, and scaling; facial distribution of German short-haired pointers; young dogs, wax and wane (see Figure 6.60).
- Cold agglutinin disease: tips of extremities most often affected; ulceration/necrosis.
- Vasculitis: idiopathic, immune mediated, FeLV associated (necrosis of ear tips and tail), neoplasm associated, drug induced, vaccination related (rabies), hereditary – juvenile polyarteritis syndrome of beagles, neutrophilic leukocytoclastic vasculitis of Jack Russell terriers, familial cutaneous vasculopathy of German shepherds, cutaneous and renal glomerular vasculopathy of greyhounds, thrombovascular pinnal necrosis of dachshunds, diabetes-associated vasculitis, rickettsial-associated vasculitis, uremia-associated vasculitis, eosinophilic (insect), rheumatoid arthritis (Figure 6.68).
- Toxic epidermal necrolysis: confluent epidermal necrosis; idiopathic, drug induced (Figure 6.69).
- Mucous membrane pemphigoid: subepidermal blistering disease; oral cavity, nasal, pinnal, anus, eyes, genitalia.
- Erythema multiforme: serpiginous or target "bull's eye" lesions; idiopathic, vaccine or drug induced; herpesvirus induced in the cat (Figure 6.70).
- Eosinophilic nasal furunculosis: acute onset; insect/spider bite possible cause; alopecia, erythema, erosive, nodular, ± pruritus/pain (Figure 6.71).
- Canine juvenile cellulitis: "puppy strangles," sterile granulomatous, pustular, erosive, ulcerative; face, pinnal, peripheral lymph nodes (Figure 6.72).
- Cutaneous histiocytosis: bridge nose, nasal mucosa, trunk, limbs; Bernese mountain dogs and golden retrievers predisposed (Figure 6.73).
- Staphylococcal bacterial folliculitis: superficial (crusted) and deep (ulcerative) (Figure 6.74).
- Deep and intermediate mycoses: sporotrichosis, blastomycosis, cryptococcosis, coccidioidomycosis (Figure 6.75).
- Atypical mycobacteriosis: trauma predisposes, feline more common, ulcerative nodules with fistulous tracts, adipose tissue thickened caused by infection with actinomycetic bacteria: *Nocardia* spp., *Actinomyces* spp., *Streptomyces* spp. (Figure 6.76).

- Pythiosis: animals exposed to stagnant water, ulcerative nodules, severe pruritus.
- Protothecosis: saprophytic algae, stagnant water, ulcerative MCJ, depigmentation.
- Paecilomycosis: saprophytic yeast-like fungus; decaying vegetation; ulcerative nodules and otitis externa.
- Leishmaniasis: protozoan parasite, zoonotic disease, exfoliative, crusting, ulcerative dermatosis (Figure 6.77).
- Feline cowpox: rare, cats become infected via bite wound, Europe, ulcerated papules and nodules.
- FeLV- and FIV-associated dermatoses: giant cell dermatosis (ulcerative, pruritic; face, neck, pinnae) and FeLV vasculitis of the pinnal tips and tail (Figure 6.78).
- Feline calicivirus-associated dermatoses: feline orofacial pain syndrome (trigeminal neuralgia, unilateral facial pruritus – Siamese and Burmese).
- Demodicosis: severe generalized cases become crusted and ulcerative.
- Sarcoptid mites: severe pruritus induces generalized excoriation and crusting.
- Flea bite hypersensitivity: caudodorsal trunk.
- Feline mosquito bite hypersensitivity: lesions are facial, erythematous, and ulcerative nodules (Figure 6.79).
- Pelodera and hookworm migration: erythema, ulceration; footpads, ventrum.
- Feline eosinophilic granuloma complex: indolent ulcer, linear granuloma, eosinophilic plaque (Figure 6.80).
- Allergic dermatitis: severe pruritus causes erosion, ulceration, crusting (Figure 6.81).
- Dermatomyositis: hereditary ischemic dermatopathy; face, ears, tail; megaesophagus, muscle disease/atrophy, dropped gait.
- Epidermolysis bullosa aquisita: young Great Danes (most common); urticaria, vesicles, ulcers – face, groin, footpads, oral cavity, mucocutaneous junctions (Figure 6.82).
- Cutaneous asthenia: skin hyperextensibility and fragility; both dogs and cats; ulcerations and scarring.
- Cutaneous xanthoma: cholesterol clefts in the dermis; yellow-pink alopecic plaques and nodules that tend to ulcerate, often associated with diabetes or idiopathic hyperlipidemia (Figure 6.83).
- Drug eruption (Figure 6.84).
- Superficial necrolytic dermatosis (hepatocutaneous syndrome): hyperkeratotic ulcerative dermatosis associated with liver disease and/or pancreatic glucagonoma.
- Calcinosis cutis: mineral deposits within the dermis associated with collagen degeneration induced by corticosteroid administration or hyperadrenocorticism; intense pruritus, erosion, ulceration (Figure 6.85).
- Epitheliotropic lymphoma: depigmentation, scale, plaques, nodules, and ulceration; slowly progressive; dogs and cats (see Figure 6.50).
- Ulcerative dermatosis of collies and shelties: may be variant of dermatomyositis or a vesicular cutaneous form of lupus erythematosus; serpiginous erythema with flaccid bullae that ulcerate; groin, axillae, genitalia, pinnae, oral mucosa, footpads.
- Feline ulcerative linear dermatosis: solitary lesion over neck and shoulder region, intense pruritus, refractory to therapy.

- Feline plasma cell pododermatitis: metatarsal and metacarpal pads, swollen and spongy, ulcerative; may be FIV associated (Figure 6.86).
- Idiopathic nodular panniculitis: subcutaneous nodules and draining tracts over the trunk; dachshunds predisposed, dorsum often more severely affected, lesions are sterile, heal with crusting and scarring (Figure 6.87).
- Erythema ab igne: radiant heat damage (Figure 6.88).
- Actinic dermatitis: erythema and scaling that progresses to nodules/erosion/ulceration; lightly pigmented skin predisposed.
- Solar, thermal, chemical burns: erythema, scale, erosion, ulceration, necrosis (Figure 6.89).
- Acral mutilation syndrome in springer spaniels: severe ulceration of extremities; self-induced, hereditary sensory neuropathy.

PIGMENTARY ABNORMALITIES

- Idiopathic leukoderma/leukotrichia (vitiligo): skin and hair affected; Belgian shepherds, German shepherds, dobermans, rottweilers predisposed; can be permanent or wax and wane (Figures 6.90, 6.91).
- Canine uveodermatologic syndrome (Vogt Koyanagi Harada-like syndrome): panuveitis, leukoderma, leukotrichia, meningoencephalitis; immune-mediated attack on melanocytes; huskies and akitas predisposed (Figure 6.92).
- Nasal hypopigmentation (Dudley nose – permanent, snow nose – transient): idiopathic; cobblestone texture of the planum nasale retained.
- Epitheliotropic lymphoma: mucocutaneous junctions are often depigmented (Figure 6.93).
- Discoid lupus erythematosus: depigmentation and ulceration of the planum nasale often clinical features (Figure 6.94).
- Systemic lupus erythematosus, bullous pemphigoid, pemphigus vulgaris, pemphigus erythematosus: immune-mediated diseases that affect the dermoepidermal junction region of the skin (melanocyte collateral).
- Dermatomyositis: collies and shelties; scarring dermatosis, megaesophagus, dropped gait, muscle weakness, depigmentation of skin and coat.
- Drug-induced pigment changes: ketoconazole induces graying of the coat.
- Lentigo: asymptomatic patches of black pigment in older dogs and orange cats; lesions are flat macules, hypermelanosis (Figure 6.95).
- Postinflammatory hyperpigmentation: normal response of the skin to inflammation, indicative of the healing process.
- Color dilution alopecia (color mutant alopecia): associated with blue or fawn coat colors.
- Melanoderma and alopecia of Yorkshire terriers: alopecia, shiny skin, hyperpigmented skin.
- Macular melanosis: associated with testicular neoplasm.

- Chediak–Higashi syndrome: Persian cats (blue smoke color), white tigers, Hereford, cattle, Aleutian mink; macromelanosomes; photophobia, immunodeficiency, bleeding disorders.
- Oculocutaneous albinism: white Persian cats with heterochromic irides and deafness.
- Canine cyclic hematopoiesis, gray collie syndrome, canine cyclic neutropenia; light-colored nose often diagnostic; hepatic and renal failure; often fatal by 2 years of age.
- Color dilution and cerebellar degeneration in Rhodesian ridgeback dogs: bluish coat color associated with Purkinje cell degeneration; lethal.
- Acquired aurotrichia of miniature schnauzers: young adults, patchy golden hairs of the trunk, unknown cause.
- Nevus/nevi: hyperpigmented macules and patches, nonsymptomatic (Figure 6.96).
- Melanoma: pigmented tumors (Figure 6.97).

CLAW AND CLAWFOLD DERMATOSES

- Special considerations for the claw/clawfold regions:
    - Symmetrical claw problems (multiple claws on multiple paws) often indicate immune-mediated, metabolic, genetic, nutritional, or viral etiologies
    - Asymmetrical distribution (one or multiple claws on one paw) is more likely to identify infections, trauma, or neoplasm.
- Fungal infections: dermatophyte, *Malassezia*, *Candida*, *Blastomyces*, *Cryptococcus*, *Geotrichosis*, *Sporothrix*.
- Bacterial infections: may be primary or secondary to trauma (Figure 6.98).
- Parasitic disease: demodicosis, hookworm dermatitis, ascarids (Figure 6.99).
- Protozoal disease: leishmaniasis.
- Viral disease: FeLV, FIV.
- Trauma: chemical (fertilizers, floor cleansers, salt), acquired arteriovenous fistula.
- Immune-mediated diseases: lupoid onychodystrophy, systemic lupus erythematosus. pemphigus foliaceus, pemphigus vulgaris, bullous pemphigoid, vasculitis, adverse drug reactions, vaccine reactions, cryoglobulinemia, eosinophilic plaque (EGC) (Figures 6.100–6.103).
- Metabolic diseases: hypothyroidism (dog), hyperthyroidism (cat), diabetes mellitus, hyperadrenocorticism, superficial necrolytic dermatitis, acromegaly (macronychia and onychogryphosis) (Figure 6.104).
- Genetic diseases: epidermolysis bullosa, dermatomyositis, seborrhea, linear epidermal nevus, anonychia, supernumerary claws, onychorrhexis in dachshunds (Figure 6.105).
- Neoplasm: squamous cell carcinoma, metatastatic bronchogenic adenocarcinoma, mast cell tumors, melanoma, keratoacanthoma, lymphosarcoma, hemangiopericytoma, osteosarcoma, myxosarcoma (Figures 6.106, 6.107).
- Miscellaneous: deficiencies, lethal acrodermatitis, zinc-responsive dermatosis, disseminated intravascular coagulopathy, idiopathic onychodystrophy, idiopathic onychomadesis, ergotism, thallotoxicosis, feline plasma cell pododermatitis.

NASAL PLANUM DERMATOSES

- Discoid lupus erythematosus: primarily affects nasal area, depigmentation, exacerbated by sunlight, loss of cobblestone architecture.
- Systemic lupus erythematosus: multisystemic disease; face, nose, mucocutaneous junctions, generalized.
- Pemphigus complex: immune-mediated skin disease, often more crusted than ulcerative, variable depigmentation; footpad crusting common (Figures 6.108, 6.109).
- Bullous pemphigoid: often associated with crusting and depigmentation; mucocutaneous junction common.
- Nasal solar dermatitis: starts at poorly pigmented junction of nasal planum and bridge of the nose, heavy sunlight exposure; differentiated from discoid lupus erythematosus by lack of involvement of the nasal planum (Figure 6.110).
- Contact dermatitis: not common; rubber dish; rare ulceration, erythema and depigmentation of the anterior nasal planum and lips (Figure 6.111).
- Dermatomyositis: nasal, facial, extremities; scarring depigmentation/ulceration; polymyositis and megaesophagus may be seen.
- Uveodermatologic syndrome: uveitis; depigmentation, ulceration nose, lips, eyelids (Figure 6.112).
- Nasal arteritis: profusely bleeding, often horizontally oriented ulcer on the nasal philtrum. Most often seen in St Bernards (Figure 6.113).
- Mucocutaneous pyoderma: focal areas of depigmentation and crusting. Usually asymmetrical (differentiation from DLE). Often on alar folds (Figure 6.114).
- Nasal pyoderma: primarily haired portions – bridge of the nose yet inflammation rarely extends onto the nasal planum.
- Vitiligo: depigmentation without inflammation or erosion/ulceration (Figure 6.115).
- Nasal hypopigmentation: light brown or tan color, may be seasonal, breed fault.
- Adverse drug reaction: topical sensitivity (neomycin) or systemic reaction.
- Epitheliotropic lymphoma: depigmentation and induration (see Figure 6.93).
- Histiocytosis: infiltrates often affect the nares and nasal turbinates; Bernese mountain dog predisposed (Figure 6.116).
- Idiopathic nasodigital hyperkeratosis: often older dogs; nasal planum and marginal footpads.
- Hereditary nasal parakeratosis: labradors, young dogs (see Figure 6.56)
- Allergy: mosquito bite hypersensitivity in cats (see Figure 6.79).
- Viral: herpes, calici (Figure 6.117).

NODULES AND DRAINING SINUS ETIOLOGY

- Bacterial:
  - Furunculosis secondary to *Staphylococcal* spp. most common
  - Actinomyces/nocardia
  - Mycobacteria

  - Foreign body
  - Feline mycoplasma abscess
  - Bacterial granulomas
  - Focal adnexal dysplasia secondary to chronic folliculitis/furunculosis.
- Fungal:
  - Majocchi granuloma/pseudomycetoma – dermatophyte granuloma
  - Sporotrichosis
  - Eumycetoma
  - Phaeohyphomycosis
  - Zygomycosis
  - Hyalohyphomycosis
  - Cryptococcosis
  - Coccidioidomycosis
  - Blastomycosis
  - Histoplasmosis.
- Parasitic:
  - Demodicosis
  - Leishmaniasis
  - Rhabditic dermatitis
  - Protista; pythiosis, protothecosis.
- Viral:
  - Viral papillomas.
- Hypersensitivity:
  - Urticaria
  - Angioedema
  - Eosinophilic granuloma
  - Arthropod bite hypersensitivity
  - Mosquito bite hypersensitivity (cat).
- Vascular:
  - Arteriovenous fistula
  - Vasculitis
  - Thrombosis
  - Clotting disorders.
- Metabolic:
  - Cutaneous xanthomatosis
  - Calcinosis cutis
  - Calcinosis circumscripta
  - Nodular cutaneous amyloidosis.
- Miscellaneous:
  - Sterile nodular panniculitis
  - Traumatic panniculitis
  - Postinjection panniculitis
  - Sterile nodular periadnexal pyogranulomatous dermatitis
  - Canine juvenile cellulitis syndrome
  - Reactive histiocytosis – cutaneous/systemic

- Nodular dermatofibrosis of German shepherd dogs
- Benign nodular sebaceous hyperplasia
- Skin tag/acrochordon
- Nevi/hamartoma (collagenous, vascular, follicular, sebaceous)
- Fibroadnexal dysplasia
- Dermoid cyst/sinus
- Cysts (follicular, epidermal, inclusion)
- Lipomatosis
- Apocrine cystomatosis.

■ Neoplasm:
- Round cell tumors: mast cell tumors, plasmacytomas, lymphomas, histiocytomas, malignant histiocytosis, histiocytic sarcomas, transmissable venereal tumors
- Melanocytic tumors: benign dermal melanocytoma, malignant melanoma
- Epithelial origin: squamous cell carcinoma, squamous papillomas, Bowenoid carcinoma *in situ*, basal cell tumor, keratoacanthoma, intracutaneous cornifying epithelioma, trichoepithelioma, pilomatrixoma, sebaceous gland/hepatoid/apocrine/ceruminous adenomas and carcinomas
- Mesenchymal: hemangiopericytomas, schwannomas, fibroma/fibrosarcomas, myxosarcoma, hemangioma/hemangiosarcomas, lymphangiomas/lymphangiosarcomas, lipomas/liposarcomas, fibropapilloma (feline sarcoid), leiomyosarcoma, dermatofibroma.

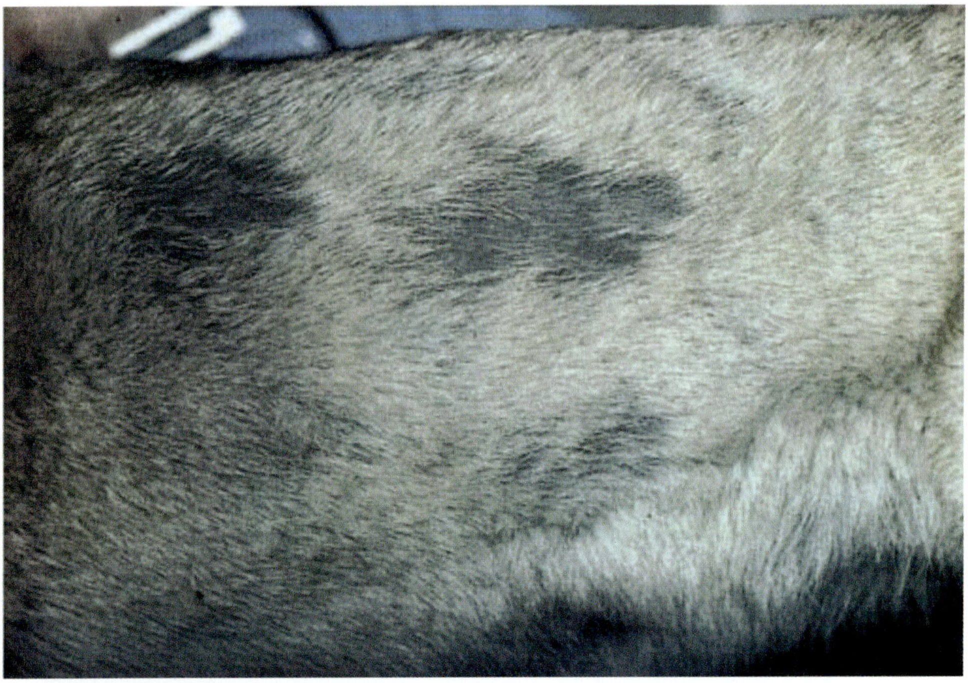

■ **Fig. 6.1.** Demodicosis characterized by multifocal patches of partial to complete alopecia.

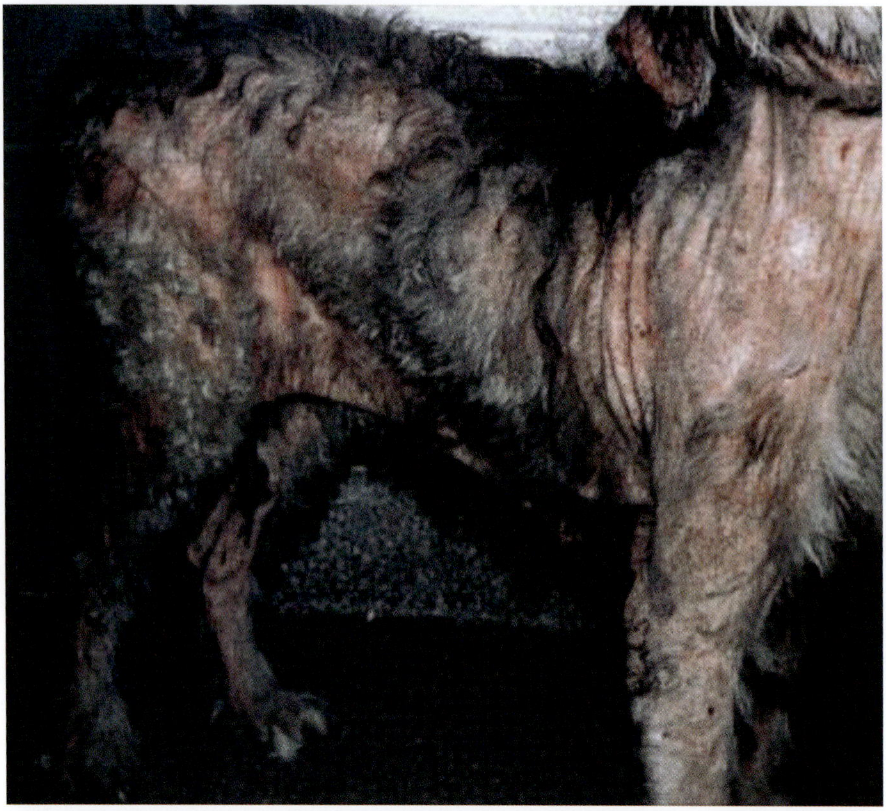

■ **Fig. 6.2.** Generalized demodicosis causing severe erythroderma, partial to complete alopecia, and crusting.

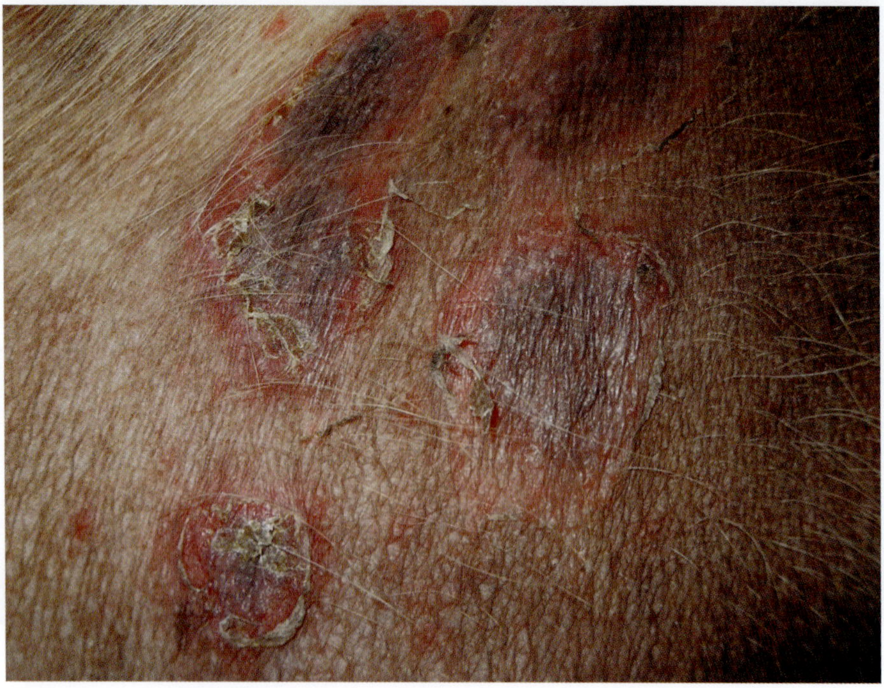

■ **Fig. 6.3.** Superficial bacterial folliculitis demonstrating alopecia and multifocal epidermal collarettes.

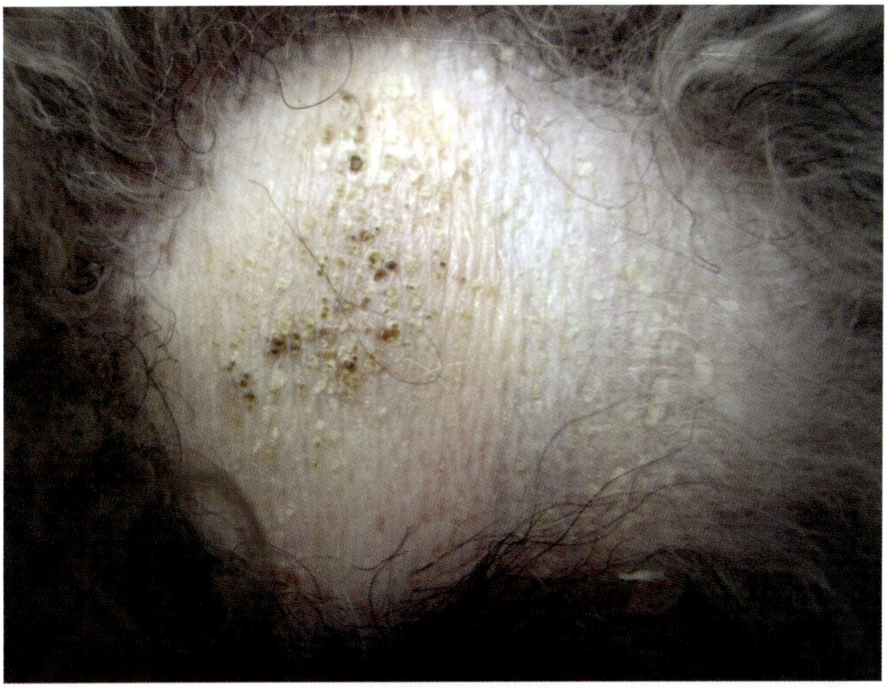

■ **Fig. 6.4.** Patch of alopecia with erythema and mild crusting over the dorsal shoulders secondary to injection of a repositol corticosteroid.

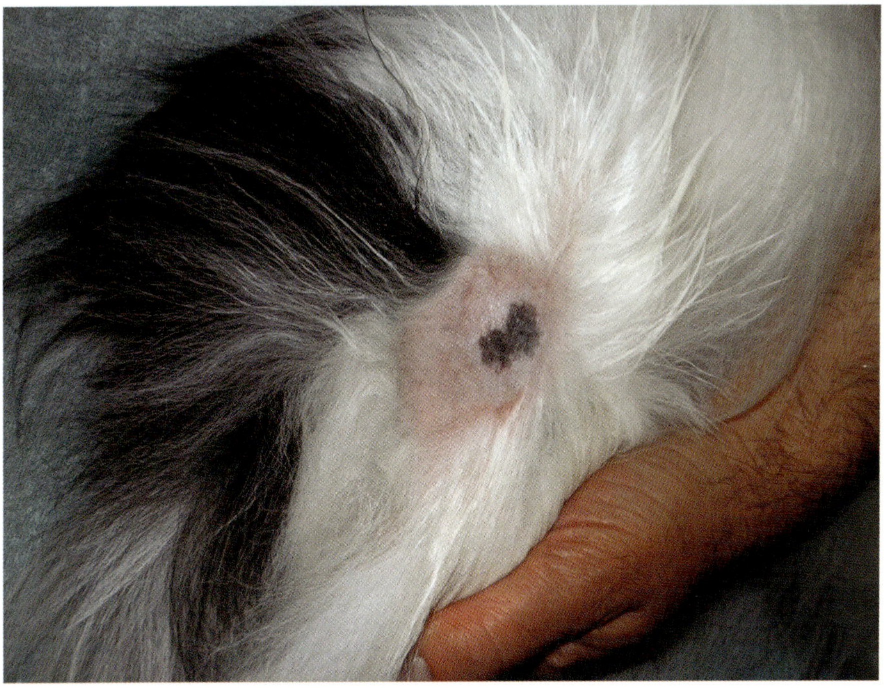

■ **Fig. 6.5.** Four-year old female-spayed pomeranian with a patch of alopecia over right lateral thigh subsequent to rabies vaccine.

(a)

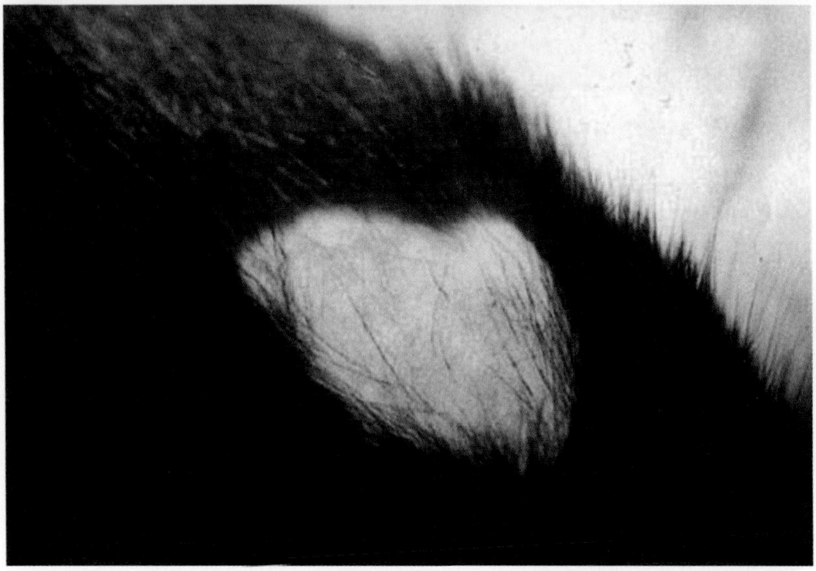

(b)

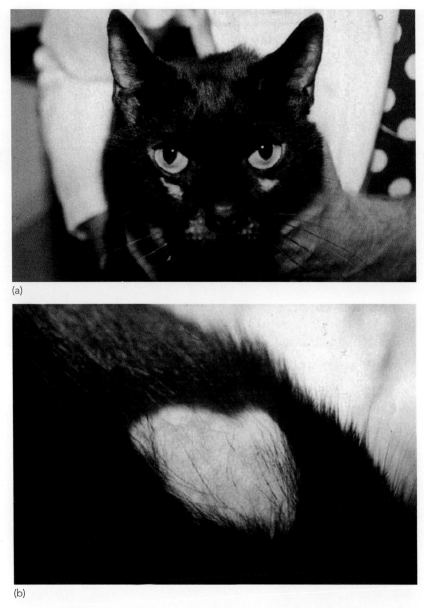

■ **Fig. 6.6.** Feline alopecia areata. (a) Noninflammatory complete alopecia in a patchy pattern. Note the areas of alopecia just below the eyes and along the muzzle and (b) on the body.

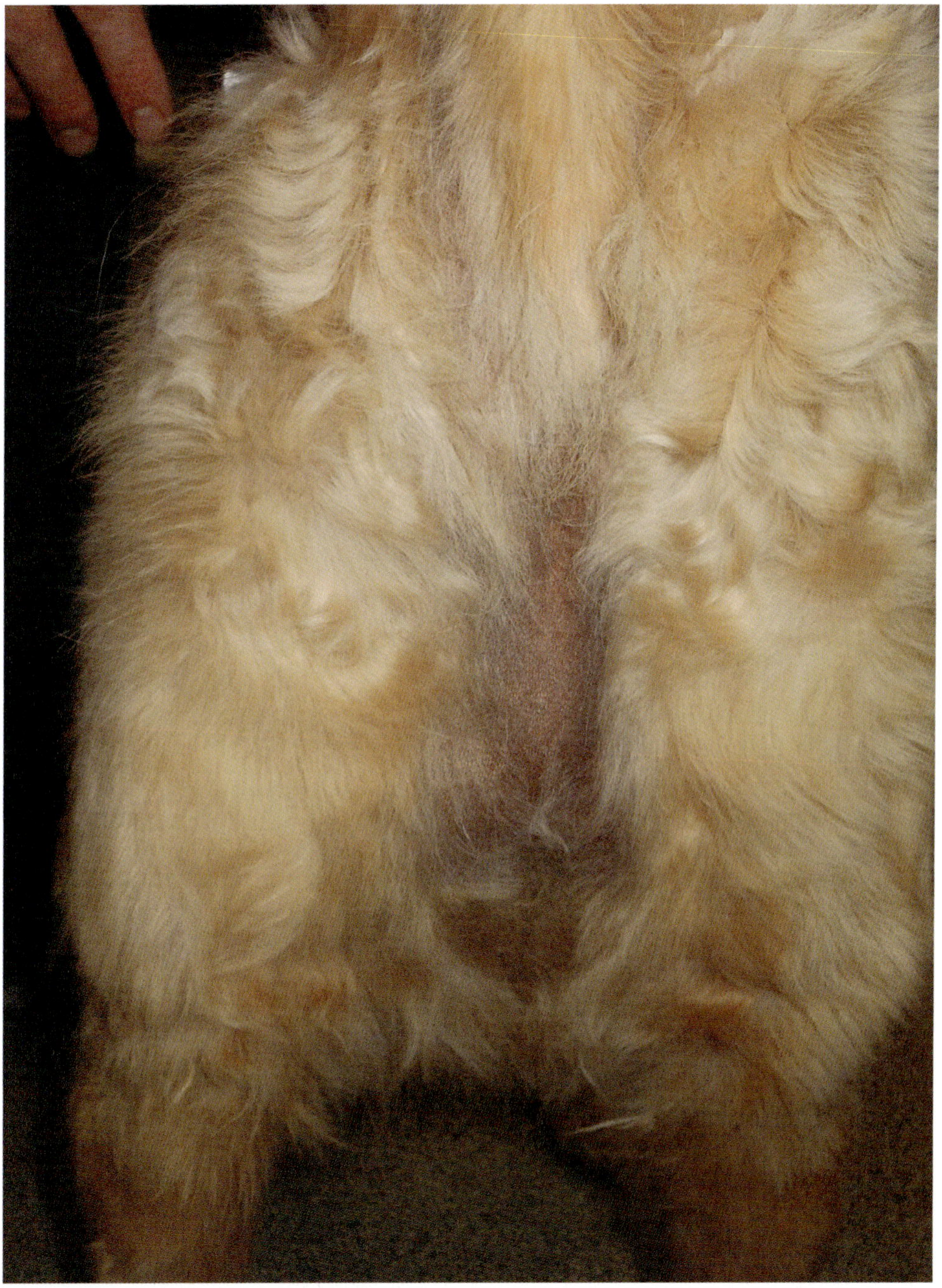

■ **Fig. 6.7.** Focal alopecia and thickening of the skin on the ventral neck in a golden retriever with scleroderma secondary to administration of cyclophosphamide.

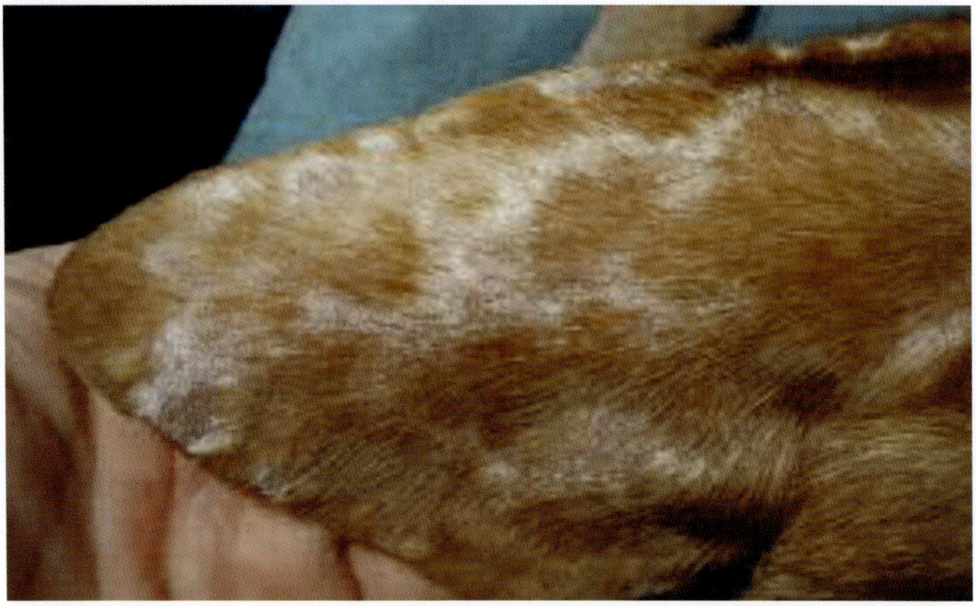

■ **Fig. 6.8.** Sebaceous adenitis (Viszla) demonstrating the polycyclic pattern of alopecia and associated light adherent scale.

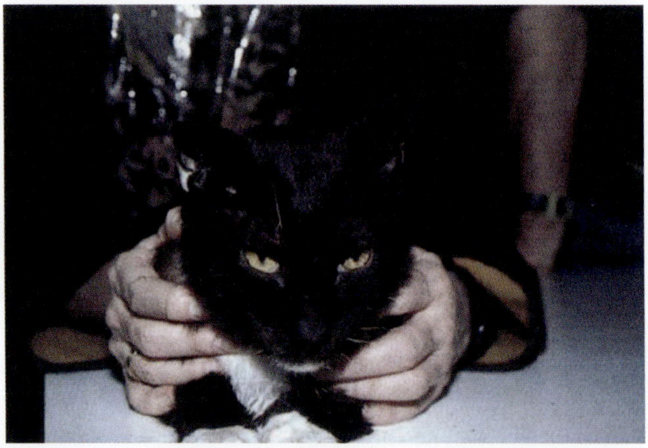

(a)

■ **Fig. 6.9.** Bowenoid *in situ* carcinoma (BISC). (a) Majority of BISC cases occur in dark-colored cats. (b) Appearance of darkly pigmented macules leading to plaques in the preauricular region of the cat in (a). (c) Slightly elevated, pigmented, slightly scaled lesions are often overlooked by the owner until an advanced stage; patches of partial alopecia with hyperpigmentation in the preauricular region of this patient. (d) Hyperpigmented macules leading to crusted plaques of BISC.

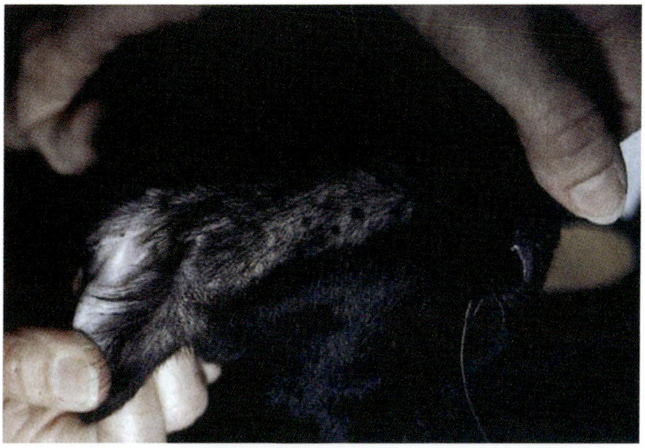

(b)

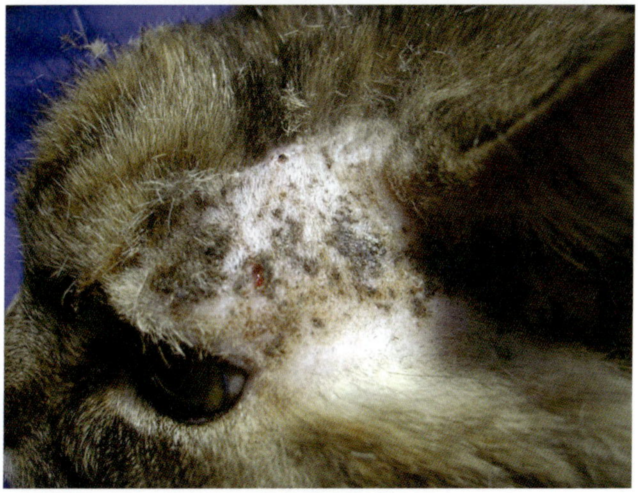

(c)

(d)

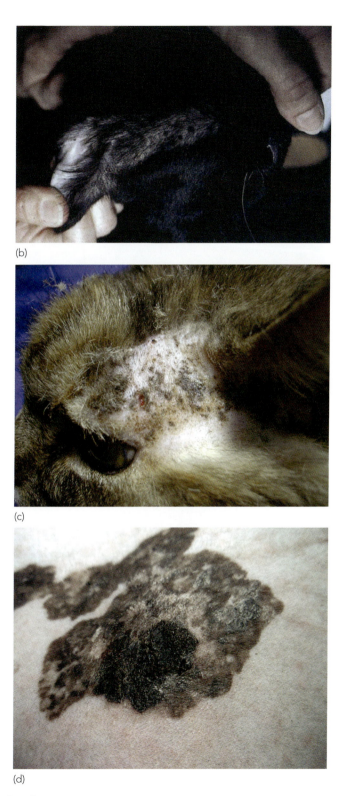

Fig. 6.9. *(Continued)*

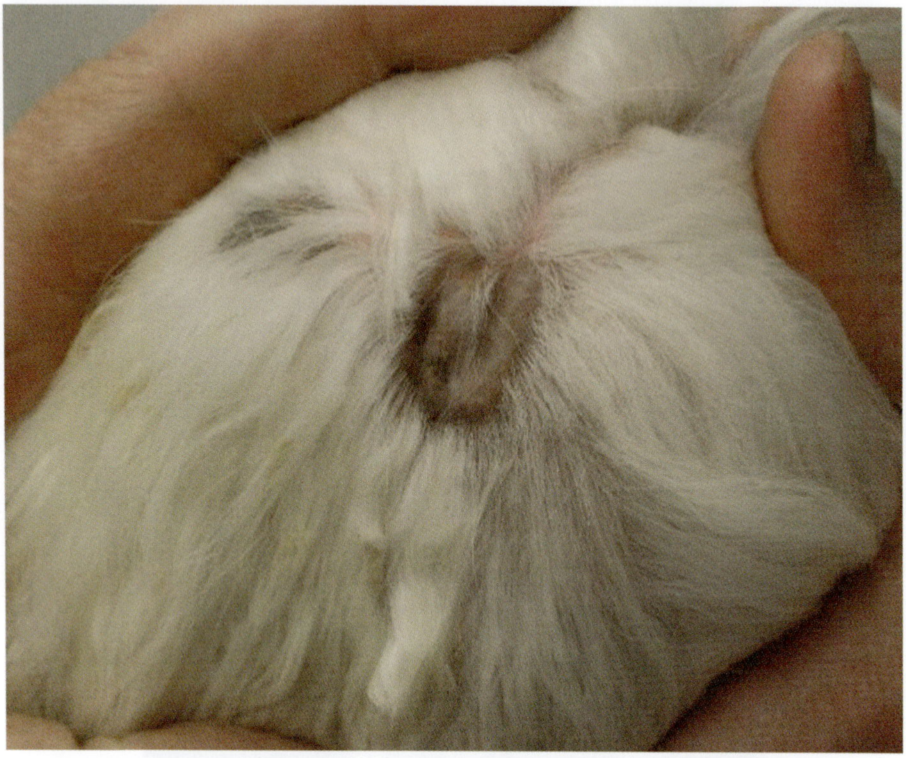

■ **Fig. 6.10.** Traction alopecia: alopecic and scarred circular patch with mild hyperpigmentation as a result of chronic irritation at the site of a hair bow on the dorsum of the head of a Maltese.

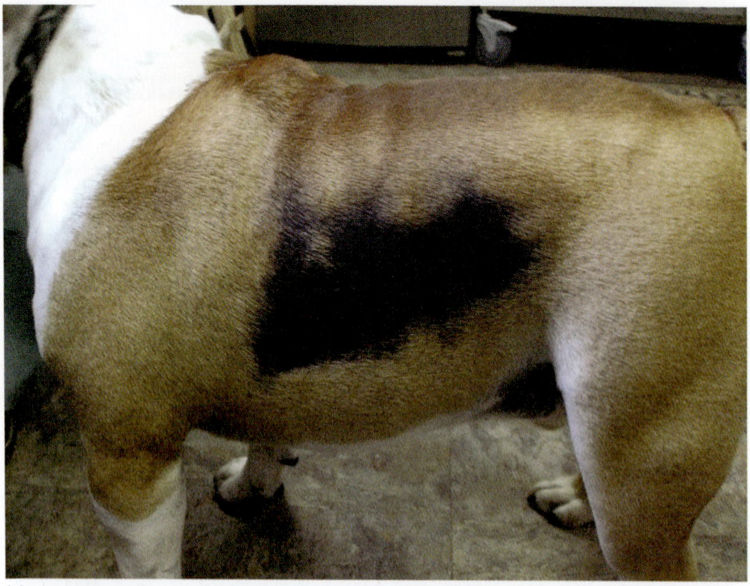

(a)

■ **Fig. 6.11.** Canine flank alopecia. (a) Alopecic patch with marked hyperpigmentation and irregular margins. (b) Dorsel view demonstrating the bilateral nature of the disorder.

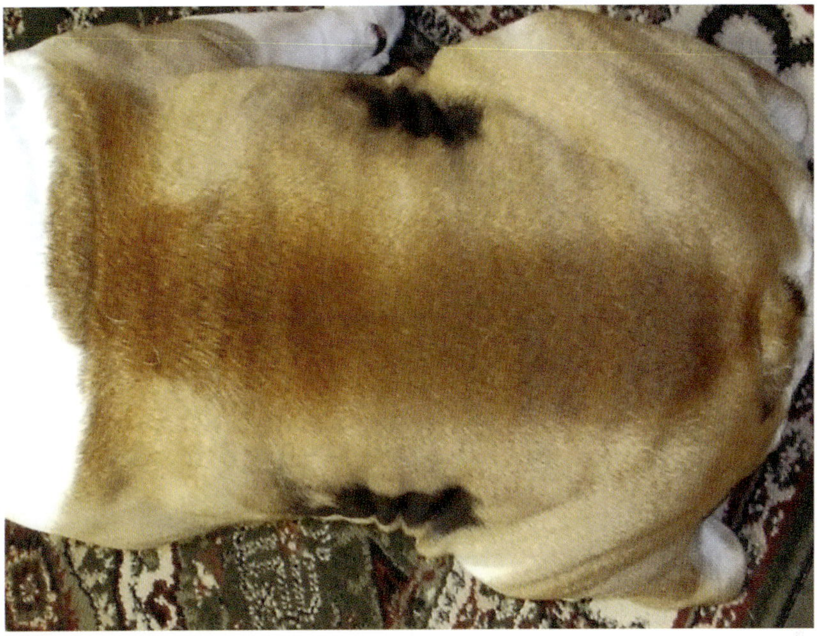

(b)

Fig. 6.11. (*Continued*)

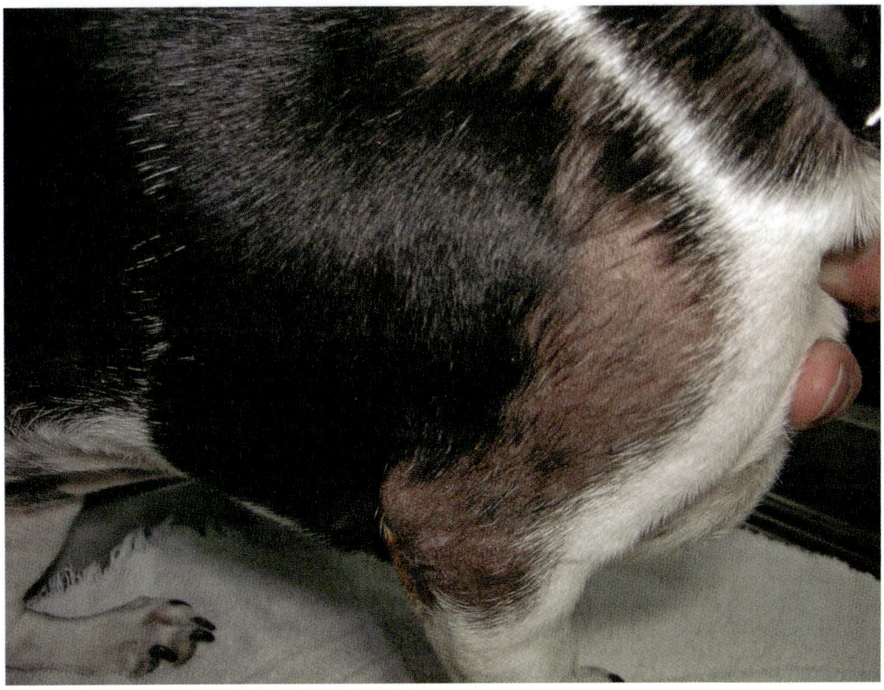

Fig. 6.12. Black follicle dysplasia: hair loss is occurring only in black-colored patches.

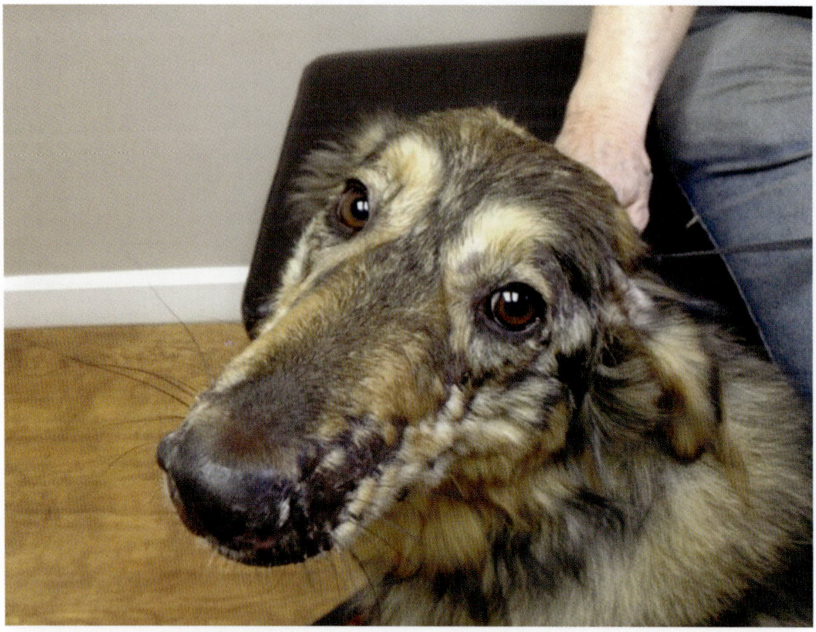

(a)

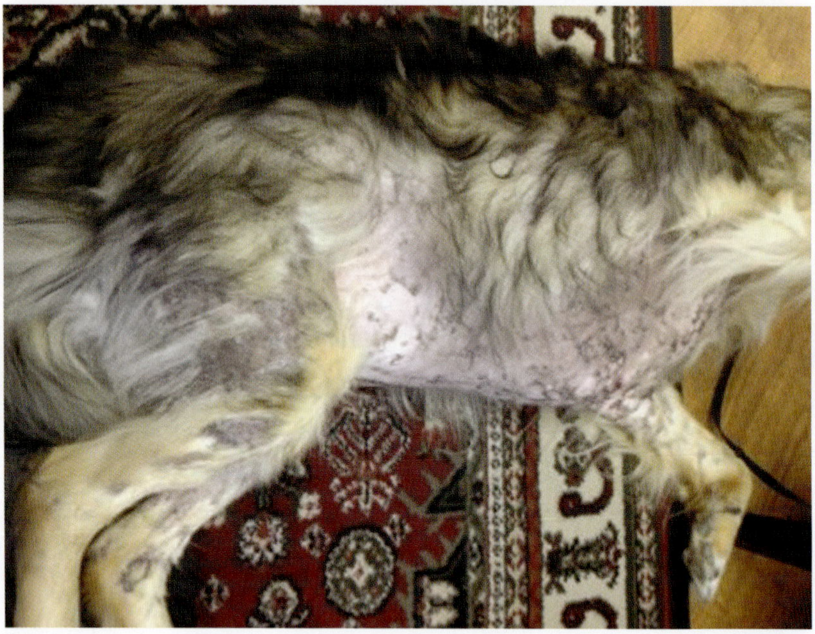

(b)

■ **Fig. 6.13.** Dermatomyositis. (a) Alopecia around the muzzle and pericular regions. (b) Multifocal patches of alopecia on the body occur in severe cases.

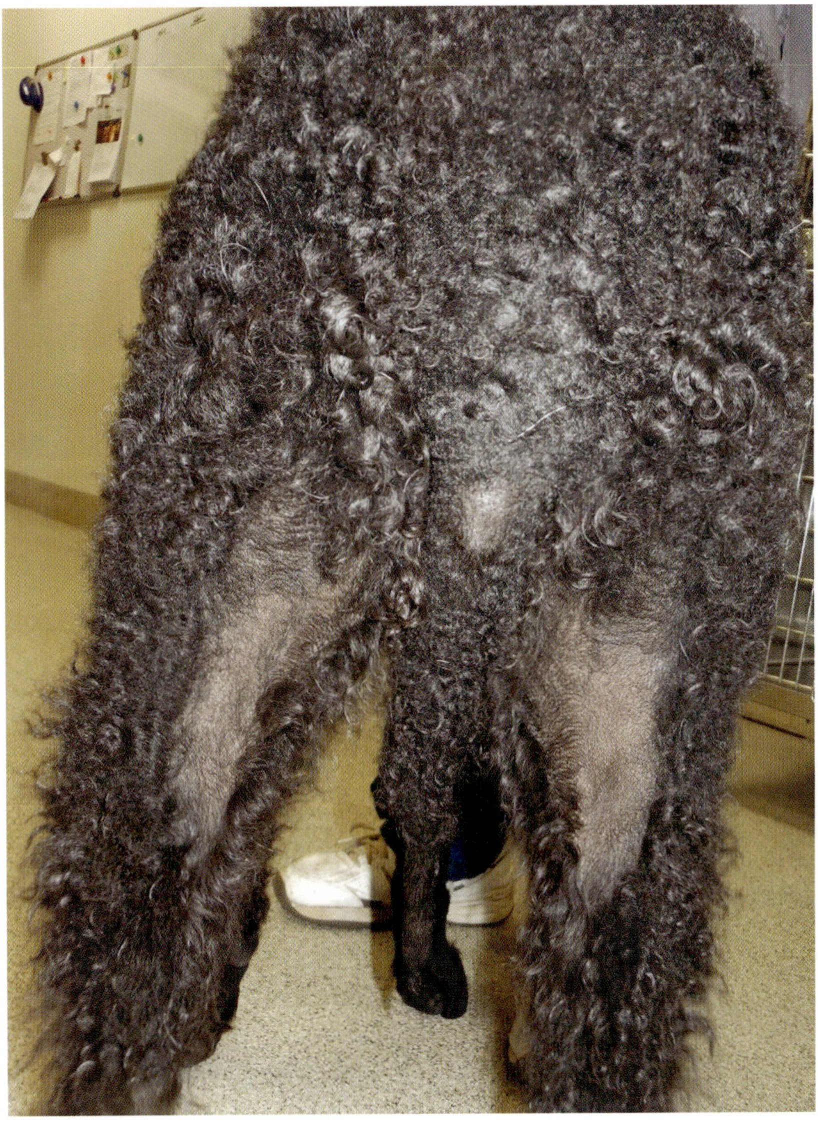

■ **Fig. 6.14.** Alopecia affecting the caudal thighs and tail of a 2-year-old male-castrate American water spaniel with pattern baldness.

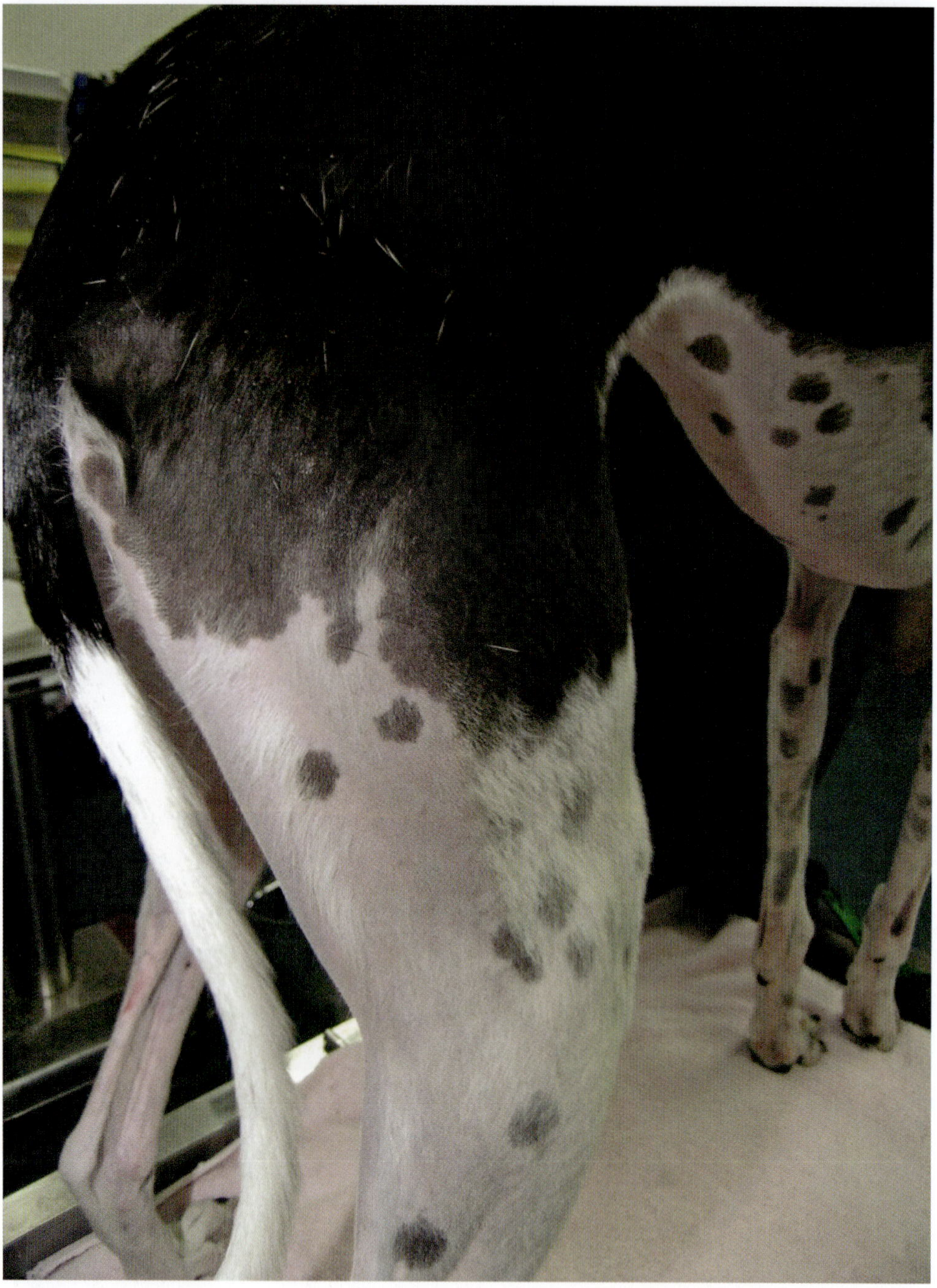

■ **Fig. 6.15.** Pattern baldness in a greyhound.

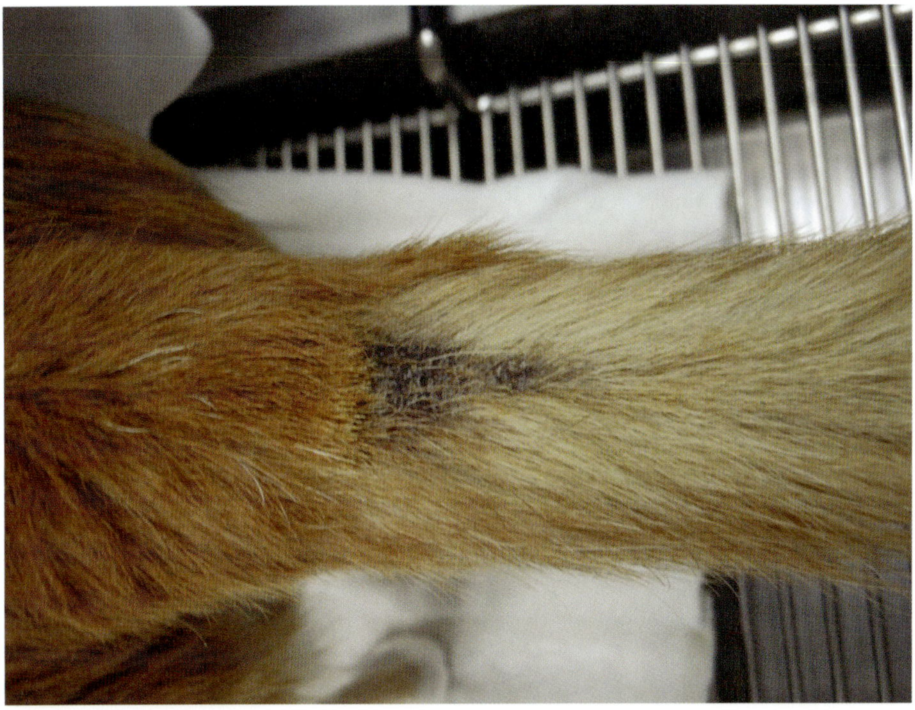

Fig. 6.16. Tail gland alopecia; an area of noninflamed hair loss on the proximal dorsal surface of the tail of a golden retriever.

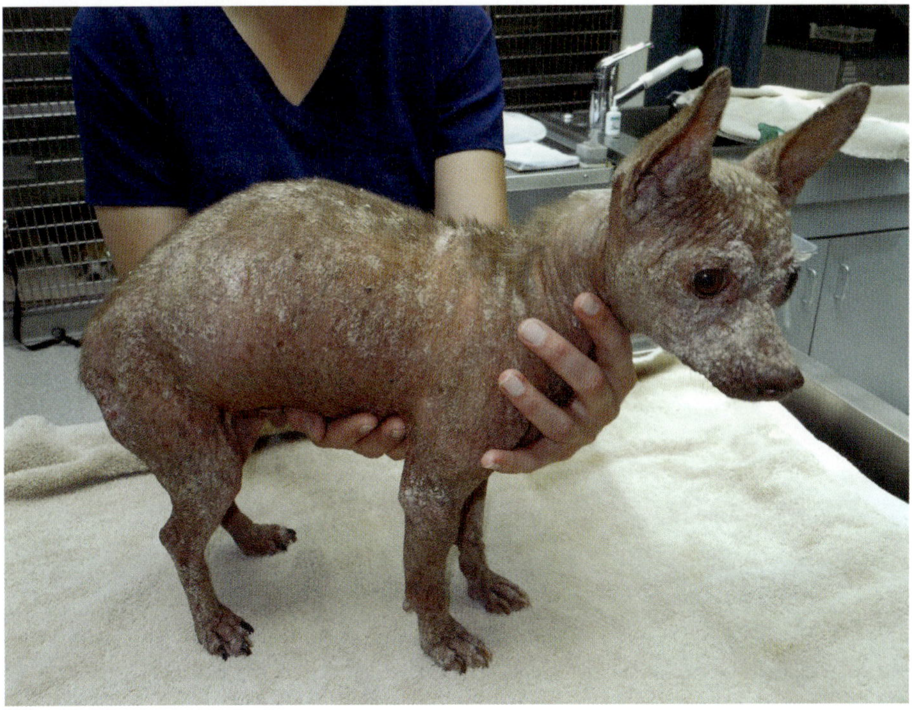

Fig. 6.17. Chronic generalized demodicosis in a 6-year-old male-castrate chihuahua.

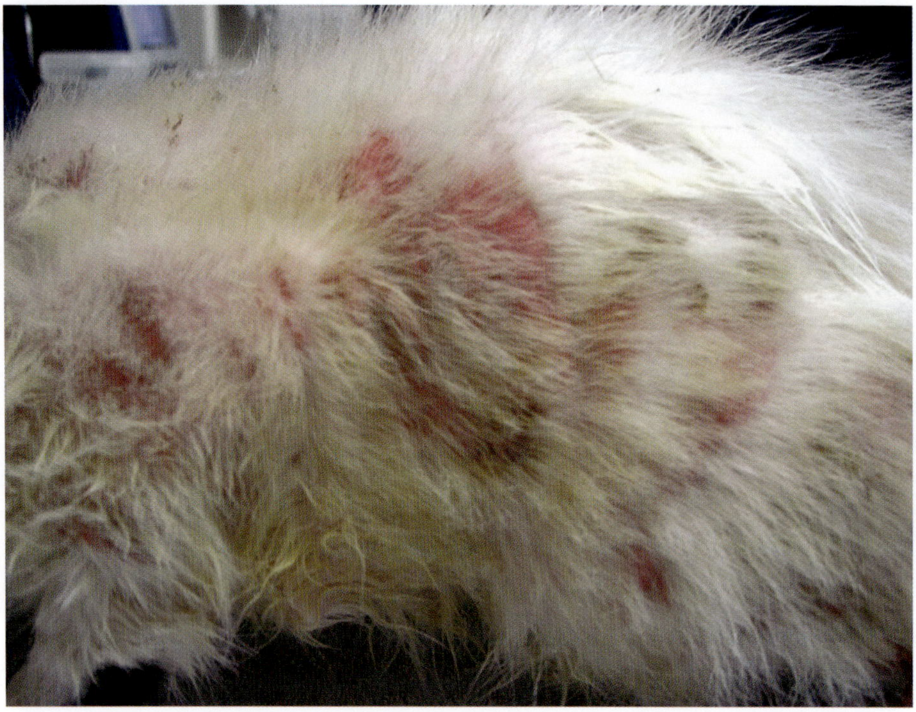

■ **Fig. 6.18.** Generalized dermatophytosis in a 1-year-old DLH.

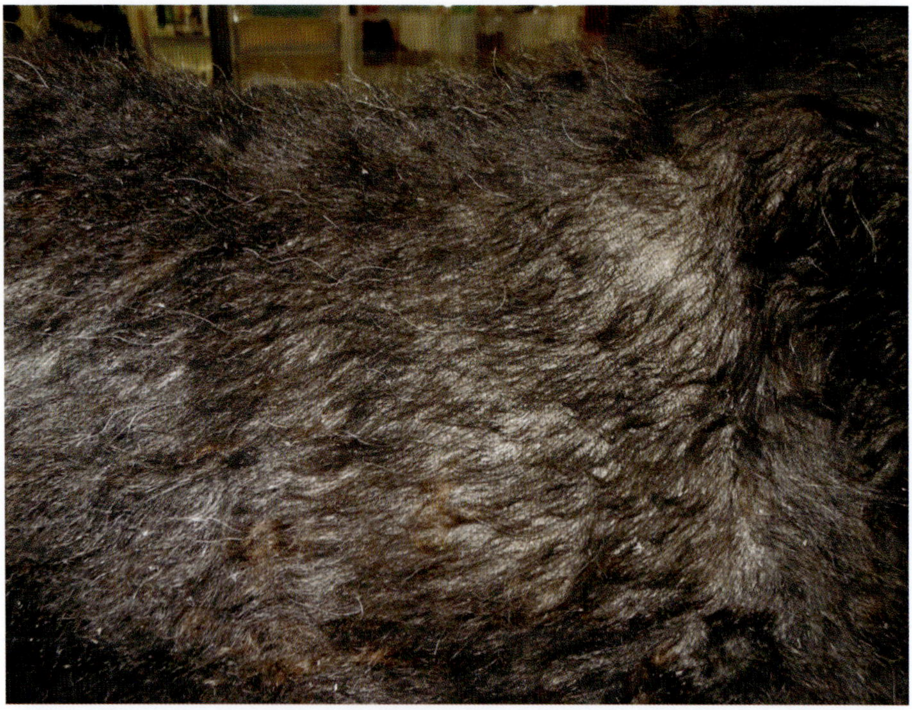

■ **Fig. 6.19.** Dorsal trunk of a standard poodle demonstrating diffuse partial alopecia with keratin collaring of the hair shafts consistent with sebaceous adenitis.

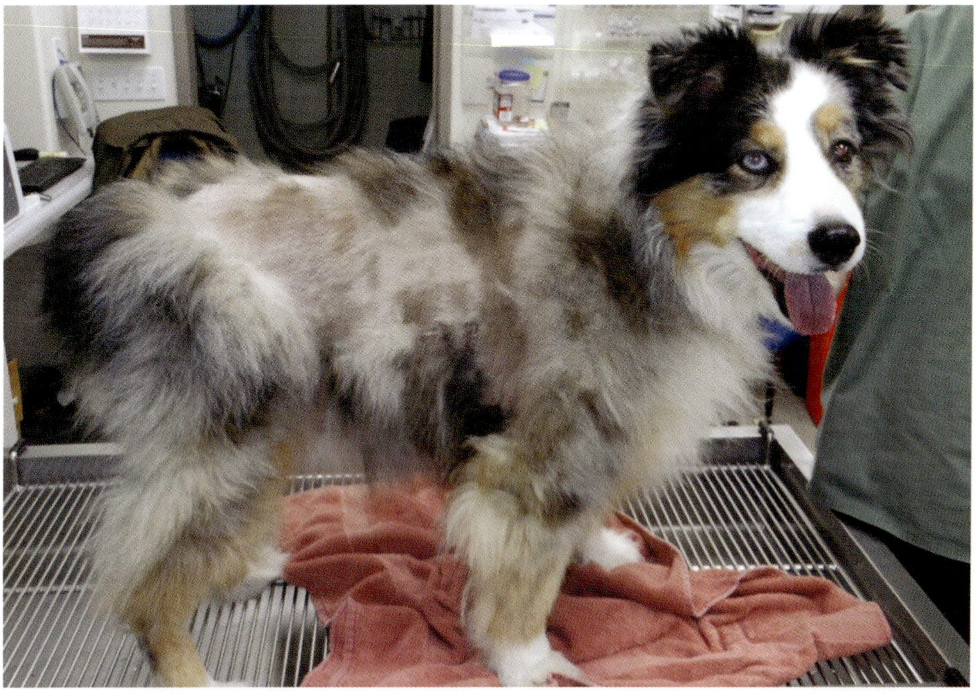

■ **Fig. 6.20.** Hyperadrenocorticism: diffuse truncal alopecia in a 14-year-old female-spayed Australian shepherd.

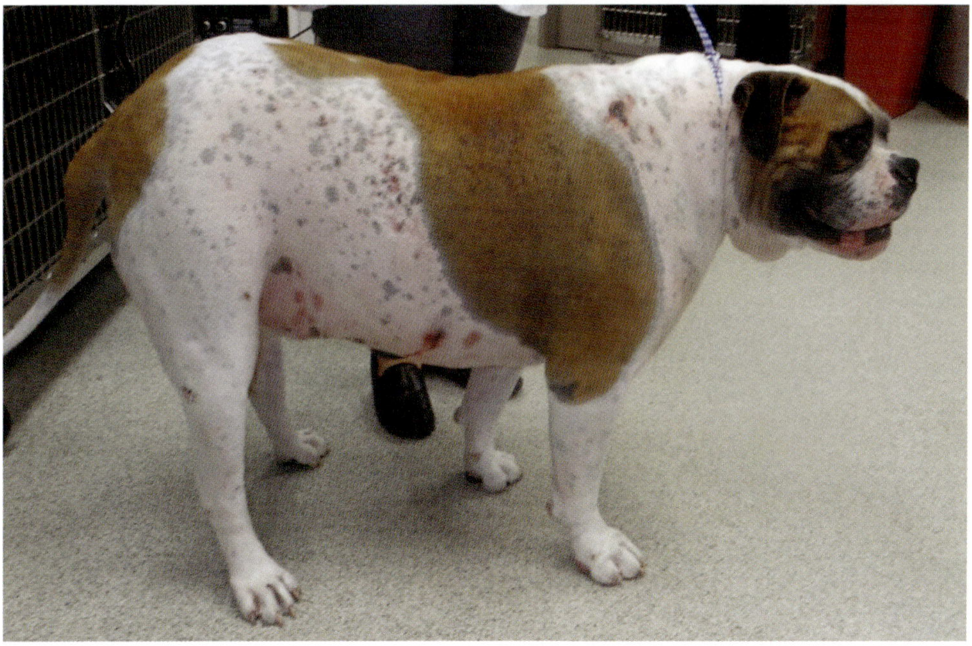

■ **Fig. 6.21.** Iatrogenic hyperadrenocorticism and secondary pyoderma in a 5-year-old male-castrate American bulldog.

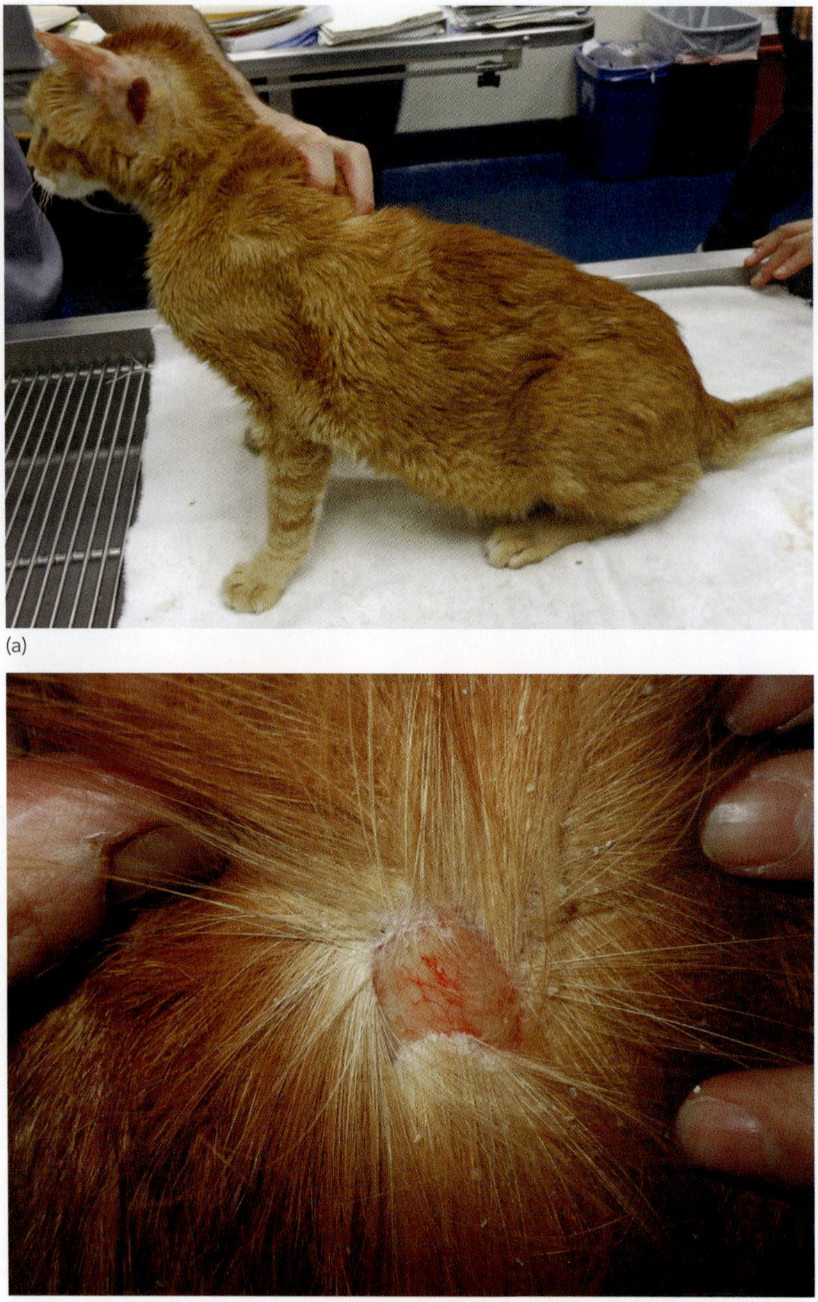

(a)

(b)

■ **Fig. 6.22.** Feline hyperadrenocorticism. (a) Note the distended abdomen, alopecia and excoriation at the base of the left pinna. (b) Atrophic skin is easily torn by traction.

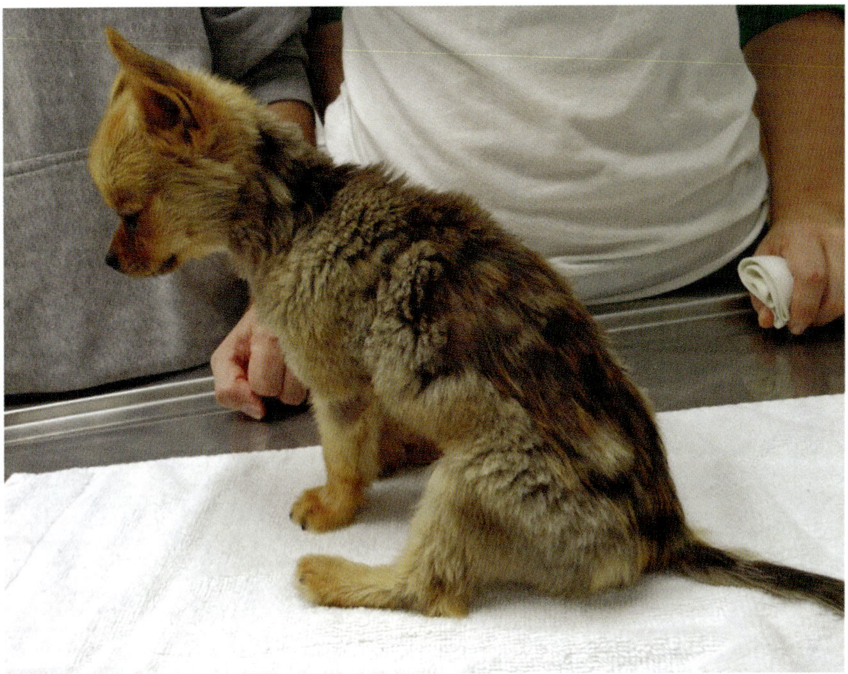

Fig. 6.23. Pituitary dwarfism and congenital hypothyroidism in a 1-year-old male-castrate pomeranian mix. Note truncal alopecia and small stature.

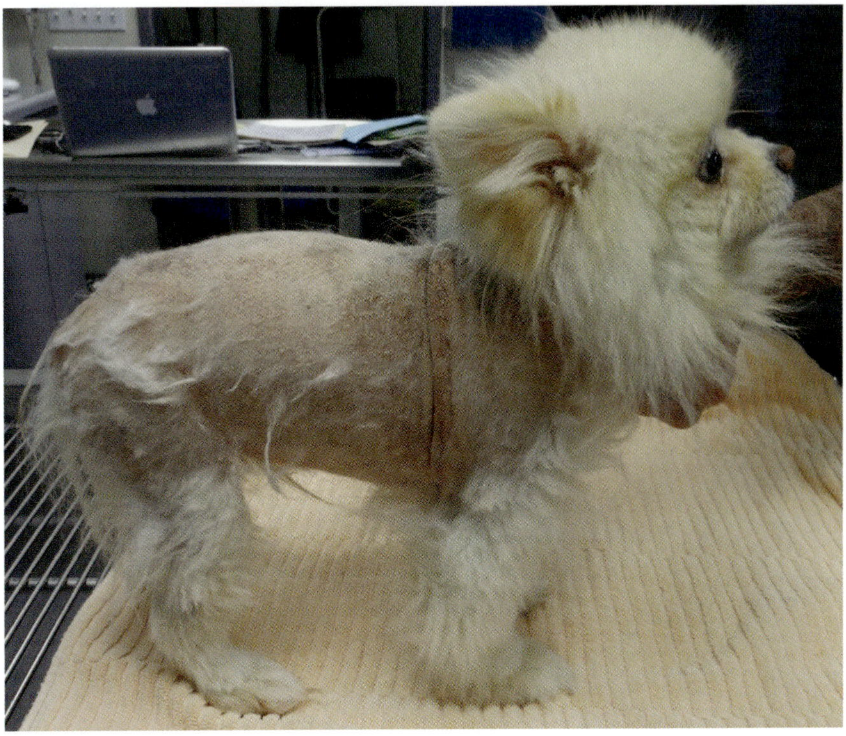

Fig. 6.24. Alopecia X (adrenal sex hormone imbalance of plush-coated breeds) in a 4-year-old female-spayed pomeranian. Alopecia affects primarily the trunk and spares the head and extremities.

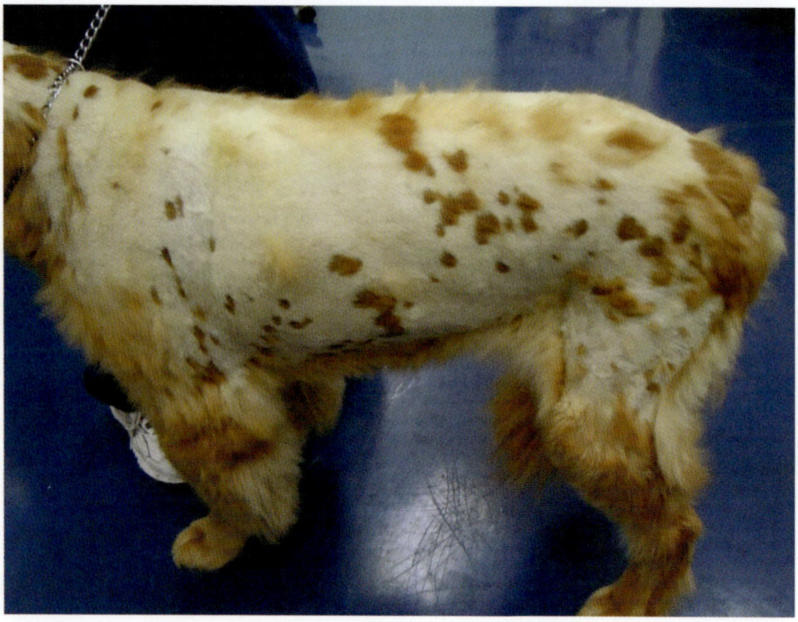

■ **Fig. 6.25.** Partial to focally complete alopecia of the trunk associated with severe hypothyroidism. (*Note:* hypothyroidism is often "overdiagnosed" as a cause for canine alopecia.)

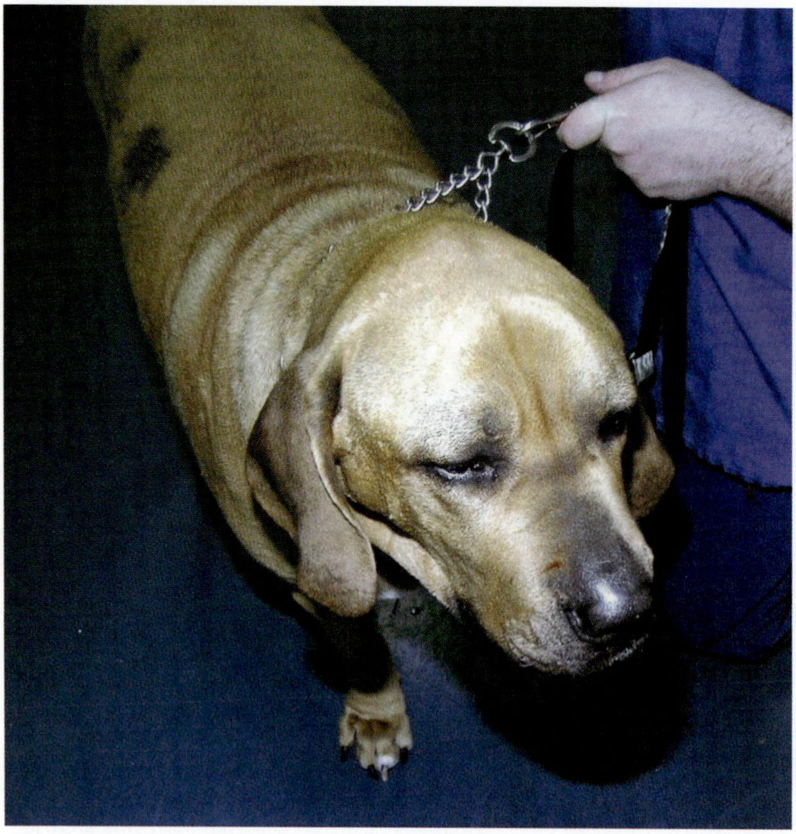

■ **Fig. 6.26.** Myxedema "tragic face" in canine hypothyroidism.

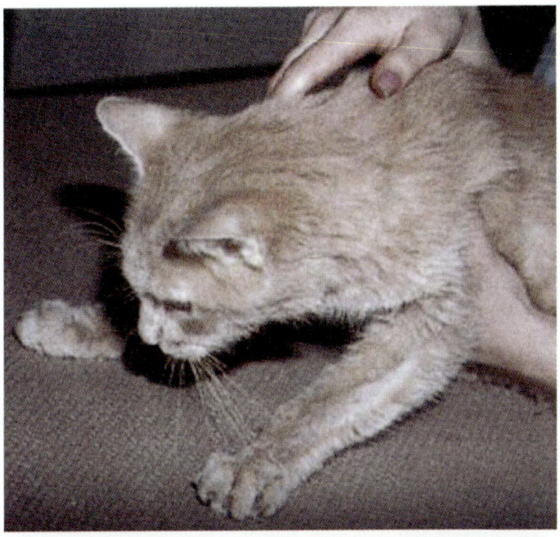

(a)

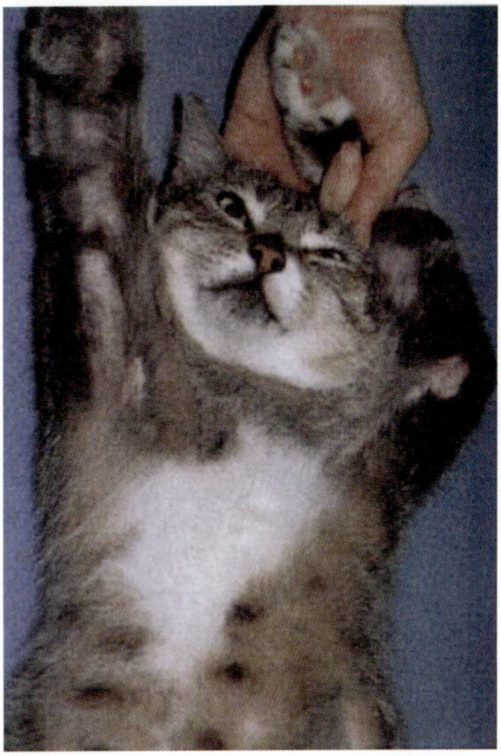

(b)

■ **Fig. 6.27.** (a) Feline hyperthyroidism is often associated with excess grooming, which may lead to focal areas of alopecia, as noted along lateral aspect of the forelimbs. (b) Nine-year-old male-castrate DSH with hyperthyroidism demonstrated by excessive grooming with alopecia along the forelimbs.

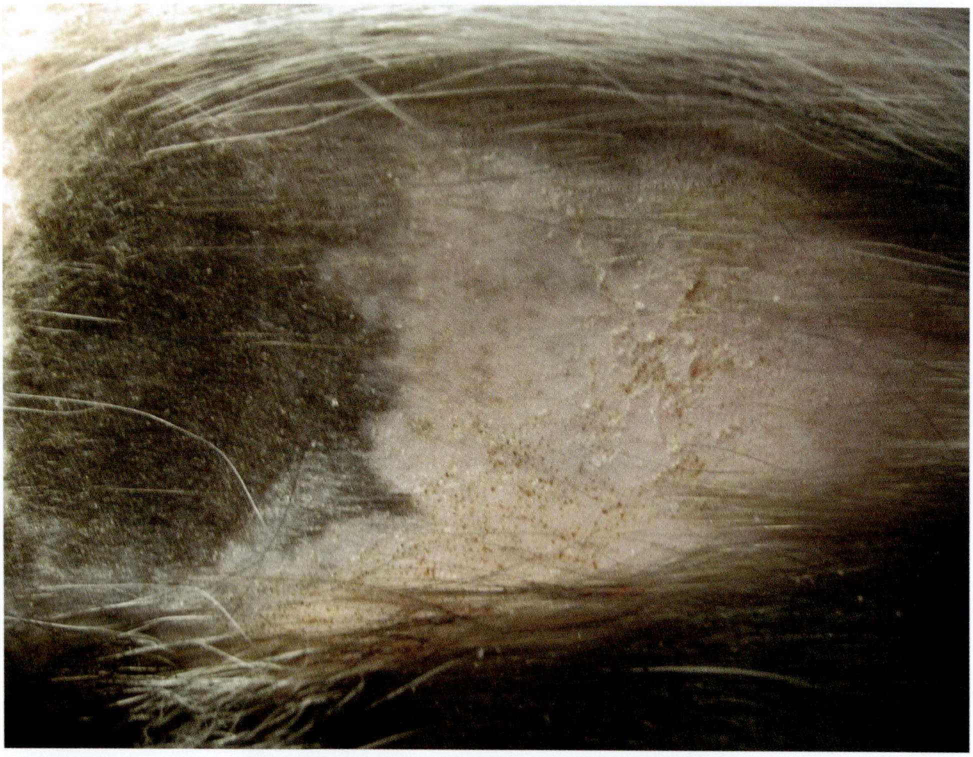

■ **Fig. 6.28.** Alopecia and scaling on the dorsum of a cat with hyperthyroidism.

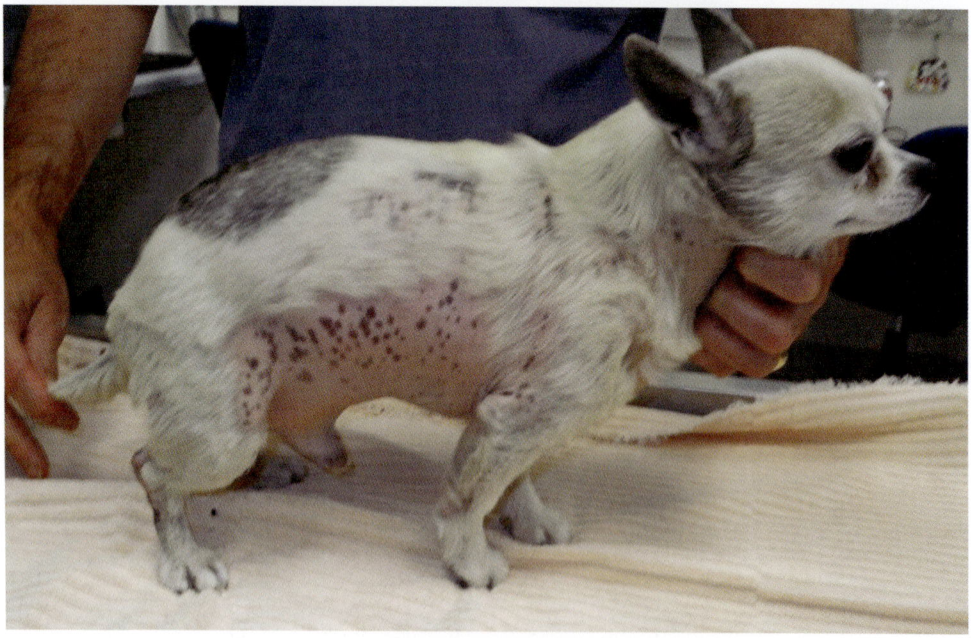

■ **Fig. 6.29.** Hyperestrogenism leading to truncal alopecia in a 5-year-old male-intact chihuahua with Sertoli cell tumor.

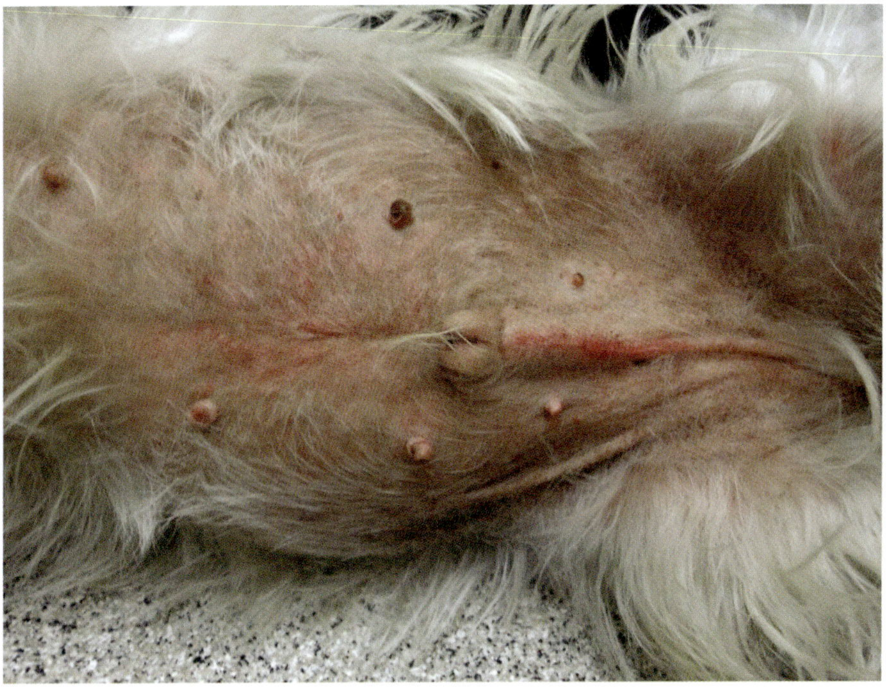

■ **Fig. 6.30.** Hyperestrogenism from exposure to topical hormone replacement therapy; note linear preputial erythema characteristic of this syndrome.

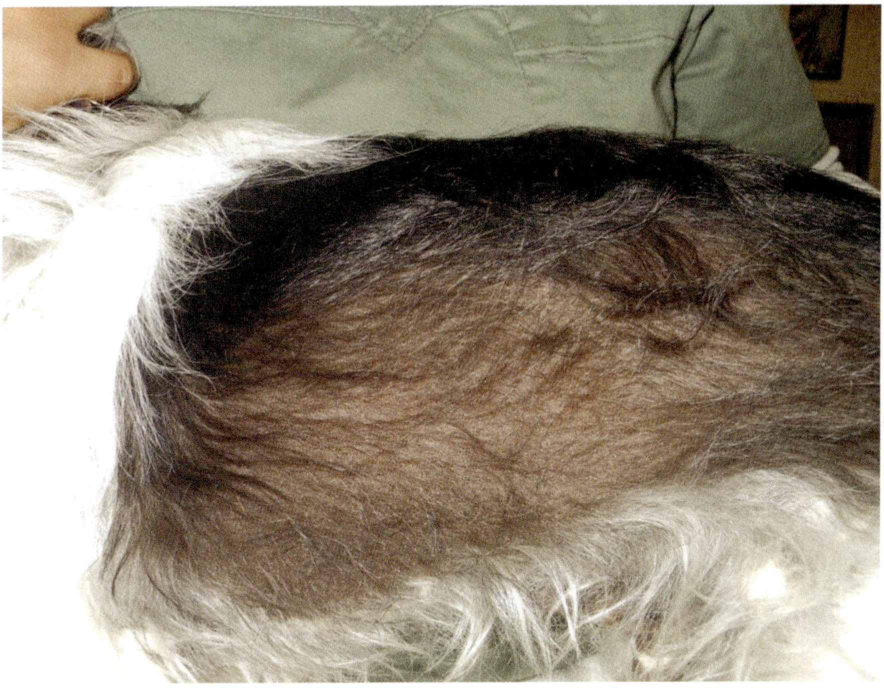

■ **Fig. 6.31.** Alopecia caused by exposure to topical hormone replacement therapy (estrogen) in a 7-year-old male-castrate shih tzu mix dog.

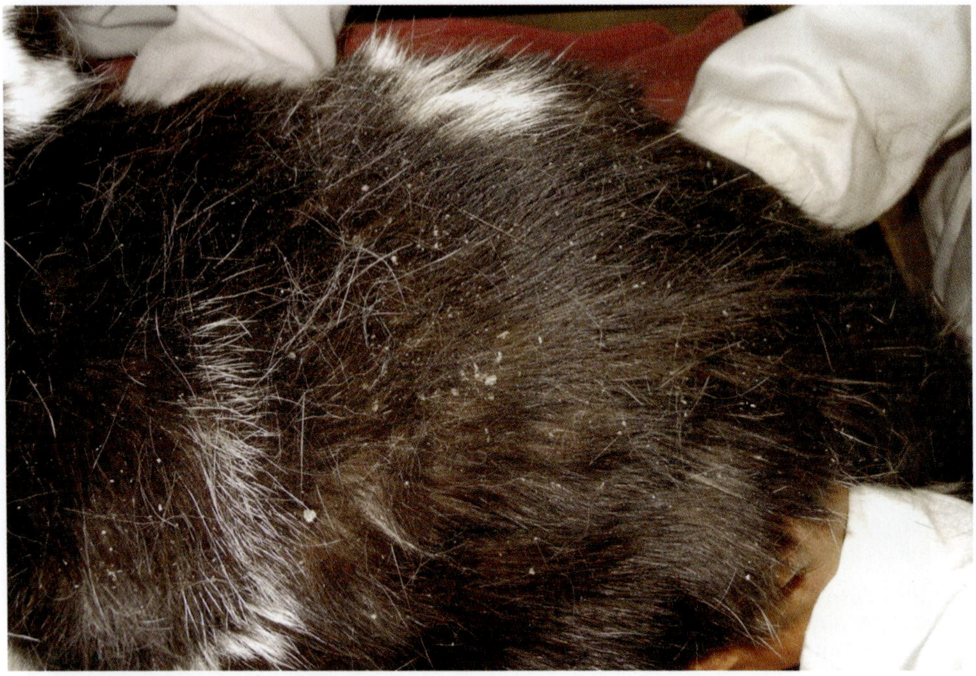

■ **Fig. 6.32.** Excessive scaling often seen in cats with diabetes mellitus.

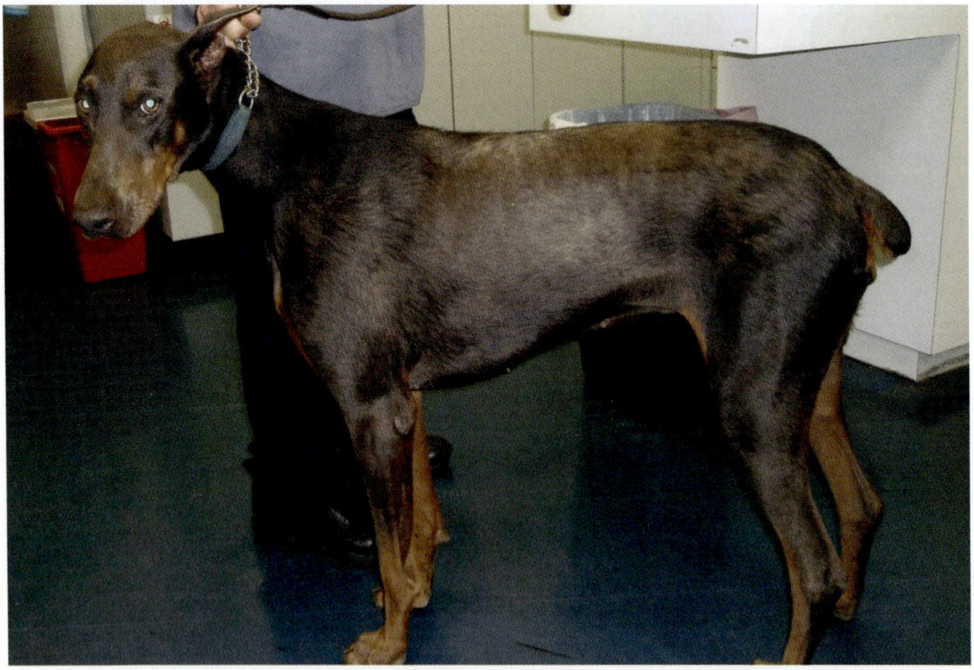

■ **Fig. 6.33.** Color dilution alopecia. Loss of a "blue" hair coat in 3-year-old female-spayed doberman pinscher.

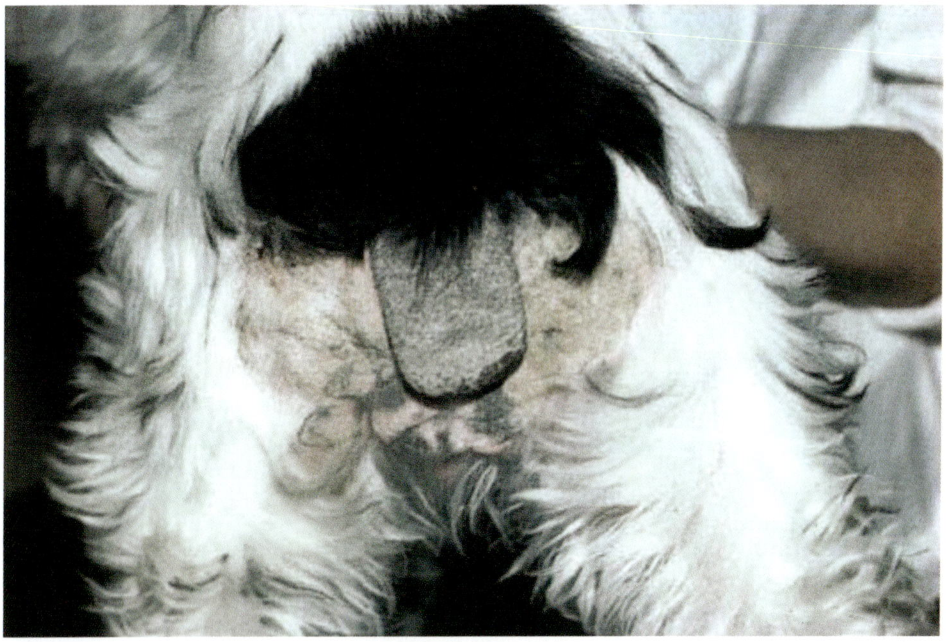

■ **Fig. 6.34.** Primary keratinization disorder with secondary yeast dermatitis of the perineum and tail region of a 6-year-old cocker spaniel.

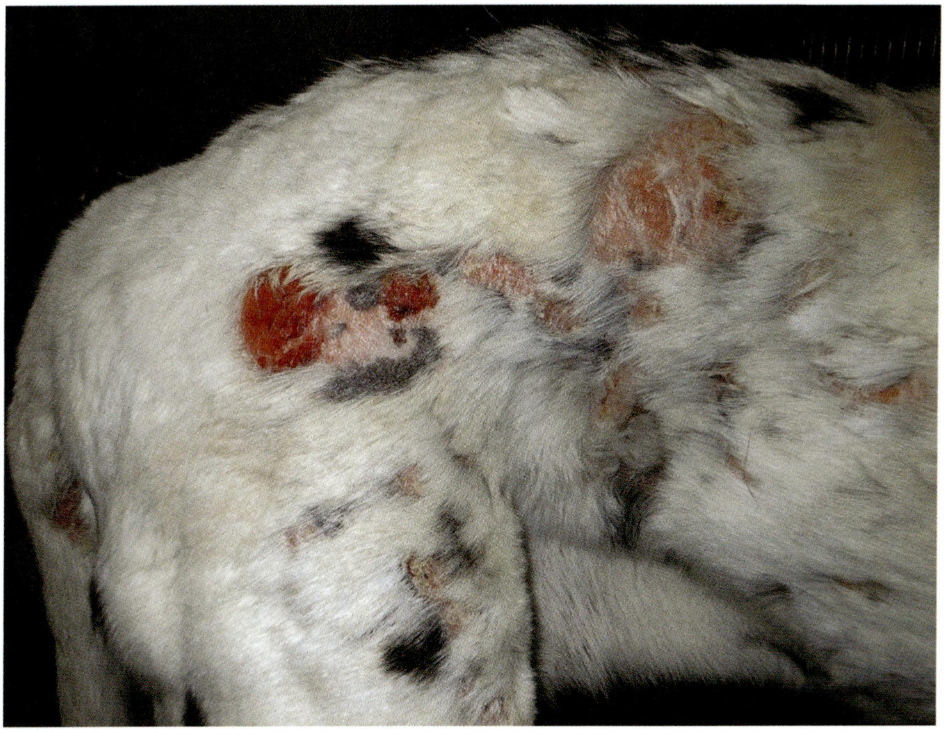

■ **Fig. 6.35.** Seventeen-year-old dalmatian with epidermotropic lymphoma; note areas of partial to complete alopecia with heavy scale and erythematous plaques.

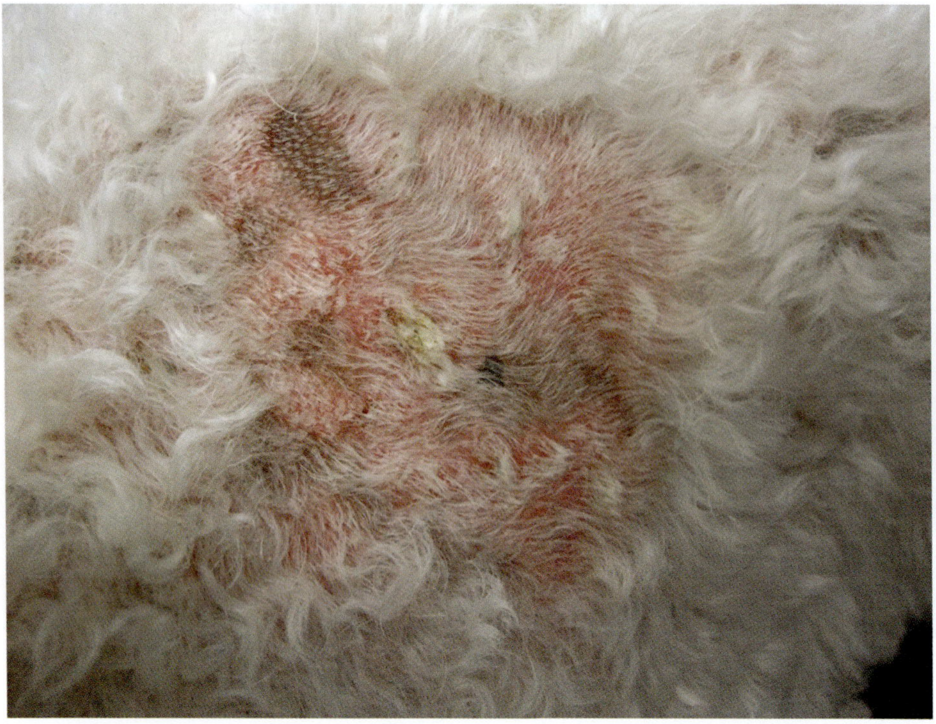

■ **Fig. 6.36.** Epitheliotropic lymphoma: note the lack of plaques and nodules. Lesions consist of multifocal patches of alopecia with adherent scale and erythroderma.

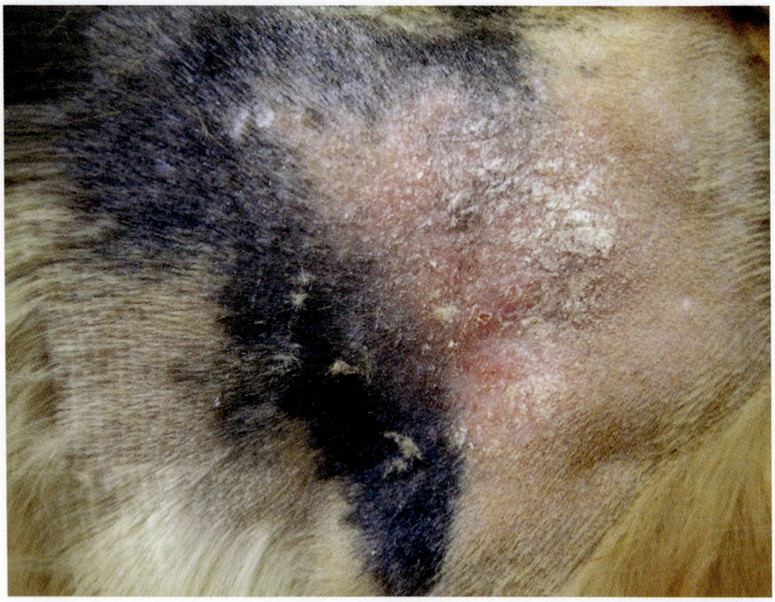

(a)

■ **Fig. 6.37.** (a) Epidermotropic lymphoma on the dorsum of a 12-year-old DSH demonstrating the partial alopecia and adherent scale characteristic of the earlier phases of the disease. (b) Advanced stage of the disease demonstrating the ulceration and exudation of the claw folds.

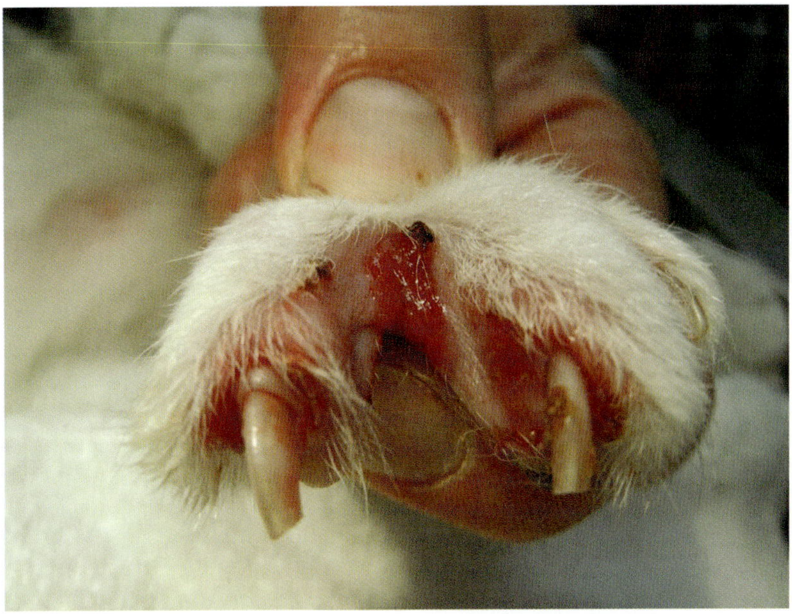

(b)

■ **Fig. 6.37.** (*Continued*)

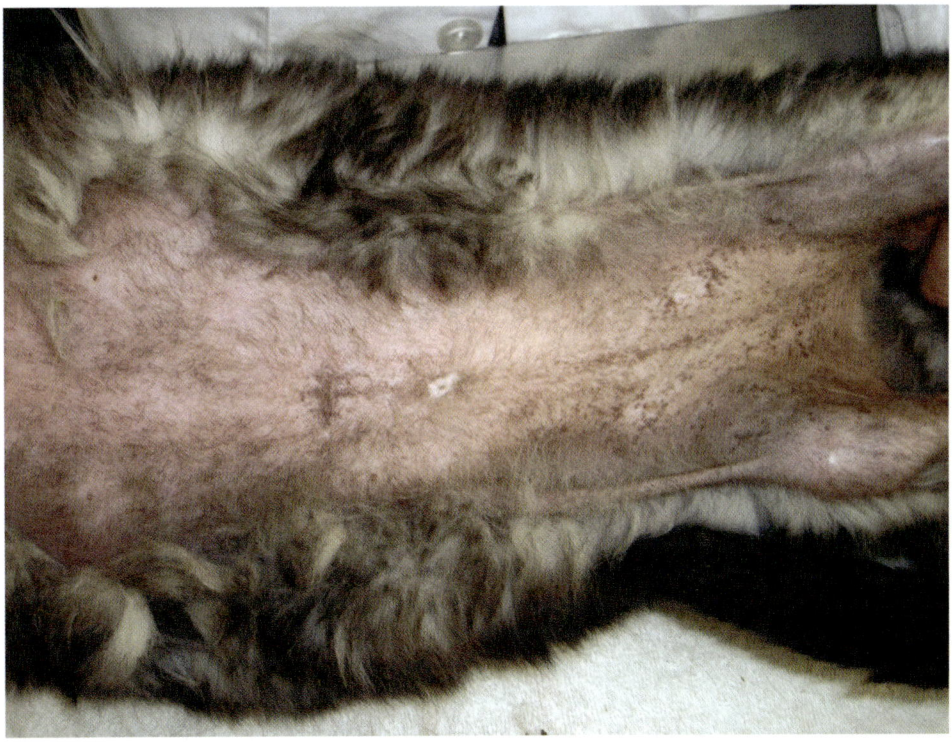

■ **Fig. 6.38.** Paraneoplastic syndrome associated with pancreatic exocrine adenocarcinoma. Note the glistening appearance of the alopecic skin on the ventrum.

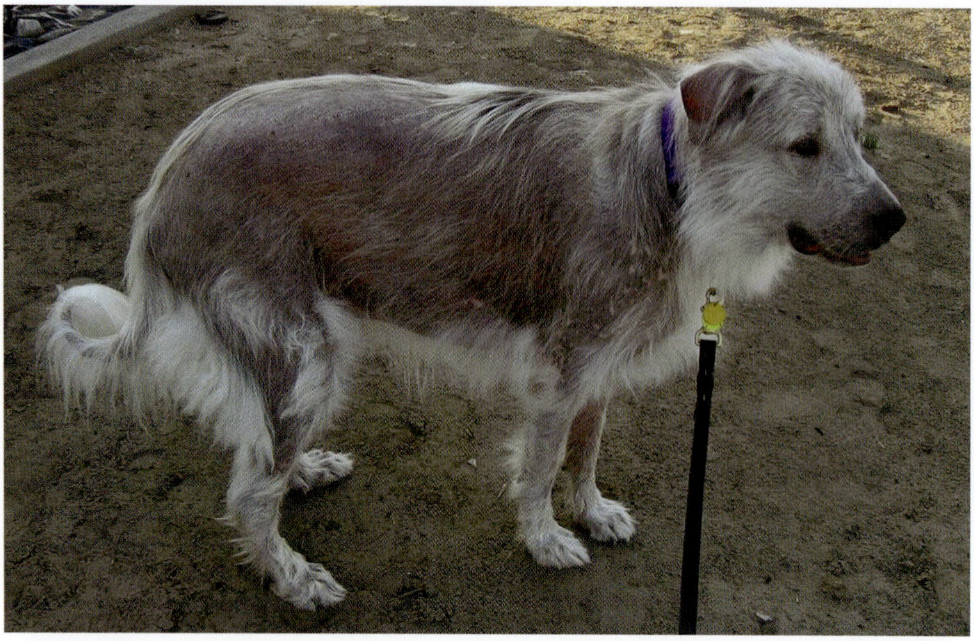

■ **Fig. 6.39.** Pseudopelade in a 2-year-old male-castrate Great Pyrenees mix producing generalized noninflammatory alopecia.

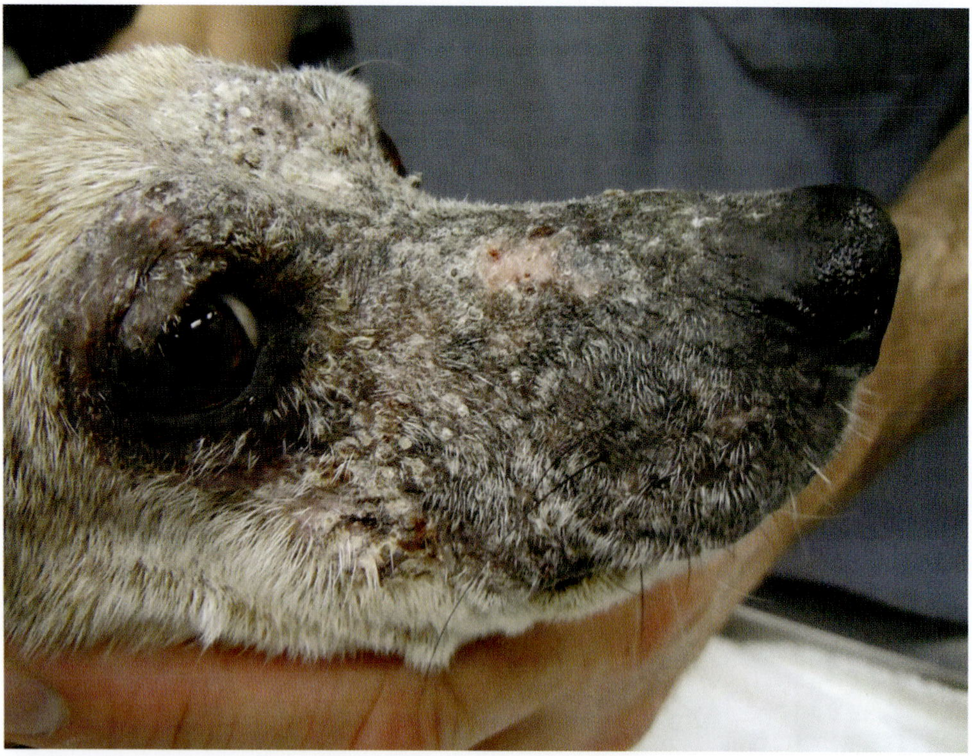

■ **Fig. 6.40.** Severe adherent scale as a result of a chronic dermatophytosis in a chihuahua mix.

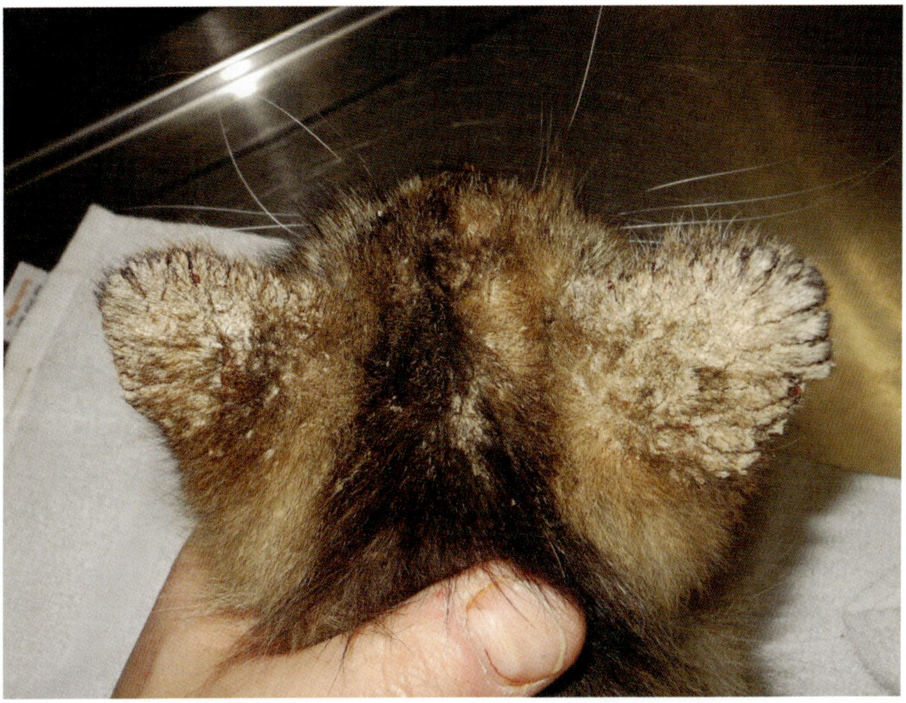

Fig. 6.41. *Notoedres* infestation manifesting as a marked hyperkeratotic disorder in a cat.

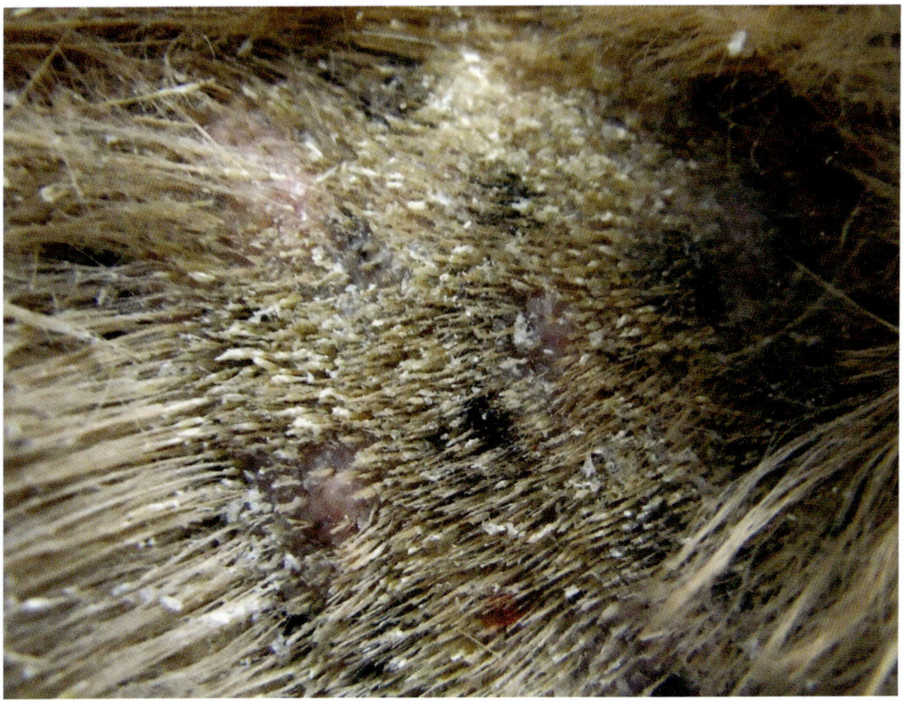

Fig. 6.42. Vitamin A-responsive dermatosis characterized by multifocal patches of excess keratin with thick adherent crusts.

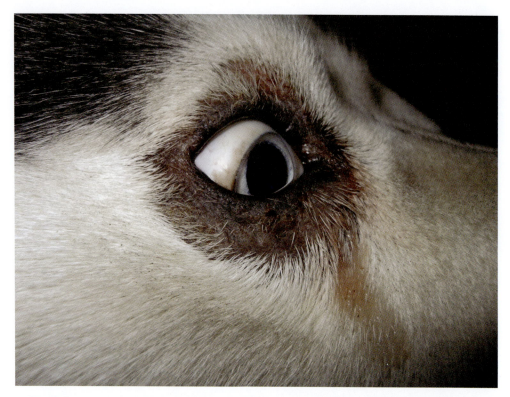

■ **Fig. 6.43.** Periocular crusting and exudation in an adult Siberian husky with zinc-responsive dermatosis.

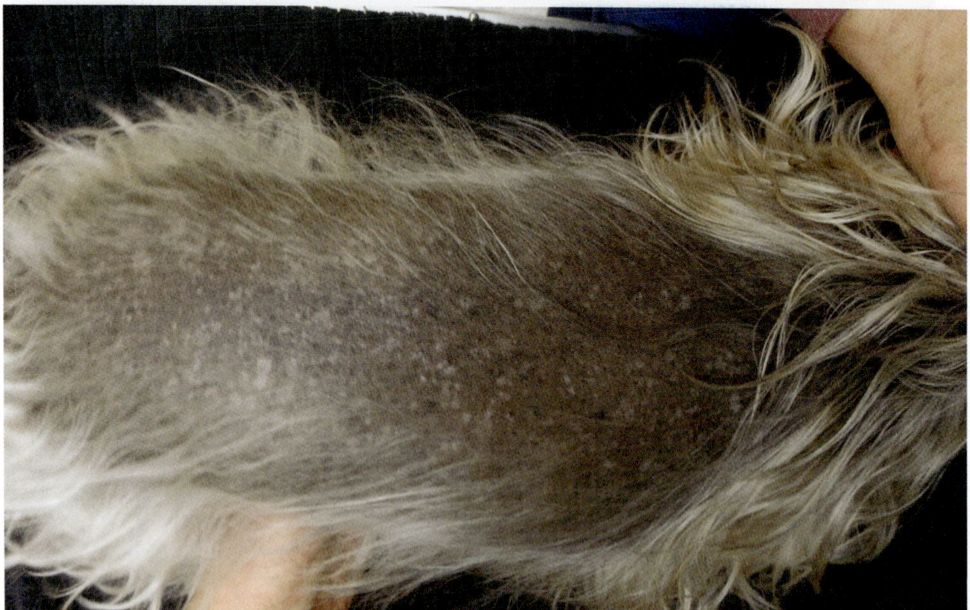

■ **Fig. 6.44.** Follicular dysplasia: moderate alopecia affecting the truncal region.

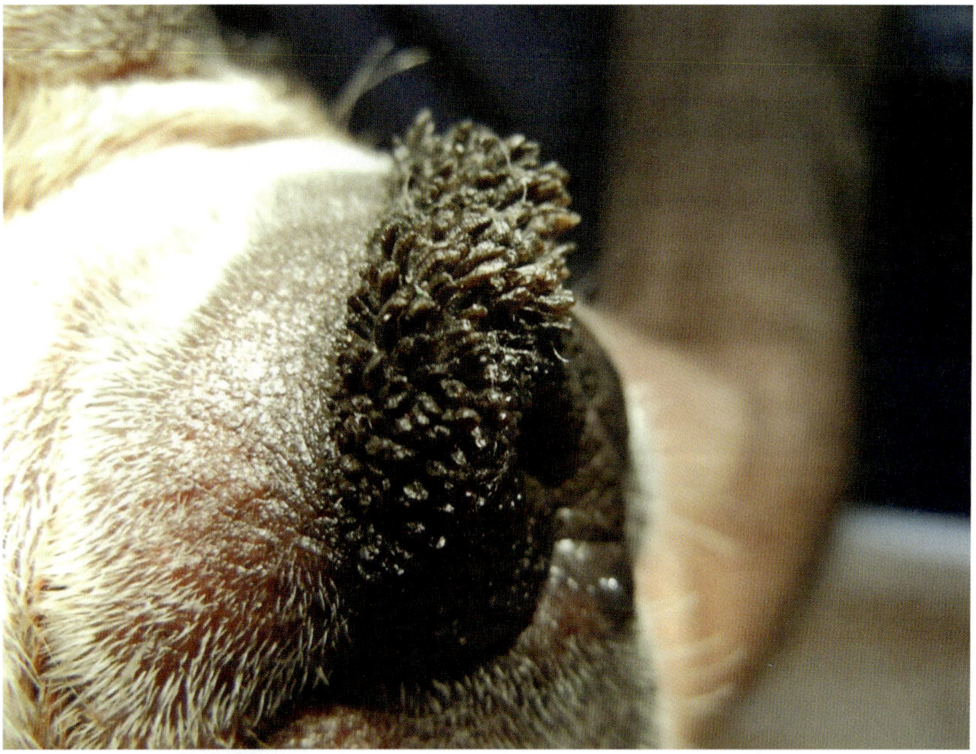

Fig. 6.45. Nasal hyperkeratosis: frond-like projections of keratin from the nasal planum.

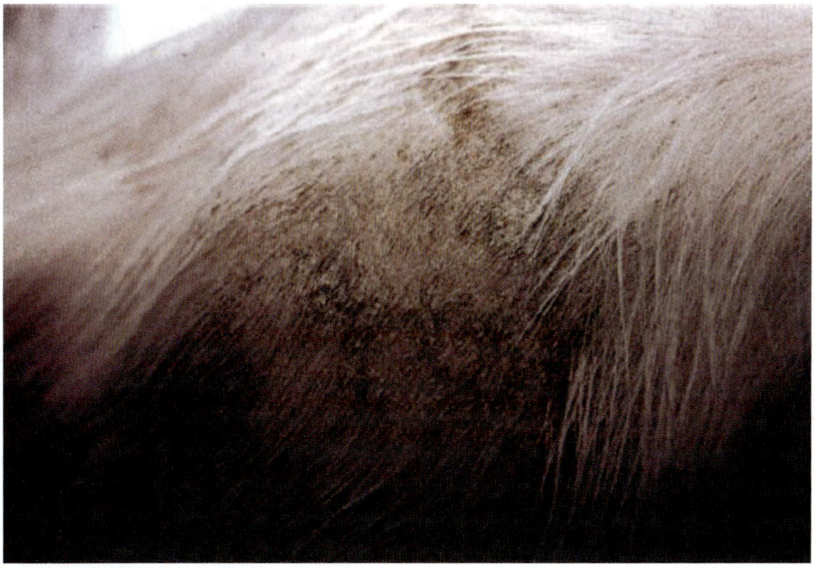

(a)

Fig. 6.46. (a) Feline sebaceous adenitis characterized by adherent scale, partial alopecia and (b) pigment accumulation along the eyelid margins.

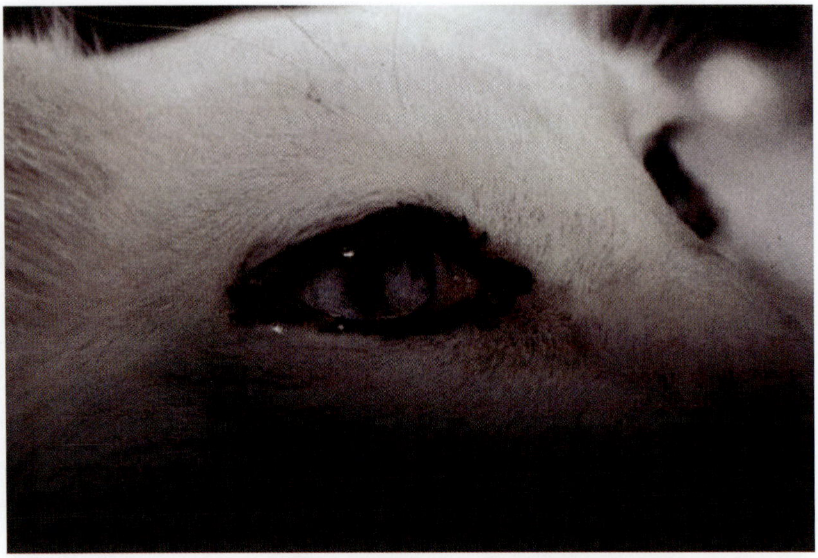

(b)

■ **Fig. 6.46.** *(Continued)*

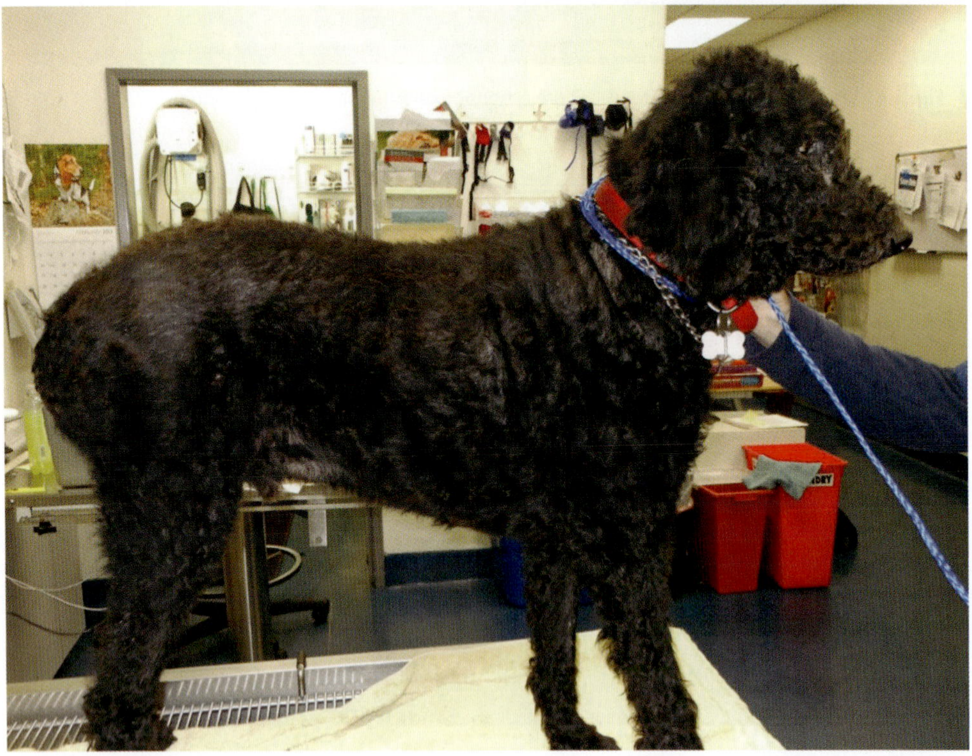

■ **Fig. 6.47.** Standard poodle with generalized granulomatous sebaceous adenitis demonstrating keratin collaring of hair shafts giving the appearance of alopecia.

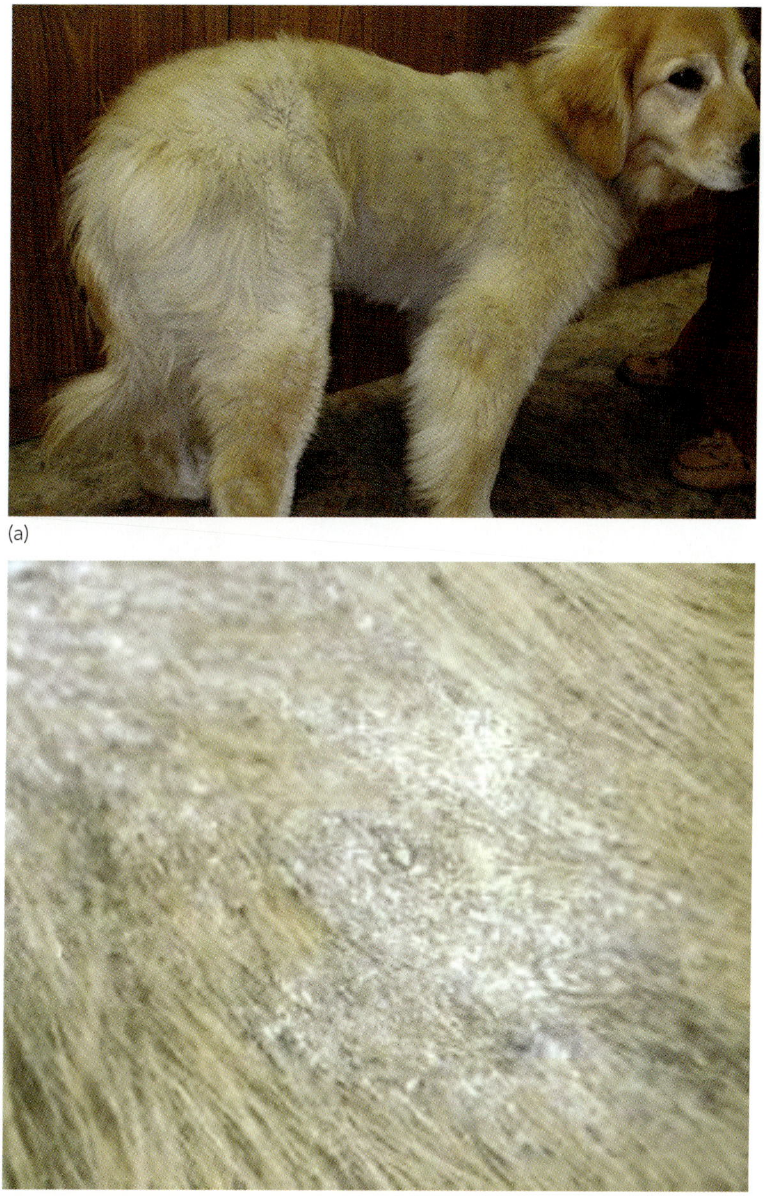

(a)

(b)

■ **Fig. 6.48.** (a) Ichthyosis in a young golden retriever showing partial alopecia with a mild surface scale and (b) tightly adherent scale along the surface of the skin.

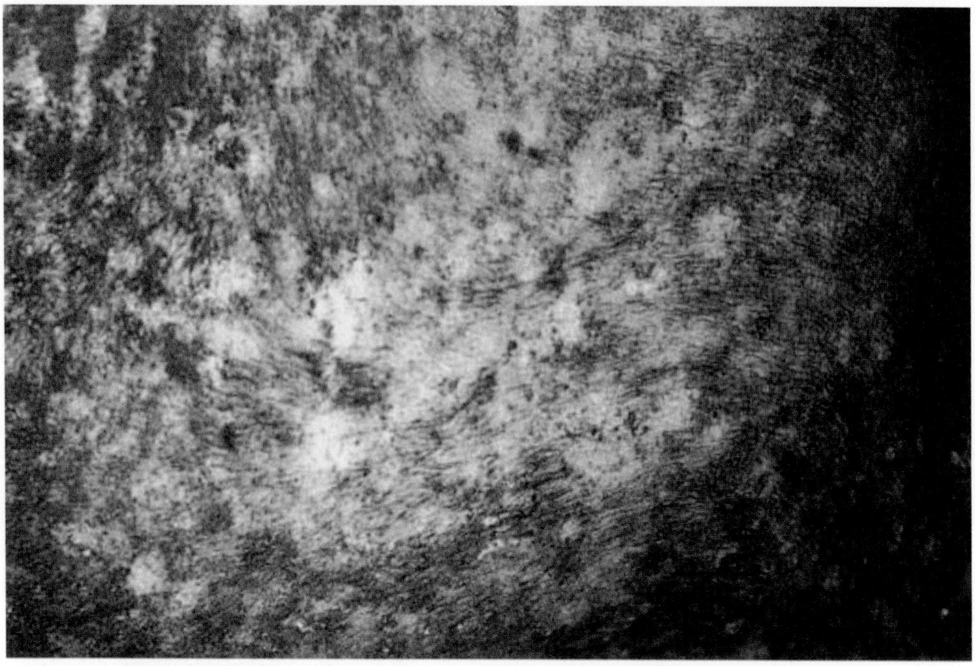

■ **Fig. 6.49.** Epitheliotropic lymphoma in a cocker spaniel. Note the areas of depigmentation and diffuse scaling on the shaved skin of this dog.

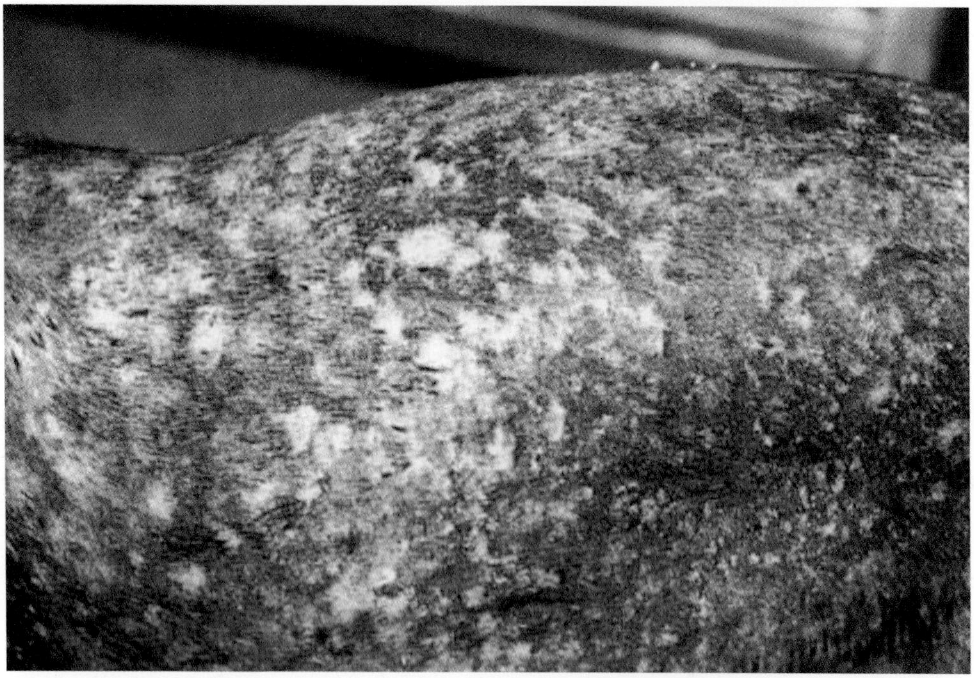

■ **Fig. 6.50.** Multifocal areas of depigmentation and diffuse scaling (shaved skin) characteristic of epitheliotropic lymphoma.

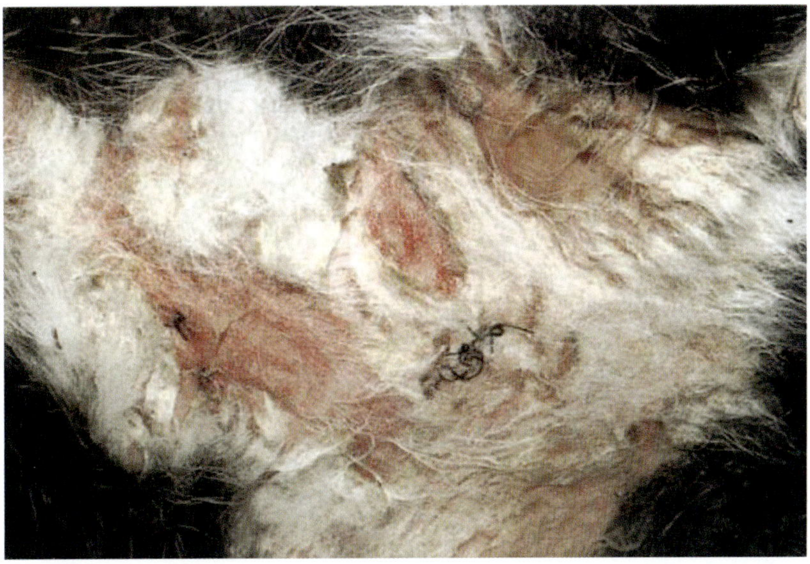

■ **Fig. 6.51.** Ventral abdominal region of a cat with epitheliotropic lymphoma revealing erythematous plaques and ulcerations associated with advanced disease.

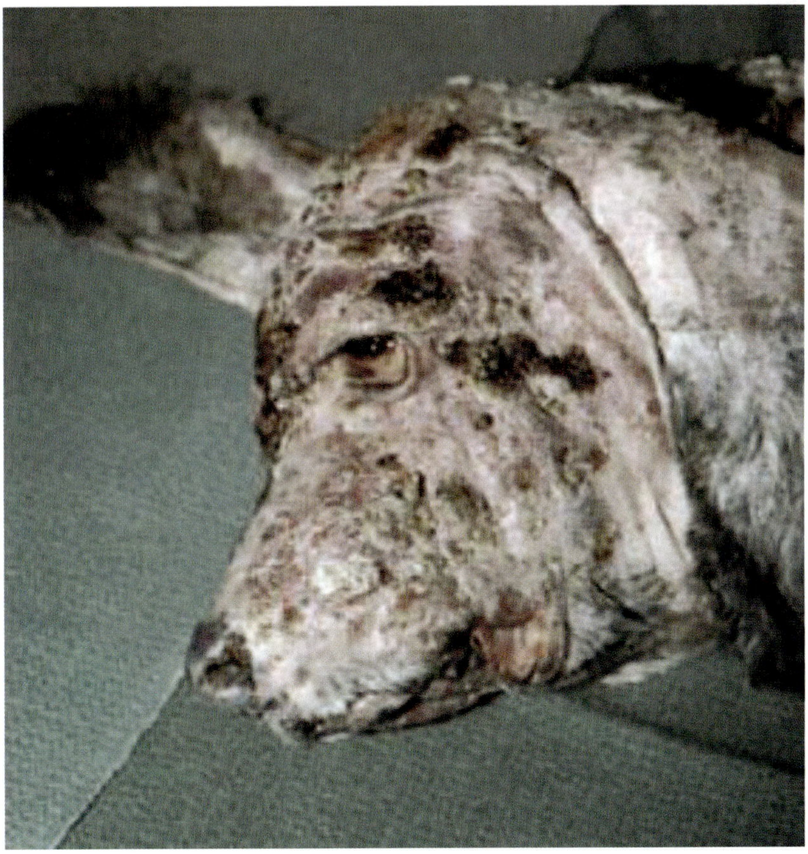

■ **Fig. 6.52.** End-stage epitheliotropic lymphoma. Note the diffuse erythema, alopecia, crusting, and depigmentation (especially the planum nasale).

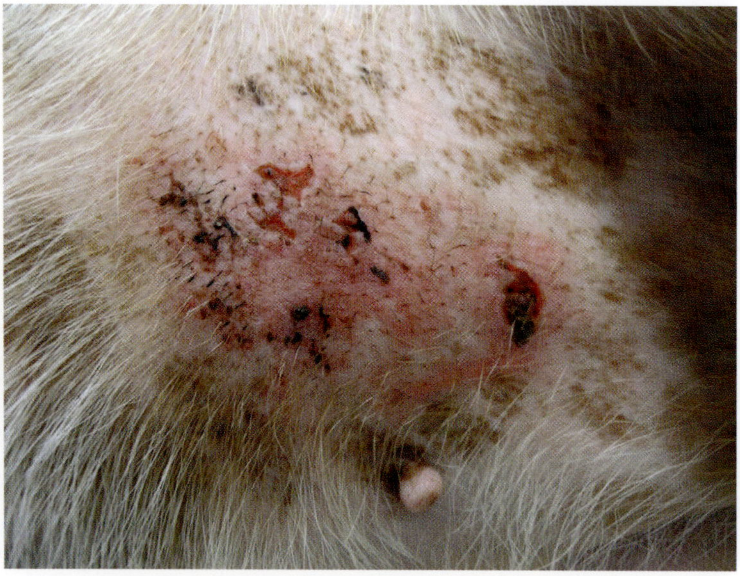

■ **Fig. 6.53.** Actinic keratoses on the ventrum of a 9-year-old female-spayed pointer mix.

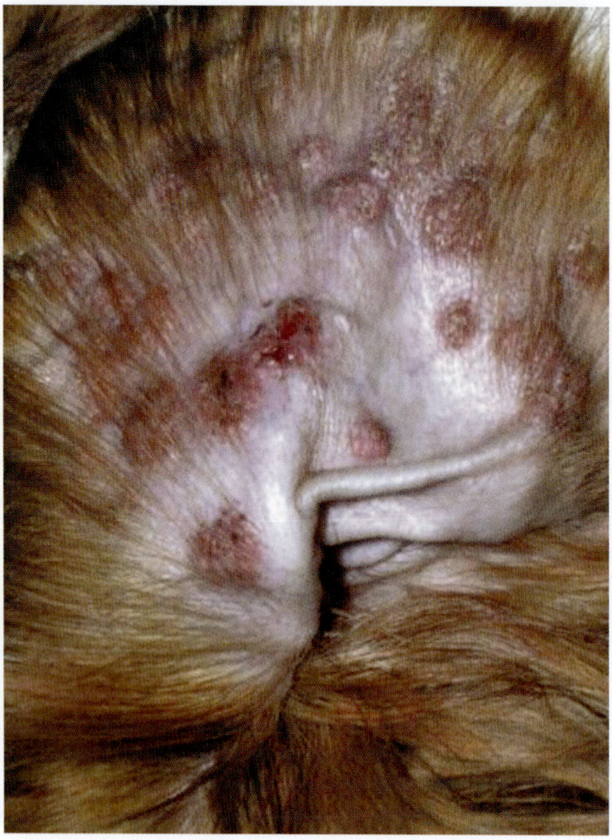

■ **Fig. 6.54.** Psoriasiform lichenoid dermatosis: raised plaque-like lesions with surface scale on the pinna.

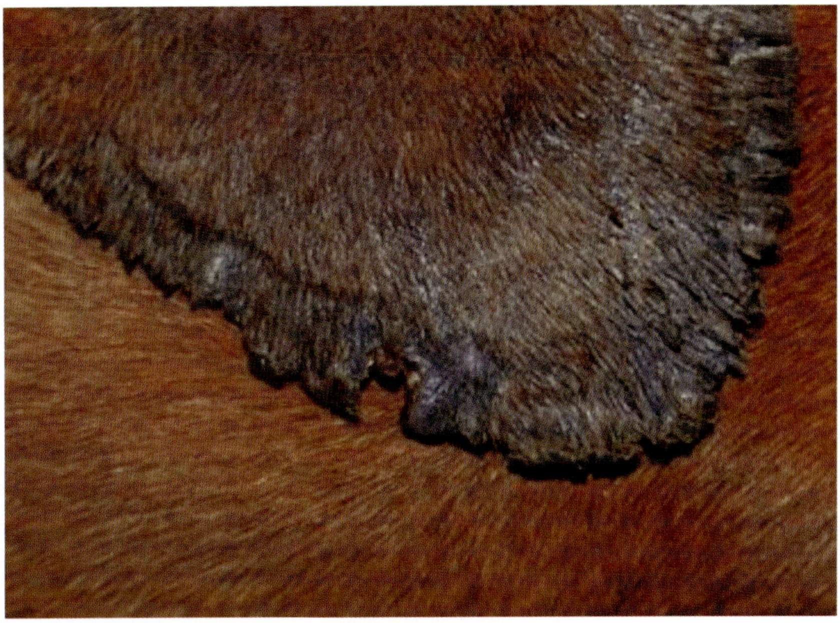

■ **Fig. 6.55.** Ear margin dermatosis: partial alopecia with marked hyperkeratosis affecting the pinnal margins with erosion and notching.

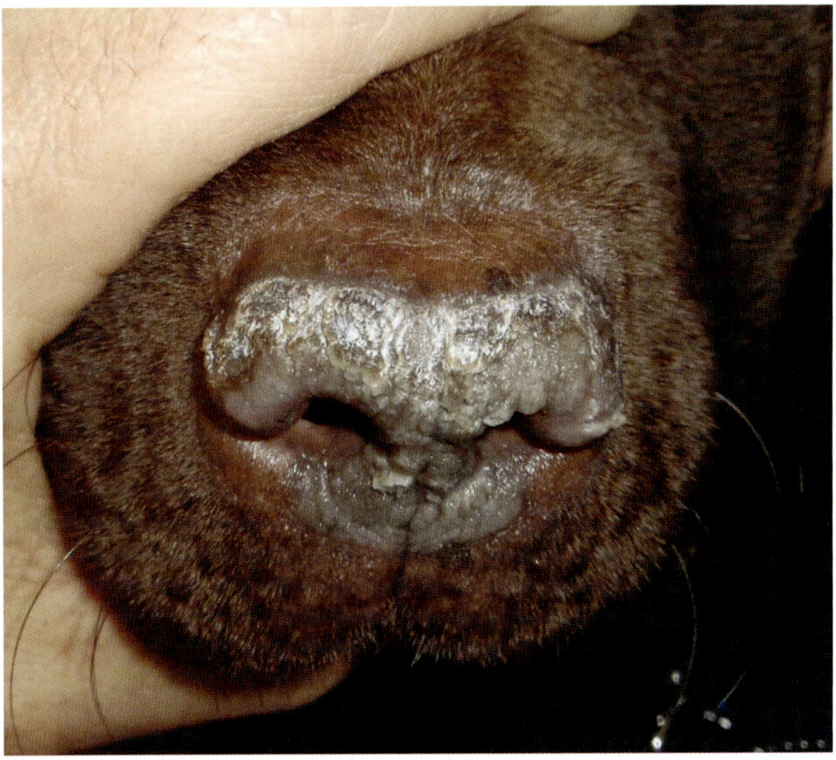

■ **Fig. 6.56.** Tightly adherent keratin with depigmentation on the nasal planum in hereditary nasal parakeratosis.

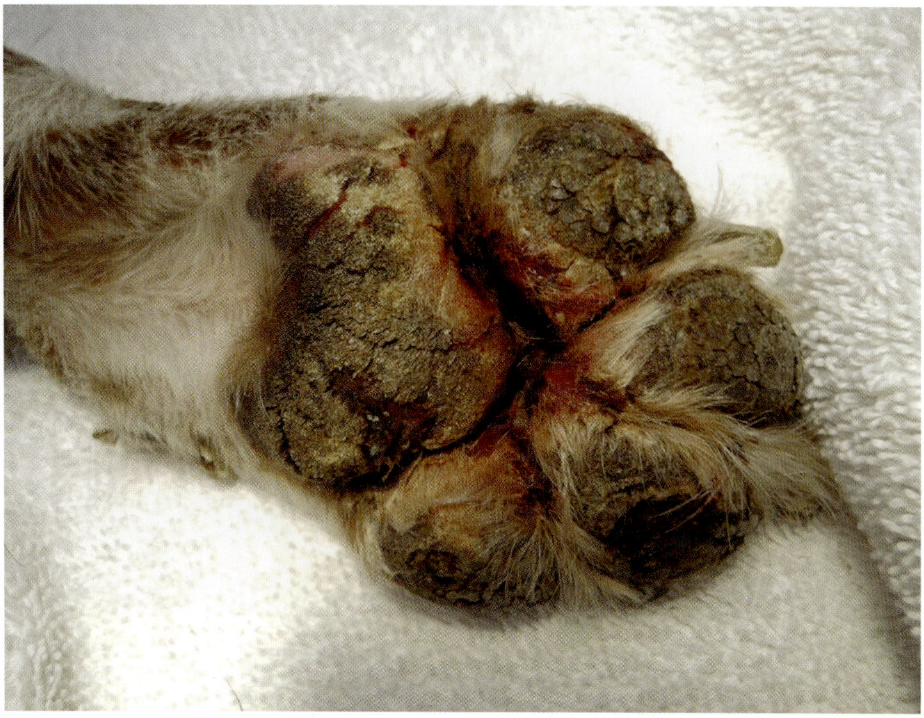

■ **Fig. 6.57.** Erosions and hyperkeratosis on the footpads of a beagle with SND.

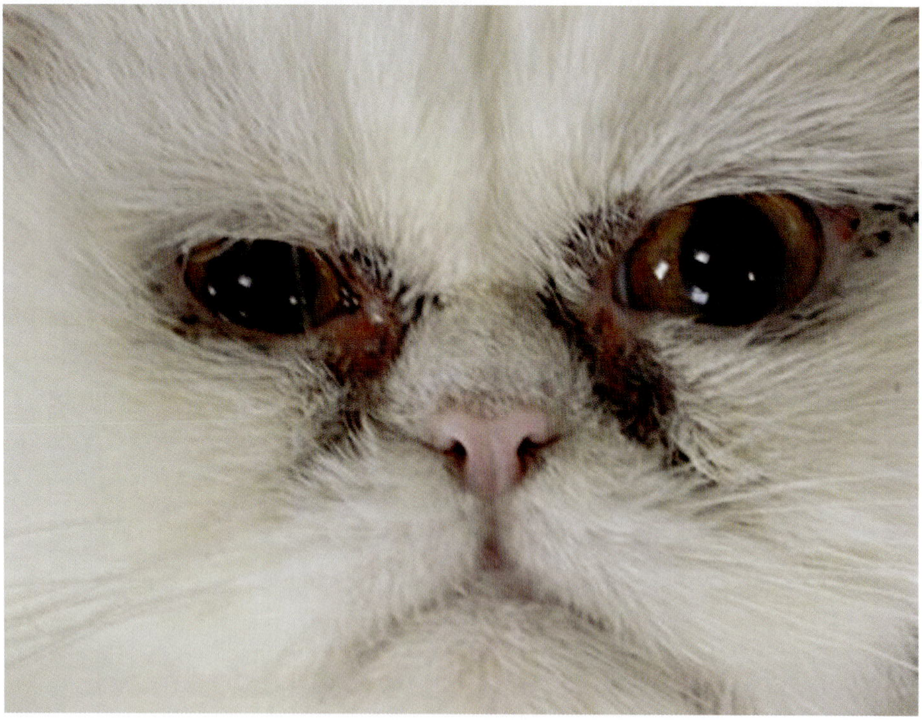

■ **Fig. 6.58.** Dirty face syndrome. Lesions can become erosive. Early cases will often present with a greasy black to brown discharge.

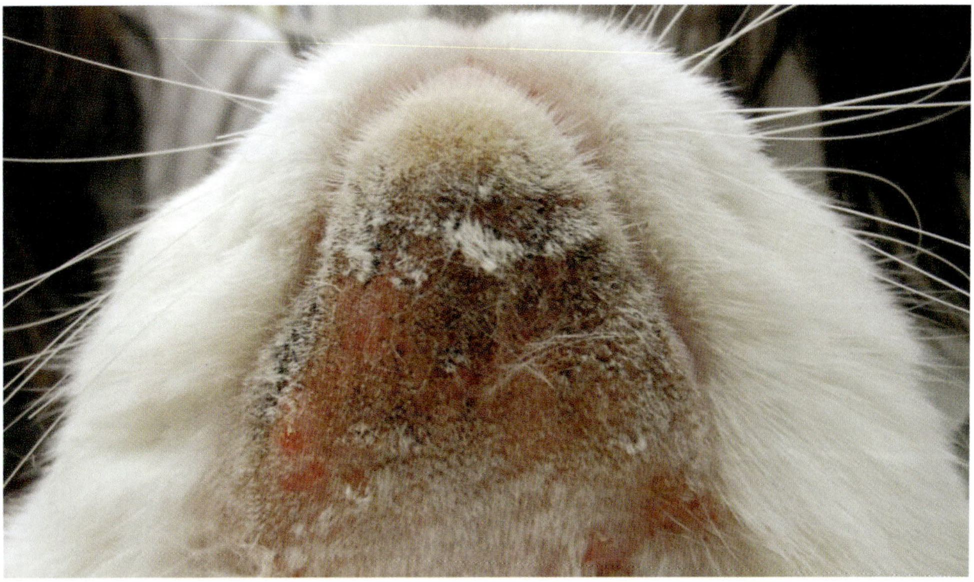

Fig. 6.59. Feline acne with crusting, comedones, and inflammation on the ventral chin.

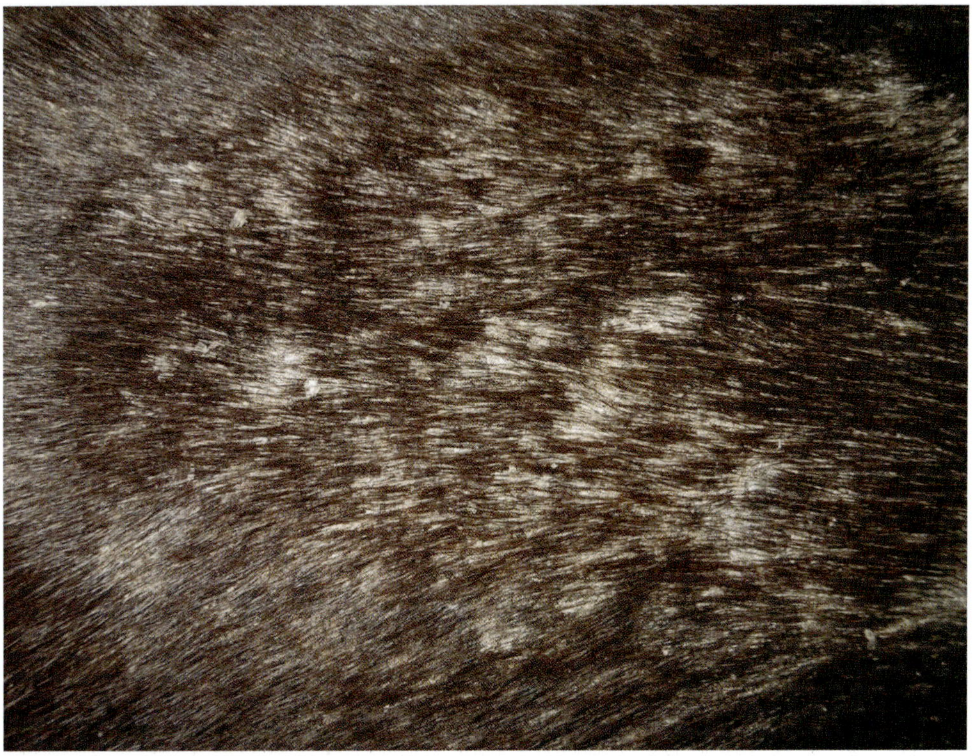

Fig. 6.60. Generalized adherent crusts with underlying erosions in exfoliative cutaneous lupus erythematosus.

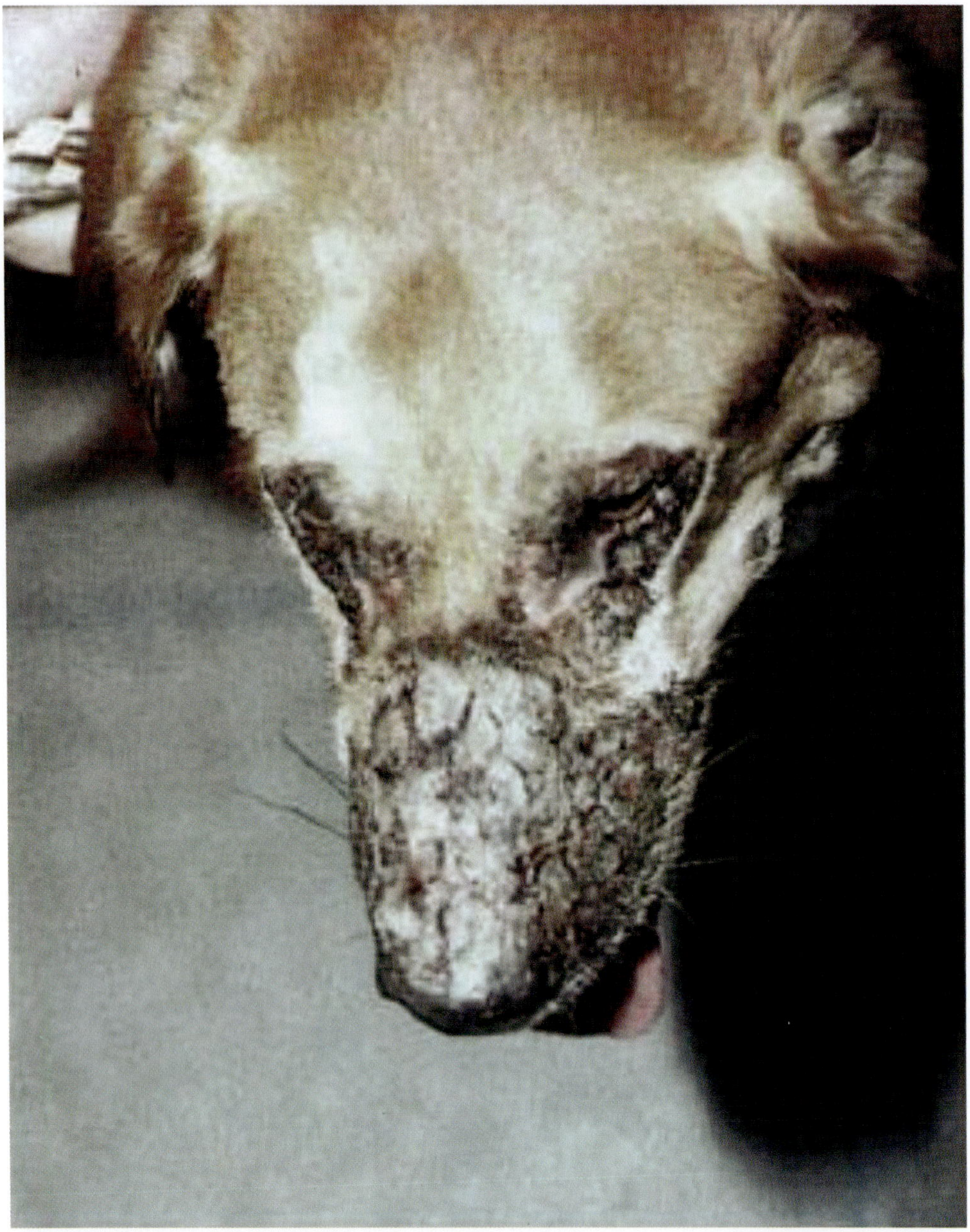

■ **Fig. 6.61.** Pemphigus foliaceus demonstrating the typical pattern of cutaneous involvement along the bridge of the nose and periocular region.

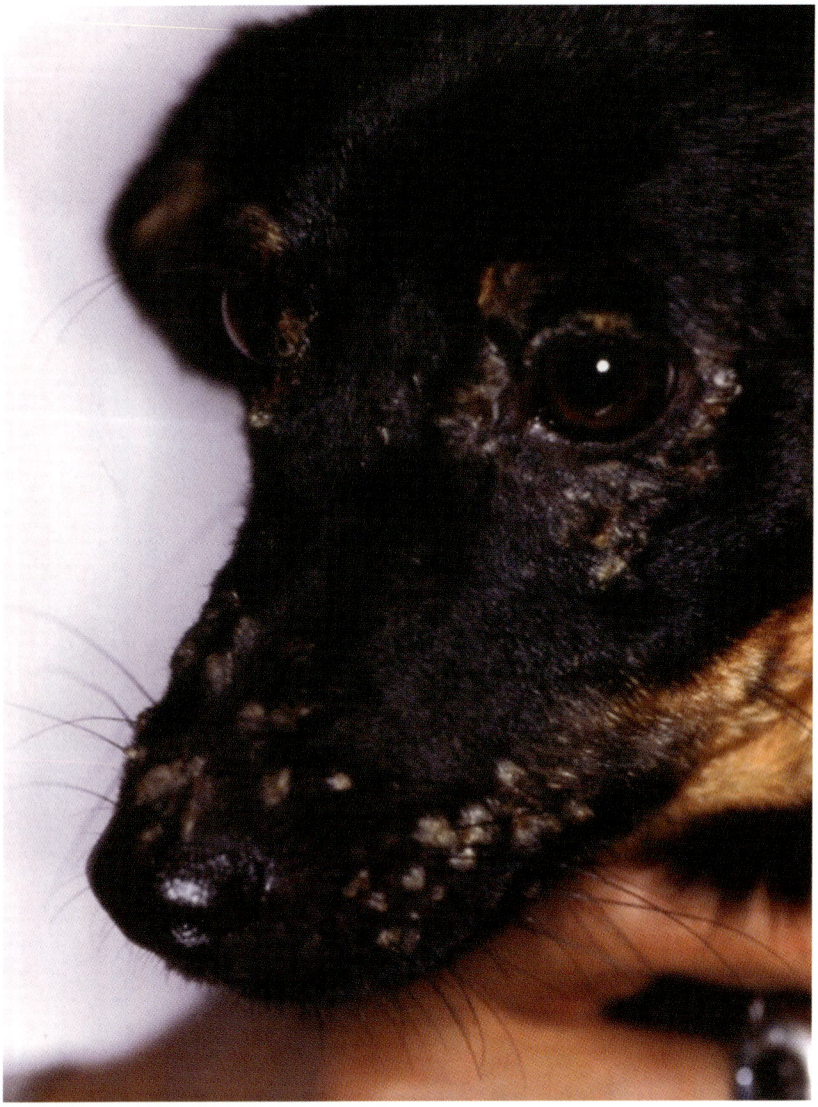

Fig. 6.62. Pemphigus foliaceus: prominent pustules along the muzzle and periocular region.

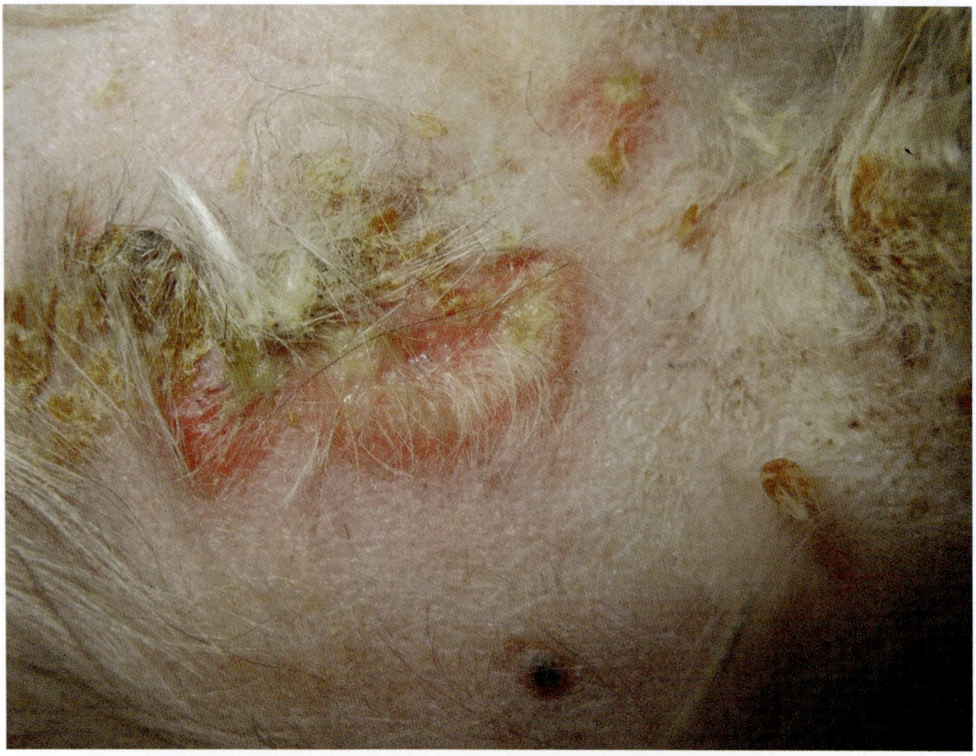

Fig. 6.63. Intact pustules on the ventrum of a dog with pemphigus foliaceus.

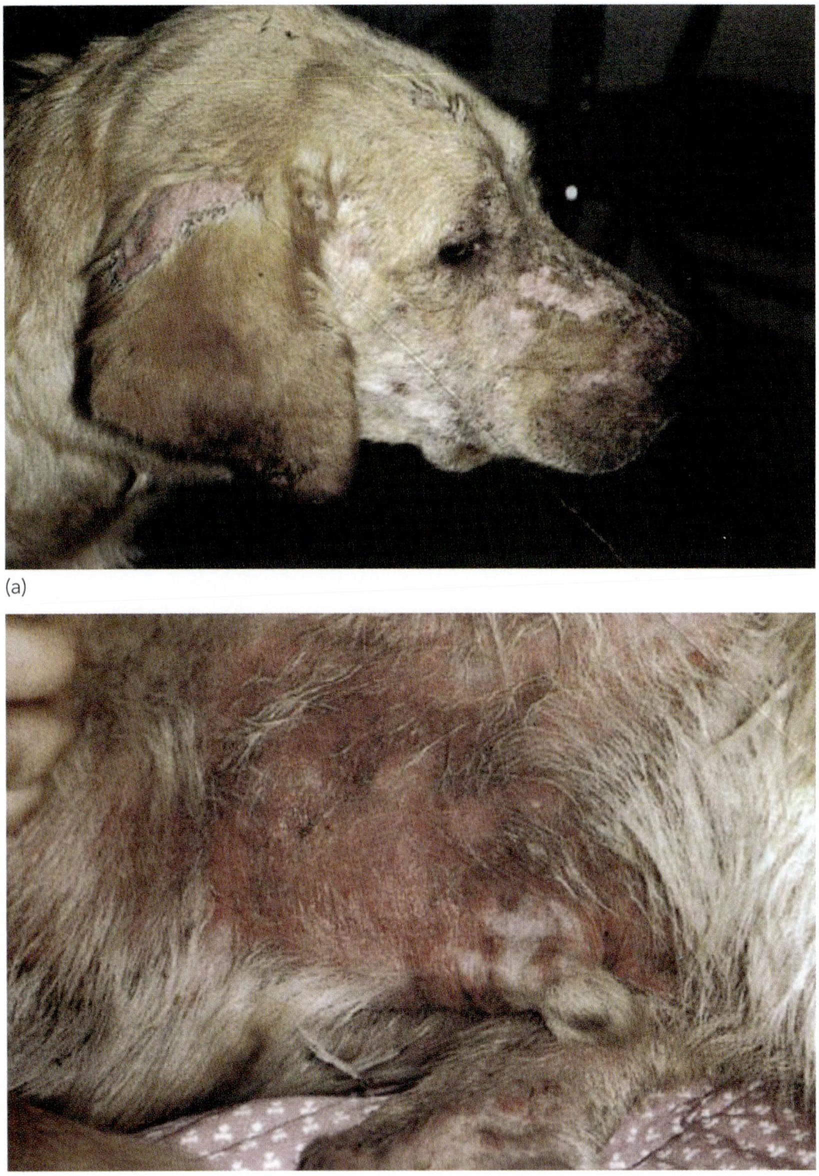

(a)

(b)

■ **Fig. 6.64.** (a) Two-year-old male golden retriever with generalized erosive facial and (b) inguinal dermatitis caused by drug-induced (cephalexin) pemphigus foliaceus.

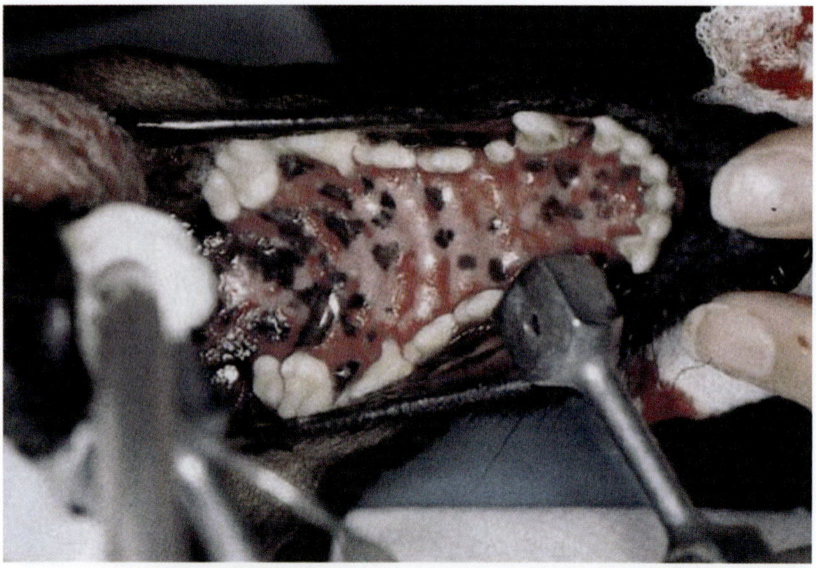

(a)

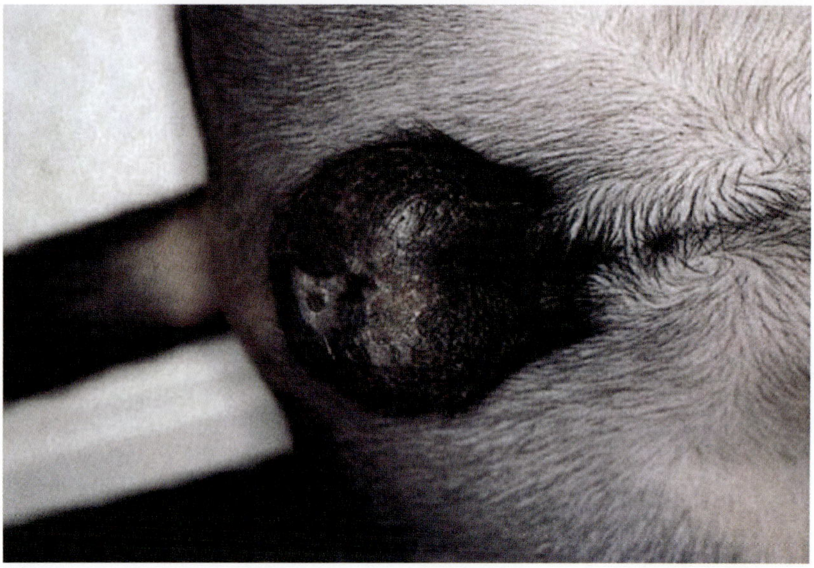

(b)

■ **Fig. 6.65.** (a) Eight-year-old male-intact mixed breed dog with pemphigus vulgaris affecting oral mucosa and (b) scrotum.

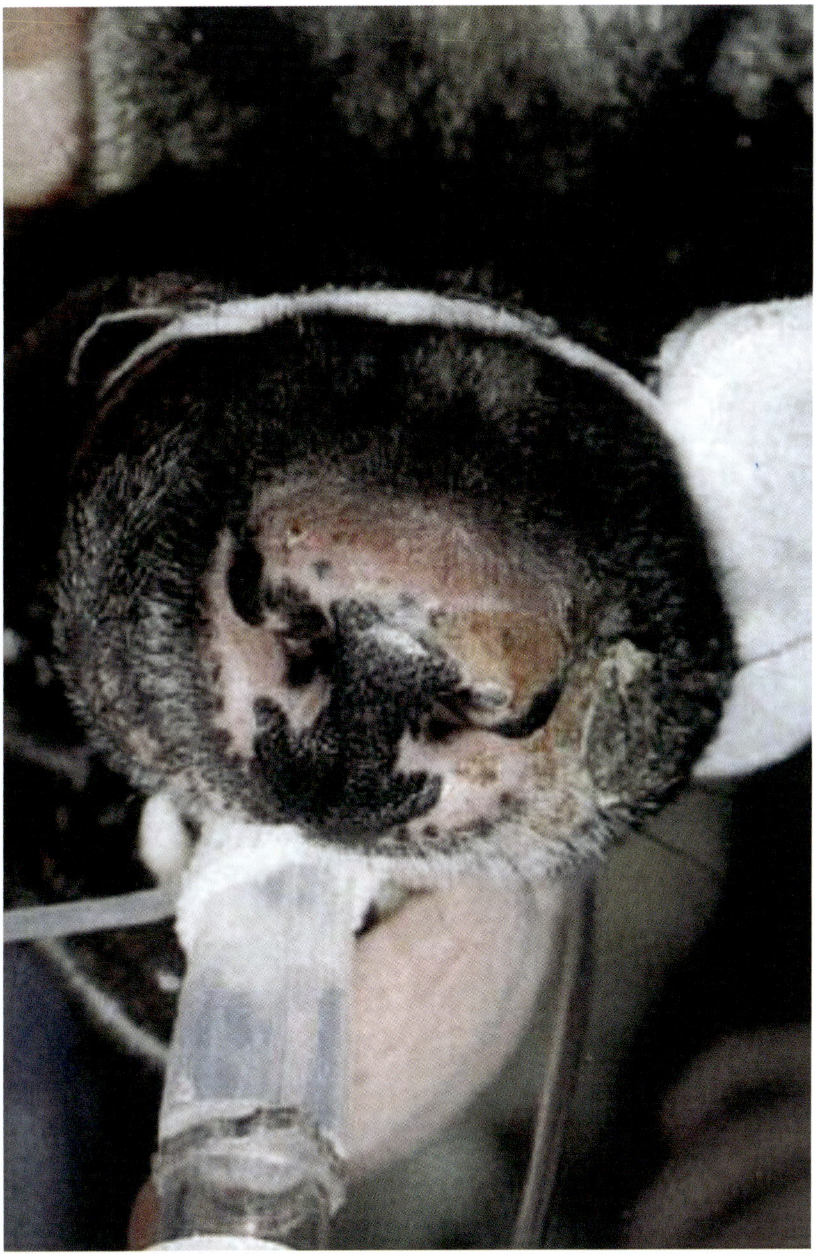

■ **Fig. 6.66.** Five-year-old male-castrate Akita with discoid lupus erythematosus.

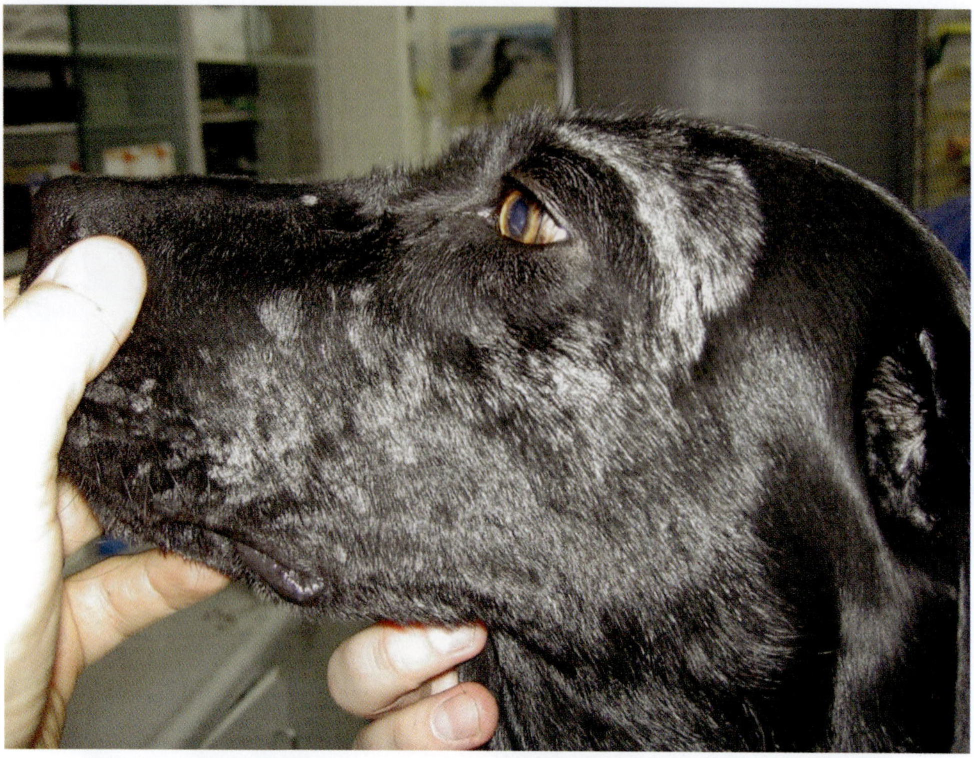

■ **Fig. 6.67.** Accumulations of crusts associated with systemic lupus erythematosus in a 12-year-old Labrador retriever.

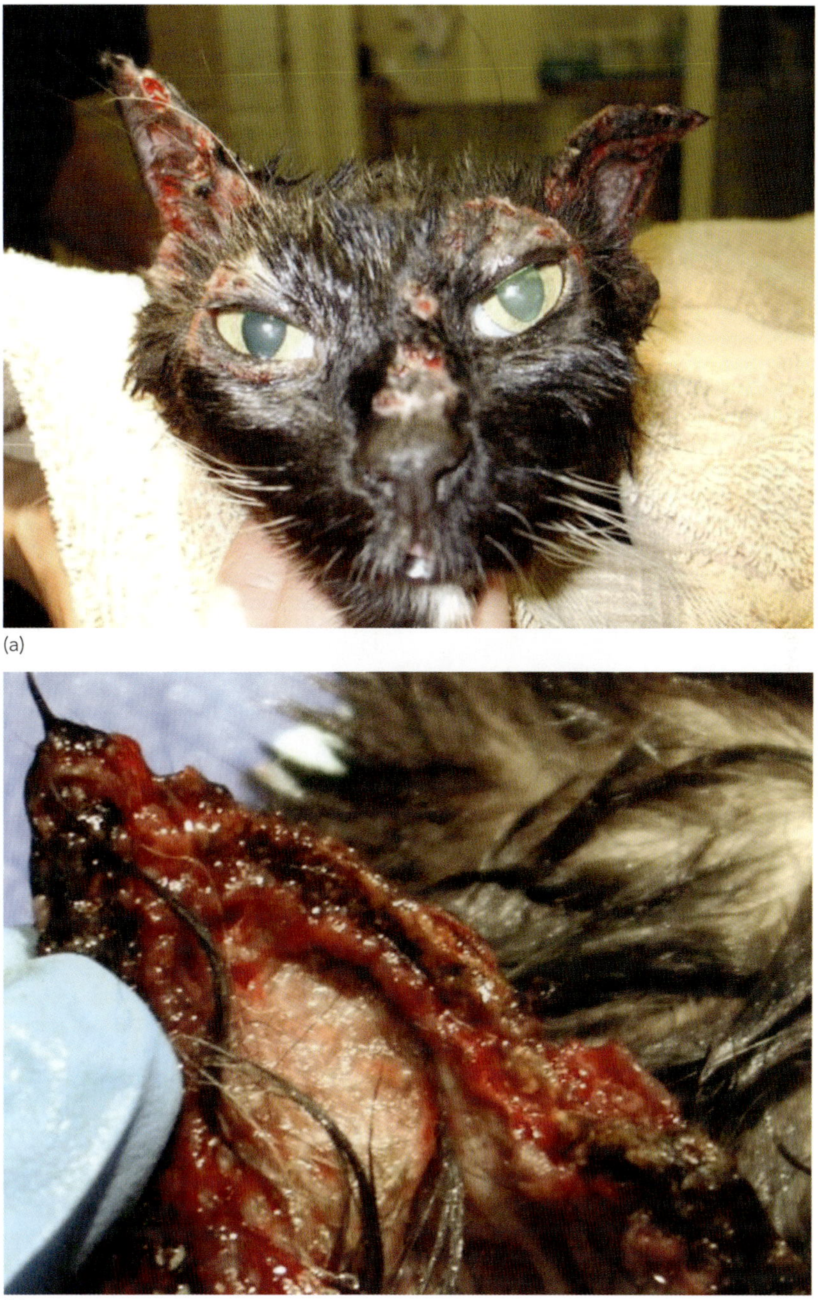

(a)

(b)

■ **Fig. 6.68.** Vasculitis. (a) Severe ulceration and disfigurement in this patient with (b) necrosis of the skin along the pinnal margin.

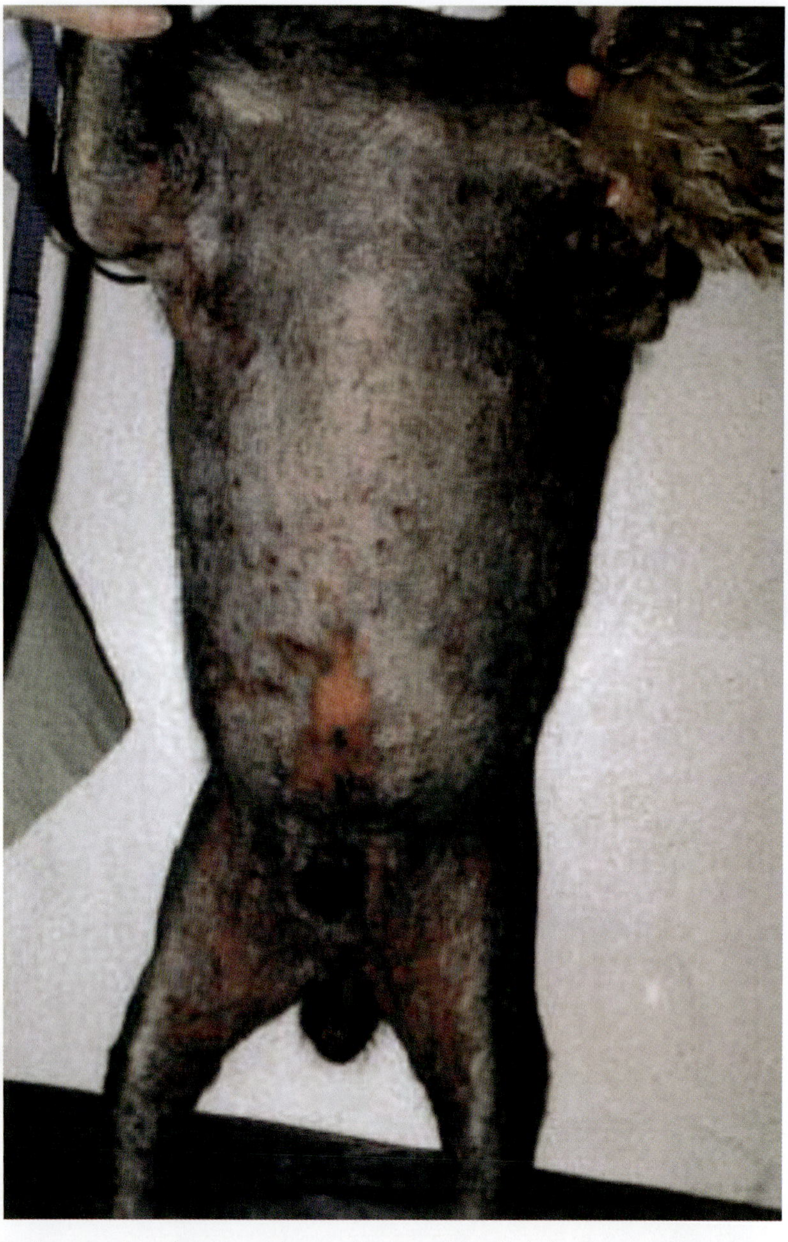

■ **Fig. 6.69.** Five-year-old male-intact miniature schnauzer with sulfa-induced toxic epidermal necrolysis.

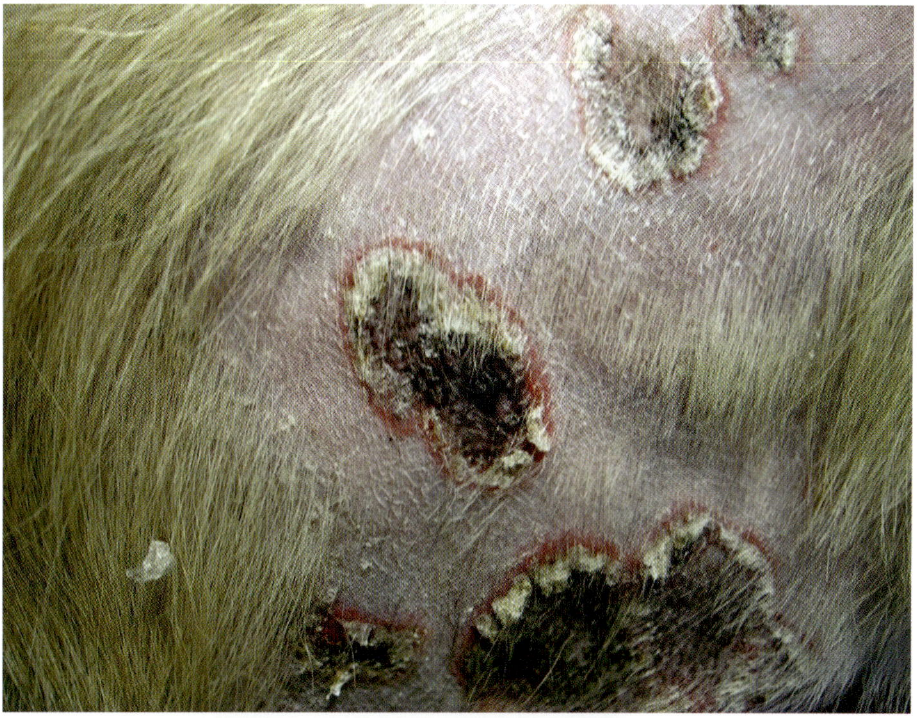

Fig. 6.70. Targetoid-like lesions characteristic of erythema multiforme.

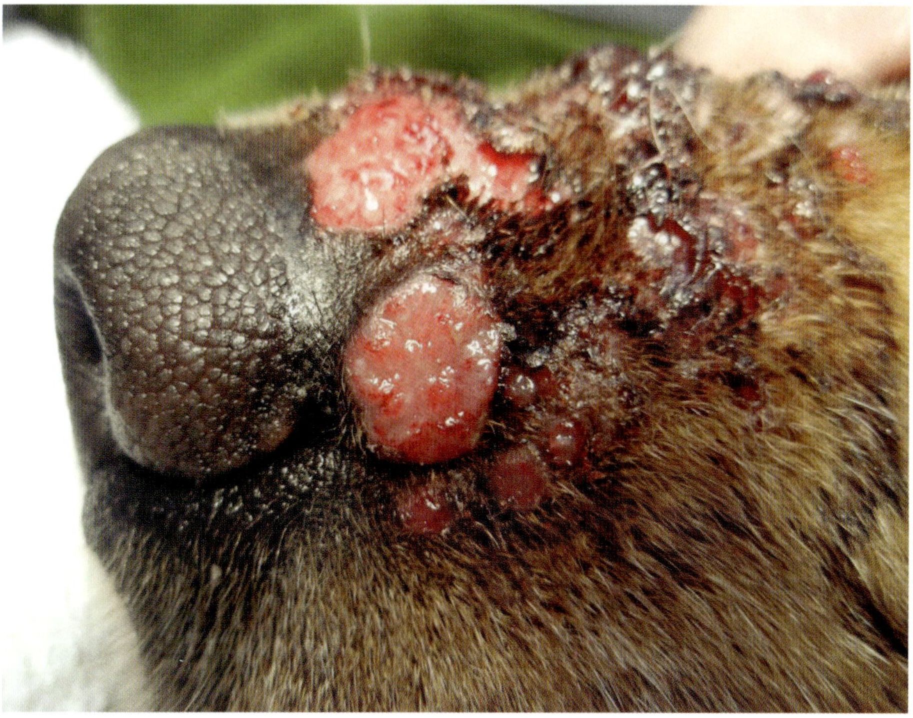

Fig. 6.71. Insect hypersensitivity resulting in an erosive dermatitis of eosinophilic nasal furunculosis.

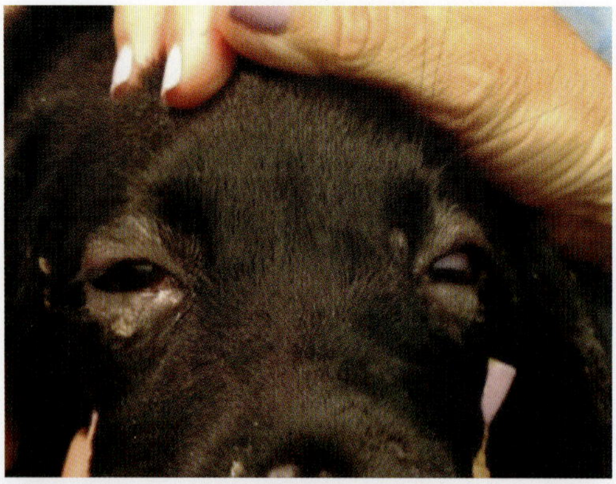

(a)

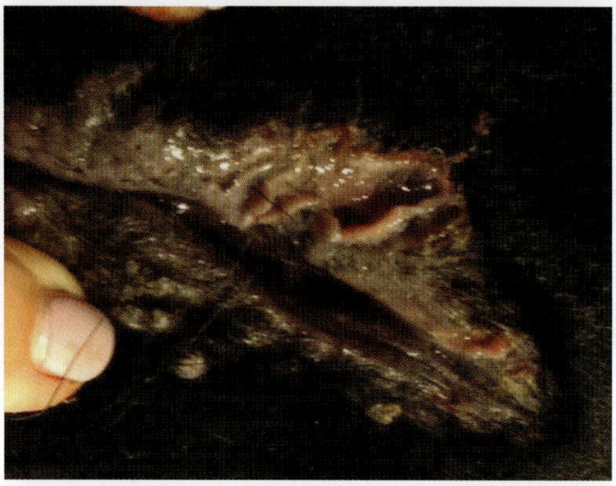

(b)

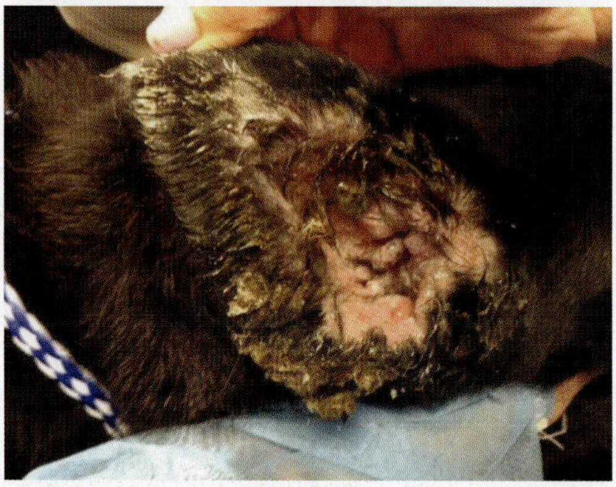

(c)

■ **Fig. 6.72.** Canine juvenile cellulitis, "puppy strangles." (a) Characteristic swollen periocular region and muzzle; peripheral lymph nodes are also usually enlarged. (b) The lip folds are markedly ulcerative and exudative. (c) Proliferative and erosive pinna and ear canal in this patient.

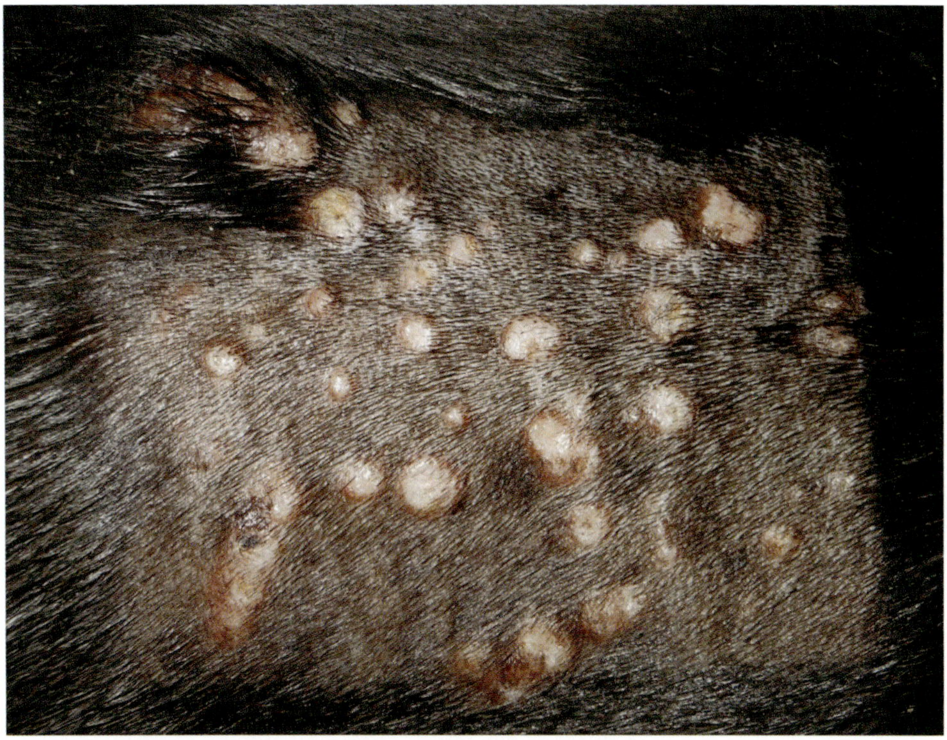

■ **Fig. 6.73.** Multiple erythematous plaques (hair coat clipped) with histiocytosis.

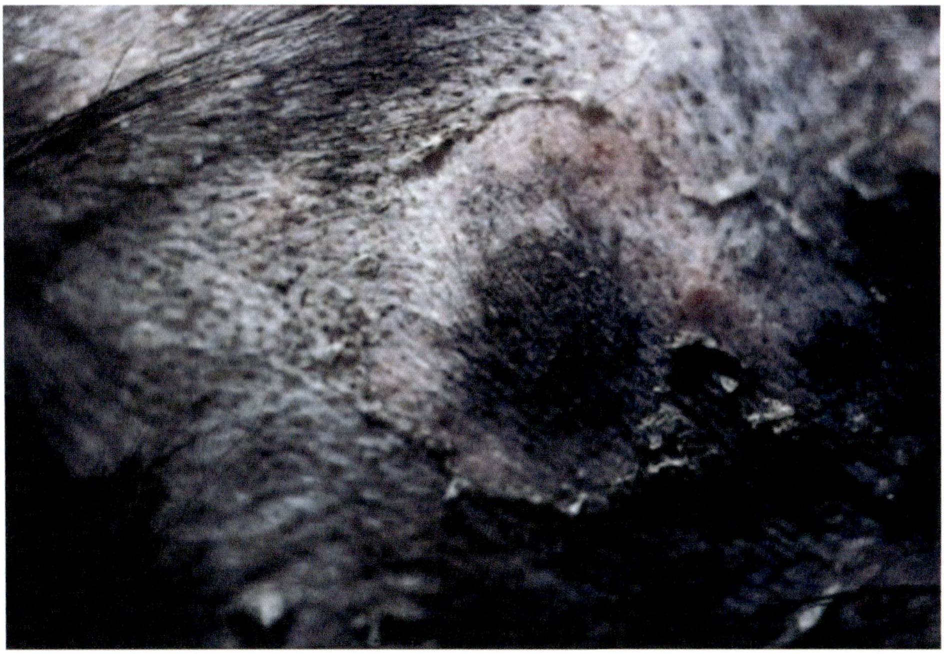

■ **Fig. 6.74.** Papules, pustules, epidermal collarettes, and hyperpigmented macule characteristic of superficial bacterial folliculitis.

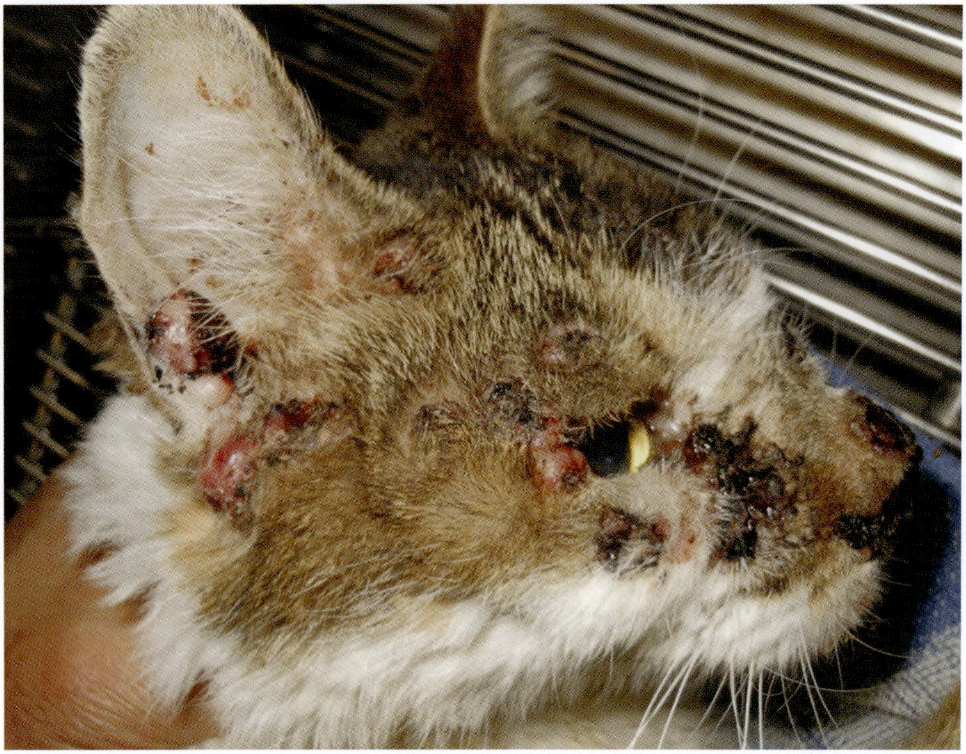

Fig. 6.75. Multiple crusted and scabbed lesions of cryptococcosis.

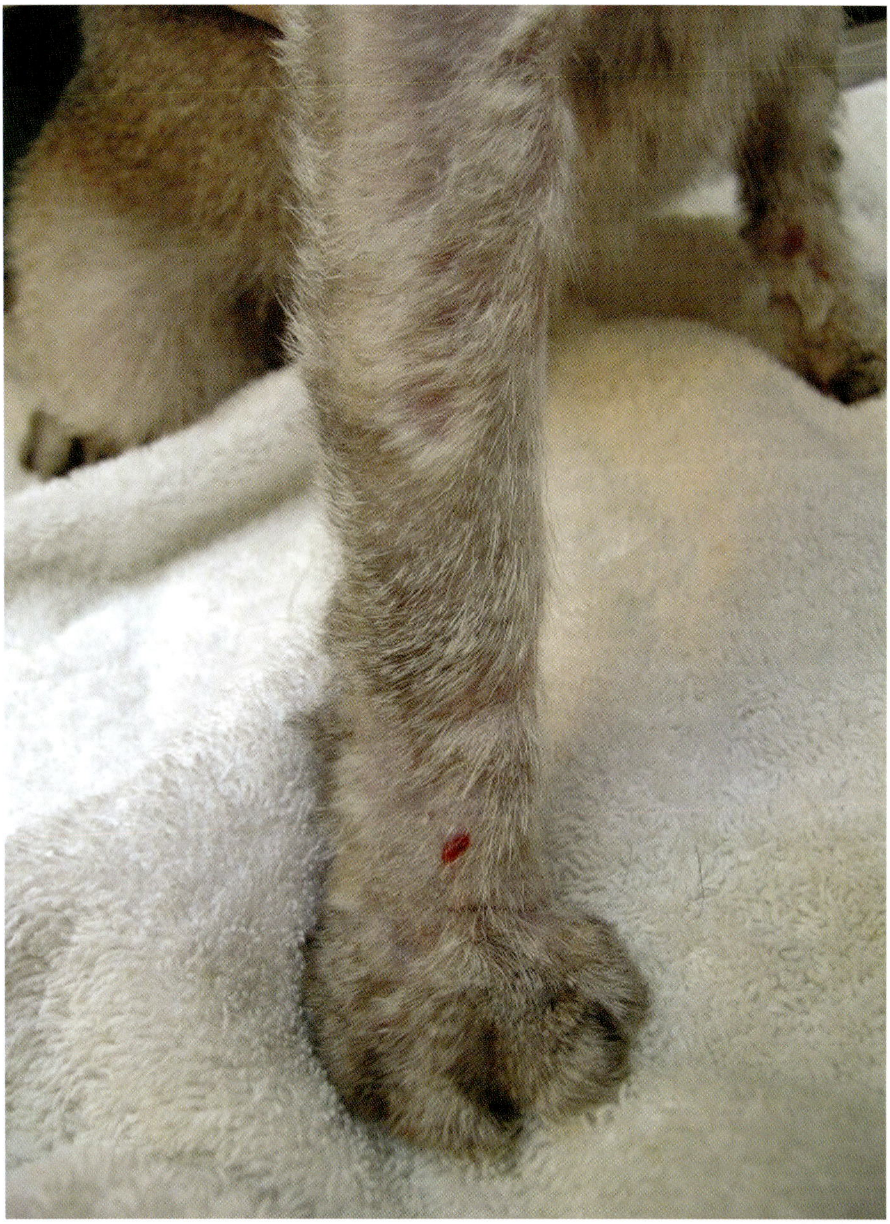

Fig. 6.76. Alopecic and draining lesions of nocardiosis.

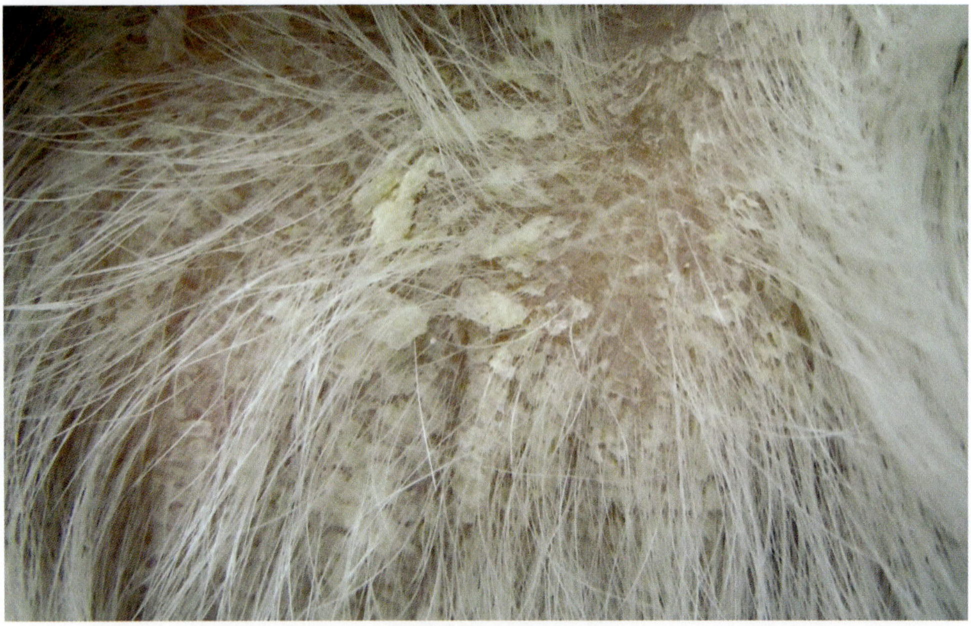

■ **Fig. 6.77.** Exfoliative lesions associated with cutaneous leishmaniasis.

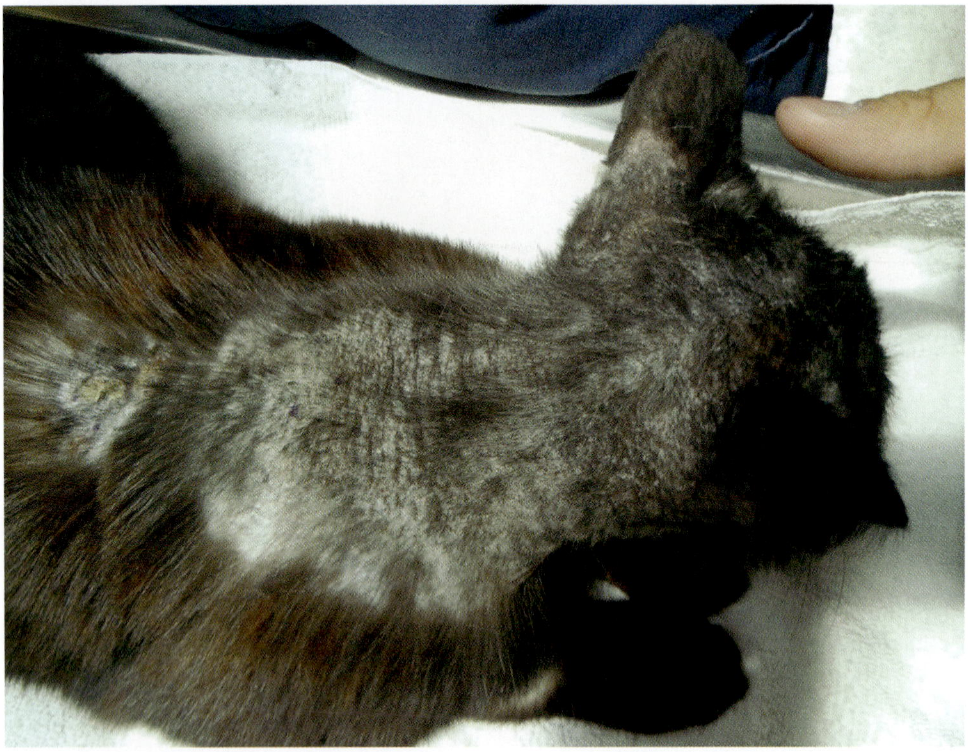

■ **Fig. 6.78.** Scaling and pruritic dermatitis associated with FIV infection.

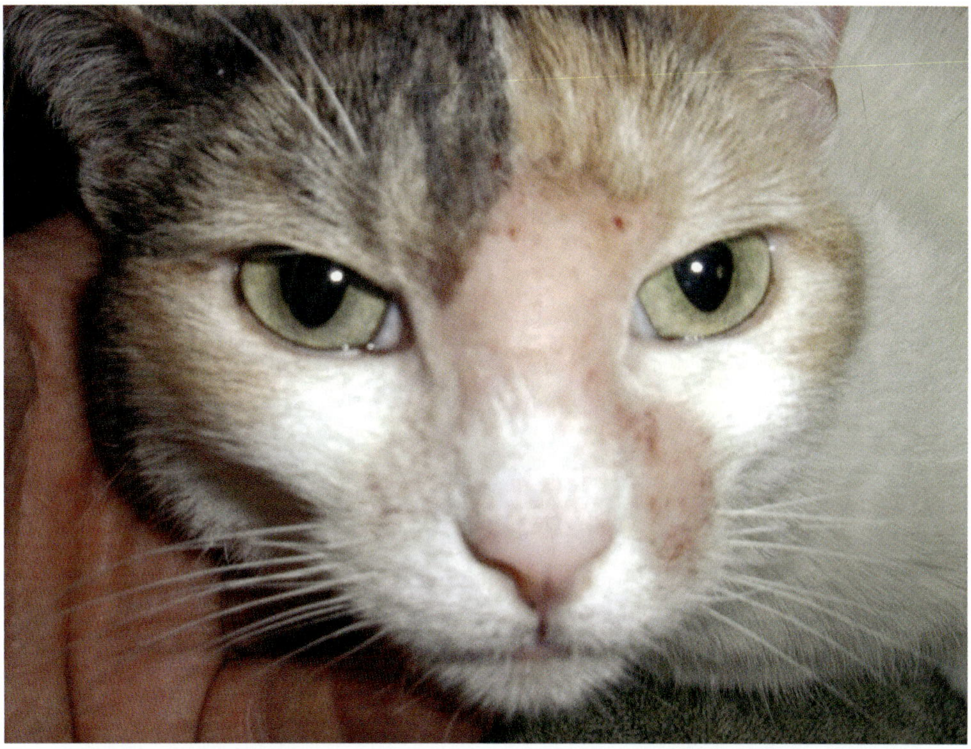

■ **Fig. 6.79.** Alopecia and erythema on the dorsal muzzle and face from mosquito bite hypersensitivity.

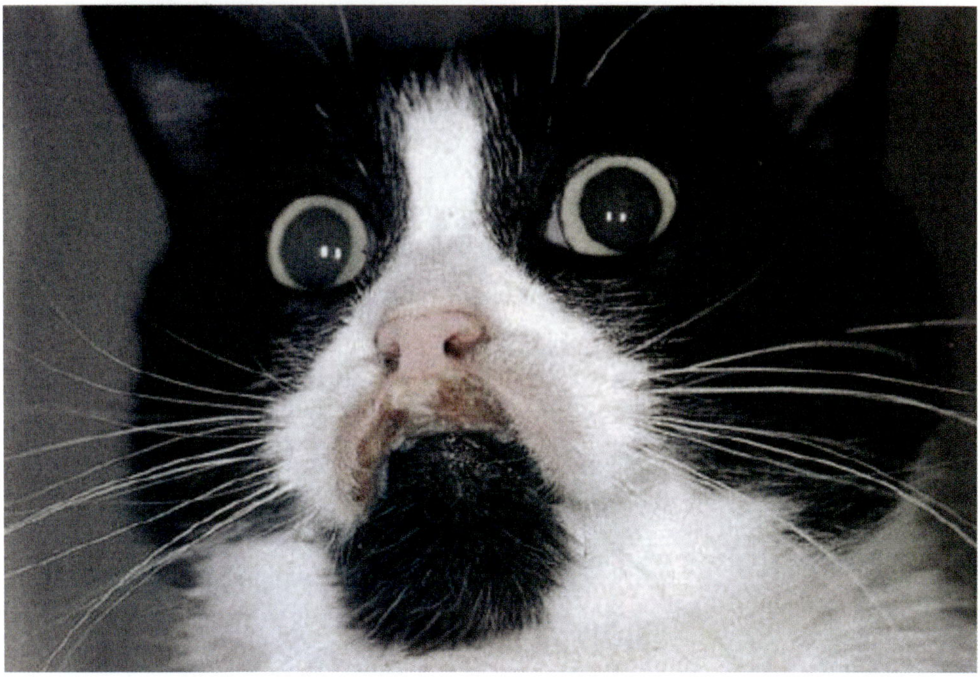

■ **Fig. 6.80.** Five-year-old male-castrate DSH with "rodent ulcer" of the upper lip.

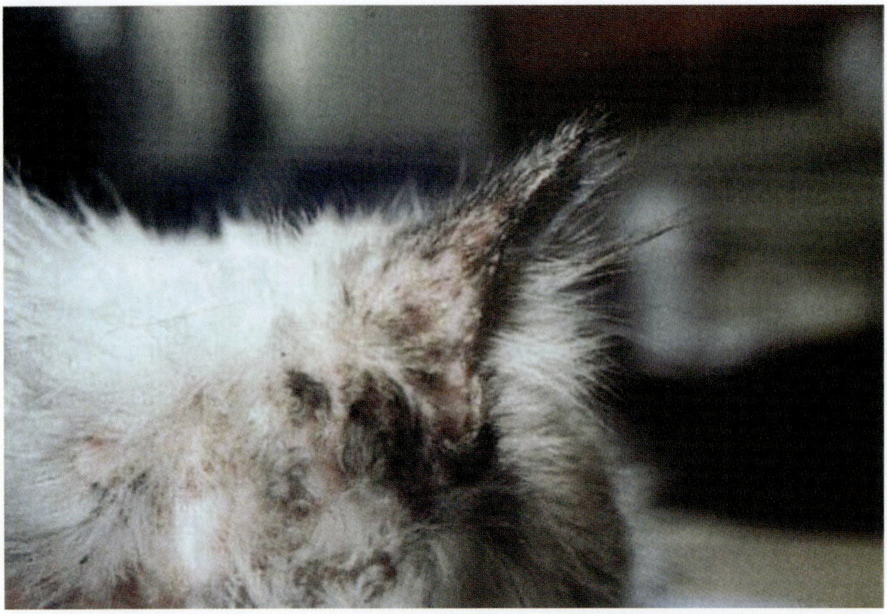

■ **Fig. 6.81.** Feline allergic dermatitis is most severe along the head and neck region. Note the excoriations along the caudal aspect of the pinnae and neck region.

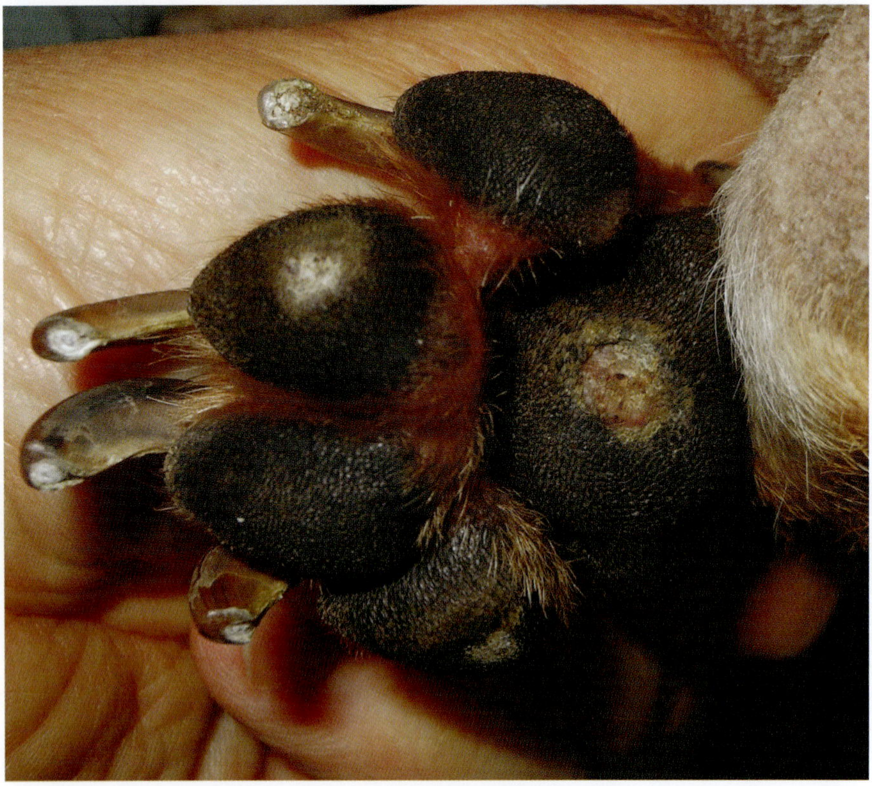

■ **Fig. 6.82.** Footpad ulcerations in a young dachshund with epidermolysis bullosa aquisita.

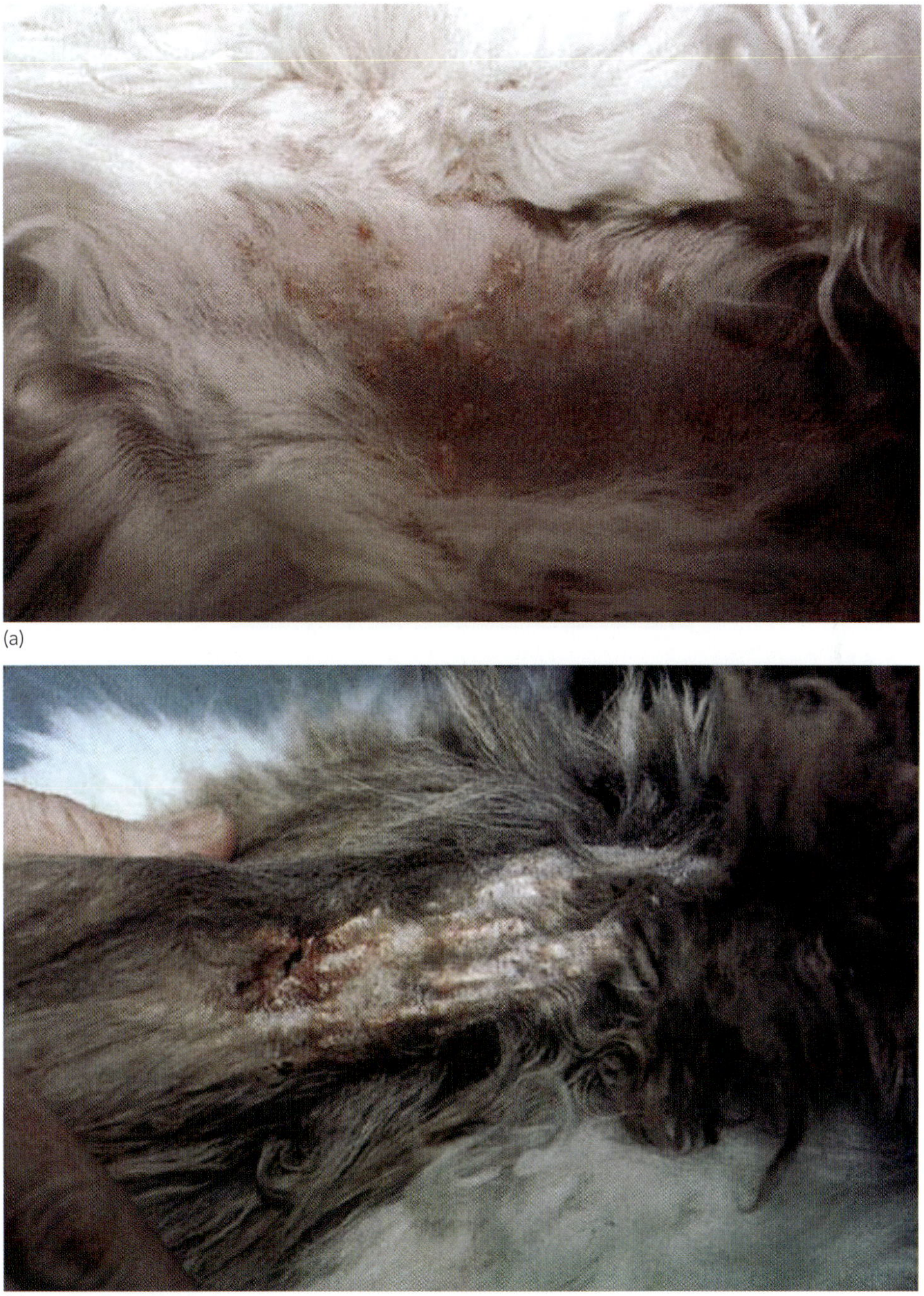

(a)

(b)

■ **Fig. 6.83.** Cutaneous xanthomatosis. (a) Associated with an endocrine imbalance (cortisol, thyroid, DM, etc.) or idiopathic hyperlipidemia. Small coalescing yellow-pink nodules and plaques along the caudal ventral trunk in a 10-year-old male-castrate DSH. (b) Linear yellow-pink lesions along the ventral region of a 7-year-old female-spayed DSH with diabetes mellitus.

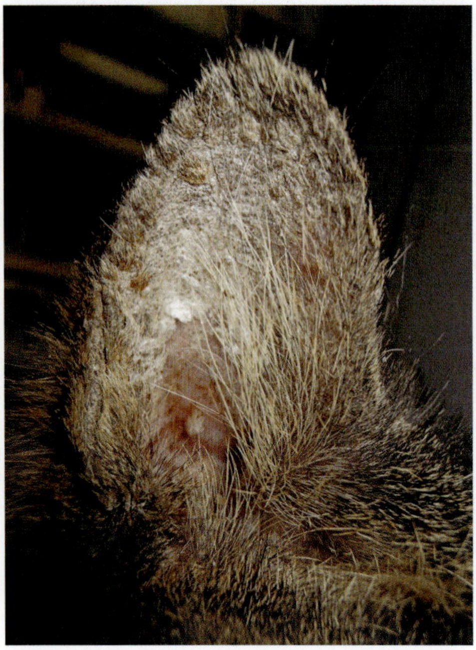

■ **Fig. 6.84.** Crusted and exudative lesions on the pinna caused by drug eruption to amoxicillin.

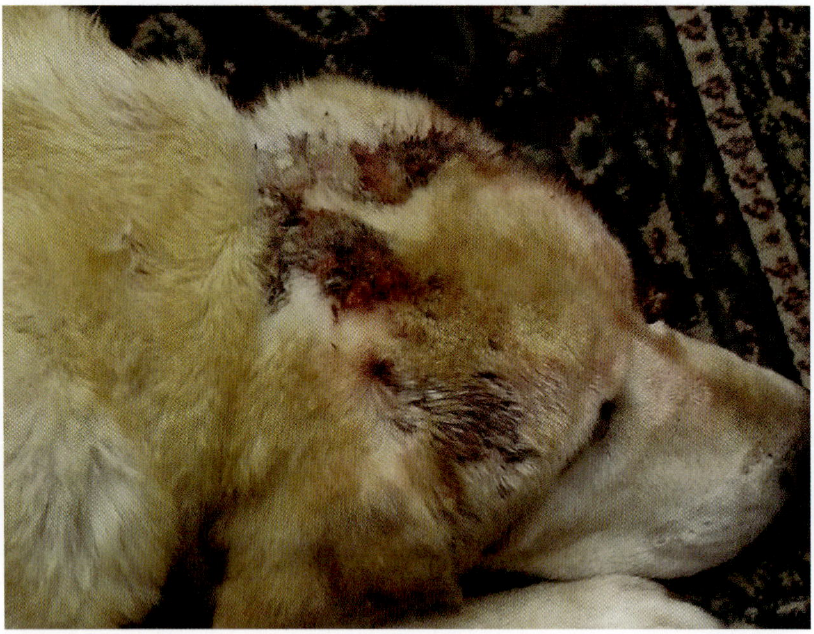

(a)

■ **Fig. 6.85.** Calcinosis cutis. (a) Accumulation of calcium in the skin causes firm plaques that can be erosive and ulcerative. (b) Thick plaque-like lesions with ulcerations along the dorsum of the trunk and (c) on the neck.

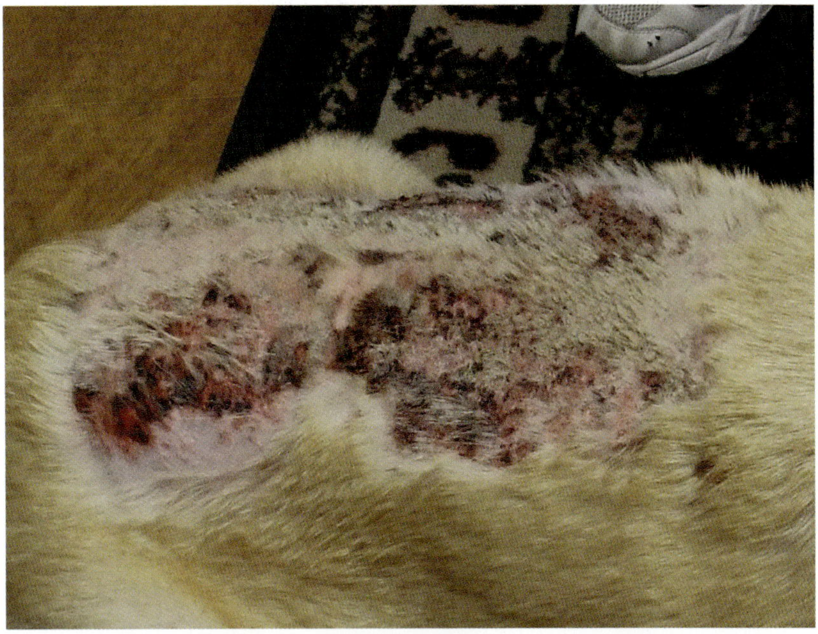

(b)

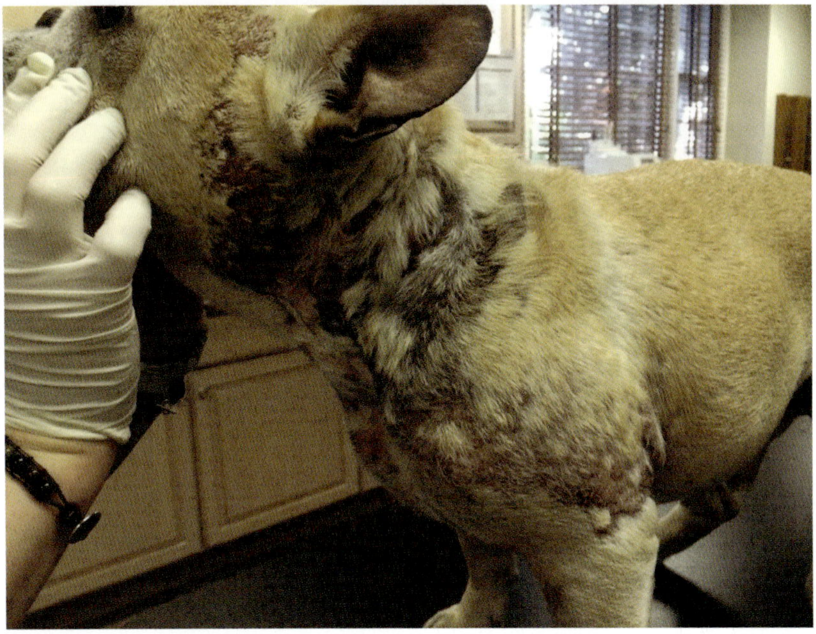

(c)

■ **Fig. 6.85.** *(Continued)*

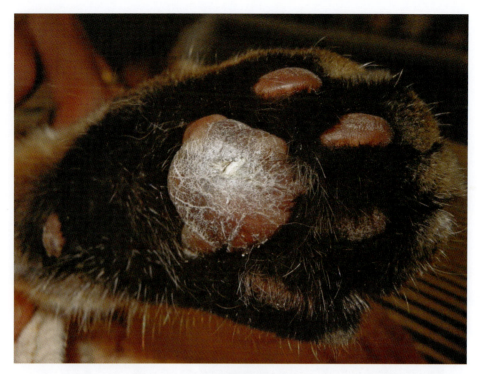

■ **Fig. 6.86.** Swollen metacarpal pad of a 7-year-old female-spayed DSH with plasma cell pododermatitis.

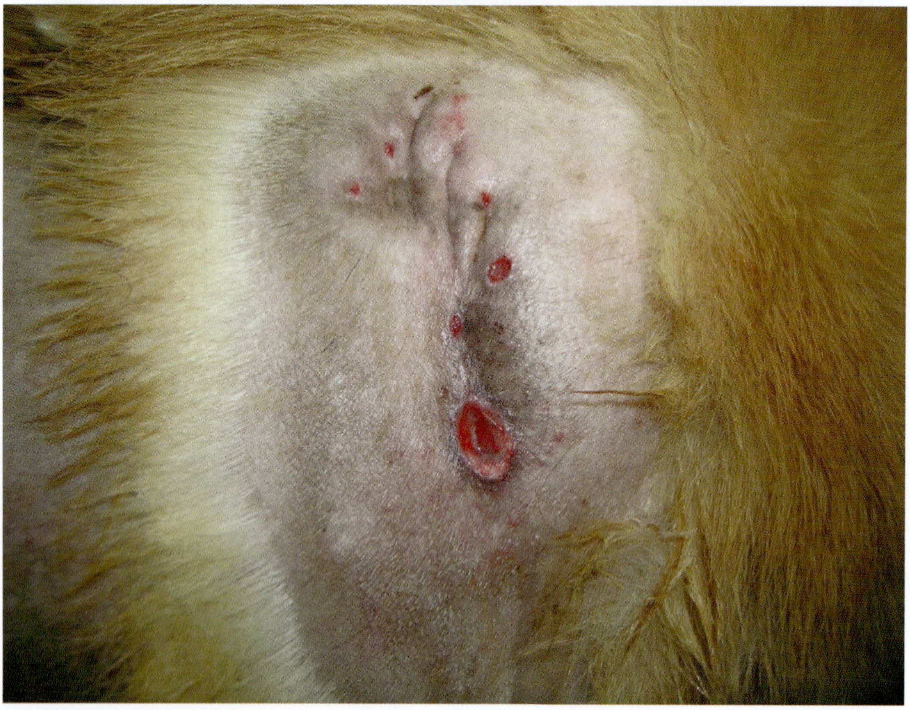

■ **Fig. 6.87.** Draining lesions on the lateral thorax of a dog with panniculitis. Exudates are often oily in appearance.

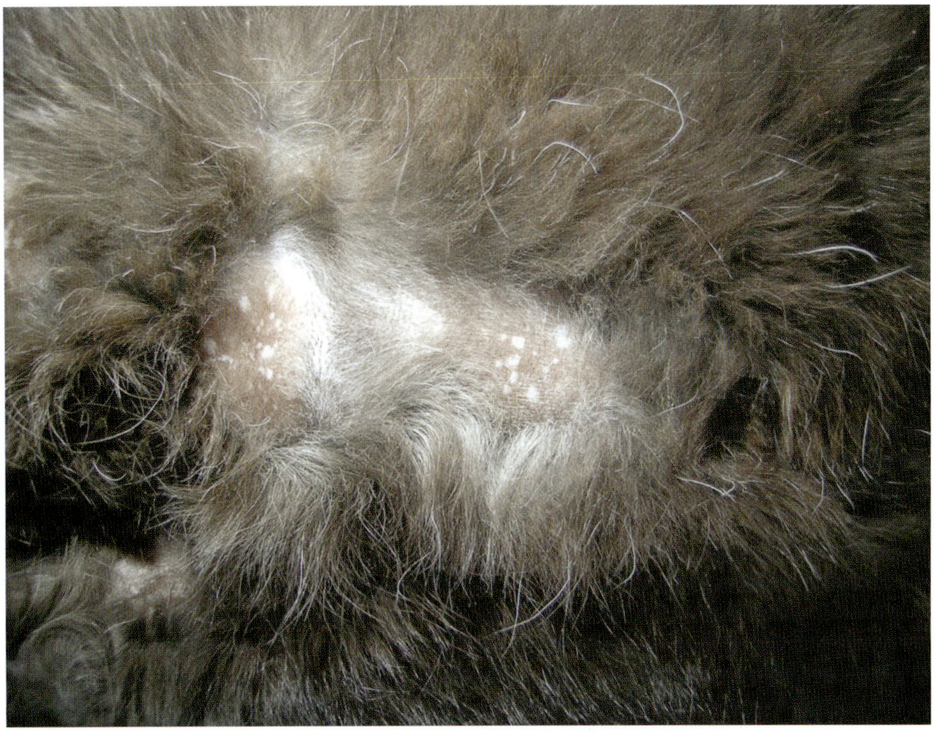

■ **Fig. 6.88.** Alopecic and erythematous plaques associated with chronic radiant heat exposure (erythema ab igne).

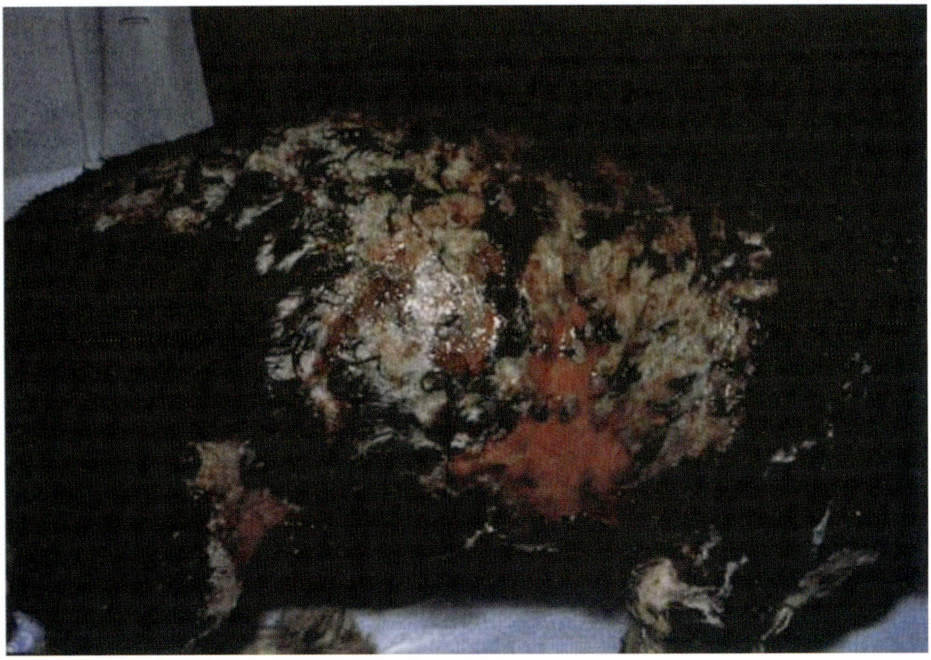

■ **Fig. 6.89.** Mixed-breed dog with a thermal burn of the dorsum resulting from heating pad injury.

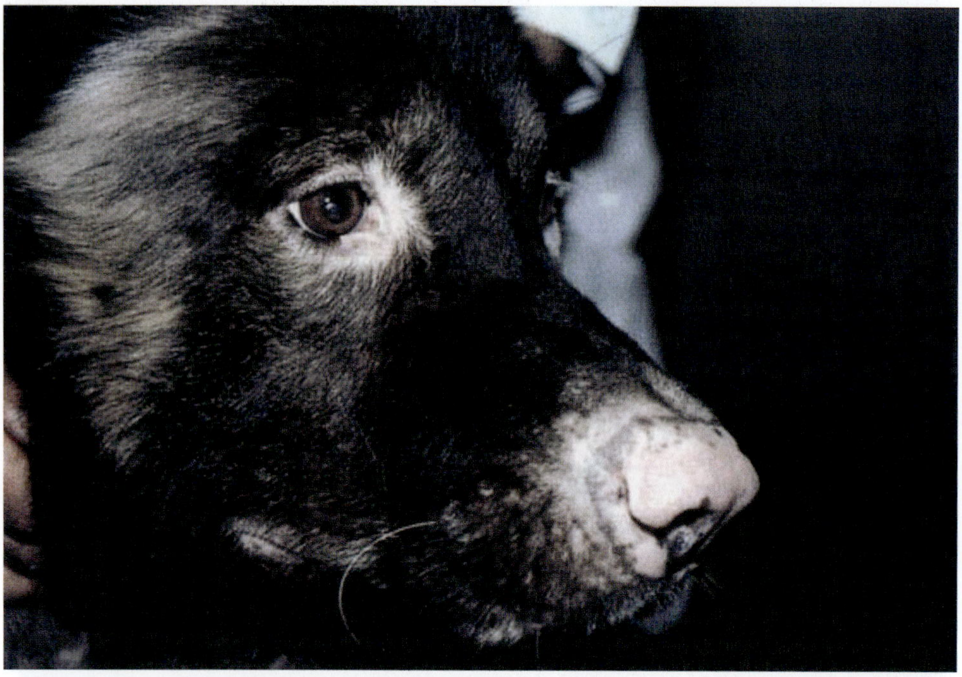

■ **Fig. 6.90.** Vitiligo (idiopathic leukoderma/leukotrichia) – progressive depigmentation with no inflammation. Rare cases may repigment spontaneously.

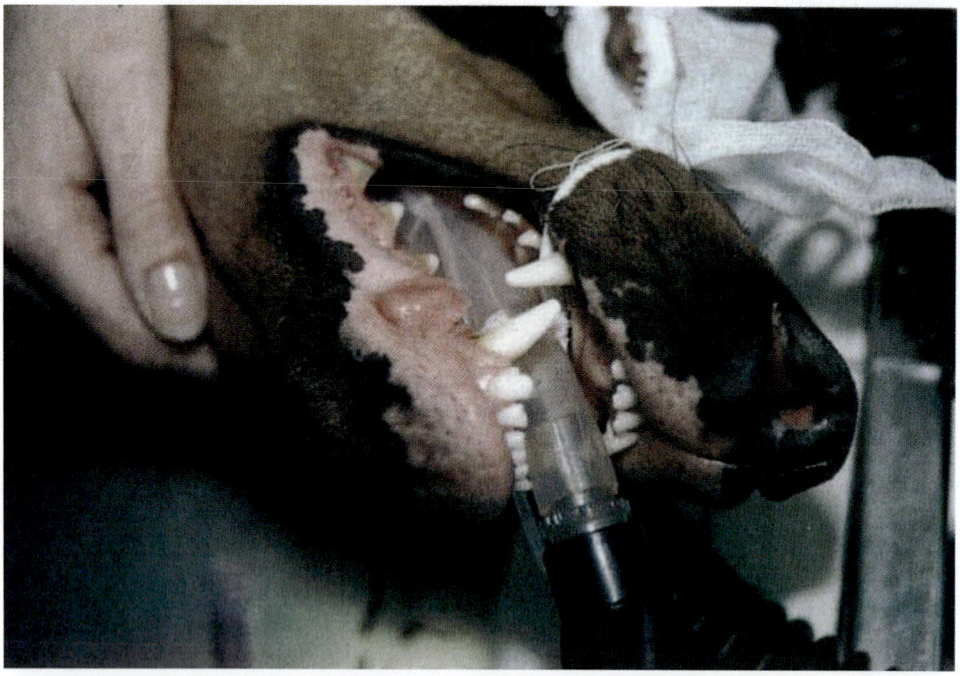

■ **Fig. 6.91.** Vitiligo (idiopathic leukoderma/leukotrichia). Note the depigmentation of the mucocutaneous junction regions.

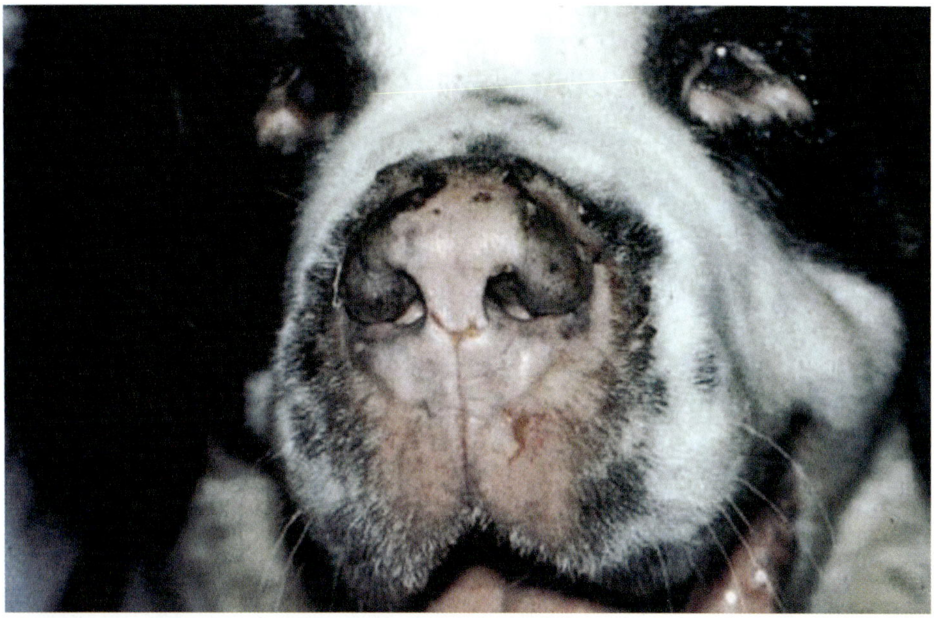

■ **Fig. 6.92.** Uveodermatologic syndrome (Vogt-Koyanagi-Harada-like syndrome). Striking depigmentation of both skin and hair, with lack of associated inflammation, is common in the early phases of the disease.

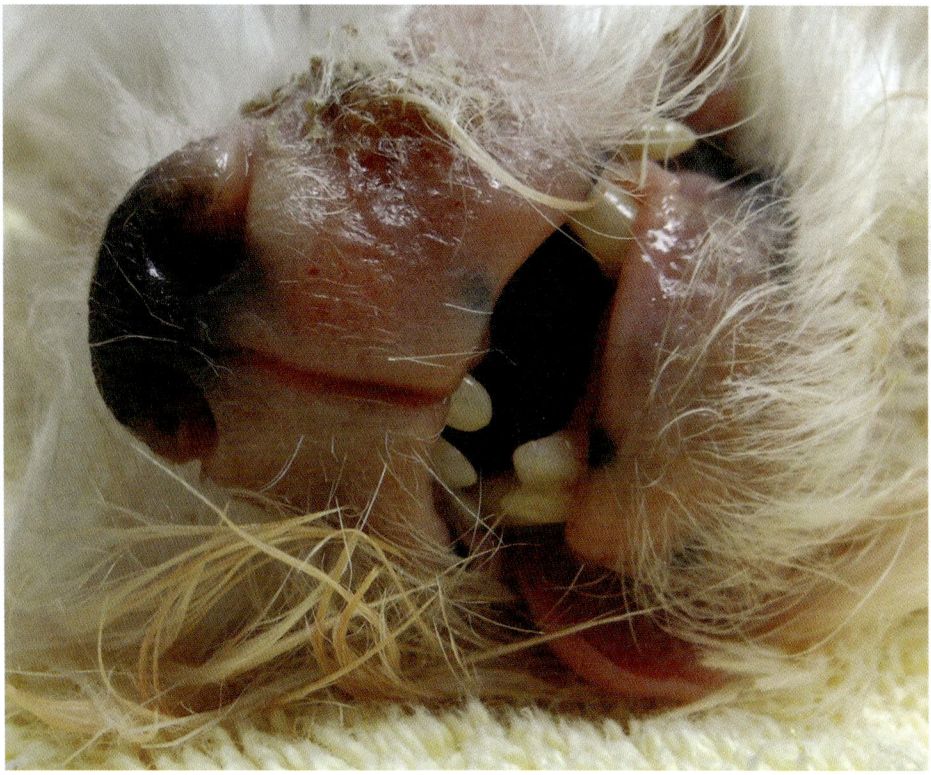

■ **Fig. 6.93.** Epitheliotropic lymphoma in an 9-year-old Maltese with depigmentation of the planum nasale and rostral muzzle.

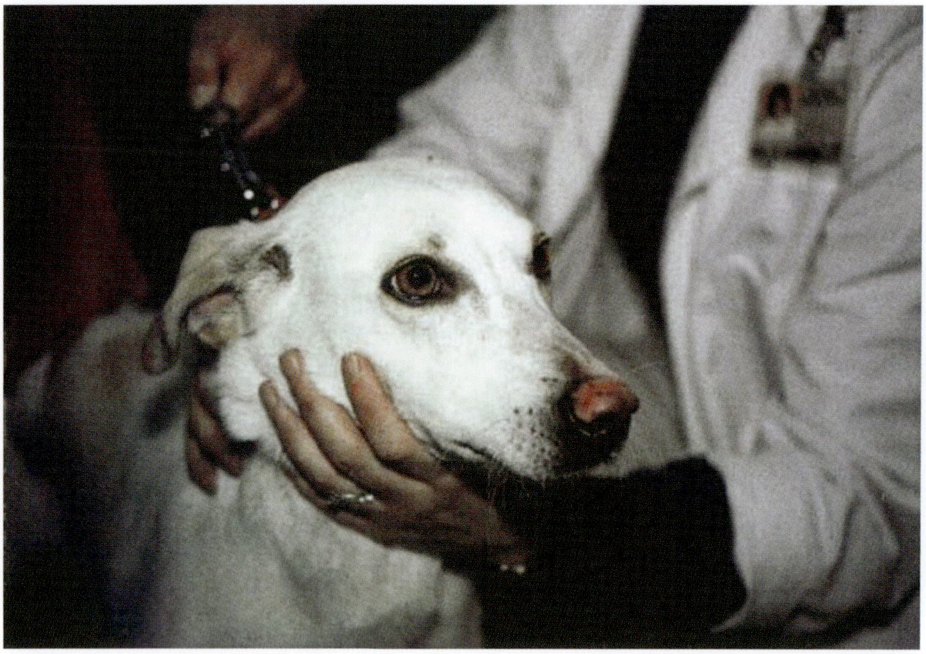

■ **Fig. 6.94.** Discoid lupus erythematosus. Three-year-old Labrador mix with progressive depigmentation with associated erythema and ulceration of the nasal planum.

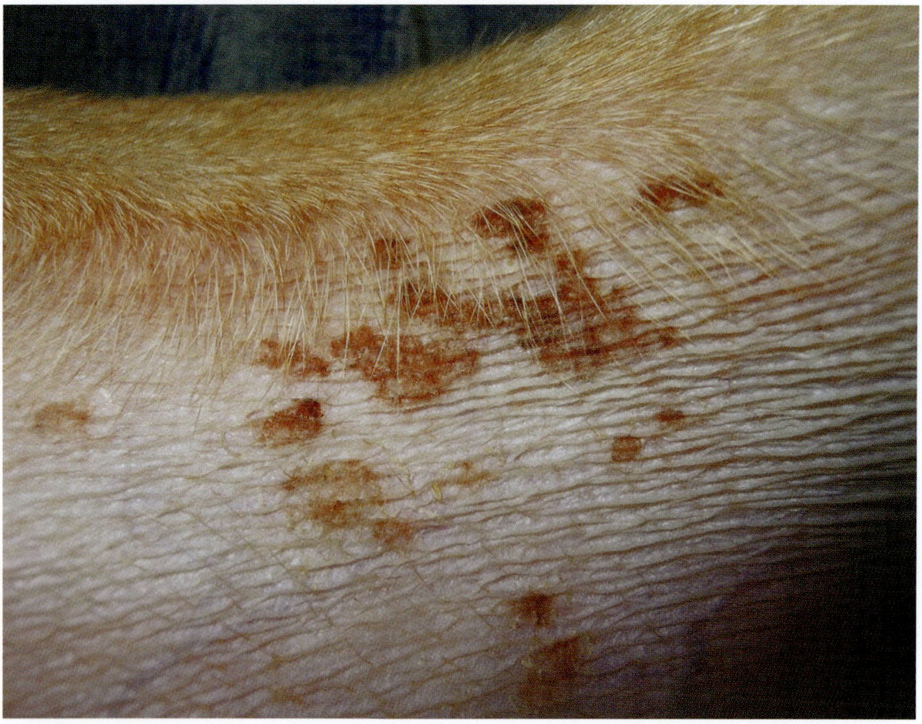

■ **Fig. 6.95.** Multiple hyperpigmented macules of lentigo in the flank region. Pigmentation change is not associated with inflammation.

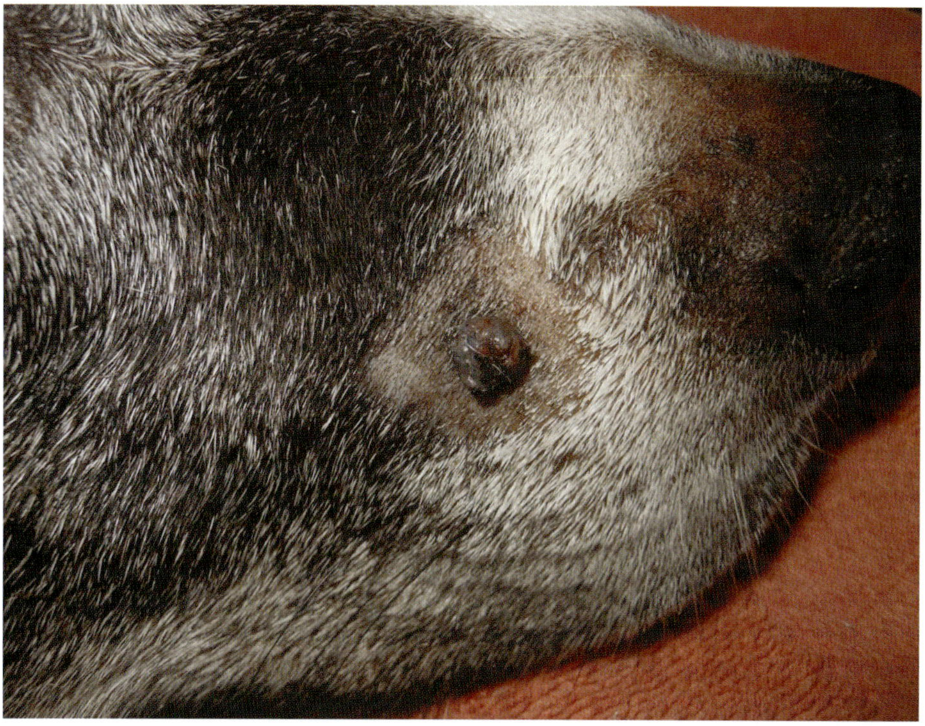

■ **Fig. 6.96.** Pigmented sebaceous nevus on face of an 11-year-old Labrador mix.

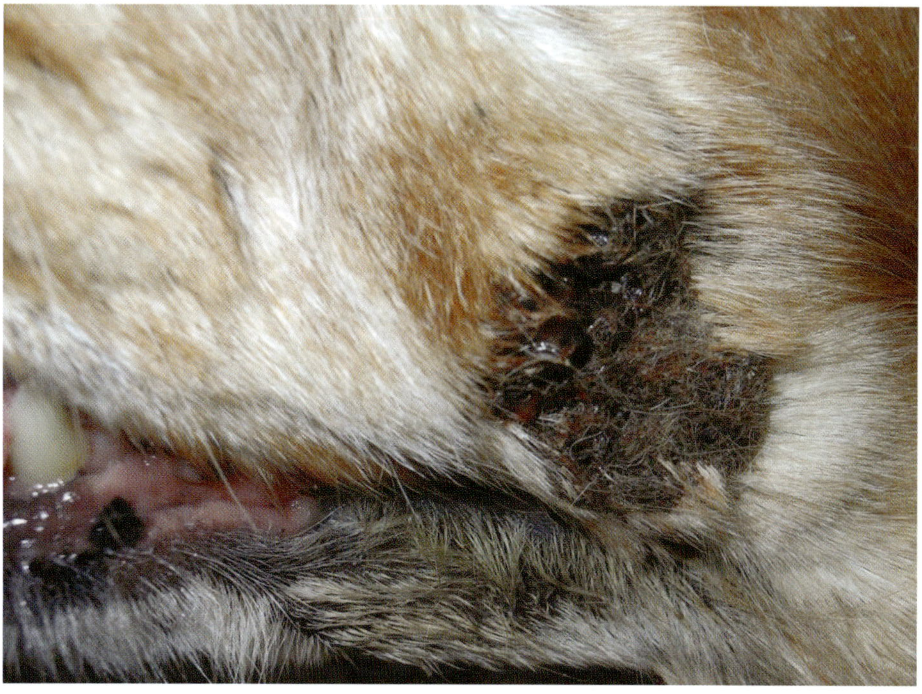

■ **Fig. 6.97.** Malignant melanoma presenting as a pigmented and eroded patch on the face and lip margins of a 12-year-old cocker spaniel.

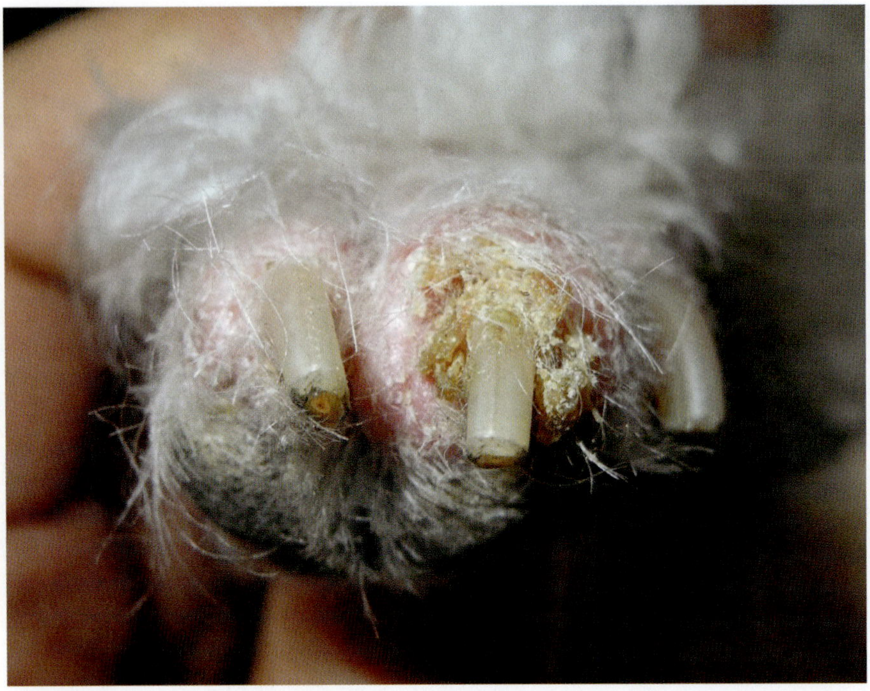

■ **Fig. 6.98.** Bacterial paronychia with exudation from within the claw fold in an 8-year-old male-castrate Maltese.

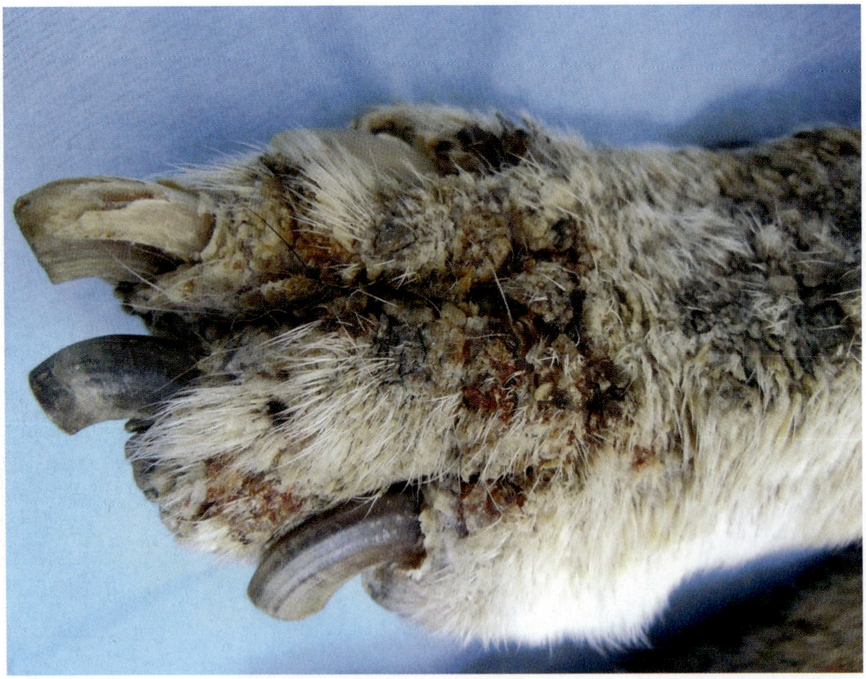

■ **Fig. 6.99.** Pododermatitis caused by bacterial folliculitis and furunculosis with demodicosis. Note the involvement of the entire digit, claw fold region, and interdigital spaces with edema of the tissues, alopecia, hyperkeratosis, and focal erosions and ulcerations.

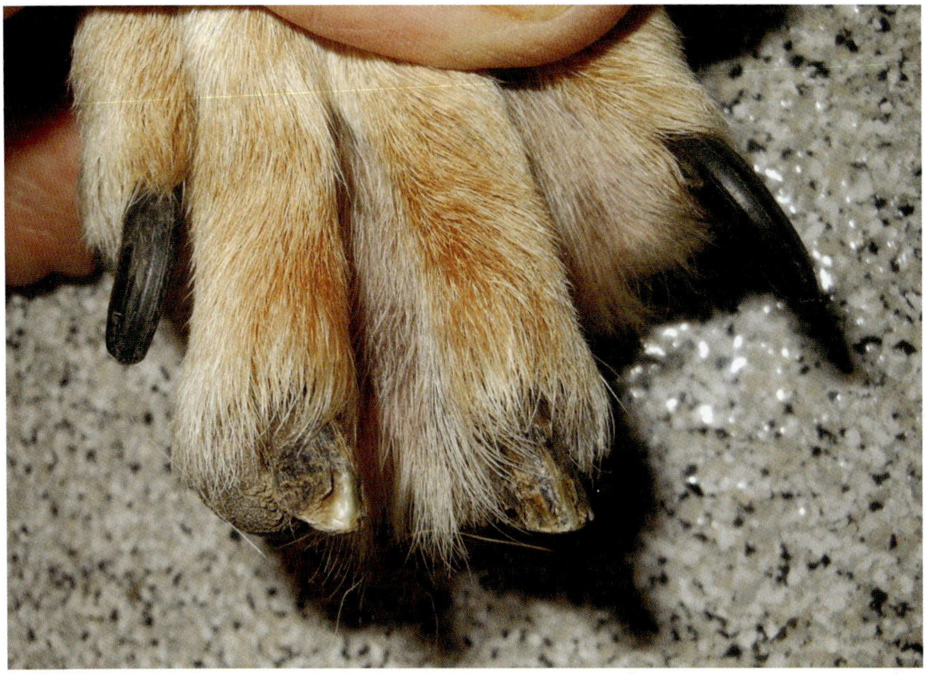

■ **Fig. 6.100.** Symmetrical lupoid onychodystrophy in a $1\frac{1}{2}$ year-old German Shepherd dog. Multiple claws on all paws are brittle, flaky, and broken.

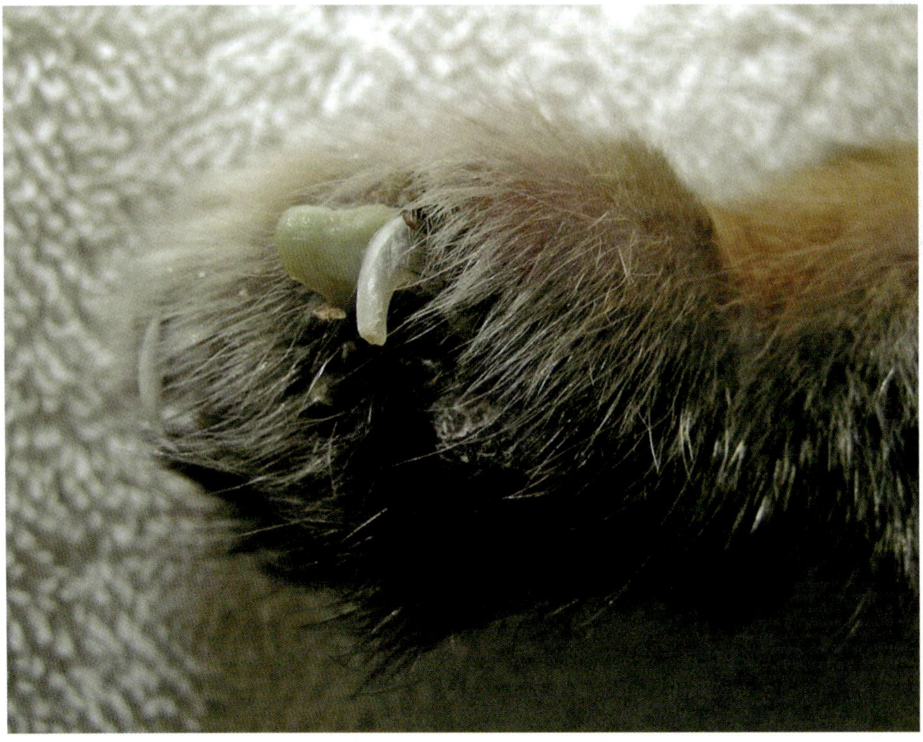

■ **Fig. 6.101.** Thick exudation from within the ungual fold of a cat with pemphigus foliaceus.

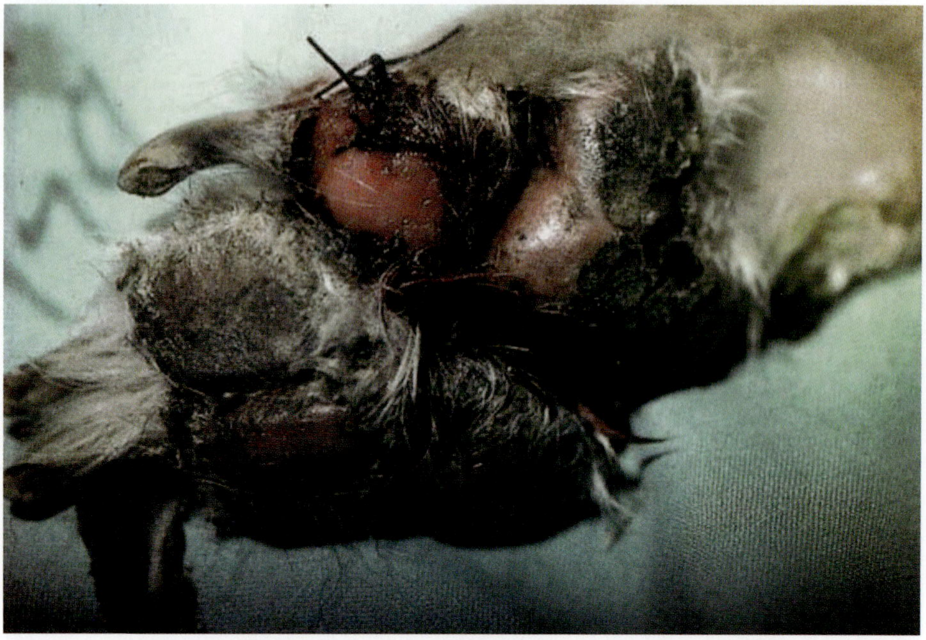

■ **Fig. 6.102.** Pemphigus vulgaris in a 9-year-old mixed breed dog. Note the marked degree of ulceration of the pads with peripheral hyperkeratosis and crusting.

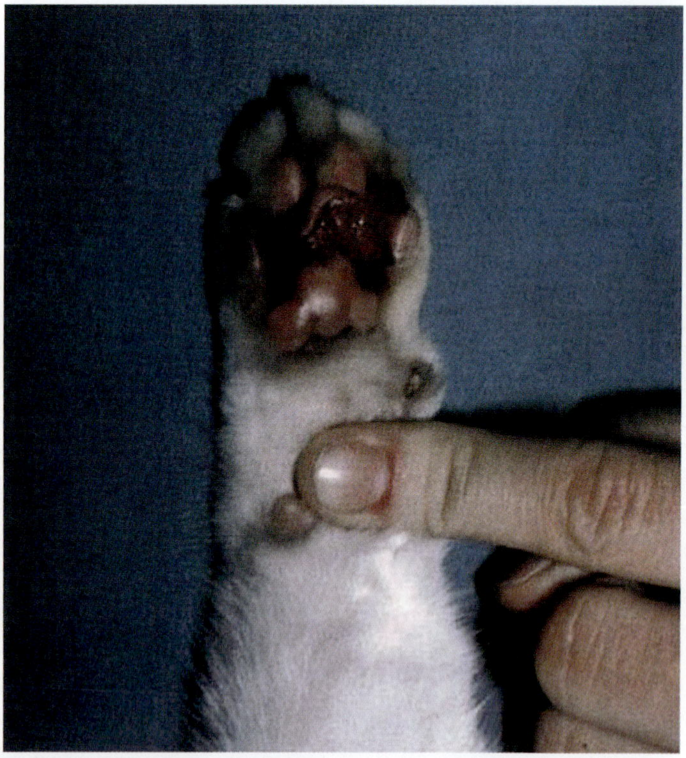

■ **Fig. 6.103.** Eosinophilic plaque (feline eosinophilic granuloma complex) involving the digital and metacarpal pads.

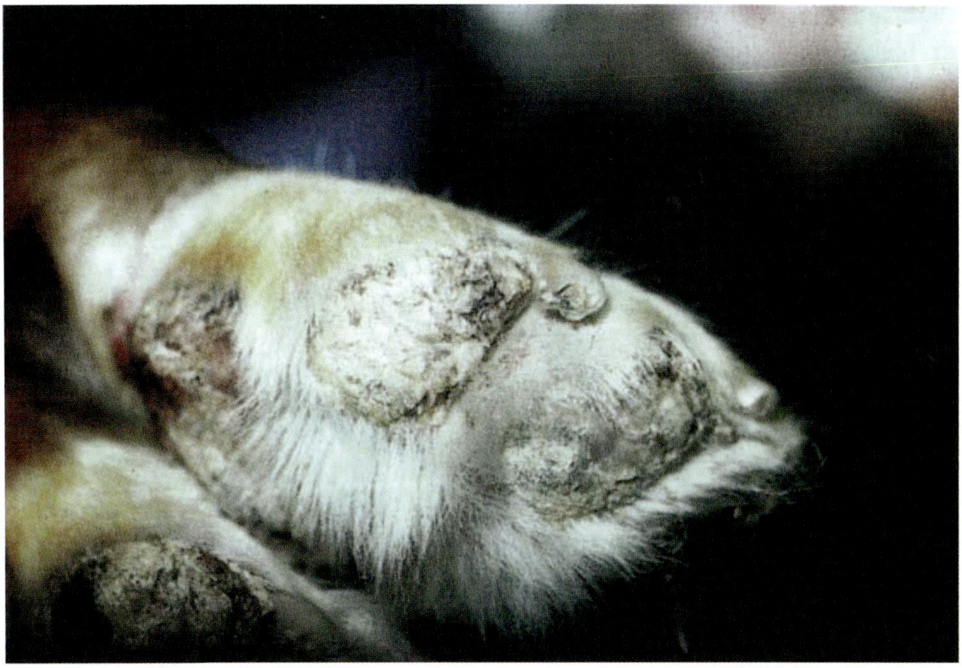

■ **Fig. 6.104.** Superifical necrolytic dermatitis (hepatocutaneous syndrome) in the dog. Note the marked degree of confluent hyperkeratosis to the footpads.

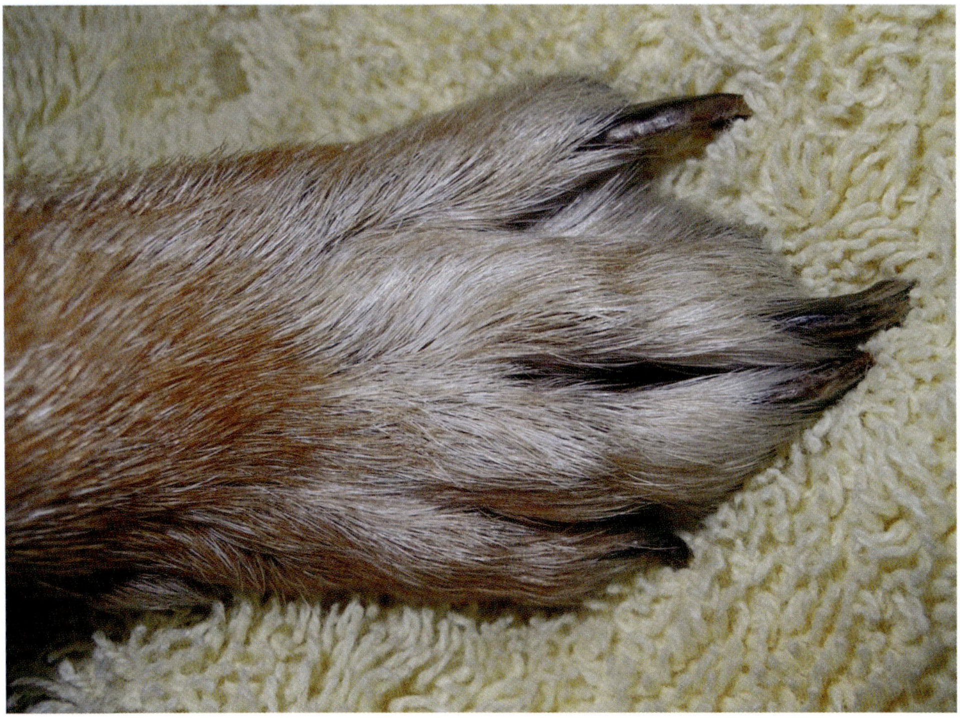

■ **Fig. 6.105.** Onychorrhexis in a dachshund. All nails are misshapen and brittle.

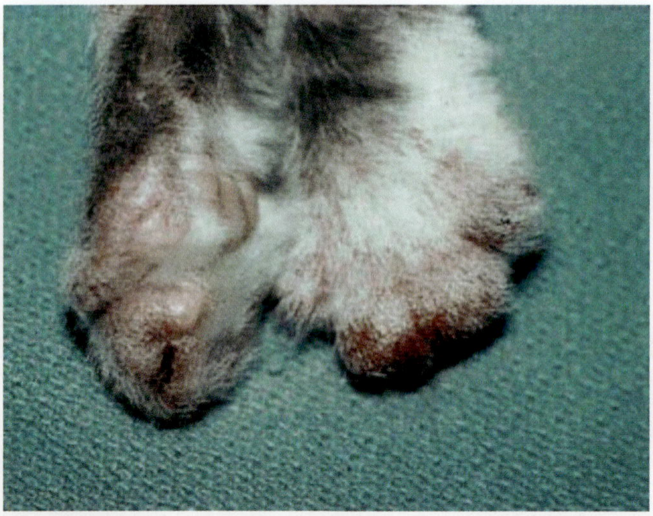

■ **Fig. 6.106.** Epitheliotropic lymphoma affecting the digits of a cat. No lesions were noted in other areas of the body.

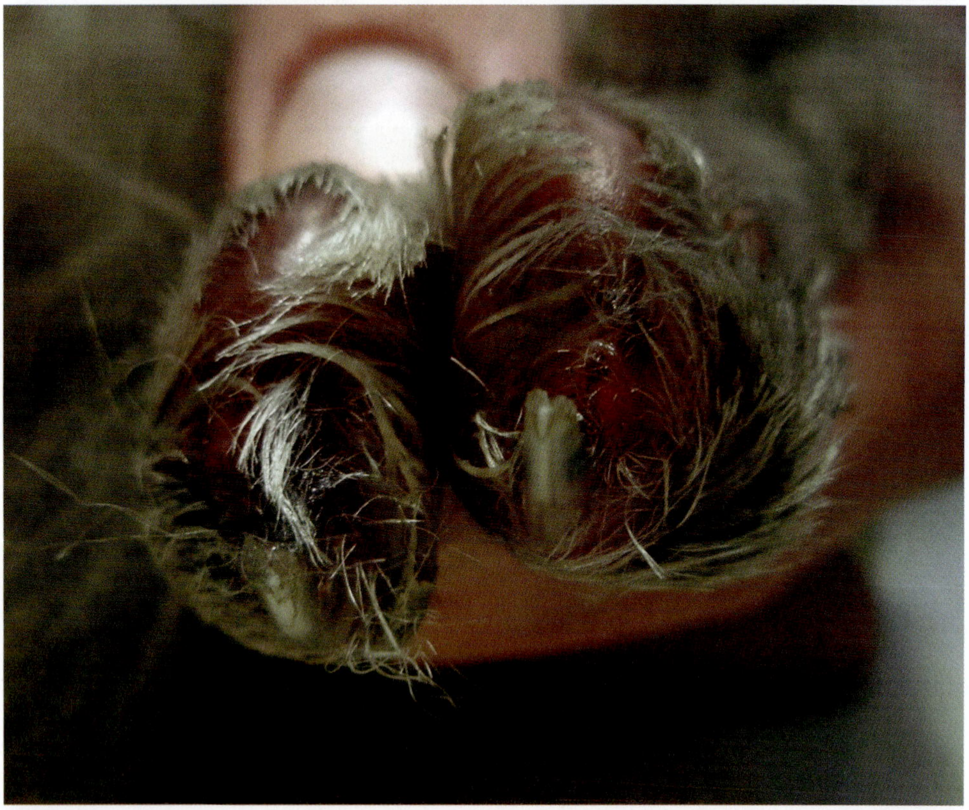

■ **Fig. 6.107.** Multifocal metastatic pulmonary adenosquamous carcinoma, "lung-digit" syndrome.

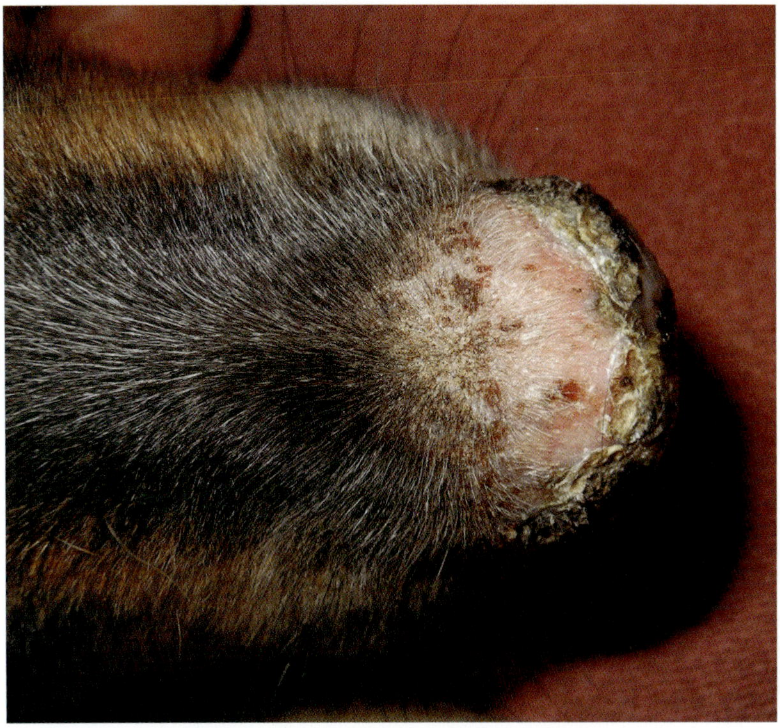

Fig. 6.108. Pemphigus erythematosus showing depigmentation, crusting, and erythema of the junction of the planum nasale and the bridge of the nose.

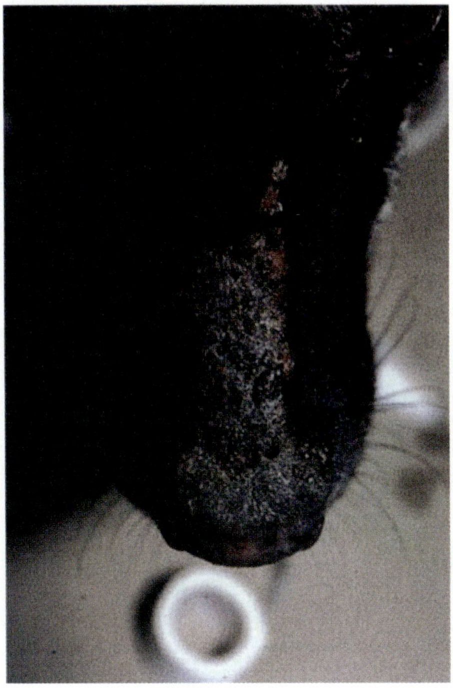

Fig. 6.109. Vesicles, erosions, ulcers, and crusts in a dog with pemphigus vulgaris.

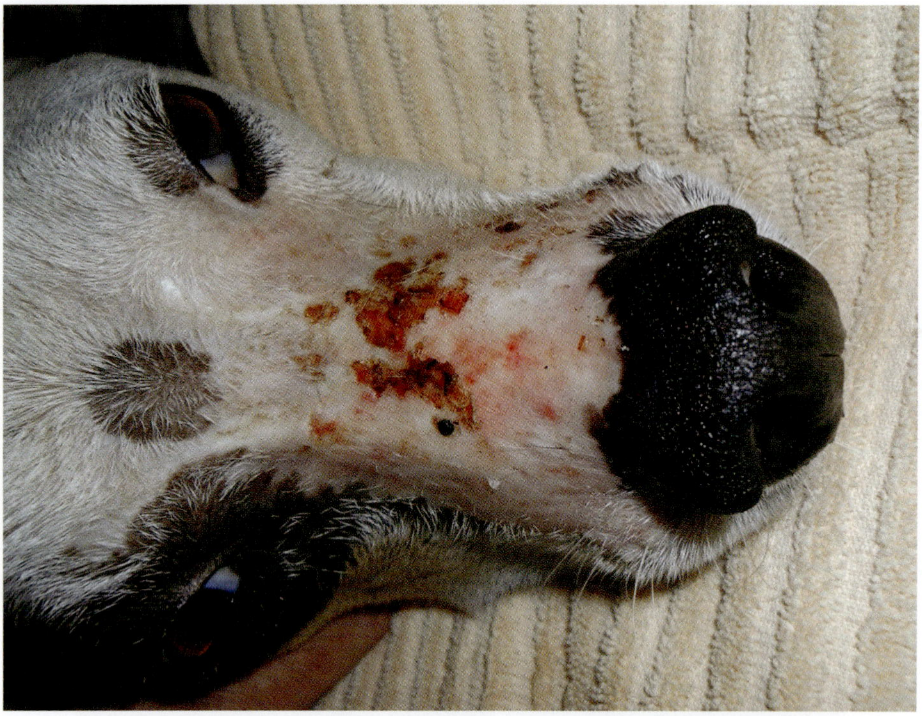

■ **Fig. 6.110.** Nasal solar dermatitis. Lesions affect the white areas of the dorsal muzzle; the pigmented nasal planum is not affected by inflammation.

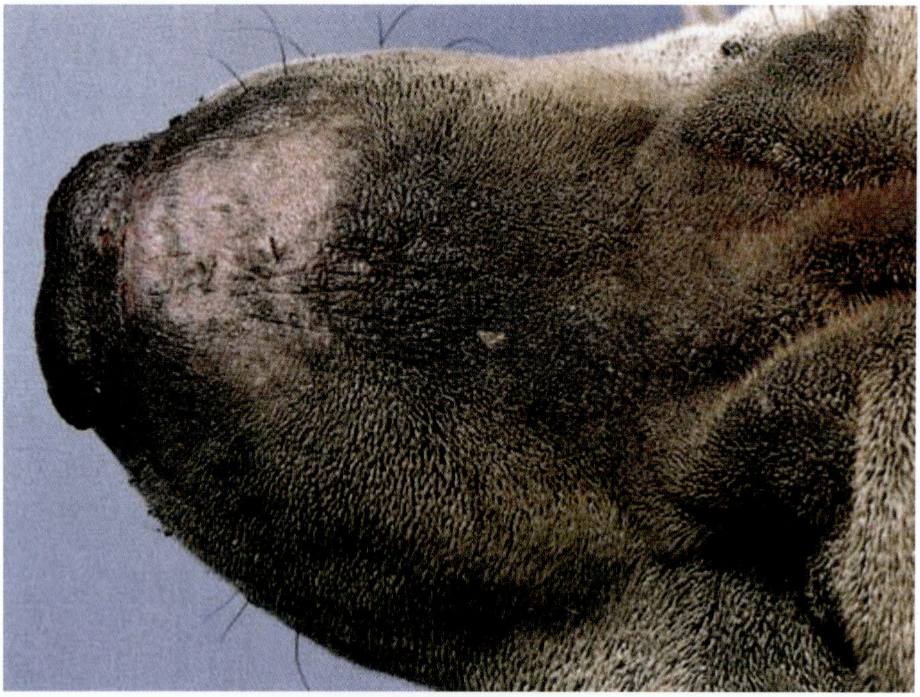

■ **Fig. 6.111.** Plastic food bowl hypersensitivity in a Chinese shar-pei.

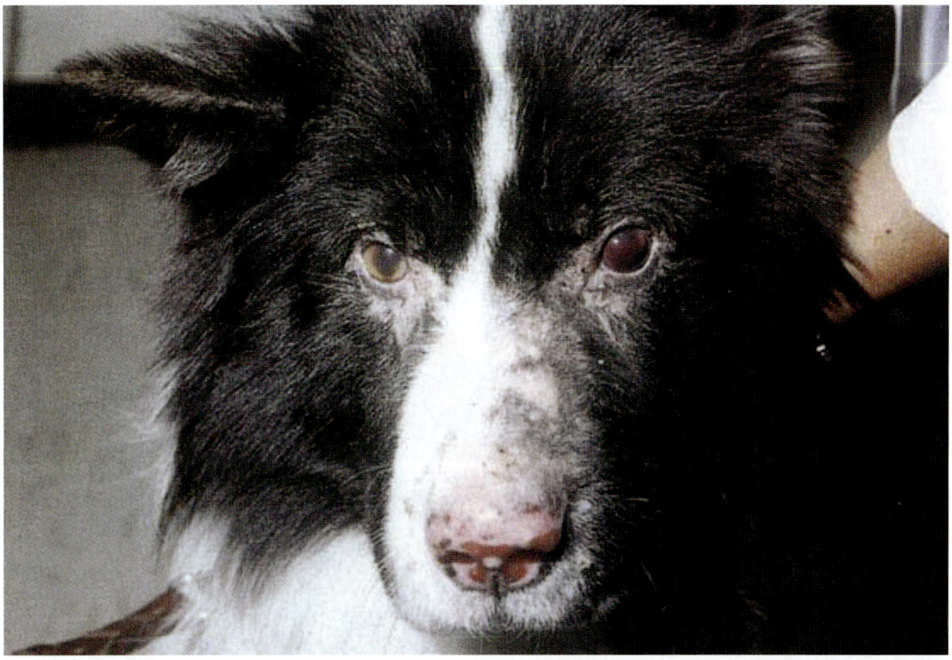

■ **Fig. 6.112.** Uveodermatologic syndrome revealing uveitis, depigmentation, mild inflammation, and focal erosions/ulcerations.

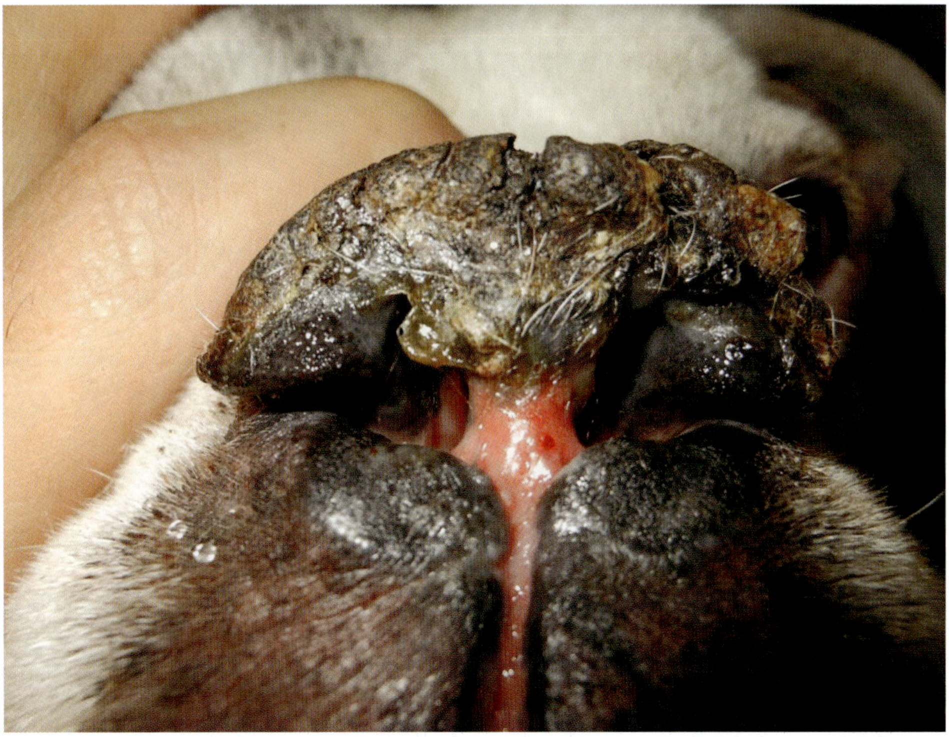

■ **Fig. 6.113.** Nasal arteritis demonstrating the deep ulceration on the nasal philtrum.

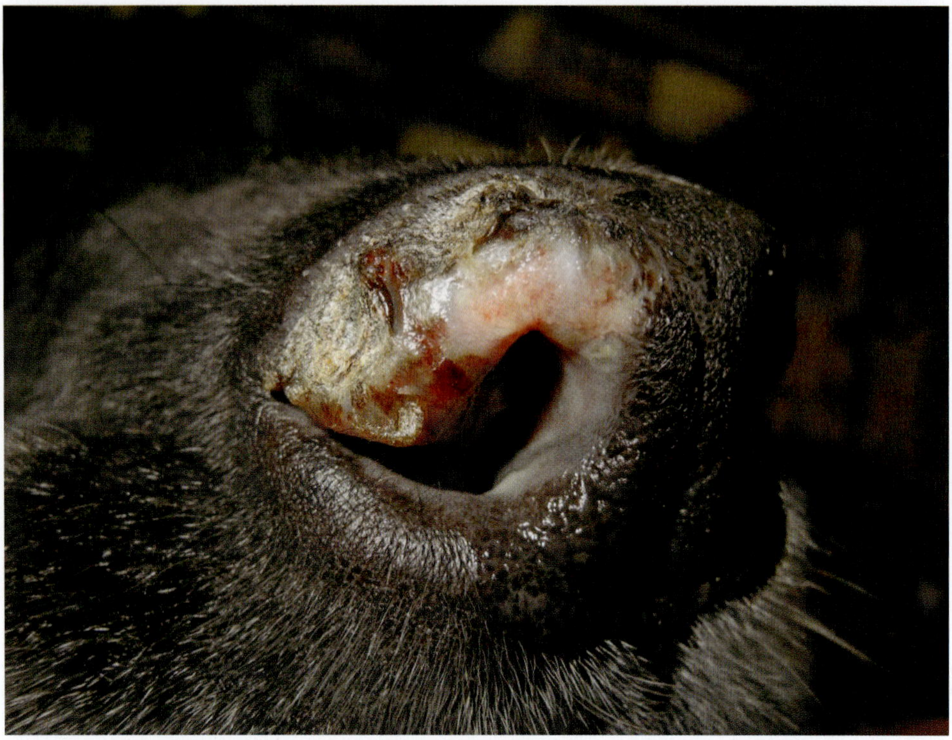

■ **Fig. 6.114.** Mucocutaneous pyoderma affecting the alar fold with crusting and depigmentation.

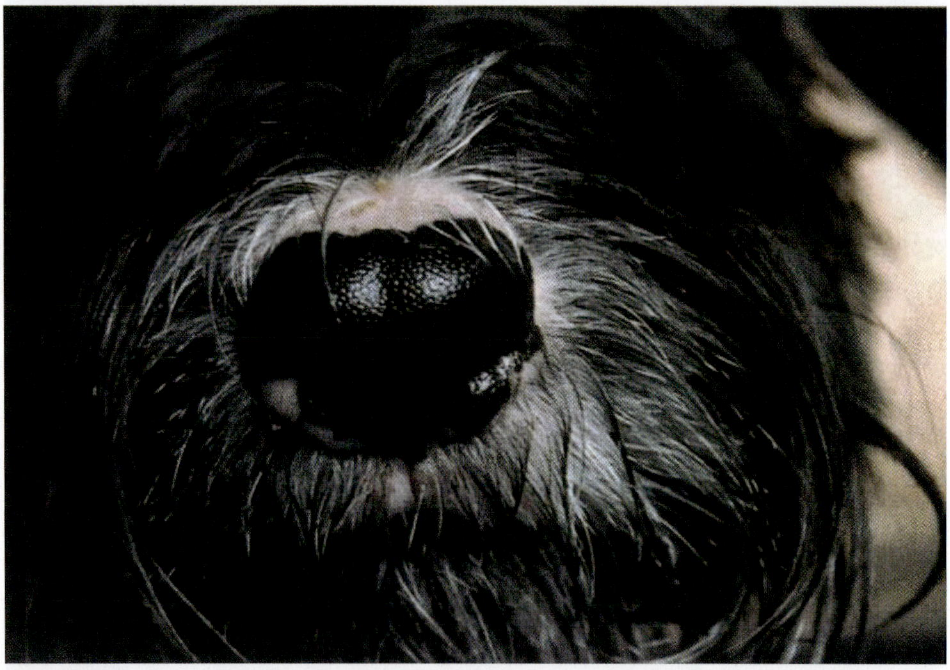

■ **Fig. 6.115.** Idiopathic leukoderma/leukotrichia (vitiligo). Loss of pigmentation is not associated with inflammation.

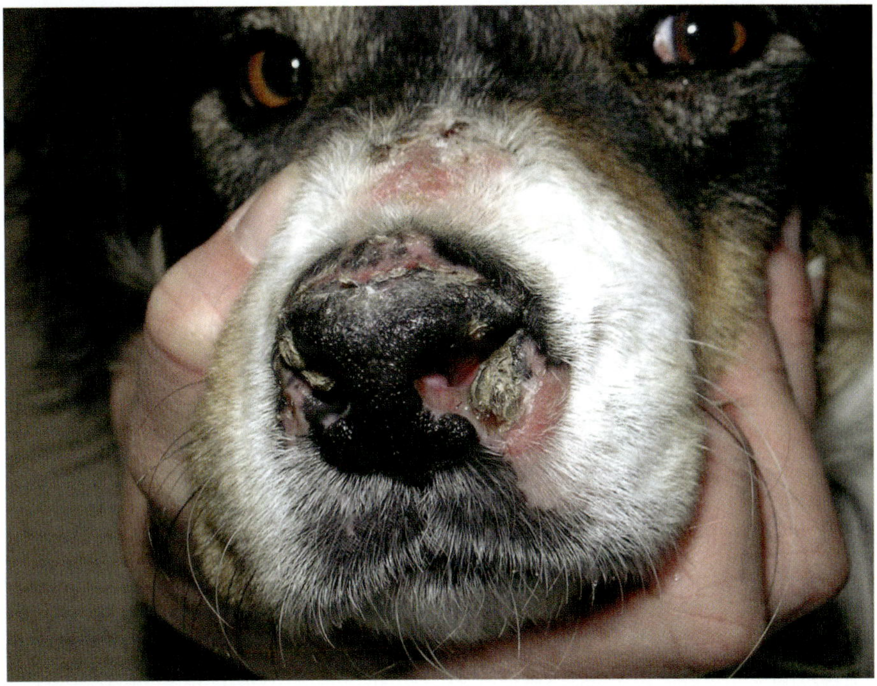

■ **Fig. 6.116.** Malignant histiocytosis causing depigmented, ulcerated nodules on the nasal planum and dorsal muzzle.

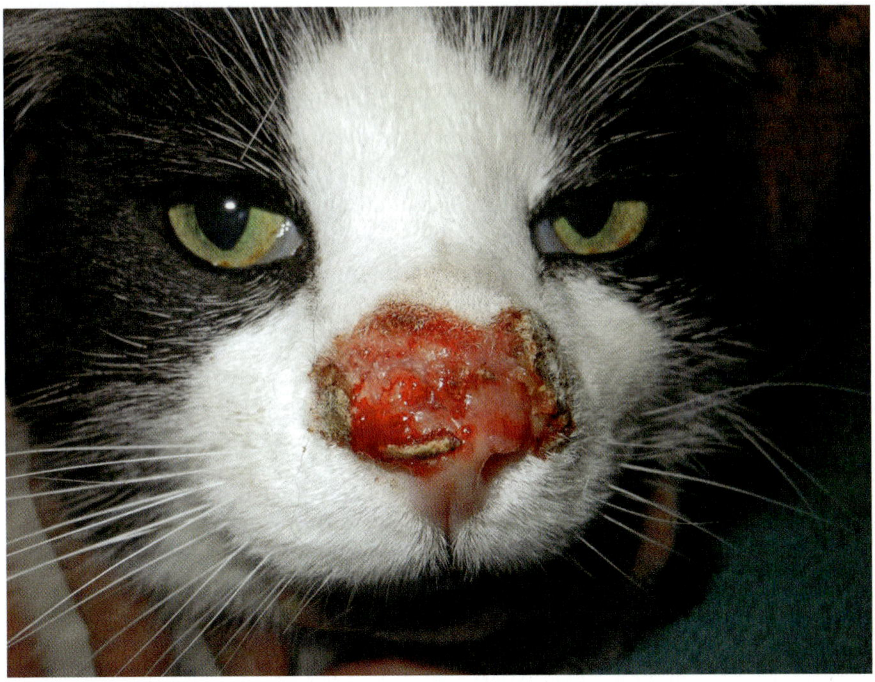

■ **Fig. 6.117.** Feline herpes virus dermatitis causing erosions and crusts on the nasal planum and dorsal muzzle in a 12-year-old DSH.

chapter 7

Antibiotic Stewardship and Emerging Resistant Bacterial Infections

EMERGING RESISTANT BACTERIA PYODERMA – OVERVIEW

- There is an emergence of bacterial infections in the dog (infrequent in the cat) that are resistant to the usual antibiotic susceptibility patterns.
- These infections pose a therapeutic challenge.
- It is imperative that primary factors be identified and that the owners be able to consistently administer the therapeutic protocol (drugs and topical therapy) for the entire treatment course in order to obtain therapeutic success and quell public health implications of antimicrobial resistance.
- Correct terminology when discussing these infections is vital to avoid alarming our clients: MRSA is, fortunately, less common in the dog than methicillin-resistant *Staphylococcus pseudintermedius* (MRSP).
- Veterinarians should practice careful antibiotic stewardship and participate in the global One Health Initiative.
- Antibiotics should be used only when necessary, selection should be based on an educated choice, dosing should be optimal, and antibiotics should be used for an appropriate length of time.
- Clients should be advised of the hazards of incomplete or partial therapy.
- Topical therapy should be considered as a "first choice" substitute for oral antibiotics in the vast majority of cases; shampoo therapy should either be chosen as a sole form of therapy or as an adjunct protocol for all cases of pyoderma: bathing mechanically removes debris and lowers surface bacterial counts; a medicated shampoo will also aid in killing microbes.
- Shampoo therapy is not only an effective protocol for treatment of active infection but will also aid in prevention of recurrence; moisturizing ingredients are vital to prevent increased transepidermal water loss (TEWL) which could exacerbate the dermatitis.
- Emperic antibiotic selection should be reserved for an initial flare of superficial pyoderma; a culture "with speciation" and susceptibility testing should be done for all recurrent or nonresponsive cases.

Blackwell's Five-Minute Veterinary Consult Clinical Companion: Small Animal Dermatology, Third Edition.
Karen Helton Rhodes and Alexander H. Werner.

ETIOLOGY

- Emerging infections include methicillin-resistant *Staphylococcus*, *Pseudomonas* sp., *Enterococcus* sp., and *Corynebacterium* sp., with staphylococcal infections being the most widespread and problematic at this time.
- The most frequently noted problematic bacterial infections include the methicillin-resistant staphylococci: MRSP (*pseudintermedius*), MRSS (*schleiferi*), and MRSA (*aureus*).
- "Methicillin resistance" implies a resistance to other antibiotics in the same beta-lactam class of drugs such as penicillin, amoxicillin, oxacillin, and cephalosporins.
- Staphylococci are gram-positive cocci that exist as part of the normal cutaneous and mucosal microflora of mammals.
- Numerous species of staphylococcus can be detected on canine skin, with the most common species being *S. pseudintermedius*.
- Coagulase-positive species have been considered to be more pathogenic than coagulase-negative species, recent data suggest that coagulase-negative species may also be pathogenic (*S. schleiferi* ssp. *schleiferi* in dogs).
- MRSA/MRSP/MRSS emergence is suspected to be associated with overuse of antibiotics; broad-spectrum antibiotics such as cephalexin, cefazolin, cefadroxil, amoxicillin, penicillin, and fluoroquinolones may hasten the development of oxacillin/methicillin resistance.
- Unnecessary prescriptions, poor client compliance in the use of antibiotics, and feed additives in livestock production are also suspect.
- Four proposed mechanisms of resistance in methicillin-resistant *Staphylococcus* organisms:
  - Penicillin-binding proteins (PBP) and the mecA gene
  - Cell wall thickening noted in all MRS organisms
  - Efflux pump
  - Biofilm production.
- PBP and mecA:
  - Transmission of the mecA gene encodes for an altered defective penicillin-binding protein (PBP2a) which is involved in cell wall peptidoglycan synthesis
  - All penicillins and cephalosporins (beta-lactams) require binding to the PBP in the bacterial cell wall to initiate the drug's activity
  - MRSA produces a defective PBP due to the presence and activation of the mecA gene
  - The mecA gene comes from a mobile genetic component called a staphyloccal chromosomal cassette (SCCmec)
  - The spread of MRSA is usually through clonal expansion rather than the normal process of mutation or plasmid transfer
  - All MRSA strains can be traced back to a single clone found in Europe in the mid-1960s.
- Cell wall thickening:
  - Increased synthesis of peptidoglycan in the cell wall of vancomycin-resistant staphylococci

  - Increased MICs associated with thickening of the cell wall possibly associated with trapping of the antibiotic within the cell wall and reduced penetration
  - Thickening is not mediated by a gene known to be related to macrolide resistance.
- Efflux pump:
  - MRS organisms often have proteins involved in active removal of antibiotics through a membrane-bound pump, which effectively limits the activity of many antibiotics that focus on internal cellular structures.
- Biofilms:
  - Biofilms are three-dimensional clusters of bacteria that are not derived from a single specific organism: they are not colonies
  - The cluster is surrounded by a protective polysaccharide coating
  - Most commonly occur in the ear canal but may be prevalent in more generalized infections and contribute to treatment failures
  - Biofilm production has become of prime importance in treating *Pseudomonas* infection in the ear canal
  - Both staphylococcal and pseudomonal organisms have the capability to produce protective biofilms that inhibit antimicrobial penetration and allow for protected reservoirs of bacteria
  - Partial antimicrobial penetration into the biofilm may increase selection pressure for mutations and resistance (treatment failure and development of therapeutic resistance)
  - One report states that 40% of canine otic *Pseudomonas* isolates, 30% of canine otic *Staphylococcus* strains, and 95% of *Malassezia* can produce biofilms
  - A second study found that *S. pseudintermedius* swabbed from the abdomen (100%) and interdigital spaces (85%) of 36 healthy dogs were able to produce biofilms.

STAPHYLOCOCCAL VIRULENCE FACTORS

Staphylococcal virulence factors aid in production of disease.

- Hyaluronidase degrades hyaluronic acid, damaging connective tissue.
- Coagulase increases production of fibrin thrombi in tissue.
- Kinase converts plasminogen to plasmin, which digests fibrin.
- Streptolysin disrupts phagocytosis.
- Streptokinase activates plasmin-like proteolytic activity.
- Beta-hemolysin destroys cells by lysis; high affinity for precursor lipids of the stratum corneum ceramides and may help penetration into the skin.
- Protein A binds IgG in a dysfunction pattern and thus avoids phagocytosis (adhesion molecule).
- Exfoliative toxin targets desmoglein 1 (a desmosomal cell-to-cell adhesion molecule) causing blistering; dermonecrotic toxin (i.e., staphylococcal scalded skin syndrome).
- Exotoxin causes local tissue damage and incites inflammation.

- Superantigens (toxic shock syndrome toxins, TSST-1) cause severe, fatal inflammation by provoking nonspecific activation of T cells and massive release of cytokines.
- Alpha toxins (cytolysin) form pores in the keratinocytes.

HISTORICAL BACKGROUND TRACKING METHICILLIN RESISTANCE

- *Staphylococcus aureus* commonly colonizes the nasal passages in 29–38% of the human population.
- Approximately 0.84% of the United States population (2 million people) have nasal colonization with MRSA with no clinical signs.
- Individuals in close contact (spouse, parent/child, caregiver) with a human patient diagnosed with MRSA infection are at a 7.5-fold greater risk of carriage than those individuals with a casual relationship (roommates, friends, etc.).
- The incidence of methicillin resistance has increased rapidly in human hospital strains of *S. aureus* since the early 1960s.
- Two main categories – hospital acquired (HA-MRSA) and community acquired (CA-MRSA):
  - HA-MRSA is the primary pathogen causing nosocomial infections in people; risk factors include immunosuppressive disease/medications, surgery, hospitalizations, etc.
  - CA-MRSA has significantly increased in recent years with at least 50% of those individuals known to be colonized with MRSA carrying the CA-MRSA strains
  - Community-acquired strains differ genetically from HA-MRSA and may express a toxin called Panton-Valentine leukocidin
  - Risk factors for the community form are crowded living conditions, military facilities, prisons, sports equipment/locker rooms, geriatric/nursing homes, daycare facilities, etc.
  - CA-MRSA is usually more sensitive to antibiotics than HA-MRSA, but life-threatening necrotizing fasciitis, necrotizing pneumonia, and sepsis can develop
  - There has been a recent shift in the traditional strain locations, with HA-MRSA being found in the community setting and CA-MRSA in hospital environments; a new term, HCA-MRSA (healthcare associated-MRSA), has evolved.
- A 2007 report by the American Medical Association (AMA) estimated that MRSA infections occurred in 95 000 Americans in 2005, with 18 650 resulting in death; the highest rate of MRSA-related deaths in human patients (58%) was found in the hospital environment.
- Methicillin resistance has been recognized in domestic animals since the early 1970s and became clinically importance in the 1990s.
- There has been a precipitous increase in reports of methicillin resistance in recent years.
- In 2005, one national laboratory reported only 19% of *S. aureus* isolates were methicillin resistant: in 2007, the percentage had increased to 42%.

- In a similar period (2004), less than 0.6% of *S. intermedius* (likely *pseudintermedius*) were methicillin resistant, increasing to 10.2% in 2007.
- Most canine cases involve MRSP and MRSS, rarely MRSA.
- Most canine clinical presentations are seen as pyoderma, otitis, and surgical wound infections (deep soft tissue, body cavities, and orthopedic repairs).
- MRSP and MRSS are most commonly associated with superficial infections (skin and ear canal) in dogs (Figures 7.1–7.5).
- MRSA in canine patients is more commonly associated with deep infections – genitourinary, respiratory, joint space, body cavity, and wounds.

TRANSFER OF INFECTION BETWEEN SPECIES: INCREASING CONCERN

- The zoonotic potential of *S. pseudintermedius*, *S. aureus*, and *S. schleiferi* is becoming increasingly concerning; all three species have the potential to cause disease in both humans and animals.
- It is important to remember that not all transfers result in actual disease and may represent only colonization: one study found MRSP in 4.5% of healthy dogs and 1.2% of healthy cats.
- As a zoonotic example, household cats have been identified with MRSA isolates that contain the staphylococcal chromosome cassette (SCC) mec element that is associated with nosocomial MRSA infections in people; these findings suggest a reverse zoonotic transmission from humans.
- Increased incidence noted with owners employed in the healthcare field, suggesting a possible mode of transmission from the person to the pet; *S. pseudintermedius* has been isolated from pet owners with and without active infection.
- *Staphylococcus schleiferi* has the ability to develop multidrug resistance and is a known cause of infection in both dogs and humans independent of interspecies transfer.
- There is concern about dogs involved in hospital visitation programs causing increased risk to both the animal and the hospitalized patient; current recommendations are to avoid contact between visiting animals and patients infected with MRS species; pets should be bathed and groomed prior to each visit.
- Transmission can happen by many paths: environment to human, human to environment, human to human, human to pet, pet to human, pet to pet, pet to environment, and environment to pet.
- Transmission is usually by direct contact with the nasal passages, throat, and skin or by indirect contact from walls, floors, counters, bedding, dishes, etc.
- Routine decolonization therapy is not recommended for humans or animals that have mucosal colonization with MRSA; there is currently no evidence that such treatment is effective, even with topical mupirocin.
- Adequate topical coverage of nasal passages, skin, or mucosa cannot be achieved.
- Most pets will clear MRSA colonization spontaneously.

RISK REDUCTION FOR ZOONOSIS/REVERSE ZOONOSIS

- Wash hands thoroughly with soap and water for at least 15 seconds (avoid bar soap).
- Use an alcohol-based hand sanitizer (62% alcohol).
- Use gloves when handling suspect patients.
- Avoid reusing contaminated clothing (lab coats, neckties, scrubs, etc.).
- Do not allow pets to share food or use the same dishes.
- Do not allow a pet to lick your face or open wounds.
- Immunocompromised individuals should take extra precautions.
- Sterilize surgical equipment.
- Sanitize all cages and equipment routinely (e.g., stethoscope).
- Launder bedding at 60 °C (140 °F).
- Clean the clinic surfaces on a routine basis (table surfaces, anesthetic machines, floors, walls, cages, keyboards, telephones, clippers, leashes, muzzles, etc.).

CLIENT EDUCATION

- www.wormsandgermsblog.com has a handout called MRSP for Pet Owners.
- www.CCAR-ccra.org provides useful clinical information, including client education handouts.

MRSA Facts

- Can be found in the environment up to 42 days in carcasses and 60 days in meat products.
- Remains viable on glass for 46 hours.
- Remains viable in direct sunlight for 17 hours.
- Remains viable on the floor for 7 days
- Can survive up to 12 months in clinic bedding and clothing.
- UVC (ultraviolet light C) is germicidal and may be an effective method for cleaning textiles in household and hospital environments.

Hand washing is the single most important act to help prevent spread of contagion

From the public domain from the Canadian Committee on Antibiotic Research *Infection Control and Best Practices for Small Animal Veterinary Clinics*, November 2008:

Hand Washing

Most transient bacteria present on the hands are removed during the mechanical action of washing, rinsing, and drying hands. Hand washing with soap and running water must be performed when hands are visibly soiled. If running water is not available, use moistened towelettes to remove all visible dirt and debris, followed by an alcohol-based hand rub.

Bar soaps are not acceptable in veterinary practice settings because of the potential for indirect transmission of pathogens from one person to another. Instead, liquid or foam soap should be used.

- Soap should be dispensed in a disposable pump dispenser.
- Soap containers should not be refilled without being disinfected, since there is a risk of contamination.
- **Antibacterial soaps should be used in critical care areas** such as ICU, and in other areas where invasive procedures are performed.

Technique

1. Remove all hand and arm jewelry.
2. Wet hands with warm (not hot) water. Hot water is hard on the skin and will lead to dryness and additional skin damage.
3. Apply liquid or foam soap.
4. Vigorously lather all surfaces of hand for a **minimum of 15 seconds**. This is the minimum amount of time required for mechanical removal of transient bacteria. Pay particular attention to fingertips, between fingers, backs of the hands and base of the thumbs. These are the most commonly missed areas. A simple way many people time their hand-washing is by singing "Happy Birthday".
5. Using a rubbing motion, thoroughly rinse soap from hands under warm running water. Residual soap can lead to dryness and cracking of skin.
6. Dry hands thoroughly by blotting hands gently with a paper towel. Rubbing vigorously with paper towels can damage the skin.
7. Turn off taps with paper towel to avoid recontamination of hands.

NOTE: If air hand dryers are used, hands-free taps are necessary, as turning taps off without using paper towel as described will result in recontamination of hands after washing.

When Hand Hygiene Should Be Performed

- Before and after contact with a patient
- Especially before performing invasive procedures
- Before and after contact with items in the patient's environment
- After any contact with or any activity involving the body fluids of a patient
- Before putting on and especially after taking off gloves
- Before eating food
- After personal body functions, such as using the toilet, or blowing one's nose.

Surface Disinfectants

TABLE 7.1. Characteristics of Selected Disinfectants (Modified from Linton et al 1987 and Block 2001). In the public domain from the Canadian Committee on Antibiotic Research (2008) *Infection Control and Best Practices for Small Animal Veterinary Clinics*, November 2008

Disinfectant Category	Activity in Presence of Organic Matter	Advantages	Disadvantages	Precautions	Comments
Alcohols: Ethyl alcohol Isopropyl alcohol	Rapidly inactivated	Fast-acting No residue Relatively nontoxic	Rapid evaporation	Flammable	Not appropriate for environmental disinfection Primarily used as antiseptics
Aldehydes: Formaldehyde Gutaraldehyde	Good	Broad spectrum Relatively noncorrosive	Highly toxic	Irritant Carcinogenic Requires ventilation	Used as an aqueous solution or as a gas (fumigation)
Alkalis: Ammonia			Unpleasant odor Irritating	Do not mix with bleach	Not recommended for general use
Biguanides: Chlorhexidine	Rapidly inactivated	Nontoxic	Incompatible with anionic detergents		Not appropriate for environmental disinfection Primarily used as antiseptics
Halogens: Hypochlorites (Bleach)	Rapidly inactivated	Broad spectrum, including spores Inexpensive Can be used on food preparation surfaces	Inactivated by cationic soaps/detergents and sunlight Frequent application required	Corrosive Irritant Mixing with other chemicals may produce toxic gas	Used to disinfect clean environmental surfaces Commonly available sporicidal disinfectant
Oxidizing Agents	Good	Broad spectrum Environmentally friendly	Break down with time	Corrosive	Excellent choice for environmental disinfection
Phenols	Good	Broad spectrum Noncorrosive Stable in storage	Toxic to cats Unpleasant odor Incompatible with cationic and nonionic detergents	Irritant	Some residual activity after drying
Quaternary Ammonium Compounds (QACs)	Moderate	Stable in storage Nonirritating to skin Low toxicity Can be used on food preparation surfaces Effective at high temperatures and pH	Incompatible with anionic detergents		Commonly used primary environmental disinfectant Some residual activity after drying

TABLE 7.2. Antimicrobial Spectrum of Selected Disinfectants (Modified from Linton et al. 1987 and Block 2001). In the public domain from the Canadian Committee on Antibiotic Research (2008) *Infection Control and Best Practices for Small Animal Veterinary Clinics*, November 2008

	Agent	Alcohols	Aldehydes	Alkalis: Ammonia	Biguanides: Chlorhexidine	Halogens: Hypochlorite (Bleach)	Agents Oxidizing	Phenols	Quaternary Ammonium Compounds
Most susceptible	Mycoplasmas	++	++	++	++	++	++	++	+
	Gram-positive bacteria	++	++	+	++	++	++	++	++
	Gram-negative bacteria	++	++	+	+	++	++	++	+
	Pseudomonads	++	++	+	±	++	++	++	±
	Enveloped viruses	+	++	+	±	++	++	++	+
Most resistant	Chlamydiae	±	+	+	±	+	+	±	–
	Nonenveloped viruses	–	+	±	–	++	+	+	–
	Fungal spores	±	+	+	±	+	±	+	±
	Acid-fast bacteria	+	++	+	–	+	±	++	–
	Bacterial spores	–	+	±	–	++	+	–	–
	Coccidia	–	–	+	–	–	–	+	–

++ Highly effective; + Effective; ± Limited activity; - No activity.

TOPICAL THERAPEUTICS FOR THE PYODERMA PATIENT

- Chlorhexidine gluconate: less irritating than benzoyl peroxide, good residual effect, good for gram-positive, poor against pseudomonads, percent concentration may be important.
- Benzoyl peroxide: oxidizing agent, lowers skin pH, can be drying and irritating, disrupts bacterial cell membranes; caution – may bleach fabrics.
- Ethyl lactate 10%: lowers skin pH, variable clinical response.
- Retapamulin (Altabax): excellent penetration, gram-positive bacteria, expensive.
- Dilute bleach formulations (shampoos, rinses, sprays, soaks): 0.00156% kills 100% of staphylococci, yeast and pseudomonads; bleach bath concentrations recommended at 0.003–0.007%.
- Accelerated hydrogen peroxide: stabilized solutions of hydrogen peroxide for extended bactericidal activity.
- N-acetyl-L-cysteine for disruption of biofilm production; used as a topical (2%) in otic preparations for infections and persistent secretory otitis media (PSOM); oral administration (600 mg/day as a mucolytic agent) may help prevent ototoxicity from medications (i.e., gentamycin, amikacin) and may help decrease mucoid accumulation in the middle ear in cases of PSOM.
- TrizEDTA and N-acetyl-L-cysteine can disrupt biofilms, facilitating their removal and enhancing penetration of antimicrobials (otitis).
- Amikacin topical 1%.
- Fusidic acid 2% cream: not available in all countries.
- Mupirocin 2% ointment: excellent penetration, mostly gram-positive sensitivity, bacteriostatic; good residual effect in reservoir locations; should be reserved for more resistant infections.
- Sucralfate (1 g/2 mL saline) and cicalfate (10% in DMSO) containing skin creams may inhibit bacterial growth; further investigation needed.
- IIS-PAA (incomplete iron salt of polyacrylic acid); ingredient may prove to be beneficial in treating resistant strains of *Staphylococcus* and *Pseudomonas* spp.
- Lactoferricin (LFcin) is a peptide under investigation for antimicrobial activity.
- Silver salts, silver nanoparticles, and micronized silver; potential antibacterial properties/lysis of the bacterial cell wall, may inhibit biofilm production/no data to support biofilm degradation.

Systemic Treatment Options for Methicillin-Resistant *Staphylococcus* Based on Culture and Sensitivity Testing

- Chloramphenicol: 25–40 mg/kg BID to TID; GI upset, bone marrow suppression and peripheral neuropathy in large breed dogs; aplastic anemia in humans.
- Potentiated sulfonamides: 10–15 mg/kg BID; keratoconjunctivitis sicca, hypersensitivity reactions, lowered serum thyroid measurement; doberman pinschers and rottweilers reported to be more sensitive.
- Amikacin injectable: 20 mg/kg q24h; painful, potential for nephrotoxicity – renal monitoring required.

- Doxycycline and minocycline: 5 mg/kg BID; GI upset; new data on breakpoints for MIC reported.
- Clindamcyin: limited use; resistance often noted with MRSP despite test results.
- Fluoroquinolones: limited use due to emerging resistance.
- Rifampin: hepatotoxic, potent inducer of cytochrome p450 hepatic enzymes.
- Vancomycin: sensitive to the vast majority of MRS spp.; nephrotoxic in dogs.
- Linezolid: excellent activity, oral or parenteral, low toxicity, very expensive; veterinary use controversial due to its being the only effective drug in "life-threatening" human cases.

Veterinarians and physicians must commit to Antibiotic Stewardship and participate in the One Health Initiative.

The emergence of bacterial resistance is a serious therapeutic challenge.

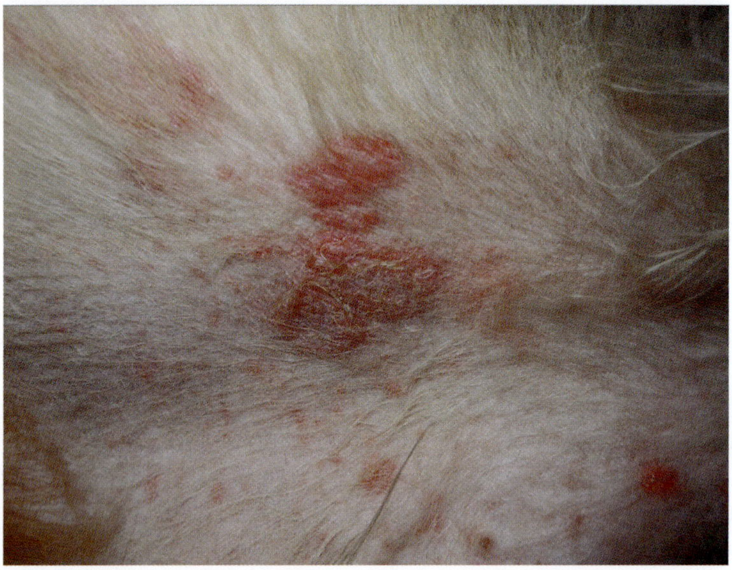

Fig. 7.1. Epidermal collarettes from MRSP on the ventrum of a 9-year-old female-spayed golden retriever. These lesions cannot be distinguished from those of MSSP without culture and sensitivity testing.

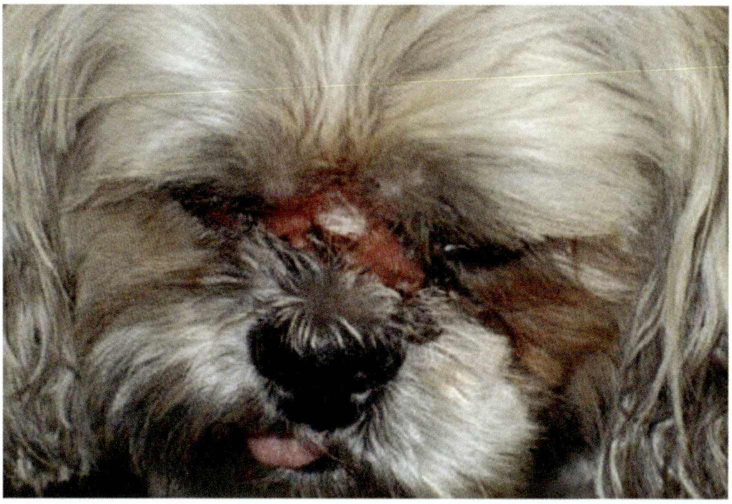

Fig. 7.2. Chronic recurrent ulceration over the bridge of the nose, secondary to MRSP infection.

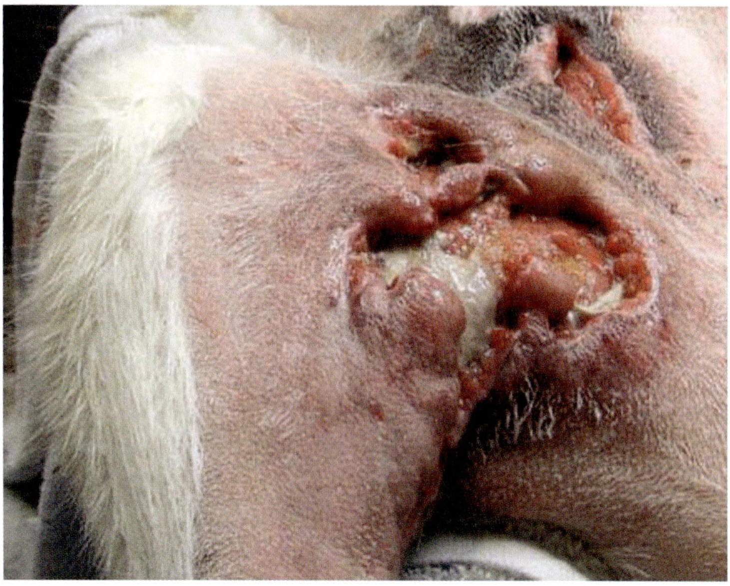

Fig. 7.3. Severe "melting" dermatitis associated with MRSP infection.

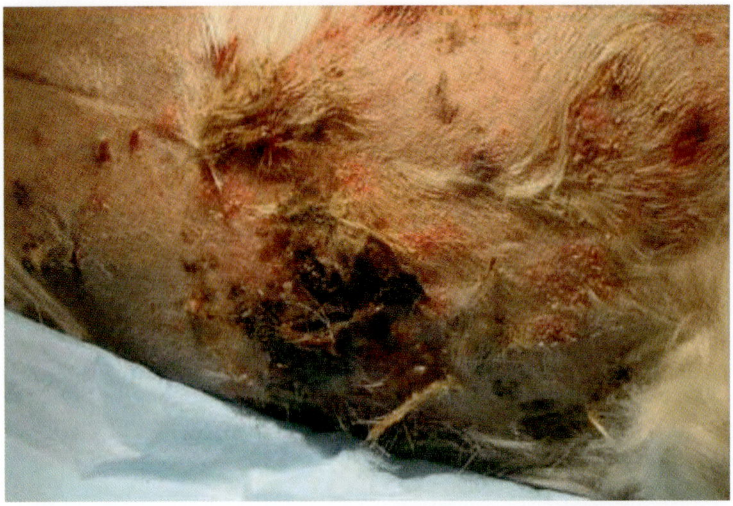

■ **Fig. 7.4.** Superficial folliculitis and focal furunculosis on the ventrum due to MRSP infection.

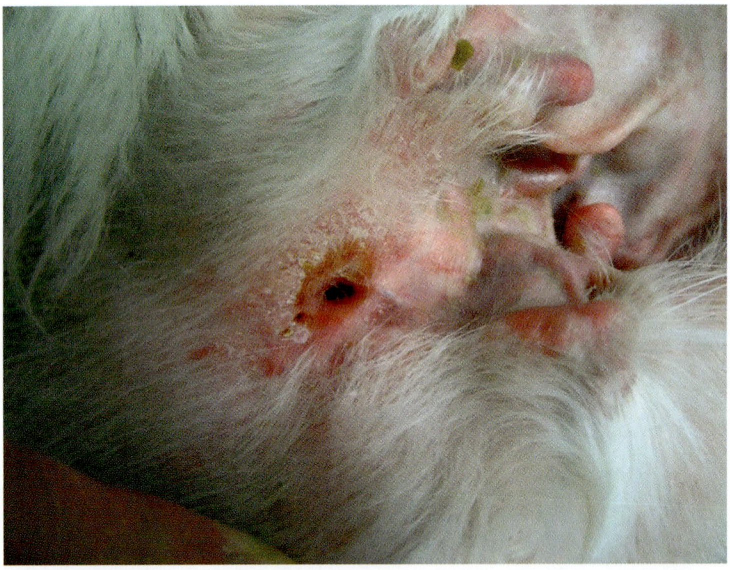

■ **Fig. 7.5.** MRSP and *Pseudomonas* infection at the postsurgical lateral ear resection site in a 6-year-old pitbull mix.

section 2

Diseases/Disorders

chapter 8

Acne (Canine and Feline)

DEFINITION/OVERVIEW

- Chronic inflammatory disorder of the chin and lips of young animals.
- Characterized primarily by abnormal follicular keratinization with secondary folliculitis and furunculosis, comedones rare in the dog/common in the cat.
- Secondary bacterial invasion is common in both dogs and cats.
- Canine:
    - Recognized almost exclusively in short-coated canine breeds
    - Also known as muzzle folliculitis/furunculosis
    - Hormones (increased androgen turnover) not a significant trigger; local trauma and genetic predisposition more important role
    - Mechanical irritation may facilitate development of lesions by causing breakage of the short hairs below the surface of the epidermis and subsequent follicular inflammation and rupture
    - Exposed keratin may trigger a foreign body inflammatory reaction.
- Feline:
    - Potential triggers include poor grooming habits, production of abnormal sebum/seborrhea, hair follicle dysplasia, viral infection, atopic disease, and immunosuppression.

SIGNALMENT/HISTORY

- Canine predisposed short-coated breeds: boxers, doberman pinschers, English bulldogs, Great Danes, weimaraners, mastiffs, rottweilers, German short-haired pointers, and pit bull terriers.
- Feline: no age, breed or gender predisposition.
- Young dogs: under 1 year of age.
- Initial stages: accentuation of follicular ostia, comedones (55% of feline cases remain in this stage), mild crusting, mild erythema, and swelling of rostral chin.
- Progression: the area may become minimally to markedly swollen with numerous erythematous papules and pustules (folliculitis); if chin swelling is noted in the cat, consider eosinophilic granuloma as a differential.
- Advanced stages: lesions may be exudative and indicate a secondary deep bacterial infection/furunculosis.

Blackwell's Five-Minute Veterinary Consult Clinical Companion: Small Animal Dermatology, Third Edition.
Karen Helton Rhodes and Alexander H. Werner.

- Lesions may be painful on palpation but are most frequently nonpainful and nonpruritic.
- Resolved lesions may remain scarred, thickened, and lichenified with follicular cysts.
- Chronic lesions predispose the site to recurrent infections.
- Regional lymphadenopathy may be prominent in both the dog and cat.

CLINICAL FEATURES

- Initial stages:
  - Accentuation of follicular ostia and follicular papules; chin may be palpated as "thickened" (Figure 8.1).
  - Comedones (55% of feline cases remain in this stage), mild crusting, erythema and swelling of rostral chin.
  - Progression to a markedly swollen region with numerous erythematous papules and pustules (folliculitis) (Figure 8.2).
- Advanced stages: exudative lesions indicate a secondary deep bacterial infection/ furunculosis.
- Lesions may be painful on palpation but are usually nonpainful and nonpruritic.
- Previously severe lesions may remain scarred, thickened, and lichenified with follicular cysts.
- Cat: eosinophilic granuloma should be considered as a differential if chin swelling is noted (Figure 8.3).

DIFFERENTIAL DIAGNOSIS

- Dermatophytosis
- Demodicosis
- Foreign body
- Contact dermatitis
- Eosinophilic granuloma
- Juvenile cellulitis
- Malassezia dermatitis

DIAGNOSTICS

- Skin scrapings: demodicosis.
- Fungal culture: dermatophytosis.
- Bacterial culture and sensitivity testing: in patients with suppurative folliculitis and furunculosis that are nonresponsive to initial antibiotic selection.
- Impression smear for *Malassezia* overgrowth.
- Biopsy: dilated keratin-filled hair follicles leading to plugging and dilatation (comedones), perifolliculitis, folliculitis and furunculosis; fibrosis in chronic cases.
- Bacteria: in the early stages, not seen and cannot be isolated from lesions.
- As disease progresses: papules enlarge and rupture, promoting a suppurative folliculitis and furunculosis.

THERAPEUTICS

- Depends on the severity and chronicity of the disease.
- Reduce behavioral trauma to the chin (e.g., rubbing on the carpet, chewing bones that increase salivation).
- Instruct owners to avoid scrubbing or manually expressing the lesions, which may cause internal rupture (furunculosis) of the papule/pustule and create marked inflammation.
- Frequent cleansing with an antibacterial shampoo, wipe, or ointment to reduce the bacterial numbers on the surface of the skin.
- Topical antibiotics (mupirocin, clindamycin, tetracycline, erythromycin, metronidazole).
- Retinoids: topical; tretinoin (Retin-A), tazarotene (Tazorac): may reduce follicular keratosis: may be irritating; oral isotretinoin (2 mg/kg/day) for severe cases.
- Corticosteroids: may be necessary to reduce inflammation.
- Antibiotics appropriate for deep bacterial infection based on culture and sensitivity results; may be required for 4–6 weeks (canine).

Precautions/Interactions

- Topicals with benzoyl peroxide: may bleach carpets and fabrics; may be irritating.
- Mupirocin ointment: greasy.
- Topical retinoids: may be drying and irritating.
- Oral retinoids: severe teratogen.
- Topical steroids: may cause adrenal suppression with repeated use.

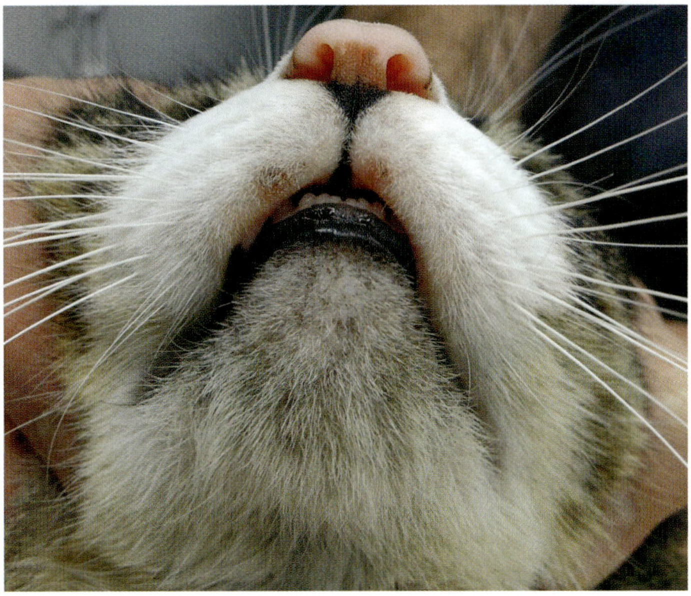

Fig. 8.1. Initial stages of feline acne: the skin palpates as thickened and there is mild alopecia.

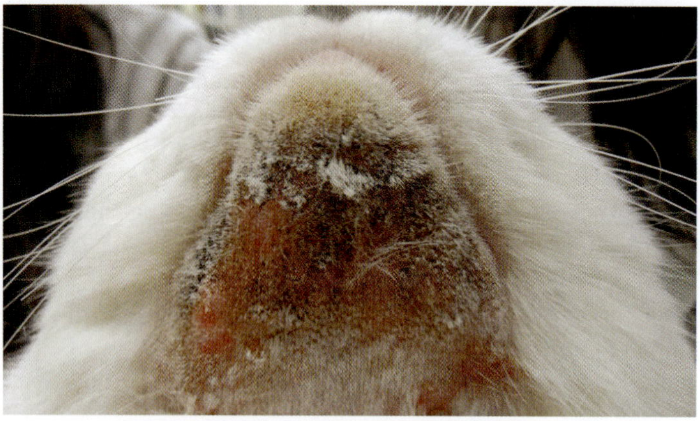

■ **Fig. 8.2.** Accumulations of crusts on the ventral chin with comedones, erythema, and mild exudation seen with chronic feline acne (area clipped prior to treatment).

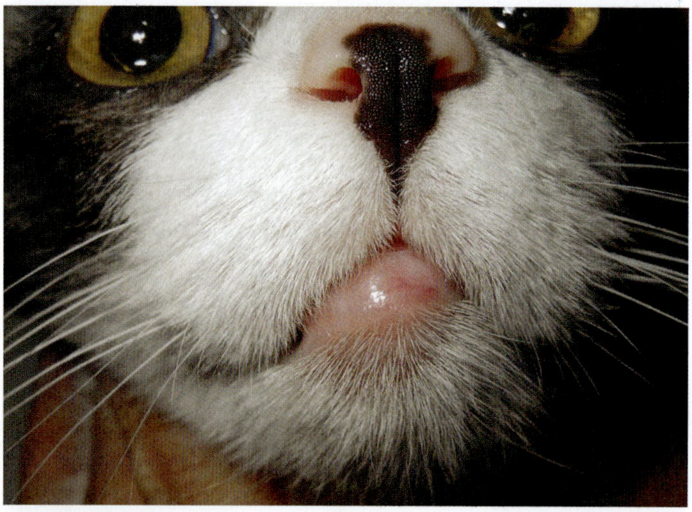

■ **Fig. 8.3.** "Pouty" chin seen with eosinophilic granuloma. Surrounding skin is not crusted or inflamed.

chapter 9

Anal Furunculosis/Perianal Fistula

DEFINITION/OVERVIEW

- Characterized as a chronic, often relapsing, inflammatory disease with multiple fistulous tracts or ulcerating sinuses involving the perianal tissues.
- Tracts may interconnect and may perforate the anus.
- Causes significant malodor, ulceration, suppuration, and pain.

ETIOLOGY/PATHOPHYSIOLOGY

- Etiology unknown; proposed causes include:
    - Multifactorial immune-mediated process (T cell mediated)
    - Impaction and infection of the anal sinuses and crypts
    - Infection of the circumanal glands and hair follicles
    - Anal sacculitis (may be a sequela)
    - Deep staphylococcal folliculitis
    - Low tail carriage and a broad tail base predisposing to inflammation and infection due to poor ventilation, accumulation of feces, moisture, and secretions
    - High density of apocrine sweat glands in the cutaneous zone of the anal canal of German shepherd dogs leading to apocrine gland inflammation (hidradenitis suppurativa).
- Epithelial-lined sinus tracts develop in the perianal tissue.
- Associated with colitis in German shepherd dogs (50%) similar to Crohn's disease in humans (possible enteral triggers).
- Excessive scar tissue formation around the anus results in tenesmus and dyschezia.
- Hidradenitis suppurativa may be associated with immune or endocrine dysfunction, genetic factors, and poor hygiene.

SIGNALMENT/HISTORY

- Dogs.
- German shepherd dog (84%) and Irish setter most commonly affected breeds.
- Mean age, 5–7 years; range 7 months to 14 years.

Blackwell's Five-Minute Veterinary Consult Clinical Companion: Small Animal Dermatology, Third Edition.
Karen Helton Rhodes and Alexander H. Werner.

- Gender predisposition reports inconsistent: higher prevalence possible in male sexually intact dogs.
- A genetic basis has been proposed but not proven.

CLINICAL FEATURES

- Vary with the severity and extent of involvement (Figures 9.1–9.5).
- Dyschezia.
- Tenesmus.
- Hematochezia.
- Ribbon-like stool.
- Constipation.
- Diarrhea.
- Malodorous anal discharge.
- Purulent anal discharge or bleeding.
- Painful tail movements.
- Licking and self-mutilation.
- Reluctance to sit, posturing difficulties, and personality changes.
- Fecal incontinence.
- Anorexia.
- Weight loss.
- Perianal sinus and fistulous tracts.
- Tracts may interconnect.
- Lesions may extend beyond the perianal tissues in severe cases (Figure 9.6).

DIFFERENTIAL DIAGNOSIS

- Chronic anal sac abscess
- Perianal infection
- Perianal adenoma or adenocarcinoma with ulceration and drainage
- Anal sac adenocarcinoma or squamous cell carcinoma
- Colitis or inflammatory bowel disease
- Rectal neoplasia
- Rectal fistula

DIAGNOSTICS

- Presumptive diagnosis: based on clinical signs and results of physical examination.
- Biopsy (primarily to rule out neoplasia): epithelial-lined tracts with pleocellular infiltrate, granulating fibrosis, and lymphoid nodules.
- Probing of tracts to determine depth and extent.
- Palpation of the anal sphincter and caudal rectum for thickening (fibrosis).

- Bacterial culture and sensitivity from sinus tracts: samples should be obtained from within the tract and not from surface debris (wipe skin surface with alcohol prior to sampling to remove fecal contamination, if possible).
- Fine-needle aspirate and cytology from thickened anal sacs (if present).
- Colonoscopy with biopsy may reveal associated colitis.

THERAPEUTICS

Basic Care

- Clip hair from the affected area.
- Daily antiseptic lavage.
- Systemic and topical antibiotics.
- Hydrotherapy.
- Elevation of the tail.
- Analgesics.
- Dietary modification: fiber-enhanced diet or stool softeners if pain/tenesmus.
- Restricted-ingredient diet trial if associated with colitis.

Surgical Options

- Surgery: no longer considered as primary treatment.
- High recurrence rate (70%) in cases treated with surgery alone.
- Adjunctive to medical management for cases with incomplete resolution.
- Primary objective of surgery is complete removal or destruction of diseased tissue while preserving normal tissue and function.
- Surgical options:
  - Electrocautery of fistulae
  - Cryosurgery
  - Surgical debridement with fulguration by chemical cautery
  - Exteriorization and fulguration by electrocautery
  - *En bloc* surgical resection
  - Radical excision of the rectal ring
  - Tail setting or amputation
  - Laser surgery.
- Anal sacculectomy should be performed.
- Postoperative complications include anal stenosis and fecal incontinence.
- Multiple procedures may be necessary for complete resolution.

Medical Options

- Cyclosporine A (5 mg/kg/day):
  - Success rate 5–96% of cases (Figure 9.7)
  - Surgery may be required due to inadequate healing or anal stricture

- Measure cyclosporine serum level in nonresponders: appropriate levels are 200–400 ng/mL (trough level); levels greater than 1000 ng/mL are toxic/immunosuppressive
- Microemulsion cyclosporine A required (Atopica®); nonmicroemulsion poorly absorbed
- Major disadvantage of cyclosporine is cost
- Maintenance therapy required; recurrence rate greater than 35%
- Routine monitoring: serum chemistry and CBC every 3–6 months
- Adverse effects: gastrointestinal distress (vomiting, diarrhea), gingival hyperplasia, viral papillomas
- Ketoconazole (2.5 mg/kg/day) given in conjunction permits 50% reduction in dosage of cyclosporine for cost savings; decreases clearance of cyclosporine by inhibition of hepatic cytochrome p450 microsomal enzymes.

- Antibiotics and analgesics may be indicated in some cases: antibiotic choice based on culture and sensitivity or empirically (initially) on effectiveness against organisms associated with the gastrointestinal tract: clindamycin (11 mg/kg q24h to BID); metronidazole 10 mg/kg BID; amoxicillin-clavulanate 12.5 mg/kg BID).
- Corticosteroids: immunosuppressive dosages (2 mg/kg q24h to BID initially; tapered to EOD); significantly less effective than cyclosporine.
- Azathioprine (1–2 mg/kg q24h initially; tapered to EOD or twice weekly).
- Restricted/novel-ingredient diet may yield partial or complete resolution (about 33% of cases); most dogs do not improve.
- Tacrolimus ointment (0.1%): apply to tissues BID initially; tapered to EOD; may reduce dosages of or replace systemic therapy for maintenance.
- Mupirocin ointment (2%): apply to tissues q24h to BID until healed.
- Mesenchymal stem cell injections: initial studies report efficacy.

Possible Treatment Complications

- Recurrence.
- Failure to heal.
- Dehiscence of surgical site.
- Tenesmus.
- Fecal incontinence.
- Anal stricture.
- Flatulence.
- The incidence of postoperative complications is directly related to severity of disease.

COMMENTS

Expected Course and Prognosis

- Guarded for complete resolution except in mildly affected patients.
- Treatment is often lifelong.
- Resolution of pain and discharge is primary goal of therapy.
- Client education and understanding of therapy goal required.

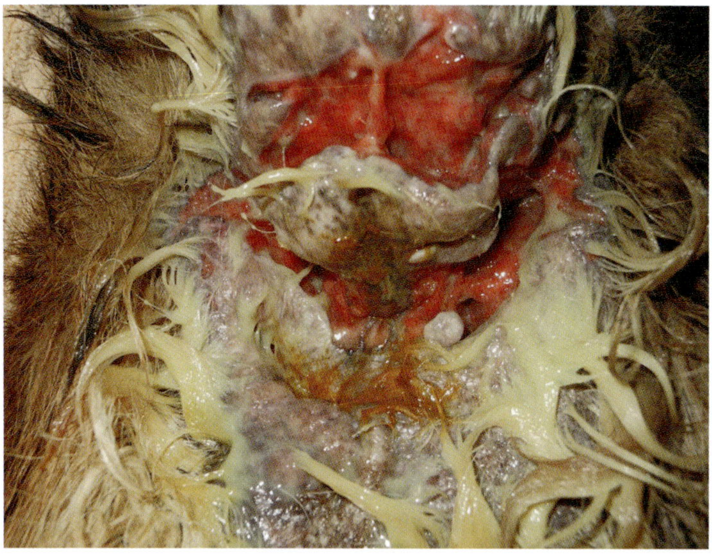

■ **Fig. 9.1.** Perianal fisulae in a 9-year-old female-spayed German shepherd dog at presentation.

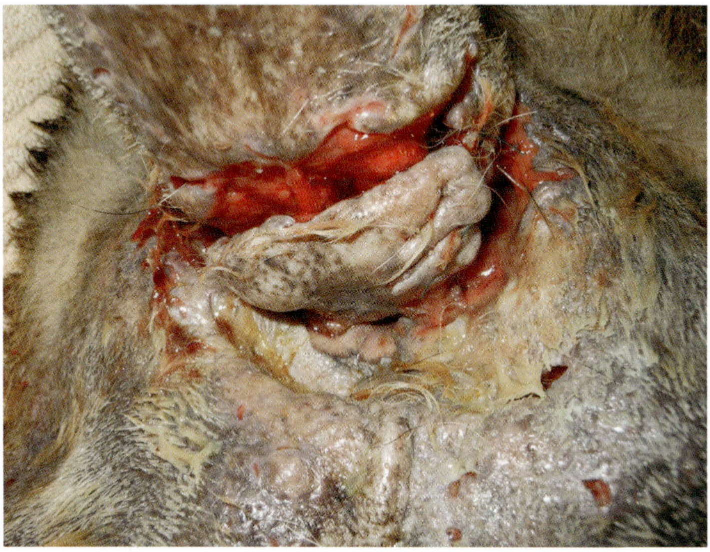

■ **Fig. 9.2.** Additional image of patient in Figure 9.1 following clipping and cleaning of affected area.

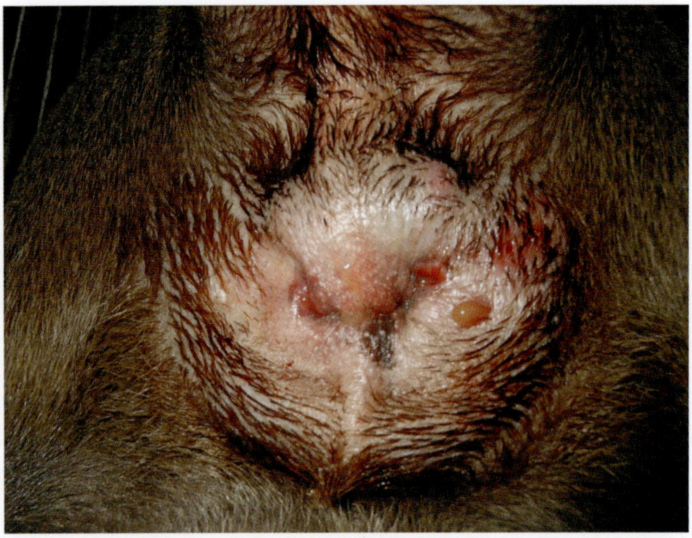

■ **Fig. 9.3.** Perianal fistulae in a 7-year-old female-spayed pit bull terrier. Punctate lesions are present most notably in the upper right quadrant of the perianal tissues. The major differential diagnosis for this case is anal sac impaction.

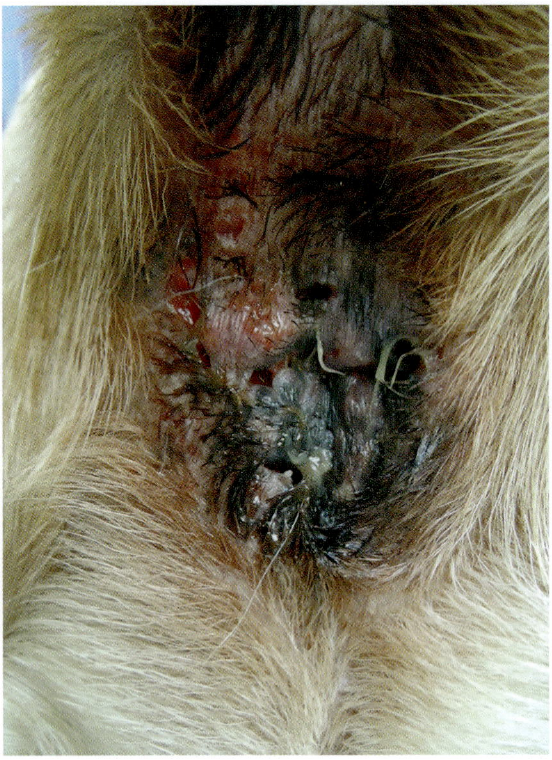

■ **Fig. 9.4.** Multiple draining tracts in a 9-year-old male-castrate pit bull mix.

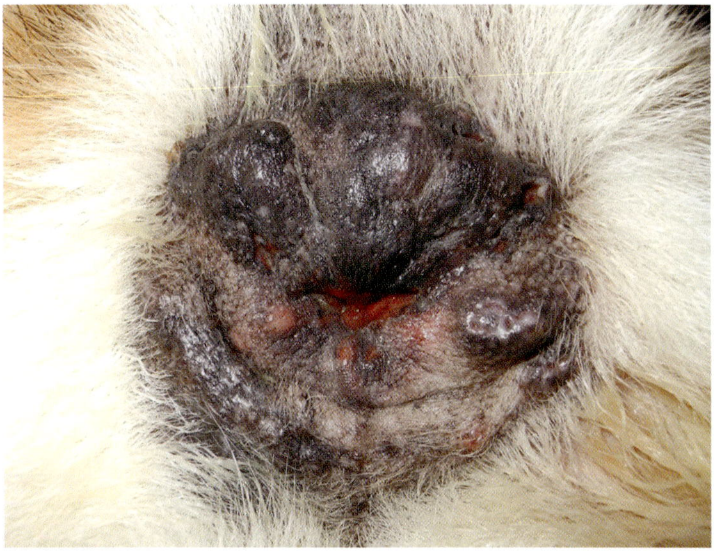

■ **Fig. 9.5.** Thickened anal ring and developing perianal fistulae in a 9-year-old female-spayed Akita.

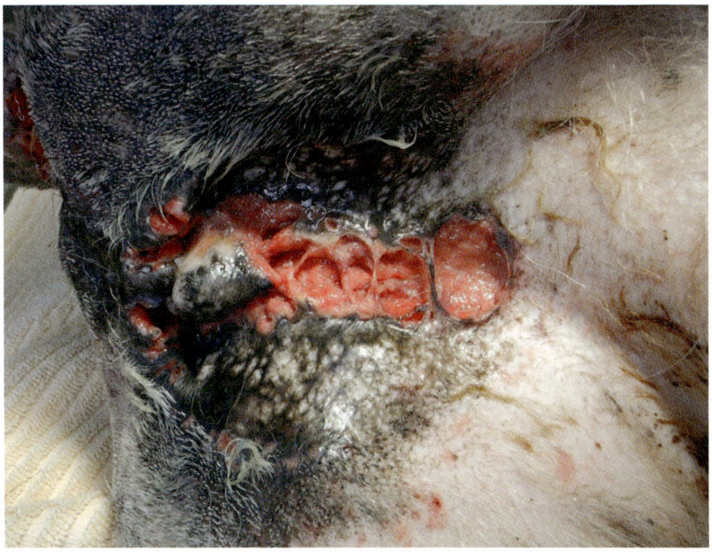

■ **Fig. 9.6.** Extension of ulcerations and tracts around the vulva and inguinal region of the patient in Figures 9.1 and 9.2.

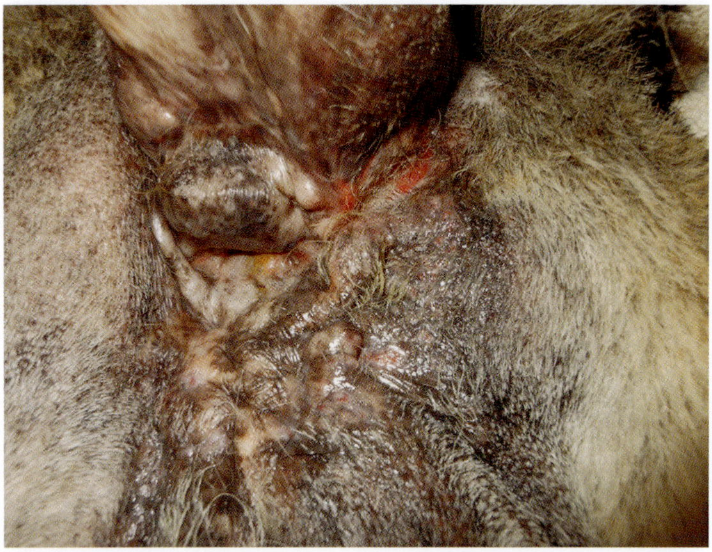

(a)

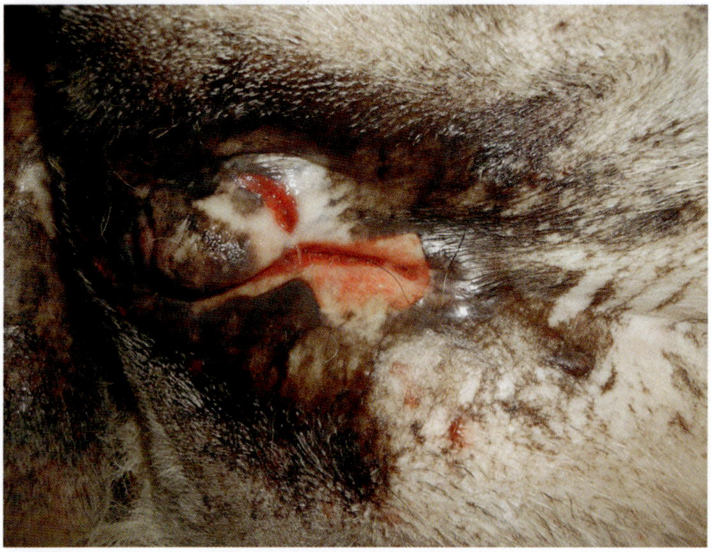

(b)

■ **Fig. 9.7.** Midtreatment images of the patient in Figures 9.1 (a) and 9.6 (b): tracts and ulcerations are healing with administration of cyclosporine A and antibiotics.

chapter 10

Anal Sac Disorders

DEFINITION/OVERVIEW

- Anal sacs are infoldings or pouches between the muscle layers of the external and internal anal sphincters; they are lined by squamous epithelium and contain large apocrine glands.
- Wide variability in color, consistency, and contents of normal and abnormal anal sac secretions.
- Function of anal sacs unknown; may be vestigial structures for marking territory.
- Anal sac diseases include impaction, inflammation (sacculitis), infection/abscessation, and neoplasia.
- Inflammatory anal sac disorders are more common in dogs than in cats.
- More common in small breed dogs, spaniels, poodles, and obese dogs and cats.
- Impaction occurs when the anal sacs fail to empty and become distended, causing discomfort/pain.
- Sacculitis is inflammation that can lead to secondary bacterial infection and abscessation; may lead to rupture and fistulation.
- Anal sac neoplasia: adenocarcinoma; rarely squamous cell carcinoma.

ETIOLOGY/PATHOPHYSIOLOGY

- The exact cause is unknown.
- Often associated with gastrointestinal disease including chronic diarrhea or constipation (dogs and cats), and anal sphincter laxity or muscle weakness.
- May be associated with hypersecretion as well as with obstruction.
- Anal sacculitis has a proposed association with food hypersensitivity.

SIGNALMENT/HISTORY

- Scooting.
- Licking or biting at the anal area (Figures 10.1, 10.2).
- Pain with defecation.
- Constipation.

Blackwell's Five-Minute Veterinary Consult Clinical Companion: Small Animal Dermatology, Third Edition.
Karen Helton Rhodes and Alexander H. Werner.

- Tenesmus.
- Involuntary leakage of malodorous contents from the anal sacs.
- Blood-tinged exudate on feces.
- Cats: excessive licking of the tail fold and tail base or perianal region.
- Anal sac abscessation: malodorous, blood-tinged secretions; pain when sitting or unwillingness to sit (Figure 10.3).
- Anal sac adenocarcinomas:
  - May secrete a parathormone-like substance that causes pseudohyperparathyroidism with hypercalcemia, causing polyuria, polydipsia, weakness, lethargy, or gastrointestinal signs (53% of cases)
  - Renal calcification may produce renal failure
  - Locally invasive
  - May be bilateral (14%)
  - Older dogs (>10 years)
  - High metastasis rate (47–96%).

DIFFERENTIAL DIAGNOSIS

- Food hypersensitivity
- Atopic dermatitis
- Flea bite hypersensitivity
- Gastrointestinal parasites
- Colitis
- Tail fold pyoderma
- Psychogenic (behavioral) perianal pruritus
- Neoplasia
- Perianal fistulae

DIAGNOSTICS

- Rectal exam.
- Expression of anal sacs; contents should evacuate without significant pressure or discomfort to patient.
- Impacted sacs may contain thick, pasty fluid; often becomes thinner with infection and accumulation of inflammatory cells (pus).
- Cytology of contents: ineffective for distinguishing between normal and affected dogs; neutrophils and bacteria common.
- Culture and sensitivity of contents or draining tract; gram-negative bacteria predominate.
- Adenocarcinoma:
  - CBC, serum chemistry: azotemia, hypercalcemia, hypophosphatemia
  - Urinalysis and sediment: hypercalciuria, urine specific gravity increased

- Radiography: pulmonary metastasis, dystrophic calcification
- Biopsy to rule out adenocarcinoma.

THERAPEUTICS

- Medical management of impaction by expression; affected dogs often require expression at approximately 3-week intervals.
- Flushing of impacted sacs followed by infusion with corticosteroids and/or antibiotics.
- High-fiber diet or fiber supplement to maintain stool consistency.
- Weight loss.
- Sacculitis: treatment based on culture and sensitivity testing; empiric treatment clindamycin (11 mg/kg/day) for at least 4 weeks; anal sac expression and lavage, followed by infusion with corticosteroids and/or antibiotics; effectiveness inconsistently reported.
- Anal sacculectomy may be necessary if medical management fails; complications include incontinence (uncommon).
- Adenocarcinoma: surgical excision, radiation, chemotherapy, radiation therapy; poor prognosis.

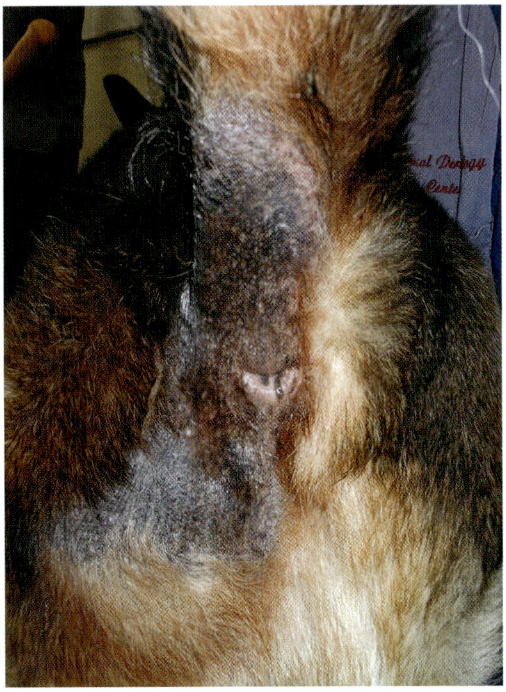

Fig. 10.1. Chronic anal sac impaction causing unilateral pruritus with alopecia and lichenification.

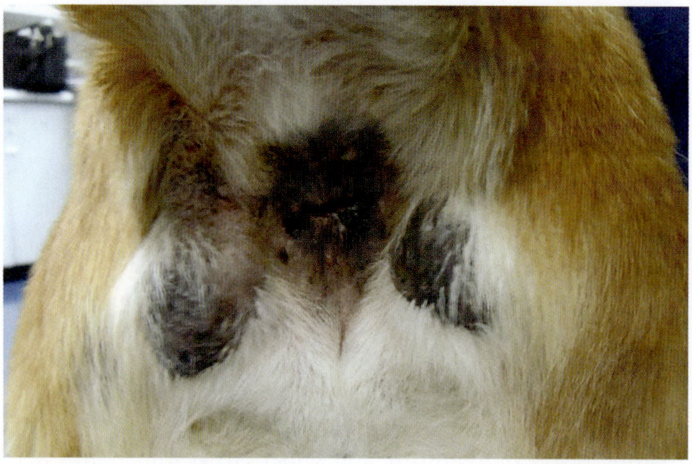

■ **Fig. 10.2.** Alopecia, lichenification, and hyperpigmentation over the anal sacs due to chronic impaction and scooting in a 14-year-old female-spayed shepherd mix.

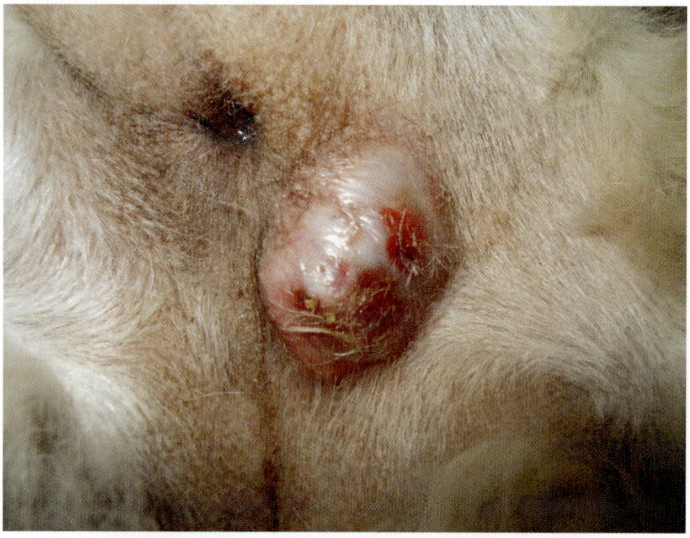

■ **Fig. 10.3.** Anal sac abscess in a 6-year-old female-spayed shih tzu.

chapter 11

Atopic Disease

DEFINITION/OVERVIEW

- Atopic disease is a predisposition to develop allergic reactions to normally innocuous substances, such as pollens (grasses, weeds, and trees), molds, house dust mites, epithelial antigens, other environmental allergens, and occasionally foods.
- Historically, atopic disease and atopy were considered synonymous.
- Atopy by definition requires the presence of environmental allergen-specific IgE; many patients with symptoms of atopic dermatitis do not have identifiable allergen-specific IgE (designated as atopic-like dermatitis).
- Dogs and cats with adverse reactions to food may demonstrate symptoms indistinguishable from classic atopy.
- The inclusive term "atopic disease" (AD) may be most appropriate.

ETIOLOGY/PATHOPHYSIOLOGY

- Our understanding of the pathophysiology of AD is constantly changing and expanding; each new study brings insight into the complexity of this disorder.
- A brief explanation of current concepts, relating to cutaneous symptoms, is attempted below for an understanding of treatment options addressing different aspects of the etiology.

Current Concept: Outside-Inside-Outside Theory

- Defects in epidermal barrier function (outside) facilitate epidermal penetration of allergens and microbes, increasing their exposure in genetically predisposed individuals.
- Increased exposure produces sensitization (inside).
- Sensitization and elicitation lead to reactions that include pruritus as well as exacerbating damage of the epidermis, furthering barrier dysfunction (outside).
    - Defects in epidermal barrier function are evidenced as:
        - □ Decreases in and disorganization of lipids within the stratum corneum

Blackwell's Five-Minute Veterinary Consult Clinical Companion: Small Animal Dermatology, Third Edition.
Karen Helton Rhodes and Alexander H. Werner.

    - Decreases in epidermal ceramides and sphingosine-1-phosphate causing increased transepidermal water loss and changes in cell signaling
    - Mutations in filaggrin (an important structural protein). Results in penetration of allergens, microbes, and PAMPs into the epidermis where both reaction to their presence and detection for immunological response are enhanced.
- Increased cellular reactivity in genetically predisposed individuals may include:
    - Increased expression by keratinocytes of TARC and TSLP, promoting a Th_2-lymphocyte response
    - Dendritic cells (DC) exposed to antigen in the presence of "danger signals," including proteases and PAMPs, become activated to promote a T cell response
    - Increased activated DC, Langerhans cells (LC) in the epidermis
    - Possible increased number of mast cells in atopic skin as well as mast cell "hyperreleasability"
    - Altered ratio of $CD4^+$ to $CD8^+$ cells promoting a Th_2 over Th_1 response: the role of T_{reg} lymphocytes in atopic dermatitis is an area of active research.
- Reexposure in a sensitized animal induces pruritus, causing epidermal damage, and elicits activated keratinocytes to release TARC, TSLP, and other cytokines, promoting the recruitment of reactive immune cells into the epidermis and furthering the inflammatory response.

The Role of IgE

- IgE has an essential role in type 1 hypersensitivity.
- Classic definition of atopy is an inflammatory dermatitis characterized by the development of IgE to environmental allergens.
- The classic definition is being challenged by findings that include:
    - Elevated levels of IgE in asymptomatic individuals and reactivity to allergens in individuals without detectable levels of IgE (atopic-like dermatitis)
    - Production of IgE is favored by Th_2-lymphocyte proliferation
    - The development of clinical disease is not predicted by the level of detectable IgE
    - Non-IgE antibodies (IgG_d) and a late-phase reaction may also be involved in development of AD.

Th_1/Th_2/Th_{17}/T_{reg} and Cytokines

- AD is an imbalance in the activity and production of cytokines by various immune (and other) cells.
- Th_2 activity (evidenced by increases in Th_2-promoting cytokines) increases production of IgE and recruitment of inflammatory cells.
- This has been used as justification for the concept of atopic disease as a Th_2-polarized immune response.

- Additional research has demonstrated increased expression of Th_1 and T_{reg} cytokines in chronic disease.
- T_{reg} cells may be induced by ASIT to promote tolerance. Cytokines reported to be pruritogenic or proinflammatory include IL-2, IL-4, IL-6, IL-13, and IL-31.

IL-31 and JAK/STAT

- Reported increased levels of cytokine IL-31 in atopic skin; IL-31 can induce pruritus in normal dogs.
- Blocking of IL-31 (by neutralizing antibody) or its receptor on neurons (JAK1 inhibitor) can reduce the symptoms of atopic dermatitis.
- The role of this cytokine in the development of hypersensitivity and inflammation (versus strictly as a pruritogenic cytokine) remains to be determined.

Summary Based on Current Knowledge

- Susceptible animals (barrier dysfunction/immune dysregulation) become sensitized to environmental allergens.
- Repeat allergen exposure (most importantly by percutaneous absorption and less so by oral exposure) causes a hypersensitivity reaction, and results in the release of mediators of inflammation that may include histamine, heparin, proteolytic enzymes, leukotrienes, serotonin, cytokines, chemokines, and perhaps many others.
- Cumulative pruritogenic factors (insect, food, environmental allergens, bacterial and yeast antigens) may lower the individual threshold (further barrier dysfunction/immune hyperreactivity), leading to persistent clinical symptoms in some patients or intermittent clinical symptoms in others (allergic threshold principle),

SIGNALMENT/HISTORY

- Risk factors reported or proposed for the development of canine AD: exposure/lack of exposure to environmental allergens ("hygiene hypothesis"), environmental proteases (e.g., house dust mite antigens), and oxidative stress (e.g., tobacco smoke).
- Canine: true incidence unknown; estimated at 3–27% of the canine population; with efficacy of newer parasiticides, AD may replace flea bite dermatitis as the most common allergic skin disease.
- Feline: unknown; generally believed to be lower than for dogs.
- Canine: any breed, including mongrels; although it may not have a simple mode of inheritance, it has been recognized more frequently in certain breeds or families.
- Canine: Boston terriers, boxers, cairn terriers, cocker spaniels, dalmatians, English bulldogs, English setters, French bulldogs, German shepherds, Irish setters, lhasa apsos, miniature schnauzers, pugs, Sealyham terriers, Scottish terriers, West Highland white terriers, wire-haired fox terriers, and golden retrievers.
- Canine: mean age at onset 1–3 years; range 3 months to 6 years; symptoms may be mild initially but are usually progressive and clinically apparent by 3 years of age.

- Feline: mean age of onset 1–5 years of age.
- Reports of sex predilection inconsistent.

Historical Findings

- Pruritus with or without skin changes.
- Most often facial, pedal, perineal, or axillary.
- Early onset.
- Increased incidence in patients living indoors.
- Family history of atopy.
- May be seasonal initially (42–75%); becomes nonseasonal in most cases (75%).
- Recurring skin or ear infections (bacterial or yeast).
- Response to glucocorticoids.
- Symptoms progressively worsen with time.

CLINICAL FEATURES

- Hallmark sign: pruritus (itching, scratching, rubbing, licking).
- Canine:
    - Primary lesions (erythematous papules and urticaria) may occur, but most cutaneous changes are believed to be produced by self-induced trauma (Figure 11.1)
    - Areas most commonly affected: interdigital spaces (dorsal as well as palmar/plantar), carpal and tarsal areas, lips, muzzle, periocular region, pinnae, axillae, flexural surfaces of the forelegs, flank folds, and perineal/inguinal areas (Figure 11.2, 11.3)
    - Erythema of the ventral skin surface between the accessory and metacarpal or metatarsal pads (Figure 11.4)
    - Lesions: vary from none to broken hairs or salivary discoloration to erythema, papular eruptions, urticaria, crusts, alopecia, hyperpigmentation, lichenification, excessively oily or dry seborrheic changes, and hyperhidrosis (apocrine sweating)
    - Altered skin bacterial microbiome with increased epidermal staphylococcal colonization and secondary pyoderma
    - Secondary yeast skin infections (Figure 11.5)
    - Chronic relapsing otitis externa
    - Conjunctivitis with secondary blepharitis
    - Rhinitis.
- Feline:
    - Miliary dermatitis
    - Self-induced alopecia (Figure 11.6, 11.7)
    - Facial excoriation (Figure 11.8)
    - Head and neck pruritus
    - Otitis externa
    - Allergic asthma
    - Eosinophilic plaque/granuloma (Figure 11.9).

DIFFERENTIAL DIAGNOSIS

- Cutaneous adverse reactions to food: may cause identical lesion distribution and physical examination findings; often nonseasonal; may occur concurrently with AD; differentiation made by response to restricted-ingredient diet.
- Flea bite hypersensitivity: may occur concurrently with AD; most often affects the dorsal lumbosacral region; differentiation made by noting lesion distribution, response to flea control.
- Sarcoptic mange: can develop at any age; causes severe pruritus of the ventral chest, lateral elbows, lateral hocks, and pinnal margins; differentiation made by positive skin scrapings and/or complete response to miticidal therapy.
- Demodicosis: not primarily pruritic; pruritus develops with secondary infection; differentiation made by positive skin scrapings and response to miticidal therapy.
- Dermatophytosis: not primarily pruritic; differentiation made by positive fungal culture and/or response to antifungal therapy.
- Pyoderma: common secondary to AD in dogs; usually caused by *Staphylococcus pseudintermedius*; characterized by follicular papules, pustules, crusts, and epidermal collarettes.
- *Malassezia* dermatitis: characterized by erythematous, scaly, crusting, greasy, lichenified dermatitis; malodor; demonstration of numerous budding yeast organisms by skin cytology, favorable response to antifungal therapy.
- Contact dermatitis (allergic or irritant): may cause severe erythema and pruritus of the feet and thinly haired areas of the ventral abdomen; history of exposure to a known contact sensitizer or irritant, response to a change of environment, and patch testing may be diagnostic; uncommon in dogs and cats.

DIAGNOSTICS

- There is no definitive test for atopic disease: presumption of diagnosis is made only after the exclusion of other causes of pruritus, appropriate symptom history, and clinical examination.
- Determination of criteria to establish the diagnosis of canine AD is evolving; the following should be used to aid the identification of potential cases:
  - Age of onset <3 years
  - Mostly indoors
  - Corticosteroid-responsive pruritus
  - Chronic or recurrent yeast infections
  - Affected front feet
  - Affected ear pinnae
  - Nonaffected pinnal margins
  - Nonaffected dorsal lumbosacral region.

- Allergy testing:
  - Neither serum nor intradermal allergy testing can discriminate between normal and allergic patients, or to make the diagnosis of AD
  - Both normal and patients with AD may have positive or negative tests
  - Serum and intradermal allergy test results rarely correlate
  - Allergy testing is necessary only for the identification of allergens to be included in allergen-specific immunotherapy
  - Studies lack documentation of the accuracy of alternative forms of "allergy testing:" these modalities are not recommended.

Serologic Allergy Tests

- Measure the amount of allergen-specific IgE antibody in the patient's serum.
- Appropriate for the selection of allergens for immunotherapy when referral for intradermal testing not possible.
- Negative/not relevant test results obtained from patients with atopic-like dermatitis (non-IgE mediated) and cutaneous adverse reaction to food.
- Advantages over IDST: availability; shaving of the hair coat not needed; sedation not necessary; no potential for anaphylactic reaction to testing material; less sensitive to medication administration (withdrawal recommendations vary by laboratory).
- Disadvantages: frequent false-positive reactions; limited number of allergens tested; inconsistent assay validation and quality control (may vary by laboratory).
- Reliability and reproducibility vary with each laboratory/test utilized; widely varying results obtained from the same patient serum sent to multiple laboratories.
- Serum testing alone often performed in cats with allergic asthma to avoid sedation.
- Often submitted in conjunction with intradermal skin test results for allergen selection (best use).

Intradermal Skin Testing (IDST)

- Small amounts of test allergens injected intradermally; wheal formation is measured.
- More accurate (and physiologically relevant) method of identifying offending allergens for possible avoidance or inclusion in allergen-specific immunotherapy.
- Results more variable and difficult to interpret in cats.
- False-negative test results may be caused by medications (glucocorticoids, antihistamines, specific tranquilizers), diluted/weakened allergens, and/or severe stresses (physiological or medical).
- False-positive test results may be caused by irritant or contaminated allergens and/or poor testing technique.
- Testing not affected by cyclosporine, oclacitinib, or neutralizing IL-31 antibody.

Skin Biopsy

- Skin biopsy is most useful in AD to reinforce the diagnosis and to exclude other likely causes of pruritus.

- Dermatohistopathologic changes include superficial perivascular dermatitis with lymphocytes, eosinophils and mast cells, mild to moderate acanthosis, foci of spongiosis with lymphocytes and histiocytes, and dilated sweat glands.
- Eosinophilic epidermal micropustules suggest direct contact with aeroallergens.

THERAPEUTICS

- Treatment of atopic disease in dogs and cats should be proactive rather than reactive.
- Focus should be on the consistent and effective management of the disease rather than "crisis management" during flare-ups.
- Newer treatment modalities have expanded the ability to reduce pruritus but are not replacements for diagnosis and resolution or control of the primary disease.
- Treatment of AD should not be considered until other causes of pruritus have been eliminated.
- Previous treatment recommendations have focused more on management of the immunologic causes of AD – the "inside-outside" model.
- More recently, restoring the skin barrier function – the "outside-inside-outside" model – has gained attention.

Skin Barrier Function

- Mechanical action of bathing, regardless of product used, can reduce pruritus.
- Topical therapies remove allergens, microbes, and inflammatory compounds from the skin, help to restore the barrier function of the skin, and deliver medications directly to areas of infection and inflammation.
- Shampoos: medicated (e.g., oatmeal as an antipruritic, chlorhexidine as an antiseptic to reduce bacterial colonization, ketoconazole to reduce yeast population); bathing once to twice weekly; shampoo should be followed with a conditioner or emollient to rehydrate the skin or to apply residual medications.
- Ceramide, phytosphingosine, essential oil, or essential fatty acid-containing spot-on, mousse, and spray products: improve barrier function of the skin and reduce transepidermal water loss.
- Topical corticosteroids: low-potency products (e.g., hydrocortisone aceponate) applied twice weekly to pruritic areas decrease frequency of "flares"; high-potency products (e.g. dexamethasone, fluocinolone) should be restricted to the short-term treatment of acute lesions.
- Essential fatty acid (specifically n-3 fatty acids) supplementation: high doses may help repair skin barrier by providing structural components of the stratum corneum deficient in AD; may reduce inflammation and pruritus by competitive inhibition and displacement of proinflammatory phospholipids; may decrease need for antipruritic medications; 40 mg/kg eicosapentaenoic acid.

Allergen-Specific Immunotherapy (ASIT)

- The only intervention to resolve AD and to prevent recurrence of symptoms in subsequent seasons.

- Administration of gradually increasing doses of the allergens identified by testing (serum and/or intradermal) as potentially contributing to symptoms to reduce sensitivity.
- Allergens selected based on allergy test results, patient history, and knowledge of local flora; immunotherapy with standard, regional-specific allergens not selected by testing of the individual patient not as effective.
- Indicated when symptoms last longer than 4–6 months per year, when nonsteroidal forms of therapy are ineffective, and/or to avoid or reduce the use of corticosteroids.
- Successfully reduces pruritus in 60–80% of dogs and cats.
- Response is gradual and may take months to induce a beneficial competitive inhibition; treatment should be continued at least 1 year to fully evaluate effect.
- ASIT may be administered by subcutaneous injection or by sublingual (oral) route.
- Both modalities are safe and effective.
- Patients that fail to respond to one modality of immunotherapy may respond to the alternative formulation.
- Client/patient compliance in treatment should be considered when choosing the modality.

Corticosteroids

- Most effective for management of acute "flare-ups" to break the itch–scratch cycle.
- Should be tapered to the lowest dosage that adequately controls pruritus.
- Prednisolone or methylprednisolone tablets: 0.2–0.5 mg/kg PO at a tapering dosage with targeted maintenance of twice-weekly administration if needed.
- Repository injectable corticosteroids should be avoided due to persistent adrenal access suppression and increased incidence of long-term adverse effects.

Cyclosporine

- Inhibits cytokine-induced activation of immune cells (specifically lymphocytes, Langerhans cells, mast cells, and eosinophils).
- Poor bioavailability; microemulsion formulation increases absorption; name-brand (Atopica®) more effective.
- Advantages: long-term experience indicates safety; steroid sparing; effective as single-therapy management of AD.
- Adverse reactions: gastrointestinal upset (vomiting, diarrhea); psoriasiform lichenoid-like dermatitis; papillomatosis; gingival hyperplasia; opportunistic infections (rare); possible increase in urinary tract infection.
- Slow onset: 4–8 weeks treatment required for control of symptoms prior to tapering of dosage.
- Dogs 5 mg/kg q24h; cats 7.3 mg/kg q24h: administered daily until control of symptoms; most patients maintained on every other day schedule.
- Reduce initial dosage if gastrointestinal upset occurs.

- Cats: cyclosporine blood level should be measured when on maintenance dosage to prevent immunosuppression; patients must be FeLV/FIV negative; initial exposure to toxoplasmosis during treatment may be fatal.
- Caution: inhibitors of cytochrome p450 activity will decrease drug clearance, requiring dose adjustment.

Janus Kinase Inhibitor (JAK)

- Oclacitinib: JAK1 inhibitor (major effect); blocks neuronal itch by inhibiting IL-31 cytokine function; additional immunomodulatory effects.
- Advantages: rapid onset; alternative to glucocorticoids during flare-ups.
- Adverse reactions associated with chronic use: demodicosis, pneumonia, dermal nodules; rare cutaneous neoplasia; nonspecific immunosuppressive effects; nonspecific bone marrow suppression; possible increase in urinary tract infection.
- May not decrease recurrences of AD-associated otitis externa or pyoderma.
- Should not be combined with immunosuppressive therapies.
- 0.4–0.6 mg/kg BID for 14 days; then once daily.
- Dogs only; not approved for use in patients under 1 year of age.

Biological Therapy

- Caninized anti-cIL31 monoclonal antibody (Loviktinab).
- Advantages: rapid onset; alternative to glucocorticoids during flare-ups; effective 4–6 weeks; no gastrointestinal side effects.
- Long-term (repeated administration) efficacy and safety information lacking; inactivation or allergic reaction theoretically possible with repeated usage; adverse effects from continuous inactivation of IL-31 unknown.
- 2 mg/kg by subcutaneous injection; repeated monthly or as needed to control symptoms.
- Dogs only.

Antihistamines

- Variable response; less effective than corticosteroids.
- May act synergistically with essential fatty acid supplements.
- Advantages: safe; inexpensive; minimal adverse effects.
- Diphenhydramine 2.2 mg/kg BID.
- Hydroxyzine 2.2 mg/kg BID.
- Chlorpheniramine 0.4 mg/kg BID.
- Cetirizine 1 mg/kg q24h.

Alternative Drugs

- Pentoxifylline (phosphodiesterase inhibitor) 10 mg/kg BID to TID.
- Tricyclic antidepressants: doxepin 0.5–3 mg/kg BID; amitriptyline 0.5–2.0 mg/kg BID; effectiveness variable.

COMMENTS

- AD is a chronic, progressive, often relapsing and lifelong disease; it can be a frustrating disease for the client as well as for the clinician.
- Treatment should be aimed at management rather than "crisis management."
- Many factors may summate to cause intermittent flares (allergic threshold principle).
- AD rarely goes into remission and cannot be cured: some form of therapy may be necessary for life.
- Regular evaluations are necessary to achieve adequate control of symptoms and to manage flares.
- Treatment monitoring is based on medications prescribed (e.g., CBC, serum chemistry profile, and urinalysis with culture recommended every 6–12 months for patients on chronic immunomodulatory therapy).
- Although some allergens identified through testing can be avoided, immunotherapy is the only treatment that may resolve the allergic response (versus symptom control).
- Minimizing other sources of pruritus (e.g., fleas, food hypersensitivity, secondary skin infections) is crucial to reduce pruritus to acceptable levels.
- Secondary pyoderma, *Malassezia* dermatitis, and concurrent flea allergy dermatitis are common.
- This is not life-threatening unless intractable pruritus results in euthanasia.
- Inadequately managed, pruritus worsens and becomes less responsive to treatment; appropriate diagnosis and intervention should be initiated early.

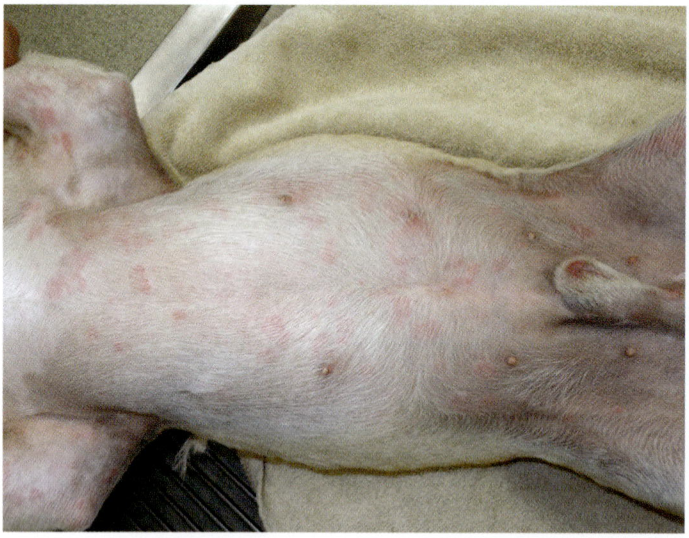

Fig. 11.1. Erythematous papules and urticaria on the ventrum of a 1-year-old MC French bulldog with AD.

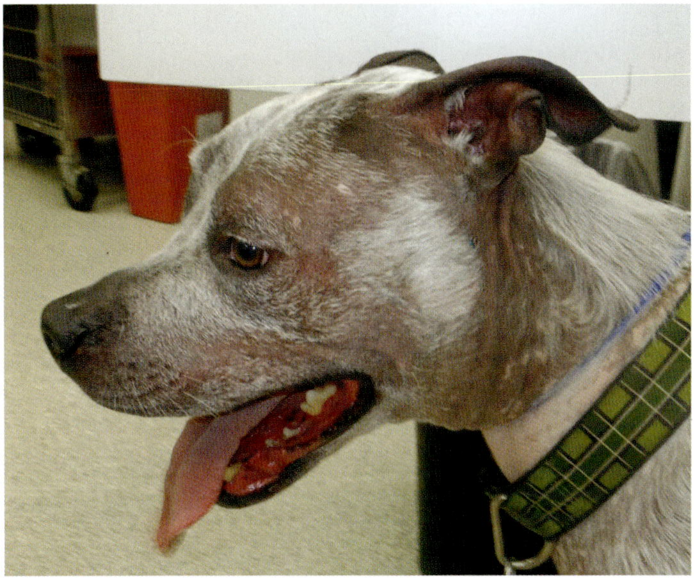

■ **Fig. 11.2.** Erythema, alopecia, and excoriations affecting the muzzle, face, and periocular areas of a patient with AD. Note erythematous pinnae.

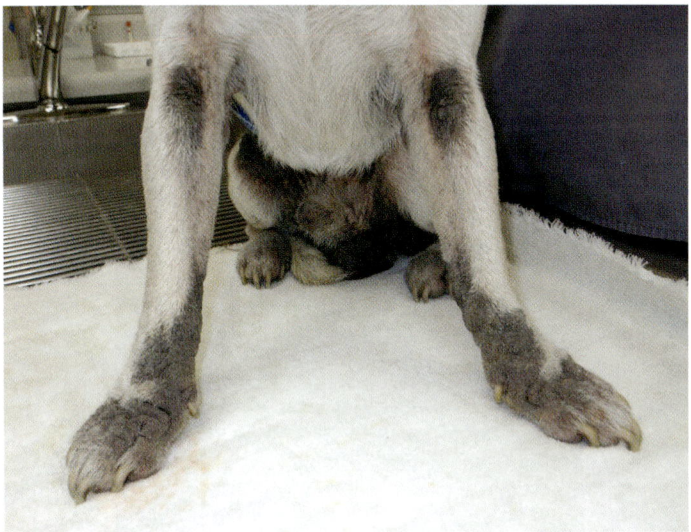

■ **Fig. 11.3.** Alopecia, lichenification, hyperpigmentation, and crusting affecting all four feet, the flexural surfaces of the forelegs, and the flank folds in a 6-year-old pug with chronic untreated AD. There was concurrent secondary pyoderma and *Malassezia* dermatitis.

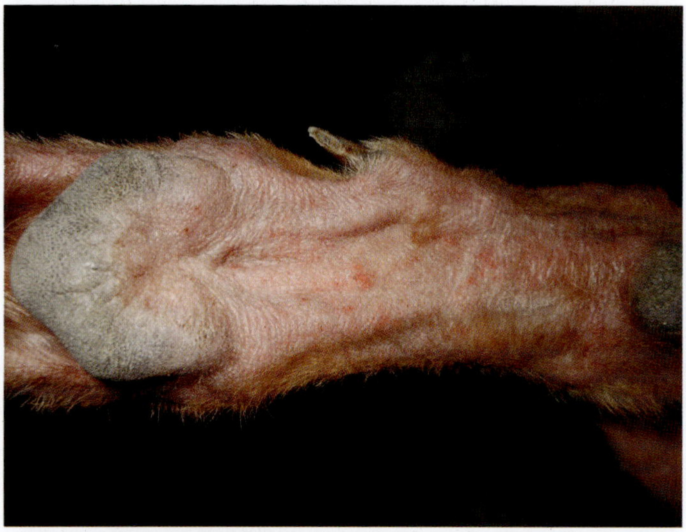

■ **Fig. 11.4.** Erythroderma with lichenification between the digital pads and between the metacarpal and accessory pads characteristic of AD.

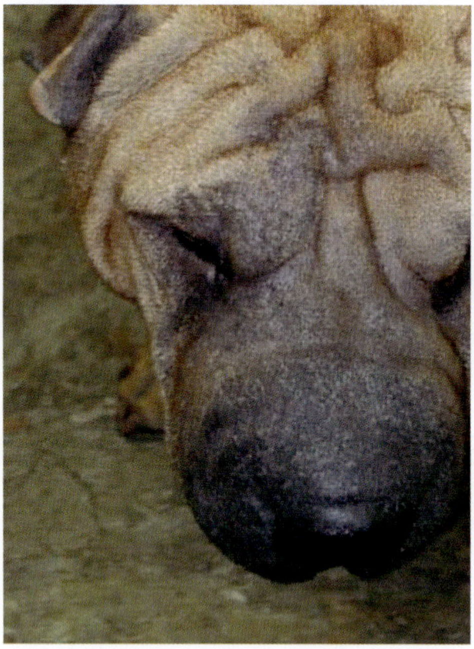

■ **Fig. 11.5.** Diffuse partial alopecia with erythema and secondary *Malassezia* hypersensitivity associated with AD.

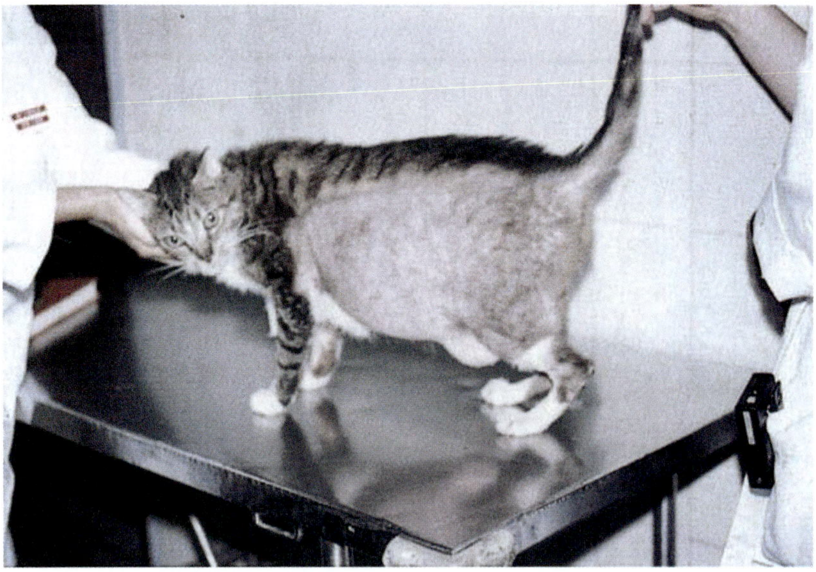

Fig. 11.6. Overgrooming/self-induced alopecia in a DSH with AD. Note the well-demarcated area of alopecia with no associated inflammation.

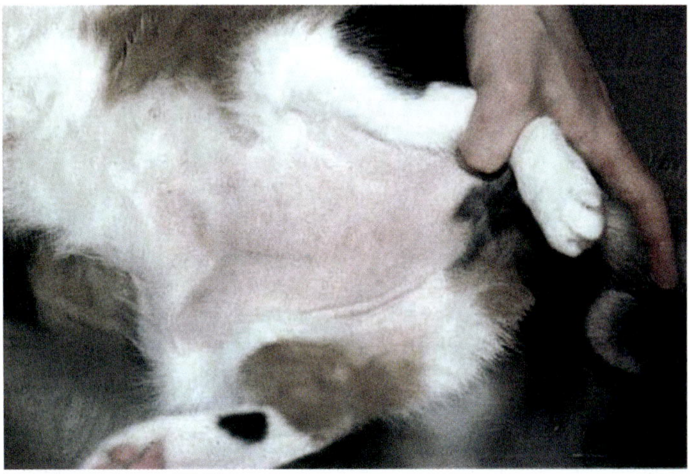

Fig. 11.7. Excessive grooming of the ventrum commonly seen in cats with AD.

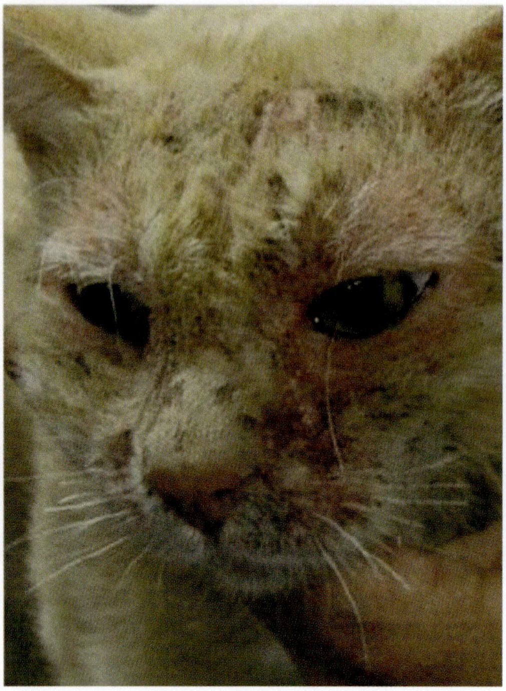

■ **Fig. 11.8.** Marked erythema, alopecia, and excoriation of the face in a DSH with AD.

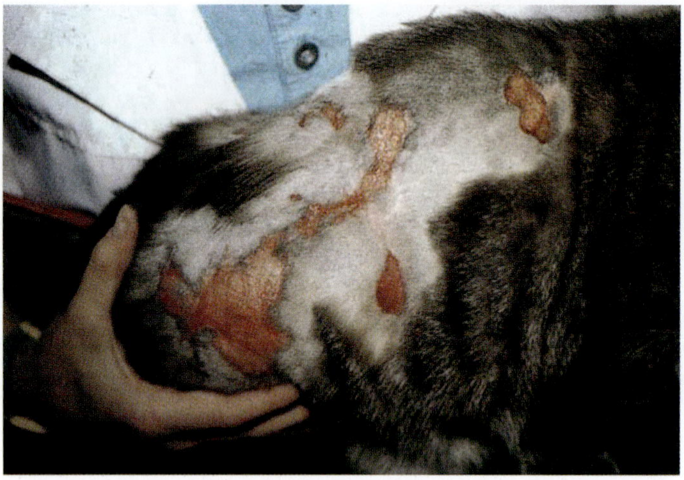

■ **Fig. 11.9.** Eosinophilic plaques: raised erythematous plaques on the body with areas of secondary excoriation from intense pruritus.

chapter 12

Autoimmune Blistering Diseases

DEFINITION/OVERVIEW

Pemphigus Complex

- Uncommon to rare autoimmune epidermal pustular dermatoses.
- Epidermal pustule and vesicle formation leads to varying degrees of erosion, ulceration, and crusting.
- Forms identified in animals:
    - Pemphigus foliaceus (PF)
    - Pemphigus erythematosus (PE)
    - Pemphigus vulgaris (PV)
    - Panepidermal pustular pemphigus/pemphigus vegetans (PEP/Pveg)
    - Paraneoplastic pemphigus (PP).

Pemphigoid Complex

- Very rare, autoimmune subepidermal blistering dermatoses (AISBD):
    - Bullous pemphigoid (BP)
    - Mucous membrane pemphigoid (MP).

Epidermolysis Bullosa Acquisita

- Chronic, very rare, autoimmune subepidermal blistering dermatosis.
- Most common AISBD.
- Also called cicatricial pemphigoid.

ETIOLOGY/PATHOPHYSIOLOGY

General Concepts

- Terminology:
    - Desmosome: major adhesion structure; creates tight connections between intracellular intermediate filaments of adjacent cells
    - Hemidesmosome: major adhesion structure on the basal keratinocytes at the epidermal-dermal junction

Blackwell's Five-Minute Veterinary Consult Clinical Companion: Small Animal Dermatology, Third Edition.
Karen Helton Rhodes and Alexander H. Werner.

- Components of desmosomes and hemidesmosomes may be targets of autoimmunity, and include:
  - Plakins (e.g., desmoplakin, bullous pemphigoid antigen 1): proteins that anchor filaments to desmosomal plaques
  - Armadillo protein (e.g., plakophilin, plakoglobin): structural and signaling proteins that share repeated amino acid sequences
  - Cadherins (e.g., desmoglein1–4, desmocollin1–3): transmembrane, calcium-dependent adhesion proteins
  - Plectin: links components of cytoskeleton (actin microfilaments, microtubules, intermediate filaments) in hemidesmosomes
  - Integrins: heterodimers with alpha and beta subunits; transmembrane receptor glycoproteins that mediate adhesion
  - Laminin (specifically laminin 5): structural glycoproteins in the extracellular matrix (with alpha, beta, and gamma chains)
  - Collagen (type VII and XVII): transmembrane structural components (anchoring fibrils) of hemidesmosomes.
- Autoimmune blistering diseases: circulating autoantibodies (most commonly IgG) bind to structural components to induce cell separation within desmosomes of the epidermis or hemidesmosomes at the basement membrane zone (BMZ).
- Acantholysis: disruption of desmosomes causing keratinocyte separation; disruption of hemidesmosomes causes blistering beneath the epidermis and thus does not cause acantholysis.
- Acantholysis may have genetic, infectious (proteolytic), or autoimmune causes.
- Binding of autoantibodies causes steric hindrance (direct interference with function), triggering of (or impaired) transmembrane signaling resulting in desmosome depletion, and/or reduction of acetylcholine-induced phosphorylation leading to abnormal desmosome production.
- Loss of intracellular cohesion produces vesicles, pustules, and/or bullae.
- Severity of erosion, ulceration, and disease: related to location of autoantibody deposition (specific structure molecule targeted) within or beneath the epidermis.

Pemphigus Complex

- PF: precise autoantibody antigen unknown but targets the superficial epidermis; some cases demonstrate anti-desmoglein (Dsg) 1 IgG.
- PE: autoantibody targets Dsg1 and antigens expressed on epidermal cells following ultraviolet light exposure.
- PV: autoantibody targets Dsg3; additional targeting of Dsg1 with mucosal lesions.
- PEP/Pveg: autoantibody targets Dsg1 (suggesting PEP is a more severe variant of PF and not PV as in humans).
- PP: autoantibody targets Dsg3, desmoplakin, and possibly plakoglobin.
- Implicated trigger factors are varied: genetics, hormones, neoplasia, drugs, nutrition, viral, emotional stress, and physical factors (burns, UV radiation).
- Pemphigus may be drug induced (directly initiate acantholysis) or drug triggered (cause symptomatic disease in predisposed individuals).

Pemphigoid Complex

- Heterogenous group of autoantibodies targeting various basement membrane zone components.
- Targets include specific (αβ) integrins, plakins (bullous pemphigoid antigen), and collagen type XVII.
- Autoantibodies in mucous membrane pemphigoid may also target laminin 5.
- Binding of autoantibodies at the BMZ leads to activation of complement and recruitment of inflammatory cells; released proteases damage the BMZ to cause blister formation.

Epidermolysis Bullosa Acquisita

- Autoantibodies target collagen VII within hemidesmosomes.
- Pathomechanism similar to pemphigoid: binding of autoantibodies at the BMZ leads to activation of complement and recruitment of inflammatory cells; released proteases damage the BMZ to cause blister formation.

SIGNALMENT/HISTORY

Pemphigus Complex

- Uncommon group of diseases.
- Usually middle-aged to old animals.
- PF:
  - Most common type
  - Dogs: Akita, chow chow, dachshund, spaniels, English bulldog; median age of onset 4 years; rarely develops in young dogs.
  - Cats: no breed or sex predisposition; median age of onset 5 years.
  - Most commonly implicated drug causes: antibiotics (sulfonamides, cephalexin), methimazole.
  - Insecticide-contact PF: amitraz-metaflumizone product; large-breed dogs (Figure 12.1).
- PE:
  - Uncommon
  - May be a more benign variant of PF or may be a cross-over syndrome of pemphigus and lupus erythematosus
  - Collie, German shepherd dog, and Shetland sheepdog
  - Aggravated by ultraviolet light exposure.
- PV:
  - Rare
  - Most severe form
  - German shepherd dog, collie; males predisposed; median age of onset 6 years.
- PEP/Pveg: rarest type; course of disease may represent a more severe variant of PF.
- PP: rare; clinical signs vary from severe to relatively benign crusted lesions.

Pemphigoid Complex

- Very rare.
- Collie, Shetland sheepdog, doberman pinscher and dachshund may be predisposed.
- Mucous membrane pemphigoid: German shepherd dog; median age of onset 6 years.

Epidermolysis Bullosa Acquisita

- Very rare.
- Great Dane; not yet described in cats.
- Male predisposition; earlier age of onset; median 15 months of age.

CLINICAL FEATURES

Pemphigus Complex

- PF:
  - Transient waves of vesicles and pustules coalescing to crusted patches (Figure 12.2)
  - Scales, crust, pustules, epidermal collarettes, erosions, erythema, alopecia, and footpad hyperkeratosis with fissuring
  - Ulcerations indicate a deeper disease and/or secondary bacterial infection
  - Dogs:
    - Facial lesions: nasal planum, dorsal muzzle, periorbital ("butterfly" pattern), and pinnae (Figures 12.3–12.5)
    - Footpad margins (Figures 12.6, 12.7)
    - Truncal patches of crusts, scales, vesicles, and pustules (Figure 12.8)
    - Mucosal and mucocutaneous lesions rare; due to secondary infection
  - Cats: facial as well as nipple and ungual fold involvement common (Figures 12.9–12.11)
  - Lymphadenopathy, edema, depression, fever, and lameness (if footpads involved) in more severe or chronic cases; however, patients are often in good health
  - Variable pain and pruritus.
- PE:
  - Similar to PF
  - Facially confined lesions; rarely footpads
  - Aggravated by ultraviolet light; seasonality possible in certain geographic locations
  - Depigmentation of the nasal planum, dorsal muzzle, lip margins, and eyelid margins common, and may precede crusting (Figure 12.12)
  - No oral or mucosal lesions
  - ANA rarely positive.
- PV:
  - Oral ulceration frequent and may precede skin lesions
  - Ulcerative lesions, erosions, epidermal collarettes, blisters, and crusts

- Vesicles and bullae may persist longer due to thickness of the overlying epidermis
- Rupture leads to deep crateriform erosions progressing quickly to ulcerations
- More severe than PF and PE; patients often ill
- Affects mucous membranes, mucocutaneous junctions, and skin; may become generalized (Figure 12.13)
- Positive Nikolsky sign (new or extended erosive lesion created when lateral pressure is applied to the skin near an existing lesion)
- Friction and trauma areas (axillae, inguinum, limb pressure points)
- Paw pads and nails may slough
- Variable pruritus and pain
- Anorexia, depression, and fever
- Secondary bacterial infections common.

■ PEP/Pveg:
- Vesicles and bullae develop in all layers of the epidermis, including follicles
- Pustule groups become eruptive papillomatous lesions and vegetative masses (thick, adherent crusts) that ooze (Figure 12.14)
- No oral or mucosal lesions
- Systemic illness associated with secondary bacterial infection.

■ PP:
- Very rare
- Blistering disease with flaccid pustules, erosions, ulcerations affecting the mucosae and mucocutaneous junctions as well as haired skin (Figures 12.15–12.17)
- Seen in conjunction with neoplasia
- Systemic signs associated both with neoplasia and cutaneous lesions
- Reported neoplasia: thymoma, thymic lymphosarcoma, splenic sarcoma.

Pemphigoid Complex

- Signs similar to PV, although blisters are less fragile.
- Chronic, clinically benign disease most common.
- Macules lead to vesicles and bullae that rupture to reveal ulcerations.
- Common sites: head, ears, axillae, ventral abdomen, inguinum.
- Uncommonly affects footpads and ungual folds (Figure 12.18).
- Scarring is common.
- Variable pruritus and pain.
- Anorexia, depression, and fever.
- Mucous membrane pemphigoid:
  - May be the more common presentation of BP
  - Symmetrical lesions
  - Vesicles rapidly lead to ulcerations of the oral cavity, lip margins, periocular, nasal and genital mucosae (Figure 12.19)
  - Over 90% of dogs exhibit erosions in more than one mucosal region.

Epidermolysis Bullosa Acquisita

- Erythematous plaques and vesicles leading to ulcerations (Figure 12.20a).
- Common sites: face, concave pinnae, axillae, ventral abdomen, inguinum.
- Lesions nearly always affect oral mucosa.
- Footpad sloughing (Figure 12.20b,c).
- Areas of pressure or trauma commonly affected (Figure 12.20d).
- Scarring is common.
- Variable pruritus and pain.
- Anorexia, depression, and fever.

DIFFERENTIAL DIAGNOSIS

Pemphigus Complex

- PF:
    - Bacterial folliculitis
    - Neutrophilic or eosinophilic furunculosis
    - Dermatophytosis
    - Demodicosis
    - Leishmaniasis
    - Sebaceous adenitis
    - Keratinization disorders
    - Discoid or cutaneous lupus erythematosus
    - Pemphigus erythematosus
    - Subcorneal pustular dermatosis
    - Drug eruption
    - Erythema multiforme
    - Zinc-responsive dermatitis
    - Dermatomyositis
    - Tyrosinemia
    - Epitheliotropic lymphoma
    - Lymphoreticular malignancies
    - Superficial necrolytic dermatosis
    - Uveodermatologic syndrome
    - Sterile eosinophilic pustulosis
    - Linear IgA dermatosis.
- PE:
    - Pemphigus foliaceus (facially oriented)
    - Systemic lupus erythematosus
    - Discoid lupus erythematosus
    - Bacterial folliculitis
    - Neutrophilic or eosinophilic furunculosis
    - Demodicosis
    - Dermatophytosis

    - Eptheliotropic lymphoma
    - Epidermolysis bullosa simplex
    - Uveodermatologic syndrome.
- PV:
    - Bullous pemphigoid
    - Systemic lupus erythematosus
    - Paraneoplastic pemphigus
    - Toxic epidermal necrolysis
    - Epidermolysis bullosa acquisita
    - Drug eruption
    - Superficial necrolytic dermatitis
    - Epitheliotropic lymphoma
    - Lymphoreticular neoplasia
    - Causes of ulcerative stomatitis
    - Erythema multiforme.
- PEP/Pveg:
    - Pemphigus vulgaris
    - Erythema multiforme
    - Bacterial folliculitis
    - Leishmaniasis
    - Pemphigus foliaceus
    - Lichenoid dermatoses
    - Cutaneous neoplasia.
- PP:
    - Pemphigus vulgaris
    - Bullous pemphigoid
    - Erythema multiforme.

Pemphigoid Complex

- Pemphigus vulgaris
- Systemic lupus erythematosus
- Drug eruption
- Erythema multiforme
- Toxic epidermal necrolysis
- Epitheliotropic lymphoma
- Lymphoreticular neoplasia
- Causes of ulcerative stomatitis

Epidermolysis Bullosa Acquisita

- Pemphigus vulgaris
- Systemic lupus erythematosus
- Drug eruption
- Erythema multiforme

- Toxic epidermal necrolysis
- Epitheliotropic lymphoma
- Lymphoreticular neoplasia
- Causes of ulcerative stomatitis

DIAGNOSTICS

CBC/Biochemistry/Urinalysis

- Neutrophilia and hyperglobulinemia.
- Abnormalities may be related to underlying pathology (i.e., neoplasia producing PP) or from chronic inflammation or infection.
- Baseline values should be obtained prior to initiating immunosuppressive therapy.

Other Laboratory Tests

- Antinuclear antibody: may be weakly positive in PE only.

Diagnostic Procedures

- Cytology of aspirates or impression smears of pustules or crusts:
    - Acantholytic keratinocytes, neutrophils and eosinophils
    - Acantholytic keratinocytes appear as rounded, darkly stained cells with prominent nuclei ("fried egg") (Figure 12.21)
    - No acantholytic cells in BP or EBA; rare in PV due to depth of clefting.
- Bacteriologic culture: identify secondary bacterial infections.
- Biopsy of lesions with dermatohistopathologic examination required for diagnosis.
- Biopsy samples should be obtained from lesional or perilesional skin.

Pathologic Findings – Pemphigus Complex

- PF: acantholytic keratinocytes in crusts; acantholysis and intraepidermal clefting; microabscess or pustule formation that spans and extends into follicles; acantholytic keratinocytes may be individual, associated together into "rafts" or adherent to the overlying epidermis ("cling-ons"); dermal inflammation mixed and perivascular neutophilic and eosinophilic (Figure 12.22).
- PE: findings similar to PF; lichenoid interface dermatitis with basal cell damage; pigmentary incontinence.
- PV: suprabasilar clefting with acantholytic keratinocytes; individual keratinocytes remain attached to the basement zone creating a "tombstone" pattern; secondary ulceration common; degree of superficial dermal inflammation variable.
- PEP/Pveg: pustules present throughout the epidermal layers and includes the follicular epithelium.
- PP: transepidermal pustulation with suprabasilar and superficial acantholysis; prominent apoptotic keratinocytes; dermal or submucosal infiltrate of lymphocytes, macrophages, and plasma cells; variable numbers of neutrophils.

- Immunopathology of biopsied skin via immunofluorescent antibody assays or immunohistochemical testing.
    - Results can be affected by concurrent or previous corticosteroid (or other immunosuppressive drug) administration.
    - Indirect immunofluorescence usually negative.
    - PF: positive staining for Dsg1 in the superficial epithelia in 50–90% of cases.
    - PE may demonstrate staining of basement membranes and intercellular spaces.
    - PV: positive staining for Dsg3 in the deep epithelia.
    - PP: positive staining for one or both Dsg1 and Dsg3 with desmoplakin.

Pathologic Findings – Pemphigoid Complex

- Subepidermal vesicle.
- Predominantly eosinophilic inflammatory infiltrate; numbers significantly lower with MP.
- No acantholytic keratinocytes: defect is subepidermal.
- Dermal and submucosal inflammation due to secondary infection or insult.
- Direct immunofluorescence positive at the BMZ.

Pathologic Findings – Epidermolysis Bullosa Acquisita

- Subepidermal vesicle.
- Predominantly acellular.
- No acantholytic keratinocytes: defect is subepidermal.
- Neutrophilic dermal infiltrate.
- Direct immunofluorescence positive at the BMZ.

THERAPEUTICS

General Considerations

- Initial inpatient supportive therapy for severely affected patients.
- Outpatient treatment with initial frequent hospital visits (every 1–3 weeks); taper to every 1–3 months when remission is achieved and the patient is on a maintenance medical regimen.
- Severely affected patients may require antibiotics based on culture and sensitivity testing.
- Hydrotherapy and soaks very helpful and soothing.
- Avoid ultraviolet light – may exacerbate lesions (especially PE).

Drugs of Choice – Pemphigus Complex

- PF and PV:
    - Corticosteroids:
        - Prednisolone: 2.2–6.6 mg/kg/day PO divided BID to achieve clinical remission; alternative pulse dose therapy: 10 mg/kg q24h for 3 days followed by standard dosing at 2.2 mg/kg/day

- Minimum maintenance: 0.5 mg/kg q48–72h
- Taper dosage at 2–4-week intervals.
- Cytotoxic agents:
  - More than half of patients require the addition of other immunomodulating drugs.
  - Synergistic with corticosteroids, allowing reduction in dose and side effects.
  - Azathioprine (2 mg/kg or 50 mg/m^2 PO q24h, then q48–72h); rarely used in cats due to marked bone marrow suppression; feline dose 1 mg/kg q24–48h
  - Chlorambucil (0.2 mg/kg daily): primary choice for cats and small dogs
  - Mycophenolate mofetil: 20–40 mg/kg/day PO divided BID to TID
  - Chrysotherapy: auranofin (0.1–0.2 mg/kg PO BID to q24h).
- Cyclosporine, microemulsion:
  - Alternative or supplemental therapy with corticosteroids
  - Initial dosage: 5–10 mg/kg/day until remission; then EOD or twice weekly.
- Tacrolimus topical (Protopic): apply to individual lesions daily to twice weekly.

- PE and PEP:
  - Cycline antibiotics: tetracycline (250 mg PO q8h dogs <10 kg; 500 mg PO q8h dogs >10 kg); doxycycline (10 mg/kg PO q24h); minocycline (5 mg/kg PO BID); often administered with niacinamide 250 mg PO for dogs <10 kg and 500 mg PO for dogs >10 kg
  - Topical corticosteroids – betamethasone diproprionate 0.05% or fluocinolone 0.1%: apply sparingly q24h for 14 days; then EOD or twice weekly; if in remission, switch to less potent product (e.g., 0.5% or 2.5% hydrocortisone)
  - Topical tacrolimus 0.1%: apply sparingly q24h for 14 days; then EOD or twice weekly
  - Prednisolone: 1–2 mg/kg PO BID initially tapered to EOD or twice weekly either alone or in combination with cytotoxic immunosuppressive drugs
  - Azathioprine: 2 mg/kg or 50 mg/m^2 PO daily until remission; then EOD or twice weekly; not for use in cats
  - Chlorambucil: 0.1–0.2 mg/kg/day until remission; then EOD or twice weekly
  - Cyclosporine, microemulsion: 5–10 mg/kg/day until remission; then EOD or twice weekly.
  - Leflunomide: 2–4 mg/kg/day or divided BID
  - Mycophenolate mofetil: 20–40 mg/kg/day PO divided BID to TID
  - Vitamin E: 10–20 IU/kg PO q12h; may help reduce inflammation.
- PP:
  - Identify underlying neoplasia and resolve or control
  - Additional treatment similar to PF/PE.

Drugs of Choice – Pemphigoid Complex

- Cycline antibiotics: tetracycline (250 mg PO q8h dogs <10 kg; 500 mg PO q8h dogs >10 kg); doxycycline (10 mg/kg PO q24h); minocycline (5 mg/kg PO BID); often administered with niacinamide 250 mg PO for dogs <10 kg and 500 mg PO for dogs >10 kg.

- Additional treatment similar to PF/PE in recalcitrant cases.
- Corticosteroid monotherapy not recommended.
- Many cases are chronic and mild, necessitating minimal intervention.

Drugs of Choice – Epidermolysis Bullosa Acquisita

- Corticosteroids:
  - Prednisolone: 2.2–6.6 mg/kg/day PO divided BID to achieve clinical remission
  - Minimum maintenance: 0.5 mg/kg q48–72h
  - Taper dosage at 2–4-week intervals.
- Cytotoxic agents:
- Azathioprine (2 mg/kg or 50 mg/m^2 PO q24h, then q48–72h)
- Mycophenolate mofetil: 20–40 mg/kg/day PO divided BID to TID
- Colchicine 0.03 mg/kg PO q24h.
- Cyclosporine:
  - Alternative or supplemental therapy with corticosteroids
  - Initial dosage 5 mg/kg PO daily.

Alternative Corticosteroids

- Use instead of prednisolone if undesirable side effects or poor response occur.
- Methylprednisolone (initial dosage 0.8–1.5 mg/kg PO BID): patients that tolerate prednisolone poorly.
- Triamcinolone (0.2–0.3 mg/kg PO BID; then 0.05–0.1 mg/kg EOD to twice weekly).
- Dexamethasone (0.1–0.2 mg/kg PO q24h; then 0.05 mg/kg twice weekly).

Topical Steroids

- Hydrocortisone cream.
- More potent topical corticosteroids: 0.1% betamethasone valerate, fluocinolone acetonide, or 0.1% triamcinonide; BID tapering to EOD or twice weekly.

COMMENTS

Patient Monitoring

- Monitor response to therapy at 2–4-week intervals initially; monitor less frequently as lesions heal and medication dosages are reduced.
- Routine hematology and serum biochemistry, especially patients on high doses of corticosteroids, cytotoxic drugs, or chrysotherapy; check every 2–4 weeks, and then every 1–3 months when in remission.
- Common side effects:
  - Corticosteroids: polyuria, polydipsia, polyphagia, temperament changes, diabetes mellitus, pancreatitis, and hepatotoxicity
  - Azathioprine: pancreatitis, bone marrow suppression

- Chlorambucil: leukopenia, thrombocytopenia, nephrotoxicity, and hepatotoxicity
- Chrysotherapy: leukopenia, thrombocytopenia, nephrotoxicity, dermatitis, stomatitis, and allergic reactions
- Cyclosporine: vomiting, diarrhea, hirsutism, psoriasiform lichenoid-like dermatitis
- Mycophenolate mofetil: vomiting, diarrhea, lymphopenia
- Colchicine: vomiting, diarrhea, rare bone marrow suppression
- Immunosuppression: can predispose animal to demodectic mange, cutaneous and systemic bacterial and fungal infection.

Expected Course and Prognosis – Pemphigus Complex

- PF, PV, PEP/Pveg:
  - Lifelong therapy with corticosteroids and cytotoxic drugs needed; remission rare
  - Routine monitoring paramount
  - Side effects of medications may affect quality of life
  - May be fatal if untreated (especially PV)
  - Secondary infections cause morbidity and possible mortality (especially PV).
- PE:
  - Relatively benign and self-limiting
  - Oral corticosteroids may eventually be tapered to low maintenance doses or may be stopped in some patients
  - Dermatitis worsens if untreated; systemic symptoms are rare
  - Prognosis fair.
- PP:
  - Grave prognosis due to underlying neoplasia.

Expected Course and Prognosis – Pemphigoid Complex

- Lifelong therapy necessary.
- In severe cases, aggressive initial intervention is usually required; some cases do not respond to treatment.
- Chronic cases may be controlled with cycline antibiotics/niacinamide and/or topical therapy.
- Morbidity is associated with secondary bacterial infection.

Expected Course and Prognosis – Epidermolysis Bullosa Acquisita

- Lifelong therapy may be necessary.
- In severe cases, aggressive initial intervention is usually required; some cases do not respond to treatment.
- Morbidity is associated with oral lesions and secondary bacterial infection.

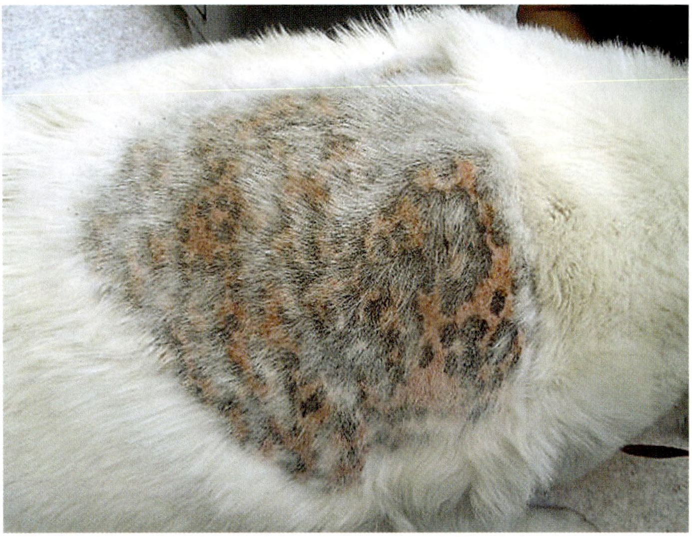

■ **Fig. 12.1.** Insecticide-induced pemphigus foliaceus: a large patch of alopecia with erythema, crusting, and thickening at the location of application (dorsal shoulder region) in a 6-year-old male-castrate Akita. Complete clinical remission was achieved with treatment.

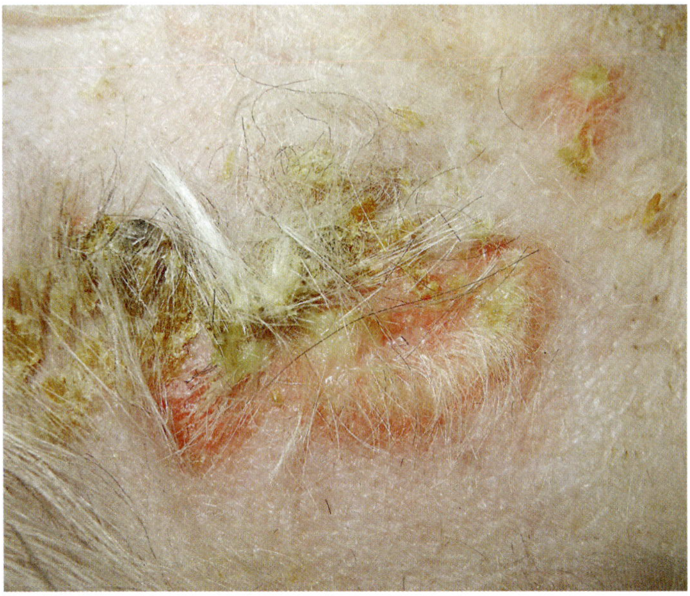

■ **Fig. 12.2.** Large, panfollicular and coalescing, flaccid pustules with secondary crusts characteristic of pemphigus foliaceus.

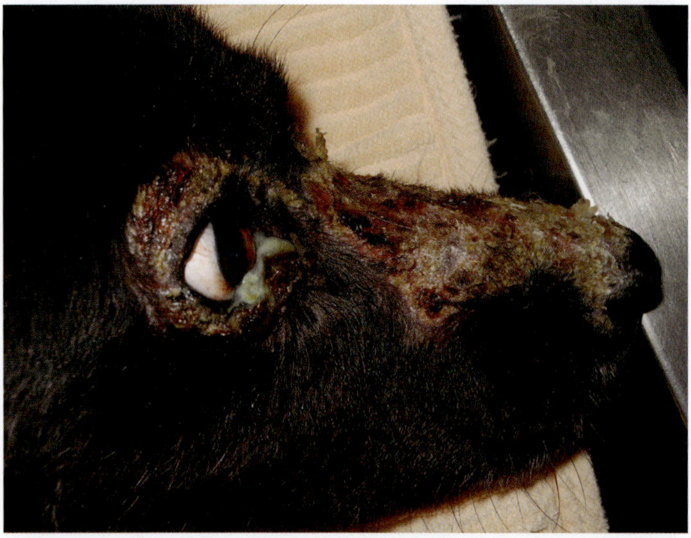

■ **Fig. 12.3.** Facial lesions in a "butterfly" pattern (around the nasal planum, up the dorsal muzzle, and around the eyes) with crusting and alopecia on the face of an 8-year-old male-castrate Labrador retriever mix with pemphigus foliaceus.

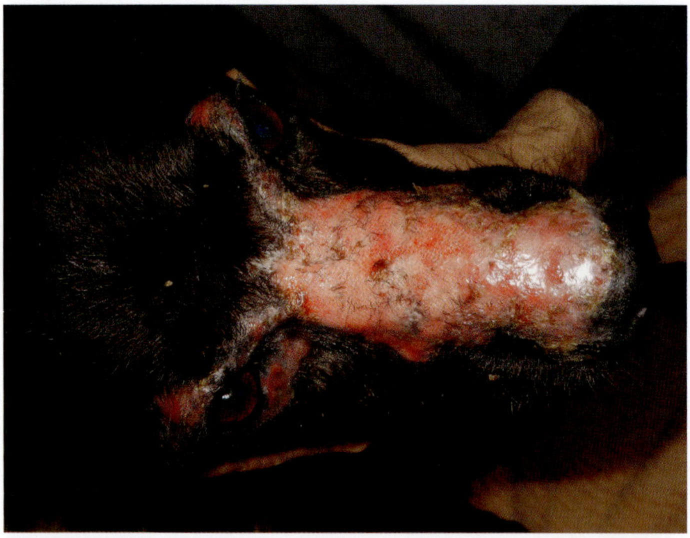

■ **Fig. 12.4.** Erosions seen after removing crusts from lesions of the patient in Figure 12.3.

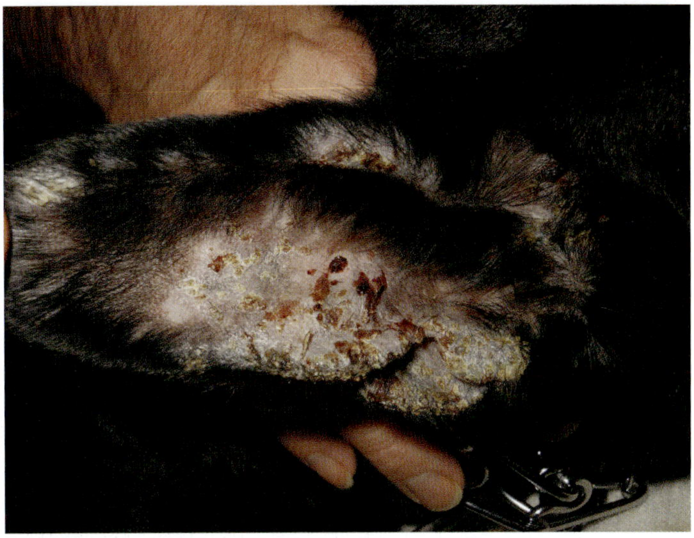

■ **Fig. 12.5.** Accumulations of crusts on the pinna of a 4-year-old male-castrate German shepherd-chow mix with pemphigus foliaceus.

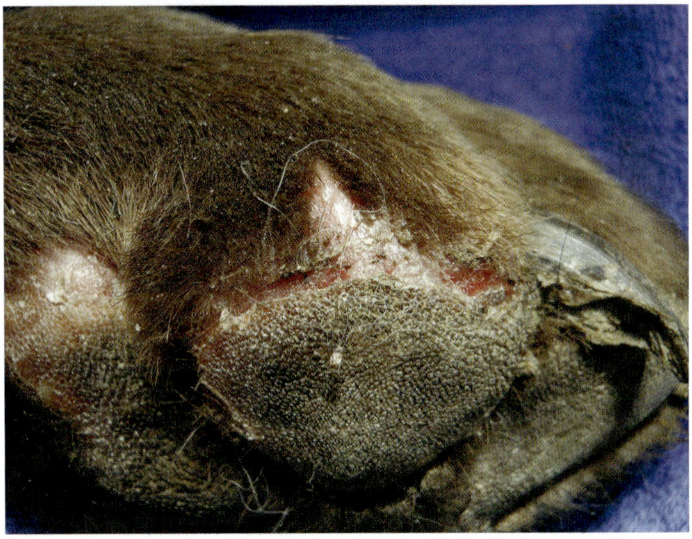

■ **Fig. 12.6.** Thickening and erosions at the margins of the footpads with pemphigus foliaceus. The adjacent nail is misshapen due to chronic inflammation in this 10-year-old male-castrate Labrador retriever.

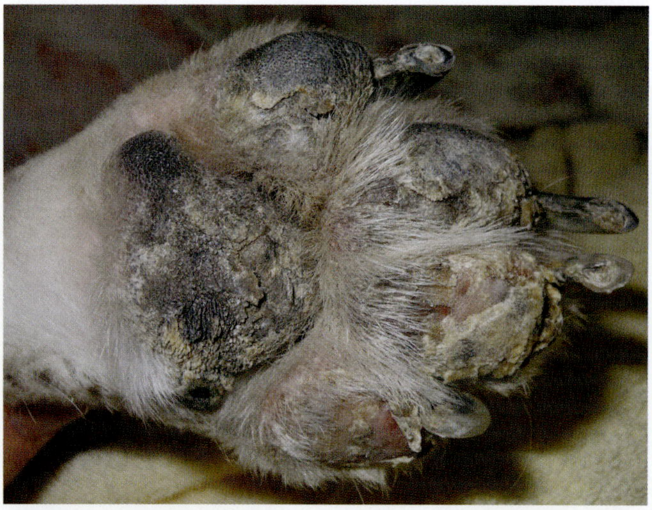

■ **Fig. 12.7.** Hyperkeratotic footpads with adherent crusts and mild erosions in a 6-year-old male-castrate English bulldog with pemphigus foliaceus.

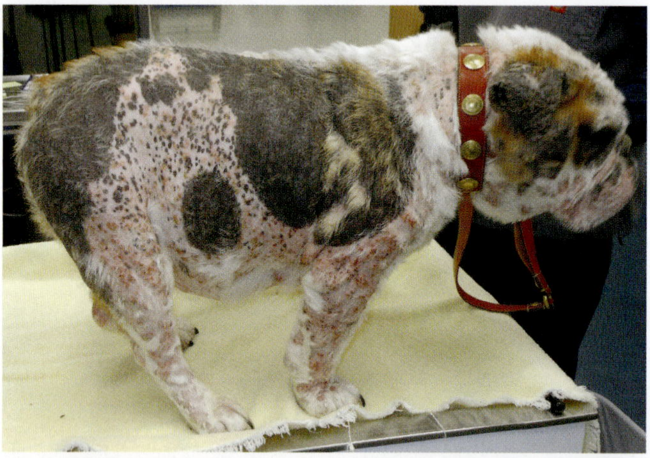

(a)

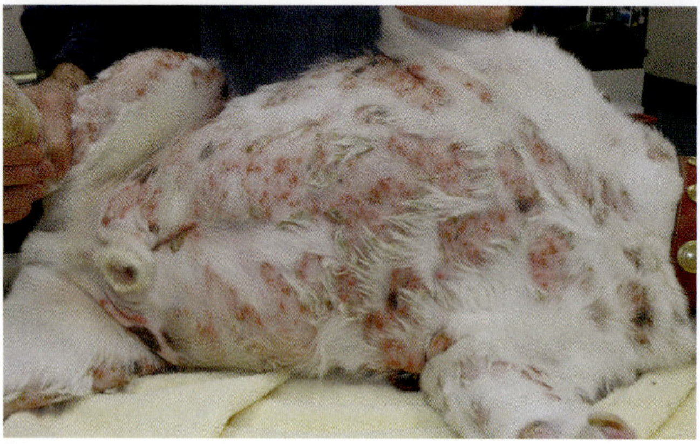

(b)

■ **Fig. 12.8.** Generalized lesions consisting of punctate pustules, crusted papules, crusts, and erythema in the patient of Figure 12.7.

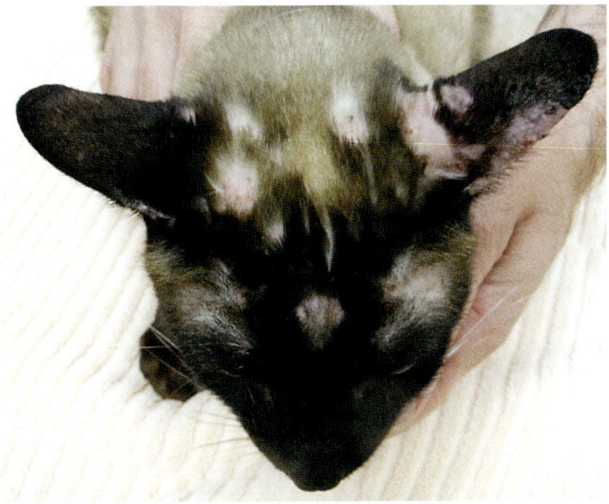

■ **Fig. 12.9.** Pemphigus foliaceus in a 7-year-old female-spayed Siamese. Lesions of alopecia and crusted are noted on the face and pinnae.

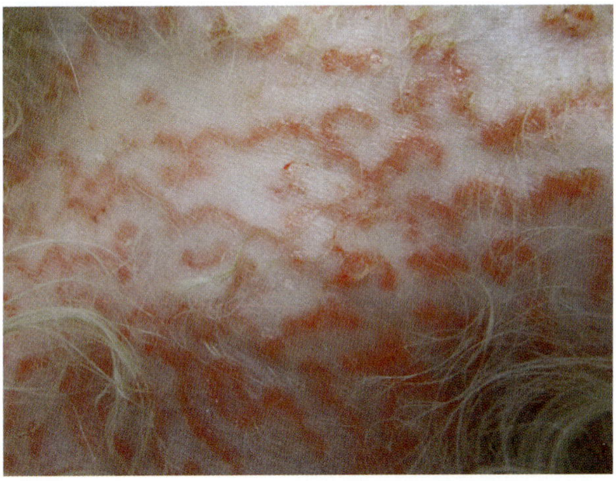

■ **Fig. 12.10.** Serpiginous erythematous and exudative lesions on the ventrum of a 13-year-old female-spayed DLH with pemphigus foliaceus.

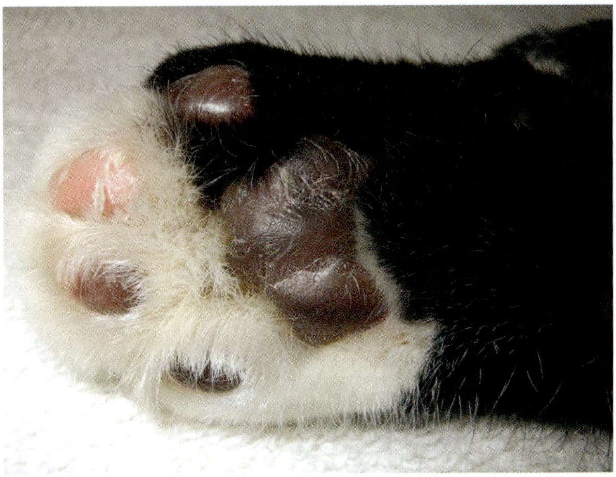

■ **Fig. 12.11.** Subtle thickening, crusting, and scaling affecting the footpads on a 1-year-old male-castrate DSH with pemphigus foliaceus.

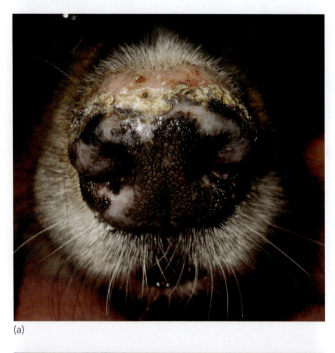

(a)

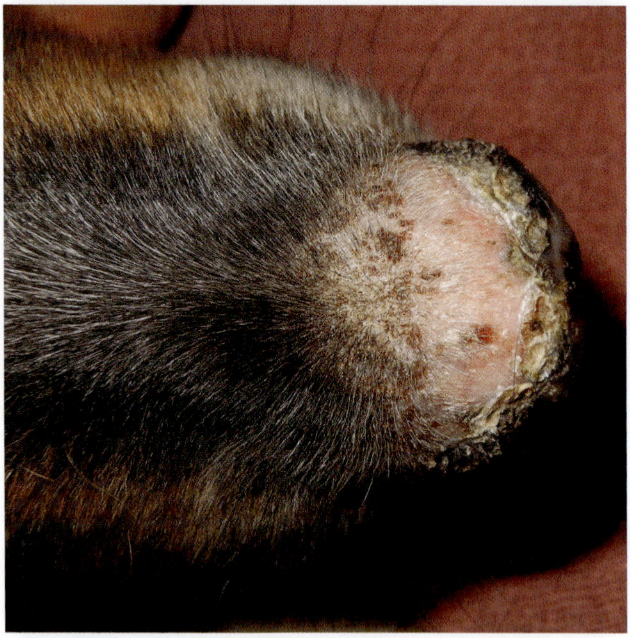

(b)

■ **Fig. 12.12.** Pemphigus erythematosus in a 7-year-old female-spayed Australian shepherd. Lesions are confined to the nasal planum and adjacent dorsal muzzle. Unlike pemphigus foliaceus, areas of depigmentation precede and are more significant than accumulated crusts.

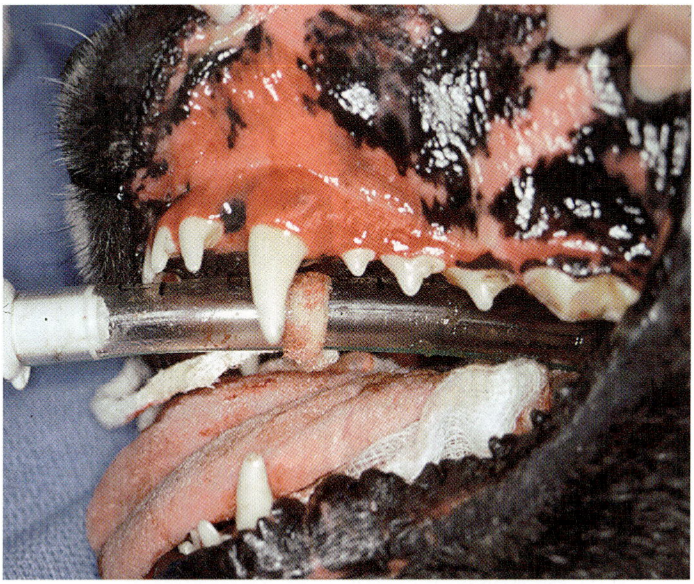

(a)

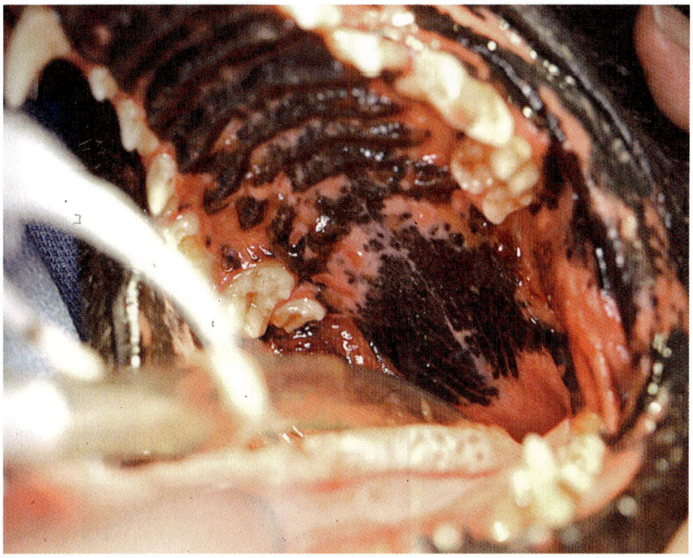

(b)

■ **Fig. 12.13.** Oral and gingival erosions and ulcerations in a patient with pemphigus vulgaris. Lesions are most evident on the hard palate surrounded by areas of depigmentation.

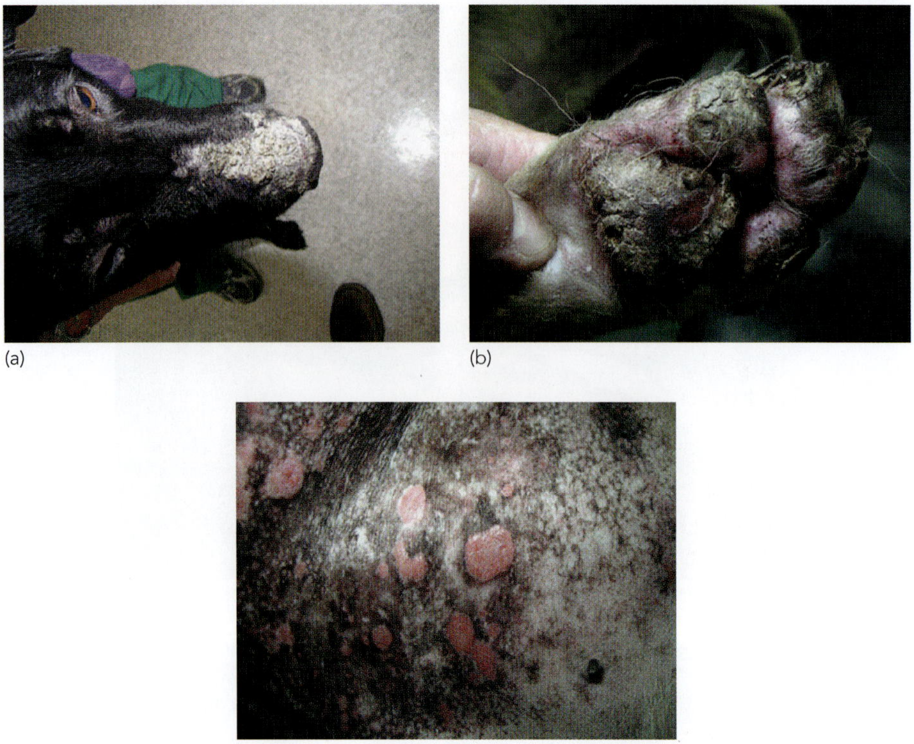

(a) (b) (c)

■ **Fig. 12.14.** Panepidermal pemphigus/pemphigus vegetans in a chow-mix. Lesions are thickly crusted with underlying erosions and inflammation.

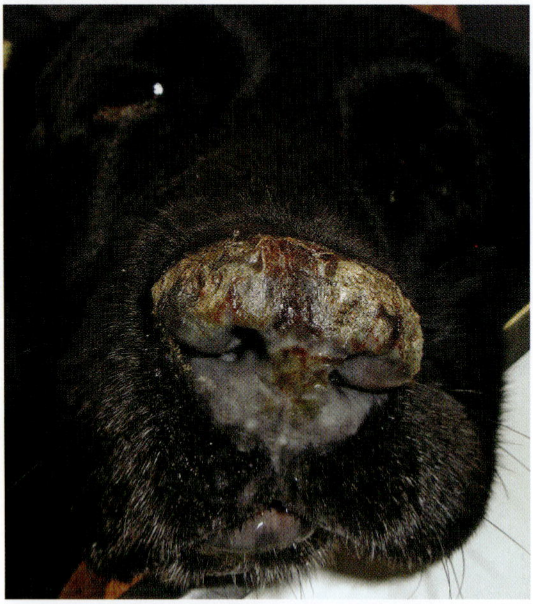

■ **Fig. 12.15.** Depigmentation, crusting, and swelling of the nasal planum in an 11-year-old female-spayed Labrador retriever with paraneoplastic pemphigus from a thoracic tumor.

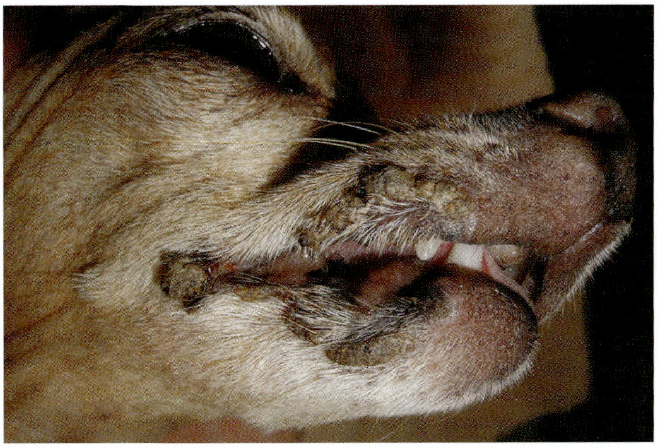

■ **Fig. 12.16.** Thick lip margin crusting with mucous membrane erosions in a 10-year-old female-spayed chihuahua diagnosed with paraneoplastic pemphigus.

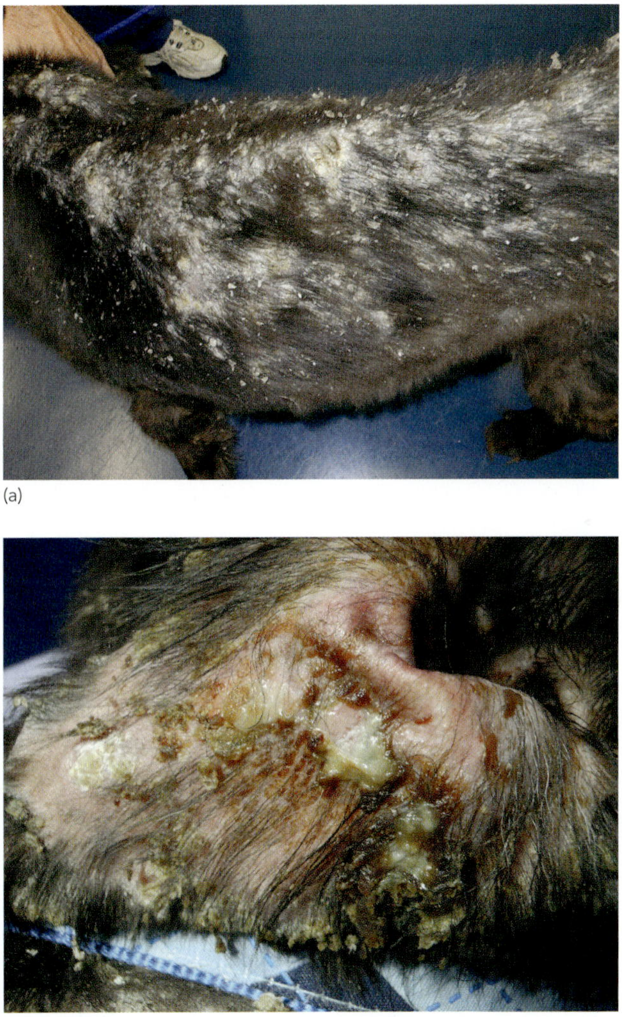

(a)

(b)

■ **Fig. 12.17.** Generalized and thick crusted lesions of paraneoplastic pemphigus with exudative purulent lesions on the pinnae in an 11-year-old male-castrate Labrador retriever-Newfoundland cross with a splenic mass.

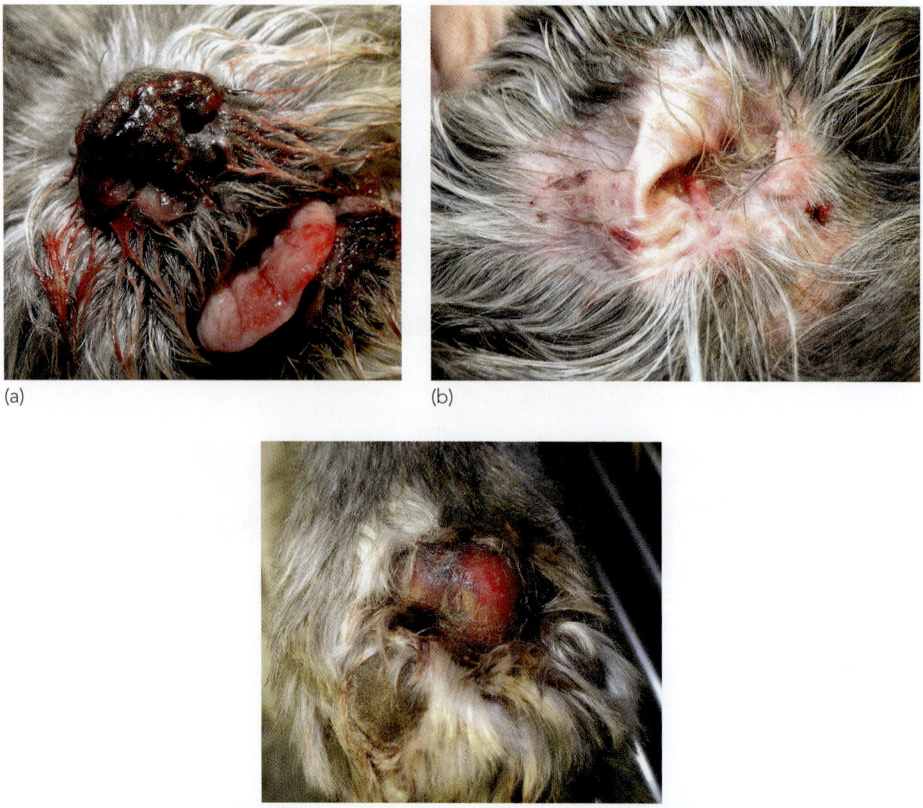
(a) (b) (c)

■ **Fig. 12.18.** Bullous pemphigoid in a 7-year-old male-castrate shih tzu. (a) Erosions on the nasal planum, tongue, and lip margins. (b) Erosions on the concave pinna. (c) Erosions affecting the footpads and interdigital regions.

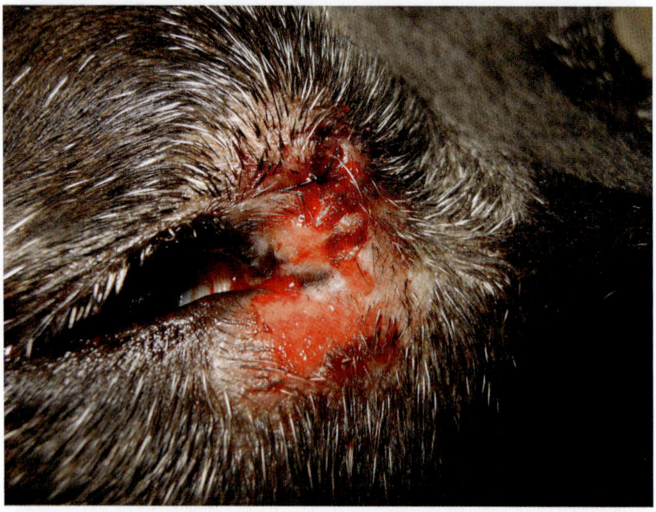

■ **Fig. 12.19.** Erosions at the medial canthus of mucous membrane pemphigoid in a 9-year-old female-spayed mixed breed dog.

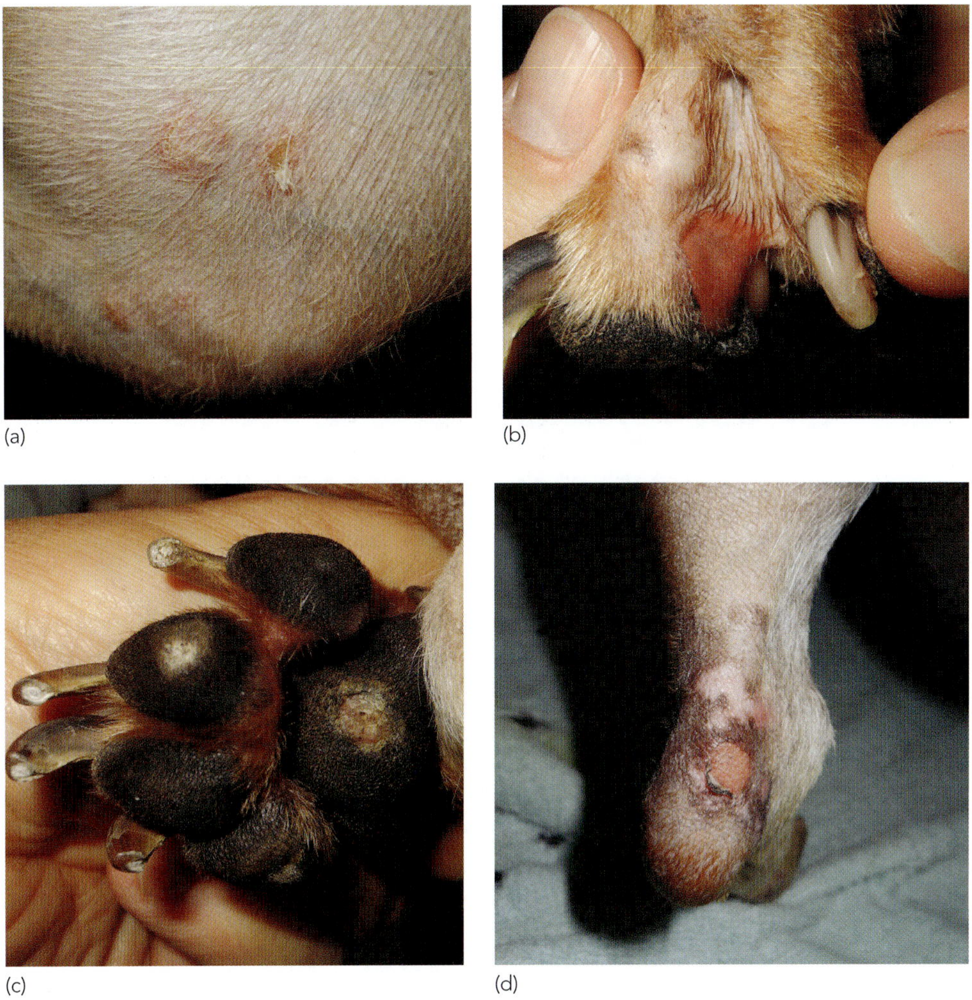

■ **Fig. 12.20.** Epidermolysis bullosa acquisita in a 1-year-old male-castrate dachshund. (a) Vesicles leading to ulcerations on the medial thigh. (b,c) Ulcerations at the footpad margin and on the footpads. (d) Vesicle leading to full-thickness sloughing of the epidermis on the caudal hock.

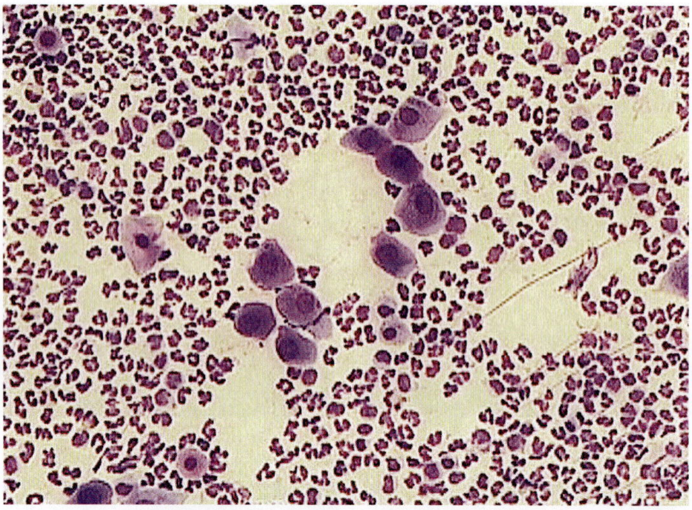

■ **Fig. 12.21.** Contents of a pustule with pemphigus folicaceus. Acantholytic keratinocytes appear as "fried eggs" surrounded by intact neutrophils.

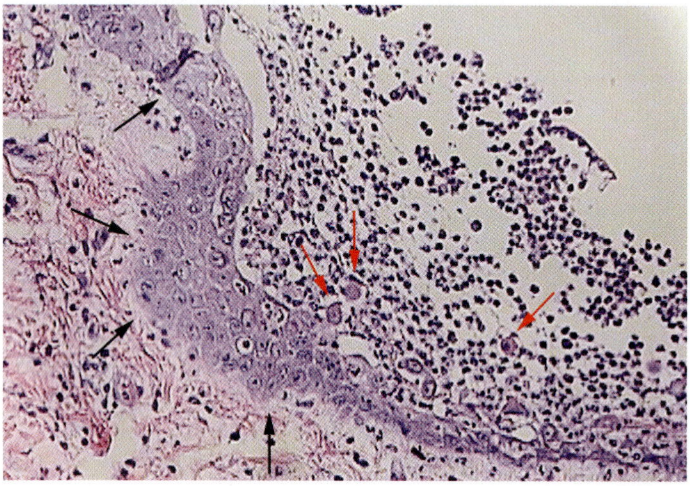

■ **Fig. 12.22.** Hematoxylin and eosin stained tissue slide of a pustule in pemphigus foliaceus. Dermal-epidermal junction (*black arrows*). Acantholytic keratinocytes separating from the underlying epidermis (*red arrows*).

chapter 13

Bacterial Pyoderma

DEFINITION/OVERVIEW

- Bacterial infections of the skin and adnexal structures.
- Microbiome: mixed population of microorganisms that colonize the skin, gut, oral cavity, and other sites: up to 90% of total cells in an individual may be microbial.
- Pyoderma is a term used to describe any skin disease that is pyogenic (has pus); commonly used in veterinary medicine to describe superficial and deep bacterial infections.

ETIOLOGY/PATHOPHYSIOLOGY

Skin infections occur when the surface integrity of the skin has been broken, the skin has become macerated (e.g., by chronic exposure to moisture), normal bacterial flora have been altered, circulation has been impaired, and/or immunocompetency has been compromised.

- Primary types of cutaneous bacterial colonies: resident and transient.
- Resident:
  - "Normal" bacteria found on "normal" skin that can multiply to establish and maintain colonies
  - Normal skin flora (microbiome) vary with body site (greater diversity on haired skin versus mucosal or mucocutaneous surfaces)
  - Serve as a component of the immune defense system (carry important functional genes responsible for synthezing numerous metabolites that influence host health)
  - Bacterial dysbiosis: alterations in the resident microbiome may influence disease (cause or effect), i.e., atopic skin has a significantly less diverse bacterial and fungal microbiome than does healthy skin
  - Alteration of the microbiome may allow for greater management of the specific disease
  - Bacteria are located in the superficial epidermis and infundibulum of the hair follicle and receive nutrients via sebum and sweat; these organisms live in symbiosis and help inhibit colonization by invading bacteria via bacteriocins

Blackwell's Five-Minute Veterinary Consult Clinical Companion: Small Animal Dermatology, Third Edition.
Karen Helton Rhodes and Alexander H. Werner.

  - The normal flora can be altered by pH, temperature, salinity, moisture, albumin, fatty acid levels, etc.; age, sex, diet, hygiene, and environment also play a role
  - Bacterial counts in the normal individual vary greatly; counts are further affected by pathology; resident populations of staphylococci play a role in the bacterial dybiosis of disease.
- Transient:
  - Bacteria that may be cultured from "normal" skin but do not multiply or establish colonies
  - Not of significance unless associated with disease (i.e., infection).
- Different strains of the same organism may be either resident or transient; non-pathogenic strains of *S. pseudintermedius* may be cultured from normal skin (resident) whereas methicillin-resistant strains of *S. pseudintermedius* may be eliminated from the skin by treatment of reservoir sites (transient).
- Infection versus colonization:
  - Infection: the organism is present and causes an immunologic reaction (degenerating neutrophils and/or phagocytized bacteria noted in a direct smear or aspirate of a pustule)
  - Colonization: the organism is present on the skin but does not produce an adverse reaction by the host.
- Primary resident bacterial microbiome of the skin surface and hair follicle:
  - Dog:
    - *Micrococcus*
    - *Corynebacterium*
    - Coagulase-negative staphylococci (*S. epidermidis*, *S. xylosus*)
    - Alpha-hemolytic streptococci
    - *Acinetobacter* spp.
    - *Clostridium perfringens*
    - *Propionibacterium* acne
    - *Staphylococcus pseudintermedius* (often identified in hair follicle)
  - Cat:
    - Alpha-hemolytic streptococci
    - *Micrococcus*
    - Coagulase-negative and -positive staphylococci (*S. pseudintermedius* and *S. aureus*)
    - *Acinetobacter* spp.

Primary Causes

- Cutaneous bacterial infections are more common in dogs compared to other mammalian species:
  - Thin compact stratum corneum
  - Relative lack of intercellular lipids in the stratum corneum
  - Lack of a lipid-squamous epithelial plug in the ostia of the canine hair follicle
  - Relatively high cutaneous pH (basic, 7.5).

Predisposing Factors

- Systemic immuno-incompetence (metabolic disease, genetically determined cellular immunodeficiency).
- Trauma/damage to the skin (e.g., pressure, licking, scratching, parasites).
- Follicular damage (e.g., *Demodex* mites, dermatophytes).
- Dermal damage (e.g., collagen disruption, extension of disease, foreign body reaction).
- Physical factors (e.g., poor grooming, maceration of the skin, heat, humidity).
- Inappropriate antibacterial therapy: too short a course, poor drug choice, inappropriate dose.

Three Categories of Bacterial Infections

- Surface (overgrowth or colonization of the epidermis by bacteria):
  - Intertrigo (skinfold "pyoderma")
  - Acute moist dermatitis ("hot spot").
- Superficial pyoderma (infection confined within the epidermis and follicles):
  - Impetigo (puppy pyoderma): nonfollicular subcorneal pustules
  - Mucocutaneous pyoderma
  - Canine exfoliative superficial pyoderma
  - "Superficial spreading pyoderma" (large coalescing epidermal collarettes due to interfollicular pustules)
  - Superficial bacterial folliculitis (superficial portion of the hair follicle)
  - Miliary dermatitis in cats.
- Deep pyoderma (ruptured hair follicle and extension of infection into the dermis and SQ):
  - Muzzle folliculitis and furunculosis (chin acne)
  - Nasal pyoderma (rapid onset, bridge of nose)
  - Pedal pyoderma and interdigital furunculosis/nodules
  - Generalized deep pyoderma/cellulitis (German shepherd dog, familial)
  - Bacterial granulomas ("acral lick dermatitis/furunculosis")
  - Pressure point pyoderma
  - Pyotraumatic folliculitis and furunculosis.

Common Bacterial Infections

- *Staphylococcus pseudintermedius*: most frequent canine; also recognize other spp. of staph. causing pyoderma – *S. schleiferi* and *S. aureus* (methicillin resistance among staphylococcal species is an emerging clinical problem in canine patients).
- *Pasteurella multocida*: an important pathogen in cats.
- Deep pyoderma (furunculosis) may be complicated by gram-negative organisms (e.g., *E. coli*, *Proteus* spp., *Pseudomonas* spp.); emerging resistance has been noted in these organisms.
- Rarely caused by higher bacteria (e.g., *Actinomyces*, *Nocardia*, mycobacteria, *Actinobacillus*).

SIGNALMENT/HISTORY

- Dogs: very common; cats: uncommon.
- Breeds with short coats, skinfolds, or pressure calluses.
- German shepherd dog folliculitis and furunculosis: severe and deep pyoderma; only partially responsive to antibiotics; frequent relapses; familial pattern; often triggered by an underlying disease; may be an exaggerated response to bacterial antigens.
- Pedal folliculitis and furunculosis: severe and deep pyoderma affecting the interdigital region; pit bull, English bulldog, Great Dane, mastiff, dalmatian, boxer, German shepherd, Labrador retriever, golden retriever.
- Acute or gradual onset.
- Variable pruritus: underlying cause may be atopic dermatitis or the staphylococcal infection itself may be pruritic (bacterial hypersensitivity or atopic-like disease).

CLINICAL FEATURES

- Acute moist dermatitis ("hot spot"): self-induced traumatic skin disease with secondary surface bacterial infection (Figure 13.1).
- Intertrigo: skinfold dermatitis caused by maceration of tissue from chronic moisture/anatomical predisposition (facial folds, interdigital, perivulvar, axillae, etc.) (Figure 13.2).
- Impetigo (nonfollicular subcorneal pustules): puppy impetigo (poor nutrition, dirty environment, etc.) and bullous impetigo in older dogs (large flaccid nonfollicular pustule often caused by *E. coli* or *Pseudomonas* on the nose or glabrous skin; older patients may be immunocompromised) (Figures 13.3, 13.4).
- Mucocutaneous pyoderma (MCP) is an idiopathic ulcerative mucosal dermatitis with crusting and variable degrees of depigmentation. Lesions often involve the lips, alar folds, perioral, perivulvar, prepuce, and anal regions (Figure 13.5).
- Superficial pyoderma: usually involves the trunk; extent of lesions may be obscured by the hair coat; papules, pustules, epidermal collarettes, and hyperpigmented macules; creates a "moth-eaten" appearance to the hair coat; usually secondary to an underlying cause such as atopic dermatitis or "atopic-like dermatitis" (Figures 13.6, 13.7).
- Idiopathic recurrent superficial pyoderma: recurrent pruritic superficial staphylococcal infection (likely subset of atopic dermatitis where atopic-induced pruritus and recurrent infection are controlled by resolution of the pyoderma).
- Canine exfoliative superficial pyoderma ("superficial spreading pyoderma"): large coalescing epidermal collarettes are noted along the lateral trunk due to interfollicular pustules; common in collie and sheltie breeds; rule out underlying metabolic disease (Figure 13.8).
- Deep pyoderma: often affects the chin, bridge of the nose, pressure points, and feet; may be generalized (Figures 13.9, 13.10); elicits a foreign body reaction due to ruptured hair follicle release of hair shaft antigen into the dermis.

- Postgrooming furunculosis (most often caused by *Pseudomonas aeruginosa*): unique presentation of deep pyoderma initiated by bathing and/or grooming; acute and extremely painful; patients often febrile. Combing, clipping, or overly aggressive bathing against the direction of growth of the hair may cause traumatic rupture of the hair follicle, inciting a foreign body reaction; dorsal midline is often the most severely affected region; lesions often occur within 24–48 hours after grooming. Short-coated breeds predisposed. Bacterial contamination of shampoos or equipment may be important in the etiology of this condition (Figure 13.11).
- Bacterial overgrowth syndrome (BOG): due to overgrowth of *Staphylococcus* species on the surface of the skin. Bacterial toxins may act as superantigens triggering non-specific inflammatory reactions. "Quorum sensing" may be a factor in this syndrome; quorum sensing occurs when a certain density level of bacteria is exceeded, causing expression of characteristics that switch bacterial metabolism from cell proliferation to toxin production. Primary clinical signs are pruritus, erythema, and lichenification in the absence of primary lesions such as papules and pustules. Often also associated with *Malassezia* overgrowth as well as underlying diseases such as atopic disease or chronic glucocorticoid therapy. Topical shampoo therapy is required for therapeutic success (Figure 13.12).

Lesions

- Papules
- Pustules
- Hemorrhagic bullae
- Serous crusts (miliary dermatitis in the cat)
- Epidermal collarettes: footprints of ruptured pustules with slow expansion in a circular pattern – both follicular and interfollicular (Figure 13.13)
- Circular erythematous or hyperpigmented macules (Figure 13.14)
- Target lesions
- Multifocal alopecia leading to appearance of a "moth-eaten" hair coat
- Scaling, follicular casts
- Lichenification
- Abscesses
- Furunculosis, cellulitis
- Draining tracts
- Greasy skin
- Malodor

DIFFERENTIAL DIAGNOSIS

- Atopic dermatitis
- Parasitic dermatitis (fleas, scabies, demodicosis, cheyletiellosis, etc.)
- Cutaneous adverse food reaction
- Neoplasia (e.g., cutaneous lymphoma)

- Metabolic disorder (e.g., diabetes, superficial necrolytic dermatitis, idiopathic and iatrogenic hyperadrenocorticism, hypothyroidism)
- Cornification/keratinization defects (e.g., seborrhea, vitamin A-responsive dermatosis, sebaceous adenitis)
- Color dilution alopecia/follicular dysplasia
- Immune-mediated diseases (e.g., pemphigus complex, cutaneous lupus erythematosus, vasculitis)
- Immunosuppression (e.g., glucocorticoids, chemotherapy, metabolic)
- Panniculitis
- Nodular dermatosis (e.g., histiocytosis)

DIAGNOSTICS

Identifying Risk Factors

- Allergy: flea; atopic dermatitis; cutaneous adverse food reaction; contact dermatitis.
- Fungal infection: dermatophytosis.
- Endocrine disease: hypothyroidism; hyperadrenocorticism; sex hormone imbalance or exposure.
- Immune incompetency: glucocorticoids; young animals, older debilitated animals.
- Seborrhea: acne; schnauzer comedo syndrome.
- Conformation: short coat; skinfolds.
- Trauma: pressure points; grooming; scratching; rooting behavior; irritants.
- Foreign body exposure: foxtail; grass awn.

Diagnostic Tests

- Complete physical examination.
- Skin scrapings, trichogram.
- Dermatophyte culture.
- Intradermal allergy testing, restricted antigen food trial.
- Endocrine tests.
- Blood screen: may be normal or reflect the underlying cause (e.g., anemia secondary to hypothyroidism; stress leukogram and high serum alkaline phosphatase consistent with Cushing's disease; eosinophilia associated with parasitism); chronicity may show leukocytosis with a left shift and hyperglobulinemia.
- Skin biopsy.
- Cytology: direct smear from intact pustule: neutrophils engulfing bacteria; differentiate bacterial infection from pemphigus foliaceus (acantholytic keratinocytes) and deep fungal infections (blastomycosis, cryptococcosis); tissue grains may identify filamentous organisms characteristic of higher bacteria.
- Culture and sensitivity: obtained as an aspirate from intact pustule, swab from the ventral surface of an epidermal collarette, tissue biopsy, or freshly expressed exudate from a draining tract or beneath a crust.

THERAPEUTICS

- Severe, generalized, deep: may require supportive care such as intravenous fluids, parenteral antibiotics, and/or daily whirlpool baths.
- Shampoos mechanically remove surface debris and lower bacterial counts; best if also antibacterial; use at least 1–2 times weekly for both treatment and prevention of recurrence.
- Whirlpool baths: deep pyoderma; remove crusted exudate; encourage drainage.
- Nutrition: avoid poor-quality diets and excessive supplementation; restricted antigen food trial if suspect pyoderma is secondary to adverse food reaction.
- Fold pyoderma may require surgical correction to prevent recurrence; treatment should primarily rely on topical therapy.
- Superficial pyoderma: use shampoo therapy as an initial protocol or adjunctive therapy with appropriate antibiotics; antibiotic choice should be based on typical regional response rates as well as level of systemic side effects; use appropriate dose and duration (minimum 21 days); emerging antibiotic resistance of great concern; topical therapy vitally important to support decreased antibiotic dependency.
- Recurrent, resistant, or deep pyoderma: antibiotic selection based on culture (with speciation) and sensitivity testing (Table 13.1).
- Multiple organisms with different antibiotic sensitivities: often best to choose antibiotic on basis of staphylococcal susceptibility; severe cases may require combination therapy.
- Antimicrobial Guidelines Working Group of the International Society for Companion Animal Infectious Diseases recommendations:
  - First tier (empiric): clindamycin, lincomycin, first-generation cephalosporins, trimethoprim-potentiated sulfonamides
  - First or second tier: third-generation cephalosporins
  - Second tier (failure of empiric choice and cultures indicate sensitivity): doxycycline, minocycline chloramphenicol, fluoroquinolones, rifampicin, aminoglycosides
  - Third tier: linezolid, vancomycin; use strongly discouraged; reserved for serious MRSA infections in humans.
- Corticosteroids: may encourage resistance and recurrence when used long term concurrently with antibiotics; may be used short term at the onset of therapy to resolve acute inflammation.
- Vaccines: immunomodulatory "staph vaccine" therapy – Staphage lysate (SPL; Delmont Laboratories), staphoid AB, or autogenous staphylococcal bacterins; inactivated suspensions of bacteria via heating, chemical inactivation, or bacteriophage lysis; goal is to improve antibiotic efficacy, decrease recurrence, and avoid long-term antibiotic therapy; beneficial effect may be due to upregulation of interferon-gamma production or an antigen-specific immunologic response.
- Antibiotics:
  - Administer for a minimum of 2 weeks beyond clinical cure

TABLE 13.1. Systemic antibiotics for pyoderma (listed alphabetically)

Drug	Mode of action	Elimination	Notes
Amikacin 15–30 mg/kg q24h IV, IM, SQ	-cidal	Renal	Renal toxicity Ototoxicity (controversial) Vestibular effects (cats) Reserved for resistant gram+/gram− Injectable Painful Close monitoring required for use Expensive
Amoxicillin/clavulanate Dog: 12.5–25 mg/kg q12h PO Cat: similar dosage or 62.5 mg q12h PO	-cidal	Renal	Expensive for large dogs Vomiting/diarrhea
Azithromycin 5–10 mg/kg q24h PO (7–14 days); pulse-dosed following induction	-static	Liver > kidney	Anaerobes, gram+ Toxoplasmosis Absorption decreased w/food Cross-resistance with erythromycin
Cephalosporin group Cephalexin 22–30 mg/kg q12h PO Cefadroxil 22–30 mg/kg q12h PO Cefpodoxime 5–10 mg/kg q24h PO Cefovecin 8 mg/kg SQ q14 days	-static	Renal	Broad spectrum Often first choice for pyoderma
Clindamycin 11 mg/kg 24h PO; 11mg/kg q24h PO for osteomyelitis/ deep infections 22 mg/kg q24h PO	-static	Liver > kidney	Gram+ and anaerobes Absorption decreased with food Esophageal lesions Vomiting/diarrhea in cats Cross-resistance with erythromycin
Chloramphenicol Dog: 40–50 mg/kg q8h PO Cat: 10–20 mg/kg q12h	-static	Liver	Gram+ and gram− spectrum Crosses blood–brain barrier Concern about human exposure (aplastic anemia) Bone marrow suppression Reversible peripheral neuropathy (hindlimb weakness/ataxia of large breed dogs) Vomiting/diarrhea Use based on culture and sensitivity testing Reserved for methicillin resistance
Doxycycline 5 mg/kg q12h PO	-static	GI>>renal>liver	Gram+ Vomiting/diarrhea Esophageal lesions Use based on culture and sensitivity testing

TABLE 13.1. (*Continued*)

Drug	Mode of action	Elimination	Notes
Erythromycin 10–20 mg/kg q8–12h PO	-static	Liver >> renal	Gram+ and mycoplasma Vomiting
Fluoroquinolone group Enrofloxacin 10–20 mg/kg q24h PO Ciprofloxacin 25 mg/kg q24h PO Orbifloxacin 2.5–7.5 mg/kg q24h PO Marbofloxacin 2.75–5.5 mg/kg q24h PO Difloxacin 5–10 mg/kg q24h PO	-cidal	Renal > liver	Good tissue penetration Broad-spectrum activity Use for deep pyoderma or mixed infections Use based on culture and sensitivity testing Blindness: cats Enrofloxacin: cartilage defects in young large breed dogs Ciprofloxacin: variable/poor bioavailability
Rifampin Dog: 5–10 mg/kg q12h Cat: 10–15 mg/kg q24h	-cidal	Liver	Use based on culture and sensitivity testing Reserve for multidrug resistance Severe hepatitis, hemolytic anemia thrombocytopenia Anorexia Vomiting/diarrhea Orange-colored sweat, urine, tears, feces, saliva Feline leprosy
Sulfonamide group Sulfamethoxazole + trimethoprim 15 mg/kg q12h PO Sulfadimethoxine + ormetoprim Dog: 27.5 mg/kg q24h PO	-cidal	Liver and renal	Gram+ KCS Drug eruptions Hepatic necrosis Vomiting/diarrhea Arthropathies/hypersensitivity Dobermans and rottweilers Altered thyroid activity

GI, gastrointestinal; IM, intramuscular; IV, intravenous; KCS, keratoconjunctivitis sicca; PO, per os (by mouth); SQ, subcutaneous.

- Typical treatment: 3–4 weeks for superficial pyoderma and 6–12 weeks for deep pyoderma
- Protocol should be considered a treatment failure if new lesions are noted within the first week of therapy: clients should be instructed to stop the medication and return for culture and sensitivity testing prior to selection of a different antibiotic.

- Routine bathing with antimicrobial, shampoos (once or twice weekly): mechanically removes microbes and lowers bacterial counts; may help to restore epidermal barrier function; both therapeutic and helps prevent recurrences.
- Pulse therapy (frequent short course with recommended full dose) with antibiotics should be avoided due to increased risk of antibiotic resistance.

- Subminimal inhibitory concentrations of antibiotics (long term/low dose) should be avoided due to increased risk of antibiotic resistance.
- Padded bedding: may reduce pressure point pyoderma.
- Topical benzoyl peroxide gel or mupirocin ointment: focal lesions/intertrigo.
- Topical sprays with chlorhexidine or sodium hypochlorite (not hypochlorous acid); residual antibacterial activity.
- Dilute bleach baths/soaks (5% solution).
- Pyoderma will be recurrent or nonresponsive if underlying cause is not identified and effectively managed.
- Impetigo: affects young dogs before puberty; associated with poor husbandry; often requires only topical therapy.
- Superficial pustular dermatitis: occurs in kittens; associated with overzealous "mouthing" by the queen.
- Pyoderma secondary to atopic disease: usually begins at 1–3 years of age.
- Pyoderma secondary to endocrine disorders: usually begins in middle adulthood.

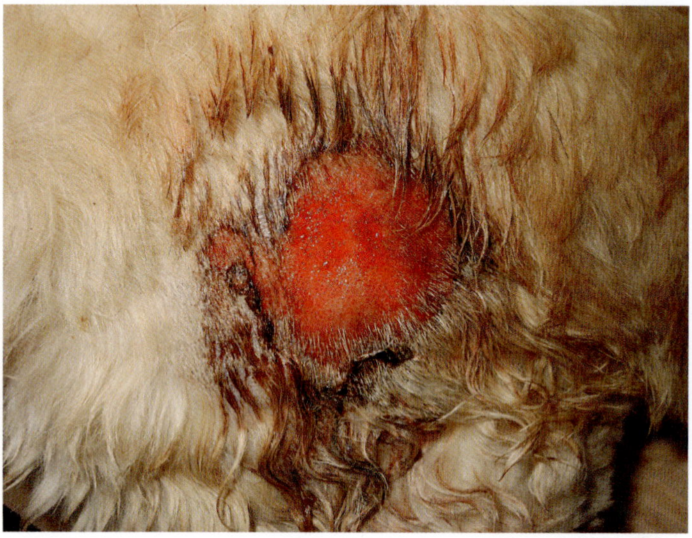

Fig. 13.1. Surface pyotraumatic dermatitis "hot spot" in a 4-year-old male-castrate cockapoo.

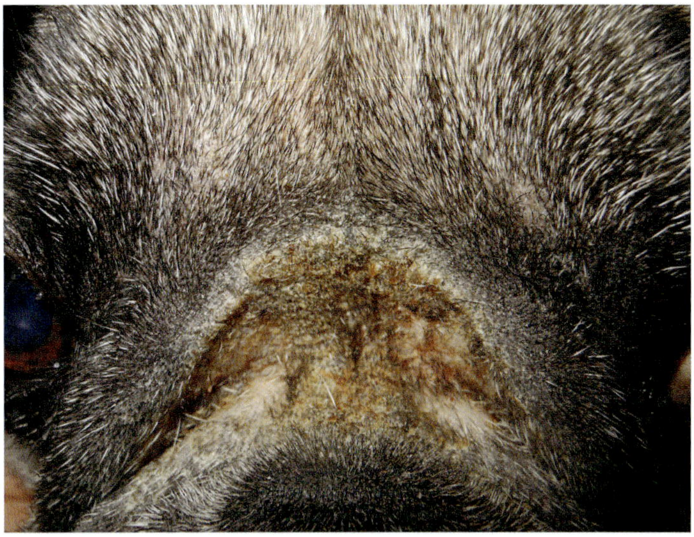

■ **Fig. 13.2.** Accumulations of dried exudate and purulent debris on the skin of a 3-year-old male-castrate pug with facial fold intertrigo.

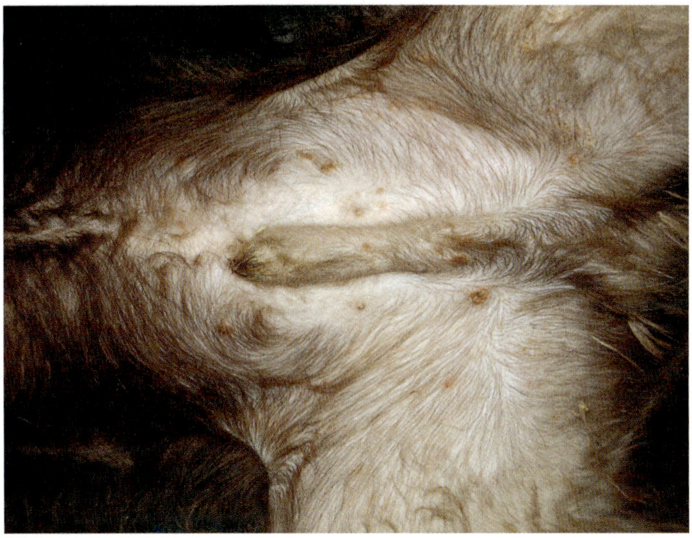

■ **Fig. 13.3.** Puppy impetigo: nonfollicular pustules on the ventral abdomen and medial thighs of a 6-month-old male goldendoodle.

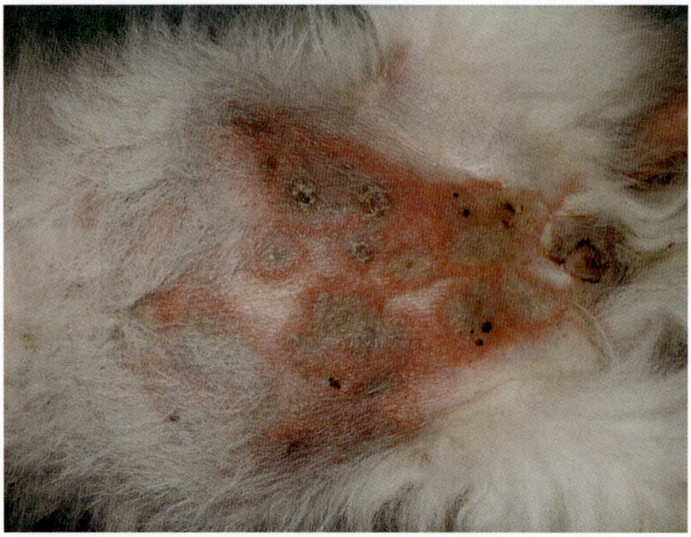

■ **Fig. 13.4.** Bullous impetigo seen as large, nonfollicular and inflammatory flaccid pustules on the glabrous skin of a 10-year-old female-spayed pomeranian treated chronically with corticosteroids for collapsing trachea.

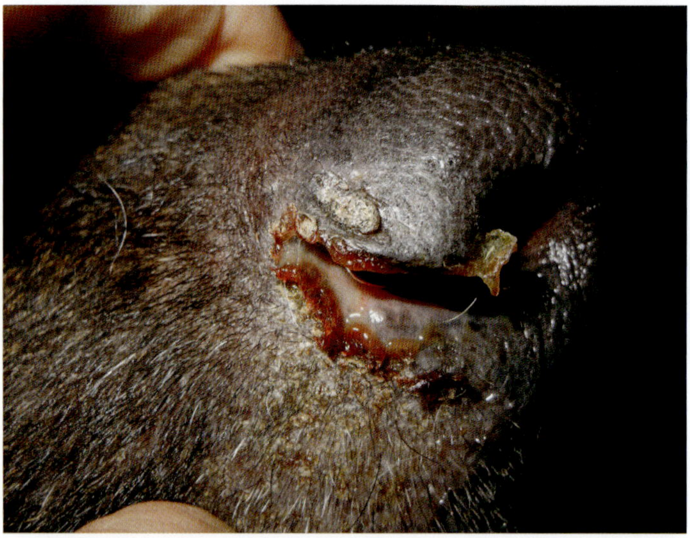

■ **Fig. 13.5.** Mucocutaneous pyoderma affecting the alar fold in a 2-year-old male-castrate German shepherd. Depigmentation is secondary to and follows inflammation from infection.

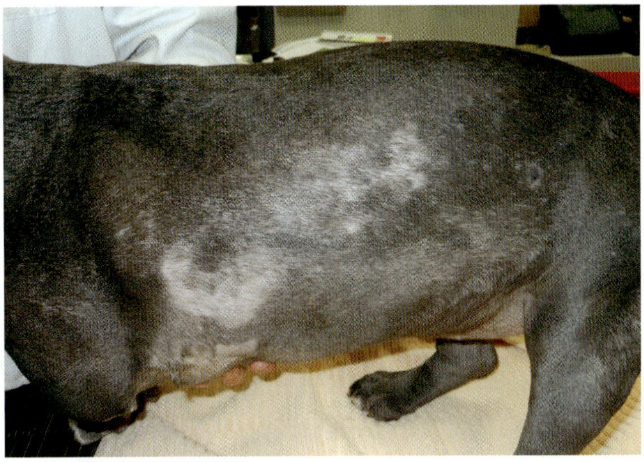

■ **Fig. 13.6.** Superficial pyoderma: coalescing circular lesions of alopecia and scales on the lateral aspect of the body of this 4-year-old female-spayed pit bull, producing a "moth-eaten" appearance to the hair coat.

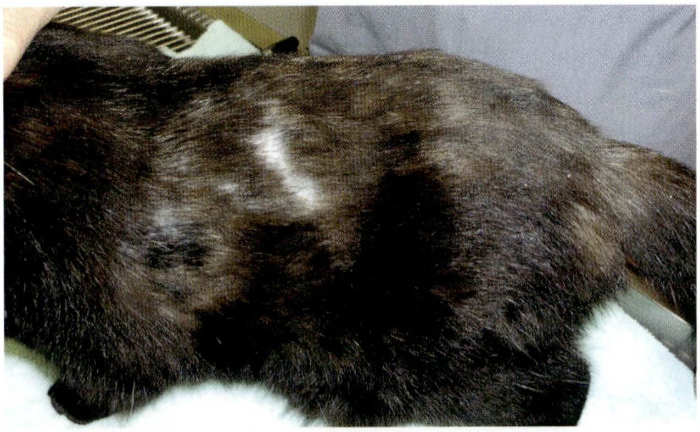

■ **Fig. 13.7.** Superficial pyoderma in a 7-year-old female-spayed DSH with similar appearance to the canine in Figure 13.6. Lesions in the cat are often initially palpated as miliary dermatitis.

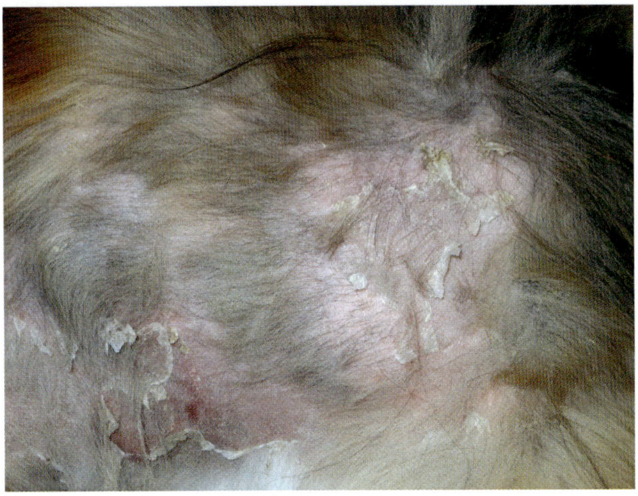

■ **Fig. 13.8.** Large, coalescing and inflammatory collarettes with peeling of the superficial epidermis in an 8-year-old male-castrate sheltie with atypical Cushing's disease.

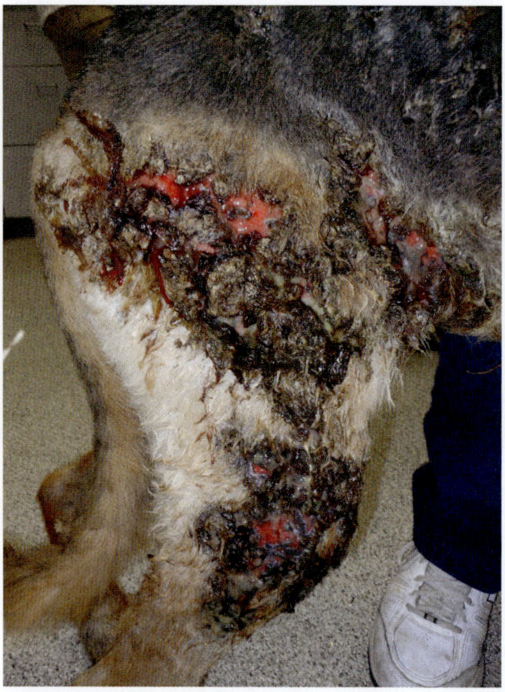

■ **Fig. 13.9.** Deep pyoderma with furunculosis and cellulitis on the lateral extremity of a 5-year-old female-spayed German shepherd dog.

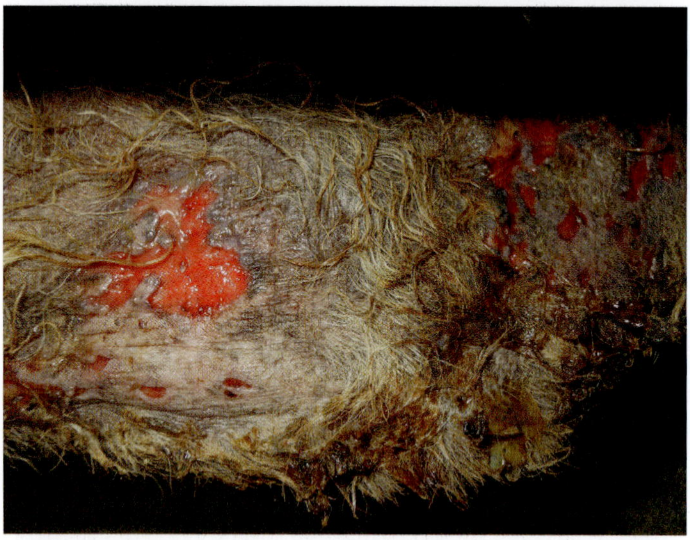

■ **Fig. 13.10.** Additional image of patient in Figure 13.9.

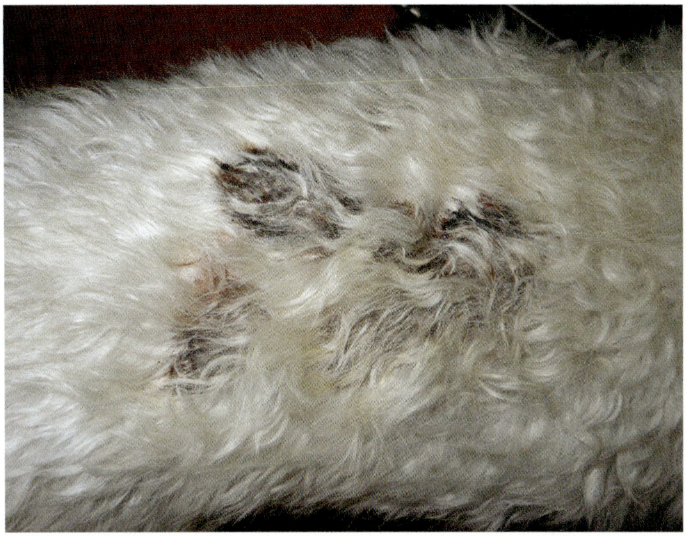

Fig. 13.11. Postgrooming pyoderma; 9-year-old male intact Maltese mix. Deep *Pseudomonas aeruginosa* infection following routine grooming or immersion in water. Lesions are often very painful and may be scarring.

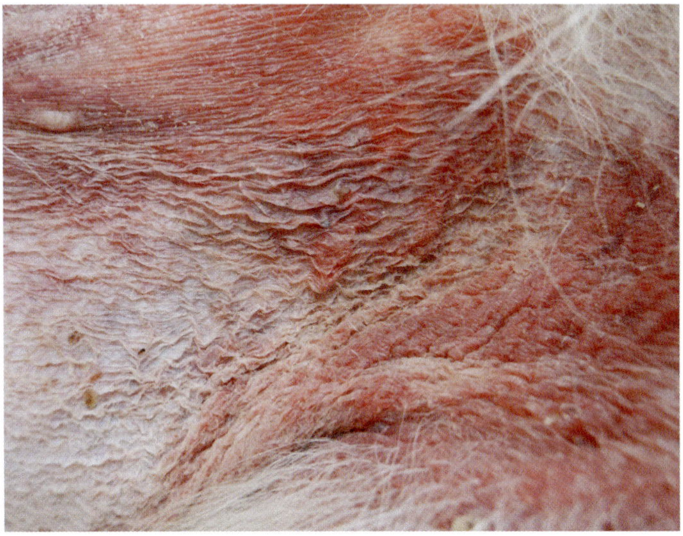

Fig. 13.12. Intense erythroderma, focal atrophy (*left*) and lichenification (*lower right*) in a 2-year-old female-spayed Great Pyrenees caused by bacterial overgrowth and toxin production. The skin appears thinned (atrophic) from previous application of a corticosteroid-containing ointment. Lesions responded completely to appropriate antibiotic administration and topical antiseptic therapy.

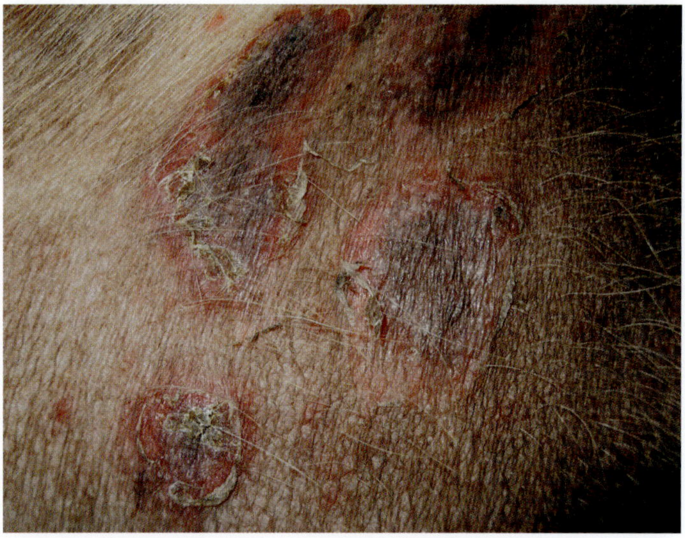

■ **Fig. 13.13.** Superficial pyoderma. Note circular crusts with erythema described as epidermal collarettes.

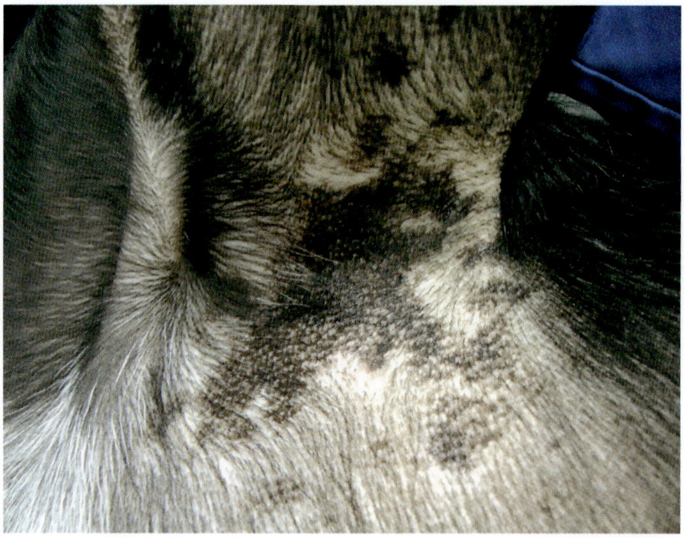

■ **Fig. 13.14.** Postinflammatory hyperpigmented macules as a resolving stage of superficial pyoderma.

chapter 14

Behavioral or Self-Injurious Dermatoses

DEFINITION/OVERVIEW

- Self-injurious behavior or compulsion refers to any voluntary action resulting in self-damage.
- Compulsive disorders are characterized by repetitive, persistent, or sustained behaviors in excess of what is required for normal function, especially if severe enough to interfere with normal function.
- The term obsessive-compulsive disorder may not be appropriate; the cognitive process producing the behavior is unknown in animals.
- Cutaneous compulsions (psychodermatoses) often have an underlying organic disease or trigger.
- Diagnosis and treatment include identifying the underlying trigger, treating secondary dermatoses, and modifying behavior to prevent recurrence; medications are a helpful adjunct if anxiety interferes with normal activities or learning.

ETIOLOGY/PATHPHYSIOLOGY

- Dermatoses may be initiated by a pathology (e.g., an allergy, an injury, arthritis, or a cutaneous growth), with subsequent self-injury causing persistence or worsening of lesions; habituation may result.
- Secondary behavioral dermatoses: effects of skin disease on a patient's wellbeing (e.g., lethargy/exhaustion from scratching); treatment of the primary cause should resolve symptoms.
- Cutaneous sensory dermatoses: self-injury produced due to abnormal sensations in the skin but in the absence of identifiable pathology or disease.
- Psychodermatoses: self-injury produced in the absence of underlying sensory, skin or other pathology; often a diagnosis of exclusion; stressful situations, however, can act as flares for pruritus and self-injurious behaviors.
- Compulsive disorders have been linked with conditions that produce frustration, fear, conflict, and anxiety.
- Skin is one of the channels of communication through which anxiety is modulated.

Blackwell's Five-Minute Veterinary Consult Clinical Companion: Small Animal Dermatology, Third Edition.
Karen Helton Rhodes and Alexander H. Werner.

- Self-injurious (especially oral) behaviors may be a coping mechanism to reduce emotional arousal; the initial stimulus may produce a ritualistic behavior that persists outside the original context.
- Neuro-immuno-cutaneous-endocrine (NICE) model: recognizes the interactions between body systems for both the production of and management of various dermatoses.
- Stress-vulnerable pathways trigger the release of neuropeptides and cytokines that mediate behavior (scratching, biting, licking) and contribute to increased sensation (pain, pruritus) through histamine release, central lowering of the itch threshold, vasodilation, and immunologic reactions.
- The resulting excoriation releases mediators of inflammation and endogenous opioids and may become a conditioned response.
- Serotonin activity has been postulated as a specific effector of compulsive disorders.
- Factors involved in the etiology of psychodermatoses include breed (emotional or nervous), lifestyle (stressful, boring, isolating), and individual personality (anxious, fearful).
- Occasionally, the owner may be able to correlate a specific physical (injury) or emotional event just before the onset of symptoms.
- Psychodermatoses primarily include acral lick dermatitis, feline symmetric alopecia, flank sucking, tail biting or chasing, and anal licking.
- The primary role of physical versus psychogenic cause is controversial, especially with acral lick dermatitis.

SIGNALMENT/HISTORY

- Acral lick dermatitis: generally younger age of onset (variable 1–12 years); no sex predilection; common in large breed dogs: Labrador and golden retriever, English and Irish setter, dalmatian, doberman pinscher, Great Dane, Akita, shar-pei, boxer, weimaraner; primarily of psychogenic origin in the Great Dane and doberman pinscher.
- Feline symmetric alopecia: variable age of onset; no sex predilection; possibly more common in Siamese, Abyssinian, and oriental breeds; majority of cases seen in indoor-only, multi-cat households.
- Flank sucking: variable age of onset; no sex predilection; seen primarily in the doberman pinscher.
- Tail biting or chasing: young (socially mature) dogs and cats; neutered males; long-tailed or herding breeds, predominantly German shepherd dog, Australian cattle dog, Staffordshire and English bull terrier.
- Anal licking: young (socially mature) dogs; predominantly poodle.

CLINICAL FEATURES

- Acral lick dermatitis (Figures 14.1–14.3):
  - Compulsive licking of the distal extremity: most often carpus or metacarpus; less commonly radius, tibia, tarsus or metatarsus

- Often a singular lesion; multiple lesions have a poorer prognosis for complete resolution
- Development of multiple lesions supportive of a primary behavioral disorder
- Early lesion: well-circumscribed area of alopecia and erythema
- Typical lesion: proliferative, eroded, crusted and firm plaque; previous lesions may heal with palpable scarring as new areas are traumatized
- Severe lesion: extensive area of ulceration and exudation; thickened and proliferative tissue may surround a central crateriform ulcer
- Severe lesions may cause lameness
- Initiating triggers include allergic dermatitis, localized trauma, arthropathy, endocrinopathy, neuropathy, and neoplasia
- Perpetuated by secondary deep bacterial infection, secondary arthritis and/or osteomyelitis, altered sensation within scar tissue, and learned behavior.

■ Feline symmetric alopecia (Figures 14.4–14.6):
- Also called feline psychogenic alopecia or neurodermatitis
- Often associated with allergic dermatitis; behavior as a primary cause is uncommon
- Skin often remains undamaged; suspect other conditions if associated with significant dermatitis
- Alopecia results from overgrooming and is less often seen as chewing or hair pulling; hair coat is barbered, resulting in short stubble emerging from follicles
- Rarely lesions of eosinophilic plaque may develop
- Behavior may be obvious or secretive to avoid a negative response; if clandestine, the owner may deny that hair loss is due to removal as opposed to lack of growth
- Evidence of self-grooming may be noted by frequent vomiting of hair balls, excessive hair in feces, and visualization of short stubble in areas of alopecia
- Well-demarcated patches of alopecia develop in accessible areas; patches may initially appear asymmetric
- Regrowing hair may appear darker in breeds with darkened "points"
- Common regions affected: ventral abdomen, thighs (medial, lateral, and caudal), ventral trunk, and dorsal aspects of the forelegs
- Diagnosis as a psychodermatosis requires exclusion of other causes; significant history may include hair coat regrowth in response to use of an Elizabethan collar or administration of a corticosteroid; see differential diagnosis list below.

■ Flank sucking:
- May occur in response to a specific trigger or be a generalized (displacement) activity
- Dogs suck or nurse on a portion of the flank fold
- Skin often remains undamaged; alopecia and lichenification may result from chronic behavior
- Secondary bacterial folliculitis and reaction to topical treatments may perpetuate the process.

■ Tail biting or chasing (Figures 14.7, 14.8):
- Most dogs chase, but do not catch, the tail
- Tail trauma may be severe in some patients

- Secondary bacterial folliculitis and pain may perpetuate the process
- Any portion of the tail may be injured; location of lesions (tail fold, area of tail gland, tail tip) may assist in determining the cause
- Behavior may be difficult to disrupt and may specifically occur in the presence of, or in the absence of, the owner
- Lesions seen as scabbed and exudative patches; extensive hemorrhage from the tail tip; extreme tenderness to the touch.

■ Anal licking (Figure 14.9):
- Alopecia and erythema affecting the tail folds and perianal area
- Lichenification and hyperpigmentation in chronic cases
- Exudation and crusting with secondary bacterial folliculitis and/or *Malassezia* dermatitis
- Behavior may be difficult to disrupt.

DIFFERENTIAL DIAGNOSIS

■ Acral lick dermatitis:
- Allergic dermatitis
- Bacterial folliculitis/furunculosis
- Dermatophytosis
- Pressure callus (appropriate location)
- Underlying osteomyelitis or arthritis
- Neuropathy or referred pain
- Focal, traumatized neoplasia (sebaceous adenoma, mast cell tumor, histiocytoma, squamous cell carcinoma)
- Foreign body reaction
- Endocrinopathy (hypothyroidism)
- Localized demodicosis.

■ Feline symmetric alopecia:
- Allergic dermatitis
- Ectoparasitism (*Cheyletiella*, *Demodex gatoi*, *Demodex cati*)
- Dermatophytosis
- *Malassezia* dermatitis
- Endocrinopathy (hyperadrenocortisolism, hyperthyroidism)
- Neoplasia (paraneoplastic alopecia).

■ Flank sucking:
- Contact dermatitis (especially topical medication)
- Trauma
- Neuropathy
- Dermatophytosis
- Bacterial folliculitis
- Psychomotor epilepsy/CNS disorder.

■ Tail biting or chasing:
- Allergic dermatitis

- Neuropathy (central or peripheral)
- Trauma
- Anal sac disorder
- Degenerative disease (arthritis, disk)
- Tail gland infection
- Tail docking neuroma
- Vasculitis/vasculopathy.

■ Anal licking:
- Anal sac disease
- *Malassezia* dermatitis
- Allergic dermatitis
- Intestinal parasitism
- Colitis/gastrointestinal disorder
- Degenerative disease (arthritis, disk).

DIAGNOSTICS

■ Basic work-up to rule out medical causes of self-injurious behavior should include evaluation for pain or pruritus, including musculoskeletal disease, neurologic disease, and/or primary dermatologic disease.

■ CBC/biochemistry/urinalysis: usually normal unless associated with a specific cause (e.g., hypothyroidism); occasional eosinophilia in cats.

■ Other laboratory tests:
- Serum thyroxine
- FeLV/FIV (feline symmetric alopecia)
- ACTH-stimulation or LDDS test.

■ Imaging:
- Radiology: evidence of osteomyelitis or arthropathy (acral lick dermatitis); degenerative disease (tail biting or chasing, anal licking).

■ Behavioral history considerations:
- Household composition (animals and people); include recent changes
- Description of patient's interactions with other animals
- Description of patient's temperament
- Daily routines (feeding, exercise, interactions)
- Patient's response to routines (i.e., separation anxiety)
- Onset and progression of symptoms; accurate description of behavior (frequency, duration, situation, triggers)
- Previous history of dermatoses
- Previous history of therapies and responses
- Owner's response to behavior.

■ Diagnostic procedures:
- Acral lick dermatitis
- Allergy work-up: adequate flea control; intradermal allergen testing; restricted-ingredient food trial

- Bacterial culture and sensitivity testing: results from surface and tissue cultures frequently differ; deep bacterial infection present in a majority of cases
- Fungal culture: exclude dermatophytosis
- Skin scraping: exclude external parasites
- Trichogram: presence of broken hairs (self-trauma); anagen follicles (active hair growth); fungal hyphae and spores (dermatophytosis); *Demodex* mites
- Diagnostic testing and evaluation for musculoskeletal disease, neuropathy or referred pain
- Dermatohistopathology: exclude neoplasia and/or infectious granuloma; severe epidermal hyperplasia with compact hyperkeratosis; hidradenitis, dermal fibrosis ("vertical streaking"), follicular thickening and elongation; mixed dermal (especially perivascular) inflammation, folliculitis, and furunculosis.

■ Feline symmetric alopecia:
- Allergy work-up: adequate flea control; intradermal allergen testing; restricted-ingredient food trial
- Trichogram: presence of broken hairs (self-trauma); anagen follicles (active hair growth); fungal hyphae (dermatophytosis); *Demodex* mites
- Skin scraping: superficial and deep
- Fungal culture
- Skin cytology: evidence of yeast and/or bacteria
- Dermatohistopathology: most often normal; mild trichomalacia; evidence of inflammation supports an underlying cause.

■ Flank sucking:
- Association with topical therapy
- Fungal culture
- Bacterial culture/sensitivity
- Neurologic assessment.

■ Tail biting or chasing:
- Allergy work-up: adequate flea control; intradermal allergen testing; restricted-ingredient food trial
- Bacterial culture and sensitivity testing (especially if tail gland affected)
- Neurologic assessment
- Orthopedic assessment
- Anal sac palpation and examination of contents (cytology, culture and sensitivity testing).

■ Anal licking:
- Anal sac palpation and examination of contents (cytology, culture and sensitivity testing)
- Skin cytology: evidence of yeast and/or bacteria
- Allergy work-up: adequate flea control; intradermal allergen testing; restricted-ingredient food trial
- Fecal parasite and ova testing
- Gastrointestinal assessment: exclude colitis or colon neoplasia
- Neurologic assessment
- Orthopedic assessment.

THERAPEUTICS

- Diagnosis and management of underlying causes required for successful control of symptoms.
- Glucocorticosteroids and antihistamines may be helpful in allergic patients; not recommended for use with acral lick dermatitis; see specific chapters regarding use of these medications.
- Response requires lengthy treatment periods.
- Relapses not uncommon; maintenance therapy necessary.
- Behavior-modifying medications are adjunctive therapy.
- Mechanical devices (e.g., collars, bandages) to prohibit further damage to the skin and allow healing often required at least initially; not a long-term solution.
- For acral lick dermatitis:
    - Bandages with embedded electric contacts may dissuade licking
    - Intralesional injections not useful for larger or multiple lesions
    - Surgical excision (including by laser): removal of exuberant tissue useful only if primary disease is identified and resolved; severe postoperative complications possible
    - Therapeutic laser therapy not supported by controlled studies.

Behavior Modification

- Reduce stress.
- Identify and remove sources of conflict, triggers, fear, boredom, or frustration.
- Provide outlets for alternative behaviors such as exercise and stimulation with toys.
- Increase calm and social interaction with owner.
- Use operant conditioning by rewarding positive behaviors; avoid punishment or attention for the self-injurious behavior.
- Increase supervision to reduce opportunities for the behavior; distract rather than punish the behavior when it occurs.

Drugs of Choice

- Acral lick dermatitis:
    - Topical:
        - Rarely effective as single therapy
        - Fluocinolone-DMSO combined with flunixin meglumine or antibiotics
        - Capsaicin: may decrease reinforcing sensation and discourage licking
        - Mupirocin ointment
    - Systemic:
        - Long-term antibiotics based on culture and sensitivity testing (e.g., cephalexin 22 mg/kg BID)
        - May be required for several months
        - Pulse-dose therapy may be necessary: see chapter on antibiotic stewardship.

- Behavior-modifying medication:
  - Analgesic/anticonvulsant:
    - □ Gabapentin – dog: 10–20 mg/kg q12h: cat: 5–10 mg/kg q12h
  - Selective serotonin reuptake inhibitors:
    - □ Fluoxetine – dog: 1.0–2.0 mg/kg q24h; cat: 0.5–1.0 mg/kg q24h
    - □ Paroxetine– dog: 0.5–1.0 mg/kg q24h; cat: 1.0–2.5 mg q24h
    - □ Sertraline: dog: 0.5–2.5 mg/kg q24h; cat: 0.5–1.0 mg/kg q24h
  - Tricyclic antidepressants:
    - □ Amitriptyline: dog: 1.0–2.2 mg/kg q12–24h; cat: 0.5–1.0 mg/kg q12–24h
    - □ Clomipramine: dog: 1.0–2.0 mg/kg q12–24h; cat: 0.5–1.0 mg/kg q24h
    - □ Doxepin: Initial dosage 1mg/kg q12h with gradual increase up to 3.0–5.0 mg/kg q8–12h (maximum 150 mg BID); cat: 0.5 mg/kg q24h.

COMMENTS

- Begin with a low dose of behavior-modifying medication and increase biweekly if there is inadequate response.
- Serotonin-enhancing medications: long-acting anxiolytics.
- Doxepin and amitriptyline are also H_1 blockers; may be useful in cases with allergy.
- Treatment goal is to interrupt the conditioned response while resolving the organic disease and/or modifying the behavior.
- Reports of success with other psychoactive medications are limited (e.g., hydrocodone, naltrexone).
- Few of these medications are FDA-approved for use in animals.
- Some medications may lower the seizure threshold; gabapentin is beneficial in seizure patients.
- Do not use with MAO inhibitors (e.g., amitraz, selegiline).
- Obtain a minimum database to ascertain the patient's ability to metabolize and excrete medications (especially hepatic disease).
- Monitor patients regularly during therapy.
- Avoid concomitant use of multiple serotonin-enhancing medications to prevent side effects including fatal serotonin syndrome.
- Use cautiously with other highly protein-bound medications (anticonvulsants, thyroid medications, nonsteroidal antiinflammatory drugs) as well as with general anesthesia, anticholinergics, antihistamines, and anticoagulants.
- Avoid use of tricyclic antidepressants in patients with cardiac conduction abnormalities or with glaucoma.
- Avoid sudden changes in dosages; gradual increases and decreases are recommended.
- Common side effects include reduced appetite and sedation, dry mouth, urine retention, constipation, reduced tear production, and increased agitation.
- Medications may take 4–8 weeks to achieve efficacy.
- Symptoms of overdose include behavioral changes (agitation, depression), tremors, ataxia, seizures, hyperthermia, and diarrhea; fatal serotonin syndrome reported.
- Treatment of toxicosis is supportive and symptomatic; cyproheptadine hydrochloride (1.1 mg/kg PO) is a nonspecific serotonin antagonist.

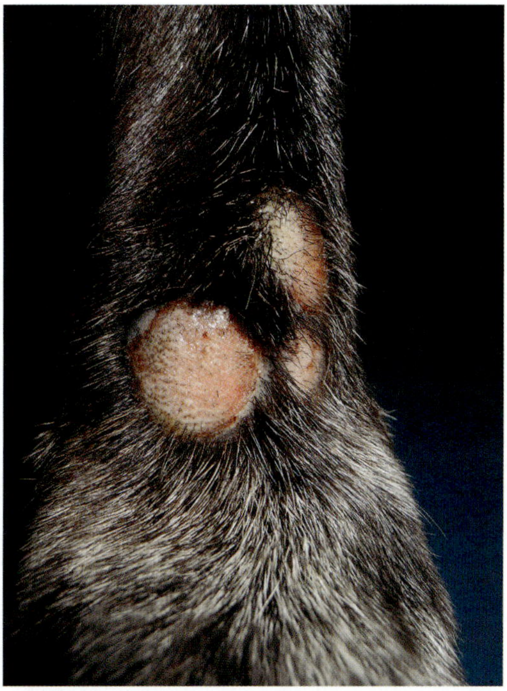

■ **Fig. 14.1.** Acral lick dermatitis on the carpus of an 11-year-old male-castrate retriever mix. The skin is palpably thickened and eroded.

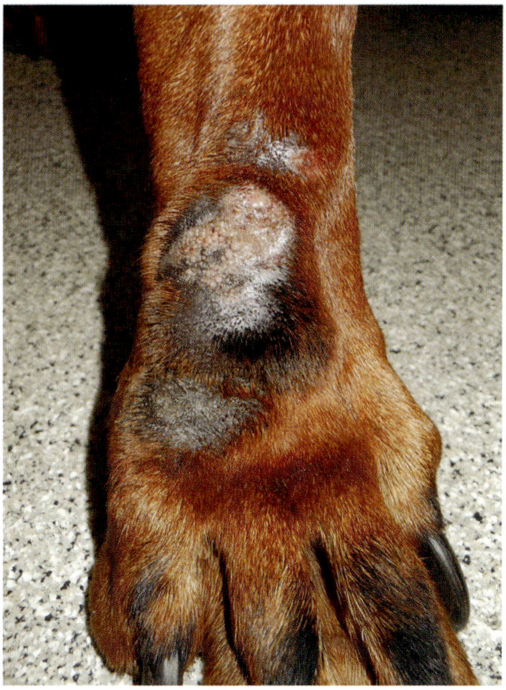

■ **Fig. 14.2.** Firm alopecic acral lick dermatitis plaque on the carpus of a 5-year-old female-spayed doberman pinscher.

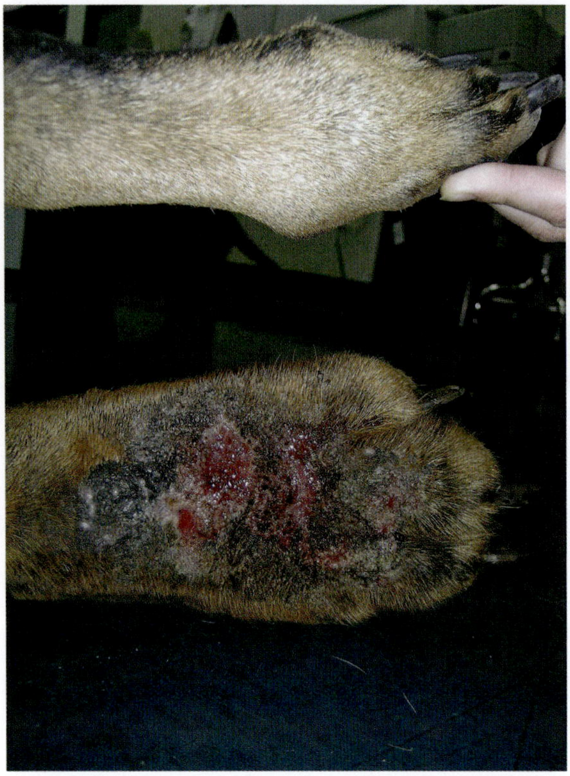

■ **Fig. 14.3.** Large acral lick lesion affecting one metatarsus (normal foot included for comparison) in an adult German shepherd dog. The lesion has a deep secondary bacterial infection.

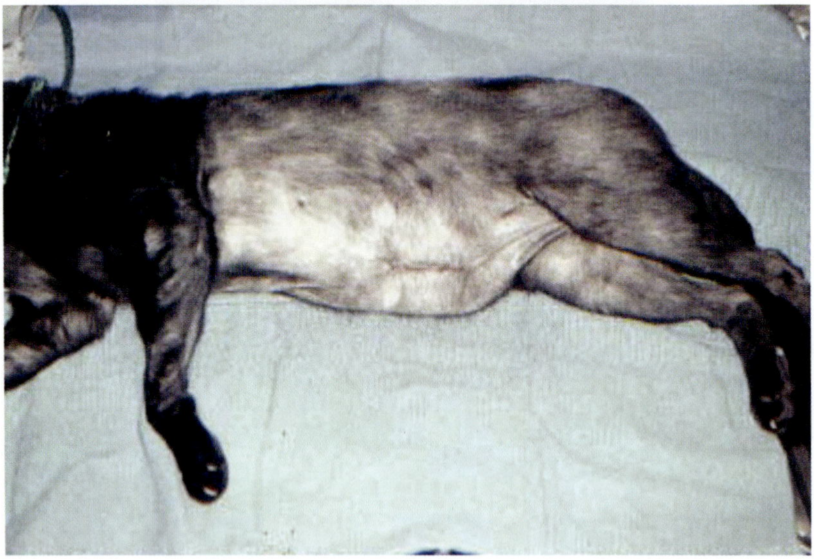

■ **Fig. 14.4.** Generalized alopecia in an adult cat; the hair coat has been barbered in areas that are accessible by overgrooming.

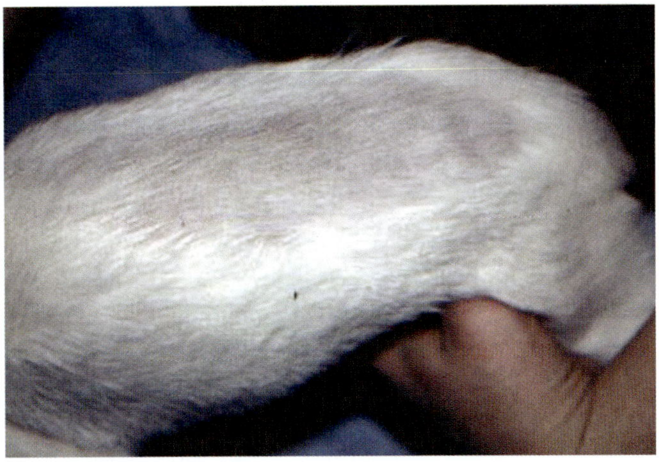

■ **Fig. 14.5.** Darker hair regrowth in overgroomed area on the dorsum of a Siamese cat.

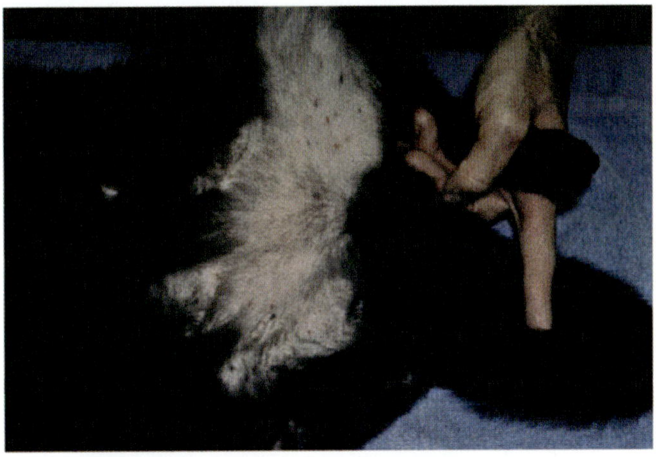

■ **Fig. 14.6.** Self-induced alopecia of the ventral abdomen and rear legs of a DLH.

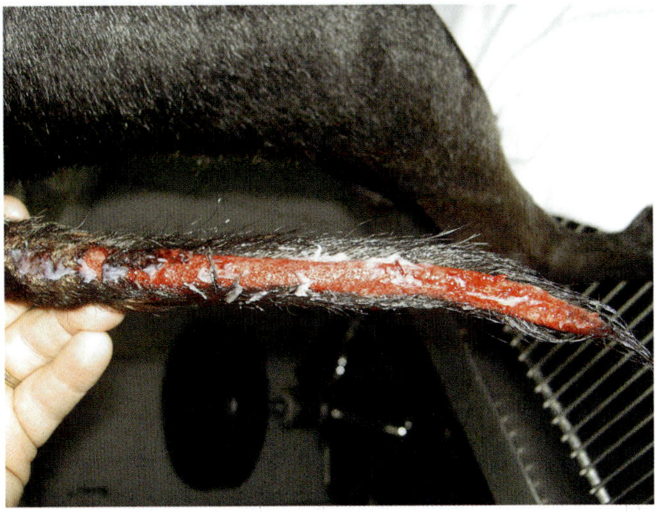

■ **Fig. 14.7.** Severe mutilation of the tail in a 5-year-old female-spayed Labrador mix.

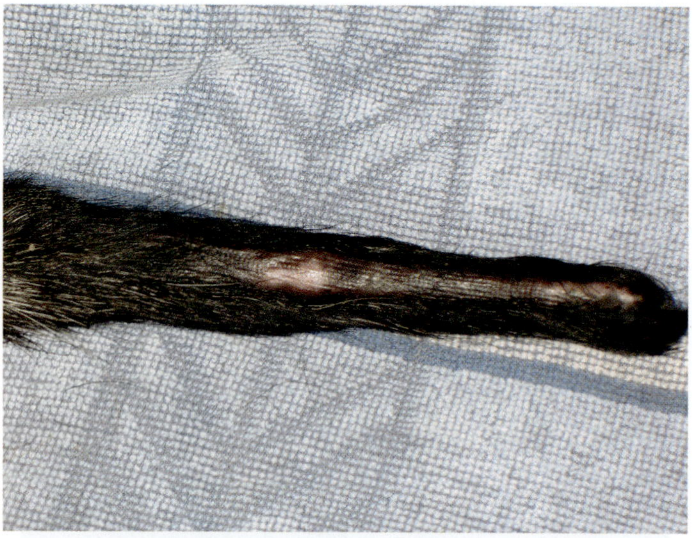

■ **Fig. 14.8.** Healed tail after treatment of patient in Figure 14.7.

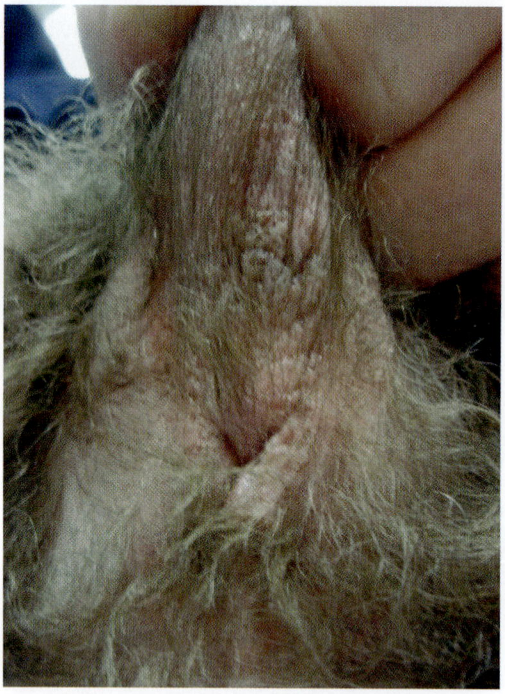

■ **Fig. 14.9.** Perianal erythema and lichenification from licking in a 6-year-old male-castrate toy poodle.

chapter 15

Biting and Stinging Insects

DEFINITION/OVERVIEW

- Insects produce dermatitis by bite, sting, or percutaneous absorption of allergens.
- Allergenic substances are present in saliva, feces, and body parts, as well as in venom.
- Atopic dogs more commonly have positive *in vitro* reactions to insect allergens than nonatopic dogs living in the same environment.
- There is significant cross-reactivity between mite and insect allergens and between the various insect allergens.
- *In vivo* reactions to these allergens may be due to direct irritation and/or injury to tissues (nonimmune-mediated response) or due to hypersensitivity (immune-mediated response).
- Insects as vectors of disease should not be underestimated.
- Of most importance to the small animal practitioner are reactions to fleas, spiders, flies, mosquitoes, ticks, and hymenoptera.
- Dermatitis caused by ants may be by direct envenomation or by absorption of allergens; symptoms may appear similar to FBD/FBH and/or atopic dermatitis.

ETIOLOGY/PATHOPHYSIOLOGY

Flea Bite Dermatitis and Hypersensitivity

- Flea bite dermatitis (FBD) and flea bite hypersensitivity (FBH) remain the most common causes of pruritic skin disease in dogs and cats, although the efficacy and convenience of flea control products have decreased the occurrence – in comparison to other allergic dermatoses – in some locations.
- Fleas are small, wingless parasites that require a blood meal to reproduce; adult fleas remain on the host although most life stages of the parasite occur in the environment.
- More than 90% of fleas found on dogs and cats are *Ctenocephalides felis felis*; other species are often associated with atypical environmental situations.
- *C. felis* demonstrates a preference to remain on the rear half of the body; correlated with a similar location for the majority of lesions in both FBD and FBH.
- *Echidnophaga gallinacea* (sticktight flea) is seen in warmer climates and associated with exposure to poultry (Figures 15.1, 15.2).

Blackwell's Five-Minute Veterinary Consult Clinical Companion: Small Animal Dermatology, Third Edition.
Karen Helton Rhodes and Alexander H. Werner.

- FBD: caused by direct irritation at the site of bites.
- FBH: caused by immediate (type I), delayed (type IV), and cutaneous basophil hypersensitivities.
- Flea saliva contains histamine-like compounds, several complete allergens, and haptens that bind to form complete antigens.

Spider Bite Dermatitis

- Medically important species include the common brown spider (*Loxosceles unicolor*), brown recluse (*Loxosceles reclusa*), black widow (*Latrodectus mactans*), and red-legged widow (*Latrodectus bishopi*).
- Bites of *Loxosceles* spp. produce localized tissue necrosis.
- Bites of *Latrodectus* spp. are more likely to produce systemic reactions.
- Spider bites occur most often on the face and forelegs.

Fly Dermatitis

- Flies can create significant dermatitis by direct damage to intact skin and subsequent irritation (fly dermatitis).
- Fly strike (myiasis) is a distinct and separate dermatitis caused by laying of eggs by dipterous flies on warm, wet skin, and subsequent larval (maggot) invasion of tissues.
- Most often caused by bites from stable flies (*Stomoxys calcitrans*) and black flies (*Simulium* spp.).
- May also be caused by horseflies and deerflies (*Tabanus* and *Chrysops* spp.).

Mosquito Bite Dermatitis and Hypersensitivity

- The hair coat usually protects dogs and cats from mosquito and gnat bites (*Culicoides* spp.).
- Dogs and cats can be irritated by mosquito bites.
- A distinct syndrome of mosquito bite hypersensitivity has been documented in cats.

Tick Bite Dermatitis and Hypersensitivity

- Dogs and cats can be irritated by tick bites.
- Ticks are vectors for bacterial, rickettsial, protozoal, and viral infections.
- Ticks are the cause of tick paralysis.
- Most dogs fail to demonstrate a delayed-type hypersensitivity.
- Seasonal incidence: warm weather; May through July.
- Ear ticks infest the ear canal, producing symptoms of otitis externa.

Hymenoptera Sting

- Order includes ants, bees, wasps, yellow jackets, and hornets.
- Only a few species of ants cause venomous reactions.
- Bees and some wasps die after a single sting; other hymenoptera can sting multiple times.

- Toxins released into the skin cause acute inflammation and pain.
- Hypersensitivity reactions can produce systemic symptoms including anaphylaxis and death.

SIGNALMENT/HISTORY

Flea Bite Dermatitis and Hypersensitivity

- FBD:
  - No age, sex, or breed predisposition
  - Related to presence of significant numbers of fleas.
- FBH, dogs:
  - Age of onset usually between 3 and 5 years
  - FBH is more likely to develop (and/or develop more severely) with intermittent (versus continuous) exposure to fleas.
- FBH, cats: no age, breed, or sex predisposition.

Spider/Fly/Mosquito/Tick Bite Dermatitis and Hypersensitivity/Hymenoptera

- No age, breed, or sex predisposition except as related to exposure to insects.

CLINICAL FEATURES

Flea Bite Dermatitis and Hypersensitivity

- FBD, dogs and cats:
  - Fleas may or may not be evident based on infestation severity and self-grooming behavior
  - Mild papular dermatitis and mild hair barbering
  - Incisors may be worn down with chronic chewing on hair coat (Figure 15.3)
  - Anemia in young or debilitated animals
  - Tapeworm infestation
  - Flea feces.
- FBH, dogs:
  - Significant pruritus of the caudal lumbosacral region (triangular patch), tail folds, caudal thighs, and inguinum (Figures 15.4, 15.5)
  - Pyotraumatic dermatitis (acute moist dermatitis or "hot spot") (Figure 15.6)
  - Pyotraumatic folliculitis (deep "hot spot") of the head and neck in golden and Labrador retrievers, and St Bernard dogs (Figure 15.7)
  - Fibropruritic nodules (Figure 15.8).
- FBH, cats:
  - Papulocrustous dermatitis (miliary dermatitis): generalized or confined to the dorsal lumbosacral region or the head and neck (Figures 15.9, 15.10)

- Hair coat barbering of the ventral abdomen and caudal thighs
- Lesions of the eosinophilic granuloma complex (Figure 15.11).

Spider Bite Dermatitis

- Dogs and cats (Figures 15.12, 15.13):
    - *Loxoceles* spp.: initial local erythema surrounding puncture marks leading to tissue necrosis and slough; lesions are painful
    - *Latrodectus* spp.: initial local erythema surrounding puncture marks leading to granulomatous nodules; systemic effects due to neurotoxin release
    - Systemic signs include salivation, vomiting, convulsions, and death.

Fly Dermatitis

- Dogs:
    - Outdoor exposure, particularly warmer weather
    - Face and ears most affected
    - Bites most frequent on the tips of erect pinnae and the exposed ridge of skin on dogs with folded pinnae
    - Initial lesions appear as punctate accumulations of dried hemorrhagic secretions that result from oozing at the site of injury/fly bite (Figure 15.14)
    - Continued irritation causes severe erythema, ulceration, scabs, and secondary infection (Figures 15.15, 15.16)
    - Thickened and scarred pinnal margins develop with chronicity
    - Lesions are often painful
    - Flies may serve as vectors for the mycobacteria seen in canine leproid granuloma (Figure 15.17).

Mosquito Bite Dermatitis and Hypersensitivity

- Dogs and cats: irritation at the site of mosquito bite(s) (Figure 15.18).
- Cats: mosquito bite hypersensitivity (Figures 15.19–15.22):
    - Outdoor exposure, specific to seasonality of mosquitoes
    - Preference for darker hair coat and skin color
    - Pruritic lesions of papules and crusts leading to erosions and scabs
    - Lesions most often affect less haired regions of the dorsal muzzle, medial pinnae, and lip margins
    - Lesions often well demarcated and symmetric
    - Medial pinnae may have a papular to nodular appearance
    - Occasional involvement of footpads with crusting
    - Lesions resolve when cat is confined/protected from mosquitoes.

Tick Bite Dermatitis and Hypersensitivity

- Tick ecology, populations, and disease transmission vary greatly by region.
- Irritation caused by direct damage to the skin by penetration of the epidermis and laceration of superficial vessels to permit feeding (Figure 15.23)

- Species of most significance (United States) include *Rhipicephalus sanguineus*, *Dermacenter andersoni*, *Dermacenter variabilis*, *Dermacenter occidentalis*, *Ixodes ricini*, *Ixodes scapularis*, *Ixodes dammini*, and *Ambylomma maculatum*.
- Salivary toxin of species of ixodid ticks produce tick paralysis.
- *Otobius megnini* (spinous ear tick): larvae and nymphs in the external canal cause irritation, pain, and infection, and potentially significant blood loss.
- Reactions may be caused from inflammatory or toxic components of tick saliva (Figures 15.24, 15.25).
- Hypersensitivity causes focal necrosis, ulceration, and pruritus.

Hymenoptera Sting

- Ants, dogs and cats:
  - Fire ants (*Solenopsis* spp.) aggressively attack when disturbed.
  - Ants attach to the skin by jaws and may sting up to 10 times; hundreds of stings may occur in one attack.
  - Stings may initially be painless.
  - Individual stings result in pruritic and erythematous urticaria and papules leading to sterile vesicles/white pustules; they may lead to focal necrosis (Figure 15.26).
  - Lesions tend to be grouped and nonfollicular.
  - Anaphylactic shock is possible.
  - Venom contains solenopsin D, an alkaloid piperidine derivative.
  - Hypersensitivity reactions to ant allergens (similar to house dust mite) are reported (Figures 15.27–15.29).
- Bees, wasps, yellow jackets, hornets: dogs and cats:
  - Animal sensitivity and number of stings determine severity of reaction
  - Single stings result in localized pain, erythema, and severe edema
  - Anaphylactic shock can result
  - Stings occur most often on the muzzle and the extremities; if on the muzzle, angioedema can result in respiratory compromise (Figure 15.30)
  - Some wasps, yellow jackets, and hornets can sting multiple times.
- Agitated behavior of dogs during an attack may stimulate further response from Africanized bees and hornets.
- Severe attacks can result in death directly from the venom.
- Venom contains melittin and phospholipase A that act on cellular membranes causing hemolysis, rhabdomyolysis, and kidney tubular necrosis.

DIFFERENTIAL DIAGNOSES

Flea Bite Dermatitis and Hypersensitivity

- Food allergy
- Atopy
- Sarcoptic/notoedric mange
- Cheyletiellosis

- Demodicosis
- Pediculosis
- Dermatophytosis
- Bacterial folliculitis
- *Malassezia* dermatitis
- Eosinophilic granuloma complex (cats)

Spider Bite Dermatitis

- Snakebite
- Localized physical, electrical, thermal or chemical trauma
- Localized abscessation
- Localized vasculitis

Fly Dermatitis

- Sarcoptic/notoedric mange
- Cheyletiellosis
- Demodicosis
- Pediculosis
- Pemphigus foliaceus/erythematosus
- Leproid granuloma
- Neoplasia

Mosquito Bite Dermatitis and Hypersensitivity

- Food allergy
- Atopy
- Demodicosis
- Dermatophytosis
- Pemphigus foliaceus
- Herpesvirus ulcerative dermatitis
- Plasma cell pododermatitis
- Squamous cell carcinoma
- Eosinophilic granuloma complex

Tick Bite Dermatitis and Hypersensitivity

- Food allergy
- Atopy
- Localized trauma
- Sarcoptic/notoedric mange
- Cheyletiellosis
- Bacterial folliculitis
- Allergic otitis externa (*Otobius*)
- Neuropathy (tick paralysis)

Hymenoptera

- Sarcoptic/notoedric mange
- Cheyletiellosis
- Bacterial folliculitis
- Demodicosis
- Pemphigus foliaceus

DIAGNOSTICS

Flea Bite Dermatitis and Hypersensitivity

- Biopsy: superficial, perivascular to diffuse inflammation with eosinophils and mast cells; eosinophilic intraepidermal microabscesses.
- Allergy testing; intradermal testing more reliable than serum testing for FBH: large number of FBH dogs are positive to flea antigen; positives may also be seen in normal patients: not reliable, especially if negative.
- Elimination of other causes of pruritus.
- Fecal identification of *Dipylidium caninum* segments.
- Response to adequate flea control.

Spider Bite Dermatitis

- Biopsy: epidermal and dermal necrosis with inflammation extending into the subcutaneous tissue; vasculopathy and mixed inflammatory infiltrate.
- Visualization of puncture marks.
- History of exposure to arachnids.

Fly Dermatitis

- Biopsy: hyperkeratosis with erosions and serocellular crusting; dermal fibrosis, often with interstitial and perivascular plasma cell and eosinophil infiltrate.
- Elimination of other causes of lesions.
- Response to appropriate fly control.

Mosquito Bite Dermatitis and Hypersensitivity

- Biopsy: severe, eosinophil-rich superficial and deep dermal infiltrate; foci of eosinophil degranulation with flame figures and eosinophilic mural folliculitis.
- Allergy testing (intradermal and/or serum) positive to culicoides antigen: not reliable, especially if negative.
- Response to application of insect repellants or being placed in a mosquito-free environment.

Tick Bite Dermatitis and Hypersensitivity

- Presence of attached ticks.
- Biopsy: leukocytoclastic vasculitis, epidermal hemorrhage and necrosis, eosinophil-rich pyogranulomatous dermatitis.
- Diagnostic testing for tick-vectored diseases.

Hymenoptera

- Biopsy: intraepidermal neutrophilic pustule with superficial and deep dermal interstitial neutrophilic dermatitis and collagen degeneration.
- Presence of stinger(s) or adherent ants.
- History of exposure.
- Intradermal allergy testing with hymenoptera antigens.

THERAPEUTICS

Flea Bite Dermatitis and Hypersensitivity

- Flea control:
    - All dogs and cats in the household must be treated
    - Flea control measures should be tailored to the individual situation
    - Multiple effective products are available including spot-ons, sprays, collars, and systemic medications
    - Client education is required for successful control of fleas both on the pet and in the environment.
- Topical corticosteroid sprays (with or without antibiotics) effective for individual lesions.
- Prednisolone (2–4 mg/kg q24h tapering dosage).
- Antibiotics only for pyotraumatic folliculitis (“deep” hotspot).
- Antihistamines rarely effective for complete control of symptoms.

Spider Bite Dermatitis

- Local infusion of early lesions with corticosteroids and/or lidocaine.
- Systemic support with antibiotics, antiinflammatory medications, and analgesics.
- Wound treatment.
- Environmental clean-up (eliminating outdoor sites and insecticide spraying).

Fly Dermatitis

- Fly avoidance.
- Application of repellants to pinnae.
- Wound treatment.
- Environmental clean-up to remove fly breeding sources.

Mosquito Bite Dermatitis and Hypersensitivity

- Mosquito avoidance.
- Application of repellants to face and pinnae.
- Topical corticosteroid sprays effective for individual lesions.
- Prednisolone (2–4 mg/kg q24h tapering dosage) or dexamethasone (0.1 mg/kg q24h tapering dosage).
- Environmental clean-up to remove mosquito breeding sources.

Tick Bite Dermatitis and Hypersensitivity

- Manual removal of ticks.
- Corticosteroids for inflammatory reactions.
- Antibiotics as indicated for secondary infection.

Hymenoptera

- Remove stinger(s).
- Antihistamines (see Appendix B).
- Corticosteroids.
- Topical corticosteroid sprays effective for individual lesions.
- Prednisolone (2–4 mg/kg q24h tapering dosage).
- Reduce exposure.
- Systemic support.
- Hyposensitization can be very effective in patients with prior incidences of anaphylaxis.
- Portable epinephrine administration devices are available for use by the owner when reexposure is unavoidable.

COMMENTS

- Insect avoidance and control should be stressed as the primary method to prevent recurrences.
- Symptoms may be seasonal and/or geographical variation dependent on insect populations.
- In situations where complete avoidance of insects is not possible, reduction in exposure will simplify and reduce medications needed to control symptoms.

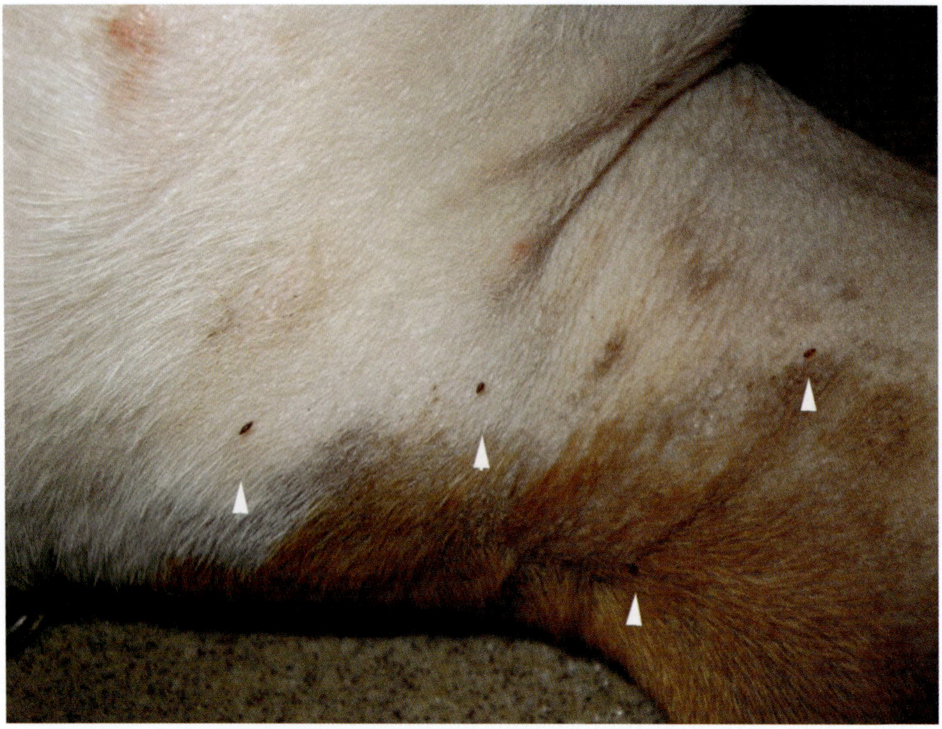

■ **Fig. 15.1.** Numerous *Echidnophaga gallinacea* (sticktight fleas) (*arrowheads*) on the medial thigh of a 3-year-old female-spayed pit bull exposed to pet chickens. Fleas remained firmly attached to the skin during examination.

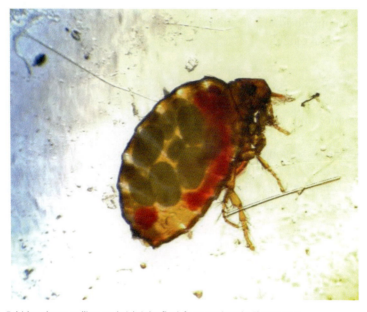

■ **Fig. 15.2.** *Echidnophaga gallinacea* (sticktight flea) from patient in Figure 15.1.

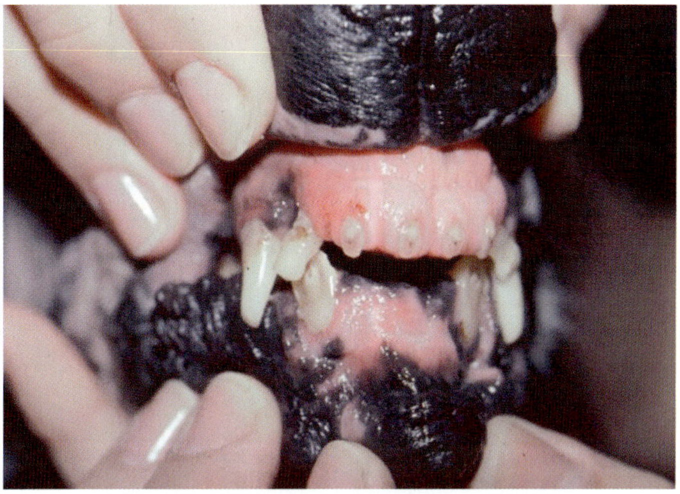

■ **Fig. 15.3.** Worn incisors from chronic self-chewing on hair coat.

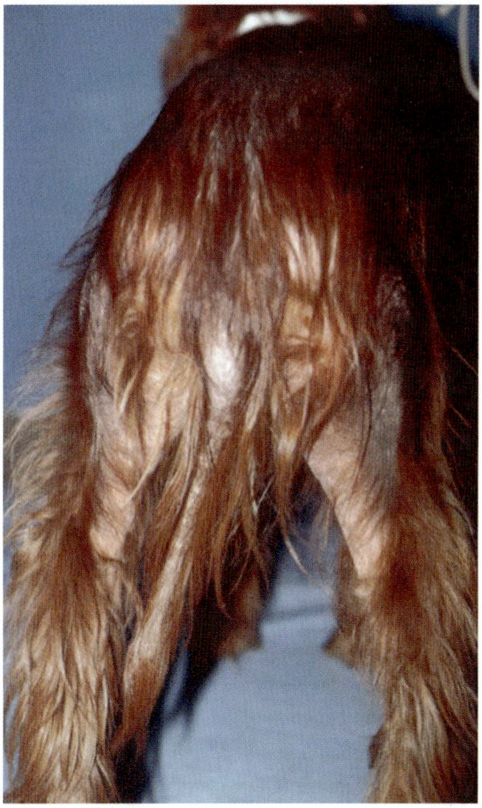

■ **Fig. 15.4.** Flea bite hypersensitivity with alopecia affecting the dorsal lumbosacral and caudal thigh regions.

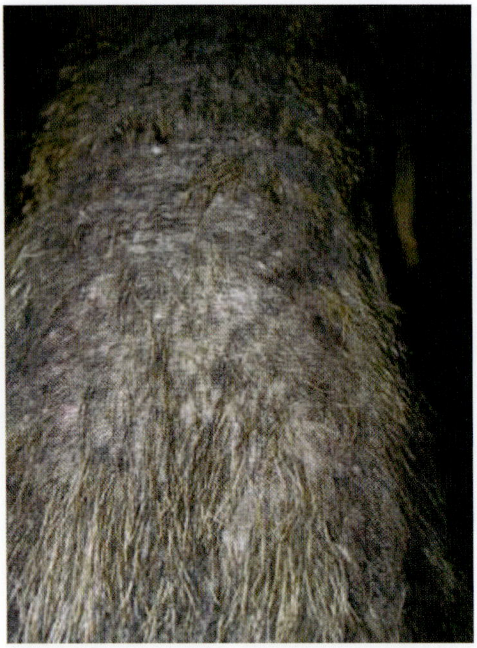

■ **Fig. 15.5.** Flea bite hypersensitivity. Significant alopecia and lichenification of the dorsal lumbosacral region of an adult German shepherd from chronic self-trauma.

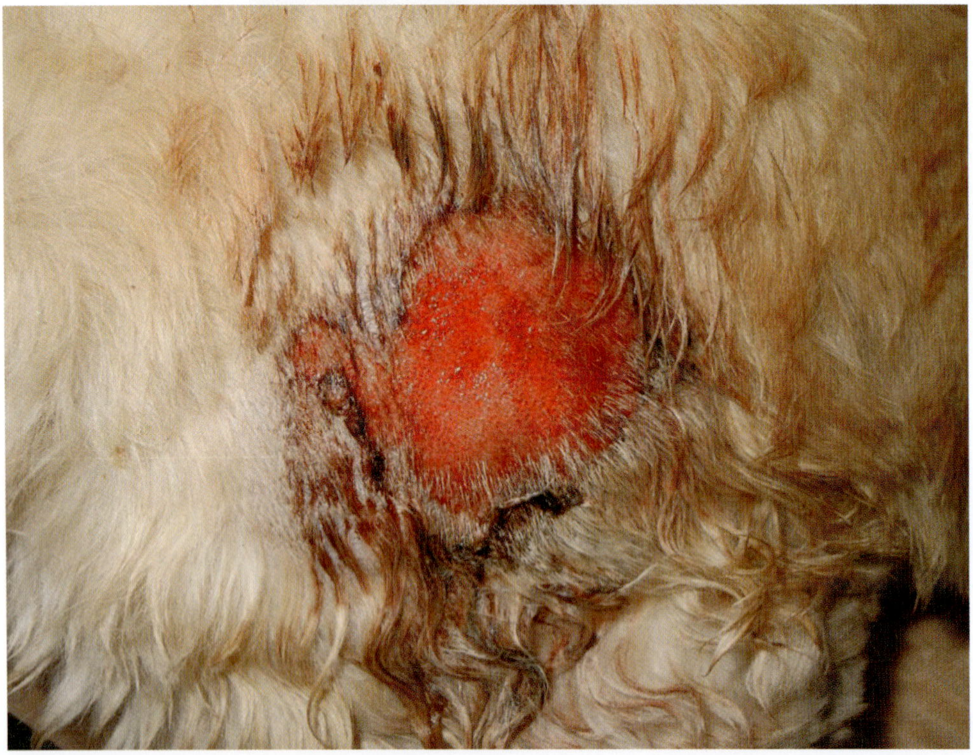

■ **Fig. 15.6.** Surface pyotraumatic dermatitis "hotspot" in a 4-year-old male-castrate cockapoo.

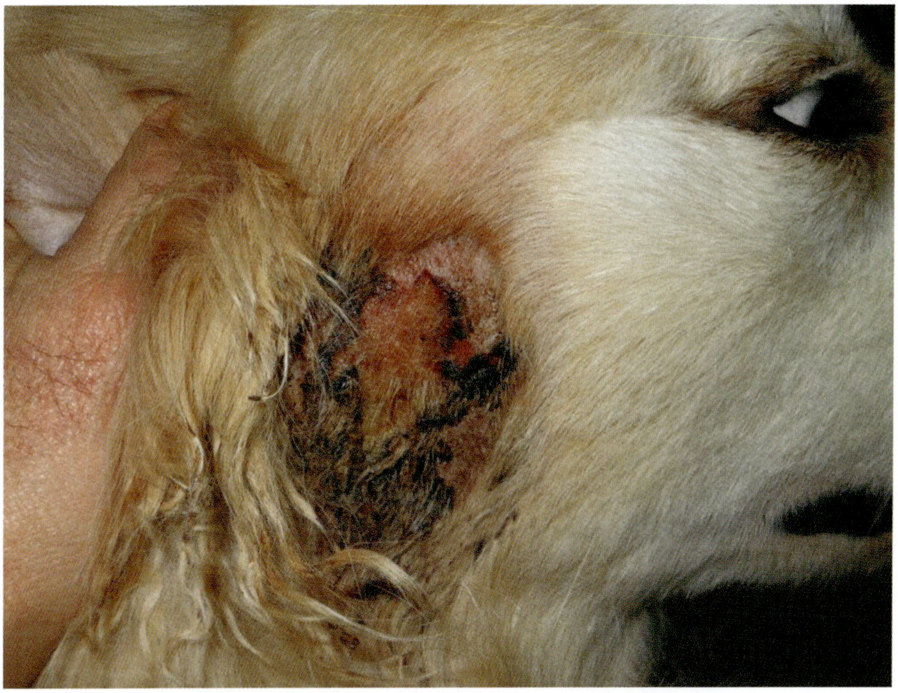

Fig. 15.7. "Deep" pyotraumatic folliculitis lesion on the neck of a 9-year-old male-castrate golden retriever.

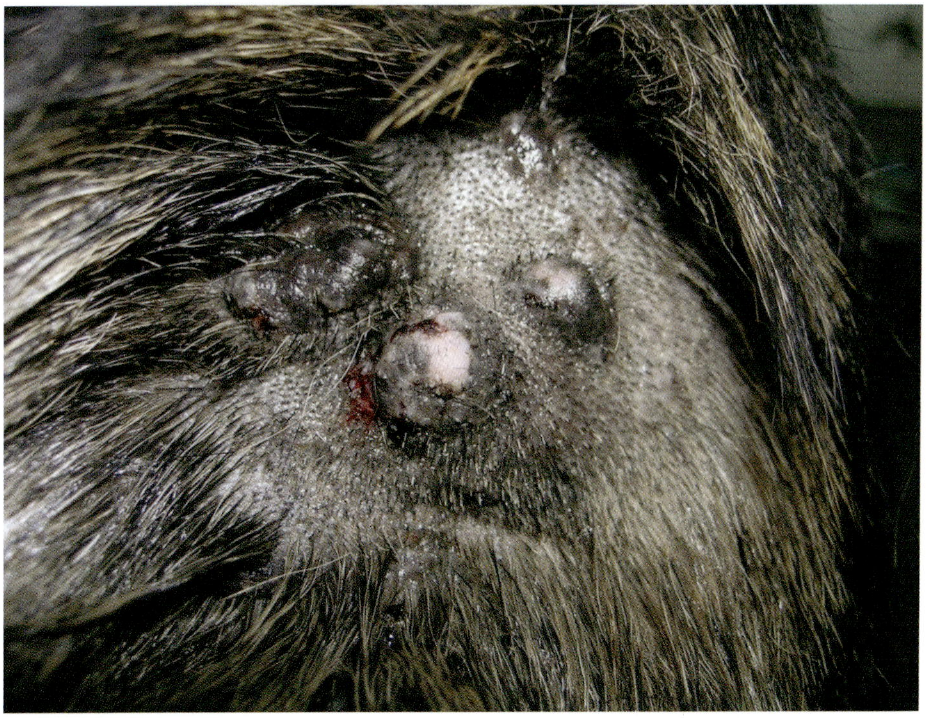

Fig. 15.8. Fibropruritic nodules: firm projections on the dorsal lumbosacral area of a 9-year-old female-spayed German shepherd dog.

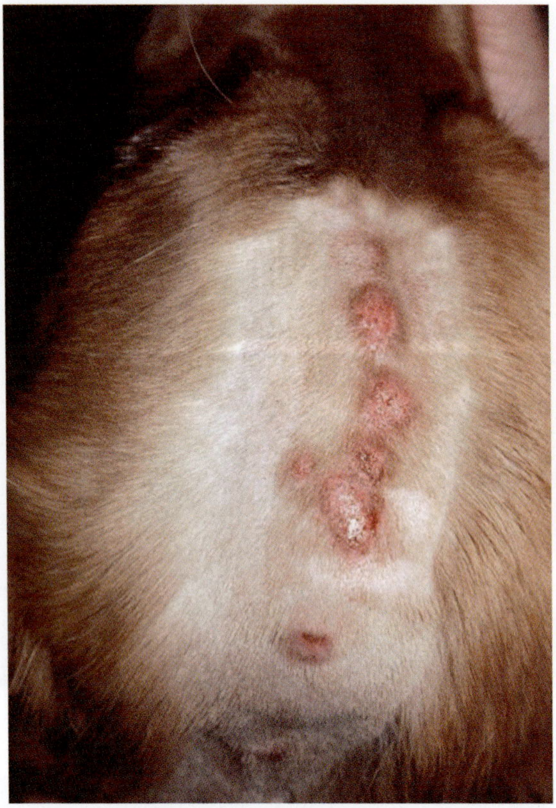

Fig. 15.9. Erythematous plaques on the dorsum of a cat due to flea bites.

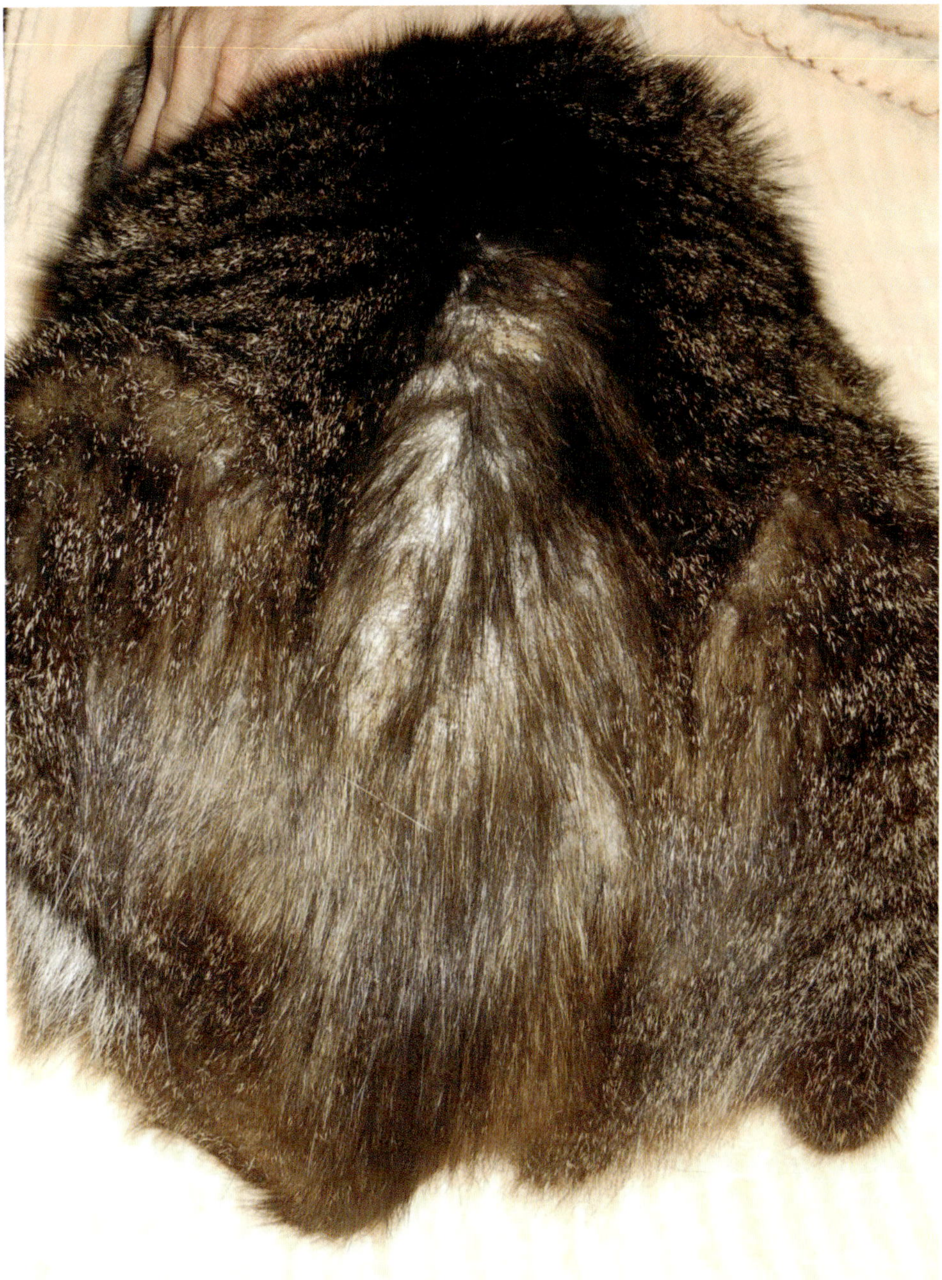

■ **Fig. 15.10.** Alopecic patches on the dorsal lumbosacral region of a 7-year-old female-spayed DSH with flea bite hypersensitivity.

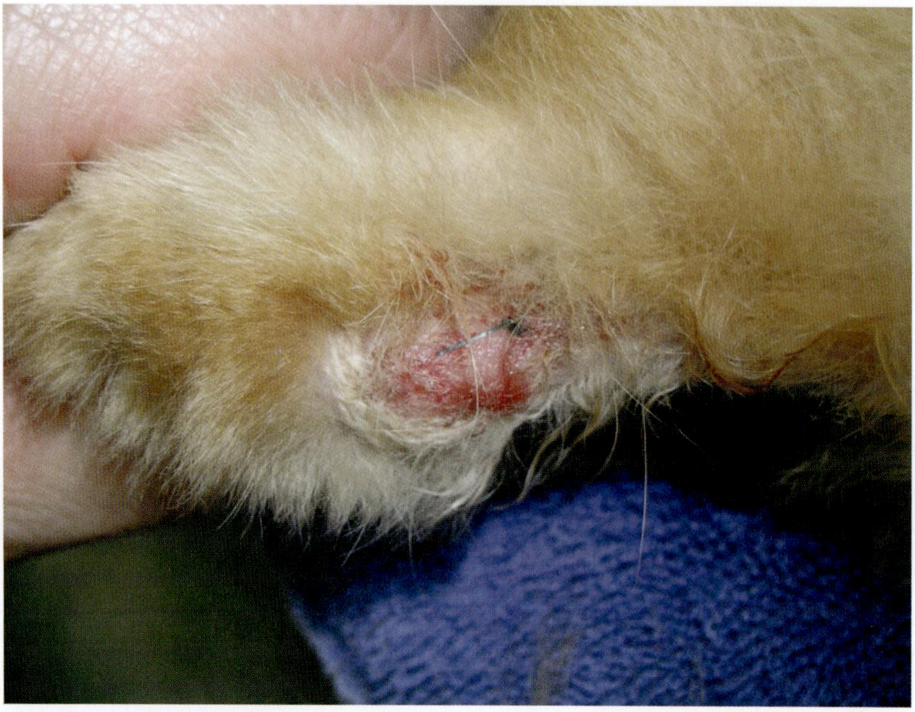

Fig. 15.11. Eosinophilic plaque on the caudal elbow of a 2-year-old male-castrate DLH secondary to flea bite hypersensitivity.

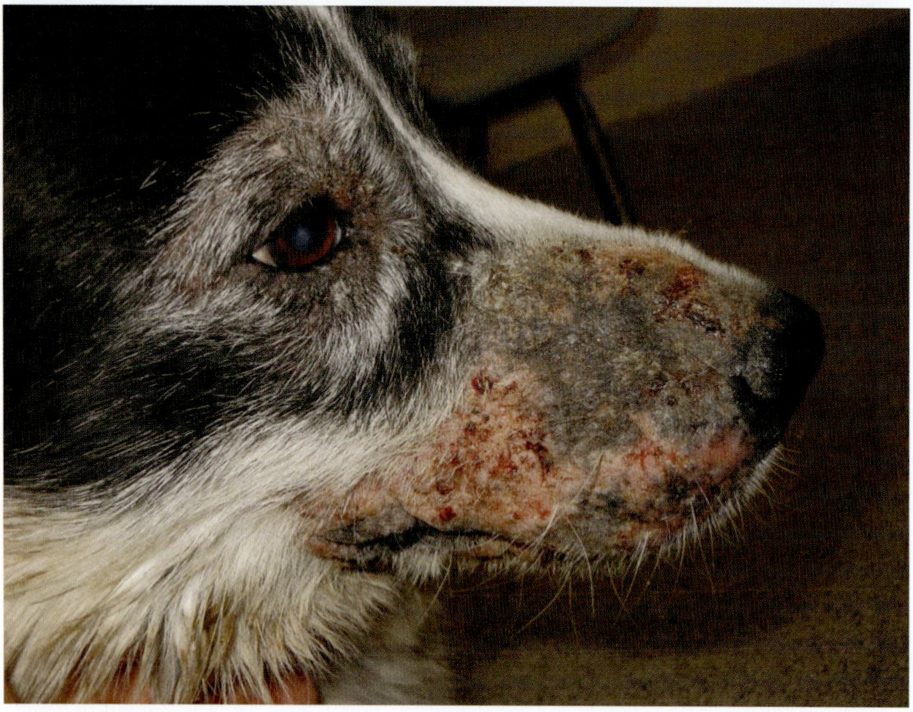

Fig. 15.12. Painful and exudative lesions on the muzzle of an Australian shepherd following a spider bite.

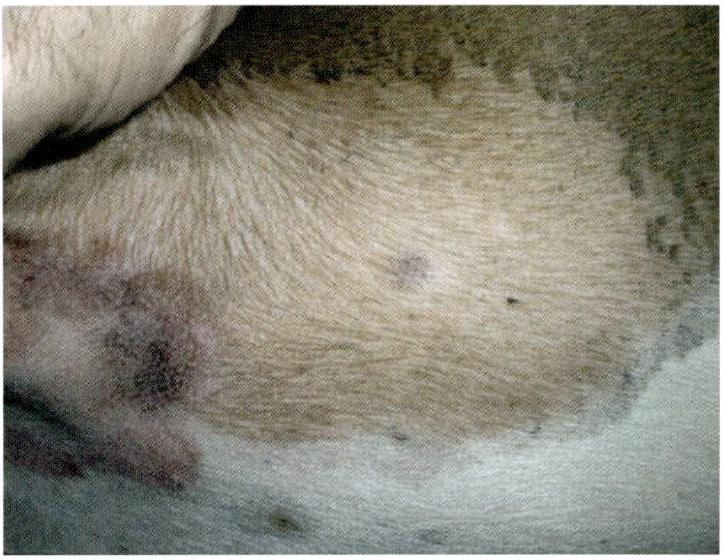

■ **Fig. 15.13.** Spider bite: the initial necrotic lesion has begun healing, leaving a central scar and surrounding zone of depigmentation caudal to the axilla.

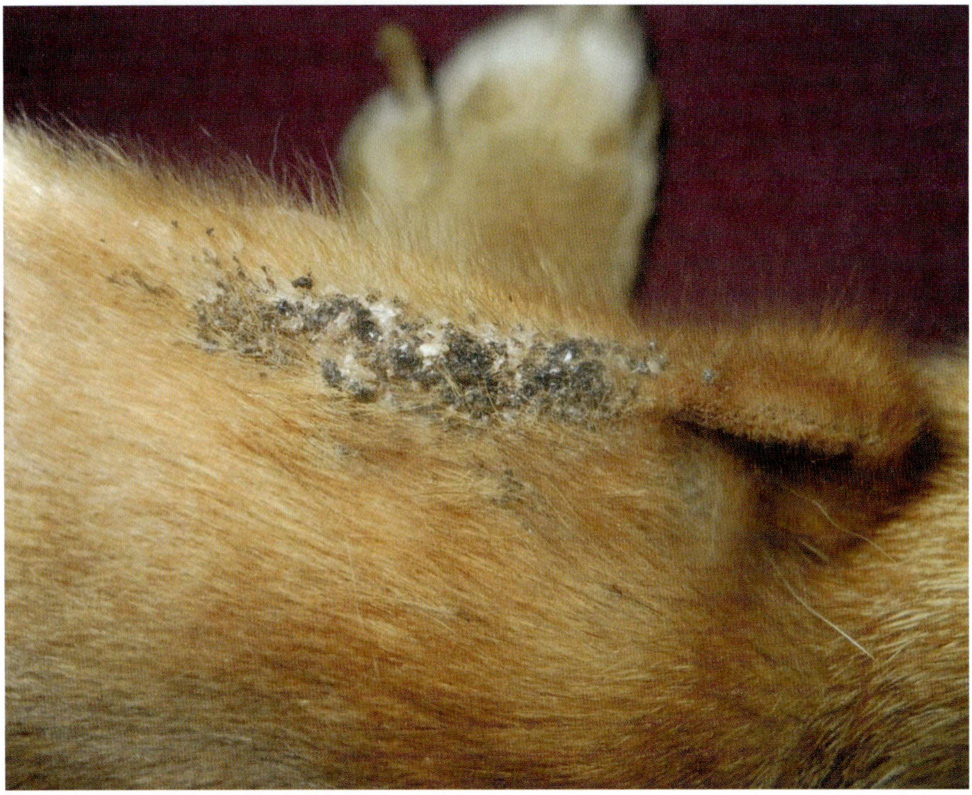

■ **Fig. 15.14.** Punctate dried hemorrhagic crusts with palpable thickening at the pinnal margin of a 2-year-old female-spayed mix breed dog from fly bites.

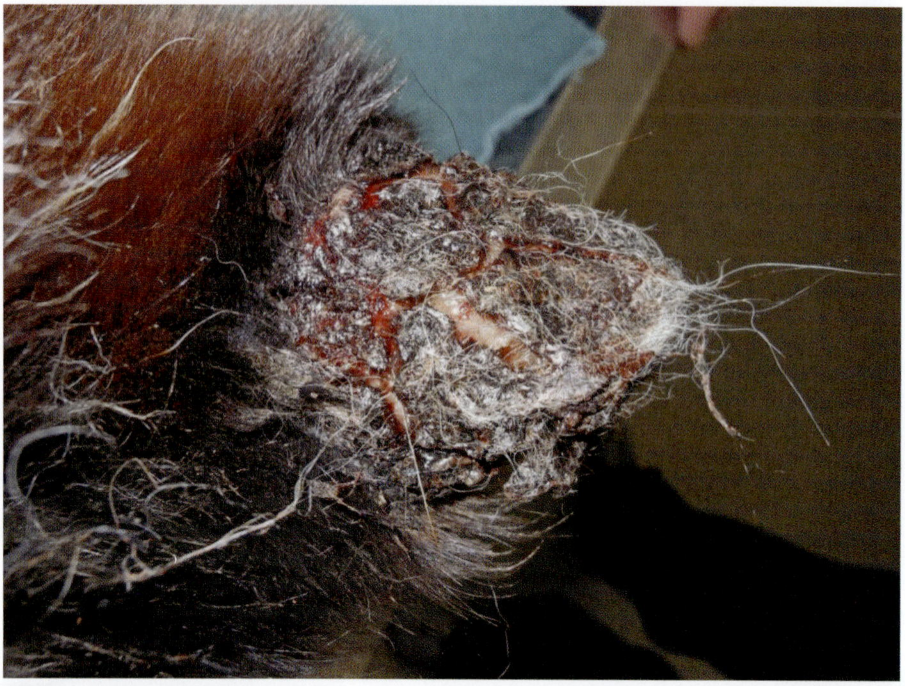

■ **Fig. 15.15.** Large accumulations of hemorrhagic debris on the pinna of a 6-year-old male-castrate malamute dog from chronic fly dermatitis.

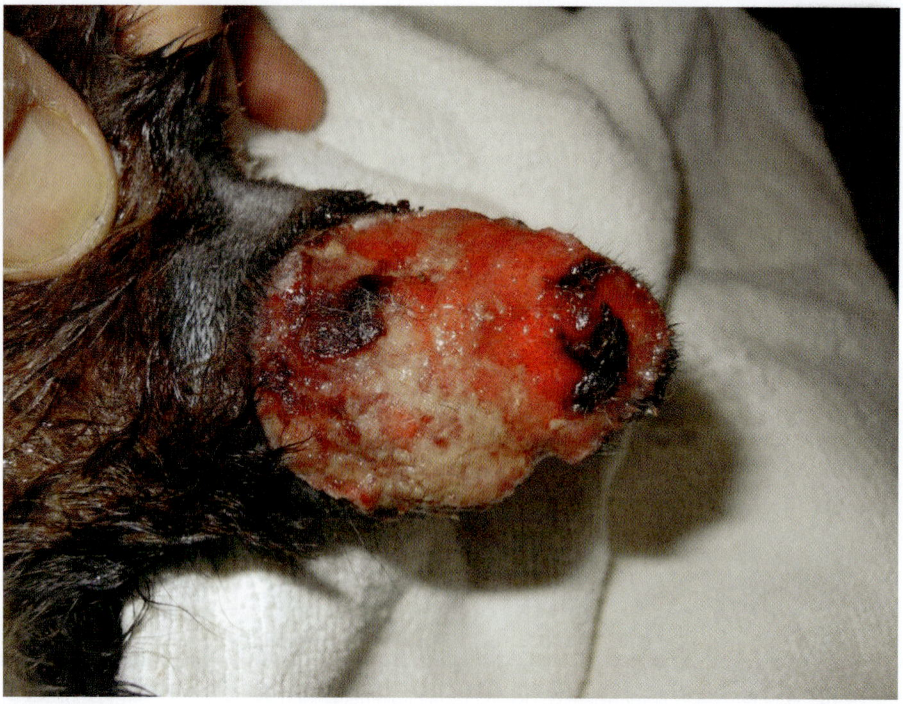

■ **Fig. 15.16.** Lesion from patient in Figure 15.15 after removal of dried exudates. The distal portion of the pinna is painful, swollen, and infected.

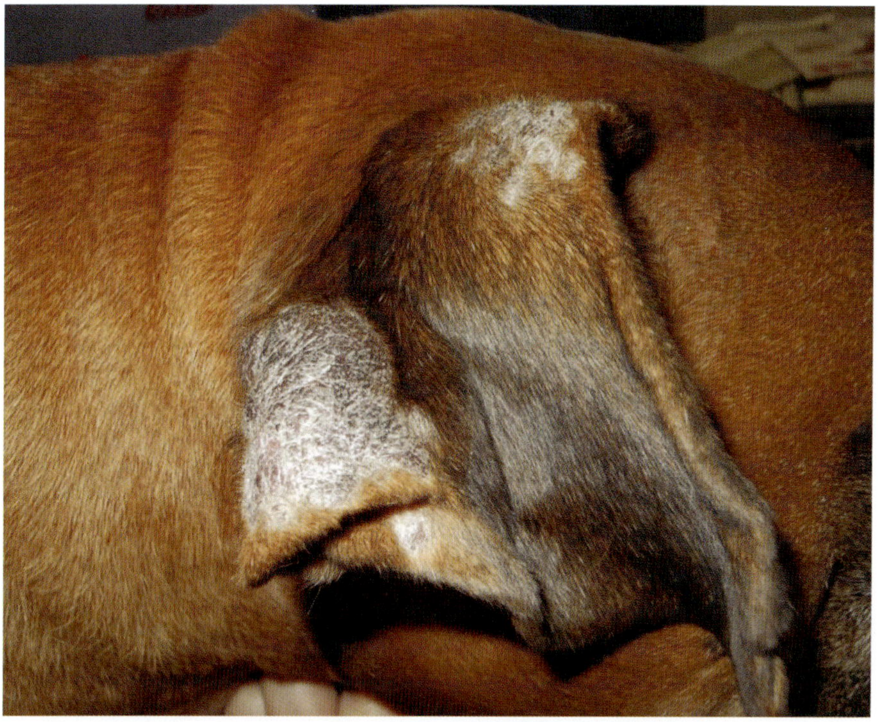

■ **Fig. 15.17.** Leproid granuloma lesions on the pinna of a 6-year-old male-castrate boxer. Note that alopecic and thickened lesions are in areas most often affected by fly bites.

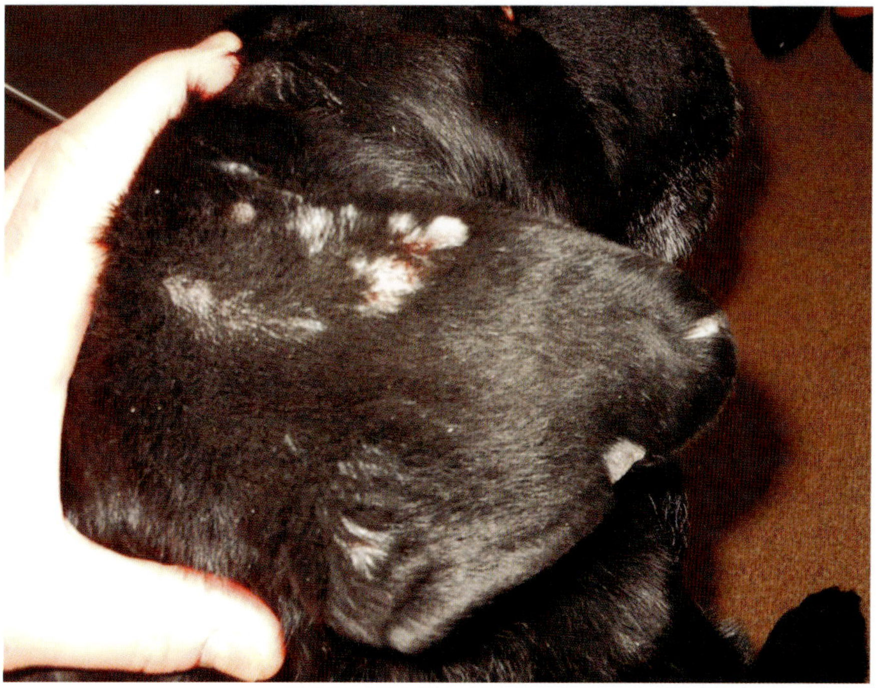

■ **Fig. 15.18.** Multiple mosquito bites on the pinna of an 8-year-old male-castrate Labrador retriever. Bites produced multifocal areas of excoriation and scabs.

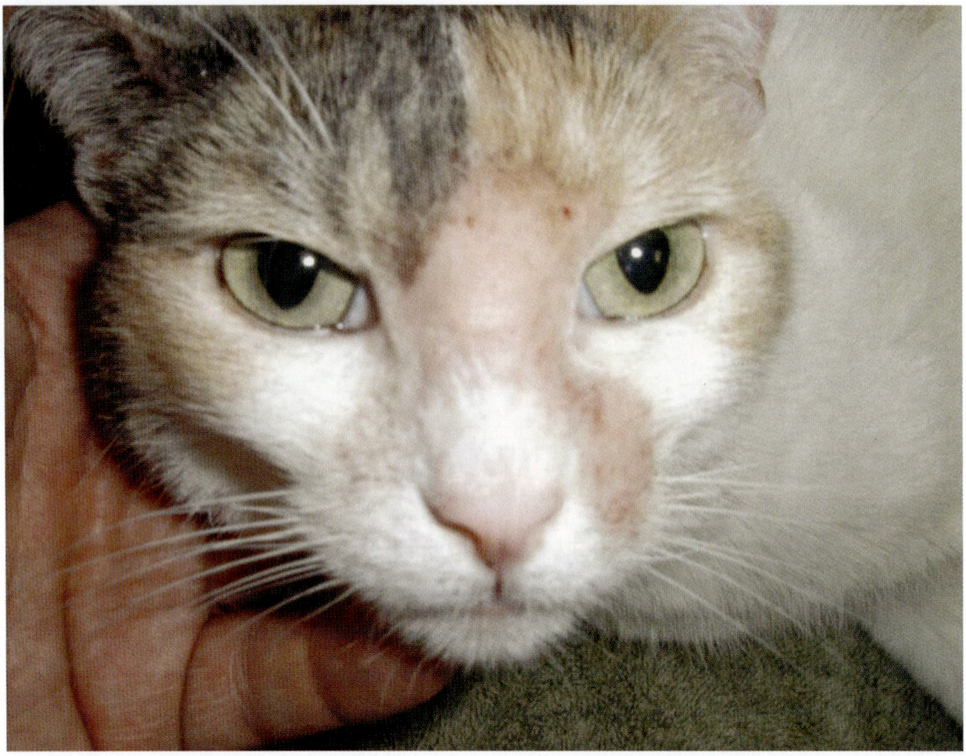

■ **Fig. 15.19.** Mosquito bite hypersensitivity producing alopecia and erythema on the muzzle and face of a 6-year-old female-spayed calico.

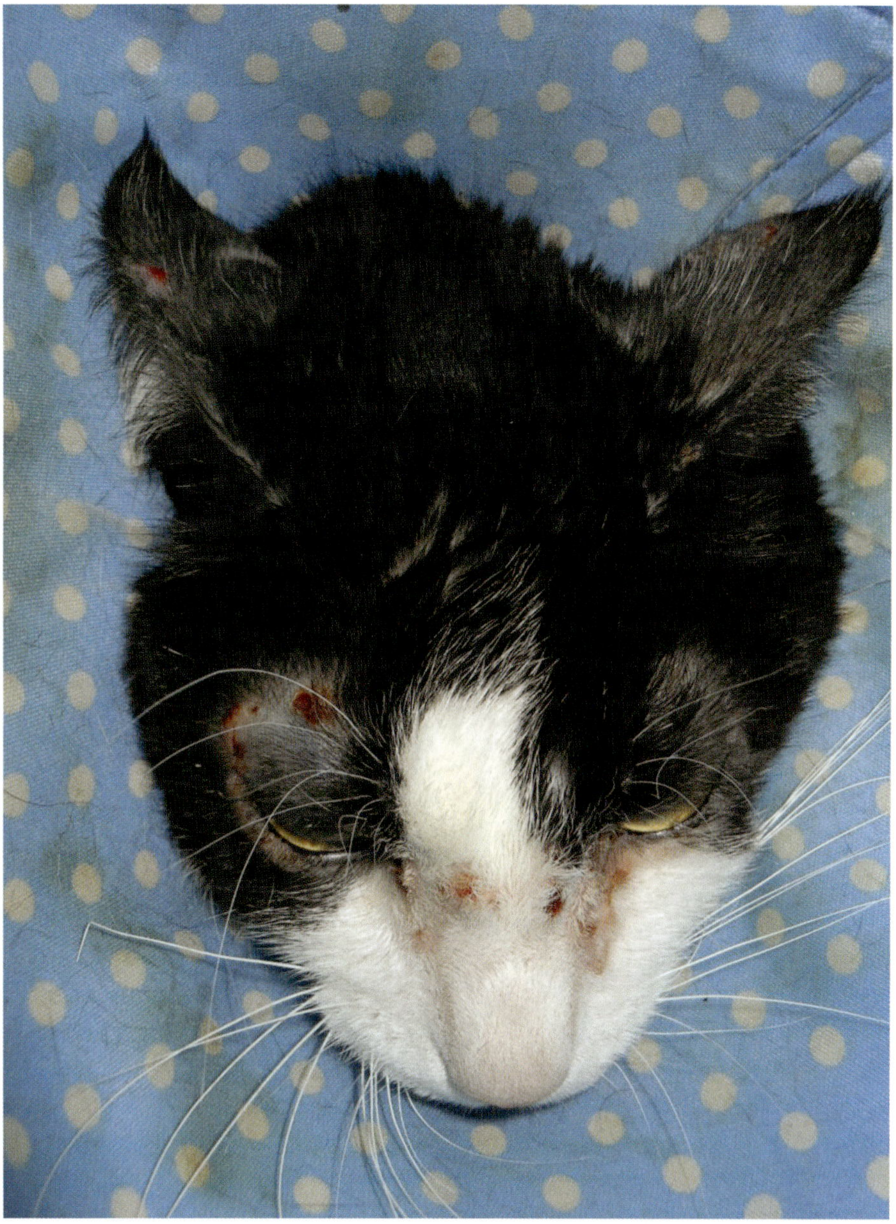

■ **Fig. 15.20.** Excoriations and punctate scabs on the dorsal muzzle, preauricular regions, and pinnae of an $11\frac{1}{2}$-year-old female-spayed DSH. Lesions of mosquito bite hypersensitivity occur most often in the less haired regions of the face, head, and pinnae.

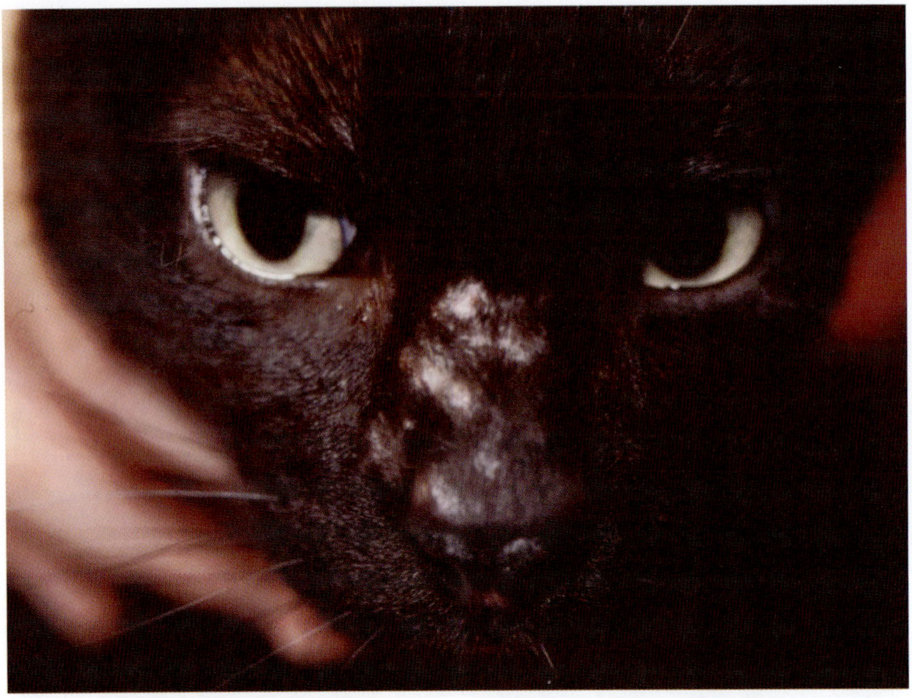

■ **Fig. 15.21.** Crusts and alopecia affecting the dorsal muzzle of a dark-coated DSH represent classic lesions of mosquito bite hypersensitivity.

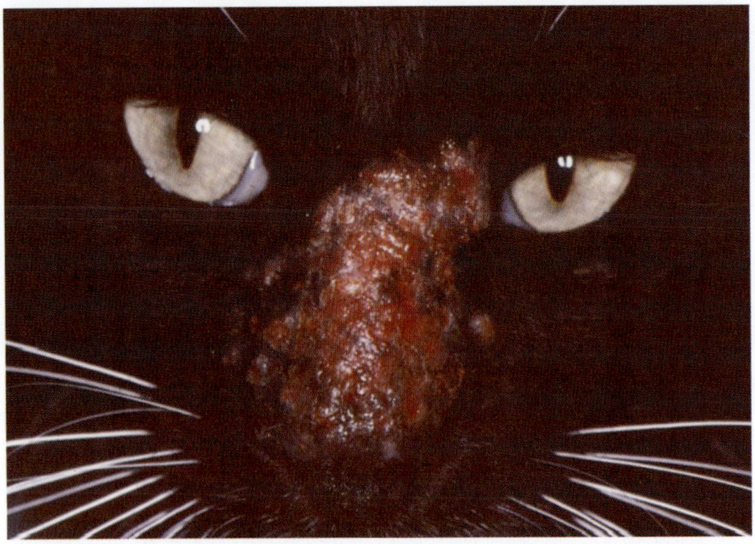

■ **Fig. 15.22.** Chronic mosquito bite hypersensitivity producing exudation and secondary folliculitis.

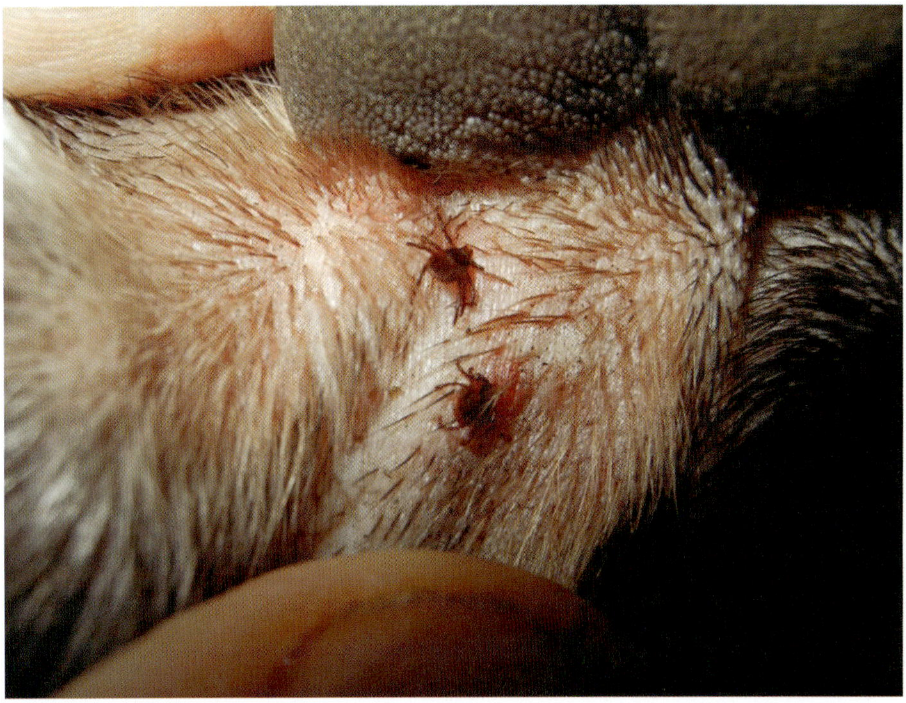

Fig. 15.23. Ticks imbedded in the interdigital space causing pedal pruritus in this cavalier King Charles spaniel.

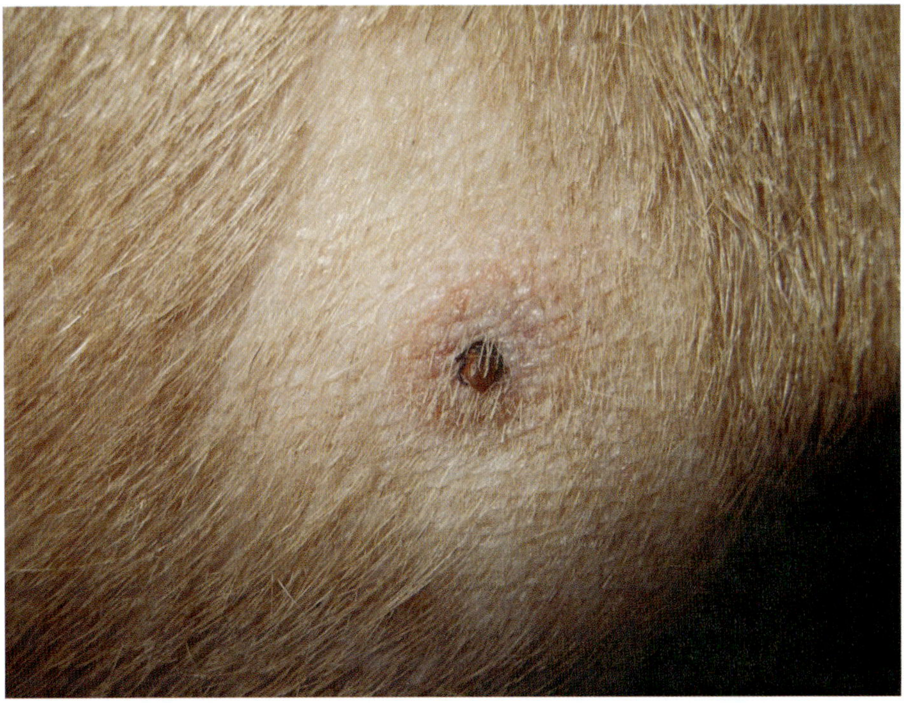

Fig. 15.24. Embedded tick on a 5-year-old male-castrate pit bull. Note the inflammation surrounding the site of tick attachment.

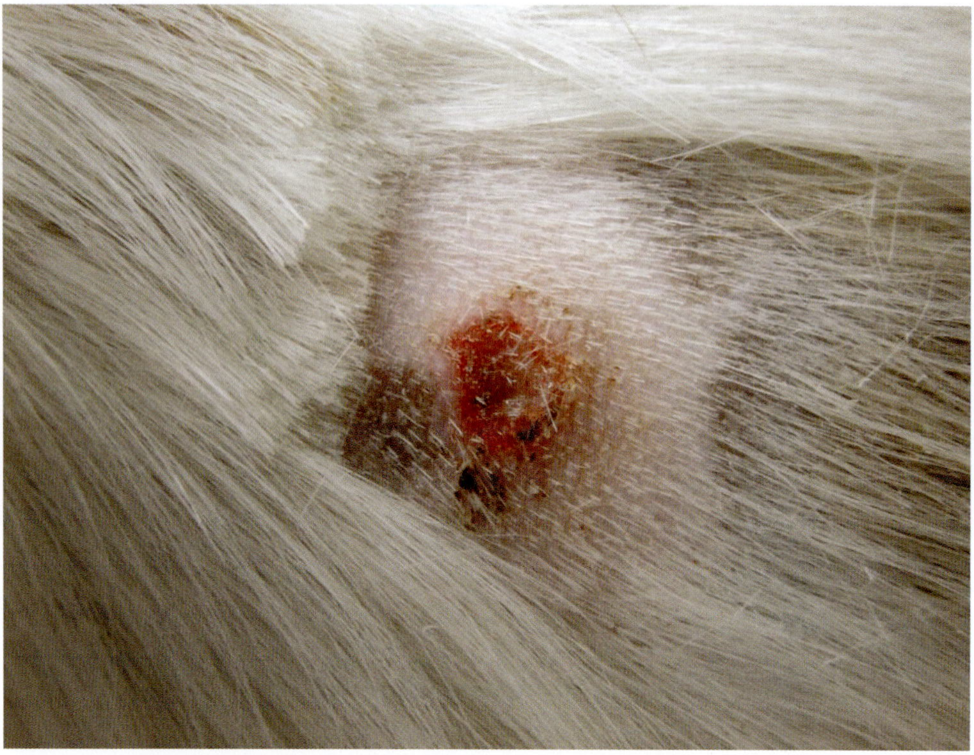

Fig. 15.25. Focal lesion of necrosis and exudation due to tick bite hypersensitivity at the site of tick attachment in a 3-year-old female-spayed pekinese.

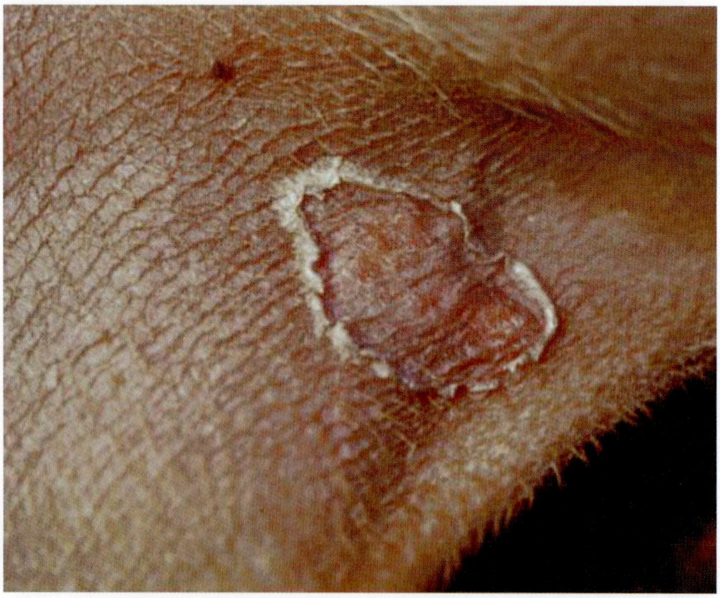

Fig. 15.26. Focal lesion of erythema and a disrupted, expanding vesicle, caused by an ant bite.

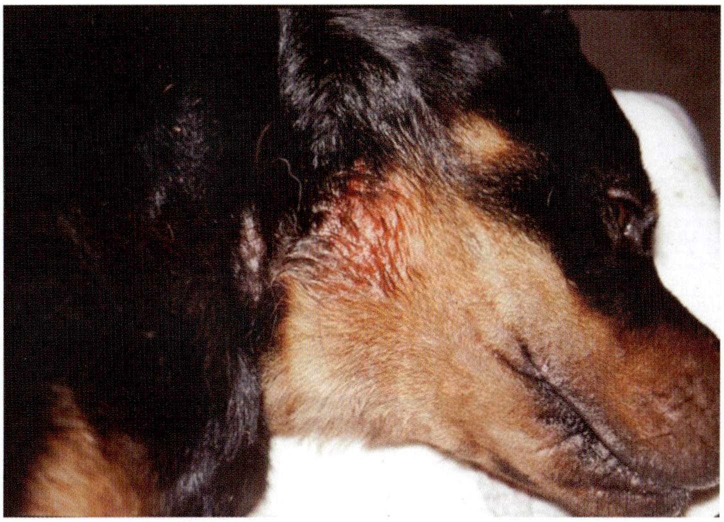

■ **Fig. 15.27.** Lesion of dermatitis on the face of a rottweiler with black ant hypersensitivity similar to pyotraumatic dermatitis seen with FBH.

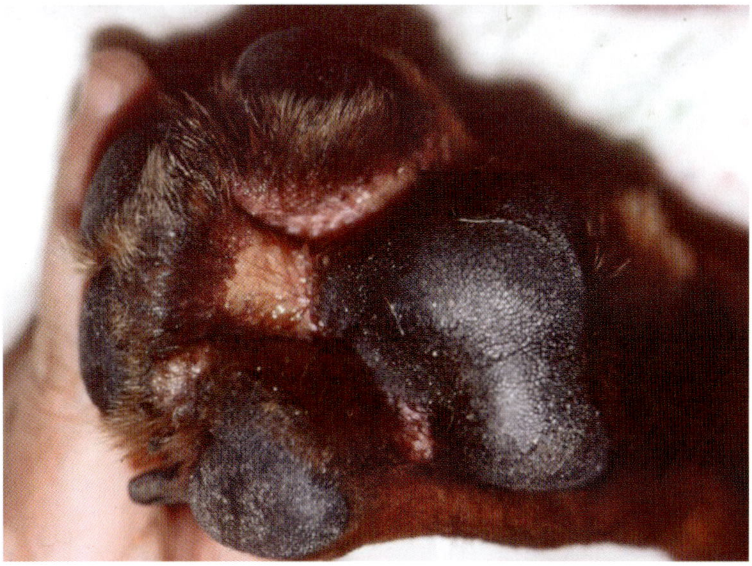

■ **Fig. 15.28.** Exudative lesion in the interdigital region of the patient in Figure 15.1; these symptoms are similar to atopic dermatitis.

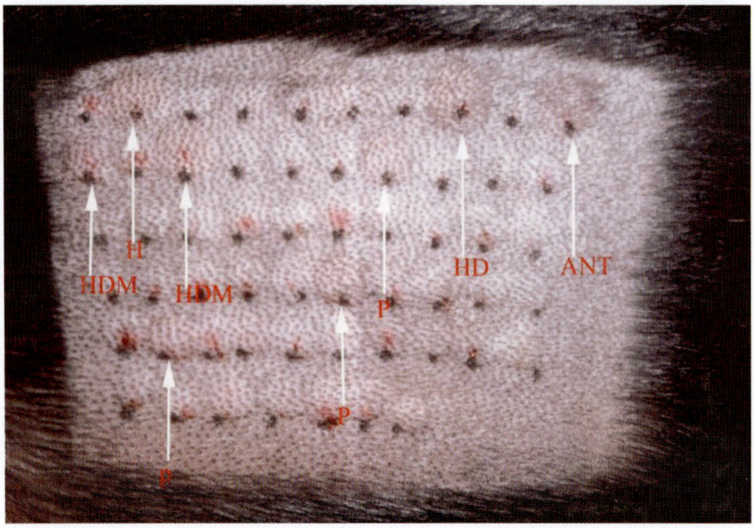

■ **Fig. 15.29.** Intradermal allergy testing of patient in Figures 15.1 and 15.2; reactions to house dust (HD), house dust mite (HDM), and pollen (P).

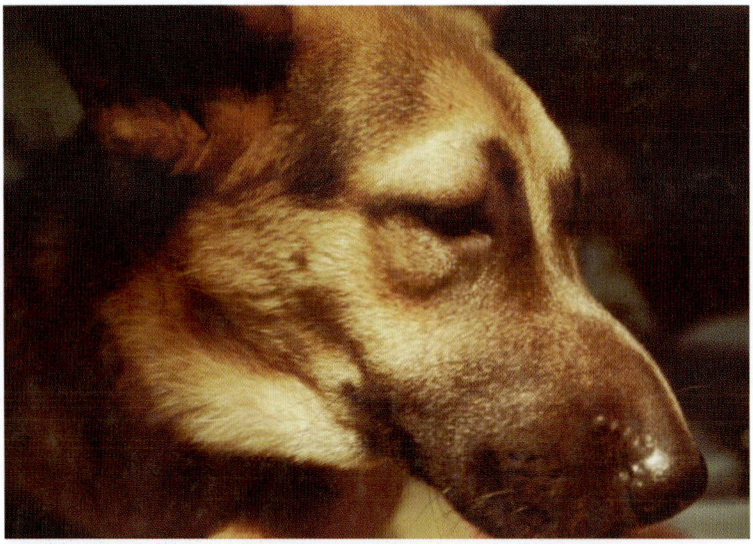

■ **Fig. 15.30.** Facial swelling due to bee sting.

chapter 16

Contact Dermatitis

DEFINITION/OVERVIEW

Irritant contact dermatitis (ICD) and allergic contact dermatitis (ACD) are two possibly different pathophysiologic syndromes with similar clinical signs resulting in an inflammatory skin response from exposure to an external substance.

ETIOLOGY/PATHOPHYSIOLOGY

- Differentiation between ICD and ACD may be more conceptual than practical.
- ICD: irritants directly damage keratinocytes, causing release of cytokines to induce an inflammatory response at the lesion site:
    - Examples of irritants include cleansers, insecticides, plants, and chemicals (e.g., fertilizers, solvents)
    - Response depends on concentration, potency, and contact time.
- ACD: a type IV (delayed) hypersensitivity requiring sensitization and elicitation:
    - Sensitizers penetrate the skin, bind to carrier proteins, are processed by dendritic cells, and lead to production of memory and effector T cells
    - During elicitation, memory and effector T cells damage keratinocytes (causing cytokine release) as well as recruiting inflammatory cells to the lesion site:
        - Examples of sensitizers include plants, topical medications, skin care products, and metals
        - Many sensitizers are also irritants.
- There are similarities between ICD, ACD, and atopic dermatitis; epidermal barrier defects as well as inflammation may encourage penetration of sensitizers/allergens to produce reactions.
- The incidence of ACD is increased in atopic animals.

SIGNALMENT/HISTORY

ICD

- Occurs at any age as a direct result of the irritant nature of the offending compound.
- Reactions may occur acutely (similar to chemical burns) or after repeated exposure.

Blackwell's Five-Minute Veterinary Consult Clinical Companion: Small Animal Dermatology, Third Edition.
Karen Helton Rhodes and Alexander H. Werner.

- Corticosteroids minimally helpful.
- Lesions resolve 1–2 days after removal of irritant.

ACD

- Rare in young animals; most animals chronically exposed to the antigen; extremely rare in cats (e.g., exposure to d-limonene-containing insecticides).
- Reported increased risk of ACD: Boston terrier, pit bull, boxer, dachshund, weimaraner, German shepherd dog, poodle, wire-haired fox terrier, Scottish terrier, West Highland white terrier, Labrador and golden retriever.
- Requires weeks to months of exposure for hypersensitivity to develop.
- Reexposure results in development of clinical signs 3–5 days following exposure; signs may persist for several weeks.
- May respond to corticosteroids applied topically at the lesion or systemically; pruritus returns after discontinuation if the antigenic stimulus persists.
- Hyposensitization: no reported efficacy.
- Prognosis: good if the allergen is identified and removed; poor if the allergen is not identified, which may then require lifelong treatment.

CLINICAL FEATURES

- Location determined by antigen contact; commonly limited to glabrous skin and regions frequently in contact with the environment (chin, lip margins, ventral neck, sternum, ventral abdomen, inguinum, perineum, scrotum, and ventral contact regions of the tail and interdigital areas) (Figures 16.1–16.3).
- Reactions to topical medications (e.g., otic preparations or spot-on insecticides) usually localized (Figures 16.4, 16.5).
- Thick hair coat of dogs can be an effective barrier against irritant and sensitizing contactants; extreme erythroderma often stops abruptly at the hairline (Figure 16.6).
- Initial erythema and swelling, leading to papules and plaques; vesicles uncommon.
- Chronic exposure leads to lichenification and hyperpigmentation (Figure 16.7).
- Generalized reactions, resulting from shampoos or insecticide sprays, less common.
- Pruritus: moderate to severe.
- Seasonal incidence may indicate a plant or outdoor antigen.
- Reported offending substances: plants, mulch, cedar chips, fabrics, rugs, carpets, plastics, rubber, leather, nickel, cobalt, concrete, soaps, detergents, floor waxes, carpet and litter deodorizers, herbicides, fertilizers, insecticides (including newer topical flea treatments), flea collars, topical preparations (especially neomycin).

DIFFERENTIAL DIAGNOSIS

- Atopy
- Food allergy

- Drug reaction
- Parasite hypersensitivity or infestation
- Insect bites
- Bacterial folliculitis
- *Malassezia* dermatitis
- Dermatophytosis
- Demodicosis
- Cutaneous lupus erythematosus
- Seborrheic dermatitis
- Solar dermatitis
- Thermal injuries
- Trauma from rough surfaces

DIAGNOSTICS

- Closed-patch testing:
  - Discontinue corticosteroids and NSAIDs 3–6 weeks before testing
  - Use materials directly from the environment or a standard patch test kit for humans applied to the skin under a bandage for 48 hours
  - After 48 hours, patch test allergens are removed from the skin. The test area should then remain protected and examined over the next 3–5 days for changes.
- Best diagnostic test: eliminate contact irritant or antigen (minimum 7–14 days); follow with provocative exposure (dechallenge/challenge testing).
- Exudate preps to examine for bacterial or yeast infection.
- Bacterial cultures to define secondary bacterial folliculitis if indicated.
- Clipping a patch of hair in a nonaffected region should result in further development of a local reaction by facilitating contact with the antigen.
- Skin biopsy:
  - Submission of samples from early lesions preferable to chronic lesions
  - Biopsy samples from areas under patch test sites particularly useful
  - Mainly nonspecific superficial perivascular dermatitis with intraepidermal vesiculation and spongiosis in both ICD and ACD
  - ICD: epidermal degeneration, polymorphonuclear cell infiltrate with leukocyte exocytosis
  - ACD: lymphocytic spongiotic or eosinophilic and lymphocytic spongiotic infiltrate progressing to vesiculation; intraepidermal neutrophilic or eosinophilic pustules.

THERAPEUTICS

- Eliminate or avoid offending substance(s).
- Bathe with hypoallergenic shampoos to remove antigen from the skin.
- Create mechanical barriers, if possible – socks, shirts, restriction from environment.

- Systemic corticosteroids: prednisolone (0.25–0.5 mg/kg PO q24h for 3–5 days; then q48h for 2 weeks; then twice weekly as needed).
- Topical corticosteroids for focal lesions.
- Topical NSAID: no reported efficacy.
- Antihistamine: no reported efficacy.
- Cyclosporine: may be effective – possibly by better management of underlying atopic dermatitis.
- Pentoxifylline 10 mg/kg PO q8–12h initially; may be reduced to q24h to maintain. May lose effect over time. May cause gastrointestinal upset or CNS excitement.

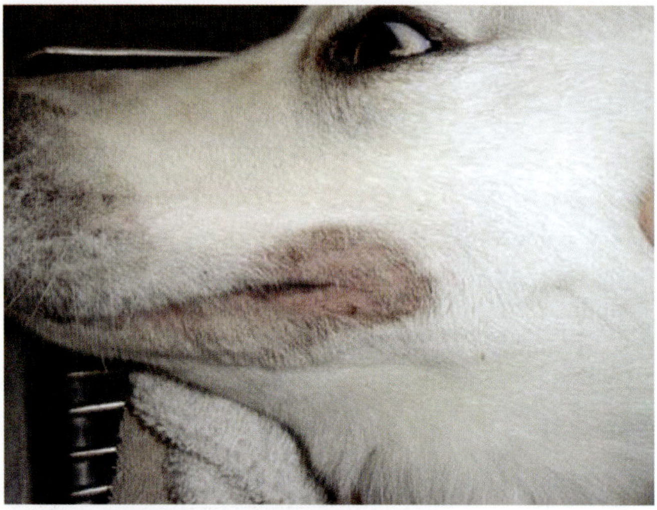

Fig. 16.1. Contact dermatitis from exposure to plants.

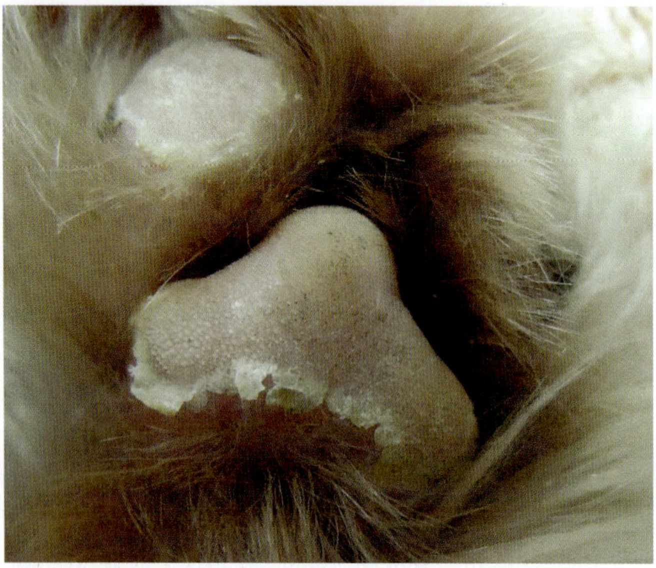

Fig. 16.2. Multiple footpad epidermal sloughing from contact with an environmental cleanser (irritant reaction).

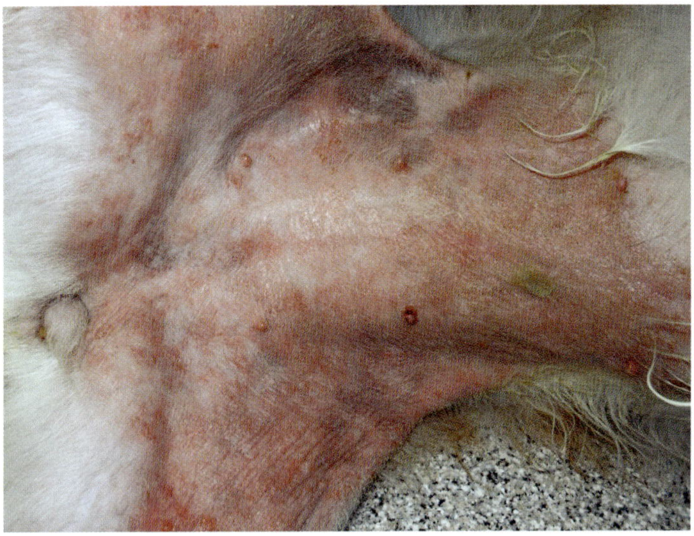

Fig. 16.3. Contact dermatitis with secondary pyoderma affecting the glabrous ventral abdomen. Lesions stopped abruptly at the hairline.

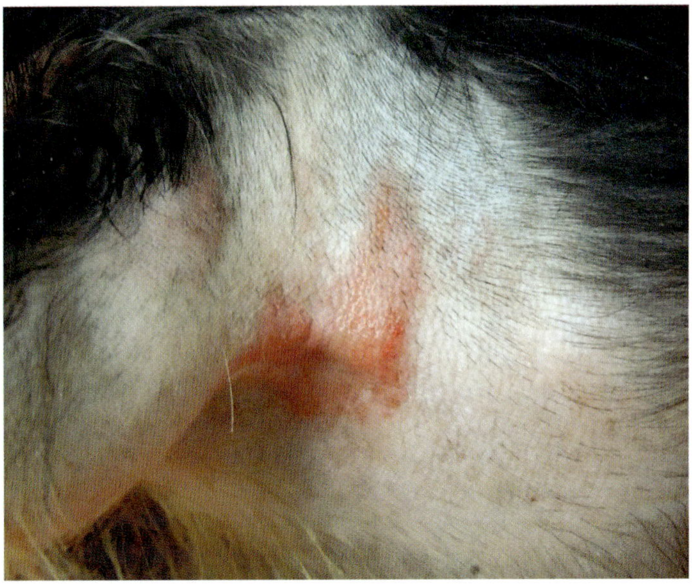

Fig. 16.4. Contact dermatitis from application of neomycin ointment to the axillary region.

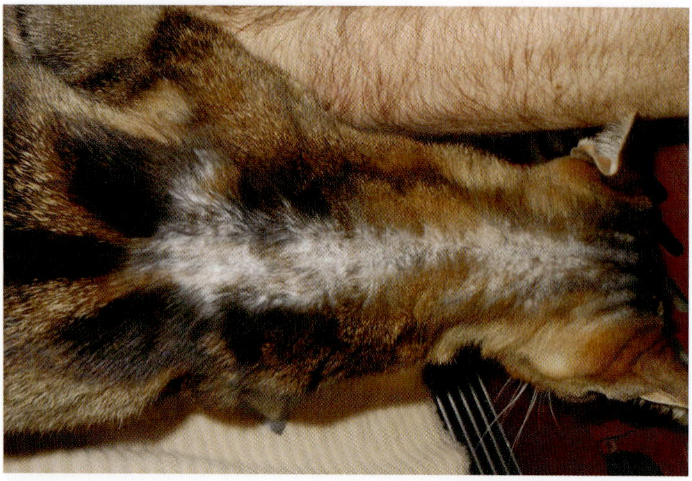

■ **Fig. 16.5.** Contact dermatitis secondary to application of a spot-on insecticide in a 10-year-old male-castrate DSH.

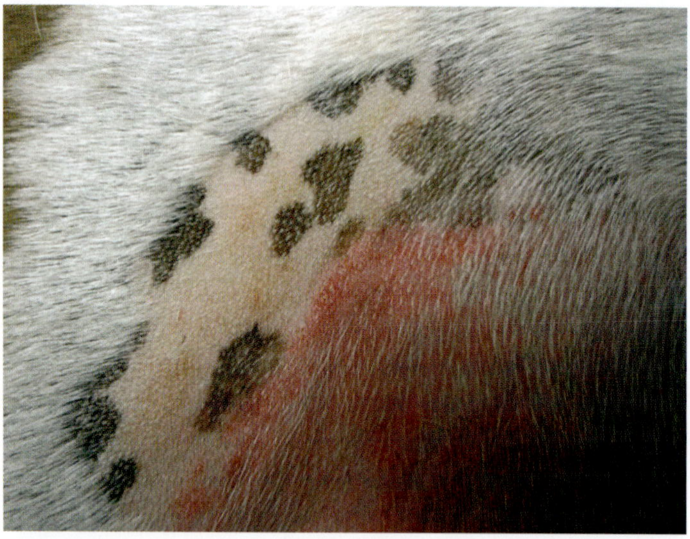

■ **Fig. 16.6.** Contact dermatitis to sunblock. Note erythema stops abruptly at hairline (edge clipped).

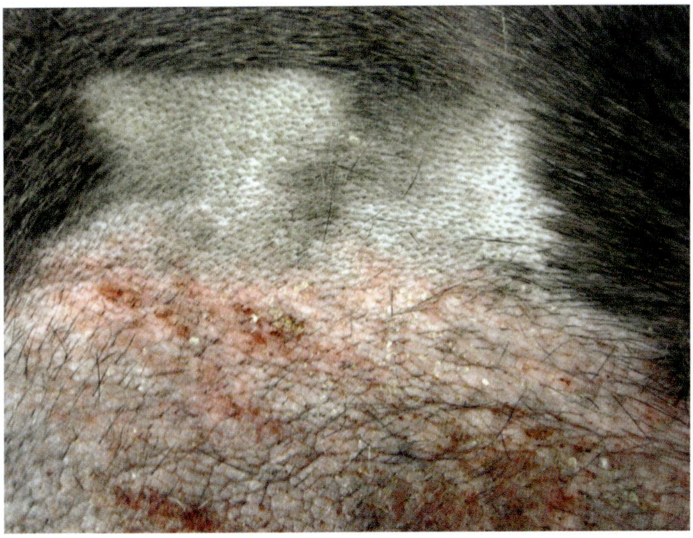

■ **Fig. 16.7.** Chronic irritant contact dermatitis leading to lichenification of the skin on the ventrum of a pit bull mix. As in previous images, lesions stop abruptly at the hairline (edge clipped).

chapter 17

Cutaneous Adverse Drug Reaction, Erythema Multiforme, Stevens–Johnson Syndrome, and Toxic Epidermal Necrolysis

DEFINITION/OVERVIEW

- A spectrum of diseases and clinical signs that vary markedly in clinical appearance and pathophysiology.
- Cutaneous adverse drug reaction (CADR) including exfoliative erythroderma: likely that many mild drug reactions go unnoticed or unreported; thus, incidence rates for specific drugs are unknown and most of the facts available on drug-specific reactions have been extrapolated from reports in the human literature; frequency estimated at 2% (dog) and 1.6% (cat).
- Erythema multiforme (EM): most often idiopathic; previously thought to be associated with drug administration (controversial).
- Stevens–Johnson syndrome (SJS) and toxic epidermal necrolysis (TEN): separate entities from EM; most likely drug-induced spectrum of dermatoses.

ETIOLOGY/PATHOPHYSIOLOGY

- CADR:
  - Drugs of any type: topical, oral, injectable
  - Exfoliative erythroderma: most often associated with shampoos and topical medications
  - Can occur after the first dose or after weeks to months of administration of the same drug; typically 5–36 days
  - Immunologic versus physiologic reaction
  - Genetic differences in susceptibility
  - May be dose related and predictable (e.g., corticosteroids and cutaneous atrophy) or idiosyncratic (immune mediated, often type 1 hypersensitivity)
  - Most common: sulfonamides, topicals, penicillins, cephalosporins (Figures 17.1–17.3).
- EM:
  - Keratinocyte is the target of an immune response resulting in apoptosis (individual keratinocyte necrosis)
  - Reported triggers include antibiotics, food ingredients, infections (bacterial and viral), and nutraceuticals (Figures 17.4–17.7)

Blackwell's Five-Minute Veterinary Consult Clinical Companion: Small Animal Dermatology, Third Edition.
Karen Helton Rhodes and Alexander H. Werner.

- Pathogenesis unclear: may involve α/β $CD4^+$ Th_1 cells and $CD8^+$ cytotoxic effector cells
- Considered to involve a variety of mechanisms such as the upregulation of expression of MHC II and ICAM-1 adhesion molecules on keratinocytes
- T cells are recruited to the epidermis and dermis and result in direct lymphocyte-mediated cytotoxicity and apoptosis
- Granulysin (released by T cells)-induced intrinsic apoptosis.

■ SJS/TEN:
- Drug molecules combine with host peptides to form immunogenic compounds
- Drug molecules trigger T cell receptors directly
- Drug molecules alter "self" antigens activating T cells
- Keratinocyte is the target of an immune response resulting in apoptosis
- Genetic differences may result in enhanced T cell activation
- Soluble cytotoxic proteins (i.e., granulysin) trigger apoptosis (not direct cell–cell interaction).

SIGNALMENT/HISTORY

■ Dogs and cats.

■ CADR: no age or sex predispositions: Shetland sheepdog, dalmatian, Yorkshire terrier, miniature poodle, miniature schnauzer, Australian shepherd, Old English sheepdog, Scottish terrier, wire-haired fox terrier, and greyhound; doberman pinschers and miniature schnauzers (sulfonamides); miniature schnauzers (shampoo-induced exfoliative erythroderma).

■ EM and SJS/TEN: no age, breed, or sex predispositions.

■ Some types of drug reactions appear to have a familial basis (e.g., rabies vaccine reactions in dogs have been diagnosed in littermates).

CLINICAL FEATURES

■ CADR:
- Wide variety of clinical symptoms reported
- Contact dermatitis (erythema, papular eruption, scaling) from topical medications
- Pruritus (resulting in excoriation), erythroderma, exfoliative dermatitis, urticaria, vasculitis most commonly described with systemic medications (Figure 17.8)
- Drug-induced pemphigus/pemphigoid; can closely mimic the autoimmune (spontaneous) forms of these diseases (Figures 17.9, 17.10)
- Focal ischemic dermatopathy/vasculitis post vaccination (Figure 17.11)
- Systemic symptoms (e.g., depression, anorexia, fever, lameness), hematologic changes
- Urticaria/angioedema: results from an immediate (type I) hypersensitivity; requires prior sensitization; increased vascular permeability leads to fluid leakage into the interstitium (Figure 17.12)

- Hypersensitivity vasculitis: inflammation of cutaneous vasculature; results in poor blood flow and anoxic injury to recipient tissue; in most cases, thought to represent a type III hypersensitivity response
- Exfoliative erythroderma: diffuse erythematous response caused by vasodilation; often leads to exfoliation (diffuse scaling) and intense erythema
- Superficial suppurative necrolytic dermatitis of miniature schnauzers: systemic symptoms and painful ulcerative patches developing within 72 hours of bathing/topical therapy.

■ EM:
- Classic "target" or "bull's-eye" lesion not a common finding; seen as annular lesions with erythematous, often scaling borders and central clearing; postinflammatory pigmentation centrally (Figure 17.13)
- EM minor: no systemic symptoms; none or only one mucosal site involvement
- EM major: systemic symptoms; more than one mucosal site involvement
- Glabrous skin of ventrum, flanks, axillae, inguinal; pinnae; mucocutaneous junctions
- Some lesions may be significantly crusted ("old dog" EM) (Figure 17.14)
- Macular and papular rashes often serpiginous and polycyclic: commonly accompany pruritus as a nonspecific sign of inflammation (EM minor) (Figure 17.15)
- Mucocutaneous ulceration/erosion, oral cavity, footpads, pinnae (EM major) (Figures 17.16–17.18)
- EM lesions may be plaque-like (palpable) or bullous
- Spontaneous resolution possible (especially if the trigger is identified/treated/removed).

■ SJS/TEN:
- Sudden onset
- Systemic symptoms (e.g., depression, anorexia, fever)
- Coalescing targetoid lesions lead to extensive necrosis and sloughing of the epidermis in sheets; results in moist and intensely inflamed ulcerations (Figures 17.19, 17.20)
- Pseudo-Nikolsky sign (separation of epidermis by shearing force)
- Generalized truncal lesions
- Mucosal lesions common
- Footpads often affected (Figure 17.21).

DIFFERENTIAL DIAGNOSIS

- Pruritus, macular/papular rashes, and urticaria/angioedema: allergic diseases (atopy, food allergy, contact allergy) and reactions to ectoparasitism (scabies, flea bite allergy, stinging insects), bacterial folliculitis, dermatophytosis.
- Exfoliative erythroderma with crusting: cutaneous T cell lymphoma, pemphigus/pemphigoid, superficial necrolytic dermatitis, zinc-responsive dermatitis, seborrhea/keratinization disorders.
- Vasculitis: infectious, neoplastic, and autoimmune diseases (especially lupus erythematosus); many cases of vasculitis are idiopathic.

- EM: respiratory infection and internal neoplasia (especially thymoma in cats).
- Thermal or chemical burns may give similar clinical appearance.

DIAGNOSTICS

- Serum biochemistry and complete blood count (especially when cutaneous vasculitis is suspected or diagnosed: potential for concurrent hepatic, renal, and gastrointestinal disease).
- Rickettsial serology, ANA.
- Cats: FIV and FeLV serology.
- Bacterial and fungal cultures and sensitivity testing (especially if pyogranulomatous inflammation is a clinical feature).
- Biopsy: CADR – may be nonspecific and/or specific to a drug-induced syndrome: EM – hyperkeratosis and parakeratosis (especially noted in "old dog" EM); cytotoxic (interface) dermatitis with apoptosis (cell death) in both suprabasilar and basilar cell layers; apoptosis with lymphocyte satellitosis is prominent in the upper layers of the epidermis as well as affecting the follicular infundibular epithelium: SJS/TEN – interfollicular and follicular infundibular cytotoxic dermatitis with apoptosis; more extensive than EM and progressing to full-thickness coagulative epidermal necrosis; separation of necrotic epidermis from the dermis; lack of dermal necrosis differentiates from thermal burn.

THERAPEUTICS

- Discontinue use of the potential offending drug.
- SJS/TEN: intensive supportive care and fluid/nutritional support because of fluid and protein exudation and risk of sepsis; pain control.
- Corticosteroids: controversial; early/high then tapering dosage.
- Cyclosporine (5 mg/kg/day).
- Oclacitinib (0.4–0.6 mg/kg q24h to BID); may reduce T cell response.
- Tacrolimus applied to lesions (feline).
- Azathioprine 50 mg/m^2/day tapering dosage (canine).
- Human intravenous immunoglobulin (IVIG) may be helpful in refractory cases.
- Pentoxifylline (Trental) may be helpful in some cases.

COMMENTS

- Inpatient: if debilitated.
- Outpatient: regular rechecks, depending on physical condition.
- Some reactions appear to activate self-perpetuating immune responses.
- Some drug metabolites may persist for days to weeks and provoke a continued response.
- Vasculitis: prognosis guarded when there are systemic complications associated with arthropathy, hepatitis, glomerulonephritis, and neuromuscular disorders, among others.
- Prognosis: EM good to poor; SJS poor to guarded; TEN guarded to grave.

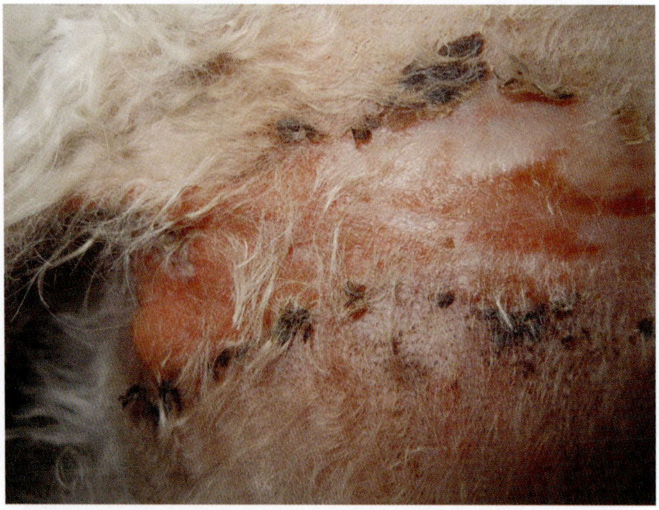

■ **Fig. 17.1.** Erythematous and eroded lesions from contact reaction to a neomycin-containing topical medication in a 9-year-old female-spayed maltipoo.

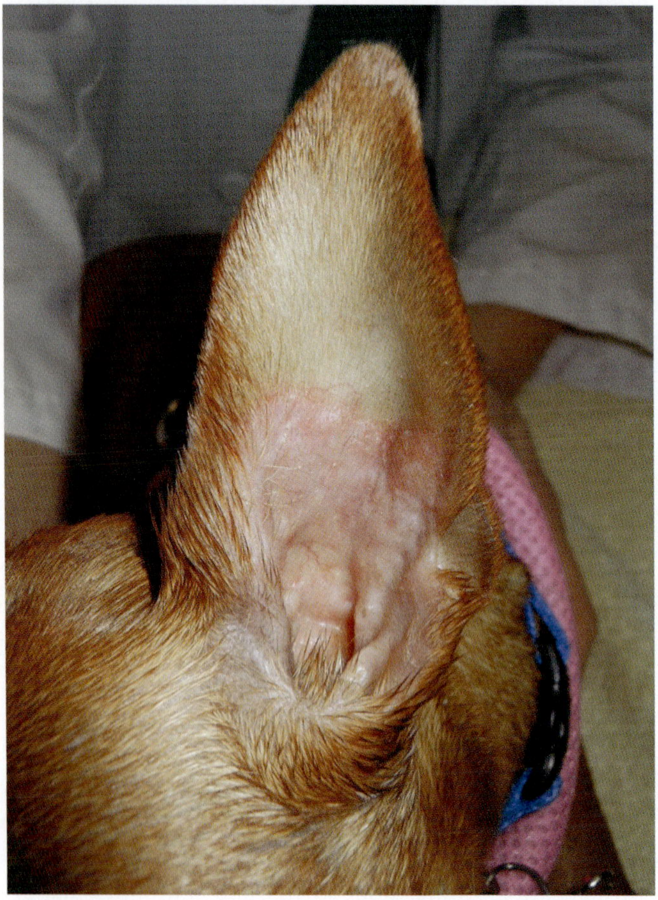

■ **Fig. 17.2.** Sharply demarcated lesion of erythema on the concave surface of the pinna secondary to an injection of cefovecin in a 2-year-old female-spayed miniature pinscher.

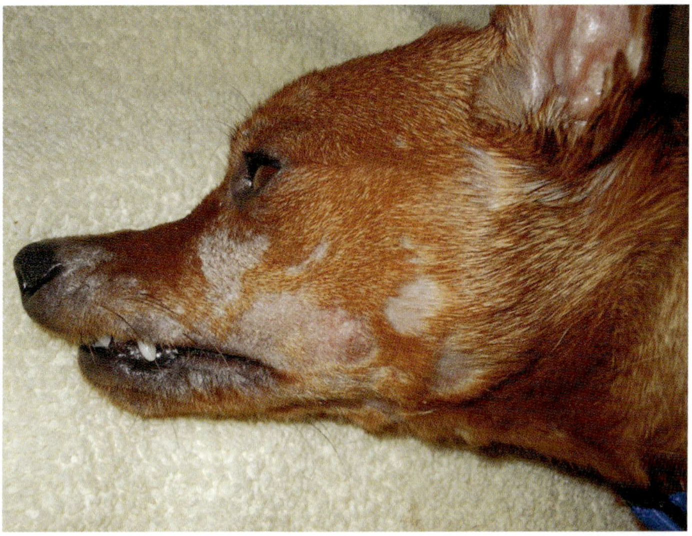

■ **Fig. 17.3.** More generalized lesions of alopecia with erythema and crusting on the face of the patient in Figure 17.2 secondary to an injection of cefovecin.

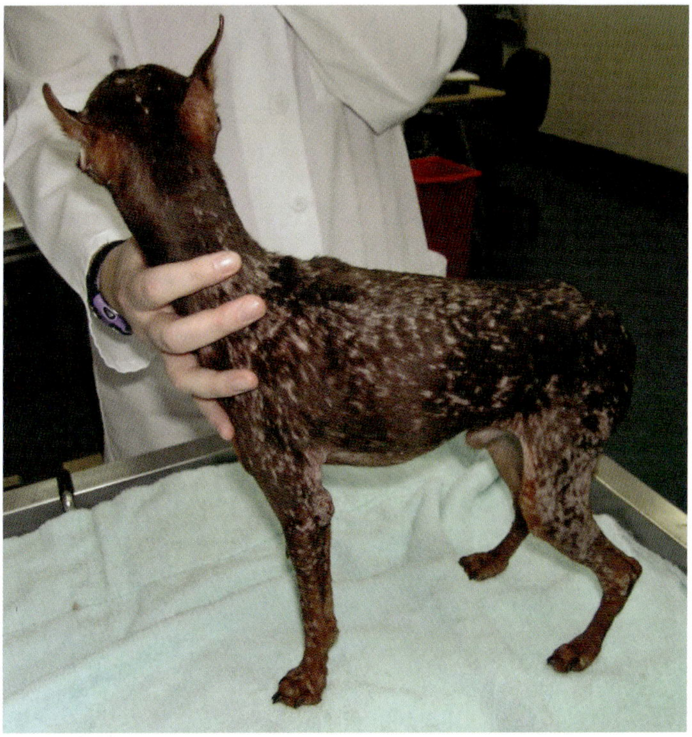

■ **Fig. 17.4.** Lesions of erythema multiforme seen as generalized erythematous and scaling dermatitis in a 6-month-old male-intact miniature pinscher that developed following an upper respiratory infection.

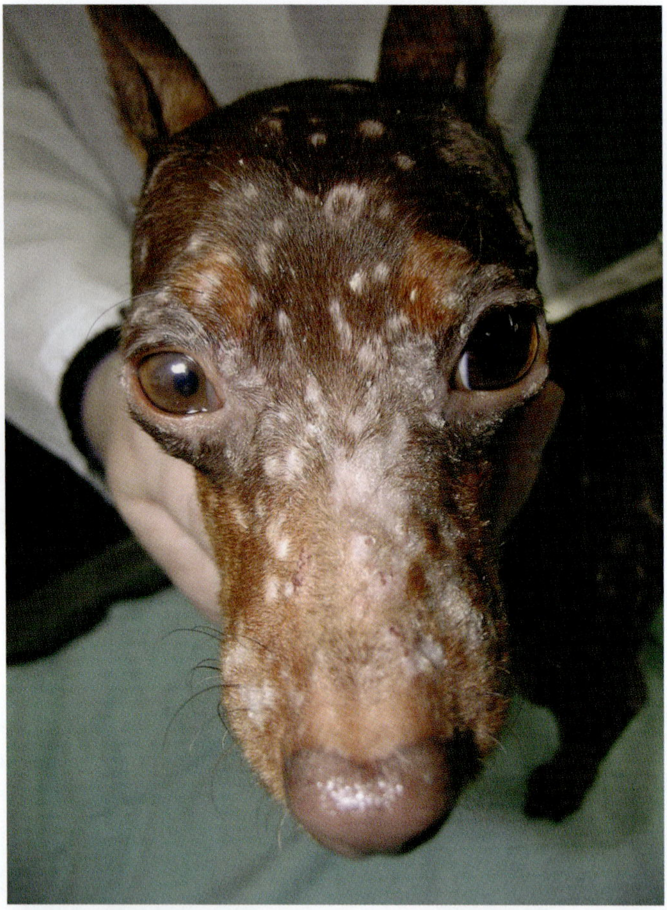

■ **Fig. 17.5.** Facial lesions of the patient in Figure 17.4.

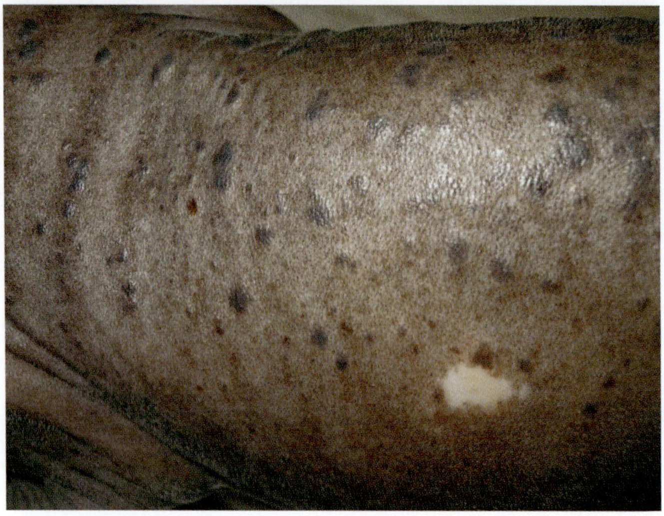

■ **Fig. 17.6.** Multifocal hyperpigmented plaques of erythema multiforme caused presumptively by herpes virus conjunctivitis in a 7-year-old female-spayed sphynx cat.

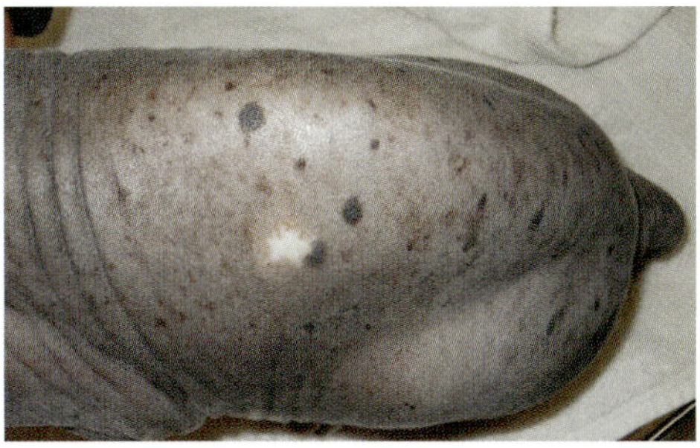

■ **Fig. 17.7.** Patient in Figure 17.6 after 30 days of treatment with famcyclovir. Pigmented plaques are healing or have resolved significantly.

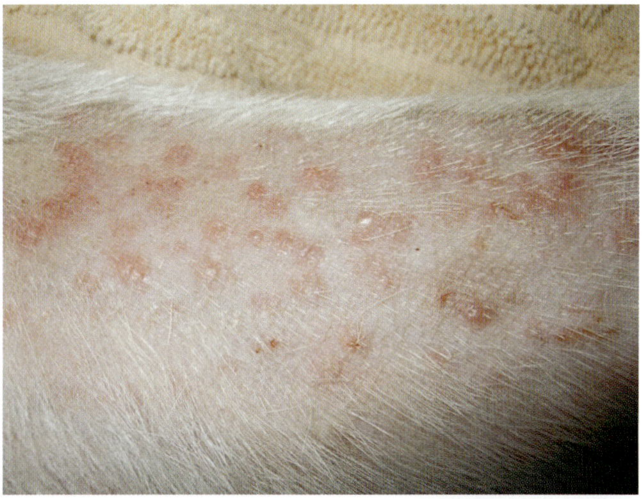

■ **Fig. 17.8.** Erythematous and papular eruption in a 4-year-old male-castrate German shepherd following administration of amoxicillin-clavulanate.

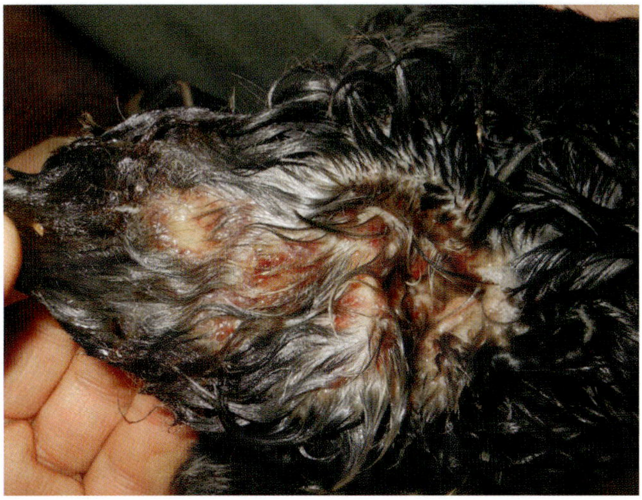

■ **Fig. 17.9.** Crusted and exudative patches on the pinna of an 11-year-old female-spayed miniature schnauzer. These are lesions of pemphigus foliaceus triggered by treatment with nitrofurantoin for recurrent urinary tract infections.

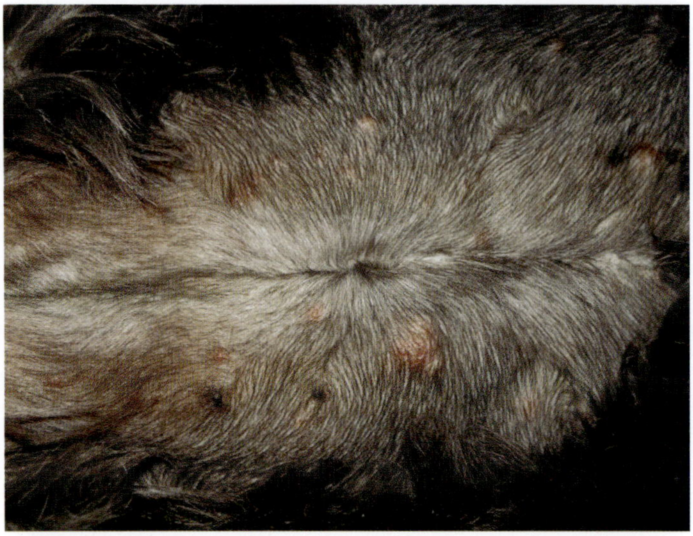

■ **Fig. 17.10.** Crusted and exudative patches on the ventrum of the patient in Figure 17.9.

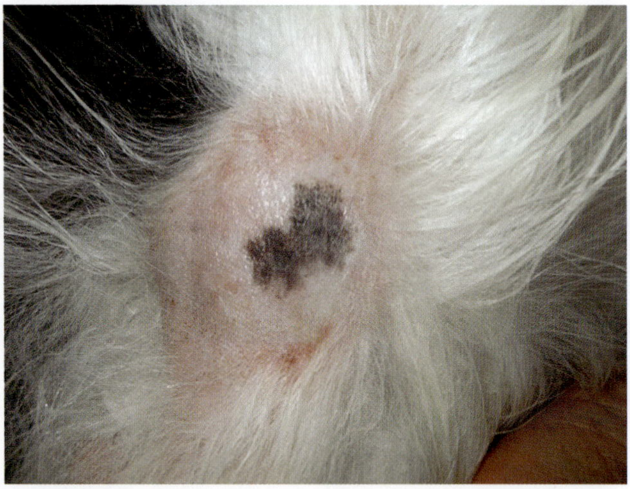

■ **Fig. 17.11.** Alopecic and scarred patch over the right lateral thigh in a 4-year-old female-spayed pomeranian secondary to rabies vaccination.

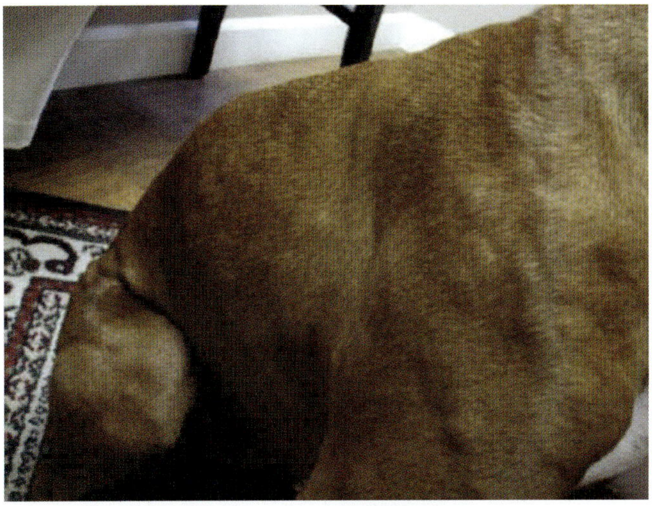

■ **Fig. 17.12.** Diffuse urticarial reaction secondary to trimethoprim-sulfamethoxazole. Lesions are characteristic of a type I hypersensitivity.

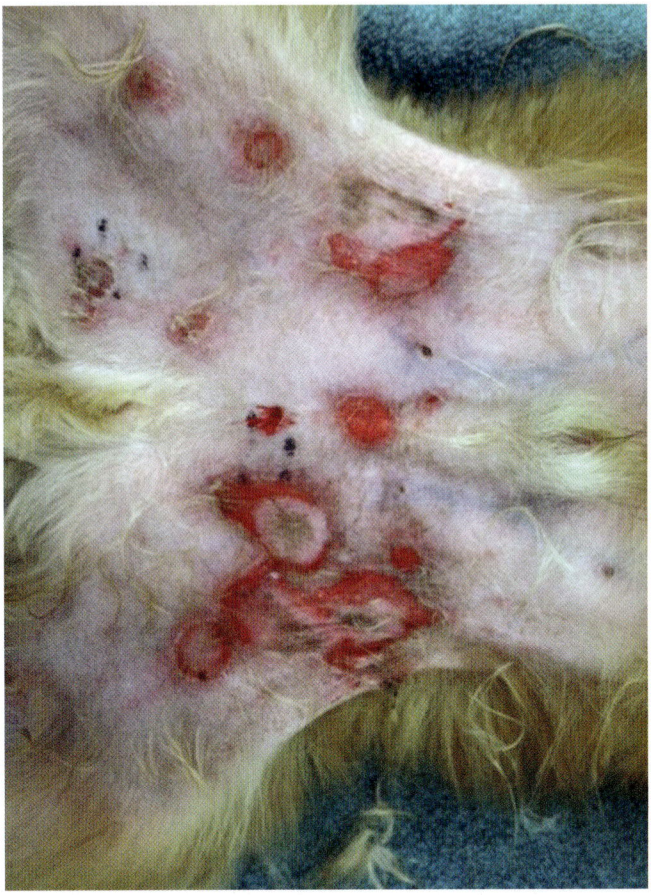

■ **Fig. 17.13.** Targetoid or "bull's-eye" lesions on the ventrum characteristic of erythema multiforme. Lesions are annular with peripheral erythema, crusting and central clearing with hyperpigmentation.

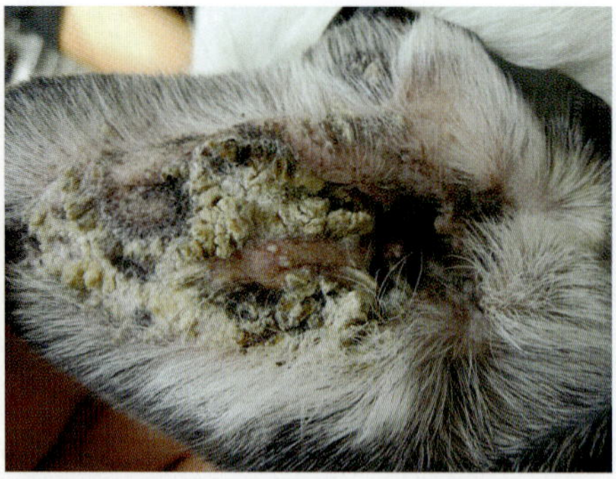

■ **Fig. 17.14.** Multiple hyperkeratotic plaques on the pinna of a 12-year-old male-castrate Jack Russell terrier with the "old dog" form of erythema multiforme.

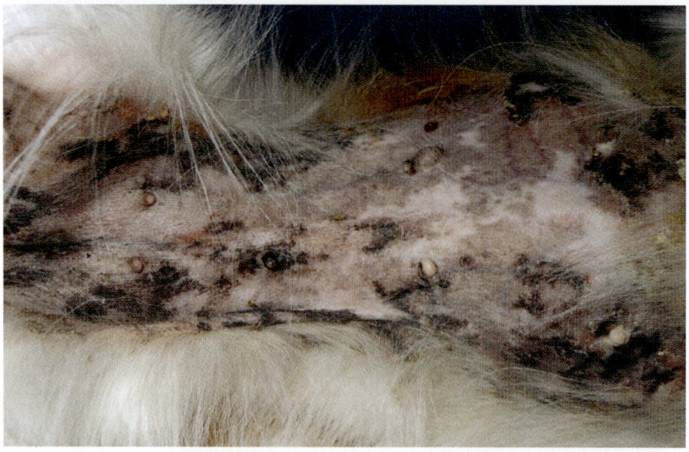

■ **Fig. 17.15.** Erythema multiforme lesions in an 11-year-old female-spayed papillon demonstrating a serpiginous and polycyclic macular and papular dermatitis affecting the entire ventrum.

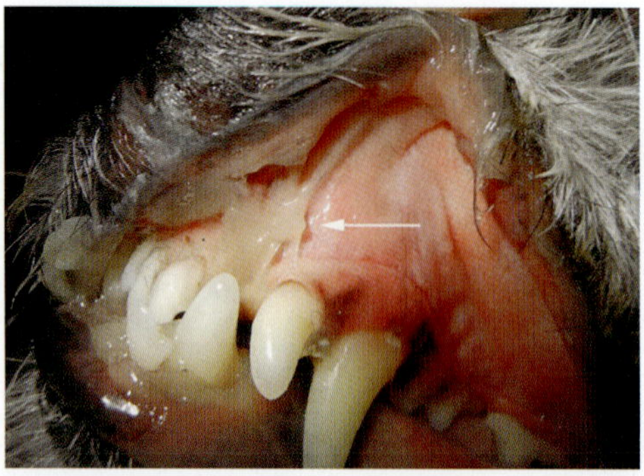

■ **Fig. 17.16.** Erythema multiforme (major) in a 7-year-old female-spayed terrier mix. Necrotic epithelium is peeling from the underlying mucosa (*arrow*), leaving ulcerations.

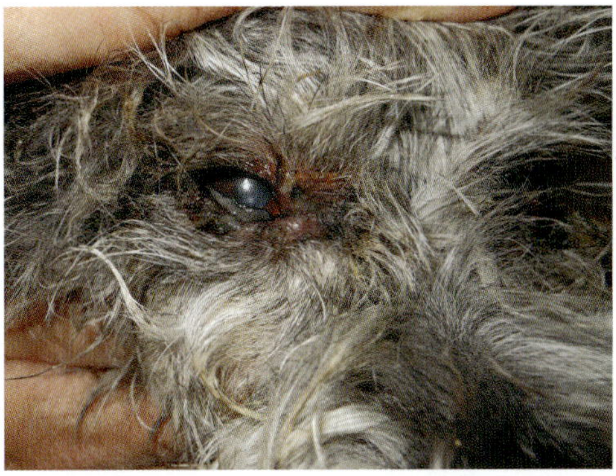

■ **Fig. 17.17.** Patient in Figure 17.16 with erosions affecting the mucosal surfaces and skin of the eyelids.

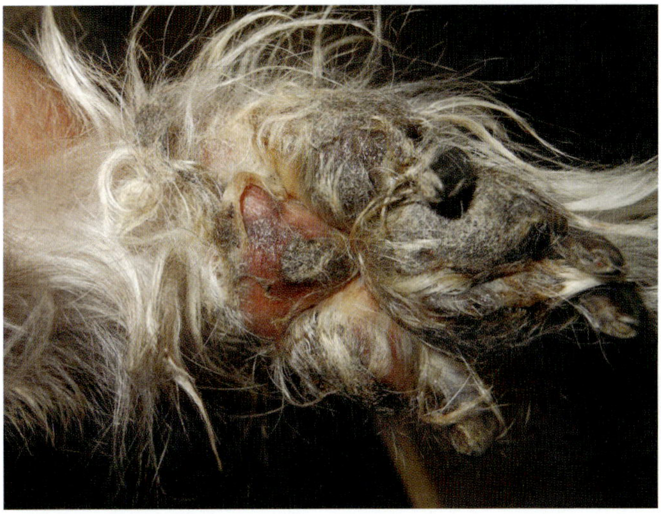

■ **Fig. 17.18.** Sloughing of footpads in the erythema multiforme (major) patient in Figures 17.16 and 17.17.

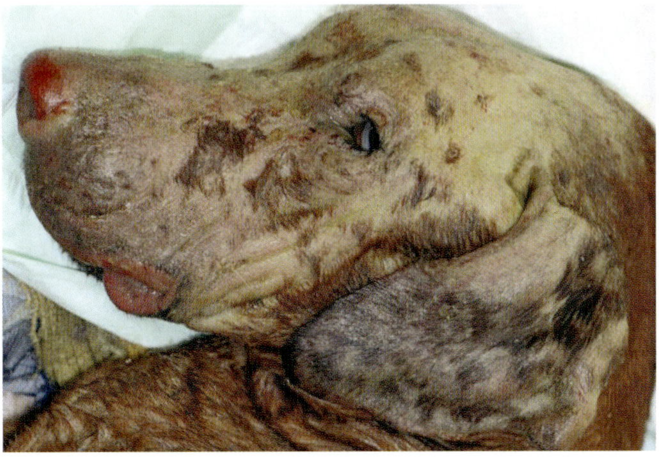

■ **Fig. 17.19.** Toxic epidermal necrolysis in a 3-year-old Rhodesian ridgeback. The epidermis of the entire head and pinnae, as well as the epithelium of the nasal planum and lip margins, is necrotic and sloughing.

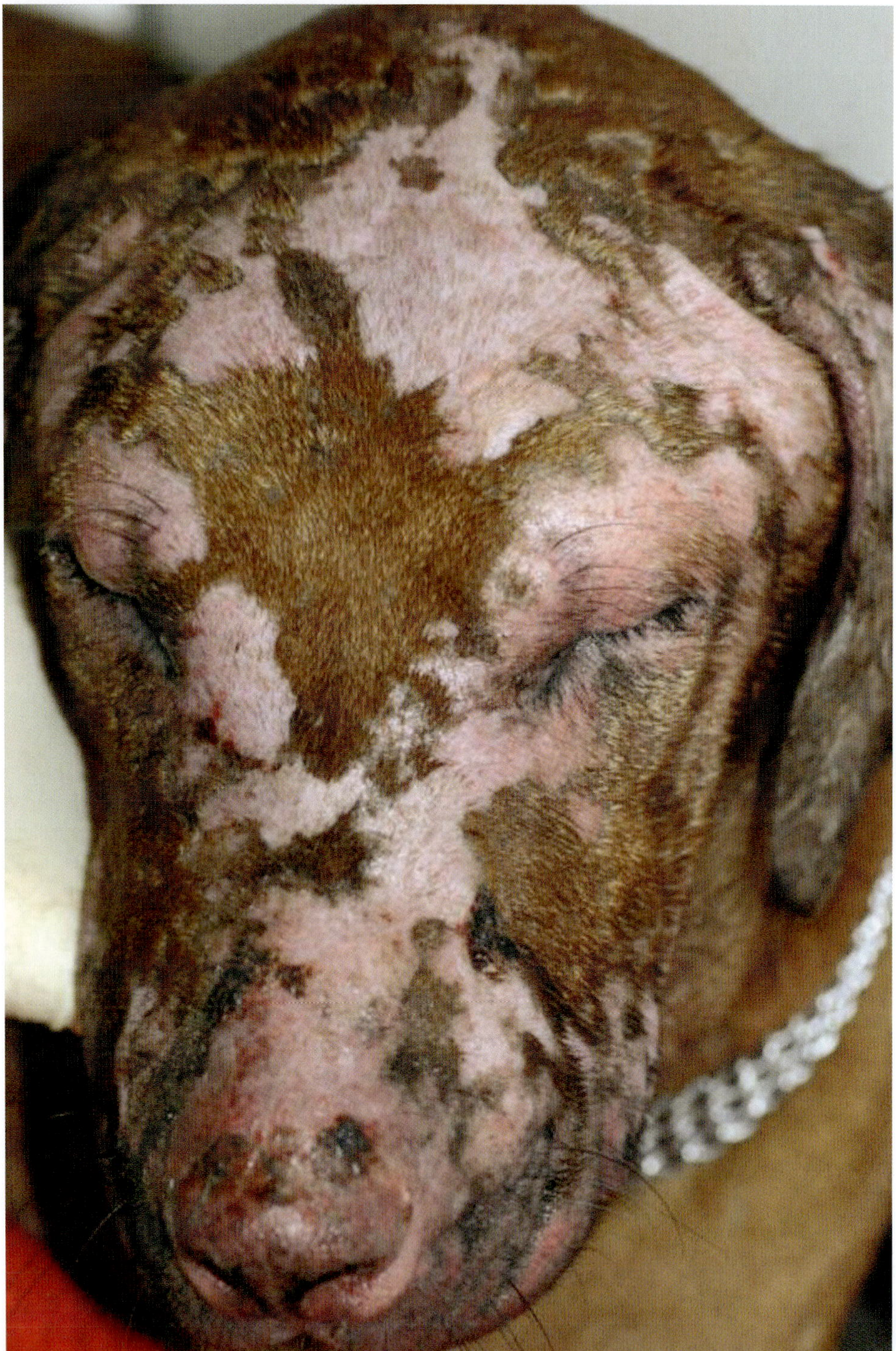

■ **Fig. 17.20.** Extensive ulcerations of the skin on the face revealed after gentle cleaning in the patient in Figure 17.19 with toxic epidermal necrolysis.

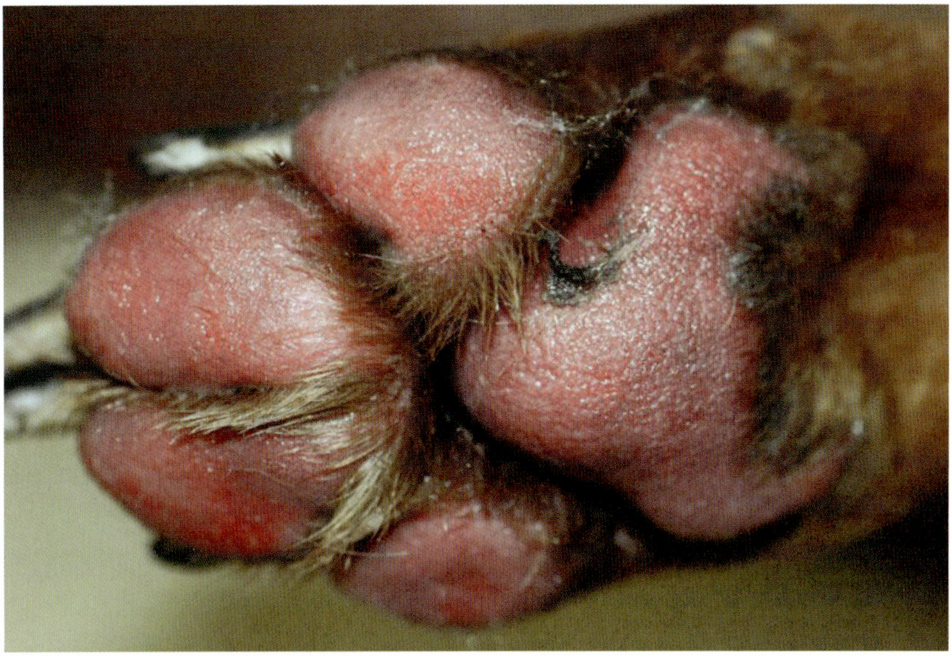

Fig. 17.21. Toxic epidermal necrolysis causing complete sloughing of the footpads of the patient in Figures 17.19 and 17.20.

chapter 18

Cutaneous Adverse Food Reactions

DEFINITION/OVERVIEW

Cutaneous adverse food reactions are pruritic, nonseasonal reactions associated with ingestion of one or more substances.

ETIOLOGY/PATHOPHYSIOLOGY

- Cutaneous adverse food reactions (CAFR) most appropriate term used; it is not easy to distinguish between immunologic and nonimmunologic reactions.
- Pathogenesis not completely understood: immunologic versus nonimmunologic.
- Immunologic (hypersensitivity):
    - Reactions to glycoproteins (allergen size range of 10–70 kD)
    - Immediate and delayed reactions to specific ingredients
    - Immediate reactions presumed to be type I hypersensitivity reactions
    - Delayed reactions due to type III or IV reactions
    - Sensitization may occur at the gastrointestinal mucosa, after the offending substance is absorbed, or both.
- Nonimmunologic:
    - Abnormal physiologic response
    - Food intolerance, idiosyncratic reaction; involves metabolic, toxic, or pharmacologic effects of offending ingredients
    - May be result of ingestion of foods with high levels of histamine or substances that induce histamine either directly or through histamine-releasing factors
    - May be induced by enzyme deficiencies, toxins, food additives, and contaminants.
- Antigens are normally broken down by the effects of gastric acid enzymes, pancreatic and intestinal enzymes in the gut lumen, and intestinal cell lysosomal activity.
- A natural state of tolerance is maintained by a number of immune functions: clonal deletion, anergy, and regulatory T (T_{reg}) cells.
- Alterations in epithelial cells, antigen-presenting cells, intercellular permeability, or any interference in the normal immune defense are likely mechanisms by which an allergic response develops instead of tolerance.

Blackwell's Five-Minute Veterinary Consult Clinical Companion: Small Animal Dermatology, Third Edition.
Karen Helton Rhodes and Alexander H. Werner.

- Intestinal parasites or intestinal infections may cause anatomic or functional damage to the intestinal mucosal barrier, resulting in the abnormal absorption of allergens and subsequent sensitization (Th_2 response) or intolerance (T_{reg} response).
- Epicutaneous exposure to food allergens via barrier-disrupted skin may promote sensitization to food proteins upon GI exposure. This method of sensitization may be clinically relevant for environmental allergens that have cross-reactivity with food allergens.

SIGNALMENT/HISTORY

- CAFR, canine: approximately 5% of dermatoses; 10–15% of all allergic diseases; prevalence in nonseasonal pruritic dogs is reported as high as 40–52%.
- CAFR, feline: approximately 1–6% of dermatoses: 10–15% of all allergic diseases.
- Percentages vary greatly with clinicians and geographic location.
- No breed or sex predilection (commonly identified in breeds predisposed to atopic disease).
- Age of onset: most often patients >7 years of age with no previous history of pruritic dermatitis; also more common in patients <1 year of age; contrasted to age of onset of atopic disease (1–3 years).
- CAFR may be a flare factor for atopic disease and may not be identified as a contributor to clinical symptoms.
- A wide range of clinical signs that can mimic any of the other hypersensitivity reactions, including atopic dermatitis (the adage of "ears and rears" is inaccurate).
- Nonseasonal pruritus of any body location.
- Gastrointestinal: vomiting; diarrhea; more frequent bowel movements; flatulence; 10–15% incidence rate in CAFR.
- Nervous: very rare; seizures have been documented with CAFR.
- Vasculitis, urticaria, and erythema multiforme have been reportedly triggered by adverse reactions to food.
- Typically poor response to antiinflammatory doses of glucocorticoids.

CLINICAL FEATURES

- Otitis externa (Figure 18.1).
- Bacterial folliculitis common in the dog; rare in the cat.
- *Malassezia* dermatitis concurrent in both dogs and cats.
- Plaques.
- Pustules.
- Erythema (Figure 18.2).
- Crusts.
- Scale.
- Self-induced alopecia (Figures 18.3, 18.4).
- Excoriation (Figure 18.5).
- Lichenification (Figure 18.6).

- Hyperpigmentation.
- Urticaria (Figure 18.7).
- Angioedema.
- Pyotraumatic dermatitis.
- Perianal pruritus.
- Facial pruritus common clinical feature; cats (Figure 18.8).
- Eosinophilic disease complex (eosinophilic granuloma complex); cats.

DIFFERENTIAL DIAGNOSIS

- Flea bite hypersensitivity: confined to the caudal-dorsal half of the body; may be seasonal.
- Atopic disease: associated with pruritus of the face, ventrum, and feet; may be seasonal or nonseasonal.
- Scabies: pruritus specific in location (ears, elbows, and hocks); mites in skin scrapings and/or response to specific therapy.
- Drug eruption/reaction: history of drug administration before the development of pruritus and resolution upon withdrawal.
- *Malassezia* hypersensitivity.
- Contact allergy/hypersensitivity.
- Seborrheic skin disease.

Food Allergen Facts

- Food allergens are typically glycoproteins with molecular weight between 10 and 70 kD.
- Most patients have been fed a diet for over 2 years prior to developing a sensitivity.
- Food allergens most often associated with adverse reaction: beef, dairy products, chicken, and wheat (canine) and beef, dairy products and fish (feline); soy, corn, eggs also reported.
- Grains (ex. corn) are not often a problem, contrary to popular belief.
- Cross-reactivity has been reported between beef, lamb, and cow's milk.
- Potential cross-reactivity between environmental allergens and foods: ragweed and apple/melon; cedar and tomatoes; birch and kiwi/apple/celery.
- Raw diets are *not* better for CAFR patients; processing and cooking do not disrupt (or produce) common food allergens; raw diets are associated with exposure to higher numbers of potentially pathogenic bacteria.

DIAGNOSTICS

Food Elimination Diet

- Most definitive test for cutaneous adverse food reactions.
- Tailored to the individual patient; a full diet history should be obtained.

- Novel food elimination diets:
  - Diet must be restricted to one protein and one carbohydrate to which the animal has had limited or no previous exposure
  - Frequently used components of a novel diet include kangaroo, lamb, white-fish, rabbit, venison, ostrich, vegetarian, oats, quinoa, rutabaga, yams, and pinto beans
  - Avoid using ground meats; they may be contaminated with other meat types
  - Over-the-counter diets are not sufficiently restrictive for the diagnosis of CAFR
  - Over-the-counter diets may be unintentionally contaminated by diet ingredients from other formulations manufactured at the same location (similar in concept to individuals sensitive to nut allergy)
  - Tofu is a potential soybean allergen
  - For home-cooked diets: canine: 1 part protein and 2 parts carbohydrate; feline: 1 part protein and 1 part carbohydrate.
- Hydrolyzed food elimination diets: ingredients processed to a molecular weight that is considered too small to be allergenic or to induce a reaction.
- Hydrolyzed food elimination diets should be considered in patients for which a diet history is unknown and/or those with concurrent gastrointestinal symptoms.
- Diet trials must be continued for up to 10 weeks to note improvement of clinical signs (8 weeks = common length of trial); noticeable improvement typically seen by the fourth week of the trial.

Diet Trial Tips

- No other foods or treats (including rawhide) are allowed during a diet trial; advise all family members and friends that pet is on a diet trial.
- Advise the owner to feed all household pets the same diet or feed them separately.
- Keep pets out of the family dining room during meals to avoid picking up dropped food.
- If pills are prescribed, only administer them in the specific diet.
- Flavored products, such as those found in medications, pill pockets, toothpaste, and certain plastic toys must be avoided during a diet trial.
- If the pet is in the habit of eating dropped food or garbage when exercised outside, keep him/her on a leash.
- Cats must not be allowed to roam free and scavenge mice, birds, etc.
- Avoid medications known to have antiinflammatory effects during the last phase of the trial; might alter the results of the diet trial.

Challenge and Provocation Diet Trials

- Used if the patient improves on the elimination diet.
- Challenge:
  - Feed the patient with the original diet
  - Return of the signs confirms that an ingredient in the diet is producing a reaction
  - Challenge period should last until the signs return but no longer than 10 days.

- Provocation:
  - If the challenge confirms the presence of a food reaction, return to the previous elimination diet until symptoms resolve
  - Add single ingredients to the elimination diet: ingredients include meats (beef, chicken, fish, pork, lamb), grains (corn, wheat, soybean, rice), eggs, and dairy products
  - Choice of ingredients may be guided by ingredients present in the previous (offending) diet
  - Provocation period for each ingredient should last up to 10 days (less if signs develop sooner; may develop within 1–2 days)
  - Results guide the selection of commercial foods that do not contain the offending substance(s) and may be tolerated.
- Some patients with CAFR must remain on prescription diets to prevent reactions.

Inaccurate or Ineffective Methods for the Diagnosis of CAFR

- Serum testing: multiple studies have confirmed a no better than random chance for the identification of CAFR; these tests cannot be used to identify either offending or tolerated diet ingredients.
- Gastroscopic testing.
- Intradermal testing with food antigens.
- Prick testing with food antigens.
- Hair analysis.
- Saliva analysis.

THERAPEUTICS

- Avoid any food substances that caused the clinical signs to return.
- Review carefully the principles of allergen avoidance with the client (and family).
- Inform client to eliminate treats, chewable toys, vitamins, and other flavored medications (e.g., heartworm preventative) that may contain ingredients from the patient's previous diet (and/or the patient has been exposed to consistently).
- Outdoor pets must be confined to prevent foraging and hunting.
- Provide handouts/instructions for clients to take home.
- Systemic antipruritic drugs may be useful during the first 2–3 weeks of diet trial to control self-mutilation.
- Antibiotics or antifungal medication may be required to relieve secondary infections; avoid those that are known to have antiinflammatory effects (e.g., tetracycline, erythromycin, and trimethoprim-potentiated sulfas) during the later phase of the elimination diet trial.
- Encourage routine bathing with a shampoo that can control/eliminate bacterial and yeast organisms as well as promote a healthy epidermal barrier function.
- Glucocorticoids and antihistamines should be discontinued during the last month of the diet trial to evaluate the animal's response.

- Encourage clients to utilize qualified nutrition websites and/or the services of a board certified veterinary nutritionist to formulate a balanced elimination and/or maintenance diet.

COMMENTS

- Examine patient and evaluate and document the pruritus and clinical signs every 4 weeks.
- Avoid intake of any of the proteins included in the previous diet.
- Treats and chewable toys should be limited to known safe substances.
- Other causes of pruritus (e.g., flea bite hypersensitivity, atopic dermatitis, and external parasites such as *Sarcoptes*, *Notoedres*, and *Cheyletiella* mites) can mask the response to the food elimination diet trial and the maintenance diet.
- Prognosis is good if food ingredients are the only cause of the pruritus and offending ingredients are avoided.
- Rarely, a dog or cat may develop hypersensitivity to a new food ingredient, requiring a new elimination diet trial.
- Concurrent hypersensitivities (flea or atopic dermatitis) must be managed for long-term success.

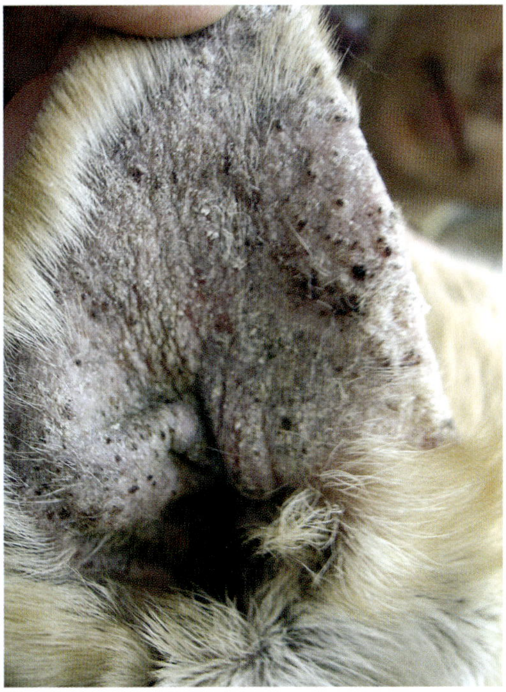

Fig. 18.1. Chronic otitis externa with *Malassezia* dermatitis on the pinna of a canine with CAFR.

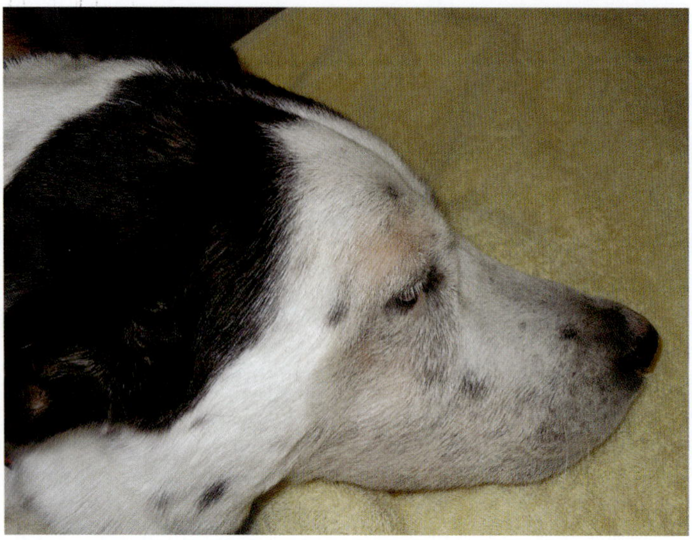

■ **Fig. 18.2.** Erythema affecting the periocular and muzzle region.

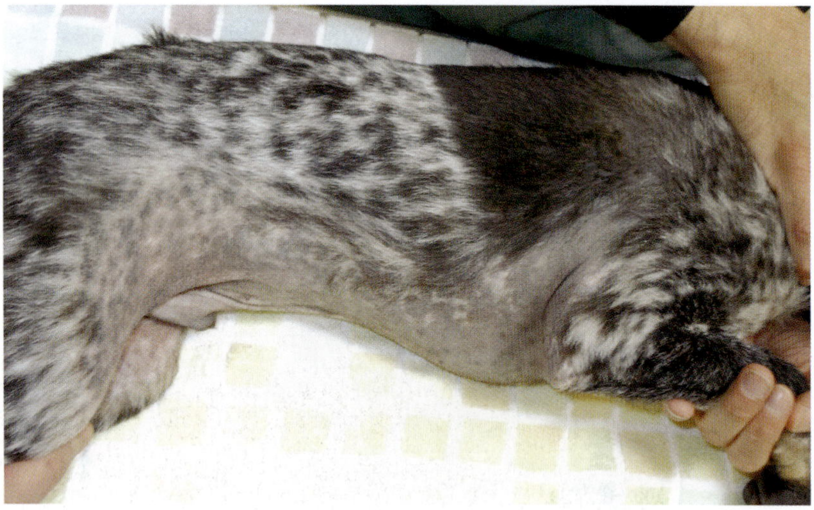

■ **Fig. 18.3.** Self-induced alopecia of the flank folds, ventrum, and axillae in an 11-month-old male-intact Australian cattle dog.

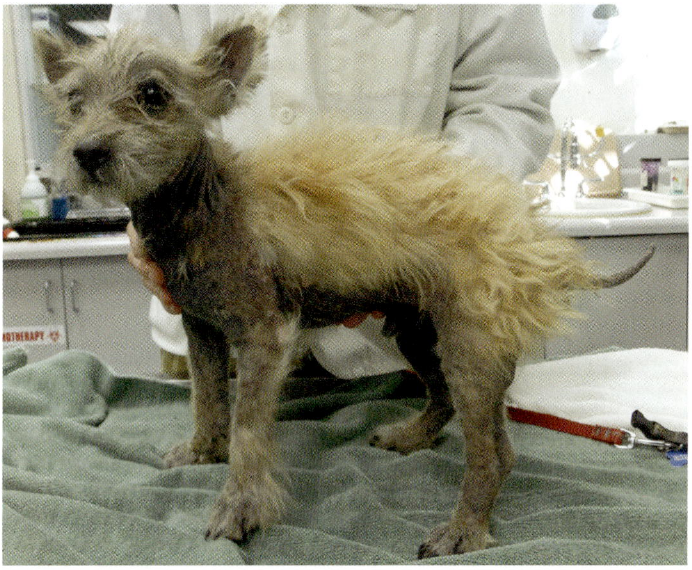

■ **Fig. 18.4.** Severe alopecia, lichenification, crusting, and secondary infection (bacterial and yeast) in a 12-year-old female-spayed cairn terrier with chronic CAFR.

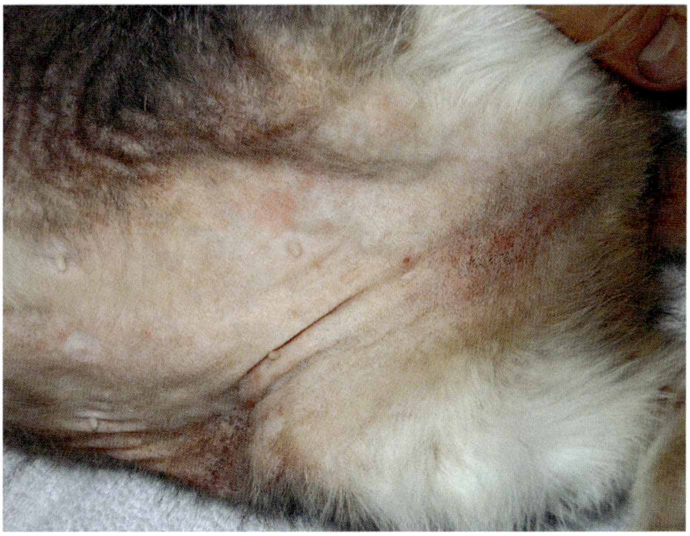

■ **Fig. 18.5.** Alopecia, erythema, and excoriations on the ventrum and lateral abdomen in a 12-year-old female-spayed DSH due to CAFR.

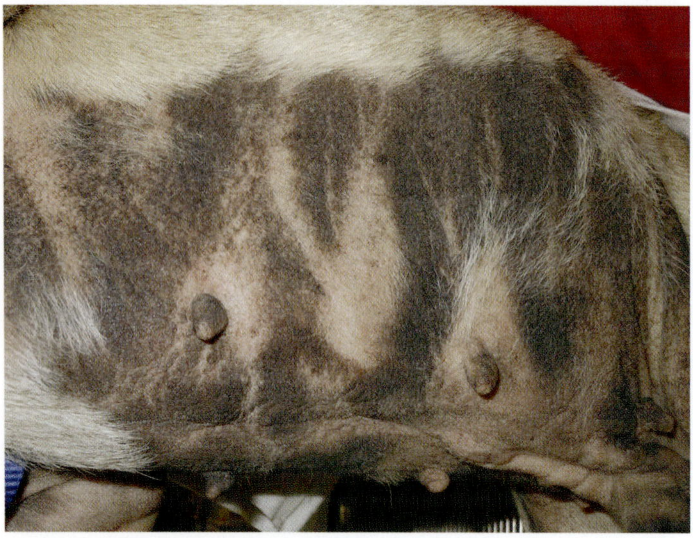

■ **Fig. 18.6.** Chronic untreated CAFR producing marked lichenification and hyperpigmentation on the ventrum and lateral body of a 3-year-old male-intact pug.

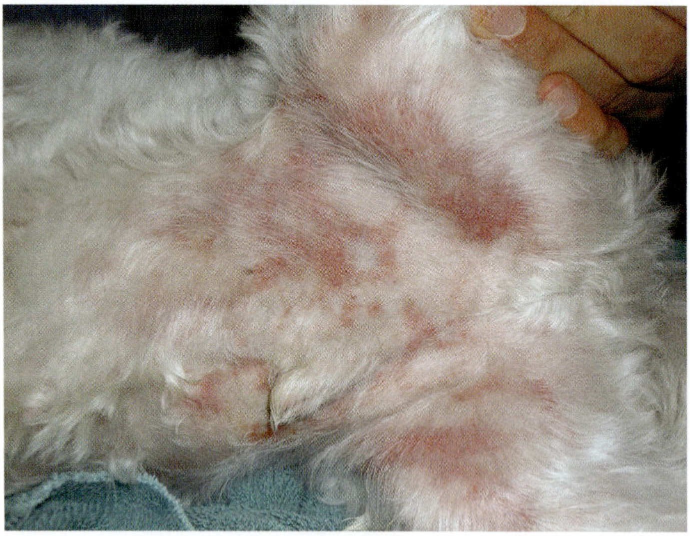

■ **Fig. 18.7.** Urticaria on the ventral abdomen of a 4-year-old male-castrate bichon frise.

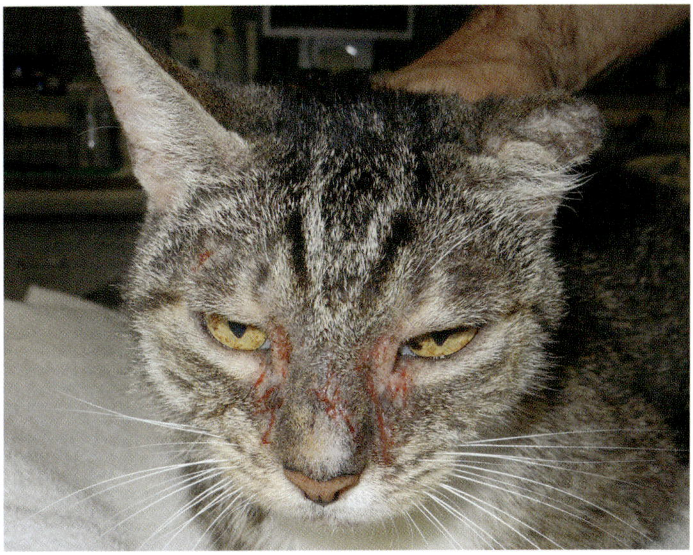

(a)

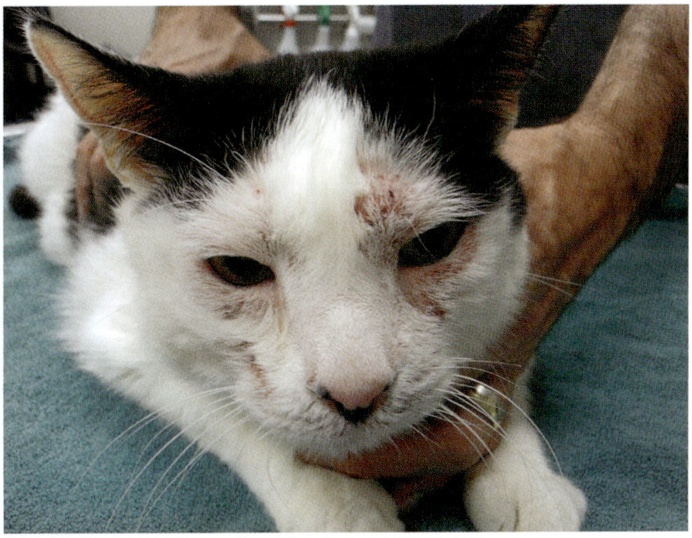

(b)

Fig. 18.8. Facial pruritus and excoriation in cats with CAFR.

chapter 19

Demodicosis (Canine and Feline)

DEFINITION/OVERVIEW

- An inflammatory parasitic disease of dogs and, less frequently, cats that is characterized by an increased number of mites in the hair follicles, adnexa, and on the surface of the skin.
- Often leads to superficial or deep folliculitis and furunculosis, and alopecia.
- May be localized or generalized.
- Juvenile-onset generalized form (dog) has a heritable basis; certain DLA haplotypes associated with disease in one study.

ETIOLOGY/PATHOPHYSIOLOGY

- Commensal organism in the dog; frequently colonizes the skin of cats.
- Normal immune system tolerates mite presence and may have an inhibitory effect on mite populations.
- Pathology develops when mites proliferate and produce inflammation within the follicle (dogs): *D. gatoi* may cause a hypersensitivity reaction (cats).
- *Demodex* mites may change from commensal to pathogenic parasite to produce disease.
- Initial proliferation of mites may be the result of a genetic or immunologic disorder.
- Mechanisms of disease include disruption of cutaneous barrier; disruption of follicular integrity (furunculosis); proliferation of bacteria; T cell exhaustion.
- Dead or degenerate mites may be found in noncutaneous sites (e.g., lymph node, intestinal wall, spleen, liver, kidney, urinary bladder, lung, thyroid gland, blood, urine, and feces) and are considered to represent drainage to these areas by blood and/or lymph.

Dogs

- *Demodex canis*: most common mite identified; transferred from bitch during nursing; typically present in small numbers; resides in the hair follicles and, rarely, in the sebaceous glands of the skin (Figure 19.1).

Blackwell's Five-Minute Veterinary Consult Clinical Companion: Small Animal Dermatology, Third Edition.
Karen Helton Rhodes and Alexander H. Werner.

- *Demodex cornei*: short-bodied *Demodex* mite; not considered a separate species: represents a morphologic variant of *D. canis;* often more found more superficially (Figure 19.2).
- *Demodex injai*: large-bodied *Demodex* sp; resides in the sebaceous glands; often associated with a seborrheic dermatitis along the dorsal midline; most often identified in West Highland white terriers and wire-haired fox terriers (Figure 19.3).

Cats

- *Demodex cati*: similar in appearance to *D. canis*; resides in the hair follicles and sebaceous glands (Figure 19.4).
- *Demodex gatoi*: resides in the stratum corneum layer of the epidermis; considered potentially contagious; may cause a hypersensitivity reaction; frequency of occurrence differs by geographic location (Figure 19.5).
- *Demodex felis* (unnamed in some publications): presumed to reside in the hair follicle (undetermined).

SIGNALMENT/HISTORY

- Dogs and rarely cats.
- Increased incidence in purebred dogs: American Staffordshire and Staffordshire bull terriers, Chinese shar-pei, Boston terrier, West Highland white terrier, and French and English bulldogs.
- Reported increased incidence in Siamese and Burmese cat breeds.
- Categorized as:
  - Juvenile onset
  - Adult onset
  - Localized
  - Generalized.
- Juvenile onset less than 18 months of age.
- Localized: usually in young dogs; median age 3–6 months.
- Generalized: both young and old animals; defined as involving the feet, an entire body region, or several remote sites; persistent or progressing.

Dogs

- Exact immunopathologic mechanism unknown.
- Studies indicate that dogs with generalized demodicosis have a subnormal percentage of IL-2 receptors on their lymphocytes and subnormal IL-2 production.
- Serum insulin-like growth factor 2 (IGF-2) is elevated in dogs with generalized demodicosis; IGF-2 is associated with regulatory functions of B and T cells.
- Genetic factors, immunosuppression, and/or metabolic diseases may predispose to disease development, including endocrinopathy, lymphoma, and autoimmune

disease; an underlying disease is identified in fewer than 50% of adult-onset generalized demodicosis cases.
- Treatment with immune-modulating medications, including oclacitinib and corticosteroids, is associated with increased incidence.

Cats

- *D. cati*: often associated with metabolic diseases (e.g., FIV, systemic lupus erythematosus, diabetes mellitus).
- Both systemic and topical immunosuppressive therapy may trigger demodicosis.
- *D. gatoi:* rarely a marker for metabolic disease; individual reports indicate that it may be transferable from cat to cat within the same household.

CLINICAL FEATURES

- Alopecia, scaling, follicular casts (keratosebaceous material adhered to the hair shaft), comedones, crust, erythema, hyperpigmentation, lichenification.
- Secondary bacterial folliculitis and furunculosis often noted in chronic canine demodicosis; produces concurrent lethargy, fever, lymphadenopathy, and pain.
- *Demodex injai* and *D. gatoi* may be associated with pruritus.
- Ceruminous otitis externa has been associated with *Demodex* mites in both dogs and cats.

Dogs

- Localized:
    - Fewer than 4–6, often well-demarcated, small (less than 2.5 cm) lesions
    - Usually mild; consists of patches of erythema and light scale
    - Juvenile form often resolves without treatment
    - Most common site is the face, especially around the perioral and periocular areas, as well as the front legs (Figure 19.6).
- Generalized:
    - Can be widespread from the onset, with multiple poorly circumscribed patches of intense erythema, alopecia, papules, comedones, and scale (Figure 19.7)
    - As hair follicles become distended with large numbers of mites, secondary bacterial infections are common, often with resultant rupturing of the follicle (furunculosis) (Figure 19.8)
    - With progression, the skin can become severely inflamed, exudative, and granulomatous (Figure 19.9)
    - Pododemodicosis: symptoms may be limited to the distal extremities; lesions associated with deep secondary bacterial infection; Old English sheepdogs reported at increased risk (Figure 19.10)
    - *Demodex injai*: most often causes an alopecic and oily patch on the dorsal midline (Figure 19.11).

Cats

- Often characterized by partial to complete multifocal alopecia of the eyelids and periocular region when localized; chin, head, forelimbs, dorsal or ventral trunk, and neck; may be generalized (Figure 19.12).
- Ceruminous otitis externa.
- Variable pruritus.
- *Demodex gatoi* infections are often indistinguishable from allergic dermatitis and psychogenic dermatoses; multiple cats in the household may be affected.

DIFFERENTIAL DIAGNOSIS

Dogs

- Bacterial folliculitis/furunculosis (from other causes)
- Allergic dermatitis (adverse reaction to food, atopic dermatitis, insect hypersensitivity)
- Dermatophytosis
- Contact dermatitis
- Pemphigus complex
- Dermatomyositis
- Systemic lupus erythematosus
- Epitheliotropic lymphoma (patch stage)

Cats

- Allergic dermatitis (adverse reaction to food, atopic dermatitis, insect hypersensitivity)
- Dermatophytosis
- Bacterial folliculitis
- Psychogenic dermatoses

DIAGNOSTICS

- May be useful for identifying underlying metabolic diseases in both dogs and cats.
- FeLV and FIV serology: identify underlying metabolic diseases in cats.
- Skin scrapings:
  - Diagnostic for finding large numbers of mites in the majority of cases
  - Intrascapular region may be the most productive site in the cat because the area is not easily groomed
  - Superficial scrapings: *D. cornei* (short-bodied *D. canis*: dog) and *D. gatoi* (cat)
  - Deep scrapings: *D. canis* (dog), *D. injai* (dog), and *D. cati* and *D. felis* (cat).
- Trichography/trichogram (hair plucks): examination of hair casts for mites; not as reliable as scrapings (Figure 19.13).

- Acetate tape preps may be used to identify *D. cornei* (short-bodied *D. canis*: dog) and *D. gatoi*.
- Otic swabs will identify *Demodex* as a cause of otitis externa.
- Fecal exams may be helpful in cats due to the grooming behavior.
- Cutaneous biopsy: may be needed when lesions are chronic, granulomatous, and fibrotic (especially on the paw); mural folliculitis, nodular dermatitis, suppurative folliculitis and furunculosis; follicles filled with mites and keratinaceous debris; useful in the shar-pei due to difficulty obtaining mites in scrapings.

THERAPEUTICS

- Localized: conservative; most cases (90%) resolve spontaneously with no treatment.
- Evaluate the general health status of dogs/cats (serum chemistry, CBC, FeLV/FIV, urinalysis, heartworm testing).
- Generalized (adult dog): frequent management problem due to expense and frustration with the chronicity; many cases are medically controlled, not cured.
- Antibiotic therapy in conjunction with adjunctive topical therapy (antibacterial shampoo/spray) frequently warranted to control secondary infections.
- Continue treatment for at least 1 month past a clinical cure and negative skin scraping.
- Regular monitoring with scrapings during the year following treatment is advisable.

Drugs of Choice: Dogs

- Amitraz:
  - FDA-approved for treating dogs over 4 months of age
  - Formamidine: inhibits monoamine oxidase and prostaglandin synthesis; an alpha 2-adrenergic agonist
  - Small dogs may exhibit marked lethargy 12–24 hours after application
  - Patients with respiratory disease or diabetes should not be treated with amitraz
  - Adverse reactions include depression, vomiting, diarrhea, ataxia, polyphagia, and polydipsia
  - Dilute as directed on the label (250 ppm); apply to the entire patient weekly to every other week until resolution of clinical signs and no mites are found on skin scrapings; do not rinse off; allow to air-dry
  - Continue rinses for at least 1 month following negative skin scrapings
  - Apply a benzoyl peroxide shampoo before application as a bactericidal therapy and to increase exposure of the mites to the miticide
  - Efficacy is proportional to the frequency of administration and the concentration of the rinse
  - Mix with mineral oil (3 mL amitraz to 30 mL mineral oil) for application to focal areas, such as pododemodicosis
  - 9% amitraz collar: success has not been established, although there are positive anecdotal reports; not recommended

- Between 11% and 30% of cases will not be cured; may need to try an alternative therapy or control with maintenance dips every 2–8 weeks.

■ Ivermectin:
- Off-label use for demodicosis
- Macrocyclic lactone with GABA agonist activity
- Binds to chloride channels in the mite's nervous system, causing paralysis and death
- Safety in mammals is due to the lack of glutamate-gated chloride channels in the peripheral nervous system and the restriction of GABA-gated channels in the central nervous system (which is protected by the blood–brain barrier)
- Contraindicated in collies, Shetland sheepdogs, Australian shepherds, Old English sheepdogs, white German shepherds, long-haired whippets, greyhounds, silken windhound, other herding breeds, and crosses with these breeds
- Ivermectin sensitivity: derived from a deletion mutation of the multidrug-resistant gene (ABCB1) resulting in a truncated nonfunctional protein called P-glycoprotein; P-glycoprotein is a transmembrane protein transporter found in the blood–brain barrier; P-glycoprotein pumps ivermectin within the brain back into the blood; testing for this mutation is available through the Washington State University Veterinary Clinical Pharmacology Laboratory (www.vetmed.wsu.edu.vcpl)
- Toxicity seen as hypersalivation, mydriasis, tremors, depression, ataxia, blindness
- Intravenous lipid emulsion therapy has shown success in the treatment of ivermectin toxicosis
- Do not use with Spinosad-containing flea control products; enhances toxicity of ivermectin
- *Demodex* otitis can be treated with 0.01% ivermectin solution
- Oral administration of the injectable formulation: 0.3–0.6 mg/kg q24h
- Administer 120 μg/kg q24h for the first 3 days to identify ivermectin-sensitive breeds (ABCB1 mutation): alternative dosing – gradual dose increase from 0.05 mg/kg on day 1; 0.1 mg/kg on day 2; 0.15 mg/kg on day 3; 0.2 mg/kg on day 4; 0.3 mg/kg on day 5: continued increases of 0.1 mg/kg daily if necessary to administer maximum dosage of 0.6 mg/kg q24h
- Treat for 60 days beyond negative skin scrapings (average 3–8 months)
- Continue rinses for at least 1 month following negative skin scrapings.

■ Milbemycin:
- Off-label use for demodicosis
- Macrocyclic lactone with GABA agonist activity
- Dosage of 1 mg/kg PO q24h cures 50% of cases; 2 mg/kg PO q24h cures 85% of cases; oral dose recommendations range between 1.5 and 3.1 mg/kg/day
- Treat for 60 days beyond multiple negative skin scrapings
- Ivermectin-sensitive breeds (ABCB1 defect) generally tolerate milbemycin
- Side effects are similar to ivermectin (depression, stupor, coma, ataxia, seizures)
- Major limitation of the drug is expense
- *Demodex* otitis can be treated with 0.1% milbemycin oxime topical.

- Moxidectin:
  - Off-label use for demodicosis
  - Macrocylic lactone with GABA agonist activity
  - Few studies available regarding oral efficacy
  - Oral administration of the injectable formulation: 0.4 mg/kg q24h
  - Do not use for ivermectin-sensitive breeds
  - Imidacloprid (10%) and moxidectin (2.5%) spot-on product: variable efficacy; most effective when applied weekly.
- Doramectin:
  - Off-label use for demodicosis
  - Macrocylic lactone with GABA agonist activity
  - Weekly subcutaneous injections at 0.6 mg/kg
  - Do not use for ivermectin-sensitive breeds.
- Isoxazolines:
  - Off-label use for demodicosis; long-term experience lacking
  - Selective inhibitor of arthropod GABA and L-glutamate-gated chloride channels
  - Afoxalaner 2.5 mg/kg every 4 weeks; approved for use in dogs over 1.8 kg and over 8 weeks of age for flea/tick control; off-label use for demodicosis; use with caution in patients with a history of seizures
  - Fluralaner 25 mg/kg every 12 weeks; approved for use in dogs over 2 kg and over 6 months of age for flea/tick control; off-label use for demodicosis
  - Sarolaner 2 mg/kg every 4 weeks; approved for use in dogs over 1.4 kg and over 6 months of age for flea/tick control; off-label use for demodicosis
  - Well tolerated; adverse effects include transient vomiting or diarrhea, and anorexia.

Drugs of Choice: Cats

- Lime sulfur dips:
  - Current treatment of choice
  - Topical 2% lime sulfur dips are the safest and most effective
  - Once weekly for at least 4–6 weeks and continuing for 1–2 months after clinical cure and negative scrapings
  - All in-contact cats should be treated in cases of *Demodex gatoi*
  - An Elizabethan collar should be used to prevent ingestion until the dip is dry, to avoid irritation.
- Amitraz:
  - Amitraz solutions (125–250 ppm): applied weekly for 4–6 treatments: risk of toxicity.
- Doramectin:
  - Anecdotal report of resolution of *D. cati* in three cats
  - Dosage: 0.6 mg/kg by subcutaneous injection once weekly for three injections.
- Ivermectin:
  - Anecdotal reports of efficacy
  - Dosage: 0.3–0.6 mg/kg q24h or every other day given orally

- Risk of neurotoxicosis and propylene glycol sensitivity
- Ivermectin use is discouraged at this time.

Drug Toxicities

- The combined use of medications (amitraz and ivermectin) is strongly discouraged and should be avoided due to potential toxicity.
- Amitraz:
  - Most common side effects: somnolence, lethargy, depression, anorexia seen in 30% of patients for 12–36 hours after treatment
  - Other side effects: vomiting, diarrhea, pruritus, polyuria, mydriasis, bradycardia, hypoventilation, hypotension, hypothermia, ataxia, ileus, bloat, hyperglycemia, convulsions, death
  - The incidence and severity of side effects do not appear to be proportional to the dose or frequency of use
  - Humans may develop dermatitis, headaches, and respiratory difficulty after exposure; apply in a well-ventilated room
  - Use of alpha 2-adrenergic antagonists can reverse signs of toxicosis. Atipamezole (Antisedan) (0.05 mg/kg intramuscularly) can reverse adverse signs in 10 minutes; may repeat every 4–8 hours
  - Yohimbine (0.11 mg/kg intravenous) administer slowly; may repeat every 4–8 hours
  - Avoid antidepressants and MAOIs, such as selegiline, in dogs receiving amitraz
  - Shampoo with mild soap to remove the topical product (dip or spot-on).
- Ivermectin and milbemycin:
  - Breed: related toxicities (see above)
  - Signs of toxicity: salivation, vomiting, mydriasis, confusion, ataxia, hypersensitivity to sound, weakness, recumbency, coma, and death
  - Ivermectin should not be given in conjunction with P-glycoprotein inhibitors: antidepressants (fluoxetine, paroxetine, St John's wort), antimicrobials (erythromycin, itraconazole, ketoconazole), opioids (methadone, pentazocine), cardiac drugs (amiodarone, carvedilol, nicardipine, quinidine, verapamil), immunosuppressants (cyclosporine, tacrolimus), miscellaneous (bromocriptine, chlorpromazine, grapefruit juice, tamoxifen, spinosad)
  - Therapy for toxicosis: supportive and symptomatic care; atropine or glycopyrrolate as needed to treat bradycardia; avoid other drugs that stimulate the GABA receptors (benzodiazepam tranquilizers).

COMMENTS

Expected Course and Prognosis

- Prognosis (dogs): depends heavily on genetic, immunologic, and underlying diseases.
- Localized: most cases (90%) resolve spontaneously with no treatment; <10% progress to the generalized form.

- Adult onset (dogs): often severe and refractory to treatment.
- Adult onset: sudden occurrence is often associated with internal disease, malignant neoplasia, and/or immunosuppressive disease; approximately 25% of cases are idiopathic over a follow-up period of 1–2 years.
- Avoid breeding dogs with the generalized form of demodicosis.

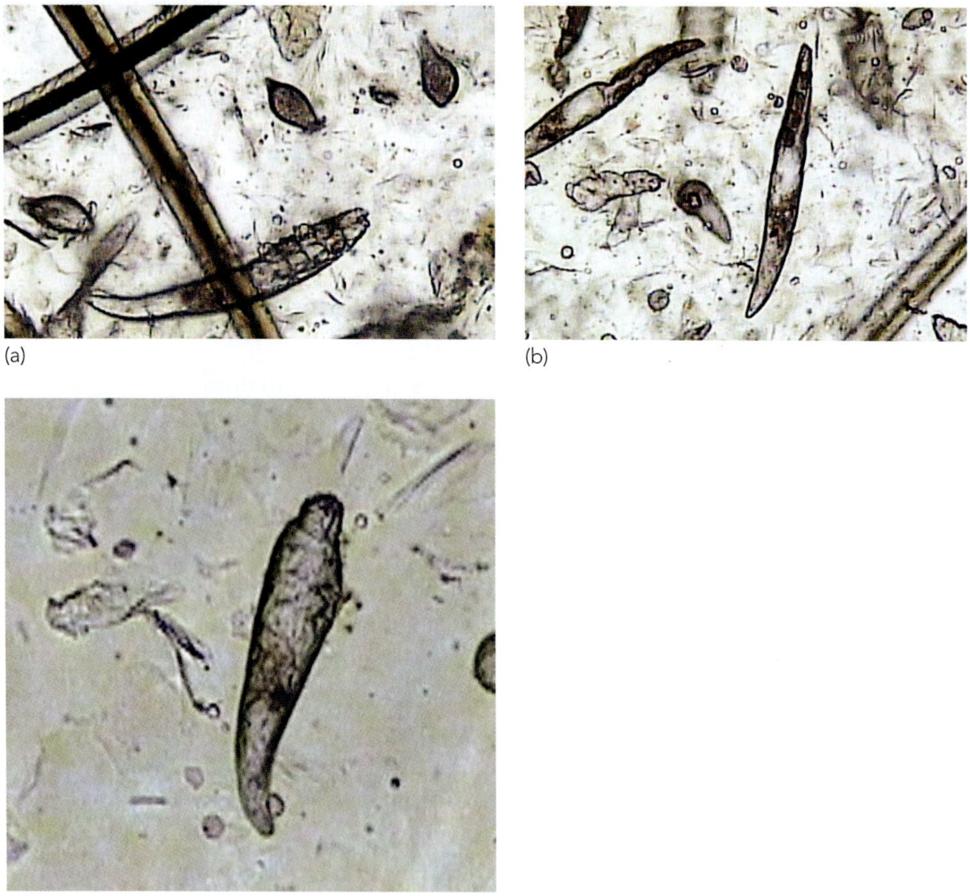

■ **Fig. 19.1.** *Demodex canis* mites from a skin scrapings. (a) Adult and eggs. (b) Nymphs. (c) Larva. Adults have a well-defined body segments with eight legs; eggs are fusiform; Nymphs have eight legs but poorly defined body segments; larva are slightly larger than eggs and have six legs.

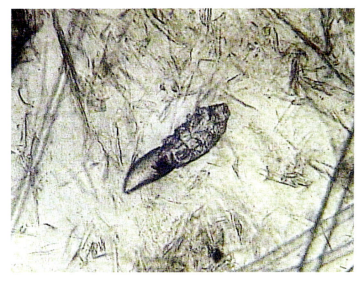

■ **Fig. 19.2.** *Demodex cornei*: considered a morphological variant of *D. canis* and is not a separate species.

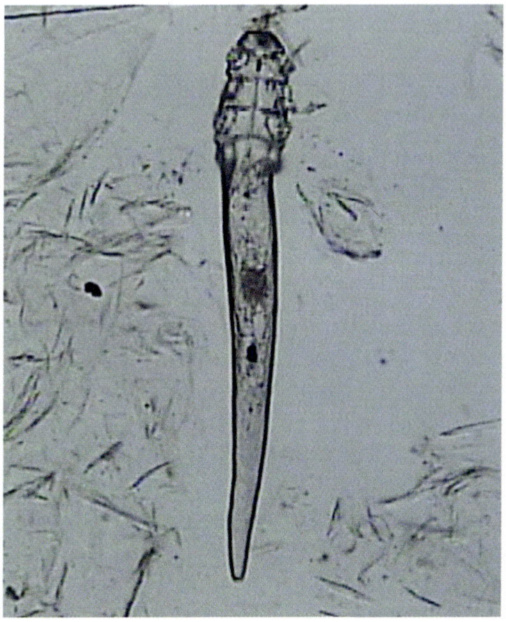

■ **Fig. 19.3.** *Demodex injai:* these mites are larger than *D. canis*, with a longer, slender tail.

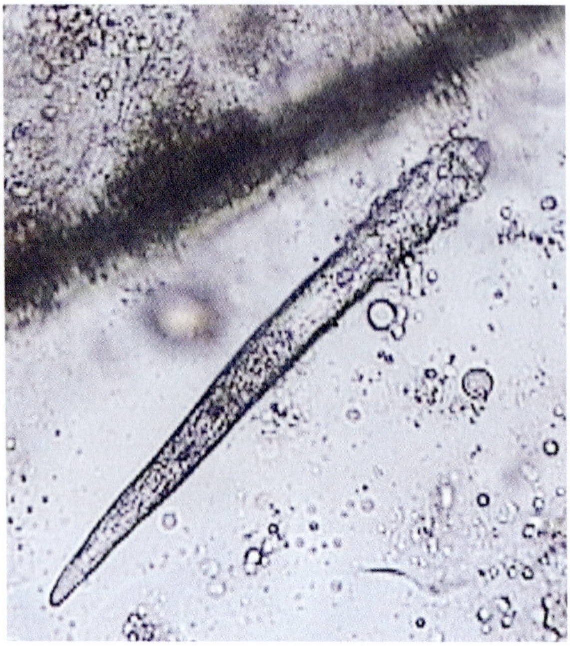

■ **Fig. 19.4.** *Demodex cati*: this mite is part of the normal skin fauna of cats and resides within the follicles and sebaceous glands. It is similar in appearance to *D. canis*, but is more slender and longer. The third feline *Demodex* mite (tentatively named *D. felis*) is smaller, but most similar to *D. cati*.

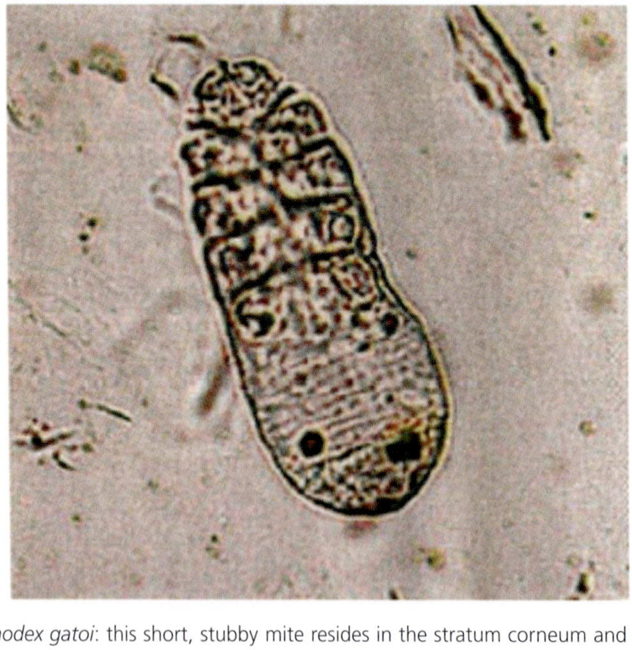

■ **Fig. 19.5.** *Demodex gatoi*: this short, stubby mite resides in the stratum corneum and is potentially contagious. Source: Reproduced with permission of Katy Tater.

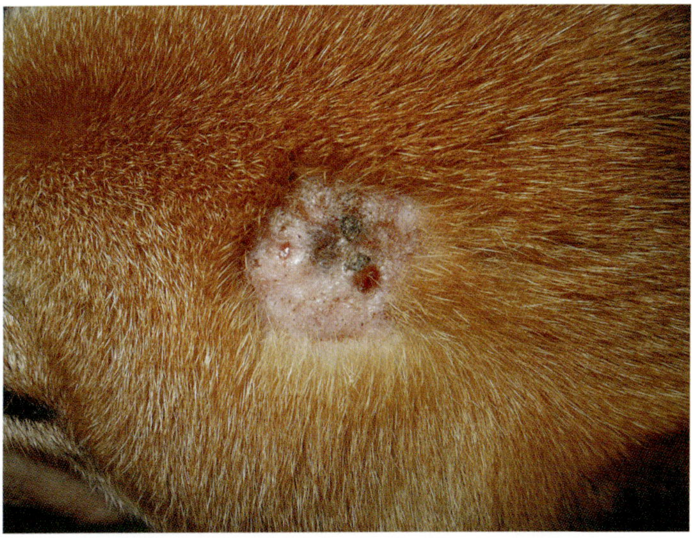

■ **Fig. 19.6.** Localized demodicosis: patch of alopecia with erythema and scaling on the forehead of a 2-year-old female-spayed shiba inu.

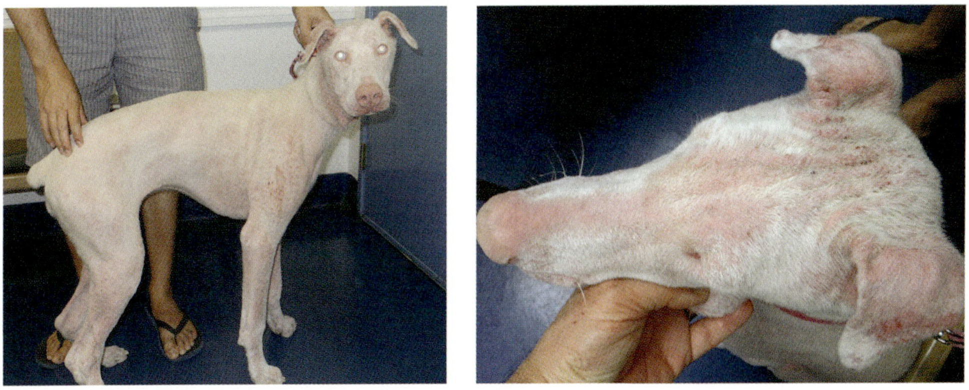

(a) (b)

■ **Fig. 19.7.** Generalized juvenile-onset demodicosis in an 8-month-old female-intact doberman pinscher with diffuse erythroderma and crusted papular dermatitis.

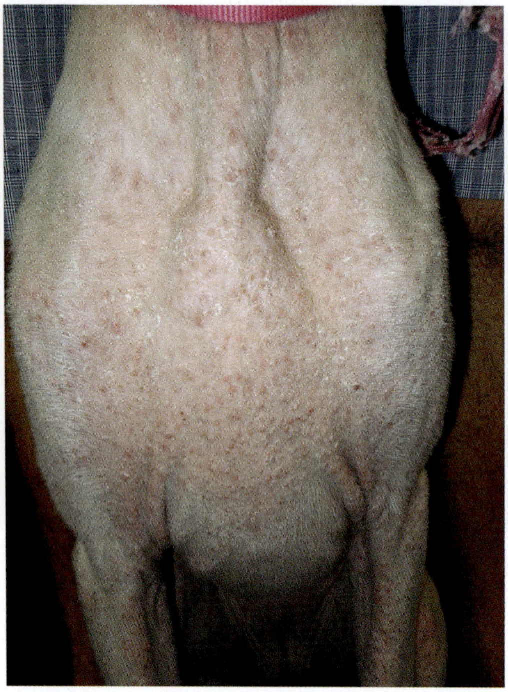

(c)

■ **Fig. 19.7.** (*Continued*)

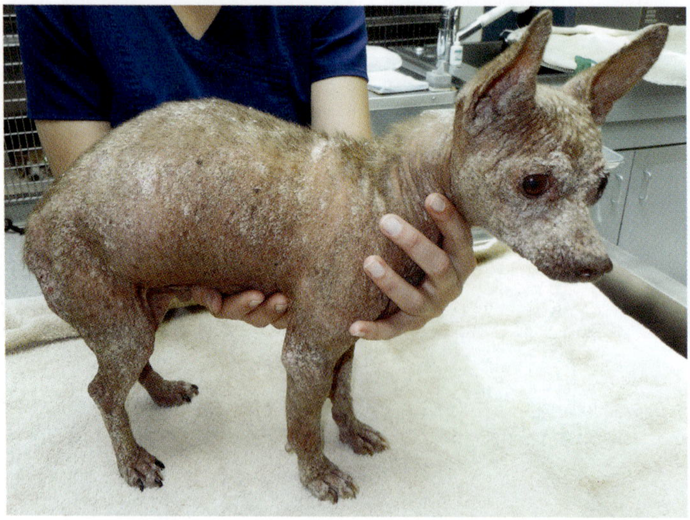

■ **Fig. 19.8.** Generalized demodicosis in a 6-year-old male-castrate chihuahua.

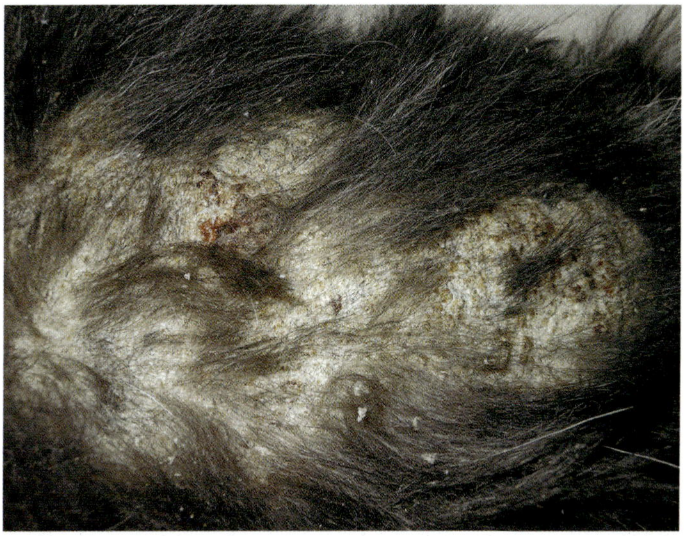

■ **Fig. 19.9.** Generalized demodicosis with severe lesions on the dorsum of an 11-year-old male-intact shih tzu with secondary *Pseudomonas aeruginosa* and *Staphylococcus simulans* infection.

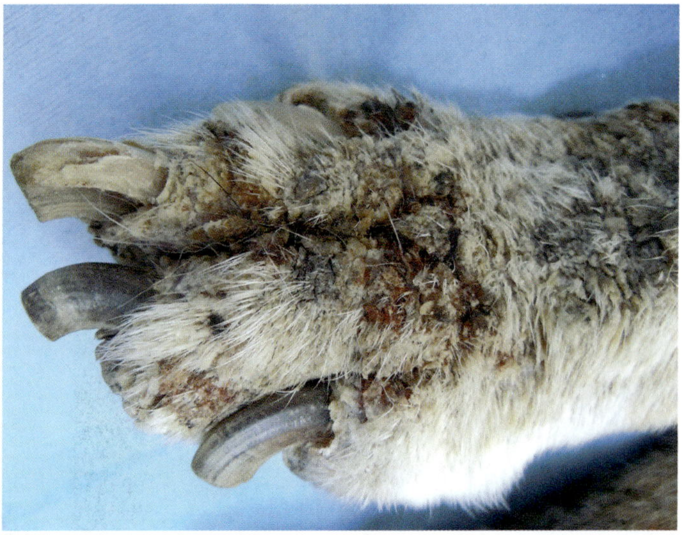

■ **Fig. 19.10.** Pododemodicosis and secondary bacterial furunculosis.

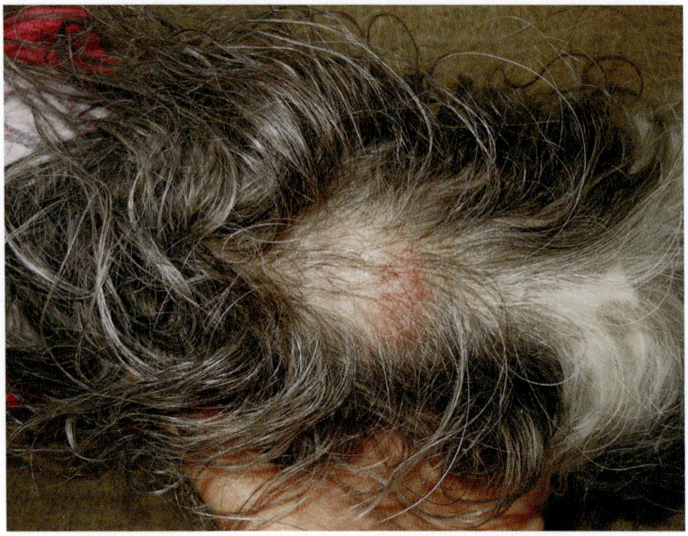

■ **Fig. 19.11.** Alopecia and oily patch on the dorsum of a 2-year-old female-spayed pekingese mix caused by *Demodex injai*.

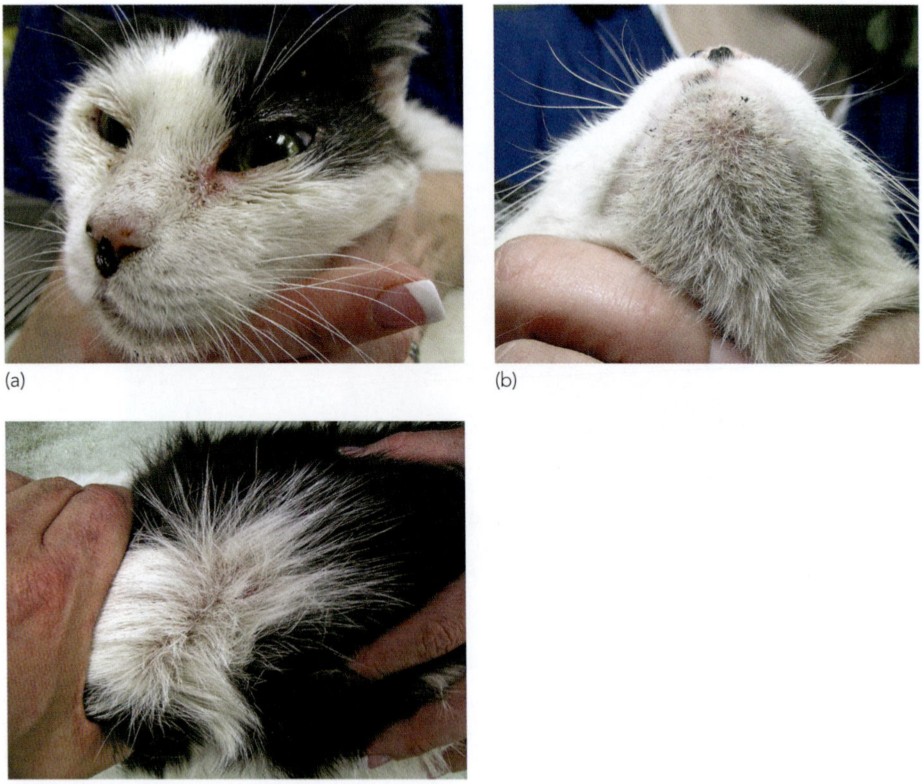

(a) (b) (c)

■ **Fig. 19.12.** Demodicosis in an adult, FIV+ DLH with erythema and erosions affecting the face, crusting on the chin, and a generalized oily skin and hair coat.

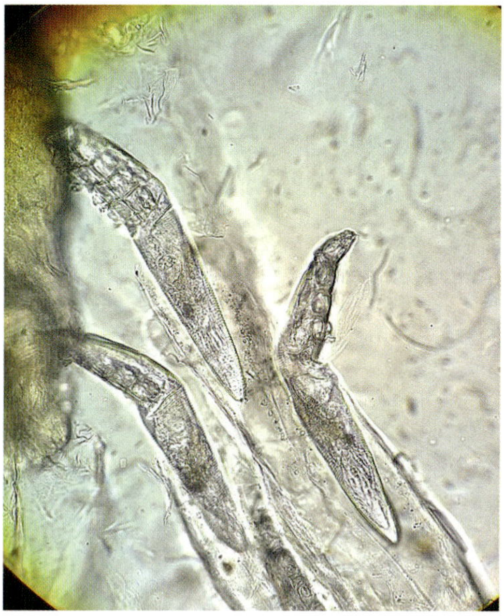

Fig. 19.13. Adult *D. canis* mites within the follicle outer root sheath from a trichogram.

chapter 20

Dermatomyositis, Canine Familial

DEFINITION/OVERVIEW

An inherited idiopathic inflammatory disorder of dogs that involves the skin and muscle (rarely, blood vessels).

ETIOLOGY/PATHOPHYSIOLOGY

- Exact pathogenesis unknown.
- Although it is well accepted that there is a genetic predisposition, an infectious agent (i.e., a virus) may act as a trigger for the development of clinical signs; an immune-mediated or autoimmune process may be involved.
- Skin: variable dermatitis on the face, ears, tail tip, and over the bony prominences of the distal extremities; may become more generalized.
- Musculoskeletal: subtle to severe; temporal and masseter muscles initial; severe cases exhibit generalized muscle disease, involvement of the esophageal muscles results in megaesophagus.
- Typically, advanced dermatitis is associated with severe myositis.
- Thought to be inherited as an autosomal dominant trait with variable expression in collies, Shetland sheepdogs, and Beauceron shepherds.

SIGNALMENT/HISTORY

Breed Predilection

- Collies, Shetland sheepdogs, Beauceron shepherds, and their cross-breeds.
- Isolated reports: Australian cattle dogs, Welsh corgis, chow chows, German shepherds, and the kuvasz.

MEAN AGE AND RANGE

- Cutaneous lesions usually develop between 7 weeks and 6 months of age.
- Mild disease: lesions may resolve in 3 months.

Blackwell's Five-Minute Veterinary Consult Clinical Companion: Small Animal Dermatology, Third Edition.
Karen Helton Rhodes and Alexander H. Werner.

- Moderate disease: lesions may persist for 6 months or more.
- Severe disease: lesions usually persist throughout life and become progressive.
- Adult-onset disease: much less common.

RISK/AGGRAVATING FACTORS

- Trauma
- Sunlight
- Estrus
- Parturition
- Lactation

CLINICAL FEATURES

- The clinical signs vary from subtle skin lesions and subclinical myositis to severe skin lesions and generalized muscle atrophy.
- Waxing and waning skin lesions particularly in areas of trauma/pressure: in dogs <6 months old; around the eyes, lips, face, inner ear pinnae, tail tip, and bony prominences of distal extremities; healing may lead to residual scarring and pigment changes; primary vesicular lesions are rare; ulceration can occur in severe cases.
- Muscle atrophy of the masseter and/or temporal muscles may be evident.
- Severe cases may exhibit difficulty eating, drinking, and swallowing; stunted growth; gait abnormalities; widespread muscle atrophy and infertility.
- Littermates may be affected; severity of the disease varies significantly among affected dogs.
- Skin lesions: characterized by papules and vesicles (rare); variable degrees of erythema; alopecia, scaling, crusting, ulceration, and scarring on the face with pigmentary changes, around the lips and eyes, in the inner ear pinnae, on the tail tip, and over bony prominences on the distal extremities (Figures 20.1–20.5).
- Footpad and oral ulcers rare.
- Myositis: variable; from nonclinical to a bilateral symmetric decrease in the mass of the temporalis muscles to generalized symmetric muscle atrophy; lameness.
- Aspiration pneumonia: secondary to megaesophagus.

DIFFERENTIAL DIAGNOSIS

- Demodicosis
- Dermatophytosis
- Bacterial folliculitis
- Juvenile cellulitis
- Cutaneous lupus erythematosus
- Systemic lupus erythematosus
- Polymyositis

DIAGNOSTICS

- CBC: nonregenerative anemia may occur with severe disease.
- Serum chemistries: creatine kinase may be normal or slightly high.
- ANA titers and lupus erythematosus tests negative.
- EMG: abnormalities in affected muscles; fibrillation potentials; bizarre high-frequency discharges; positive sharp waves.
- Muscle biopsy: difficult because pathologic changes may be mild, multifocal, or (in early states) absent; ideally, use EMG to select affected muscles; otherwise, biopsy atrophied muscles:
    - Variable multifocal accumulations of inflammatory cells, including lymphocytes, macrophages, plasma cells, neutrophils, and eosinophils
    - Myofibril degeneration characterized by fragmentation, vacuolation, and increased eosinophilia of the myofibrils
    - Myofiber atrophy and regeneration.
- Skin biopsy: choose papules, vesicles, or lesions that show alopecia and erythema; avoid infected and scarred lesions:
    - Scattered necrotic basal cells (colloid bodies) or vacuolated individual basal cells
    - Occasionally, vesicles that contain small amounts of RBCs
    - Superficial, mild, diffuse dermal inflammatory infiltrates composed of lymphocytes and histiocytes with variable numbers of mast cells and neutrophils (especially perifollicular)
    - Follicular basal cell degeneration and follicular atrophy
    - Secondary epidermal ulceration and dermal scarring
    - Combination of perifollicular inflammation, epidermal and follicular cell degeneration, and follicular atrophy strongly supports the diagnosis.

THERAPEUTICS

- Nonspecific symptomatic therapy, including gentle soakings of crusts and treatment of secondary pyoderma.
- Avoid activities that may traumatize the skin.
- Keep indoors during the day to avoid exposure to intense sunlight.
- Estrus may exacerbate the disease; neutering intact females is recommended.

Drugs of Choice

- Therapeutic efficacy of medical treatment can be difficult to assess because the disease tends to be cyclic and is often self-limiting.
- Vitamin E: 100–400 IU PO BID to q24h.
- Prednisolone: 1–2 mg/kg PO BID until remission; then alternate-day administration; use the lowest dosage possible for long-term control.

- Pentoxifylline: 10–20 mg/kg with food PO BID to TID: proposed to increase microvascular blood flow and tissue oxygenation by lowering blood viscosity, inhibit platelet aggregation, increase RBC deformability, and reduce serum fibrinogen levels; beneficial in some dogs.
- Cyclosporine, modified: 5–10 mg/kg PO q24h as an intitial dose and then tapered; reserved for severe cases with an active inflammatory component.

Precautions/Interactions

- Pentoxifylline should not be used in dogs that are sensitive to methylxanthine derivatives (e.g., theophylline).
- Pentoxifylline can cause gastric irritation; animals with prolonged clotting times and those receiving anticoagulant therapy should be monitored carefully.
- Glucocorticoids: discuss possible side effects with the owner.
- Cyclosporine: monitor serum chemistry for potential side effects.

COMMENTS

- Discuss the hereditary nature of the disease.
- Note that affected dogs should not be bred.
- Inform owner that the disease is not curable, although spontaneous resolution can occur.
- Discuss prognosis and possible complications, especially in severely affected dogs.
- Advise that medications may not help.

Client Education

- Prevention/avoidance.
- Minimize trauma and exposure to sunlight.
- Spay intact females to prevent estrus, parturition, and lactation (all precipitating causes of active dermatomyositis).
- Do not breed affected animals.

Possible Complications

- Secondary pyoderma.
- Mild to moderate disease: residual foci of alopecia, hypopigmentation, and hyperpigmentation in areas of previously active skin lesions; occurs most frequently on the bridge of the nose and around the eyes.
- Severe disease: extensive scarring; trouble chewing, drinking, and swallowing if the masticatory and esophageal muscles are involved; megaesophagus may develop, predisposing the dog to aspiration pneumonia.
- Generalized myositis: growth may be stunted.

Expected Course and Prognosis

- Long-term prognosis: varies, depending on the severity.
- Minimal disease: prognosis good; tends to resolve spontaneously with no evidence of scarring.
- Mild to moderate disease: tends to eventually resolve spontaneously, usually with residual scarring.
- Severe disease: poor prognosis for long-term survival; dermatitis and myositis are severe and lifelong; may lead to crippling lameness and/or recurrent aspiration pneumonia from megaesophagus.

Associated Conditions

- Vesicular cutaneous lupus erythematosus (idiopathic ulcerative dermatosis) of Shetland sheepdogs and collies: poorly understood disease; described in adult collies and Shetland sheepdogs; characterized by well-demarcated serpiginous ulcers in the intertriginous areas of the groin and axillae; may occur alone or concurrently with dermatomyositis; originally considered a subgroup of dermatomyositis; likely a variant of lupus erythematosus.

Pregnancy

- Disease is inheritable; do not breed affected dogs.
- Pregnancy exacerbates clinical symptoms.

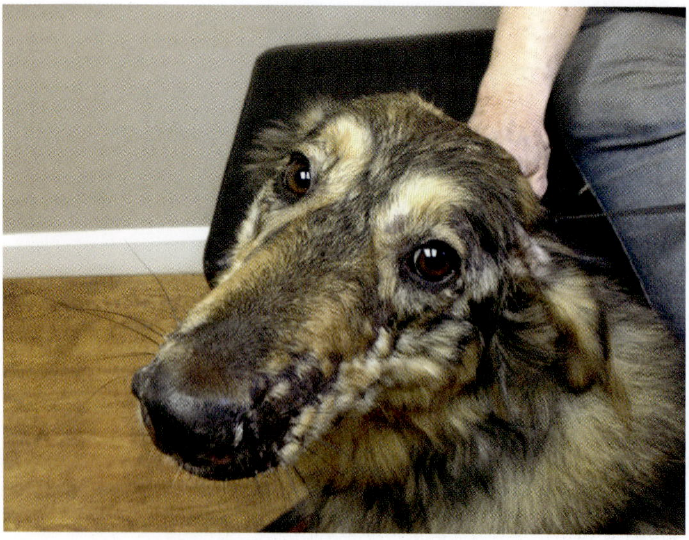

Fig. 20.1. Dermatomyositis in a collie mix with lesions of alopecia, crusting, and scarring of the face.

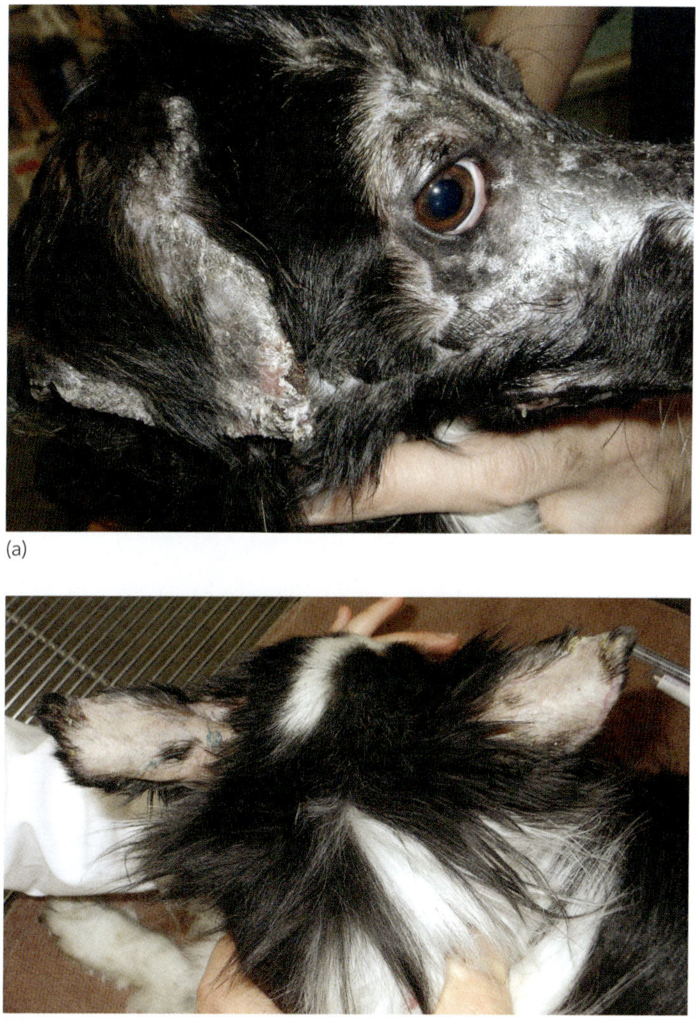

(a)

(b)

■ **Fig. 20.2.** Skin lesions on the pinnae and face consisting of crusts and alopecia with significant scarring. The facial lesions are characteristic of dermatomyositis.

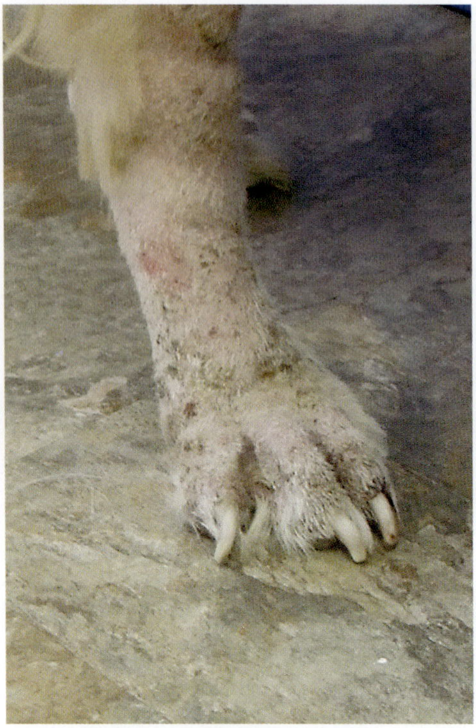

Fig. 20.3. Crusting alopecic lesions on the distal extremities (post clipping).

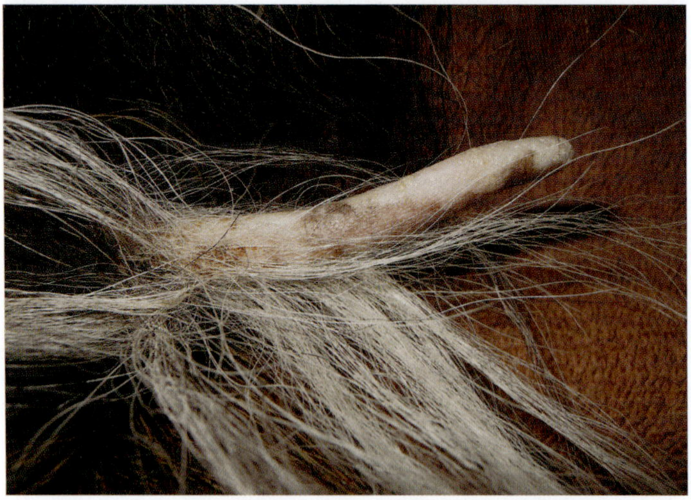

Fig. 20.4. Characteristic tail tip lesions of dermatomyositis often consist of alopecia and crusting.

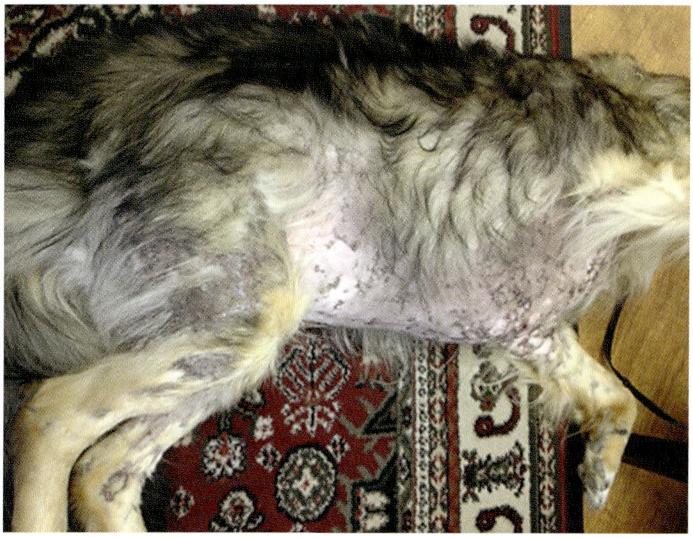

■ **Fig. 20.5.** Dermatomyositis in a collie mix. Note the areas of scarring and hypopigmentation of the ventrum and extremities.

chapter 21

Dermatophytosis

DEFINITION/OVERVIEW

- Cutaneous fungal infection affecting the cornified regions of hair and claws and the superficial layers of the skin (ringworm).
- Commonly isolated organisms: *Microsporum canis*, *Trichophyton mentagrophytes*, and *Microsporum gypseum*.
- Source of *M. canis* is usually an infected cat.
- Source of *T. mentagrophytes* is often direct or indirect contact with rodents.
- Source of *M. gypseum* is from soil – digging in contaminated areas.
- Dermatophytosis is a zoonotic disease.

ETIOLOGY/PATHOPHYSIOLOGY

- Exposure to or contact with a dermatophyte does not necessarily result in an infection.
- Infection may not result in overt clinical signs.
- Dermatophytes grow in the keratinized layers of hair, claws, and skin; do not thrive in living tissue or persist in the presence of severe inflammation; incubation period is 1–4 weeks.
- Affected animals may remain asymptomatic carriers for a prolonged period of time; some animals never become symptomatic.
- Corticosteroids can modulate inflammation and prolong the infection.

Incidence/Prevalence

- Lesions can mimic many dermatologic conditions.
- Infection rates vary widely, depending on the population studied.
- Catteries and shelters are at risk.
- Incidence of asymptomatic carriage as well as clinical infection is higher in hot and humid regions.
- Incidence rates of geophilic dermatophytes vary geographically.
- Dermatophytes spread between animals and people via direct contact with infected hair and/or scale (directly or by fomite).

Blackwell's Five-Minute Veterinary Consult Clinical Companion: Small Animal Dermatology, Third Edition.
Karen Helton Rhodes and Alexander H. Werner.

SIGNALMENT/HISTORY

- Cats: more common in long-haired breeds with increased persistent subclinical infection.
- Clinical signs are more common in young and older animals.
- Lesions begin as focal alopecia or a poor hair coat.
- A history of previously confirmed infection, exposure to an infected animal or environment (e.g., a cattery) increases risk of disease.

Causes

- Cats: *M. canis* most common organism.
- Dogs: *M. canis*, *M. gypseum*, and *T. mentagrophytes*; incidence of each organism varies geographically.

Risk Factors

- Immunocompromised condition caused by disease or medications (corticosteroids).
- FIV infection (three times higher prevalence).
- High population density (shelters).
- Poor nutrition.
- Poor management practices.
- Lack of an adequate quarantine period.
- Excessive bathing and grooming.

CLINICAL FEATURES

- Varies from a nonclinical carrier state to patchy alopecia, which may rapidly progress to generalized lesions (Figures 21.1–21.5).
- Lesions may resolve spontaneously as hair follicles enter telogen.
- Classic circular area of erythema, alopecia, and scale: common in people, rare in animals (Figures 21.6, 21.7).
- Scales, erythema, hyperpigmentation, and pruritus: variable.
- Granulomatous lesions (pseudomycetoma) or kerions may occur (often *M. gypseum*) (Figure 21.8).
- Folliculitis (Figure 21.9).
- Miliary dermatitis in cats.
- Clawbed inflammation and claw deformity (Figure 21.10).
- Facial folliculitis and furunculosis may mimic an autoimmune disease.
- Zoonotic (Figures 21.11, 21.12).
- Acantholytic dermatophytosis; mimics pemphigus complex; often *Trichophyton* spp. (Figure 21.13).

DIFFERENTIAL DIAGNOSIS

- Dermatophytosis may mimic many scaling and alopecic dermatoses in the dog (e.g., bacterial folliculitis, demodicosis, hyperkeratotic disorders, endocrine dermatoses) and cat (e.g., allergy, lymphocytic mural folliculitis, cutaneous lymphoma) and must be ruled in/out during an initial diagnostic plan.
- Acantholytic dermatophytosis mimics clinical lesions consistent with pemphigus complex.

DIAGNOSTICS

Wood's Lamp Examination

- Variable screening tool; poor confidence in this test may be due to inadequate equipment and diagnostic techniques; some pathogenic dermatophytes do not fluoresce.
- Fluorescence is due to a pigment on the hair and is not associated with arthrospores or the infection itself. As the infection resolves, the pigment will be lost in the proximal portion of the hair shaft while the tips may demonstrate residual fluorescence.
- Spontaneously occurring feline *M. canis*: 72% of cats fluoresce.
- False fluorescence is common; medications, keratin associated with epidermal scales, and sebum may all produce false-positive fluorescence yet the color is different from that seen in dermatophytosis.
- Topical therapy will not remove fluorescence.
- Plug-in lamps are more effective than battery-operated lamps.
- A true positive reaction associated with *M. canis* consists of apple-green fluorescence of the hair shafts (Figure 21.14).

Microscopic Examination of Hair

- Examination of plucked hairs placed in mineral oil can help provide a rapid diagnosis. Positive and negative predictive values are as high as 93% with an educated investigator. KOH preparation is not necessary.
- Infected hairs often appear broken or misshapen due to ectothrix invasion of the cuticle (Figure 21.15).
- Use hairs that fluoresce under Wood's lamp illumination to increase the likelihood of identifying the fungal hyphae associated with the hair shaft.
- Saprophytic fungal spores may be visualized microscopically (dermatophytes do not form macroconidia in tissue but may demonstrate a yeast form in cytology) (Figure 21.16).

Fungal Culture with Identification

- Hairs that exhibit a positive apple-green fluorescence under Wood's lamp examination are ideal candidates for culture.

- Pluck hairs from the periphery of an alopecic area.
- Use a new toothbrush to collect hairs from an asymptomatic animal (Figure 21.17).
- Dermatophyte test media: Sabouraud's dextrose agar with phenol red indicator: dermatophyte growth changes media color from yellow to red as it becomes alkaline; dermatophytes produce color change simultaneously with the early growing phase of the culture; saprophytes may cause color change after significant colony growth, so it is important to examine the media daily to match growth with potential color change (Figure 21.18).
- Microscopic examination of the culture growth for microconidia and macroconidia is necessary to confirm a pathogenic dermatophyte; identify genus and species to help identify the source of infection; *Trichophyton* spp. are often more difficult to identify (Figure 21.19).
- Dermatophyte colonies are white to buff in color; contaminants are often blue, green, black, or dark brown (Figure 21.20).
- Positive culture indicates presence of a dermatophyte; organisms may be transient (i.e., geophilic dermatophytes on the feet).

Skin Biopsy

- Not usually required for diagnosis.
- Can be helpful in confirming true invasion and infection, or to diagnose suspicious cases with negative fungal culture.
- Most helpful in cases of granulomatous dermatophytosis (kerion, pseudomycetoma).
- Histopathology results: folliculitis, perifolliculitis, or furunculosis are common; hyperkeratosis, intraepidermal pustules, and pyogranulomatous reaction pattern may occur.
- Fungal hyphae may be observed in H&E-stained sections; special stains allow easier visualization of the organism (Figure 21.21).

THERAPEUTICS

Drugs of Choice

- Itraconazole: dogs: 3–5 mg/kg PO q24h, refractory cases 10 mg/kg PO BID; cats: 3–5 mg/kg PO q24h alternating dose (week on/week off) may be used after the first week of daily dose; available in 100 mg capsules and as 10 mg/mL liquid containing cyclodextrin; liquid preferred over compounded formulations due to absorption variability; best for small dogs and cats.
- Griseofulvin: no longer a drug of choice: microsized formulation: 25–60 mg/kg PO BID to q24h for 4–10 weeks; ultramicrosized formulation: 2.5–15 mg/kg PO BID to q24h; absorption increased by dividing the dose twice a day and giving with a fatty meal; higher doses are associated with an increased likelihood of toxicity and should be used with extreme caution; gastrointestinal upset is the most common side effect – alleviate by reducing the dose or dividing the dose for more frequent administration;

not recommended for cats – associated with idiosyncratic toxicity (bone marrow suppression).

- Ketoconazole: efficacy unknown – dogs: 10–15 mg/kg PO divided BID to TID; anorexia and vomiting are the most common side effects; not recommended in cats; best for medium to large dogs.
- Fluconazole: dogs: 5–10 mg/kg PO BID; cats: 10 mg/kg PO BID; less effective than itraconazole.
- Voriconazole: dogs: 5–6 mg/kg PO BID; cats: 4 mg/kg PO as a loading dose followed by 2 mg/kg every other day; associated with neurotoxicity in cats at high doses (10 mg/kg); miosis and hypersalivation common at therapeutic doses.
- Terbinafine: dogs and cats: 30–40 mg/kg PO q24h; alternate weekly dosing after the first 2 weeks of daily dosing is an option.

Topical Therapy

- Scissor clipping often recommended in long-coated patients; may help prevent environmental contamination and allow easier application of topical therapy.
- Lime sulfur (1:16 dilution or 8 oz per gallon of water) rinses; twice weekly; odiferous and can stain; commercial rose garden sprayer can be used to saturate the skin and hair coat.
- Enilconazole 10% emulsion: environmental treatment or sponged directly on the animal at 0.2% solution (dilute from 10% emulsion to 0.2%) applied every 3–4 days; not currently available in the United States.
- Miconazole 2%: available in both shampoo and "leave-on" preparations.
- Chlorhexidine 2%: when used alone, the response to chorhexidine is variable; works synergistically with other antifungals (e.g., miconazole) to increase effectiveness.
- Bleach (Na hypochlorite) – dilute solutions applied topically as a rinse.
- Elizabethan collar, particularly in cats, is recommended to prevent ingestion of topical products.

Precautions

- Griseofulvin:
  - Highly teratogenic; do not administer to pregnant animals
  - Bone marrow suppression (anemia, pancytopenia, and neutropenia) can occur as an idiosyncratic reaction or with prolonged therapy
  - Neutropenia: fatal reaction in cats; persists after discontinuation of drug; can be life-threatening in cats with FIV or FeLV infection
  - Neurologic side effects.
- Ketoconazole:
  - Reduces metabolism of many drugs, requiring dosage alteration
  - Hepatopathy has been reported and may be severe
  - Inhibits endogenous production of steroid hormones in dogs
  - Vomiting and diarrhea
  - Rare thrombocytopenia in dogs

- Rare cataract formation in dogs
- May lighten coat color
- Use with food for best absorption.

- Itraconazole:
  - Vasculitis and necroulcerative skin lesions reported in 7.5% of dogs treated for blastomycosis with itraconazole at doses of 5 mg/kg q12h. Lesions were not noted in patients receiving 5 mg/kg q24h
  - Hepatotoxicity has been reported in both dogs (10–15% of treated cases) and cats (unknown %); monitor liver enzymes
  - Vasculitis has been reported in both the dog and cat
  - Use with food for best absorption.
- Lime sulfur solution, topical:
  - Ingestion of lime sulfur may lead to oral mucosa irritation; an Elizabethan collar should be placed on animals (especially cats) while drying.

Alternative Drugs

- "Ringworm vaccine": no longer available in the US; decreased clinical signs; may encourage development of inapparent carrier states.
- Lufenuron: a chitin synthesis inhibitor used in flea control; proven not effective in controlled studies.
- Effective topical products include ketoconazole, miconazole, miconazole/chlorhexidine, climbazole, accelerated hydrogen peroxide rinse (3.5% diluted 1:10), 1% clortrimazole, dilute sodium hypochlorite; essential oils (*Thymus serpillum*, *Origanum vulgare*, *Rosmarinus officinalis*) may have some benefit; minimal studies.

COMMENTS

Treatment Goals ("CCATS," Moriello)

- **Confinement**: affected animals should be confined to a specific area of the home.
- **Cleaning**: cleaning will help prevent false-positive fungal culture results on the animal; fungal spores do not "live" in the environment/spores only live in keratin; fungal spores are easily removed by mechanical cleaning and washing with a detergent and water; spores do *not* represent a respiratory risk; transmission of the disease from a contaminated environment to a person in the absence of contact with an animal is rare; bleach and hot water are not more effective than cold water in the laundry – the most important factor is to avoid overfilling the machine; accelerated hydrogen peroxide products are as effective as household bleach for hard surfaces in the home; carpets should be vacuumed, disinfected, and repeatedly washed with a carpet shampooer.
- **Assessment**: monitoring for a clinical response to therapy; examination for the presence or absence of lesions, Wood's lamp, and fungal culture results (coupled with the numbers of colony forming units per plate); routine serum chemistry and complete blood count to monitor therapy.

- **Topical therapy**: Combing of the hair coat prior to treatment to remove broken or fragile hairs followed by full body shampoo or rinses 2–3 times per week; body clipping can facilitate the spread of disease to other areas of the body; if clipping is warranted due to a long hair coat, use rounded blunted scissors rather than an electric clipper.
- **Systemic therapy**.

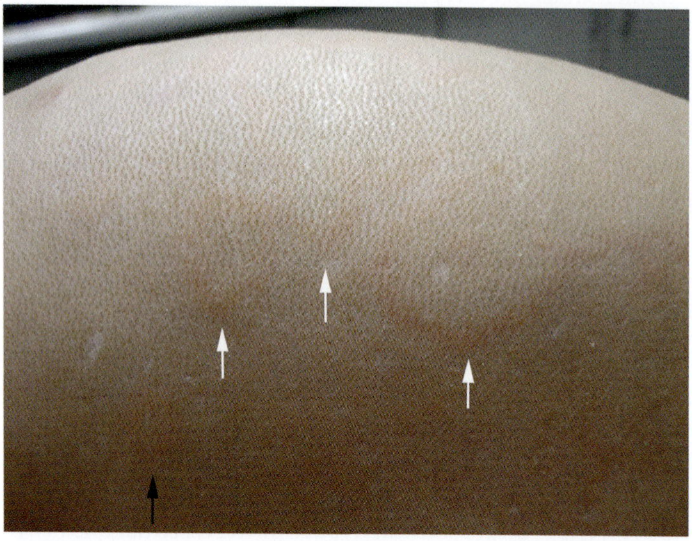

■ **Fig. 21.1.** Subtle lesions of *Microsporum canis* in a 6-year-old male-castrate sphynx cat. The lack of a thick hair coat creates lesions similar to those seen in humans. Lesions are polymorphic and appear as annular (*black arrow*), progressing to form irregular lesions with serpiginous and erythematous margins (*white arrows*).

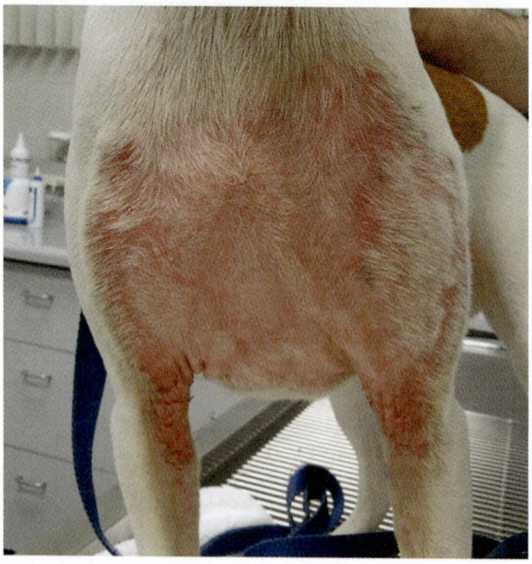

■ **Fig. 21.2.** Large patch of erythema and exudation with *Microsporum gypseum* in a 2-year-old male-castrate Jack Russell terrier.

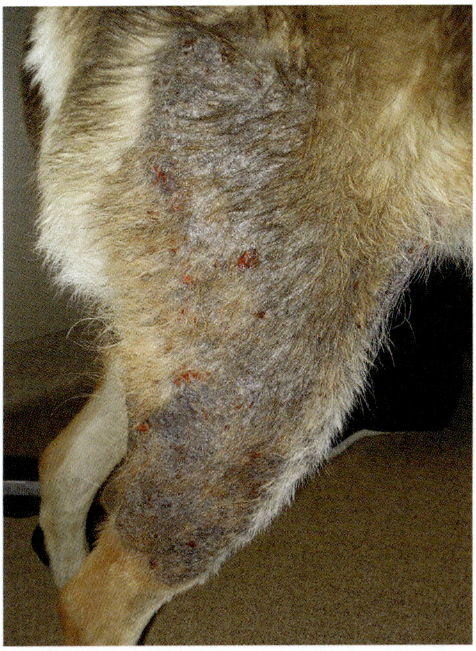

■ **Fig. 21.3.** *Trichophyton mentagrophytes* producing large patches of alopecia with exudation in a 10-year-old female-spayed German shepherd treated with oclacitinib and prednisolone for presumptive eosinophilic furunculosis.

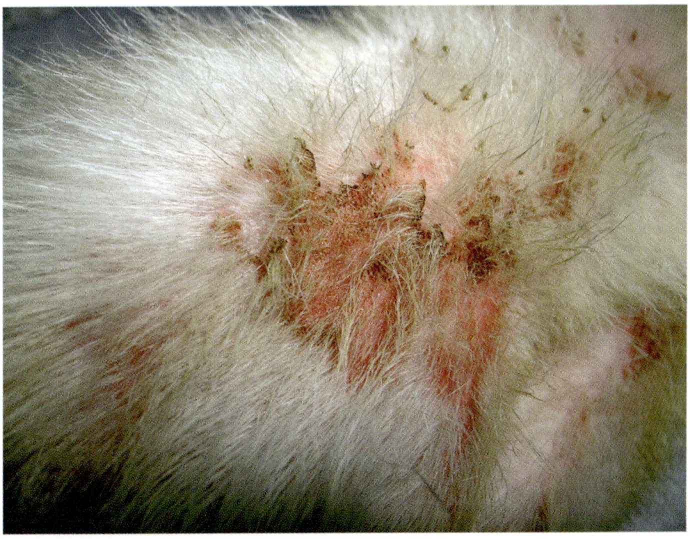

■ **Fig. 21.4.** Inflammatory lesions of *Microsporum canis* on the lateral thorax and foreleg of a 1-year-old female-spayed DMH.

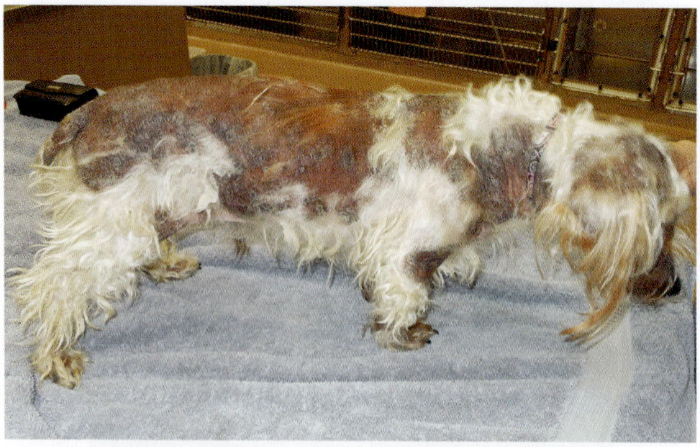

■ **Fig. 21.5.** Generalized lesions of *Microsporum canis* in a patient with hypothyroidism.

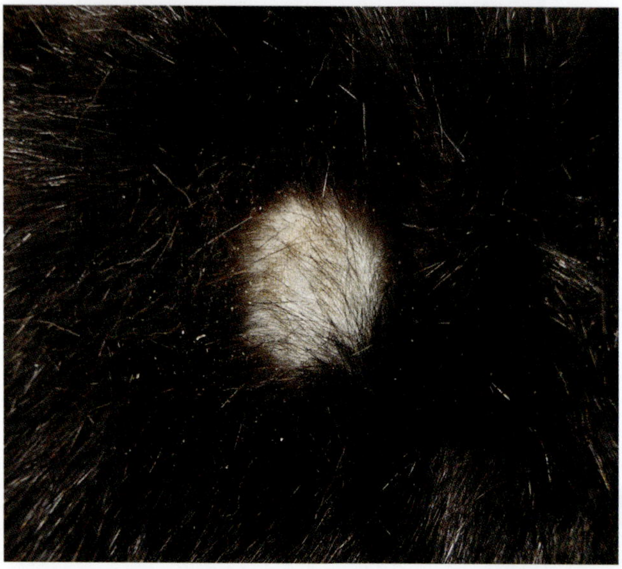

■ **Fig. 21.6.** "Classic" circular lesion of alopecia and scale with *Microsporum canis* in an 8-year-old male-castrate DSH.

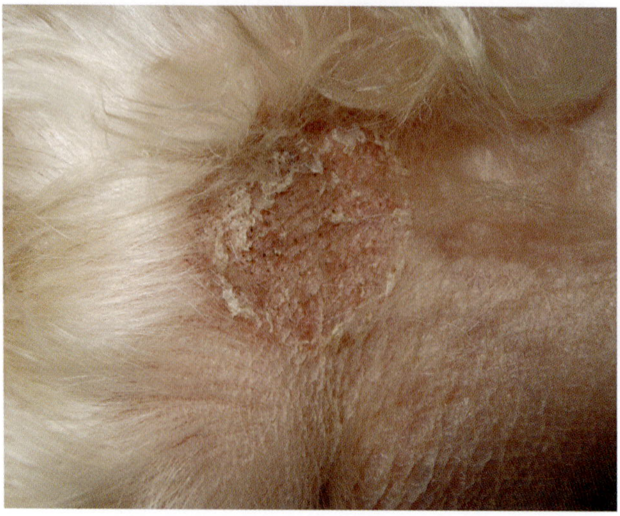

■ **Fig. 21.7.** "Classic" circular lesion of alopecia and scale with *Trichophyton mentagrophytes* in an 11-year-old male-castrate Yorkshire terrier.

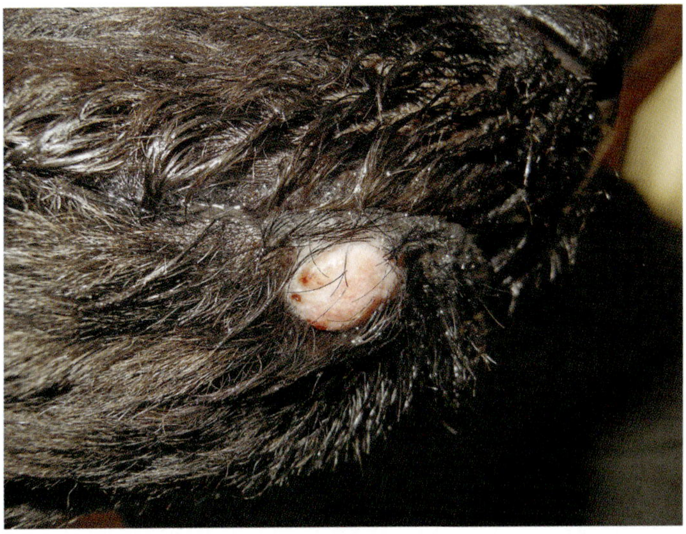

■ **Fig. 21.8.** Kerion form of dermatophytosis in a 1-year-old female-spayed toy poodle. Lesion is a "boggy" or exudative nodule on the lip margin.

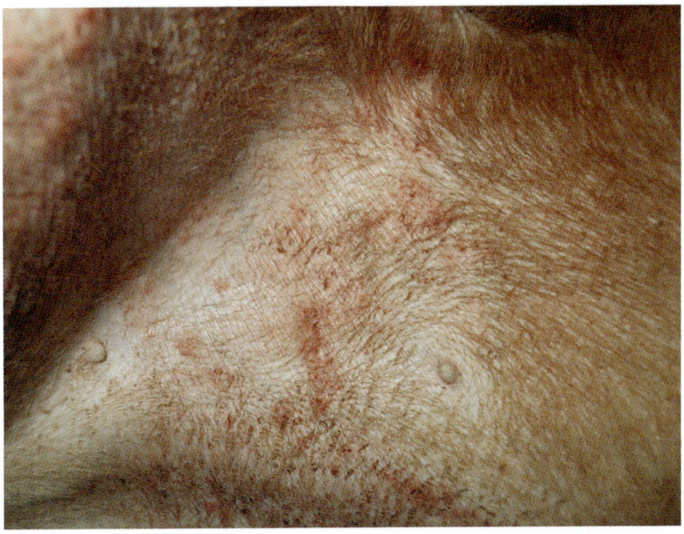

■ **Fig. 21.9.** Vesicular inflammatory dermatophytosis in a 3-year-old female-spayed pit bull mix. Lesions mimic those of bacterial folliculitis.

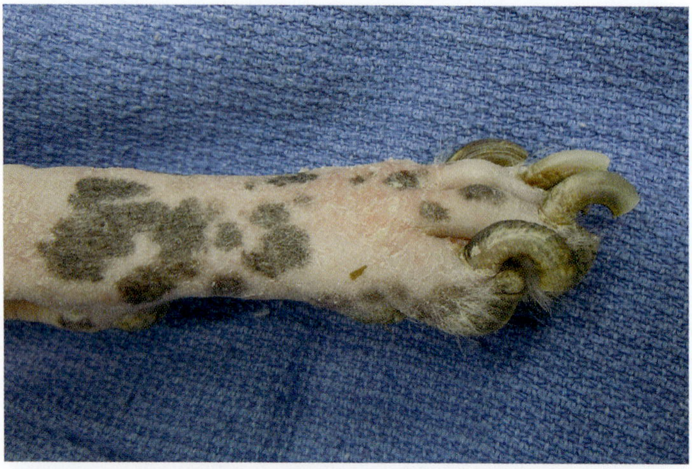

■ **Fig. 21.10.** Alopecia with paronychia and onychodystrophy from *Trichophyton mentagrophytes* in a 15-year-old male-castrate Jack Russell terrier.

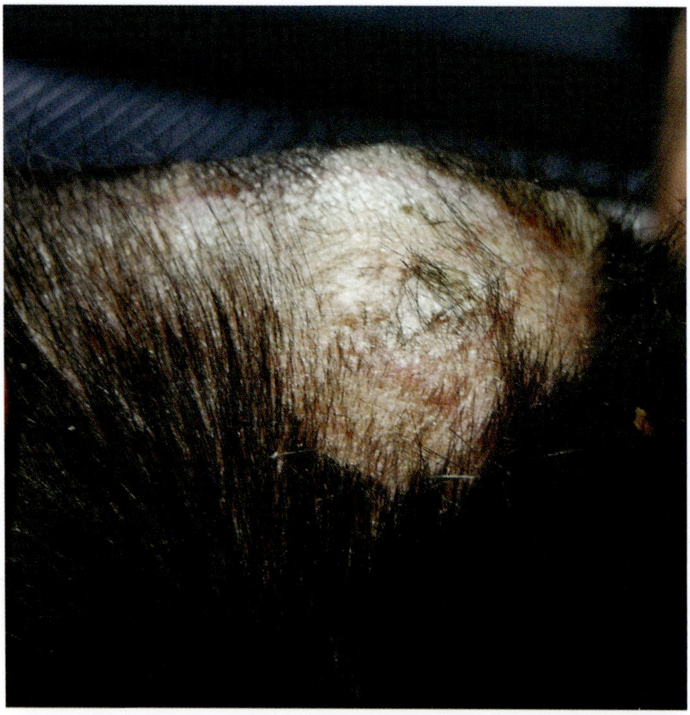

■ **Fig. 21.11.** *Microsporum canis* lesion on pinnal margin in a 9-year-old male-castrate DSH. The owner was diagnosed with tinea faciei corporis.

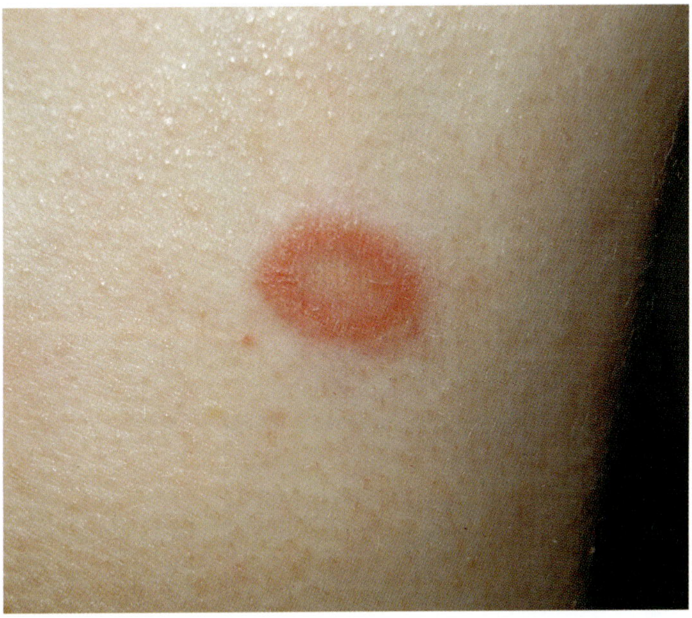

■ **Fig. 21.12.** Slowly expanding, annular lesion of erythema and scale forming the "classic" ringworm lesion seen in this owner infected with *Microsporum canis*.

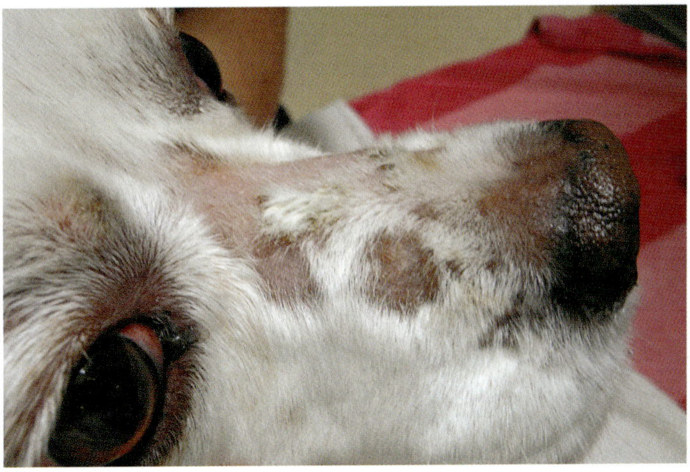

■ **Fig. 21.13.** Acantholytic dermatophytosis. Lesions in this 5-year-old female-spayed cocker spaniel mimicked clinical lesions of pemphigus foliaceus.

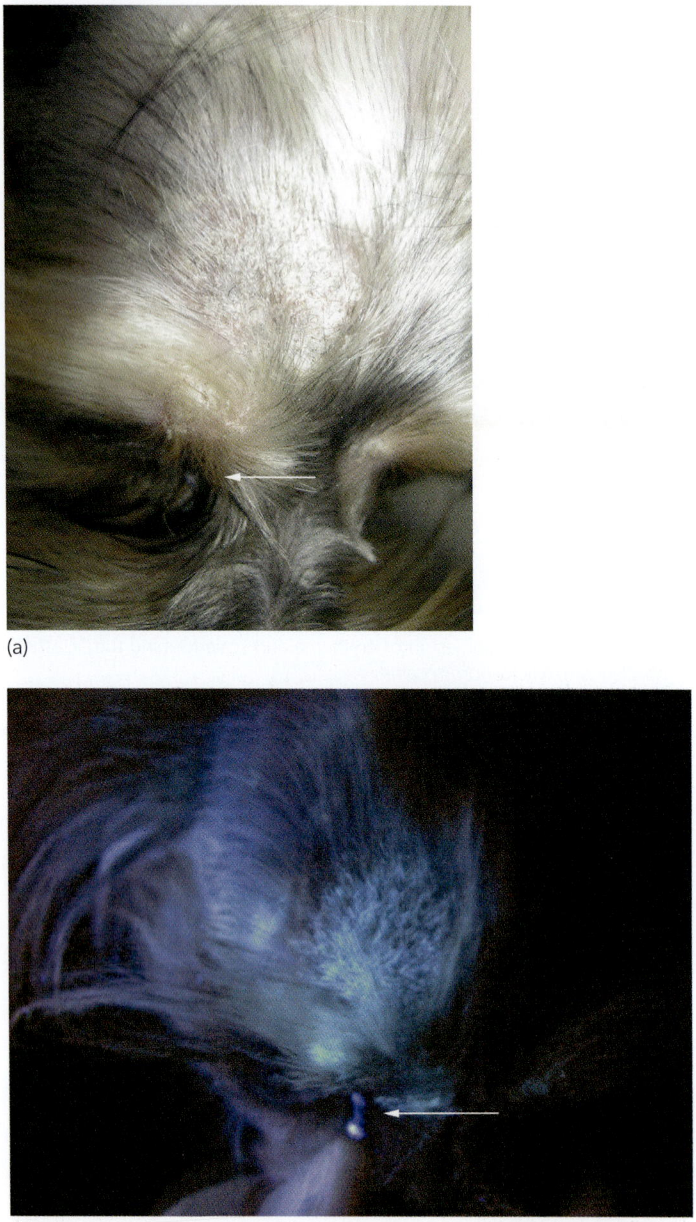

(a)

(b)

■ **Fig. 21.14.** Alopecic and scaly lesions on the forehead of a 16-week-old male-intact Yorkshire terrier: (a) normal light and (b) Wood's lamp. Positive fluorescence is seen as apple-green color on the hair shafts. Note false fluorescence of the mucoid discharge at the medial canthus (*arrows*).

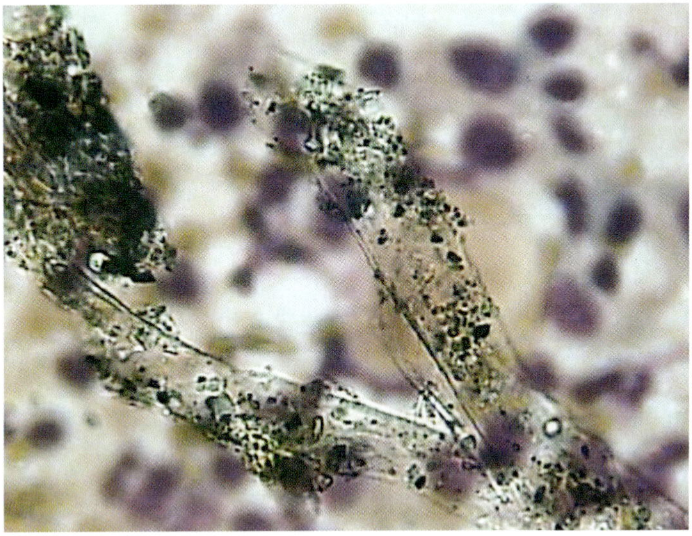

■ **Fig. 21.15.** Ectothrix invasion appears as dark dots invading the irregularly shaped hair shafts.

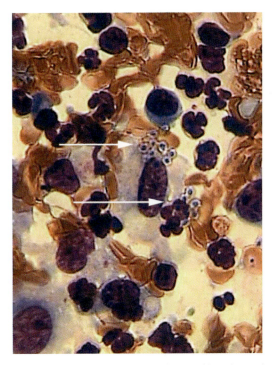

■ **Fig. 21.16.** Yeast form of *Microsporum canis* in cytological preparations (*arrows*).

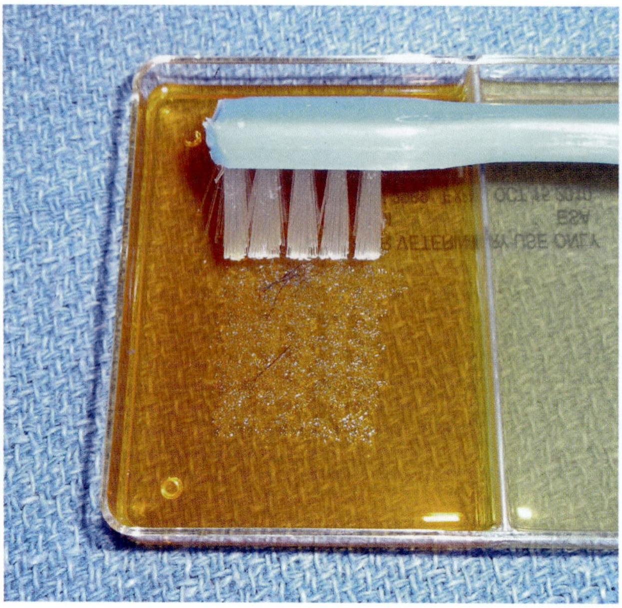

■ **Fig. 21.17.** Toothbrush sampling technique: after brushing through hair coat, bristles are lightly tapped on the surface of the culture medium; deep embedding of loosened scale and hair should be avoided.

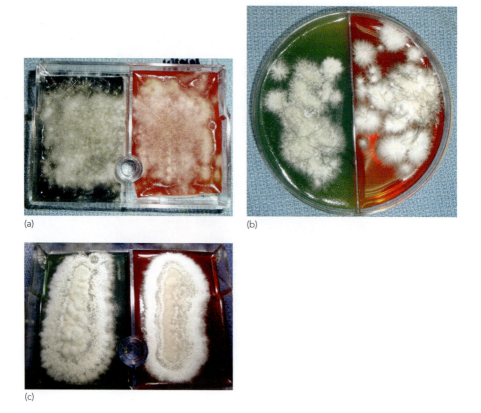

(a) (b) (c)

■ **Fig. 21.18.** (a) *Microsporum canis* colonies appear white/cottony. (b) *Microsporum gypseum* colonies appear ivory/granular. (c) *Trichophyton mentagrophytes* colonies appear white/powdery.

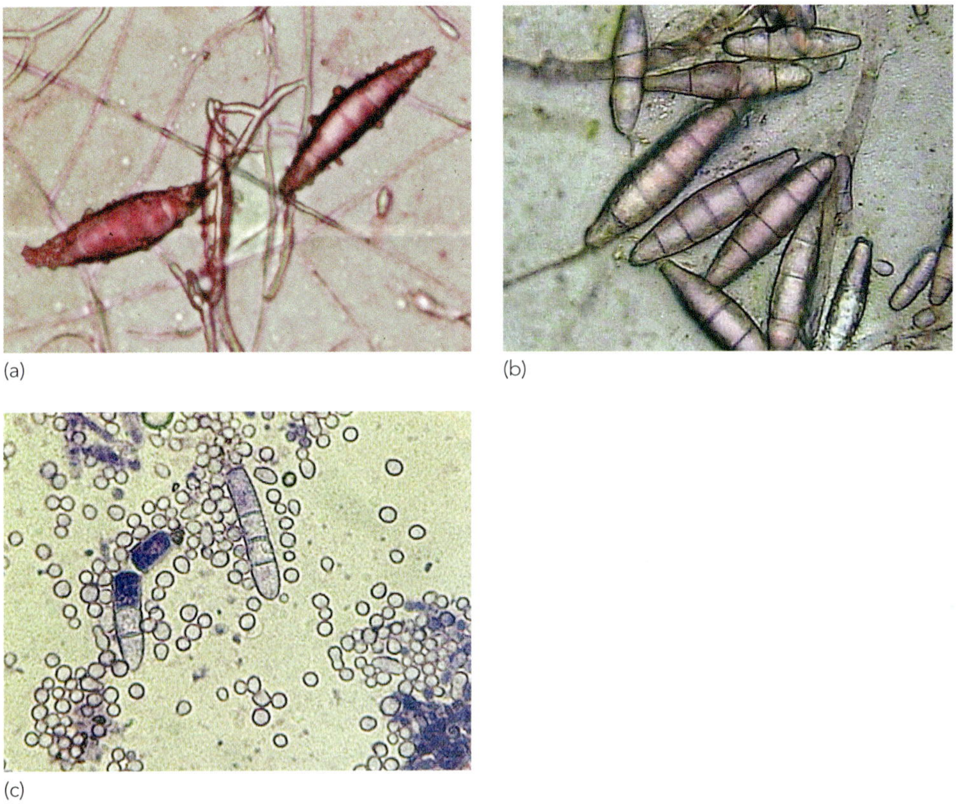

■ **Fig. 21.19.** (a) *Microsporum canis*: macroconidia are spindle shaped and thick walled with a terminal knob. (b) *Microsporum gypseum*: macroconidia are spindle to cigar shaped and thin walled. (c) *Trichophyton mentagrophytes*: abundant microconidia common; cigar-shaped macroconidia uncommon.

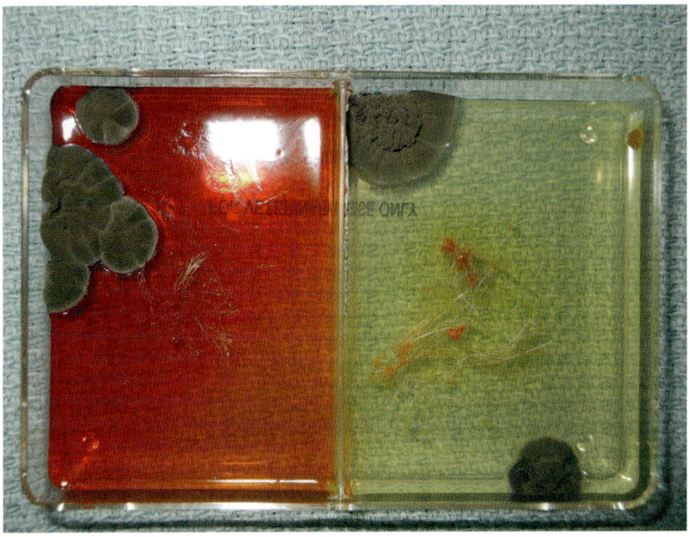

■ **Fig. 21.20.** Dermatophyte colonies on culture are not pigmented; pigmented cultures are contaminants.

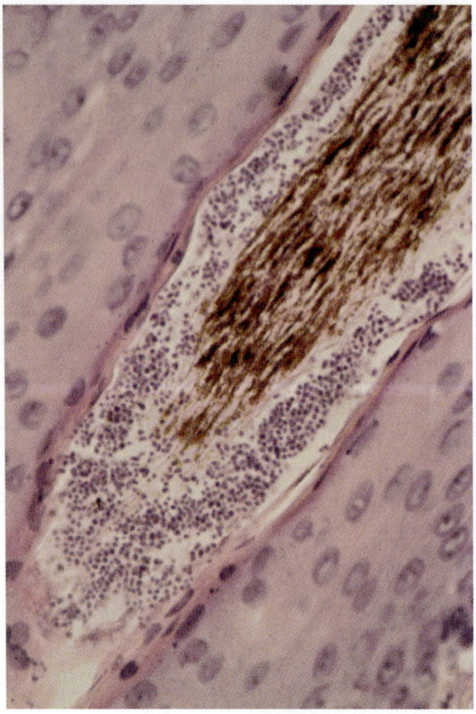

■ **Fig. 21.21.** Ectothrix invasion in hematoxylin and eosin-stained tissue preparations appear as dark dots invading the hair shaft within the follicle.

chapter 22

Endocrinopathies, Atypical

DEFINITION/OVERVIEW

- Most common canine disorders affecting the hair coat and skin are hyperadrenocorticism and hypothyroidism (discussed elsewhere).
- Multiple disorders produce similar patterns of alopecia affecting the trunk but sparing the head and distal extremities.
- Hair coat and skin abnormalities may be recognized prior to the development of nondermatologic symptoms.
- Uncommon disorders associated with abnormal hair follicle cycling and arrest include sex hormone-related dermatoses and alopecia X.
- Feline endocrinopathies such as diabetes mellitus and hyperthyroidism may have secondary effects on the skin and hair coat due to metabolic derangement or changes in grooming behavior.

ETIOLOGY/PATHOPHYSIOLOGY

- The hair follicle cycle is influenced by both hormones and nonhormonal factors.
- Endocrinopathies most often cause noninflammatory and symmetric alopecia.
- Abnormalities may be the result of primary or secondary hyperfunction of, hypofunction of, or exogenous exposure to hormones.
- Imbalances in sex hormones, especially elevations, can affect the hair cycle; sex hormones and their precursors have intrinsic glucocorticoid actions and affinity for glucocorticoid receptors, and may suppress the hypothalamic-pituitary-adrenal axis (HPA).
- Abnormalities in the HPA axis may produce elevations in glucocorticoid precursor hormones (notably androgens), with or without measured elevations in glucocorticoids.
- Alterations of hormones, in the absence of causality, may temporarily affect hair follicle cycling; these changes often do not persist.

Blackwell's Five-Minute Veterinary Consult Clinical Companion: Small Animal Dermatology, Third Edition.
Karen Helton Rhodes and Alexander H. Werner.

CLINICAL FEATURES

Diabetes Mellitus and Hyperthyroidism

- Diabetes mellitus and hyperthyroidism are common endocrinopathies in the cat.
- Changes in the hair coat and skin are caused by alterations in metabolism as well as by changes in grooming behavior.
- Metabolic alterations may result in increased incidence of pyoderma and seborrheic dermatitis.
- Diabetic cats will often have excessive scales and a dull, disheveled-appearing hair coat (Figure 22.1).
- Xanthomatosis: excessive accumulation of lipid in the skin; associated with diabetes mellitus in the cat (rarely dog) (Figure 22.2).
- Hyperthyroidism may result in overgrooming, causing patches of hair loss, as well as seborrheic dermatitis (Figure 22.3).

Alopecia X

- Synonyms: growth hormone (GH)-responsive alopecia; adrenal sex hormone imbalance of plush-coated breeds; castration-responsive dermatosis; pseudo-Cushing's syndrome; adrenal hyperplasia-like syndrome; and atypical Cushing's syndrome.
- May be caused by elevated levels of progesterone or androgen or their intermediaries causing direct effects on the hair follicle or decreased GH production.
- Hyposomatotropism is an inconsistent finding.
- Adrenal sex hormone imbalance of plush-coated breeds and adrenal hyperplasia-like syndrome may result from adrenal 21-hydroxylase enzyme deficiency producing excessive secretion of steroid hormone precursors.
- Genetic factors and hair follicle receptor defects (and/or stimulation) are current concepts in the development of and treatment for hair cycle arrest in these patients.
- Predisposed breeds: miniature poodle and plush-coated breed such as pomeranian, chow chow, Akita, samoyed, keeshonden, Alaskan malamute, and Siberian husky (Figures 22.4, 22.5).
- Occurs primarily between 1 and 5 years of age.
- Intact or neutered male and female dogs.
- Usually asymptomatic lack of hair coat growth and loss of primary hairs.
- Noninflammatory and symmetric hair loss that spares the head and extremities (see Figures 22.4, 22.5).
- Often accompanied by striking melanoderma.
- Secondary bacterial folliculitis and *Malassezia* dermatitis uncommon.
- Hypopituitary dwarfism: distinct from the syndromes considered in alopecia X; defect in or destruction of secretory capability of the adenohypophyseal cells; may be associated with other hormone deficiencies; seen in German shepherds, spitz, miniature pinscher, carnelian bear dog; noted by 3 months of age (Figure 22.6).

Estrogen Imbalances

- Estrogen is produced by ovarian follicles and cysts, Leydig and Sertoli cells of the testes, and zona glomerulosa and fasciculata of the adrenal gland.
- Estrogen is an inhibitor of anagen initiation in dogs (stimulates scalp hair growth in human beings) and potentiates the action of androgens in the prostate and progesterone in the endometrium.
- Animals with normal serum estrogen concentrations may have increased numbers of estrogen receptors in the skin.
- Peripheral conversion of estrogen and/or excess androgens, as well as regulation of hormone receptors, is affected by growth factors; abnormalities may cause estrogen excess or deficiency.
- True estrogen deficiency is uncommon; it is primarily seen following ovariohysterectomy; serum estradiol concentrations may be normal.
- Younger intact female dogs (ovarian cysts) (Figure 22.7).
- Older intact female dogs (granulosa cell tumor, other ovarian tumor, ovarian cysts).
- Older intact male dogs: testicular tumors (Sertoli cell tumor, seminoma, or interstitial cell tumor); boxer, Shetland sheepdog, weimaraner, German shepherd, cairn terrier, pekingese, collie; increased risk in cryptorchid dogs (Figures 22.8, 22.9).
- Intact or altered female and male dogs (exogenous administration of diethylstilbestrol) (Figure 22.10).
- Exposure to topical hormone replacement therapy by owner (Figures 22.11, 22.12).
- Hyperestrogenism associated with:
    - Enlargement of nipples, mammary glands, vulva, prepuce
    - Linear preputial dermatitis; testicles may palpate normal or irregular in size
    - Petechiae due to thrombocytopenia
    - Pyrexia due to neutropenia.

Hyperandrogenism and Hyperprogesteronemia

- Elevated level of progesterone has been associated with alopecia; most often caused by exogenous administration – megestrol acetate or exposure to topical hormone replacement therapy by owner (Figure 22.13).
- Progesterone effect likely due to binding of glucocorticoid receptors and/or conversion to cortisol within canine hair follicles.
- Castration-responsive alopecia as well as testosterone-responsive alopecia may result from proximate relative changes in hormone levels; response may not persist.
- Hyperandrogenism (primarily males): uncommon to rare cause of alopecia in middle-aged to old intact dogs; may cause tail gland hyperplasia (Figure 22.14).
- Exposure to topical hormone replacement therapy by owner (Figure 22.15).

SIGNALMENT/HISTORY

- Hair coat: dry or bleached because hairs are not being replaced; lack of normal shed; usually diffuse and bilaterally symmetrical truncal alopecia sparing the head and distal extremities; primary coat lost first, resulting in patchy retention of the undercoat; complete alopecia eventually develops.

- Variable secondary seborrhea, pruritus, bacterial folliculitis, and comedones.
- Epidermal and dermal atrophy; mild lichenification and scaling.
- Systemic signs (polyuria/polydypsia/polyphagia) usually not present; urinary incontinence may occur in estrogen-responsive cases.

DIFFERENTIAL DIAGNOSIS

- Hypothyroidism
- Hyperadrenocorticism
- Bacterial folliculitis
- Demodicosis
- Follicular dysplasia: color dilution alopecia, black hair follicular dysplasia
- Pattern alopecia: dachshund, Boston terrier, greyhound, water spaniel, chihuahua
- Cyclical flank alopecia: boxer, English bulldog, Airedale
- Postclipping alopecia
- Telogen defluxion
- Keratinization disorder

DIAGNOSTICS

- CBC/biochemistries/urinalysis: normal except as associated with hypothyroidism or hyperadrenocorticism; anemia and/or bone marrow hypoplasia or aplasia with hyperestrogenism.
- Serum sex hormone concentrations: often normal; treat according to suspected diagnosis based on clinical signs and ruling out other disorders.
- Serum estradiol: sometimes elevated in male dogs with testicular tumors or female dogs with cystic ovaries; normal daily fluctuations of estradiol make interpretation of estradiol concentrations difficult; prolonged elevation demonstrated by repeated tests more conclusive.
- Exposure to human topical hormone replacement therapy may or may not cause serum estradiol, progesterone, or testosterone levels to be elevated above normal despite having dramatic effects on the skin.
- ACTH stimulation test or LDDS test: exclusion of hyperadrenocorticism.
- Serum thyroxine, fT4, and TSH: exclusion of hypothyroidism.
- ACTH stimulation test with measurement of adrenal sex hormones: may indicate overproduction of cortisol precursors.
- Dermatohistopathologic changes commonly associated with endocrine dermatoses: telogenization of hairs, follicular keratosis, tricholemmal keratinization (flame follicles), epidermal and dermal atrophy, sebaceous gland atrophy; usually distinct from changes associated with pattern baldness and follicular dysplasia.
- Abdominal ultrasound: adrenal gland hyperplasia or neoplasia, and gonadal neoplasia.

THERAPEUTICS

General Considerations

- Frequent bathing with antiseborrheic shampoos to reduce scaling, comedones, and bacterial folliculitis.
- Treatment of secondary bacterial folliculitis with appropriate antibiotics.
- With exception of tumors, conditions are cosmetic, resulting in hair coat loss and hyperpigmentation; consider risk of treatment before initiating therapy.

Alopecia X

- Melatonin: 3 mg PO BID for small breeds and 6–12 mg PO BID for large breeds; hair regrowth should occur within 3 months; effective in approximately 40% of cases; once hair regrowth has occurred, discontinue treatment; begin supplementation again if hair loss redevelops.
- Melatonin at high doses can cause insulin resistance; use with caution in diabetic patients.
- Mitotane: 15–2 mg/kg PO q24h as induction: followed by twice-weekly maintenance; hair regrowth occurs in a portion of dogs; use of this drug can result in an addisonian crisis; electrolytes and ACTH stimulation testing should be monitored regularly.
- Trilostane: dosages as described for treatment of Cushing's syndrome; hair regrowth occurs in a portion of dogs; use of this drug can result in an addisonian crisis; electrolytes and ACTH stimulation testing should be monitored regularly.
- Reported but not recommended treatments include synthetic growth hormone 0.15 IU/kg subcutaneously twice weekly for 6 weeks: may cause diabetes mellitus; deslorelin 4.7 mg implant every 6 months (intact male dogs); methyltestosterone; fulvestrant; medroxyprogesterone acetate.
- Microneedling (tiny pinpoint perforations to stimulate hair growth): recent reported success in stimulating hair regrowth.

Sex Hormone Imbalances

- Diagnose and surgically excise ovarian cysts or tumors and abdominal or scrotal testicular tumors.
- Neutering of intact animals may stimulate hair coat regrowth (usually temporary).
- Methyltestosterone 1 mg/kg (maximum dosage of 30 mg/dog) every other day until hair regrowth, then once every 4–7 days; can result in behavioral changes, cholangiohepatitis, and seborrhea oleosa; monitor hepatic chemistries.
- Diethylstilbestrol 0.1–1 mg/kg PO q24h for 14–21 days; discontinue 7 days; repeat until hair coat regrowth, then administer 2–3 times weekly; monitor blood count frequently.

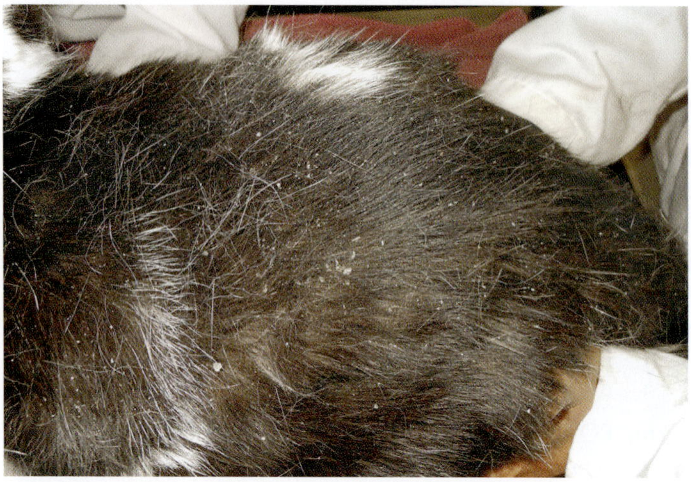

■ **Fig. 22.1.** Disheveled hair coat and excessive accumulations of scale in a 7-year-old female-spayed DLH with diabetes mellitus.

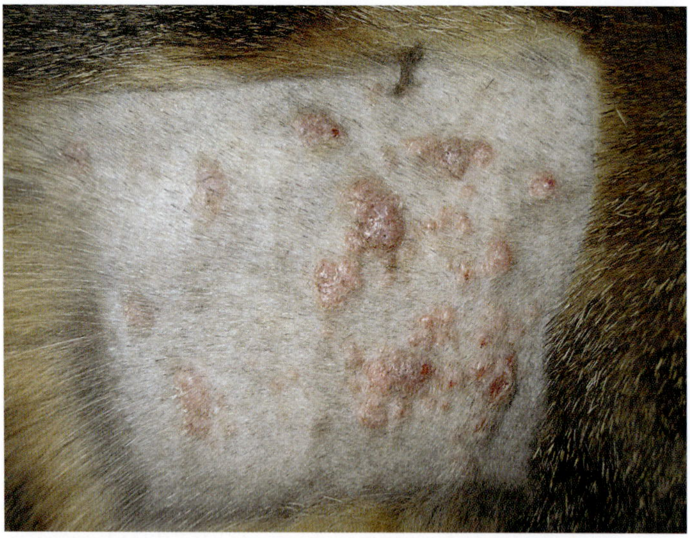

■ **Fig. 22.2.** Accumulations of lipid in the skin causing pink to cream-colored plaques in the skin of an 11-year-old female-spayed DSH with diabetes mellitus.

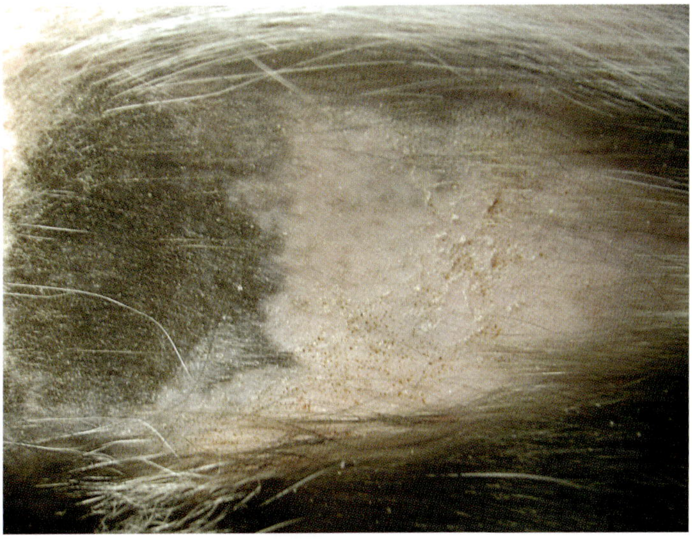

■ **Fig. 22.3.** Alopecia from excessive grooming and adherent scales on the skin of a 9-year-old female-spayed DSH with hyperthyroidism.

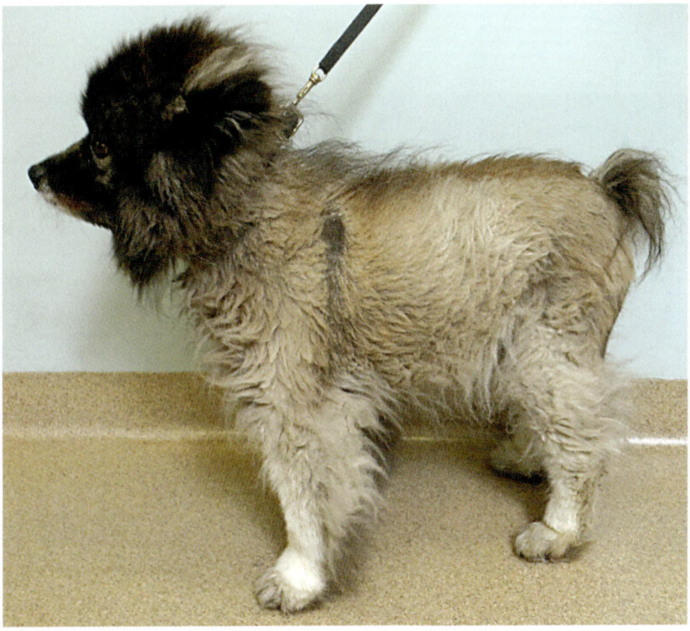

■ **Fig. 22.4.** Adult male keeshond with alopecia X. A dull, dry hair coat with lack of primary hairs and patches of alopecia are noted. The head and the distal extremities are not affected.

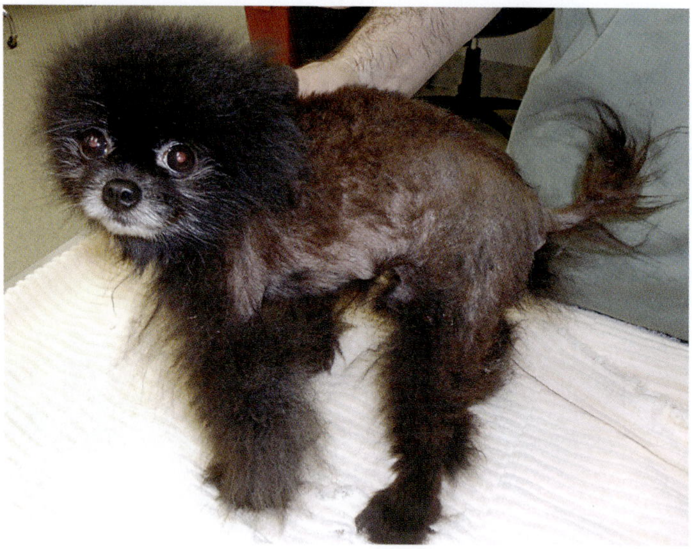

■ **Fig. 22.5.** Alopecia X in a 7-year-old male-castrate pomeranian with similar findings as the patient in Figure 22.4. Alopecic regions of skin are becoming hyperpigmented.

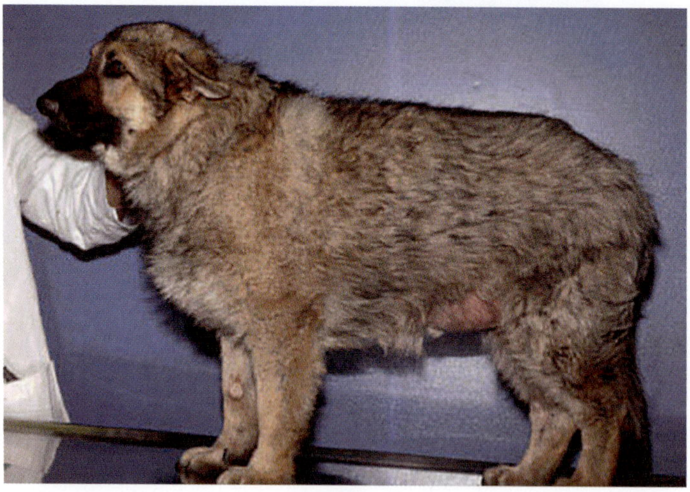

■ **Fig. 22.6.** Pituitary dwarfism.

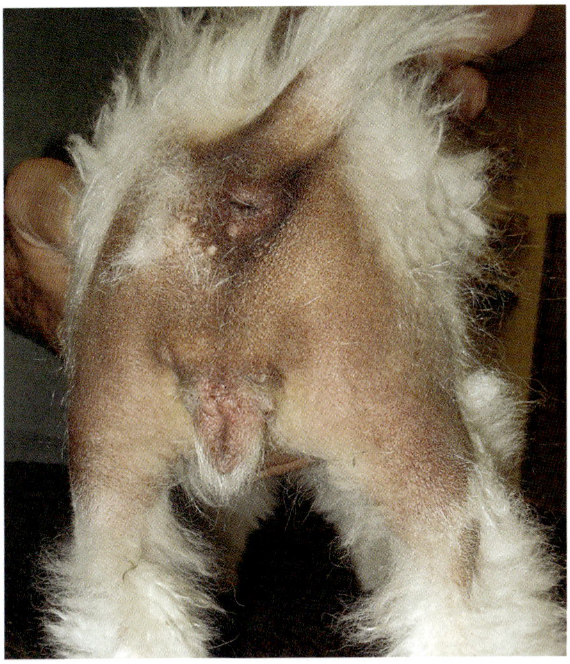

■ **Fig. 22.7.** Perianal, perineal, and caudal thigh alopecia in a 2-year-old female pomeranian. Hair coat regrew completely following ovariohysterectomy.

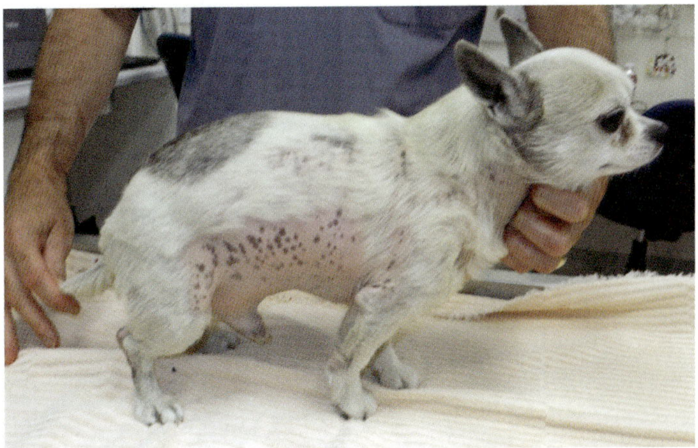

(a)

■ **Fig. 22.8.** Alopecia affecting the tail, entire ventrum, neck, and lateral aspects of the body in a 9-year-old male-intact chihuahua with a Sertoli cell tumor. Note comedones and mild linear erythema affecting the preputial skin. The right testicle palpated as larger than the left.

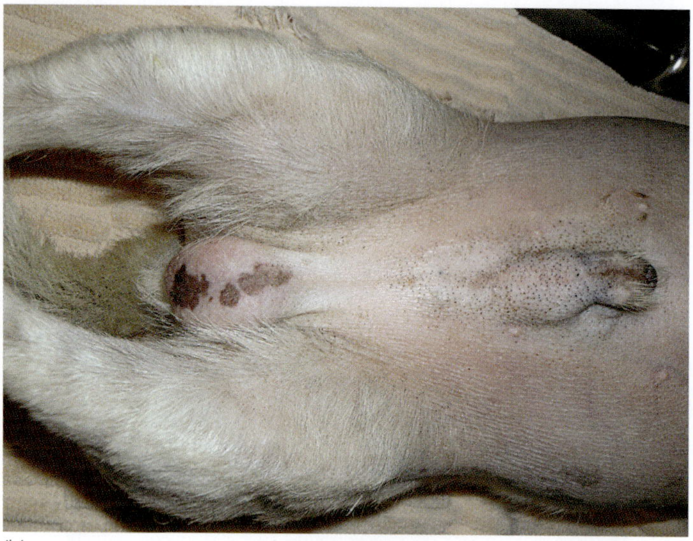

(b)

■ **Fig. 22.8.** (*Continued*)

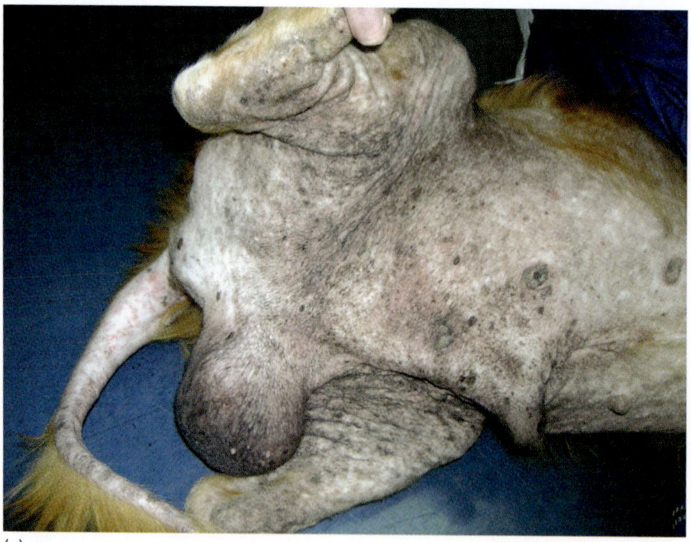

(a)

■ **Fig. 22.9.** Alopecia and lichenification on the ventral abdomen and medial thighs of a 13-year-old male-intact golden retriever with Sertoli cell tumor. The affected testicle was significantly enlarged and the other testicle appeared atrophied.

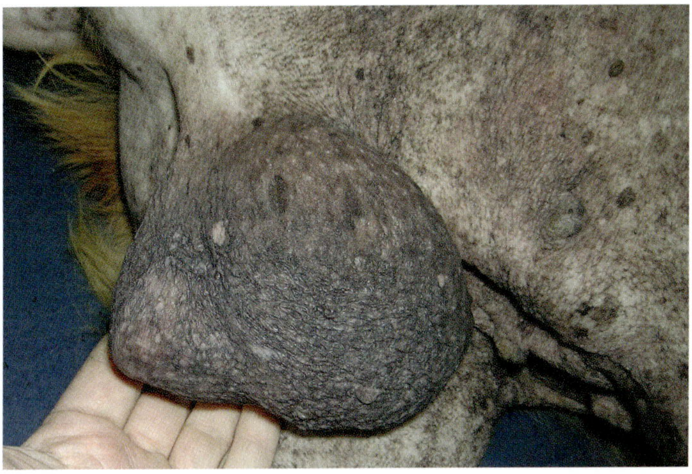

(b)

■ **Fig. 22.9.** (*Continued*)

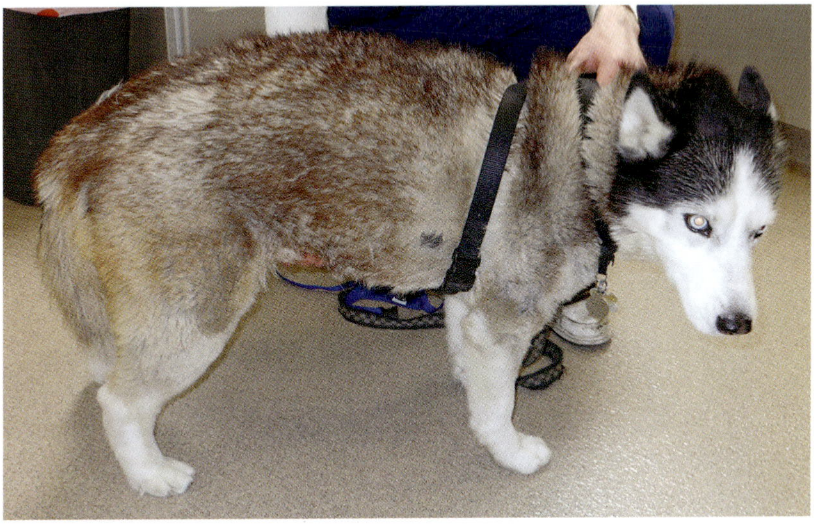

■ **Fig. 22.10.** Diethylstilbestrol supplementation causing thinning and lightening of the hair coat in this 12-year-old female-spayed Siberian husky. Note normal coloration to the hair coat on the head.

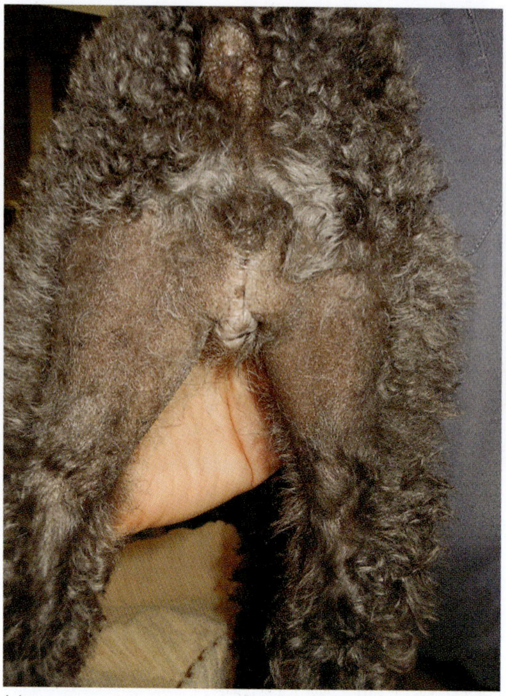

(a)

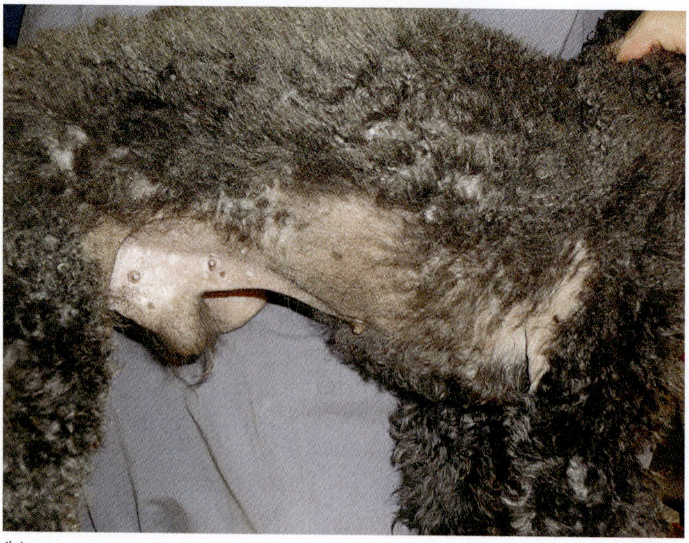

(b)

■ **Fig. 22.11.** Exposure to human topical hormone replacement therapy (estradiol). (a) Perianal, perineal, and caudal thigh alopecia similar to the patient in Figure 22.7. (b) Alopecia affecting the ventrum and lateral aspects of the body similar to the patient in Figure 22.8.

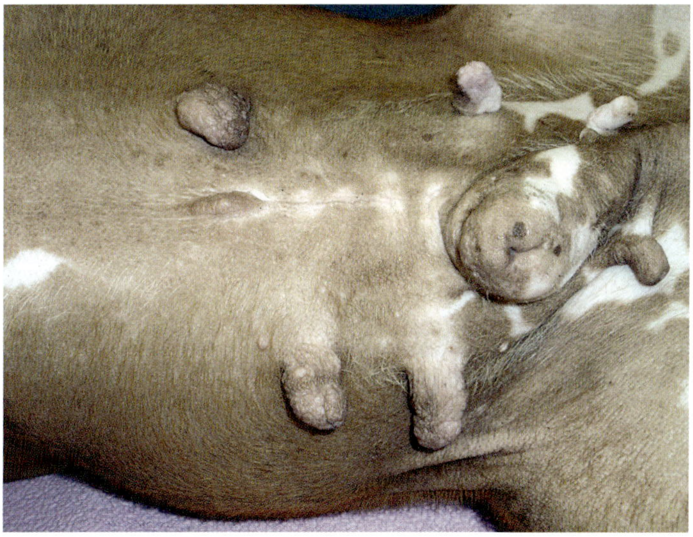

■ **Fig. 22.12.** Enlarged mammary nipples in a 2-year-old male-castrate pit bull mix exposed to estradiol cream.

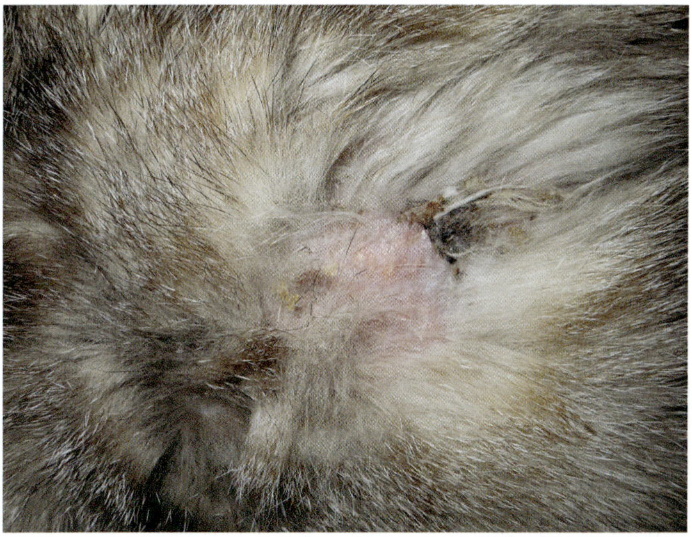

■ **Fig. 22.13.** Atrophy and alopecia affecting the ventral abdomen of a 10-year-old female-spayed Siamese cat after administration of megestrol acetate.

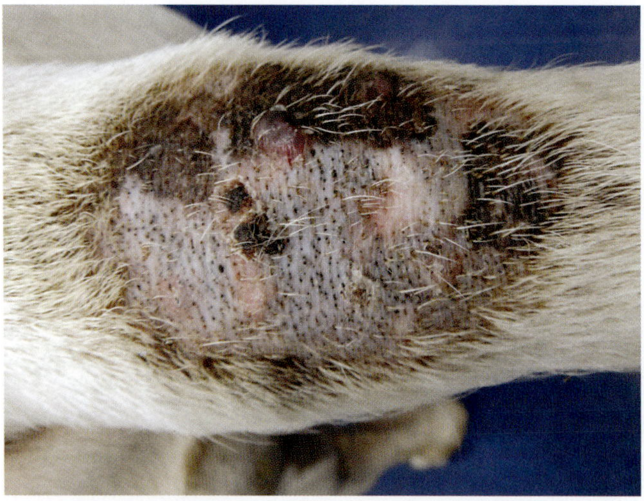

■ **Fig. 22.14.** Tail gland hyperplasia with secondary folliculitis and furunculosis in a 7-year-old male-intact American bulldog.

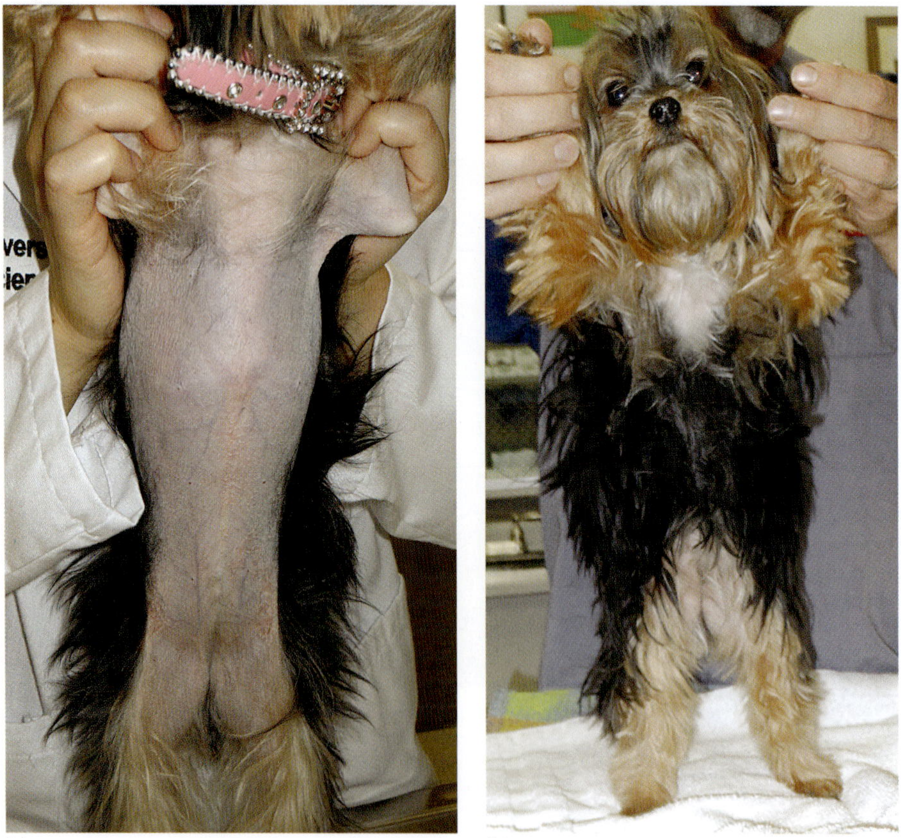

(a) (b)

■ **Fig. 22.15.** Alopecia caused by exposure to human testosterone topical hormone replacement therapy at the time of diagnosis (a) and 6 months after exposure discontinued (b) in a 3-year-old female-spayed Yorkshire terrier.

chapter 23

Eosinophilic Disease (Granuloma) Complex

DEFINITION/OVERVIEW

- Cats: Feline eosinophilic dermatitis or eosinophilic granuloma complex (EGC) is often a confusing term for four distinct syndromes grouped primarily according to their clinical similarities as a disease complex, their frequent concurrent (and recurrent) development, and their positive response to antiinflammatory therapeutics. EGC is a description, not a diagnosis:
  - Eosinophilic plaque
  - Eosinophilic granuloma
  - Indolent ulcer
  - Allergic miliary dermatitis.
- Dogs: canine eosinophilic granuloma (CEG) uncommon; not part of a disease complex; specific differences from cats are listed within the text.

ETIOLOGY/PATHOPHYSIOLOGY

- Eosinophilic plaque: hypersensitivity reaction, most often to insects (fleas, mosquitoes), food or environmental allergens; exacerbated by mechanical trauma.
- Eosinophilic granuloma: multiple causes; idiopathic, genetic predisposition, and hypersensitivity.
- Indolent ulcer: may have both hypersensitivity and genetic causes.
- Allergic miliary dermatitis: not always included within the EGC; very common hypersensitivity reaction, most often to fleas.
- Eosinophil: major infiltrative cell for eosinophilic granuloma, eosinophilic plaque, and allergic miliary dermatitis, but not indolent ulcer; most often associated with allergic or parasitic conditions, as well as a more general role in the inflammatory reaction.
- Several reports of related affected individuals and a study of disease development in a colony of specific pathogen-free cats indicate that genetic predisposition may be a significant component for development of eosinophilic granuloma and indolent ulcer.
- A heritable dysfunction of eosinophil regulation has been proposed.
- CEG (dogs): may have both a genetic predisposition and a hypersensitivity cause; insect bite often incriminated.

Blackwell's Five-Minute Veterinary Consult Clinical Companion: Small Animal Dermatology, Third Edition.
Karen Helton Rhodes and Alexander H. Werner.

SIGNALMENT/HISTORY

Cat

- No breed predilection.
- Eosinophilic plaque: 2–6 years of age.
- Genetic/idiopathic eosinophilic granuloma: less than 1 year of age.
- Allergic disorder: greater than 1 year of age.
- Indolent ulcer: no age predisposition.
- Predilection for females reported.
- Lesions of all four syndromes may develop spontaneously and acutely; lesions of more than one syndrome may occur simultaneously.
- Development of eosinophilic plaques may be preceded by periods of lethargy.
- Waxing and waning of clinical signs is common.
- Seasonal incidence in some geographic locations may indicate insect or environmental allergen exposure.
- Distinguishing among the syndromes depends on both clinical signs and dermatohistopathologic findings.

Dog

- CEG: Siberian husky (76% of cases), cavalier King Charles spaniel; also reported in German shepherd dogs, boxers, labradors, and Irish setters.
- Usually less than 3 years of age; also reported in older dogs (>10 years).
- Males may be predisposed: 72% of cases.

CLINICAL FEATURES

Cat

- Eosinophilic plaque: alopecic, erythematous, erosive patches or well-demarcated, steep-walled plaques; usually occur in the inguinal, perineal, lateral thigh, ventral abdomen, and axillary regions; frequently moist or glistening; regional lymphadenopathy common; secondary infection common (Figures 23.1–23.3).
- Eosinophilic granuloma: five, occasionally overlapping, presentations:
    - Distinctly linear orientation (linear granuloma) along the caudal thigh (Figure 23.4)
    - Individual or coalescing plaques located anywhere on the body; ulcerated with a "cobblestone" or coarse pattern; white or yellow, possibly representing collagen degeneration (Figures 23.5–23.8).
    - Lip margin and chin swelling ("pouting") (Figure 23.9).
    - Footpad swelling, pain, and lameness (most common in cats under 2 years of age) (Figure 23.10).
    - Oral cavity ulcerations (especially on the tongue, palate, and palatine arches); cats with oral lesions may be dysphagic, have halitosis, and drool (Figure 23.11).

- Indolent ulcer (rodent ulcer): classically concave and indurated ulcerations with a granular, orange-yellow color, confined to the upper lips adjacent to the philtrum; secondary infection common (Figures 23.12, 23.13).
- Allergic miliary dermatitis: multiple brown/black crusted and erythematous papules; lesions more often palpated than visualized; may be associated with alopecia; usually associated with pruritus; frequently affects the dorsum (Figures 23.14, 23.15).

Dog

- CEG: ulcerated plaques and masses; dark or orange color; most often affects the tongue and palatine arches; also reported firm, nonpruritic, erythematous, alopecic, and often ulcerative, dermal nodules on the digits, face (nasal planum, cheek, eyelid), pinnae, flanks, and prepuce (Figures 23.16, 23.17).

DIFFERENTIAL DIAGNOSIS

- Includes the other diseases in the complex.
- Herpesvirus – dermatitis.
- FeLV- or FIV-associated dermatitis.
- Unresponsive lesions:
  - Pemphigus foliaceus
  - Dermatophytosis or deep fungal infection
  - Demodicosis
  - Bacterial folliculitis
  - Neoplasia (especially metastatic adenocarcinoma, squamous cell carcinoma, and cutaneous lymphosarcoma).
- CEG (dog): neoplasia (mast cell tumor, lymphoma), histiocytosis, infectious granuloma (bacterial/fungal), insect/arthropod bite reaction, foreign body reaction, aberrant parasite migration, trauma.

DIAGNOSTICS

- Cat and dog: CBC: mild to moderate eosinophilia; serum chemistries and urinalysis usually normal.
- Cat: FeLV and FIV serum testing.

Diagnostic Procedures

- Impression smears from lesions: large numbers of eosinophils (Figure 23.18); bacteria commonly found with eosinophilic plaques and indolent ulcers.
- Insect hypersensitivity: parasite control (especially flea) to assist in excluding flea or mosquito bite hypersensitivity.
- Cutaneous adverse reaction to food: restricted-ingredient food trial: challenge to induce development of new lesions.

- Atopy: intradermal testing (preferred) or serum testing followed by allergen-specific immunotherapy.
- Dermatohistopathologic diagnosis: required for definitive diagnosis and distinguishing the EGC syndromes:
  - Eosinophilic plaque: severe epidermal and follicular spongiosis and mucinosis with eosinophilic exocytosis; intense perivascular to diffuse dermal eosinophilic infiltrate; eroded or ulcerated epidermis
  - Eosinophilic granuloma: epidermal acanthosis with scattered apoptotic keratinocytes; distinct foci of eosinophilic degranulation and collagen degeneration ("flame figures"); nodular to diffuse granulomatous inflammation; eosinophilic and giant cell infiltrate
  - Indolent ulcer: severe ulceration of the epidermis or mucosa with fibrosing dermatitis and neutrophilic inflammation; significant eosinophilic infiltration unusual
  - Allergic miliary dermatitis: discrete foci of epidermal erosion and necrosis with brightly eosinophilic crusts; dermal perivascular to interstitial eosinophil-rich infiltrate.
- CEG (dog): foci of palisading granulomas and flame figures surrounding collagen fibers; eosinophilic infiltrate mixed with multinucleated giant cells, macrophages, reactive mast cells, plasma cells, and lymphocytes.

THERAPEUTICS

General Considerations: Cats

- Adequate flea control measures paramount to manage a majority of cases.
- Outpatient unless severe oral disease prevents adequate fluid intake.
- Identify and eliminate offending allergen(s) before providing medical intervention.
- Allergen-specific immunotherapy in cats with atopic dermatitis; successful in a majority of cases; preferable to long-term corticosteroid administration.
- Deter patient from damaging lesions by excessive grooming with behavior modification techniques and/or distraction.

General Considerations: Dogs

- Individual lesions may be surgically excised or ablated via CO_2 laser if being mechanically traumatized and medically unresponsive.

Drugs of Choice

- Eosinophilic plaque and indolent ulcer: may improve with antibiotics: trimethoprim-sulfadiazine 10–15 mg/kg PO BID, cephalexin 22 mg/kg PO BID, amoxicillin trihydrate-clavulanate 12.5 mg/kg PO BID, or clindamycin 5.5 mg/kg PO BID.

- Injectable methylprednisolone: 20 mg/cat by subcutaneous route; repeat in 2 weeks (if needed); tachyphylaxis common with repeated administration; not advised for long-term therapy; increased risk for diabetes mellitus with repeated administration.
- Prednisolone (2–4 mg/kg PO), dexamethasone (0.1–0.2 mg/kg PO) or triamcinolone (0.1–0.2 mg/kg PO); initial daily dosage tapered to minimal dose and frequency required to control lesions; tachyphylaxis may occur and may be specific to the drug administered.
- Cyclosporine: 7.5 mg/kg PO initial daily dosage tapered to minimal dose and frequency required to control lesions.
- Topical: fluocinolone/DMSO (Synotic lotion) to individual lesions; not practical and/or may cause systemic effects in patients with large numbers of lesions.

Alternate Drugs

- Chlorambucil: 0.1–0.2 mg/kg PO q48h to q72h.
- Indolent ulcer: alpha-interferon: 300–1000 IU PO q24h in cycles of 7 days on, 7 days off; limited success; side effects rare; no specific treatment monitoring required.
- Doxycycline: 5–10 mg/kg PO q24h.
- Megestrol acetate: 2.5–5 mg PO every 2–7 days; significant incidence of side effects (diabetes, mammary cancer, epidermal atrophy) preclude use in all but severe, recalcitrant cases (Figure 23.19).

CEG (dog)

- Oral prednisolone: 0.5–2.2 mg/kg PO q24h initially; then taper gradually (78% of cases responsive to corticosteroids as a sole therapeutic).
- Intralesional corticosteroids: 5 mg/lesion methylprednisolone.
- Chlorambucil: 0.1–0.2 mg/kg PO q24h to q48h initial dosage.
- Azathioprine: 1 mg/kg PO q24hrto q48h initial dosage.
- Cyclosporine: 5 mg/kg PO BID to q24h initial dosage.
- Cessation of therapy without recurrence is common.
- Surgical excision of appropriate lesions/carbon dioxide (CO_2) laser ablation of the site.

COMMENTS

Patient Monitoring

- Treatment monitoring is based on medications prescribed (e.g., CBC, serum chemistry profile, and urinalysis with culture recommended frequently during treatment induction and then every 6–12 months for patients on chronic immunomodulatory therapy).
- Cats: patients must be FeLV/FIV negative; initial exposure to toxoplasmosis during treatment with cyclosporine may be fatal.

Expected Course and Prognosis

- Lesions should resolve permanently if a primary cause can be identified and controlled.
- Most lesions wax and wane, with or without therapy; an unpredictable schedule of recurrence should be anticipated.
- Drug dosages should be tapered to the lowest possible level (or discontinued, if possible) once the lesions have resolved.
- Lesions in cats with the inheritable disease may resolve spontaneously after several months to years.
- CEG (dog): lesions may be recalcitrant to medical intervention and require excision.

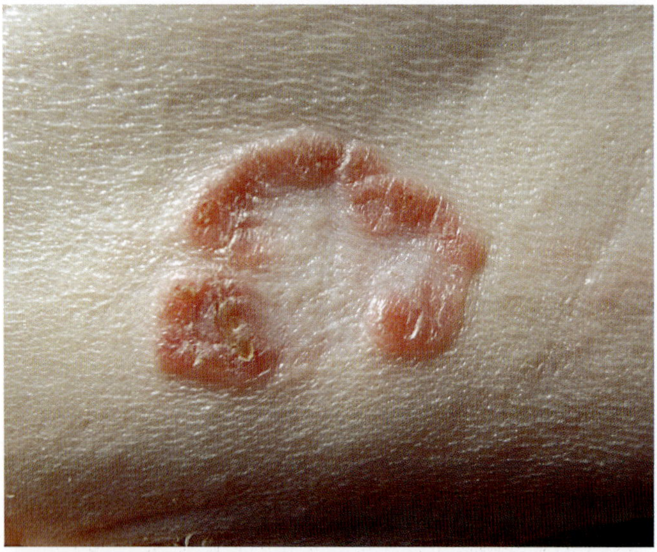

■ **Fig. 23.1.** Well-demarcated, erosive, and coalescing eosinophilic plaques on the ventral abdomen of a 6-year-old male-castrate sphynx cat.

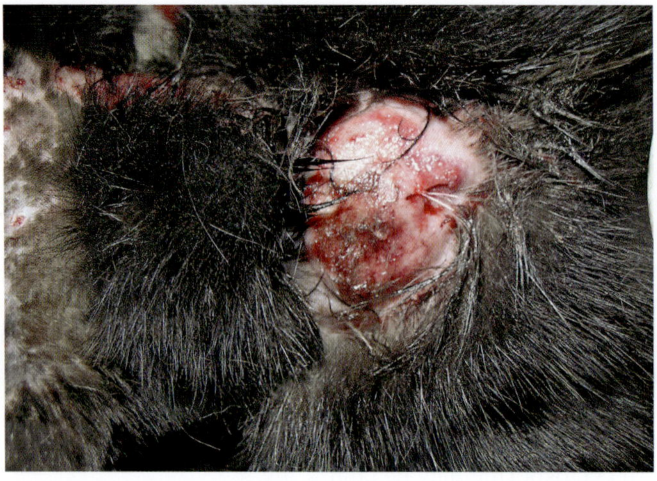

■ **Fig. 23.2.** Eosinophilic plaque on the neck of a 4-year-old DSH secondary to food allergy.

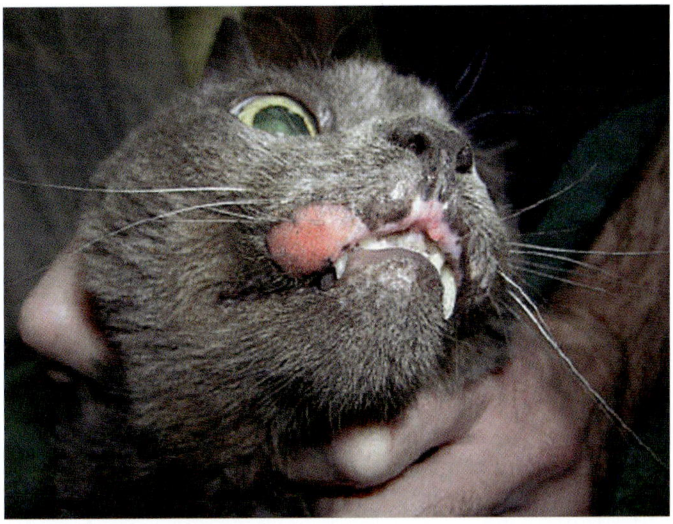

■ **Fig. 23.3.** Large erythematous eosinophilic plaque at the lip margin.

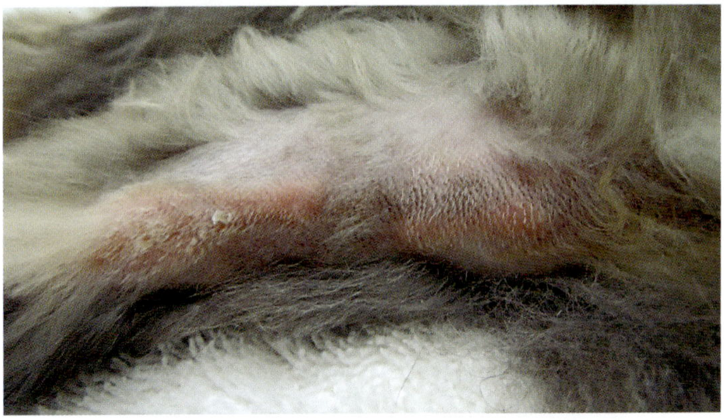

■ **Fig. 23.4.** Linear granuloma on the caudal thigh of a 2-year-old DLH.

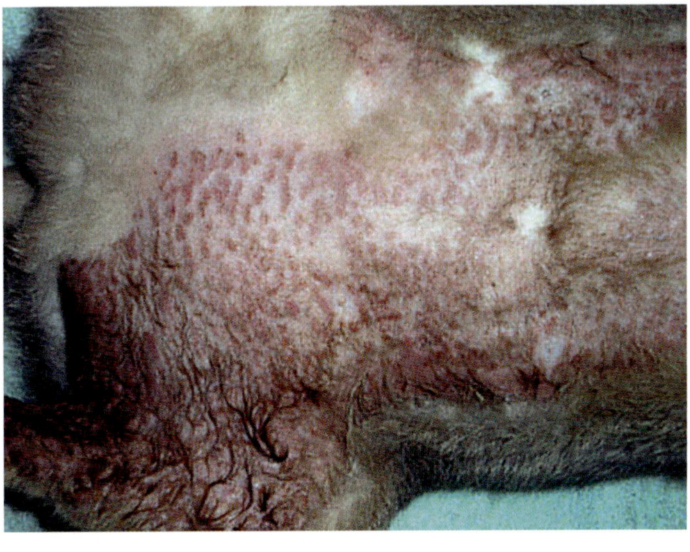

■ **Fig. 23.5.** Eosinophilic granuloma. Coalescing punctate erythematous plaques.

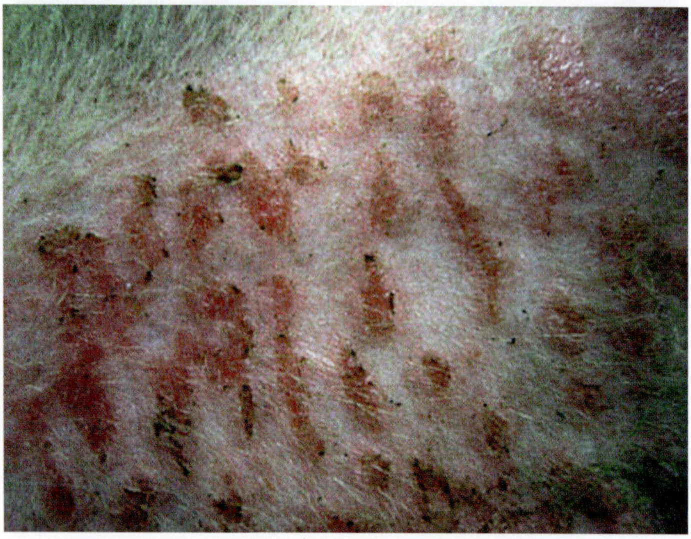

■ **Fig. 23.6.** Eosinophilic granuloma affecting the patient in Figure 23.5; plaques produce a "cobblestone" appearance.

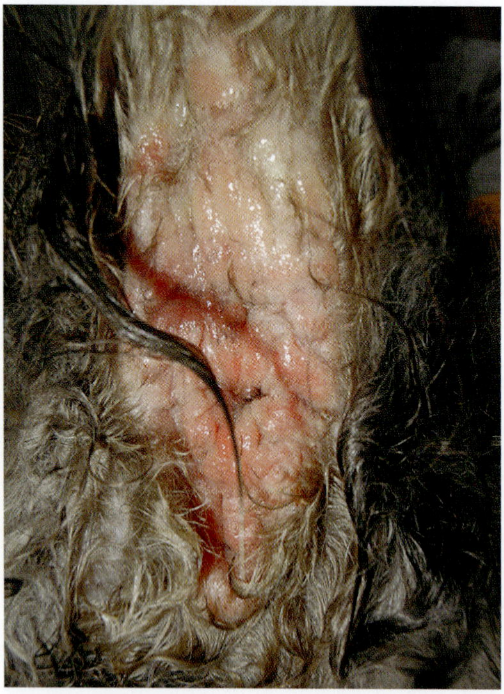

■ **Fig. 23.7.** Eroded and exudative perianal lesions in an 18-year-old female-spayed DSH with eosinophilic granuloma.

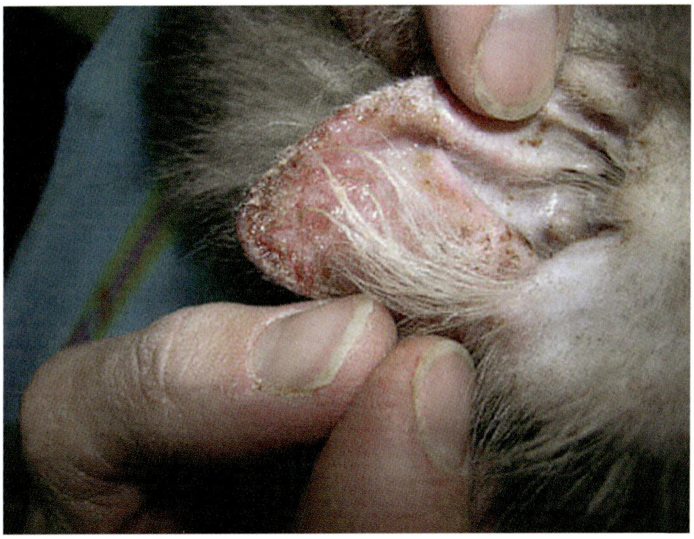

■ **Fig. 23.8.** Eosinophilic granuloma with exudation on the pinnal margin.

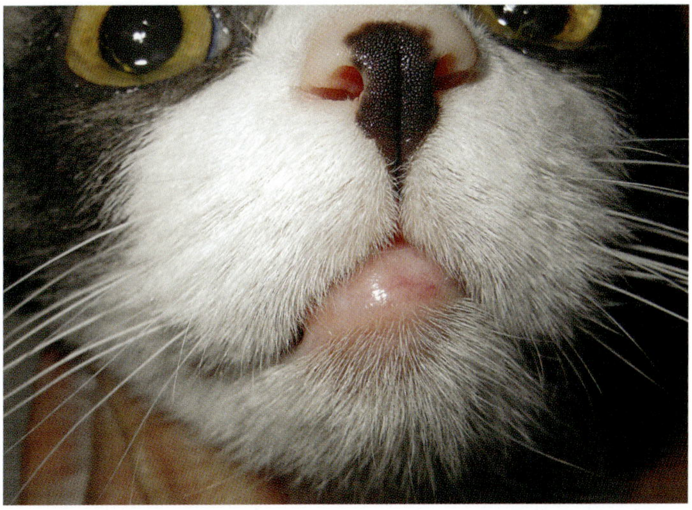

■ **Fig. 23.9.** Swollen rostral chin ("pouting") form of eosinophilic granuloma.

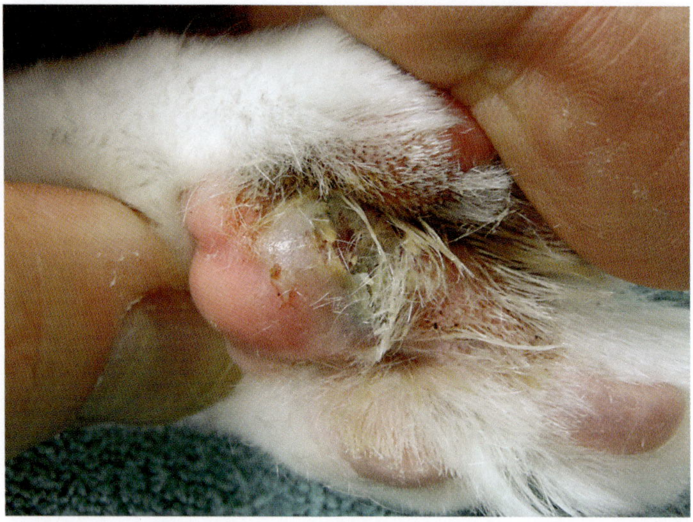

■ **Fig. 23.10.** Eosinophilic granuloma at margin of metacarpal pad in a 5-year-old Norwegian forest cat.

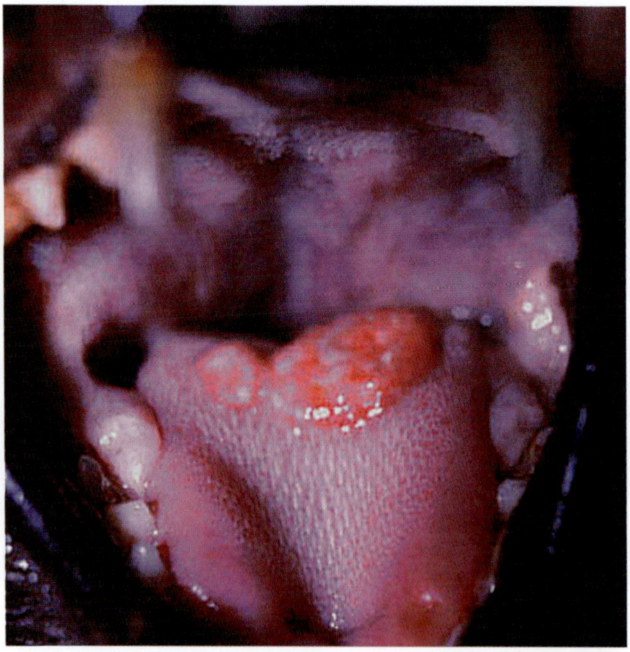

■ **Fig. 23.11.** Eroded and well-demarcated eosinophilic granuloma on the tongue.

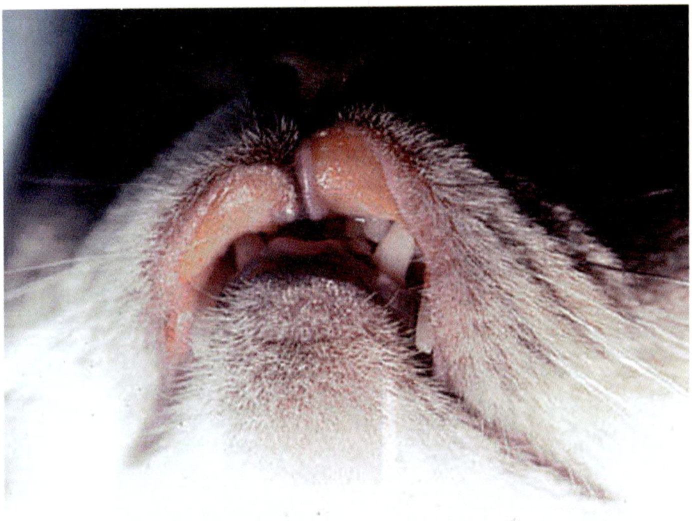

■ **Fig. 23.12.** Indolent ulcer causing swelling of the upper lips with erosions and an "orange" color to tissues.

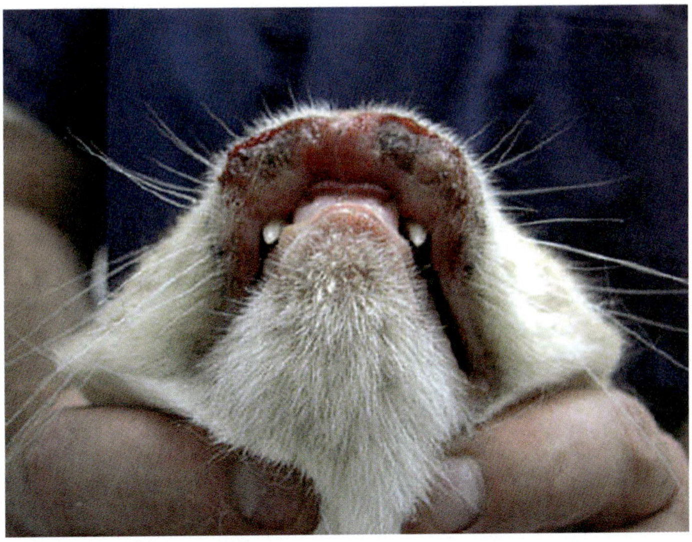

■ **Fig. 23.13.** Indolent ulcer-scabbed surface as a result of self-trauma.

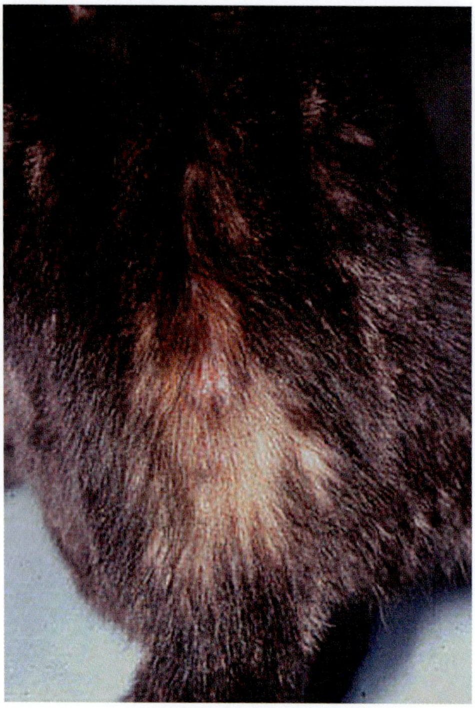

■ **Fig. 23.14.** Allergic miliary dermatitis on dorsal lumbosacral region.

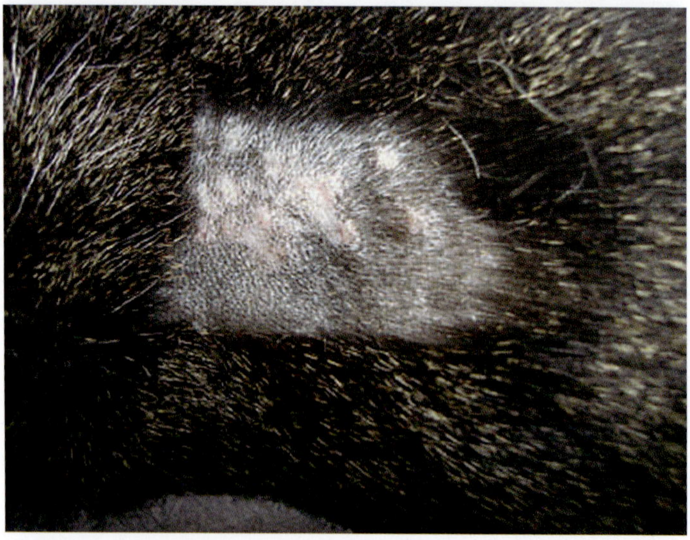

■ **Fig. 23.15.** Allergic miliary dermatitis with multiple crusted papules on the dorsum.

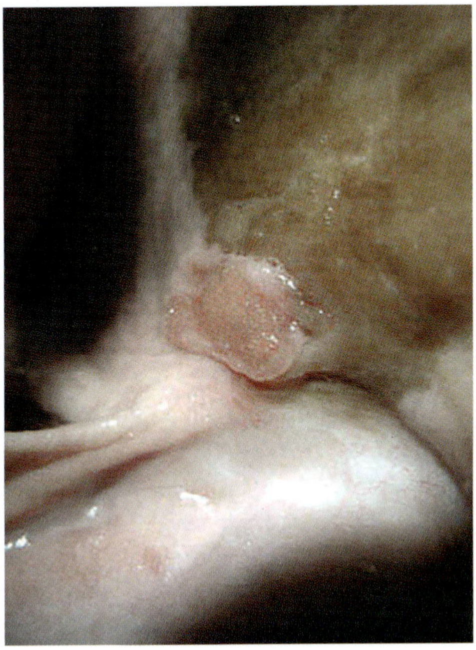

■ **Fig. 23.16.** Canine eosinophilic granuloma plaque in caudal pharynx.

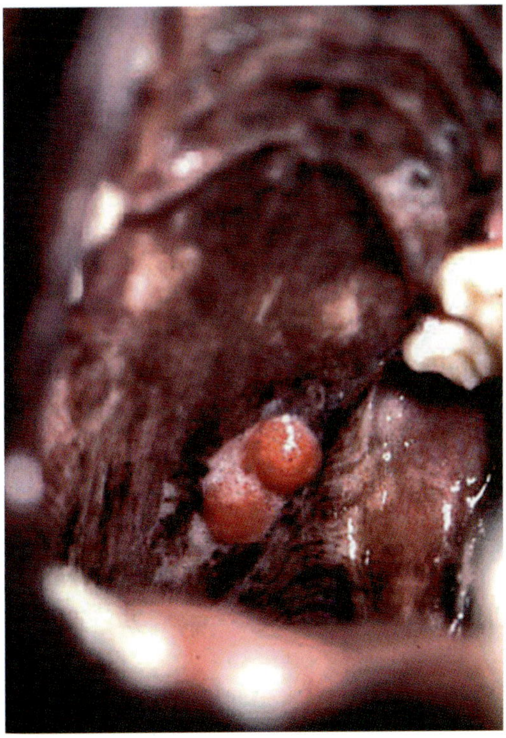

■ **Fig. 23.17.** Canine eosinophilic granuloma, dog. Erythematous plaques on caudal pharynx.

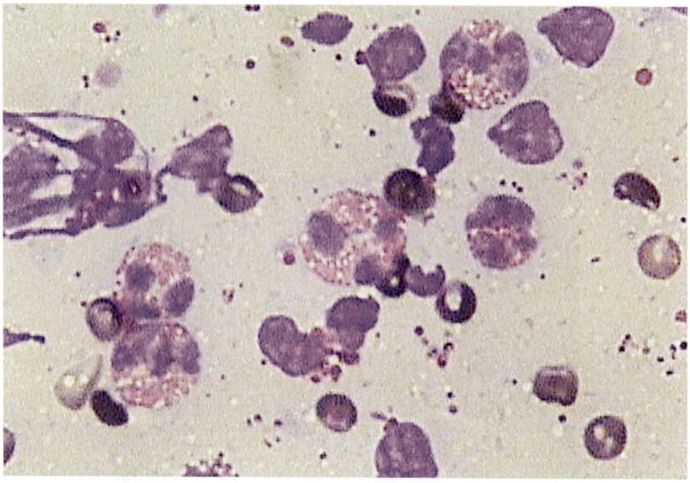

■ **Fig. 23.18.** Exudate from eosinophilic plaque demonstrating large numbers of eosinophils (cells with multiple red intracellular granules), 400×.

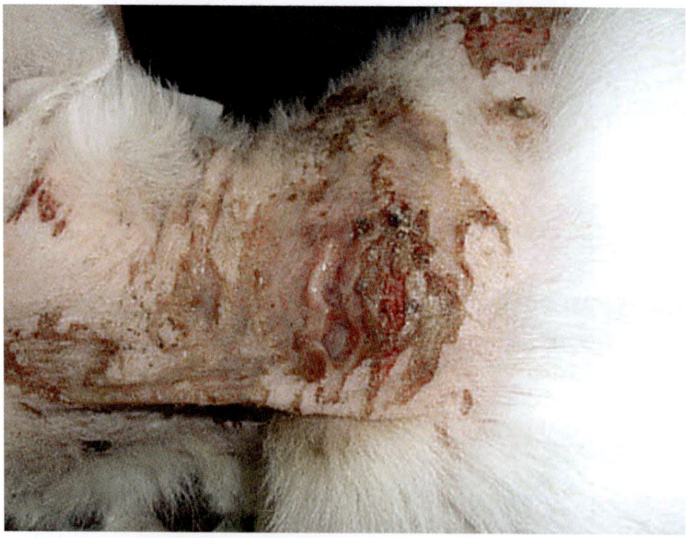

■ **Fig. 23.19.** Severe epidermal atrophy, tearing, and secondary infection from administration of megestrol acetate and application of a topical corticosteroid.

chapter **24**

Epitheliotropic (Cutaneous) Lymphoma

DEFINITION/OVERVIEW

- Cutaneous T-cell lymphoma (CTCL), both epitheliotropic and nonepitheliotrophic, is an uncommon cutaneous neoplasia affecting many species, including dogs and cats.
- Heterogeneous group of diseases with a prevalence of less than 1% of skin tumors in dogs.
- The majority of CTCL cases are epitheliotropic (CEL) characterized by infiltration of the epidermis and adnexal structures with malignant T cells.

ETIOLOGY/PATHOPHYSIOLOGY

- Cutaneous nonepitheliotrophic lymphoma (CnEL): caused by either B cells or T cells; more often T cell in cats.
- Most often associated with $CD3^+$ lymphocytes.
- CnEL: large cell lymphoma characterized by infiltration of the dermis and subcutis with heterogeneous groups of malignant cells; may be associated with FeLV in cats.
- Cutaneous epitheliotropic lymphoma, or "classic" MF (mycosis fungoides): most common T cell lymphoma in dogs.
- Caused by epitheliotropic gamma delta T cells in 70% of cases (100% in pagetoid form).
- Most often associated with $CD4^-/CD8^+$ cytotoxic T cells: differs from disease of human beings (predominantly $CD4^+/CD8^-$ helper T cells).
- COX-2 is not expressed by neoplastic infiltrates in CEL; differs from disease in human beings (significant expression of COX-2 by neoplastic lymphocytes).
- In one study, dogs with atopic dermatitis were at 12 times higher risk of developing CEL than dogs without atopic dermatitis.
- Allergic skin disease producing chronic T cell activation and proliferation leading to clonal expansion of neoplastic cells may be a cause; initial lesions often develop in areas associated with atopic dermatitis.
- Peripheral lymphocytes with skin-homing receptors may be preferentially sequestered in skin lesions.
- Spread of malignant cells to lymph nodes and organs occurs in the late tumor stage.

Blackwell's Five-Minute Veterinary Consult Clinical Companion: Small Animal Dermatology, Third Edition.
Karen Helton Rhodes and Alexander H. Werner.

- Sézary syndrome: rare form of CEL; cutaneous lesions: invasion of peripheral lymph nodes by neoplastic lymphocytes; leukemia develops simultaneously.
- Pagetoid reticulosis: rare form of CEL; lymphoid infiltrate confined to the epidermis and adnexal structures in the early stages of the disease and extends to the dermis in the late stages.

SIGNALMENT/HISTORY

- CnEL: older dogs and cats.
- CEL:
  - Dogs: age range 6–14 years; mean 8.6 years
  - Cats: age range 12–17 years
  - No apparent breed or sex predilection.

Historical Findings

- CnEL can be acute and progress rapidly.
- CEL:
  - Chronic skin disease: months before diagnosis
  - Mimics other inflammatory dermatoses
  - Pruritus is uncommon except in Sézary syndrome (severe)
  - Initial findings include erythema, scaling, depigmentation, alopecia, and crusting
  - Lesions commonly begin in areas associated with allergic conditions, mucocutaneous junctions, and oral cavity
  - Progression to nodular and tumor stages may be rapid; clinical course typically range 3 months to 4 years.

CLINICAL FEATURES

- CnEL:
  - Firm, dermal or subcutaneous nodules
  - Rarely affects the mucous membranes
  - Usually erythematous to purpuric irregular nodules to plaques (Figures 24.1–24.3)
  - Most often multicentric with rapid progression.
- CEL: overlap of four clinical categories of presentation:
  - Exfoliative erythroderma: generalized erythema, scaling, depigmentation, alopecia; lesions begin predominantly on the body; often pleomorphic and initially static to slowly progressive (Figures 24.4–24.6)
  - Mucocutaneous: erythema, erosion, and ulceration affecting facial mucocutaneous junctions; depigmentation may be extensive, leading to leukoderma; single, multiple, and bilaterally symmetrical patches appear; additional mucocutaneous junctions may be affected (Figure 24.7)

- Tumoral: solitary or multiple erythematous plaques, nodules, and masses; lesions often scaly or crusted, may ulcerate; lesions may rarely cycle (Figures 24.8, 24.9)
- Oral cavity ulceration: severe ulceration of gingiva, palate, and/or tongue (Figures 24.10, 24.11):
  - Majority of lesions disseminated on the body (83.3%), localized on the head (63%), footpads (26.6%), pruritus (40%), or lymph nodes (20%) (Figures 24.12–24.14)
  - Depigmentation caused by displacement and/or damage of melanocytes
  - Lesions throughout the skin; marked tendency for involvement of mucocutaneous junctions (lip, eyelids, nasal planum, anorectal junction, or vulva) or oral cavity (gingiva, palate, or tongue); lesions can be limited to the mucocutaneous junctions or oral mucosa.

- Exfoliative erythroderma; progression to the tumor stage is very rapid in dogs compared to human beings.
- Mucocutaneous and oral mucosa forms merge with chronicity.
- Rarely the nodular form develops without a preexisting patch or plaque stage (*d'emblee* form).
- Nodular stage may occasionally progress to a disseminated form with lymph node involvement, leukemia, and (rarely) other organs.
- Sézary syndrome: rare; leukemic variant with simultaneous development of cutaneous lesions, invasion of peripheral lymph nodes by neoplastic lymphocytes, and circulating tumor cells; generalized and severe erythroderma, scaling, alopecia, and severe pruritus reported; visceral involvement causes systemic illness.
- Pagetoid reticulosis: rare; neoplastic lymphocytic infiltrate is confined to the epidermis and adnexal structures in the early stages of the disease and extends to the dermis in the late stages; exfoliative erythroderma without nodules and masses; mucocutaneous junctions and footpads predominantly affected; exclusively gamma delta T cells (Figure 24.15).

DIFFERENTIAL DIAGNOSIS

- Dermatophytosis
- Demodicosis
- Dermatoses, i.e., Feline thymoma-associated exfoliative dermatoses
- Allergic dermatitis
- Ectoparasitism (especially sarcoptid mites)
- Cutaneous forms of lupus erythematosus
- Erythema multiforme
- Pemphigus vulgaris
- Bullous pemphigoid
- Vasculitis
- Nonneoplastic chronic stomatitis (infectious)
- Other cutaneous neoplasia: histiocytoma, cutaneous histiocytosis, mass cell tumor

DIAGNOSTICS

- Laboratory abnormalities: vary depending on the stage and form of cutaneous T cell lymphoma, and whether disease has disseminated.
- Sézary cells: small (8–20 μm) neoplastic lymphocytes with convoluted nucleus and cerebriform appearance are present in peripheral blood of patients with Sézary syndrome.
- Flow cytometry for detection of T cell lineages in blood.
- Generally unremarkable if only the skin or mucosa is affected.
- Radiographs and ultrasound: not commonly used in the early stages; imaging is eventually necessary to confirm systemic disease and/or for tumor staging.

Diagnostic Procedures

- Skin scrapings and fungal culture: rule out demodicosis and dermatophytosis, if applicable.
- Cytology: increased numbers of atypical lymphocytes with large and infolded nuclei (Figure 24.16).
- Skin biopsy: definitive diagnosis; sample multiple different-appearing lesions, avoid eroded/ulcerated and infected lesions.

Pathologic Findings

- CnEL:
    - Sheets of neoplastic lymphocytes produce diffuse and dense invasion of the dermis and subcutaneous tissues
    - Infiltration of the epidermis is lacking.
- CEL:
    - Hallmark finding: trophism of neoplastic cells for the epithelium (epidermal and mucosal)
    - Infiltrate of neoplastic lymphocytes: into epidermis and epithelium of hair follicles and adnexal structures; distributed diffusely or clustered together to form discrete Pautrier microaggregates within the epithelium
    - Follicular and adnexal structures can be obliterated by infiltrate
    - Keratinocyte apoptosis may be mild to marked
    - Interface dermatitis mimics inflammatory processes in early stages; CEL may be difficult to distinguish from reactive lymphocytic inflammation; reactive lymphocytes migrate throughout the epidermis and are associated with spongiosis whereas neoplastic lymphocytes tend to accumulate in the lower portion of the epidermis
    - Dermal-epidermal junction becomes obscured by neoplastic lymphocytes in later stages
    - Tumor cells are typically larger than normal with infolded nuclei and increased cytoplasm

- Dermal infiltrate: polymorphous; in the patch and plaque stages, limited to the superficial dermis; in the nodular stage, extends to the deep dermis and subcutis
- Epitheliotrophism of neoplastic lymphocytes: usually remains prominent throughout all stages
- Immunohistochemistry for CD3 expression and T cell antigen receptor gene rearrangement analysis staining may be required to differentiate CEL from reactive cutaneous histiocytosis.

THERAPEUTICS

Drugs of Choice

- CnEL:
  - Cyclophosphamide-doxorubicin-vincristine-prednisolone (CHOP) protocols
  - L-asparaginase-CHOP protocols
  - Vincristine-cyclophosphamide-prednisolone (COP) protocols
  - Vinblastine
  - Chlorambucil-prednisolone
  - Lomustine (CCNU)
  - Consultation with a veterinary oncologist for treatment options recommended.
- CEL:
  - Lomustine (CCNU): several studies published in the veterinary literature indicate an overall response rate of 80%, with complete remission achieved in about 25% of cases (60–70 mg/m^2 PO every 3–4 weeks for a mean of 3–5 treatments); myelosuppression and hepatoxicity (Figures 24.17, 24.18)
  - High-dose linoleic acid (e.g., sunflower oil): 3 mL/kg PO twice weekly demonstrated improvement in seven of 10 dogs for up to 2 years
  - Dacarbazine (1000 mg/m^2 intravenous over 4–8 h every 2–3 weeks) for three treatments; gastrointestinal toxicity; myelosuppression
  - CHOP protocols
  - Topical chemotherapy: mechlorethamine (nitrogen mustard) some success in managing early lesions but lack of long-term efficacy; carcinogenic potential for human beings
  - Corticosteroids: topical and/or systemic may result in symptomatic relief
  - Retinoids: isotretinoin (3 mg/kg PO q24h) or acitretin (2 mg/kg PO q24h) may be beneficial; cost can be a limiting factor; extreme teratogen; do not use in intact females because of severe and predictable teratogenicity and the extremely long withdrawal period; women of child-bearing age should not handle this medication
  - Imiquimod: a topical immunomodulator with antineoplastic and antiviral effects; may be useful for localized disease; no published reports in veterinary literature

- VDC-1101: double prodrug of PMEG; administered with prednisone in 12 dogs demonstrated efficacy to induce remission or to reduce lesions
- Consultation with a veterinary oncologist or dermatologist for treatment options recommended.

COMMENTS

- Prognosis for CnEL: remission may be achieved in 80% of dogs; median survival time depends on type/form of lymphoma; range 2 months to years.
- Prognosis for CEL: guarded to grave; cure is extremely unlikely unless a solitary, early lesion can be surgically excised: median survival time for dogs depends on stage of disease at diagnosis, therapeutic choice, and response to therapy; varies from weeks to longer than 18 months; dogs and cats may live for longer than 2 years after diagnosis (rarely).
- The goal is to maintain a good quality of life for as long as possible.
- Radiation therapy: total skin electron beam therapy (TSEBT) or orthovoltage radiation is well tolerated and may be beneficial in some cases.
- Death is usually the result of euthanasia.

Synonyms

- Lymphoma, epidermotropic
- Mycosis fungoides

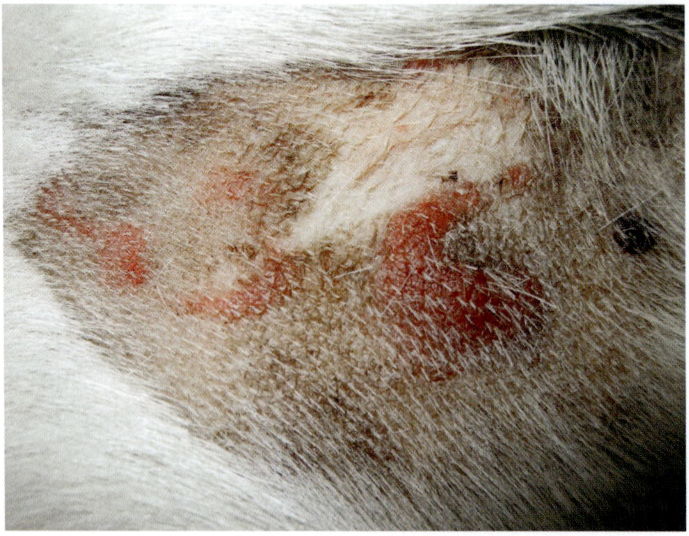

Fig. 24.1. Multiple irregular to arciform, erythematous to purpuric nodules, characteristic of CnEL, in a 14-year-old female-spayed Jack Russell terrier.

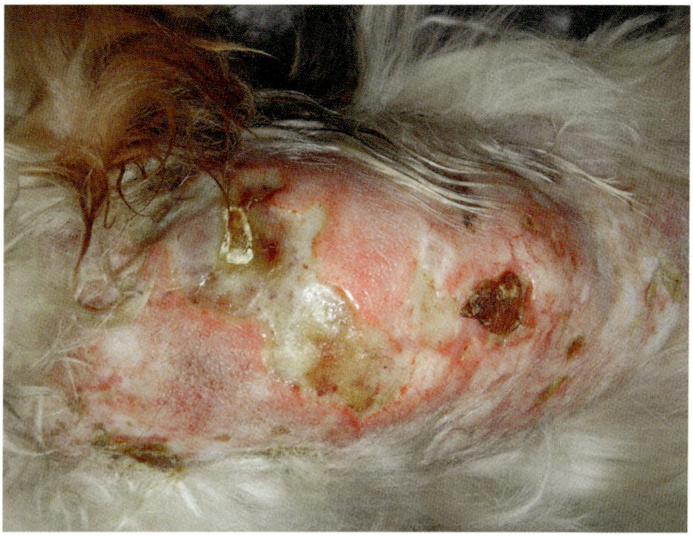

■ **Fig. 24.2.** Firm, inflamed, and necrotic plaques on the sternum of a 9-year-old female-spayed cavalier King Charles spaniel with large cell CnEL.

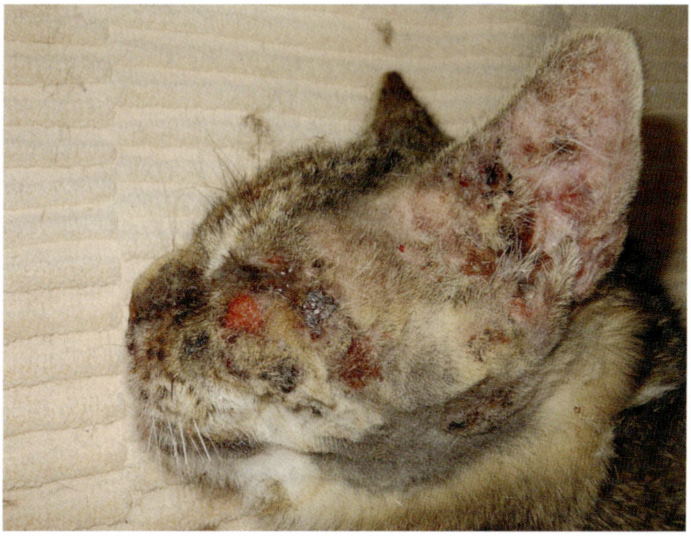

■ **Fig. 24.3.** Multiple purpuric and eroded plaques in a 12-year-old female-spayed DSH with CnEL. Lesions were generalized and progressed rapidly.

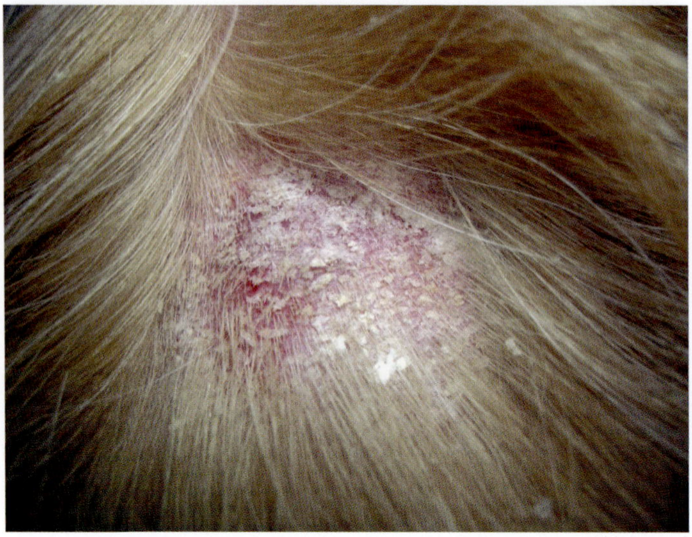

■ **Fig. 24.4.** Exfoliative erythroderma in a 14-year-old female-spayed Shetland sheepdog. There was generalized intense erythema as seen on the dorsum of the body in this image.

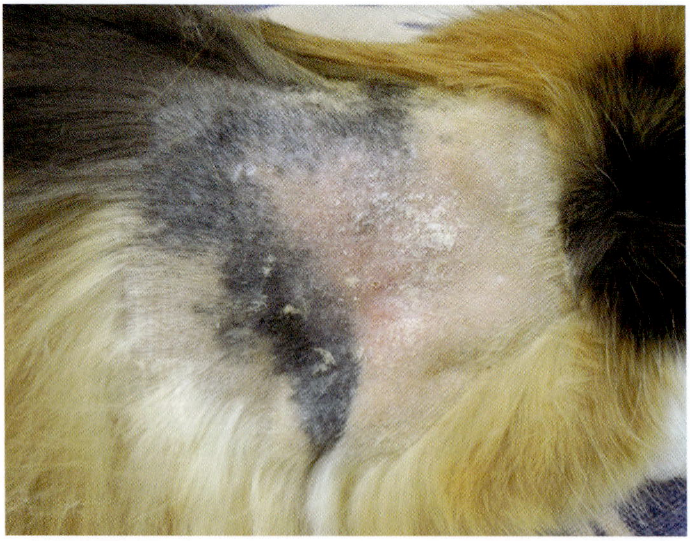

■ **Fig. 24.5.** Exfoliative and erythematous patch of CEL in a 14-year-old female-spayed DSH. Multiple patches were present and initially diagnosed as dermatophytosis.

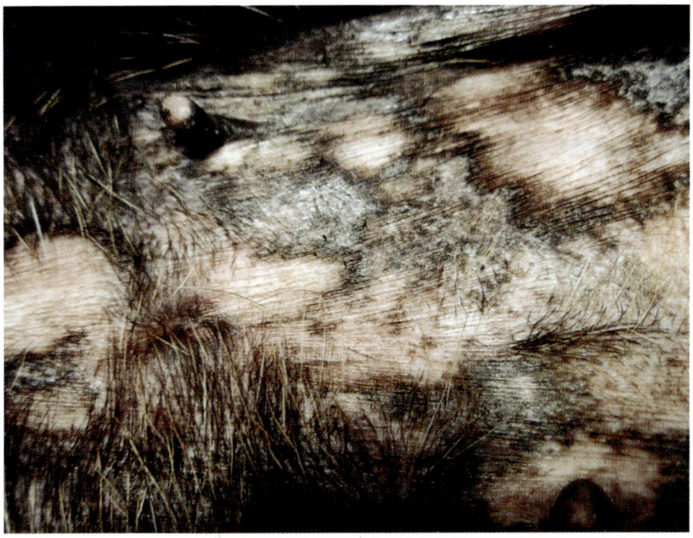

■ **Fig. 24.6.** Reticulated pattern of depigmentation and erythema on the ventral abdomen of an 11-year-old female-spayed rottweiler. These lesions are characteristic of CEL.

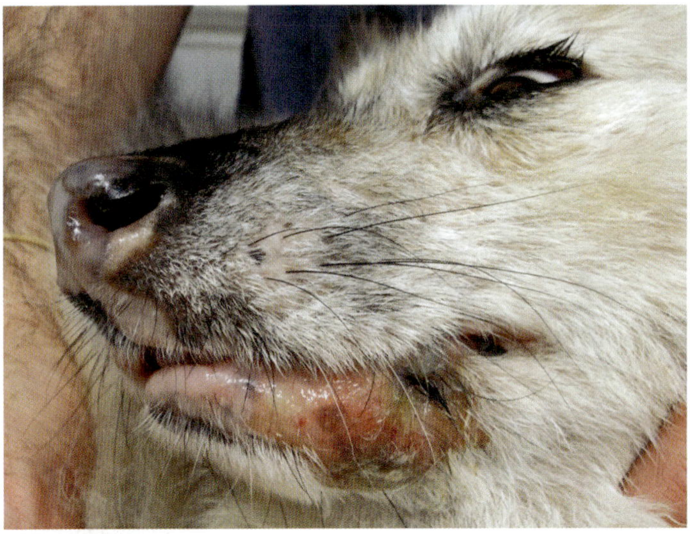

■ **Fig. 24.7.** Swelling, depigmentation, and erythema with the mucocutaneous presentation of CEL in a 10-year-old female-spayed corgi mix.

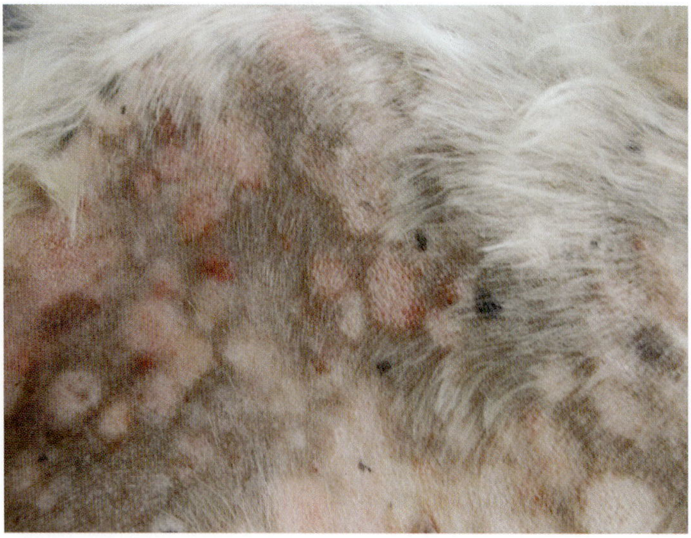

■ **Fig. 24.8.** Multiple erythematous and coalescing plaques on the ventrum of a 2-year-old male-castrate terrier with CEL. Lesions were palpably thickened.

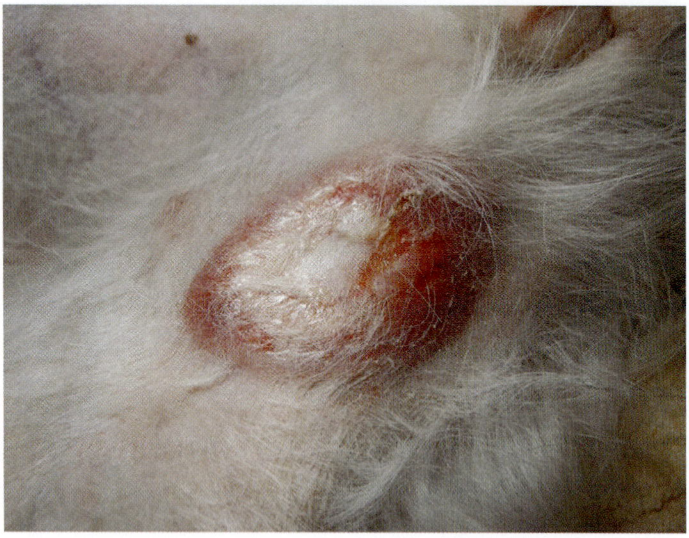

■ **Fig. 24.9.** Solitary tumor of CEL in a 10-year-old female-spayed Maltese.

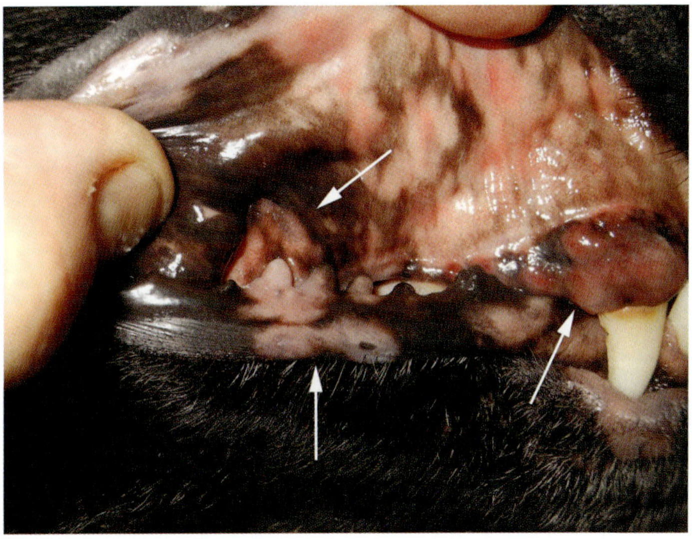

■ **Fig. 24.10.** Oral lesions of CEL in a 6-year-old female-spayed Labrador retriever. Arrows note areas of depigmentation, progressing to erosions and plaques of neoplastic tissue on the lip margins and gingiva.

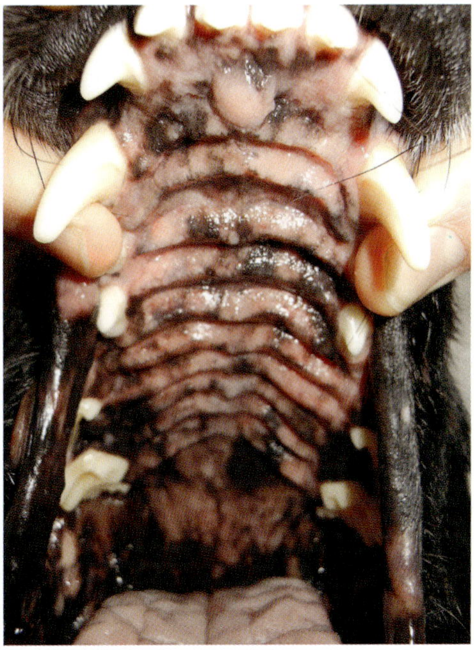

■ **Fig. 24.11.** Depigmented and eroded lesions on the hard palate of the patient in Figure 24.10. Small erosions are also present on the tongue.

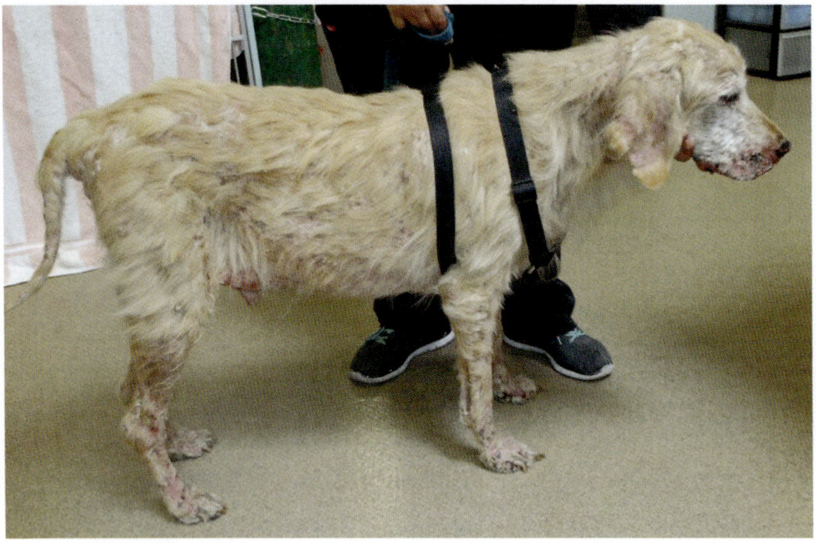

■ **Fig. 24.12.** Generalized and severe scales, crusts, and erythroderma of CEL in a 9-year-old male-castrate golden retriever.

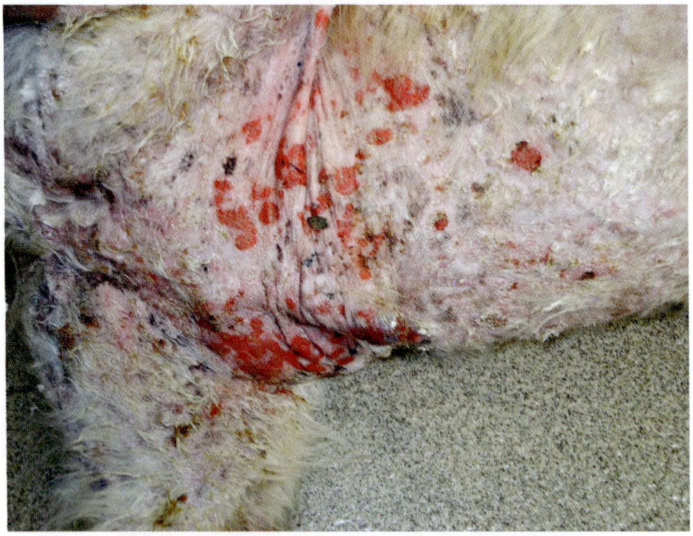

■ **Fig. 24.13.** Lesions on the ventrum of the patient in Figure 24.12. With progression, neoplastic infiltration has produced significant erosions with exudation.

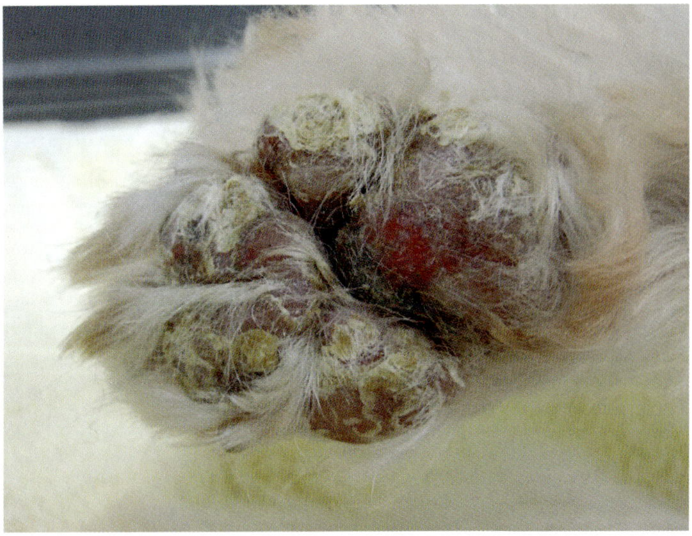

■ **Fig. 24.14.** Footpad lesions of CEL with swelling, depigmentation, and crusts in a 9-year-old female-spayed Maltese.

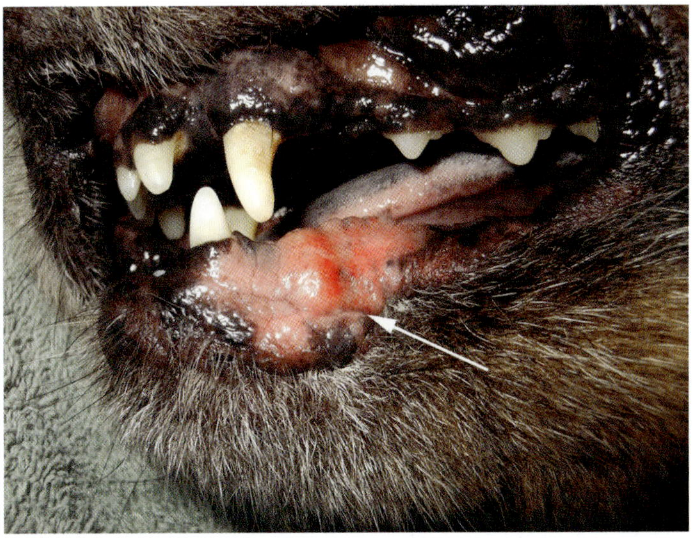

■ **Fig. 24.15.** Pagetoid reticulosis lesion in a 14-year-old female-spayed chow mix. A plaque of depigmentation and thickening (*arrow*) on the lip margin was a solitary lesion and was successfully removed by wide surgical resection.

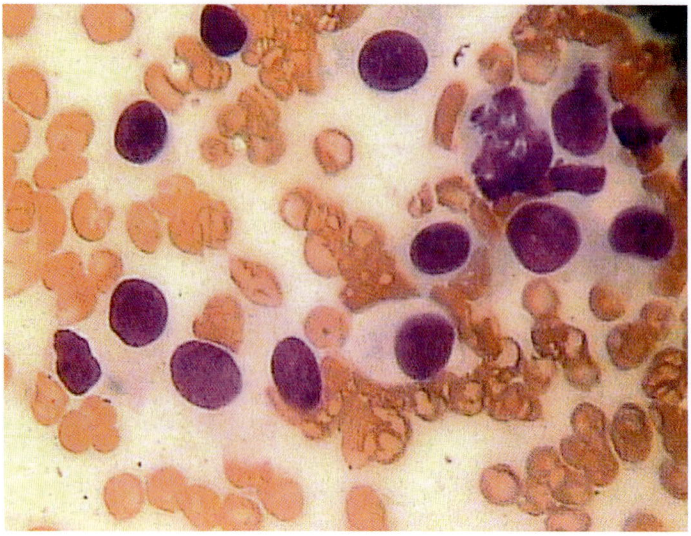

■ **Fig. 24.16.** Increased numbers of large, atypical lymphocytes in a touch-prep from tissue in a patient with CEL.

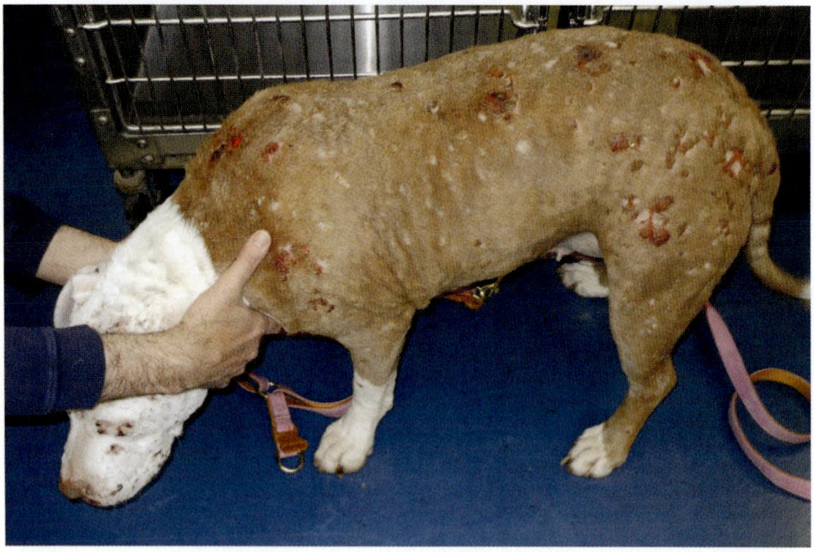

■ **Fig. 24.17.** CEL in a 4-year-old female-spayed pit bull mix prior to treatment with lomustine.

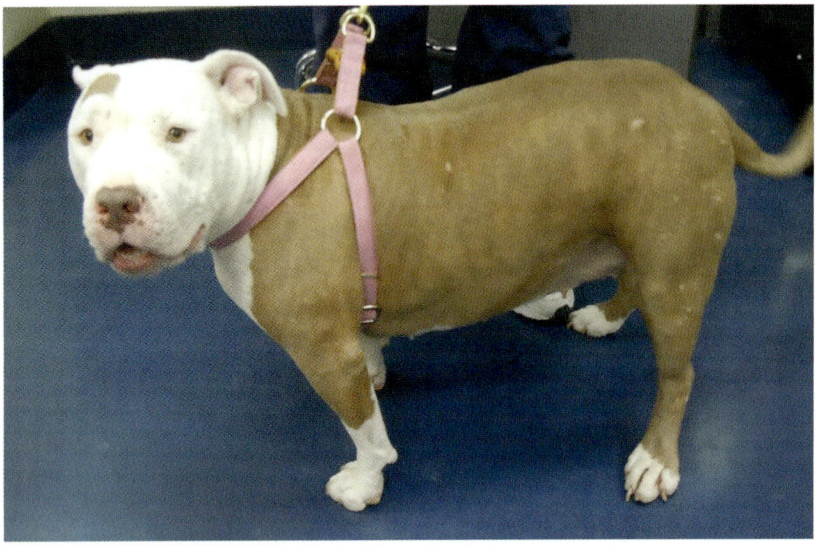

Fig. 24.18. Patient in Figure 24.17 after 8 months of therapy. A 2-year remission was achieved prior to recurrence of treatment-nonresponsive disease.

chapter 25

Histiocytic Proliferative Disorders

DEFINITION/OVERVIEW

- Disorders resulting from proliferation of cells from the monocyte/macrophage lineage, Langerhans cells of the skin and dendritic cells ("antigen-presenting cells" of the lymph nodes, thymus, and spleen).
- Histiocytic proliferative disorders include both neoplastic and nonneoplastic (reactive inflammatory granulomatous disorders secondary to dysregulation of proliferation) disorders.
- Includes cutaneous histiocytoma, reactive histiocytosis (reactive cutaneous histiocytosis, reactive systemic histiocytosis), histiocytic sarcoma (localized histiocytic sarcoma, disseminated histiocytic sarcoma, malignant histiocytosis), and malignant fibrous histiocytoma.
- Organ systems affected include skin, hemic/lymphatic, nervous, ophthalmic, and respiratory.
- Reactive histiocytoses occur in dogs; feline progressive histiocytosis is reported.

ETIOLOGY/PATHOPHYSIOLOGY

- Cutaneous histiocytoma:
  - Common benign neoplasm of the dog
  - Considered reactive hyperplasia rather than true neoplasm
  - Langerhans cell is the proliferating cell
  - Categorized as an epidermotropic Langerhans cell histiocytosis.
- Reactive cutaneous histiocytosis:
  - Dysregulation of dendritic "antigen-presenting" cells producing a benign reactive perivascular proliferation
  - Single or multiple nodules
  - Infiltration of skin and subcutaneous tissue
  - May wax and wane over years.

Blackwell's Five-Minute Veterinary Consult Clinical Companion: Small Animal Dermatology, Third Edition.
Karen Helton Rhodes and Alexander H. Werner.

- Reactive systemic histiocytosis:
  - Dysregulation of dendritic "antigen-presenting" cells producing a reactive perivascular proliferation
  - Slowly progressive disease.
- Familial disease of Bernese mountain dogs:
  - Polygenic mode of inheritance
  - Heritability of 0.298; accounts for up to 25% of all tumors in this breed
  - Characterized by multiple cutaneous, ocular, and nasal mucosa nodules
  - Other organ systems (lung, spleen, liver, bone marrow) may also be affected.
- Histiocytic sarcoma (localized histiocytic sarcoma, disseminated histiocytic sarcoma, malignant histiocytosis):
  - Malignant transformation of dendritic cells
  - Rapidly progressive, multisystem disease
  - Disease affects the skin (nodules) and subcutis, spleen, lymph nodes, lung, bone marrow
  - Usually leads to death in a matter of weeks.
- Malignant fibrous histiocytoma:
  - Uncommon in cats; rare in dogs
  - Solitary, firm, poorly circumscribed soft tissue sarcomas.

SIGNALMENT/HISTORY

- Cutaneous histiocytoma:
  - Young dogs; most under 3 years of age
  - Breeds predisposed: bull terrier, Boston terrier, boxer, Shetland sheepdog, dachshund, cocker spaniel, Great Dane.
- Reactive cutaneous histiocytosis:
  - Middle-aged to older dogs; range 2–13 years
  - Possible male predisposition
  - Breeds predisposed: Bernese mountain dog, beagle, collie, golden retriever, and Shetland sheepdog.
- Reactive systemic histiocytosis:
  - Young adult to middle-aged dogs; mean age at onset 4 years
  - Male predisposition
  - Polygenic mode of inheritance in Bernese mountain dog
  - Breeds predisposed: rottweiler, basset hound, Irish wolfhound, golden retriever, and Labrador retriever.
- Histiocytic sarcoma complex:
  - Older male dogs; mean age at onset 7 years
  - Most common in Bernese mountain dog
  - Breeds predisposed: Labrador retriever, rottweiler, golden retriever, and flat-coated retriever.
- Malignant fibrous histiocytoma:
  - Uncommon (cats); rare (dogs)
  - Middle-aged to older cats.

CLINICAL FEATURES

- Cutaneous histiocytoma:
  - Solitary cutaneous mass; may be multiple (<1% of cases) especially in the Chinese shar pei (Figure 25.1)
  - Dome-shaped, erythematous and alopecic nodule ("button cell tumor") (Figures 25.2, 25.3)
  - Usually less than 2 cm diameter
  - Predominantly develop on head, pinnae, limbs
  - Rapid development (days to few weeks)
  - Occasional regional lymph node involvement
  - Majority of cases spontaneously resolve within 3 months.
- Reactive cutaneous histiocytosis:
  - Multiple dermal and subcutaneous, erythematous nodules or plaques (Figure 25.4)
  - Nodules/plaques may be alopecic or ulcerated (Figure 25.5)
  - Nodules range in size from 1 to 5 cm
  - Not pruritic or painful
  - Number of lesions variable: may range from few to hundreds
  - Occur most frequently on the head, neck, perineum, scrotum, and extremities (Figure 25.6)
  - Tend to wax and wane
  - Nasal mucosa involvement may occur (producing a "clown nose")
  - Systemic and lymph node involvement does not occur in this form.
- Reactive systemic histiocytosis:
  - Cutaneous manifestations identical to reactive cutaneous histiocytosis:
    - Multiple, nodular, and well circumscribed (Figure 25.7)
    - Often ulcerated, crusted, or alopecic
    - Often extend into the subcutis
    - Occur most frequently on the muzzle, nasal planum, eyelids, flank, and scrotum (Figure 25.8)
    - Not painful or pruritic
  - Ocular manifestations:
    - Conjunctivitis
    - Chemosis
    - Scleritis
    - Episcleritis
    - Episcleral nodules
    - Corneal edema
    - Anterior and posterior uveitis
    - Retinal detachment
    - Glaucoma
    - Exophthalmos
  - Lethargy
  - Anorexia

- Weight loss
- Respiratory stertor
- Coughing
- Dyspnea
- Dogs with systemic disorder may not have signs of systemic illness
- Marked predilection for skin and lymph nodes
- Moderate to severe peripheral lymphadenomegaly often present
- Abnormal respiratory sounds and/or nasal mucosa infiltration (Figure 25.9)
- Organomegaly occurs with systemic involvement
- Lesions may develop in the lung, liver, spleen, bone marrow, and nasal cavity
- May have alternating episodes of exacerbation and remission.

- Histiocytic sarcoma complex:
  - Pallor
  - Weakness
  - Lethargy
  - Weight loss
  - Primary pulmonary disease; dyspnea with abnormal lung sounds
  - Lameness, joint swelling
  - Neurologic signs (e.g., seizures, central disturbances, and posterior paresis) common
  - Moderate to severe lymphadenomegaly
  - Hepatic, splenic, renal, and pulmonary involvement common
  - Occasionally, masses are palpated in the liver and/or spleen
  - Eyes and skin are rarely affected
  - May be localized: rapidly growing soft tissue mass most often on extremities (Figure 25.10)
  - Highly metastatic (91%)
  - Multiple firm dermal to subcutaneous nodules that may be alopecic or ulcerated; lesions occur anywhere on the body.
- Malignant fibrous histiocytoma:
  - Soft tissue sarcomas
  - Predilection for the shoulder and paw
  - Locally invasive to bone, muscle, organs
  - Widespread metastasis common
  - May present as an injection site sarcoma.

DIFFERENTIAL DIAGNOSIS

- Histiocytic (nonepitheliotrophic) lymphoma: differentiation and definitive diagnosis often require special staining for immunohistochemical markers.
- Lymphomatoid granulomatosis: extensive pulmonary infiltrate of lymphocytes, plasma cells, histiocytes, and atypical lymphoreticular cells; affects young to middle-aged dogs, with respiratory disease as the chief complaint; lack of lymph node, organ, or bone marrow involvement.

- Periadnexal multinodular granulomatous dermatitis: benign, well-demarcated cutaneous nodules, commonly on the muzzle and may affect the eye; histologically distinct granulomas and variable numbers of inflammatory cells; may be indistinguishable from cutaneous histiocytosis.
- Granulomatous infectious diseases (e.g., nocardiosis, actinomycosis, and mycotic diseases): may have nodular pulmonary opacities.
- Hemophagocytic syndrome (histiocytosis): benign histiocytic proliferation secondary to infectious, neoplastic, or metabolic disease; can affect bone marrow, lymph nodes, liver, and spleen; causes cytopenia of at least two cell lines.
- Anaplastic carcinoma or sarcoma: histopathologic findings in dogs with histiocytosis may indicate a poorly differentiated tumor; immunostaining for tissue-specific markers will differentiate.

DIAGNOSTICS

- Histiocytoma: no abnormalities on routine diagnostic tests.
- Reactive histiocytosis: anemia (regenerative or nonregenerative), thrombocytopenia, monocytosis, lymphopenia.
- Histiocytic sarcoma: anemia (regenerative or nonregenerative), thrombocytopenia, monocytosis, lymphopenia, pancytopenia, hypoalbuminemia, elevated liver enzymes.
- Biochemistry results reflect the degree of organ involvement; hypercalcemia reported.
- Serum ferritin: may be a tumor marker for malignant histiocytosis; one affected dog had very high serum ferritin concentration, suggesting secretion by neoplastic mononuclear phagocytes.
- Thoracic radiographs: well-defined, nodular pulmonary opacities (single or multiple), pleural effusion, lung lobe consolidation, diffuse interstitial infiltrates, mediastinal masses, and sternal and bronchial lymphadenomegaly.
- Abdominal radiographs: hepatomegaly, splenomegaly, abdominal effusion.
- Biopsy of affected organs and/or lymph nodes.
- Fine-needle aspirate cytology of histiocytoma: pleomorphic round cells with basophilic cytoplasm and round to slightly indented nuclei (Figure 25.11)
- Cytologic examination of bone marrow aspirate or biopsy reveals histiocytic infiltration.
- Immunohistochemistry: results of cytologic/histologic examinations not always definitive; cytochemical staining useful in determining the histiocytic origin of the cells.

Histopathologic Findings

- Histiocytoma:
  - Trophism of histiocytes towards the dermis and epidermis may result in nests of cells within the dermis; similar in appearance to epitheliotropic lymphoma.
  - Diffuse dermal and subcutaneous pleocellular histiocytic infiltrate.

- Mitotic index variable but often high.
- Creates a "top-heavy" pattern.
- Regression mediated by and associated with infiltration of CD8+ T cells.

- Reactive cutaneous histiocytosis:
  - Distinguished from histiocytoma by lack of epidermal trophism
  - Diffuse or periadnexal/perivascular pleocellular histiocytic infiltrate
  - Discrete perivascular infiltrate may coalesce in the deeper dermis
  - Creates a "bottom-heavy" pattern (Figure 25.12)
  - Vascular involvement may lead to thrombosis and infarction.
- Reactive systemic histiocytosis:
  - Similar pattern as for cutaneous form
  - Perivascular and nodular infiltrates of histiocytes, neutrophils, and lymphocytes in other organ systems
  - Histiocytic infiltrates fail to demonstrate the bizarre cytologic characteristics of the mononuclear cells typical of malignant disorder
  - Histiocytes appear to target small blood vessels
  - Multinucleated giant cells are rarely seen
  - Immunohistochemistry: special stains for histiocytic markers such as lysozyme or cr-1-antitrypsin may be required for a definitive diagnosis.
- Histiocytic sarcoma:
  - Cytologic atypia is a characteristic hallmark
  - Histiocytes are large and pleomorphic/anaplastic with foamy cytoplasm
  - Mitotic index generally high and abnormal mitotic figures may be present
  - Multinucleated giant cells are often seen
  - Classically, erythrophagocytosis by neoplastic histiocytes evident
  - Occasionally, leukophagocytosis and thrombophagocytosis.
- Malignant fibrous histiocytoma:
  - Histiocytic round cells, fibroblastic cells, and multinucleated giant cells
  - Locally invasive.

Immunohistochemical Markers

- Summary overview:
  - CD18: all histiocytic cells
  - CD11c: epithelial and interstitial dendritic cells
  - CD11d: macrophages
  - CD90 (Thy-1): dermal interstitial dendritic cells
  - E-cadherin: epithelial dendritic cells
  - CD4: activated dendritic cells
  - CD204: macrophages, interstitial dendritic cells (not epithelial or interdigitating dendritic cells).
- Cutaneous histiocytoma:
  - Formalin fixed tissue: CD18+, E-cadherin +/−, MHC class II +
  - Frozen section: CD1a+, CD11c+, CD90 (Thy-1)−.

- Reactive cutaneous histiocytosis:
  - Formalin fixed tissue: CD18+, MHC class II +, CD90(Thy-1)+, E-cadherin-
  - Frozen section: CD1a+, CD11c+, CD4+, CD90(Thy-1)+.
- Reactive systemic histiocytosis:
  - Formalin fixed tissue: CD18+, MHC class II+, CD90(Thy1)+
  - Frozen: CD1a+, CD11c+, CD4+, CD3+
  - Enzyme markers: TCR alpha and and beta +, acid phosphatase, lysozyme (cr-1-antitrypsin)+.
- Histiocytic sarcoma:
  - Formalin fixed tissue: CD18+, CD204+, MHC class II+
  - Frozen section: CD1a+, CD11c+.

THERAPEUTICS

- Histiocytoma:
  - Observation without treatment; most nodules will resolve within 3 months
  - Nodules often appear more inflamed, crusted, or scabbed during involution (see Figure 25.10)
  - Excisional biopsy is curative
  - Multiple tumors: may respond to prednisolone 1 mg/kg PO q24h; tapered until lesions resolve
  - Pruritic nodules may respond to the topical application of corticosteroids in DMSO.
- Reactive cutaneous histiocytosis:
  - 50% respond to corticosteroids
  - Prednisolone 1 mg/kg PO q24h tapering dosage; treatment lasting from 4 to 18 months
  - Spontaneous remission can occur
  - Cycline antibiotics: tetracycline (250 mg PO q8h for dogs <10 kg; 500 mg PO TID dogs >10 kg); doxycycline (10 mg/kg PO q24h); minocycline (5 mg/kg PO BID); often administered with niacinamide 250 mg PO for dogs <10 kg and 500 mg PO for dogs >10 kg
  - Cyclosporine: 5–10 mg/kg PO q24h; dose may be tapered slowly over time; maintenance therapy usually necessary; liver enzymes must be monitored for hepatotoxicity; vomiting is the most common side effect
  - Alternatives: vitamin E, essential fatty acids.
- Reactive systemic histiocytosis:
  - Cyclosporine: 5–10 mg/kg PO q24h; dose may be tapered slowly over time; maintenance therapy usually necessary; liver enzymes must be monitored for hepatotoxicity; vomiting is the most common side effect
  - Leflunomide: 2–4 mg/kg PO q24h; trough levels of 20 mg/mL may be optimum; variability in drug metabolism, trough levels must be monitored;

lymphopenia and anemia are uncommon side effects; most common side effect is vomiting
- Azathioprine: 2 mg/kg or 50 mg/m2 PO q24h until remission; then EOD or twice weekly.

- Histiocytic sarcoma (malignant histiocytosis):
  - Typically nonresponsive
  - Rapidly progressive, and fatal
  - Fails to respond to therapy
  - Chemotherapy often trialed including corticosteroids, cyclophosphamide, vincristine, and doxorubicin-based protocols
  - Fluid therapy or blood transfusions may be required depending on clinical findings.
- Malignant fibrous histiocytoma:
  - Surgical excision if possible
  - Poor prognosis due to local invasion and tendency to metastasize.

COMMENTS

- Effectiveness of treatment is determined by repeated physical examinations, CBC and biochemistry profiles, and diagnostic imaging.
- Patients with systemic disorder have a fluctuating debilitating disease that can be characterized by multiple clinical episodes and asymptomatic periods.
- Prognosis for malignant disorder is extremely poor; death usually occurs within a few months of diagnosis.

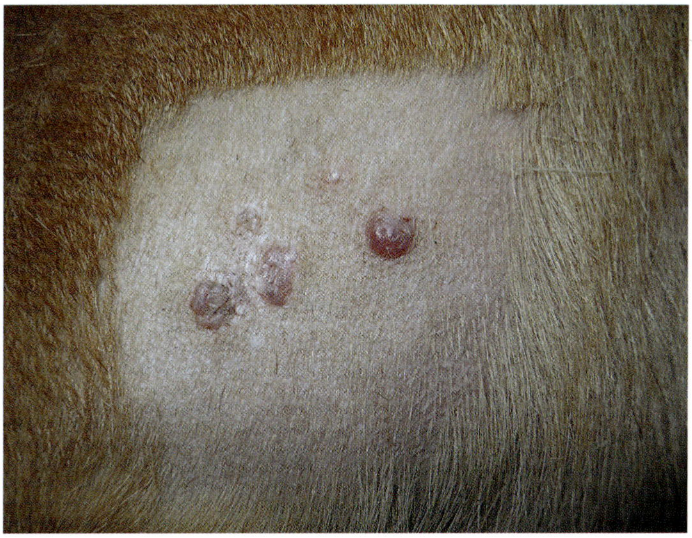

■ **Fig. 25.1.** Multiple cutaneous histiocytomas in a 2-year-old male-castrate Chinese shar pei. Additional nodules were noted over most of the body.

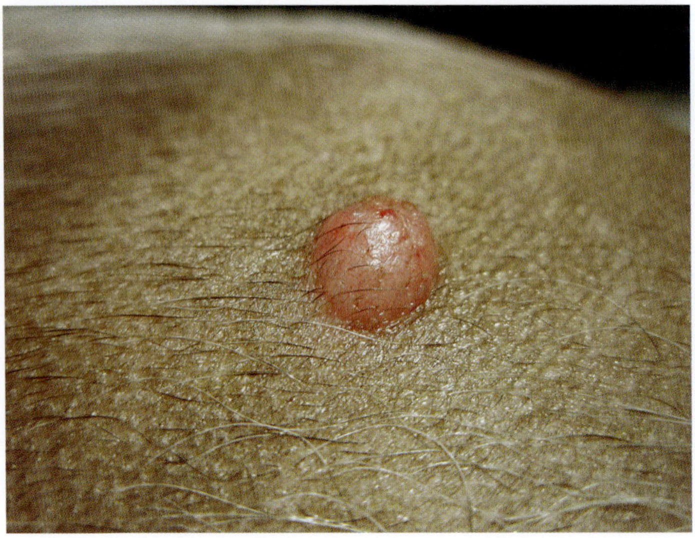

■ **Fig. 25.2.** Erythematous, dome-shaped nodule characteristic of a cutaneous histiocytoma in a 5-year-old male-castrate pug.

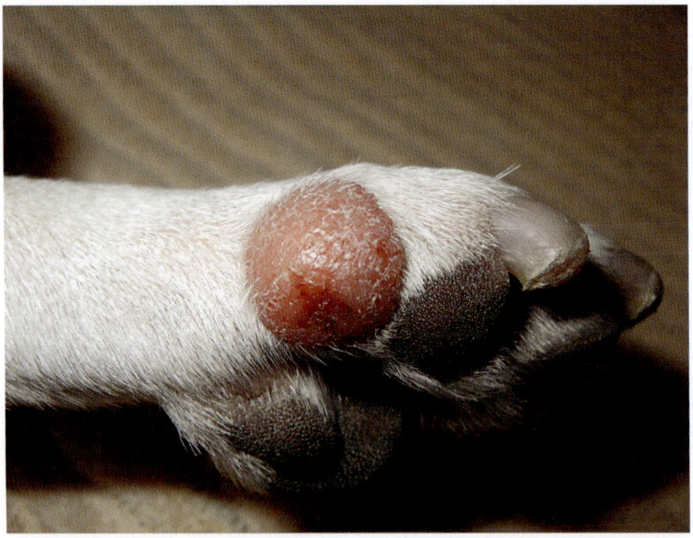

■ **Fig. 25.3.** Large erythematous cutaneous histiocytoma on the foot of a 4-year-old female-spayed French bulldog.

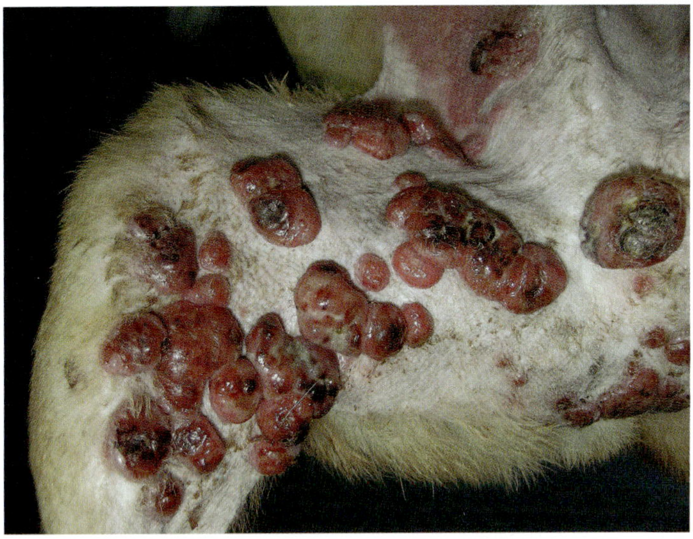

■ **Fig. 25.4.** Multiple erythematous and ulcerated nodules on the medial aspect of the rear leg of a mixed-breed dog with reactive cutaneous histiocytosis.

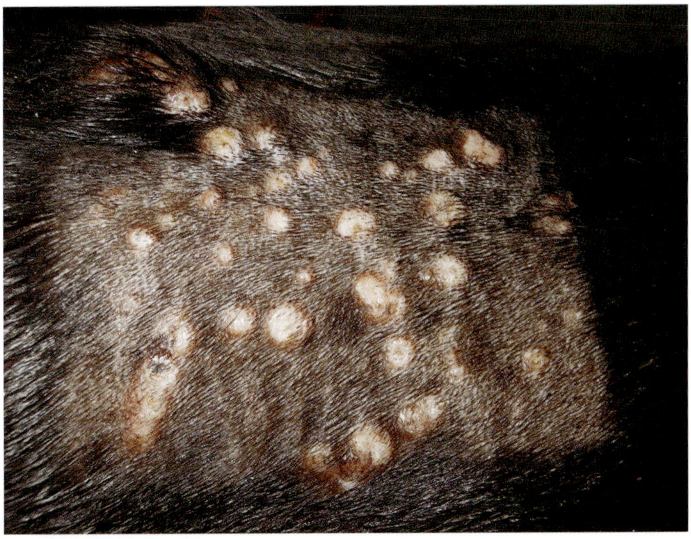

■ **Fig. 25.5.** Reactive cutaneous histiocytosis: multiple erythematous and alopecic plaques and nodules on the body of a 14-year-old female-spayed pit bull mix.

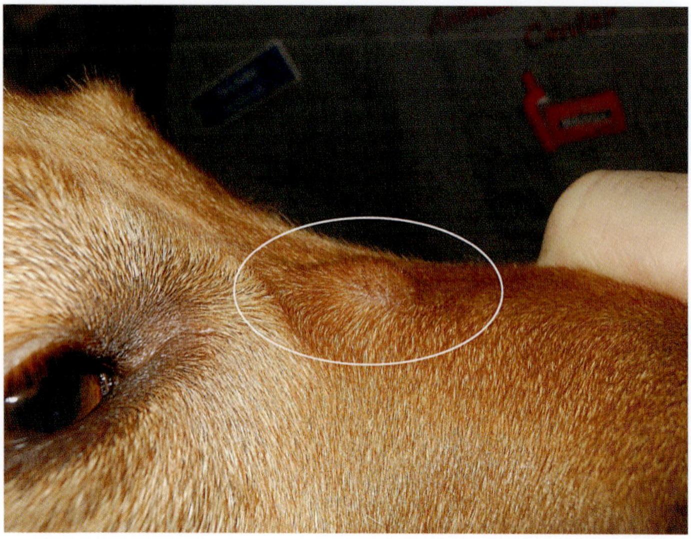

■ **Fig. 25.6.** Reactive cutaneous histiocytosis. Swelling on the dorsal muzzle (within ellipse) of a 2-year-old female-spayed golden retriever.

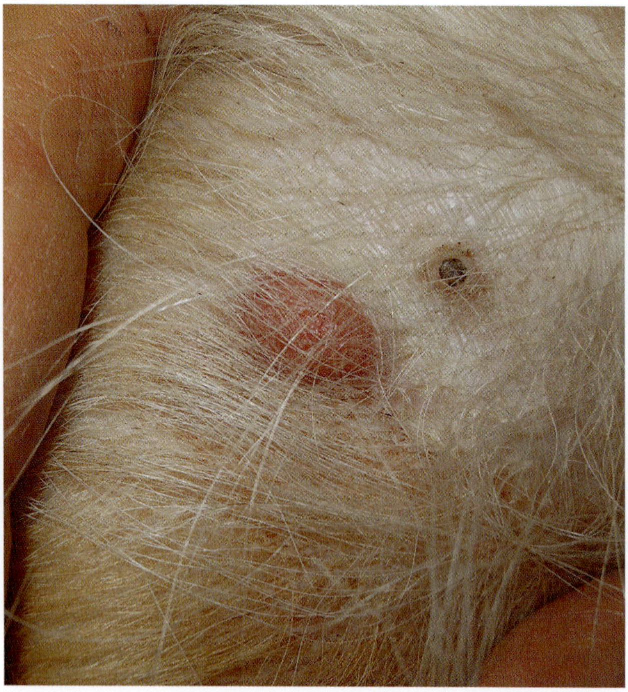

(a)

■ **Fig. 25.7.** Malignant histiocytosis in a 5-year-old female-spayed Bernese mountain dog. Erythematous nodules were generalized on the body, including (a) on the ventrum and (b) interdigitally.

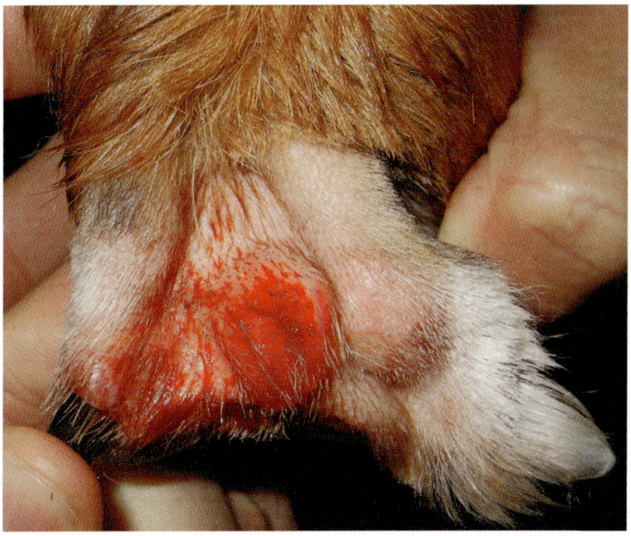

(b)

Fig. 25.7. *(Continued)*

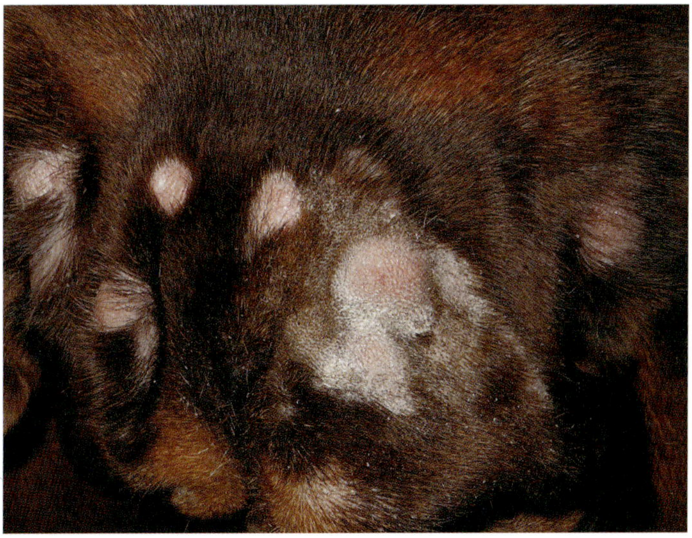

Fig. 25.8. Systemic cutaneous histiocytosis: multiple erythematous and alopecic plaques and nodules on the head of a 5-year-old male bloodhound.

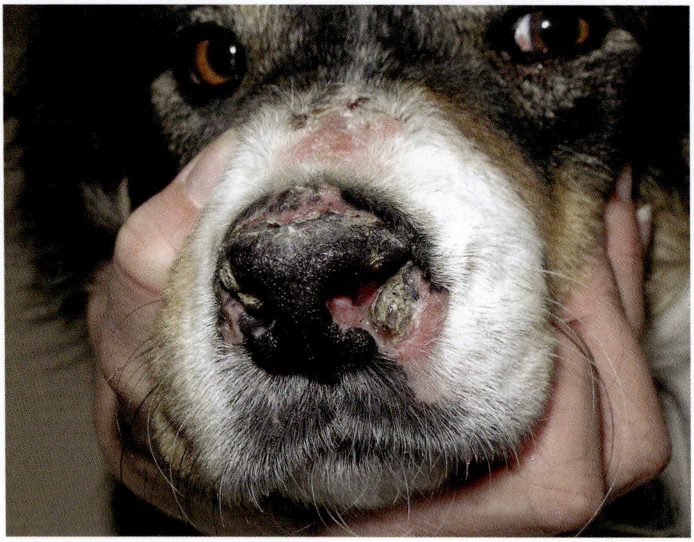

■ **Fig. 25.9.** Eroded and crusted plaques affecting the muzzle and nasal planum of an adult Australian shepherd mix with systemic cutaneous histiocytosis.

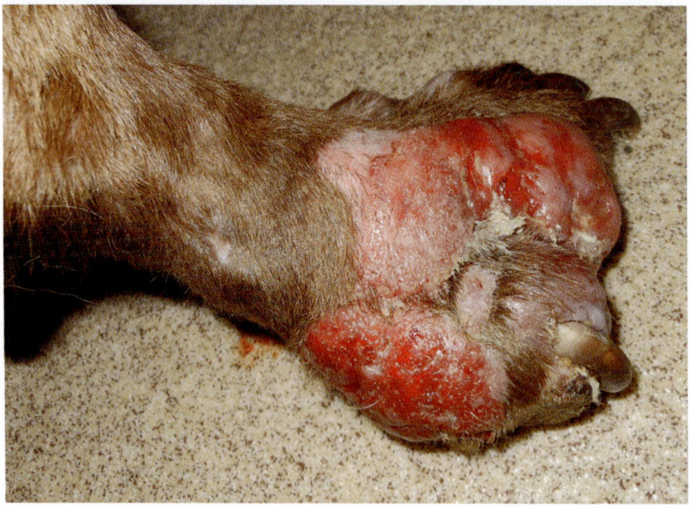

■ **Fig. 25.10.** Histiocytic sarcoma affecting the digits of a 2-year-old male-castrate Labrador retriever.

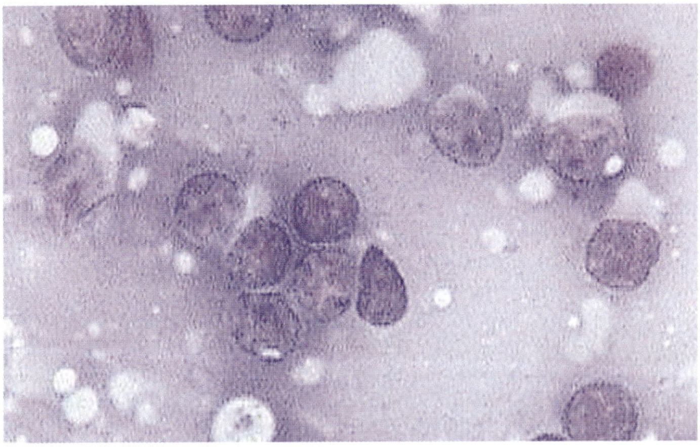

■ **Fig. 25.11.** Fine-needle aspirate cytology of a histiocytoma: pleomorphic round cells with basophilic cytoplasm and round to slightly indented nuclei.

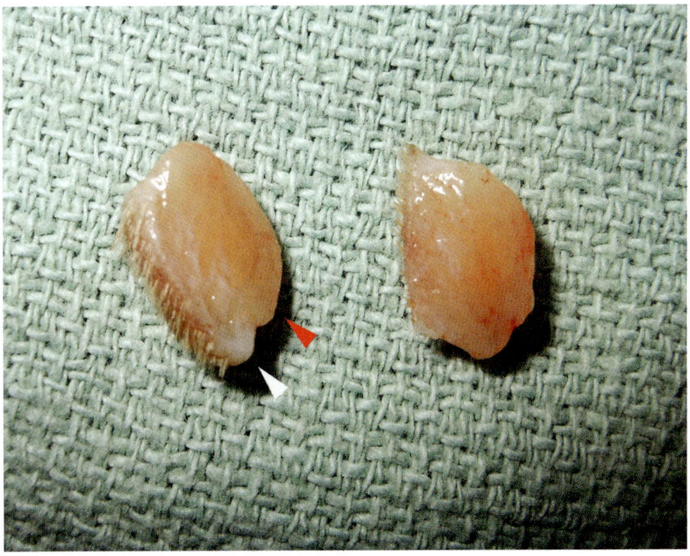

■ **Fig. 25.12.** Biopsy tissue of a nodule from the patient in Figure 25.6 with reactive cutaneous histiocytosis. Note that grossly, inflammation appears to spare the epidermis (*white arrowhead*) and predominantly affects the deeper dermis (*red arrowhead*), creating a "bottom-heavy" appearance.

chapter 26

Hyperadrenocorticism, Canine

DEFINITION/OVERVIEW

- Spontaneous hyperadrenocorticism (HAC): disorder caused by excessive production of cortisol by the adrenal cortex.
- Two forms of spontaneous hyperadrenocorticism: pituitary dependent (PDH) and adrenal dependent (ADH).
- Iatrogenic hyperadrenocorticism results from excessive exogenous administration of glucocorticoids.
- Clinical signs are a result of the deleterious effects of elevated circulating cortisol concentrations on multiple organ systems.

ETIOLOGY/PATHOPHYSIOLOGY

- PDH:
  - 85–90% of cases of naturally occurring HAC
  - Caused by uncontrolled proliferation (tumor) of the basophilic or chromophobic cells of the pars intermedia and the pars distalis of the pituitary gland, resulting in hypersecretion of adrenocorticotrophic hormone (ACTH)
  - Hypersecretion of ACTH causes bilateral adrenocortical hyperplasia
  - Most tumors are small (microadenomas); approximately 15% are macroadenomas
  - Clinical signs are similar; macroadenomas may have associated central nervous system signs due to a space-occupying mass effect.
- ADH:
  - 10–15% of cases of naturally occurring HAC
  - Caused by a cortisol-secreting adrenocortical neoplasia (cortical adenoma/carcinoma)
  - Approximately 50% of tumors are malignant
  - Contralateral "normal" adrenal gland atrophies because of excessive cortisol production by the adrenal tumor.

Blackwell's Five-Minute Veterinary Consult Clinical Companion: Small Animal Dermatology, Third Edition.
Karen Helton Rhodes and Alexander H. Werner.

- Iatrogenic HAC:
  - Clinically indistinguishable from the naturally occurring disease
  - Results from excessive or prolonged exogenous administration (systemic and/or topical, including otic) of glucocorticoids
  - Causes bilateral adrenal atrophy and suppressed ACTH levels.
- HAC is a multisystemic disorder; the degree to which each system is involved varies considerably; in some patients, signs referable to one system may predominate; others have multiple systems affected.
- Urinary tract and/or dermatologic abnormalities are most often the first to be noticed.

SIGNALMENT/HISTORY

- Considered one of the most common endocrine disorders in dogs.
- Dogs: poodles, dachshunds, Boston terriers, boxers, and beagles are reportedly at increased risk.
- Predominantly female.
- HAC is usually a disorder of middle-aged to older animals.

CLINICAL FEATURES (Figures 26.1–26.9)

- Polyuria and polydipsia: occur in 85–95% of cases; glucocorticoids interfere with antidiuretic hormone (ADH) release, resulting in compensatory polyuria and polydipsia.
- Polyphagia: direct stimulatory effect on the appetite.
- Abdominal distension ("pot belly") occurs due to redistribution of fat, wasting of the abdominal muscles, and hepatomegaly.
- Hepatomegaly: accumulation of glycogen.
- Hair loss: bilateral and symmetric truncal alopecia with sparing of the head and extremities; atrophy of the hair follicles, epidermis, and adnexal structures; may see alopecia along the bridge of the nose.
- Atrophy of the skin: decreased epidermal turnover/regeneration; decreased elasticity.
- Phlebectasia: small, red, slightly raised areas that represent abnormal vessel dilation, extension, or duplication.
- Demodicosis: proliferation of *Demodex* mites due to immunosuppression; rare.
- Poor wound healing: excessive glucocorticoids suppress the inflammatory response, fibroblast proliferation, and collagen deposition.
- Comedones: plugged follicular ostia with keratin, black or white; sometimes associated with demodicosis.
- Calcinosis cutis: accumulation and deposition of calcium in the dermis and/or subcutis and along the follicular epithelium, which is palpable as firm gritty nodules or plaques, yellow-pink in color; subsequent foreign body reaction; large coalescing plaques are typically prominent in the dorsal neck region, milder cases are often most pronounced in the ventral intertriginous areas (axillae, groin).

- Bacterial folliculitis (pyoderma): excess glucocorticoids predispose to skin infections from bacterial overgrowth and poor immune response.
- Dystrophic mineralization may occur in tissues other than the skin: renal pelvis, skeletal muscles, gastric walls, bronchial walls, heart muscle, blood vessels, and liver.
- Muscle weakness and atrophy: excessive protein catabolism and muscle wasting; cruciate ruptures can occur with little stress; high levels of cortisol may cause myotonia characterized by stiff extensor muscles.
- Anestrus: glucocorticoids exhibit a negative feedback on pituitary gonadotrophin secretion.
- Testicular atrophy and decreased libido: glucocorticoids exert a negative feedback on pituitary gonadotrophin secretion, which causes a decrease in testicular androgen production.
- Clitoral hypertrophy: excess androgen production; major source of androgen production in the female is the adrenal gland.
- Perianal gland adenomas: females and neutered males; overproduction of androgens.
- Panting: common finding and may be due to wasting of the muscles of respiration as well as reduced capacity for thoracic expansion from the distended abdomen; other possible causes include pulmonary hypertension and decreased compliance, primary CNS disturbance, or pulmonary mineralization.
- Dyspnea: uncommon; associated with pulmonary thromboembolism; life-threatening complication of HAC; may occur secondary to a hypercoagulable state, erythrocytosis, and/or hypertension.
- Hyperpigmentation: possibly due to the similarity of ACTH to melanocyte-stimulating hormone (MSH).
- Blindness and papillary light reflex changes: pressure exerted on the optic chiasm by macroadenomas.
- Central nervous system signs: seizures, pacing, head pressing, circling, behavioral change (timid/aggressive), impaired thermoregulation (unexplained fever or hypothermia), ataxia, coma, death; usually due to pituitary macroadenoma and space-occupying effect; can occur after initiation of antiadrenal therapy due to lack of negative feedback and subsequent tumor expansion (Nelson's syndrome).

DIFFERENTIAL DIAGNOSIS

- Hypothyroidism
- Sex hormone dermatoses
- Acromegaly
- Diabetes mellitus
- Hepatopathies
- Renal disease
- Other causes of polyuria/polydipsia
- Follicular dysplasias
- Alopecia X/atypical hyperadrenocorticism

DIAGNOSTICS

- Hemogram: eosinopenia, lymphopenia, neutrophilic leukocytosis, erythrocytosis, thrombocytosis.
- Serum chemistry: elevated alkaline phosphatase in over 80% of cases, mild increase in ALT, hypercholesterolemia, hypertriglyceridemia; 5–10% of dogs may have hyperglycemia (diabetes), decreased blood urea nitrogen (BUN) concentration; thyroid values may be low.
- Urinalysis: may reveal decreased specific gravity (<1.018), proteinuria secondary to glomerulopathy/glomerular sclerosis, hematuria, pyuria, or increased numbers of bacteria in urine.
- Urine cortisol-creatinine ratio (UCCR): highly sensitive test; not specific (nonadrenal diseases may cause an elevated UCCR).
- Abdominal radiographs: may show hepatomegaly; approximately 50% of adrenal tumors will be mineralized and visible on radiographs.
- Thoracic cavity radiographs: may show bronchial calcification or metastasis from an adrenal adenocarcinoma; osteopenia may also be identified.
- Ultrasonography/CT/MRI: useful for differentiating PDH from ADH and for staging ADH.
- CT and MRI: often useful for demonstrating macroadenomas.
- Pathology (PDH): gross examination reveals normal-sized pituitary to pituitary macroadenoma and bilateral adrenocortical enlargement; microscopic – evaluation for pituitary corticotroph hyperplasia or adenoma of pars distalis or pars intermedia and adrenocortical hyperplasia.
- Pathology (ADH): gross examination reveals variable-sized adrenal mass, atrophy of contralateral gland (rarely, bilateral tumors), and metastasis in some patients with adrenal carcinoma; microscopic – evaluation for adrenocortical adenoma or carcinoma.

Screening Tests

- Screening tests for HAC: ACTH stimulation test, LDDST, and UCCR.
- ACTH stimulation test:
  - Used to diagnose HAC: cannot distinguish between PDH and ADH
  - ACTH stimulation test assesses adrenocortical reserve
  - Best test for monitoring response to adrenolytic therapy or adrenal enzyme blockers
  - ACTH stimulation test: PDH cases; sensitivity 80–83%, specificity 59–93%
  - Inferior (due to low sensitivity) as a screening test for spontaneous HAC to low-dose dexamethasone suppression test (LDDST)
  - ACTH stimulation test often performed as a first step because of a shorter time to complete the test (1–2 hours versus 8 hours for LDDST)
  - Postpone testing if the patient has a concurrent serious illness to minimize false-positive test results

- "Gold standard" for diagnosis of iatrogenic HAC: baseline cortisol levels will be below normal and will not increase with stimulation
- Best test for diagnosis of spontaneous Addison's disease (hypoadrenocorticism).
- Glucocorticoids, progestagens, and ketoconazole may suppress cortisol secretion; phenobarbital does not appear to influence test results
- Testing methodology:
  - Fasted patient: hemolysis and lipemia may affect values
  - Promptly spin and separate the serum or plasma before refrigeration
  - Baseline cortisol sample
  - Inject 5 µg/kg IV or IM of cosyntropin or tetracosactrin (use of compounded ACTH is discouraged)
  - Second blood sample at 1 hour post injection
- Test interpretation:
  - Poststimulation cortisol >22 µg/dL consistent with HAC (check laboratory standard values)
  - Poststimulation cortisol <15 µg/dL not consistent with HAC: 20–30% of patients with HAC stimulate below the cut-off
  - Nonadrenal illness may yield a false-positive result
  - Both pre- and postcortisol values are blunted – consider iatrogenic HAC.

■ LDDST:
- 95% sensitive, 44–73% specific
- Screening test to identify HAC
- Testing methodology:
  - Fasted patient: hemolysis and lipemia may affect values
  - Promptly spin and separate the serum or plasma before refrigeration
  - Baseline cortisol sample
  - Inject 0.01 mg/kg of dexamethasone intravenously (dilute in 0.9% sodium chloride solution for accuracy in dosing)
  - Second sample at 4 hours post administration
  - Third sample at 8 hours post administration
- Test interpretation:
  - Normal: suppression <50% of baseline and <1.5 µg/dL at 8 hours
  - Lack of suppression to <50% baseline and <1.5 µg/dL at 8 hours confirms HAC; if no suppression is noted, cACTH measurement or abdominal ultrasound is recommended
  - Suppression to <50% baseline and <1.5 µg/dL at 4 hours but lack of suppression at 8 hours is most consistent with PDH
  - Lack of suppression does not confirm an adrenal tumor; 25% of dogs with PDH fail to suppress <1.5 µg/dL; nonadrenal illness can affect the test.

■ Urine cortisol-creatinine ratio:
- UCCR provides a reflection of cortisol production; day-to-day variation
- Screening test to be used in conjunction with LDDST
- Cannot be used to monitor treatment
- Negative result means HAC is unlikely; positive result indicates need for confirmatory testing

- Can potentially demonstrate both increased cortisol production and decreased sensitivity to glucocorticoid feedback
- Sensitivity 75–100%; specificity 20–25% in random sampling of hospital patients
- Sensitivity 99%; specificity 77% in patients exhibiting physical and biochemical changes consistent with HAC.

Tests to Differentiate PDH from ADH

- PDH and ADH treatment options and prognosis differ; several tests are used to distinguish the exact etiology: HDDST, HDDST with UCCR, endogenous ACTH, and abdominal ultrasound.
- HDDST:
  - 75% of dogs with PDH will demonstrate suppression of cortisol levels; 25% of dogs with PDH do not suppress with HDDST (likely due to a large pituitary tumor or tumor developing from the pars intermedia)
  - Nearly 100% of dogs with ADH will not demonstrate suppression of cortisol levels
  - PDH: high dose of corticosteroid (dexamethasone) results in a decrease in ACTH release from the pituitary and a resultant decrease in plasma cortisol
  - ADH: tumor secretes cortisol autonomously, suppressing ACTH production; dexamethasone has no effect on plasma cortisol because ACTH is already suppressed
  - Testing methodology: same as for LDDST except the dose of dexamethasone is higher at 0.1 mg/kg given intravenously; the 4-h sample is omitted
  - Testing interpretation: an 8-h cortisol of less than 1.0–1.4 μg/dL is consistent with PDH.
- Endogenous ACTH:
  - Canine ACTH (cACTH) is secreted episodically from the pituitary gland
  - Concentrations of cACTH do not differ from normal dogs and PDH patients (not a viable screening test for HAC)
  - Most accurate stand-alone test for differentiating PDH from ADH (normal or elevated concentrations of cACTH = PDH; suppressed levels = ADH)
  - Very accurate but highly susceptible to sample mishandling causing the ACTH levels to be falsely low and giving the false impression that the dog has ADH; use of a preservative in EDTA tubes called aprotinin may result in fewer handling errors (follow reference laboratory guidelines)
  - PDH cases have normal to high levels of endogenous ACTH
  - ADH cases have low to undetectable levels of endogenous cACTH because the adrenal tumor produces high levels of cortisol, suppressing cACTH production by the pituitary gland.
- Abdominal ultrasound:
  - Evaluate adrenal size (normal width should be less than 7 mm), symmetry, and invasion of adjacent structures
  - Some adrenal tumors are mineralized
  - Often used in place of HDDST or endogenous ACTH testing.

THERAPEUTICS

Surgical Considerations

- Hypophysectomy: described, but generally not recommended for treatment of PDH because of the difficulty of the procedure and the need for intensive monitoring and life-long hormonal supplementation.
- Adrenalectomy is a demanding procedure not generally used for the treatment of PDH in dogs.
- Surgery is probably the treatment of choice for adrenocortical adenomas and small carcinomas unless the patient is a poor surgical risk.

Radiation Therapy for Pituitary Tumors

- Radiation therapy successful for pituitary tumors; availability limited.

Drugs of Choice

- Mitotane (o, p'-DDD):
  - Cytotoxic drug causing progressive necrosis of the zona fasciculata and zona reticularis of the adrenal gland
  - Medical management of both PDH and ADH in dogs
  - Mitotane destroys adrenocortical cells
  - Adverse effects are common and include lethargy, weakness, vomiting, diarrhea, ataxia, head pressing, blindness, and iatrogenic hypoadrenocorticism
  - Incidence rate of side effects may be as high as 25–30%
  - Give with food to increase absorption
  - Monitor ACTH stimulation test cortisol levels every 1–6 months as a maintenance protocol
  - Mitotane does not suppress estradiol
  - Phenobarbital enhances the metabolism of mitotane, making it less effective
  - PDH:
    - Initial loading dose of 25–50 mg/kg PO divided and administered BID for approximately 3–8 days
    - Observe for subtle changes in appetite or thirst
    - Repeat ACTH stimulation test until both basal and post-ACTH cortisol levels are in the normal resting range (2–6 μg/dL)
    - Maintenance dosage: 50 mg/kg per week divided and administered twice weekly; dosage requirements may vary; dosage adjustments are based on ACTH stimulation test results
    - If relapse occurs, as indicated by cortisol levels outside the normal resting range, reload for 5–7 days and increase weekly maintenance dose by approximately 50%
    - Prednisone (0.2 mg/kg PO q24h) may be given during initial and subsequent loading periods

- ADH:
  - □ Administer mitotane at highest tolerated dosage beginning with 50 mg/kg q24h as a loading dose
  - □ Administer prednisone at 0.2 mg/kg PO q24h during induction
  - □ Monitoring similar to PDH.
- Trilostane:
  - Inactive steroid analog that competitively inhibits 3-beta-hydroxysteroid dehydrogenase
  - Prevents production of cortisol and aldosterone
  - Competitive inhibition is reversible and dose dependent
  - Side effects include lethargy, anorexia, vomiting, dehydration, weakness, and hyponatremia/hyperkalemia
  - Irreversible acute adrenal necrosis may occur
  - Anecdotal reports of acute death shortly after initiating therapy
  - Give with food for maximum absorption
  - Do not use in pregnant or nursing bitches, animals intended for breeding, or patients with renal or hepatic disease or evidence of anemia
  - Trilostane may block estrogen receptors, thus causing increased levels of adrenal sex hormones. Do not use in breeding animals
  - Dosage guidelines: 3–6 mg/kg PO q24h; many dogs are controlled with a lower dose of 1.3–3 mg/kg PO BID
  - Dosage based on body weight: large dogs (>30 kg) may require a lower dose compared to small dogs (<15 kg):
    <3 kg body weight = starting dose of 10 mg q24h
    >3 kg and <10 kg = starting dose of 30 mg q24h
    >10 kg and <20 kg = starting dose of 60 mg q24h
    >20 kg and <40 kg = starting dose of 120 mg q24h
    >40 kg = starting dose of 180 mg q24h
  - Doses can be given once daily or divided twice daily; some dogs may require three times daily administration
  - Dose is adjusted based on ACTH stimulation test cortisol levels
  - Most patients show clinical improvement within 7 days
  - Repeat ACTH stimulation test 1–2 weeks after starting medication (4–6 hours post pill; some endocrinologists recommend 2–4 hours post pill)
  - Monitor levels by ACTH stimulation test at 1 month, 2 months, 3 months, 6 months post initiation of medication and then every 3–6 months if the levels are stable
  - Basal serum cortisol concentrations or post-ACTH stimulation test cortisol levels may be used for monitoring response
  - Ideal target range for basal serum cortisol: 1.3–2.9 µg/dL (35–80 nmol/L) or less than or equal to 50% of the pretreatment baseline cortisol concentration
  - Ideal target range for cortisol concentrations post ACTH stimulation: 1.45–5.4 µg/dL (40–150 nmol/L)

- Must maintain daily (or BID) dosing for maintenance therapy, as opposed to twice weekly for mitotane
- Monitor sodium and potassium levels in treated dogs.

- L-deprenyl (selegiline hydrochloride):
  - Monamine oxidase inhibitor/dopamine agonist
  - May be used as an alternative treatment for PDH
  - Decreases pituitary ACTH secretion by increasing dopaminergic tone to the hypothalamic-pituitary axis, decreasing serum cortisol concentrations
  - Indicated only for the treatment of uncomplicated PDH
  - Not recommended for treatment of PDH in dogs with concurrent illnesses such as diabetes mellitus
  - Cannot be used to treat cortisol-secreting adrenocortical neoplasia
  - Medication effective in 20–30% of patients with pars intermedia disease
  - Initiate therapy with 1 mg/kg PO q24h and increase to 2 mg/kg PO q24h after 2 months if the response is inadequate
  - If this dose is also ineffective, discontinue and institute alternative therapy
  - Disadvantages include the need for life-long daily administration, the expense of the medication, and the frequent lack of clinical response
  - Side effects are uncommon and include vomiting, diarrhea, and hyperactive behavior
  - Do not use with other monoamine oxidase inibitors, tricyclic antidepressants, serotonin reuptake inhibitors, amitraz, dobutamine, meperidine, linezolid, or tramadol.
- Ketoconazole:
  - Inhibits mammalian steroidogenesis by blocking the cytochrome p450 enzyme system, which is responsible for both androgen and cortisol production
  - Also inhibits ACTH secretion from pituitary corticotrophs
  - Dosage: 10 mg/kg PO BID initially; up to 20 mg/kg BID in some dogs
  - Indicated for dogs unable to tolerate mitotane or trilostane at doses necessary to control HAC and preoperative control of HAC in dogs with ADH scheduled for adrenalectomy
  - May be useful for palliation of clinical signs of HAC in dogs with AT
  - Over one-third of dogs reportedly fail to respond adequately to this drug
  - Adverse effects include anorexia, vomiting, diarrhea, lethargy, decreased libido/reproductive hormones, and an idiosyncratic hepatopathy
  - Avoid concurrent use with ivermectin (increased ivermectin toxicity by decreased clearance and enhanced penetration across the blood–brain barrier) and antacids.

Alternative Therapies with Minimal or Unknown Effectiveness

Melatonin, flax seed oil with lignins, metyrapone, LC1699 (similar to metyrapone), mifepristone, bromocriptine, cyproheptadine, cabergoline, aminoglutethimide, COR-003 (enantiomer of ketoconazole), retinoic acid, gefitinib (EGFR antagonist).

COMMENTS

Patient Monitoring (*see each drug*)

- Response to therapy.
- Use periodic ACTH stimulation test; test after the initial 7–10 days therapy to ensure adequate response.
- Repeat at 1, 3, and 6 months of maintenance therapy and every 3–6 months thereafter.
- Adequacy of any necessary reloading period is monitored with an ACTH stimulation test before higher maintenance dose initiated.
- Depending on the cause (PDH versus ADH), clinical signs resolve within several days to months of appropriate therapy.
- L-deprenyl therapy: current label recommendations are to evaluate efficacy solely on the basis of resolution of clinical signs of HAC; the ACTH stimulation test is not indicated for assessing the response to treatment.
- Some clinicians perform a low-dose dexamethasone suppression test every 4–6 weeks to evaluate for normalization (or improvement) of the pituitary-adrenal axis.

Expected Course and Prognosis

- Untreated HAC: generally a progressive disorder with a poor prognosis.
- Treated PDH: good prognosis; the average survival time for a dog is 2 years; at least 10% survive 4 years; dogs living longer than 6 years tend to die of causes unrelated to HAC.
- Macroadenomas with neurologic signs: poor to grave prognosis.
- Adrenal adenomas: usually a good to excellent prognosis.
- Small carcinomas (not metastasized): fair to good prognosis.
- Large carcinomas and ADH with widespread metastasis: generally poor to fair prognosis; response to high doses of mitotane is occasionally seen.

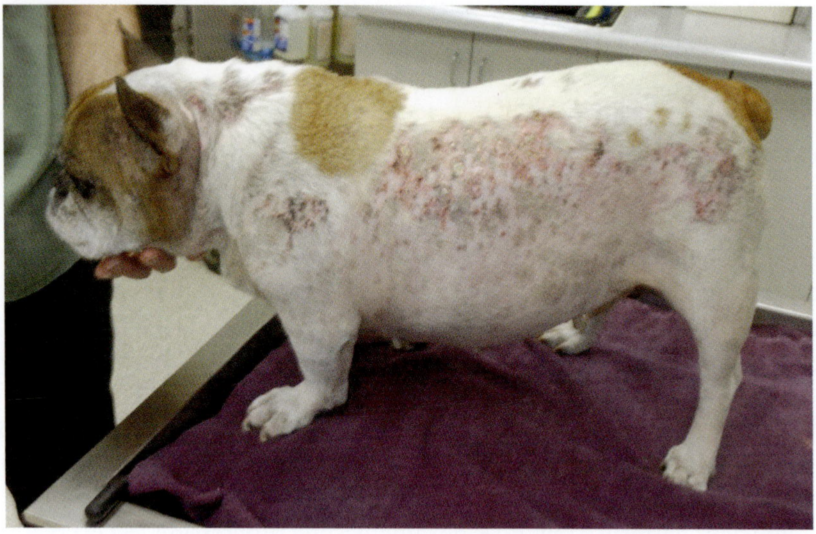

■ **Fig. 26.1.** Naturally acquired hyperadrenocorticism in a 9-year-old female-spayed French bulldog. Note distended belly appearance to the abdomen, sway-back, and diffuse alopecia characteristic of chronic disease. Patches of calcinosis cutis are evident on dorsal-lateral aspect of the body and dorsal neck.

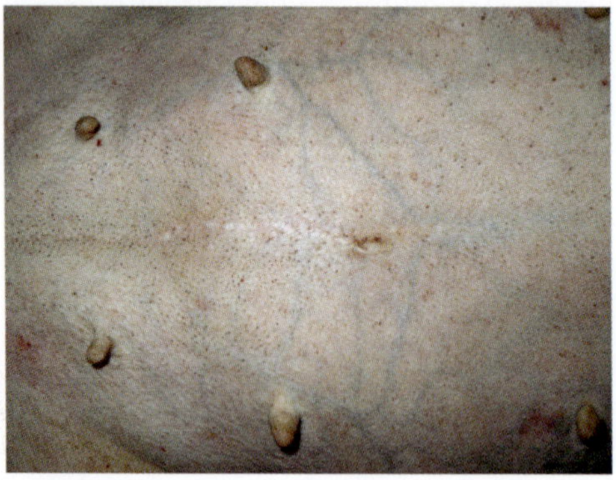

■ **Fig. 26.2.** Ventral abdomen of patient in Figure 26.1: the skin is excessively thin, with comedones and prominent subcutaneous vasculature.

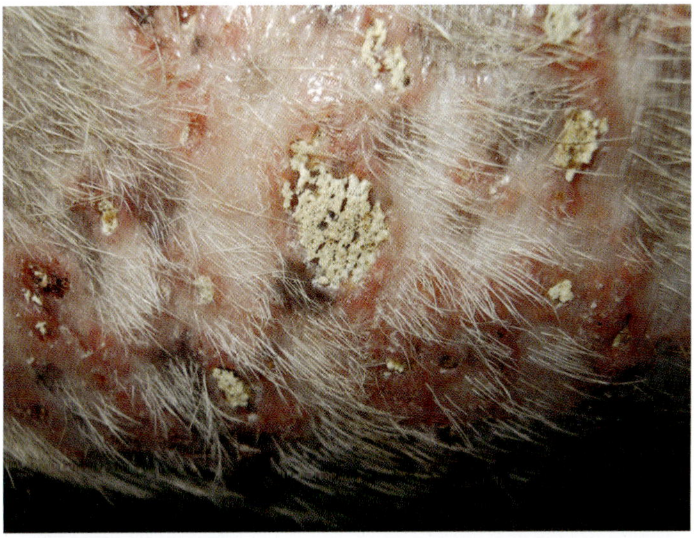

(a)

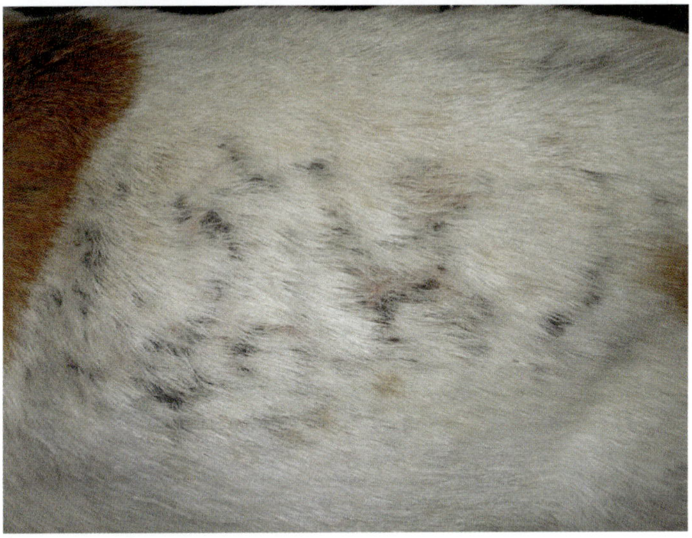

(b)

Fig. 26.3. (a)Lesions of calcinosis cutis of patient in Figures 26.1 and 26.2 at diagnosis. Lesions are palpably firm plaques with a creamy-white exudate representing calcium being extruded from follicular ostea. (b) Lesions resolving after 4 months of treatment.

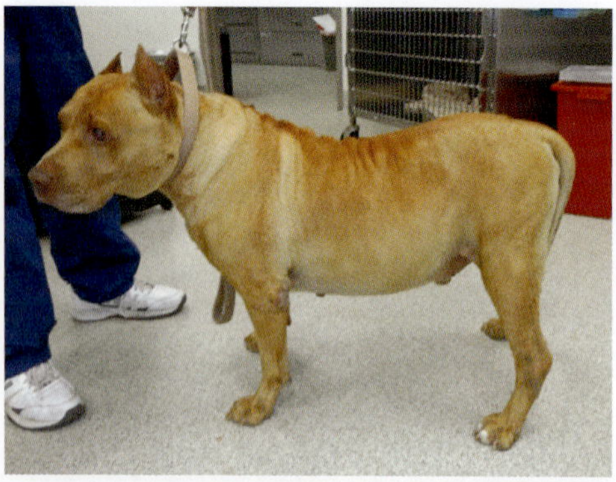

■ **Fig. 26.4.** Naturally acquired hyperadrenocorticism in a 10-year-old, male-castrate pit bull. Body conformation is similar to that of the patient in Figure 26.1 with a distended abdomen and sway-back.

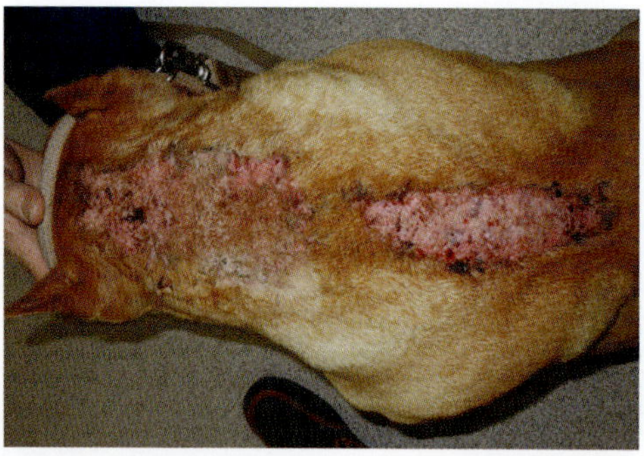

■ **Fig. 26.5.** Large patches with plaques of calcinosis cutis over the dorsal neck and shoulders of the patient in Figure 26.4. Lesions are palpably firm, alopecic and erythematous, with hemorrhagic exudation.

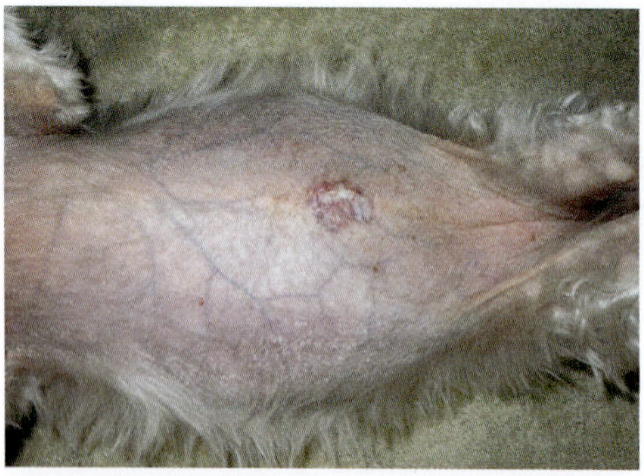

■ **Fig. 26.6.** Diffuse alopecia with alopecia, mild scaling, and prominent vasculature seen through the atrophic epidermis and dermis on the ventrum of a 9-year-old female-spayed Maltese.

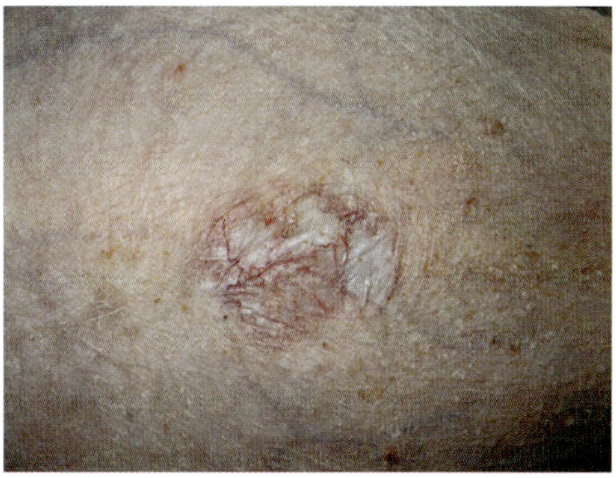

■ **Fig. 26.7.** Focal patch of severe epidermal atrophy on the ventrum of the patient in Figure 26.6. The skin palpates as paper-thin, with fragile vessels and phlebectasia.

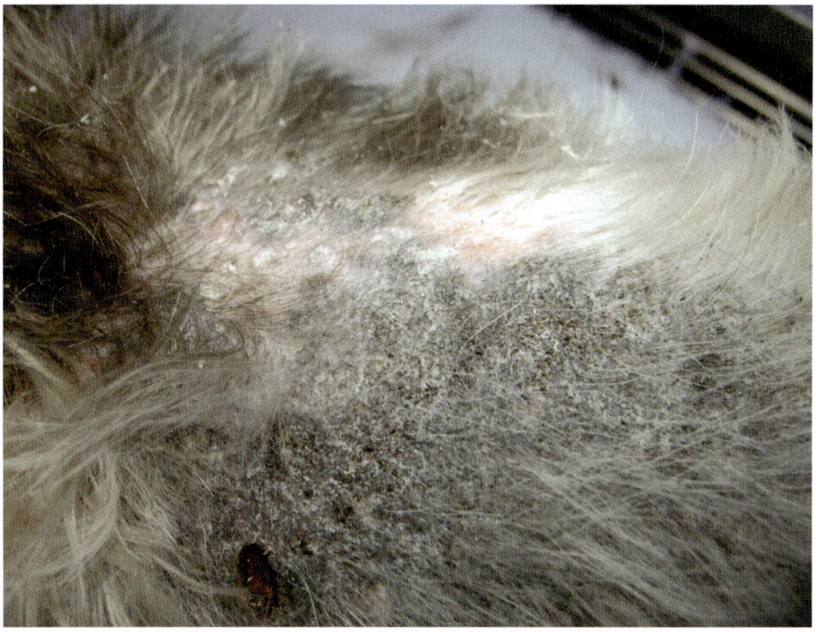

■ **Fig. 26.8.** Demodicosis and bacterial folliculitis secondary to hyperadrenocorticism in a 13-year-old female-spayed shih tzu. Hyperpigmentation and crusting are frequent findings with demodicosis.

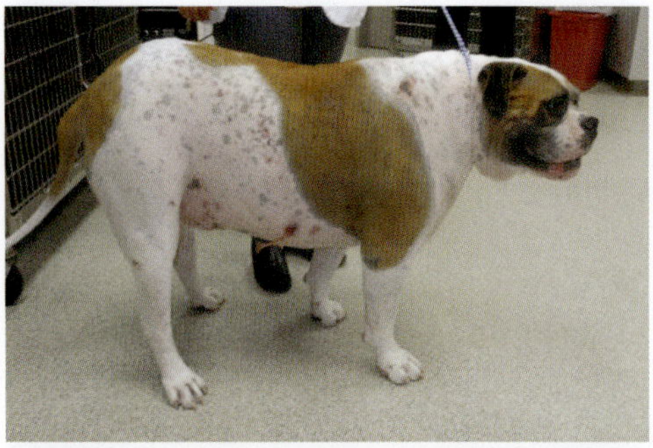

(a)

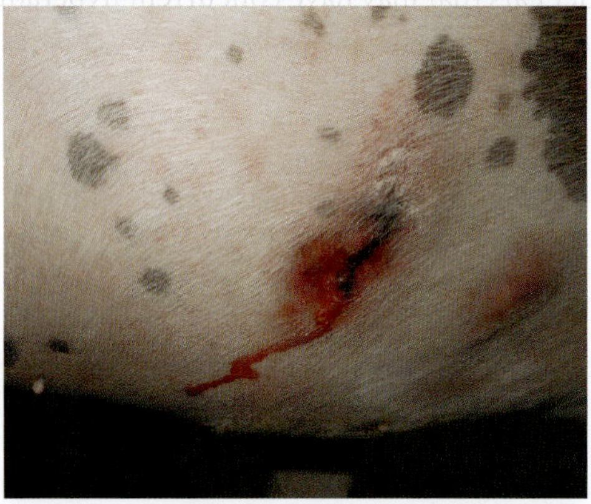

(b)

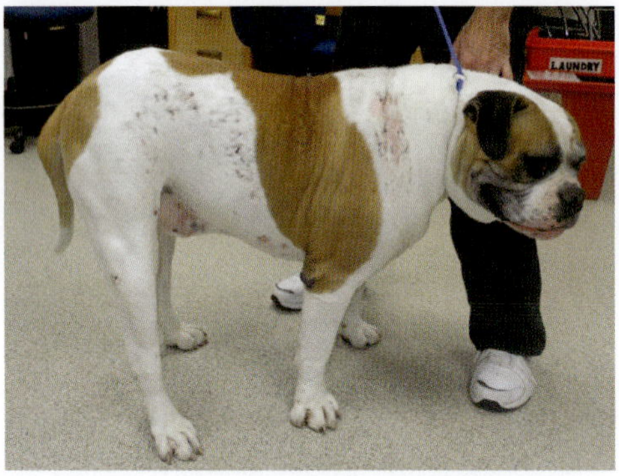

(c)

■ **Fig. 26.9.** (a) Body conformation changes, diffuse alopecia, and (b) secondary deep bacterial folliculitis secondary to chronic corticosteroid administration in a 5-year-old male-castrate American bulldog at the time of diagnosis and (c) 6 months after corticosteroid withdrawal. Note normalization of body conformation, regrowth of hair coat, and healing of infection (with scarring).

chapter 27

Hyperadrenocorticism, Feline Skin Fragility Syndrome

DEFINITION/OVERVIEW

- A disorder of multifactorial causes characterized by extremely fragile skin.
- Tends to occur in older cats that may have concurrent hyperadrenocorticism, diabetes mellitus, by excessive use of megestrol acetate or other progestational compounds, or as a paraneoplastic syndrome.
- A small number of cats have no evidence of biochemical abnormalities.

SIGNALMENT/HISTORY

- Rare, naturally occurring disease tends to be recognized in older cats (median age 10–11 years) with females slightly overrepresented.
- Iatrogenic cases have no age predilection.
- No breed predisposition.

Risk Factors

- Hyperadrenocorticism (HAC): pituitary (PDH) or adrenal dependent (ADH).
- HAC: PDH 75–80%, ADH 20–25% (75% benign adenomas).
- Iatrogenic cases: secondary to excessive corticosteroid or progestational drug administration.
- Diabetes mellitus (DM): rare, unless associated with hyperadrenocorticism (80–90% of hyperadrenocorticism cases experience late-phase DM).
- Possibly idiopathic or paraneoplastic syndrome.

Historical Findings

- Gradual onset of clinical signs.
- Polyuria and polydipsia most often reported.
- Progressive alopecia (not always present).
- Often associated with weight loss, lusterless coat, poor appetite, and lack of energy.

Blackwell's Five-Minute Veterinary Consult Clinical Companion: Small Animal Dermatology, Third Edition.
Karen Helton Rhodes and Alexander H. Werner.

CLINICAL FEATURES

- May be associated with rat tail, pinnal folding, pot belly appearance (Figure 27.1).
- Seborrheic coat.
- Skin becomes markedly thin (atrophic) and fragile; easily torn with normal handling (Figures 27.2–27.6).
- Skin bleeds minimally upon tearing (Figure 27.7).
- Multiple both new and healing lacerations; may become secondarily infected (Figure 27.8).
- Partial (thinning) to complete alopecia of the truncal region may be noted (Figure 27.9).
- HAC cases: polyphagia, polyuria, polydipsia, lethargy, weight change (gain or loss), unkempt coat, coat color change, recurrent infections, muscle atrophy, bruising, peripheral neuropathy, CNS abnormality (circling, vocalization, obtundation, blindness, incoordination).
- Iatrogenic HAC: risk for corticosteroid-associated congestive heart failure.

DIFFERENTIAL DIAGNOSIS

- Cutaneous asthenia
- Trauma/recurrent skin injury
- Hyperthyroidism
- Feline paraneoplastic syndrome: pancreatic neoplasia, hepatic lipidosis, cholangiocarcinoma

DIAGNOSTICS

CBC/Biochemistry/Urinalysis

- HAC: inconsistent increases in serum ALT, alkaline phosphatase and cholesterol; mild proteinuria.
- Approximately 80–90% of cats with hyperadrenocorticism have concurrent diabetes mellitus (hyperglycemia, glucosuria).

Other Laboratory Tests

- Urine cortisol-creatinine ratio: screening test as in dogs; may be elevated in cats with HAC; may be used as a diagnostic test to distinguish between ADH and PDH.
- ACTH stimulation test: up to 70% of cats with hyperadrenocorticism have an exaggerated response; false positives due to systemic illness; best test to distinguish between spontaneous and iatrogenic HAC; suppressed response may be due to iatrogenic HAC

or a sex hormone-secreting adrenal neoplasia; cortisol levels measured before and 30 minutes after administration of intravenous 0.125 mg synthetic corticotropin.
- LDDST: requires use of 0.1 mg/kg dexamethasone IV (10× higher dose than dogs).
- HDDST: requires 1 mg/kg dexamethasone IV; unreliable for discriminating between ADH and PDH – 50% of PDH cases will fail to suppress.
- Endogenous plasma ACTH levels: must be collected on EDTA and immediately chilled; high levels expected with PDH, low levels expected with ADH.

Imaging

- Abdominal ultrasonography: bilateral symmetric adrenal glands (normal to increased size) with PDH; unilateral adrenomegaly with ADH – adrenal masses are often small until end-stage disease; may be useful to assess for abdominal metastases and tumor expansion into the vena cava in cases of ADH.
- CT and MRI: small pituitary tumors (microadenomas) may be difficult to visualize; MRI may be more successful.

Pathologic Findings

- Histopathology: variable results suggestive but not diagnostic: decreased dermal collagen; atrophic epidermis and dermis; attenuated collagen fibers.

THERAPEUTICS

- Underlying metabolic disease should be ruled out.
- Many patients are debilitated and require supportive care.
- Surgical correction of the lacerations is not helpful because the tissue cannot withstand pressure from sutures.
- Protect skin: clothing, reduce activities that can traumatize the skin, remove sharp edges from the environment, prevent damage from interaction with other animals.
- Hyperadrenocorticism: adrenalectomy may be the preferred treatment.
- Radiation therapy: variable success in the treatment of pituitary tumors.

Drugs of Choice

- Medical management: may be useful for preparing patient for surgery and for minimizing postoperative complications (e.g., infections and poor wound healing).
- No known effective medical therapy for feline hyperadrenocorticism.
- o,p'-DDD (mitotane): 12.5–50 mg/kg PO BID; typically poor response; side effects include anorexia, vomiting, and diarrhea.
- Ketoconazole (Nizoral): 5–10 mg/kg PO BID to TID; typically poor response.
- Metyrapone: 65 mg/kg PO BID.
- Trilostane: 0.5–12 mg/kg PO q24h to BID; begin with 10 mg q24h and gradually increase (as needed) to 10 mg/kg q24h based on ACTH stimulation testing; some cats

are better managed with divided twice-daily dosing; if receiving insulin twice daily, trilostane should be given to coincide with insulin administration; effective in cats with no reported side effects; decreases clinical signs of HAC; improves regulation of diabetes but may not resolve diabetes.

Precautions/Interactions

- Hyperadrenocorticism: closely monitor diabetic cat; adjust insulin to prevent hypoglycemia when the cortisol levels fall.

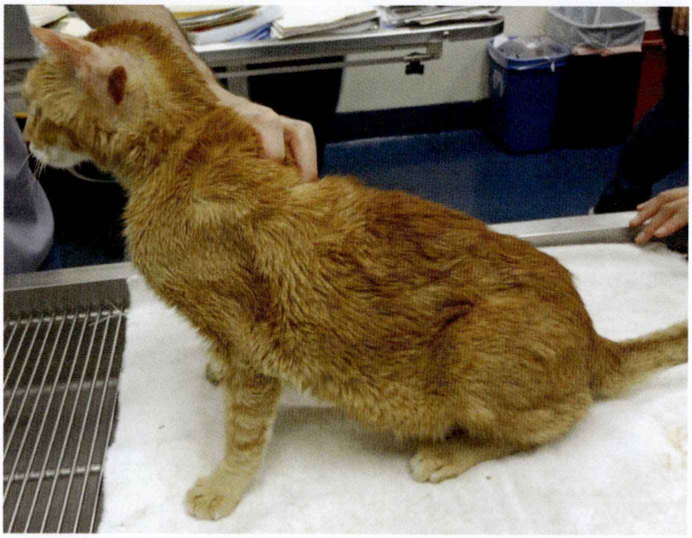

■ **Fig. 27.1.** Generalized poor hair coat and distended belly appearance of a 16-year-old male-castrate DSH with naturally acquired hyperadrenocorticism. Note alopecia of and epidermal injury at the base of the left pinna.

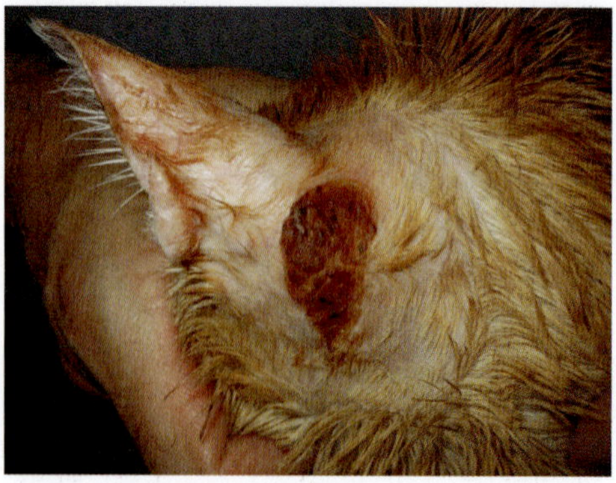

■ **Fig. 27.2.** Closer image of alopecia and a healing epidermal tear at the base of the left pinna of patient in Figure 27.1.

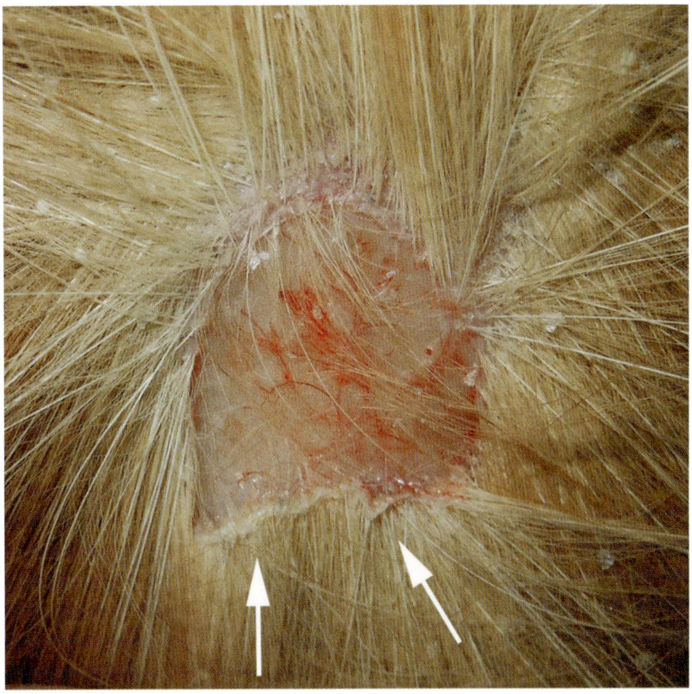

■ **Fig. 27.3.** Skin torn by simple combing of patient in Figures 27.1 and 27.2. Peeling of the epidermis is most evident at the lower margin (*arrows*).

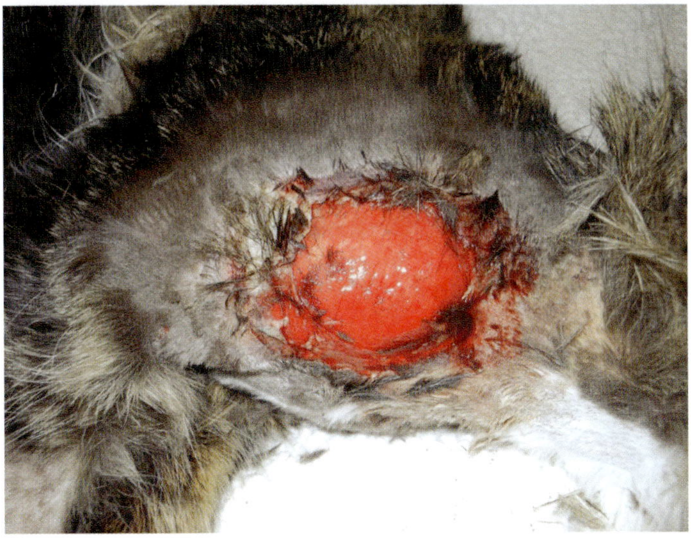

■ **Fig. 27.4.** Large skin defect on the neck of a 1-year-old male-castrate DMH from iatrogenic hyperadrenocorticism.

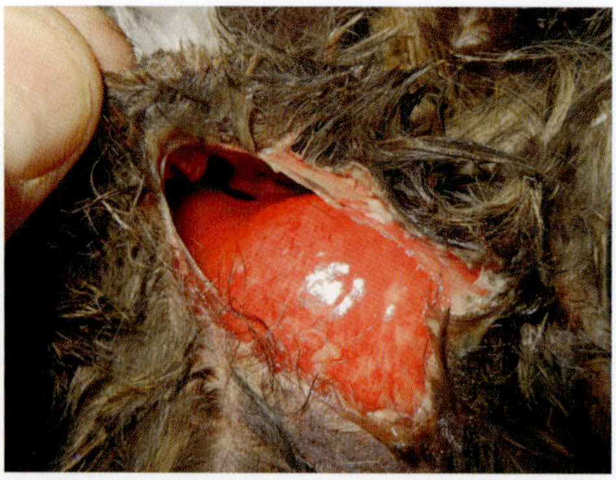

■ **Fig. 27.5.** The skin is easily pulled away from the underlying tissues of patient in Figure 27.4. Note bruising of the skin at the lower edge of the defect.

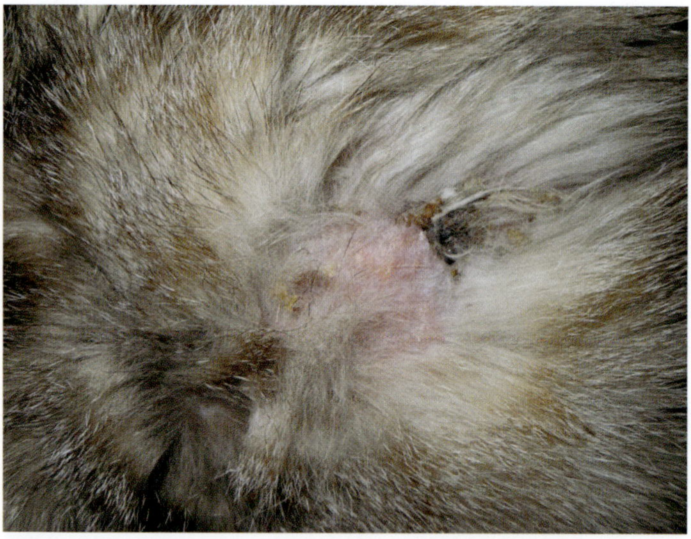

■ **Fig. 27.6.** Skin tear similar in appearance to lesions of hyperadrenocorticism caused by administration of megestrol acetate to a 10-year-old female-spayed Siamese.

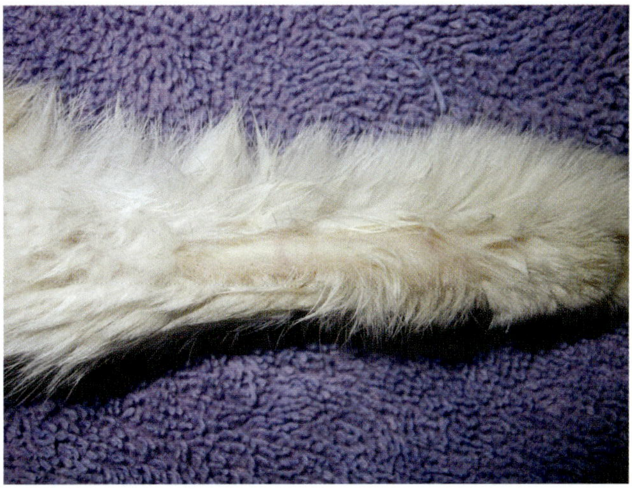

■ **Fig. 27.7.** Fragility of the skin resulting in tearing on the extremity of a 17-year-old female-spayed DLH treated with oral corticosteroids for inflammatory bowel disease. Note that despite the large defect, there is no accompanying hemorrhage.

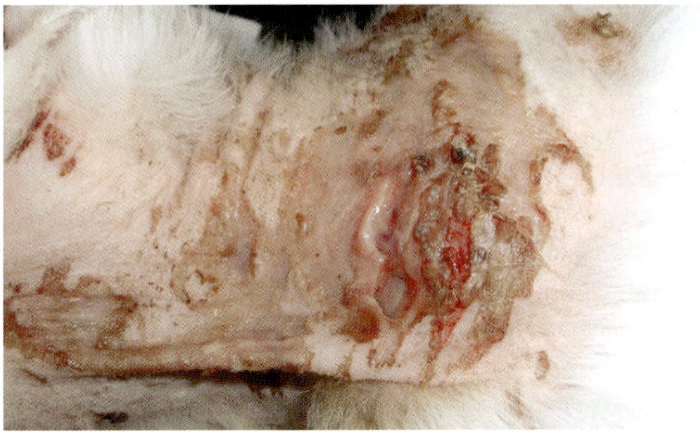

■ **Fig. 27.8.** Multiple healing and new skin tears with secondary bacterial infection in a 6-year-old male-castrate DSH from chronic use of corticosteroids for treatment of eosinophilic granuloma.

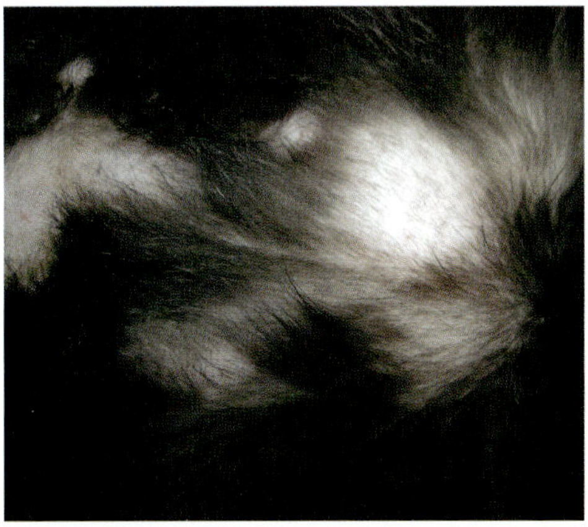

■ **Fig. 27.9.** Patchy to diffuse thinning of hair coat on the ventrum of a 6-year-old male-castrate DSH due to chronic administration of corticosteroids.

chapter 28

Hypothyroidism

DEFINITION/OVERVIEW

- Decreased production of thyroid hormones (tetraiodothyronine – T_4; triiodothyronine – T_3) by the thyroid gland.
- Thyroid hormones are essential for normal growth and development: inadequate thyroid hormone affects many metabolic processes and nearly every organ system.
- Thyroid hormones are necessary for the normal maturation of skin and initiation of the anagen phase of the follicle cycle.
- Hypothyroidism is the most common endocrine disorder in dogs; hypothyroidism is also the most overdiagnosed endocrinopathy in dogs due to the lack of a single readily available and reliable test for hypothyroidism.
- Clinical signs of hypothyroidism mimic those of other causes of alopecia.
- Dermatologic signs include lack of hair coat growth, dull dry brittle coat, initial alopecia in areas of wear (bridge of nose, elbows, tail), becoming more widespread along the entire trunk in a symmetric distribution, myxedema, hyperpigmentation, seborrhea, and recurrent bacterial folliculitis.
- Treatment is by thyroid hormone (T_4) supplementation.

ETIOLOGY/PATHOPHYSIOLOGY

- Thyrotropin (TSH) released by the pituitary gland is the major modulator of hormone secretion by the thyroid gland; T_3 inhibits TSH secretion.
- Effect of thyrotropin-releasing hormone from the hypothalamus on overall activity of the thyroid gland unclear; tertiary hypothyroidism not documented in dogs or cats.
- Thyroid hormones in plasma primarily protein bound; less than 1% is "free" in circulation; pituitary-thyroid axis functions to maintain free T_4 (fT_4) levels.
- T_3 is the metabolically active hormone; T_4 is primarily a prohormone.
- T_4: over 80% of secreted hormone; biologic activity upregulated by conversion to the active form (T_3) in peripheral tissues; conversion to reverse T_3 (rT_3) reduces activity.
- Only unbound hormone penetrates cells and has biologic activity.

Blackwell's Five-Minute Veterinary Consult Clinical Companion: Small Animal Dermatology, Third Edition.
Karen Helton Rhodes and Alexander H. Werner.

- Primary hypothyroidism is a defect in thyroid tissue causing a decrease in the secretion of thyroid hormone.
- Two forms of primary canine hypothyroidism: (naturally occurring and acquired):
  - Naturally occurring/congenital
    - Rare congenital thyroid agenesis
    - Dysgenesis
    - Dyshormogenesis (typically results in early death)
  - Acquired:
    - More than 90% of cases
    - Thyroid tissue is replaced or destroyed
    - Lymphocytic thyroiditis – most common form of canine hypothyroidism
    - Immune-mediated destruction of the thyroid gland
    - Idiopathic thyroid atrophy considered an end stage of lymphocytic thyroiditis rather than a distinct disorder
    - Autoantibodies to thyroid antigens (antithyroglobulin antibodies).
- Naturally occurring secondary canine hypothyroidism: failure of the pituitary gland to secrete TSH; often associated with pituitary dwarfism and pituitary neoplasia (Figures 28.1, 28.2)
- Acquired secondary canine hypothyroidism (impaired TSH secretion): caused by pituitary tumors, medications (glucocorticoids, sulfonamides, phenobarbital) or concurrent illness, including naturally occurring hypercortisolism
- Hypothyroidism due to dietary iodine deficiency is rare
- Alternative proposed causes include impaired conversion to active T_3 and/or increased conversion to rT_3 due to steroid hormone abnormalities (corticosteroid or estrogen) or poor absorption of replacement supplementation
- Hypothyroidism in cats most often follows bilateral thyroidectomy or radioactive iodine therapy for thyroid neoplasia.

SIGNALMENT/HISTORY

- Most common endocrinopathy of dogs: prevalence 1:250.
- Primary congenital reported in toy fox terrier, giant schnauzer, bullmastiff, Scottish deerhound, German shepherd, Abyssinian cat.
- Heritable: beagle, borzoi, Great Dane, doberman pinschers, German short-haired pointer.
- Predisposed breeds: mostly medium and large breed dogs; golden retriever, Great Dane, doberman pinscher, Irish setter, Airedale terrier, Old English sheepdog, dachshund, miniature schnauzer, Brittany and cocker spaniel, shar-pei, chow chow, poodle, Irish wolfhound, English bulldog, Newfoundland, malamute, and boxer.
- Peak age of onset at 5 years (mean 7 years); younger age of onset seen in larger breeds.
- No sex predilection; neutered male and female dogs have an increased risk over intact dogs.

CLINICAL FEATURES

- Early symptoms are nonspecific: slow progression of clinical signs often delays diagnosis.
- Systemic symptoms primarily associated with decreased metabolic function.
- Initial symptoms:
  - Malaise
  - Mental dullness; rare seizures, ataxia, coma
  - Exercise and cold intolerance
  - Behavior change
  - Obesity
  - Intact animals may demonstrate reproductive dysfunction (e.g., decreased fertility, failure to cycle).
- Nondermatologic symptoms reported with moderate frequency:
  - Peripheral neuropathy (occasionally acute)
  - Cranial nerve deficits (Horner's syndrome)
  - Generalized myopathy (weakness)
  - Megaesophagus
  - Laryngeal paralysis
  - Corneal lipidosis
  - Recovery with supplementation may be rapid for neuropathy and myopathy but is not consistent with megaesophagus or laryngeal paralysis.
- Dermatologic changes:
  - Hair coat changes seen in greater than 40% of cases:
    - Dull, brittle hair coat (Figure 28.3)
    - Change in coat quality – preferential loss of primary guard hairs, leaving the fine undercoat more visible and giving the appearance of a "puppy" coat (Figure 28.4)
    - Easily epilated hairs
    - Failure to regrow hair coat after clipping; seen initially as loss of coat in areas of friction or pressure (e.g., collar, lateral elbows, lateral hocks) (Figure 28.5)
    - Reduced hair coat growth following shedding; hypertrichosis has been described in boxers and Irish setters due to retention of dead hair coat
    - Hair coat color change (most often lightening), especially at the tips of the hair
    - Initial alopecia may be patchy and asymmetric.
- Advanced cutaneous symptoms:
  - Bilaterally symmetric alopecia; usually truncal, sparing head and extremities (Figure 28.6)
  - Pinnal alopecia and scaling
  - Alopecic or "rat" tail (Figure 28.7)
  - Edematous appearance to skin (myxedema and mucinosis) (Figures 28.8, 28.9)

- "Tragic" facial expression
- Significant hyperkeratosis/seborrheic dermatitis
- Hyperpigmentation, lichenification, and comedones in alopecic regions
- Bacterial folliculitis (Figure 28.10).

- Recurrent pyoderma: caused by decreased T cell function and humoral immunity as well as by alterations in the local epithelial environment.
- *Malassezia* dermatitis.
- Demodicosis.
- Otitis externa.
- Poor wound healing.
- Bruising.
- Pruritus uncommon unless associated with secondary infection.

DIFFERENTIAL DIAGNOSIS

- Hyperadrenocortisolism: often associated with other systemic symptoms; exogenous or endogenous source.
- Sex hormone abnormalities (adrenal, extraadrenal, and gonadal).
- Follicular dysplasia.
- Telogen effuvium.
- Alopecia due to systemic illness or secondary to medical therapy.
- Pattern alopecia including cyclic flank alopecia.
- Primary keratinization disorder.

DIAGNOSTICS

CBC/Biochemistries

- Normocytic, normochromic, nonregenerative anemia (approximately 30% of cases).
- Fasting hypercholesterolemia (greater than 75% of cases).
- Fasting hypertriglyceridemia; gross lipemia.

Thyroid Hormone Concentration

- Total T_4:
  - Reports both protein-bound and free T_4
  - Usually below normal range in hypothyroidism
  - Tests ability of the thyroid gland to produce hormone
  - Low T_4 measurement must be associated with appropriate clinical signs for presumption of hypothyroidism; additional tests (e.g., fT_4, TSH measurement) recommended to aid diagnosis
  - Autoantibodies to T_4 will affect results
  - Lower ranges in certain breeds (e.g., greyhound)
  - Wide fluctuations occur in normal dogs.
  - Declines noted with age, estrus, pregnancy, obesity, and malnutrition

- Sick euthryoid syndrome: low serum T_4 due to nonthyroidal illness
- Specific diseases known to decrease baseline T_4: renal failure, hepatic failure, systemic and cutaneous infection, diabetes mellitus, hyperadrenocortisolism, and hypoadrenocorticism
- Specific medications known to decrease baseline T_4: glucocorticoids, sulfonamides, nonsteroidal antiinflammatory drugs, phenobarbital, and tricyclic antidepressants
- In-house (ELISA) tests may be less reliable than radioimmunoassay tests.

■ fT_4:
- Measures active hormone
- Recommend measure by equilibrium dialysis to remove effect of antithyroglobulin antibodies
- Less affected by concurrent diseases (with the exception of hyperadrenocortisolism)
- Not recommended as a stand-alone test; many experts prefer measurement of both total T_4 and fT_4 as the protocol for diagnosis of hypothyroidism.

■ Total T_3/fT_3/rT_3:
- Total T_3 levels fluctuate widely; measurement not an accurate indicator of thyroid gland status
- Hypothyroid dogs often have normal T_3
- No elevation in reverse T_3 levels in canine sick-euthyroid conditions as seen in human patients
- Autoantibodies to T_3 will affect results.

■ TSH:
- High specificity, low sensitivity; useful as a confirmatory test, not as a stand-alone test for diagnosis of hypothyroidism
- Hypothyroid dogs may have normal TSH results; normal dogs may have elevated TSH results
- Elevated TSH in conjunction with low T_4 consistent with diagnosis of hypothyroidism
- Further evaluation for thyroiditis or repeat measurement of values in 1–3 months warranted for incongruent results.

■ Antithyroglobulin antibodies:
- Found in more than 50% of hypothyroid dogs
- Can occur in euthyroid dogs (25–35%)
- May indicate developing thyroiditis in dogs with normal thyroid hormone levels; may interfere with tests to falsely elevate total T_4
- May be useful in dogs with equivocal thyroid hormone levels
- May interfere with hormone assays resulting most often in increased test results.

■ TSH stimulation test:
- Determines thyroid function
- Baseline and post administration of TSH measurement of T_4
- Euthyroid: post-T_4 result within or above high normal range for T_4
- Nonthyroidal illness (sick-euthyroid): blunted response, but post-T_4 result within normal range for T_4

- Hypothyroid: pre- and post-T4 results below normal range
- Requires 8-week withdrawal period for dogs currently on T_4 supplementation for accurate TSH stimulation testing
- TSH stimulation testing can be run concurrently with corticotropin stimulation testing or a dexamethasone suppression test with no compromise in accuracy
- Recombinant human TSH can be used but is prohibitively expensive.

- Additional tests:
  - TRH stimulation test: response variable and smaller than with TSH; not practical; may help differentiate primary hypothyroidism from secondary or tertiary hypothyroidism
  - Thyroid gland biopsy: definitive diagnostic test; impractical with potential complications; pathologic findings in lymphocytic thyroiditis include infiltration of lymphocytes, macrophages and plasma cells with eventual destruction of thyroid parenchyma and replacement with fibrous connective tissue
  - Thyroid gland ultrasound: useful; euthyroid and sick-euthyroid dogs will have normal thyroid gland size; decreased thyroid gland size in hypothyroid dogs
  - Therapeutic trial: unreliable for diagnosis of hypothyroidism based on dermatologic abnormalities; thyroid hormone supplementation produces similar initial effects (e.g., hair growth, increased activity) in both euthyroid and hypothyroid dogs; prompt measurement of post-pill T_4 levels may reveal significantly elevated results in euthyroid dogs
  - Dermatohistopathology: often not specifically diagnostic for hypothyroidism; more indicative of endocrinopathy; epidermal and follicular infundibular hyperplasia and hyperkeratosis (epidermal atrophy more commonly noted in other endocrinopathies); predominance of telogen follicles; sebaceous gland hyperplasia; mucinosis/myxedema, vacuolated arrector pili muscle, frequent finding of bacterial folliculitis.

THERAPEUTICS

General Considerations

- Diet: reduced fat as indicated by abnormalities in serum lipid measurements.
- Life-long treatment necessary.
- Response to therapy: within 7 days for neuropathy and severe systemic signs; 4–6 weeks for laboratory abnormalities and general systemic signs; 1–3 months for dermatologic conditions (Figure 28.11).
- Thyrotoxicosis: seen as tachycardia, diarrhea, polyuria, polydypsia, polyphagia, pruritus, and anxiousness or behavioral changes.

Drugs of Choice

- Synthetic L-thyroxine (levothyroxine sodium): supplement of choice.
- Bioavailability may vary between formulations and with generics.

- Synthetic T_3 (liothyronine; 4–6 µg/kg TID) administration is not recommended unless impaired absorption of T_4 is suspected (very rare); thyrotoxicosis more likely with T_3 supplementation.
- Levothyroxine: serum half-life 12–16 hours; peak concentration 4–6 hours after administration.
- Initial dosage of levothyroxine: 15–20 µg/kg BID; this dosage is considerably higher than standard dosages for humans and may confuse pharmacists.
- Lowered initial dosage required for patients with congestive heart failure, renal disease, diabetes mellitus, seizure conditions, and hypoadrenocortisolism; initial dosage 10 µg/kg BIDto prevent destabilization by increased metabolic rate and cardiac demands.
- Thyroxine binds to soy and calcium; it should be given 1 hour before or 3 hours after a meal.
- Glucocorticoids, NSAIDS, and furosemide may increase absorption; low-dose corticosteroid administration may be used to increase absorption of T_4 in patients with poor response to levothyroxine administration.

Monitoring of Therapy

- Initial measurement 4–6 weeks after initiation of supplementation.
- Sample collection 4–6 hours after levothyroxine administration; consistency in monitoring is required for proper management.
- Total T_4 level should be within the normal range; reported parameters for treatment monitoring vary by laboratory; results near the middle of the reference range preferred.
- Alternative method of monitoring: T_4 measurement of trough (just prior to administration of levothyroxine) and 4–6 hours post administration; trough level should be at the low end and peak level should be at the upper end of the reference range; particularly useful for cases supplemented only once daily.
- Repeat measurements 4 weeks after each dosage change.
- Measurement of stable patients recommended at 6-month intervals.
- TSH levels, if elevated prior to supplementation, should return to normal to low with therapy; interpretation of adequate supplementation cannot currently be based solely on measurement of TSH levels.

Alternative Therapy Options

- Twice-daily supplementation considered standard.
- Once-daily supplementation may be attempted when symptoms of hypothyroidism have resolved; if attempted, monitor for return of symptoms indicating that twice-daily administration is required in a particular patient.
- Variability of drug absorption may not permit effective once-daily treatment.
- Determination of success of once-daily treatment based on continued resolution of clinical symptoms of hypothyroidism.
- Intravenous L-thyroxine (4–5 µg/kg BID) used to treat hypothyroid crisis (myxedema coma).

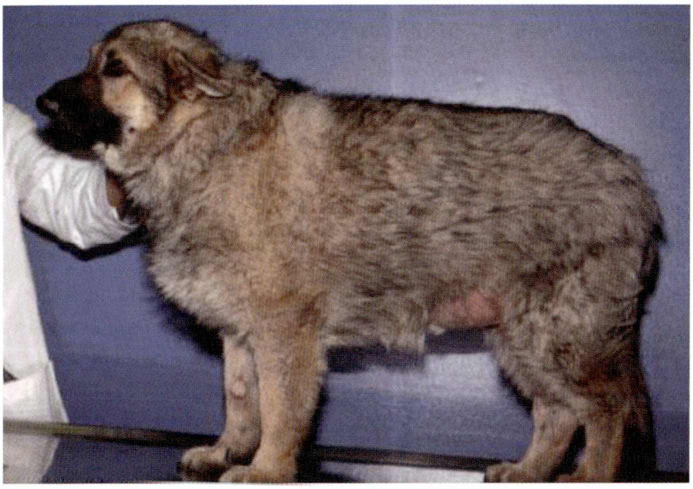

■ **Fig. 28.1.** Pituitary dwarfism in a young German shepherd.

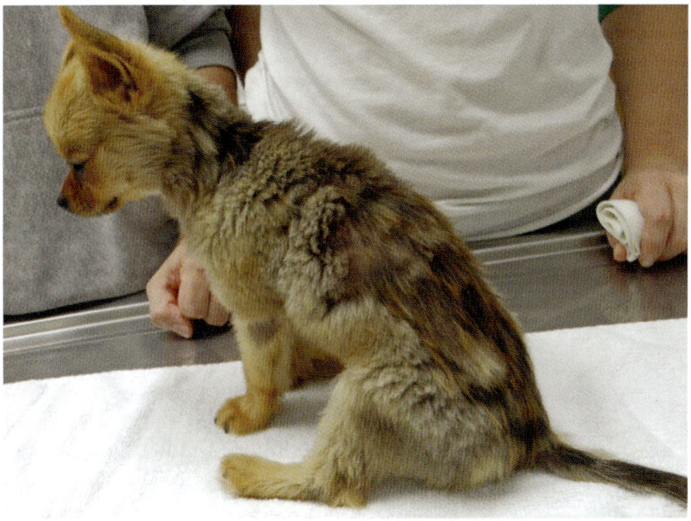

■ **Fig. 28.2.** Pituitary dwarfism with hypothyroidism in a 1-year-old male-castrate pomeranian.

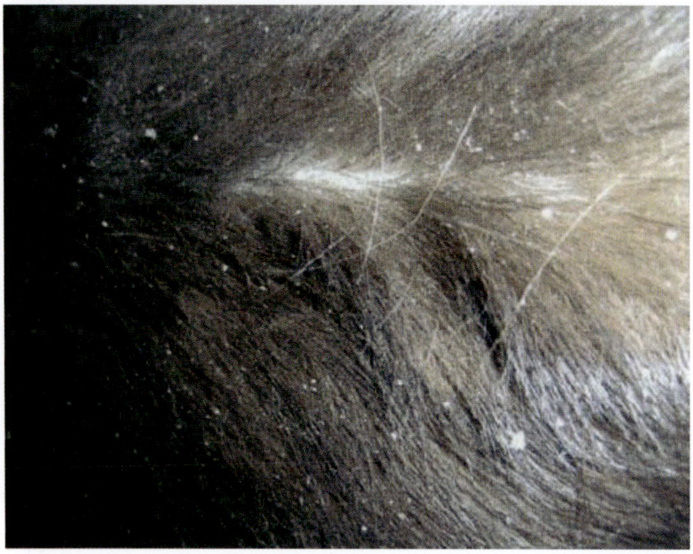

■ **Fig. 28.3.** Excessive scaling with dull brittle hair coat commonly seen with hypothyroidism.

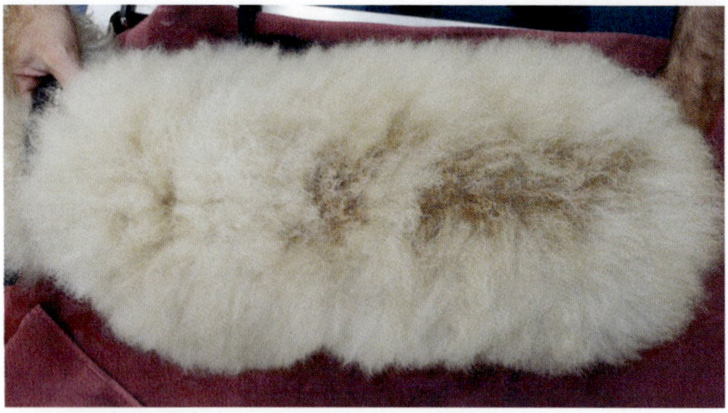

■ **Fig. 28.4.** Hair coat color and quality change in hypothyroidism. The darker and thicker primary hair coat has thinned and been replaced by the lighter colored and thinner secondary hair coat in this 5-year-old male-castrate poodle mix.

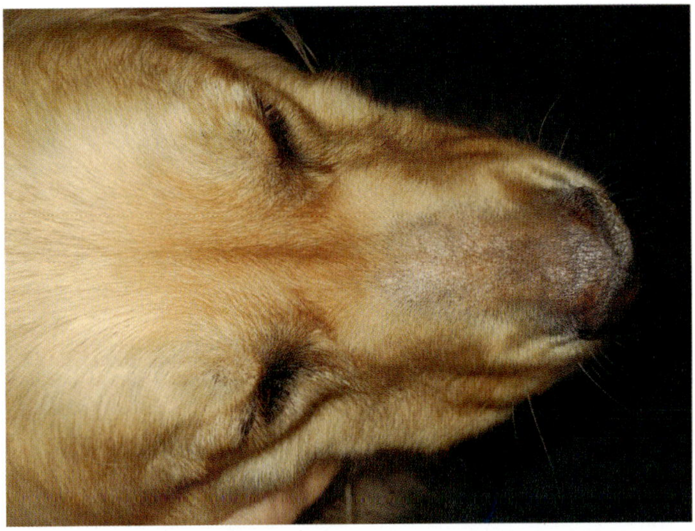

■ **Fig. 28.5.** Alopecia and mild myxedema of the face in a 4-year-old male-castrate golden retriever. The hair coat has been worn thin on the dorsal muzzle.

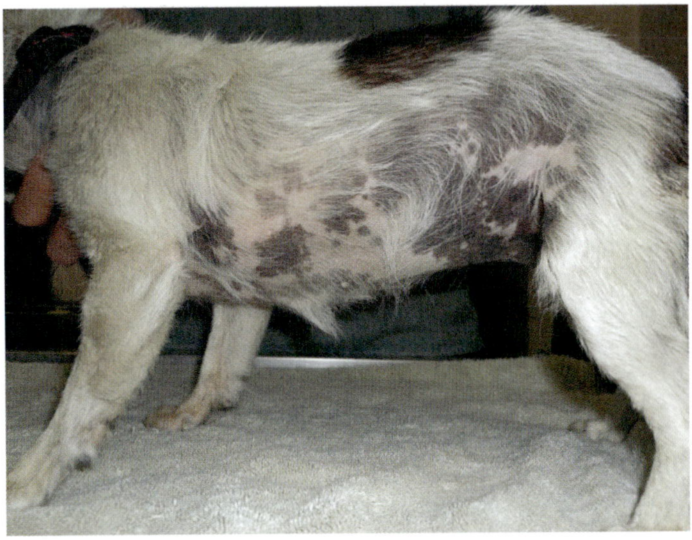

■ **Fig. 28.6.** Generalized thinning of the hair coat in a classic "endocrine" pattern on the body of an 8-year-old female-spayed chihuahua.

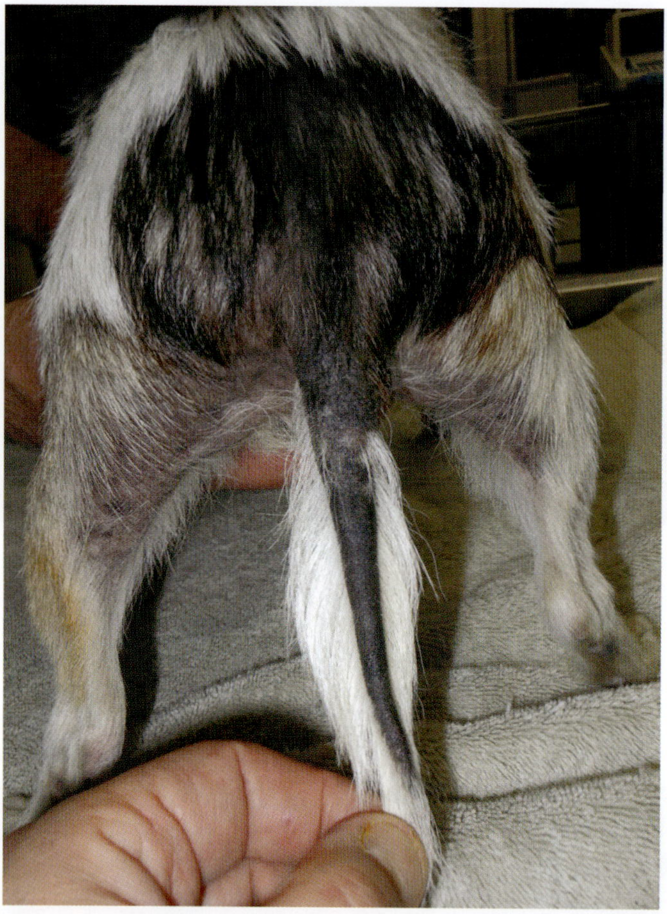

■ **Fig. 28.7.** Caudal image of the patient in Figure 28.6 demonstrating a "rat" tail appearance with alopecia and hyperpigmentation on the dorsum of the tail as well as on the caudal thighs.

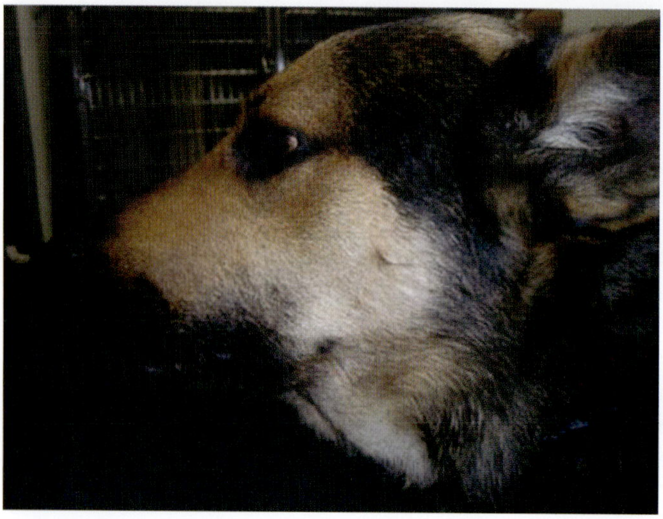

■ **Fig. 28.8.** Facial myxedema due to hypothyroidism in a 6-year-old female-spayed German shepherd mix.

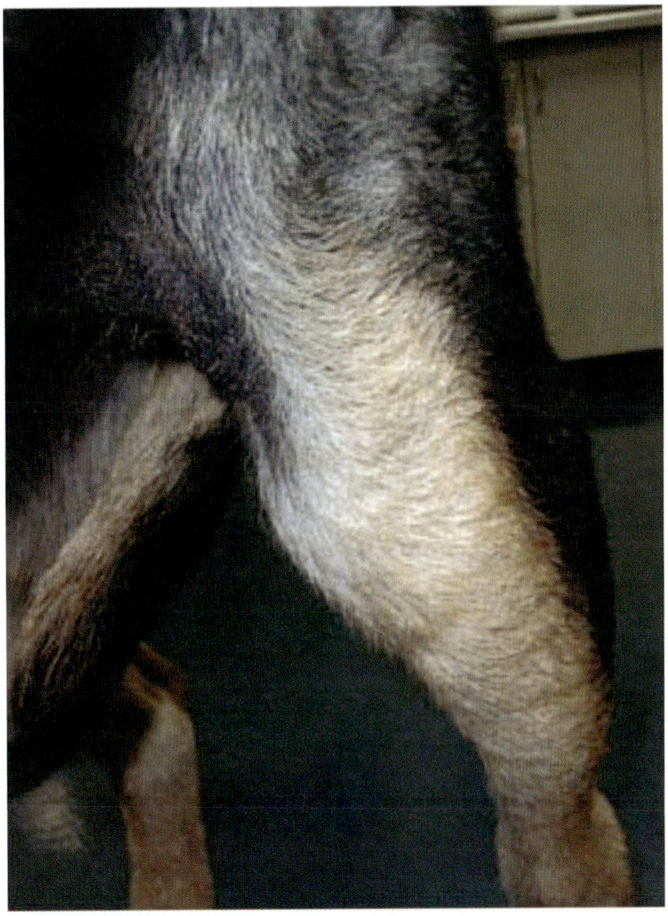

■ **Fig. 28.9.** Myxedema of the extremity of the patient in Figure 28.8.

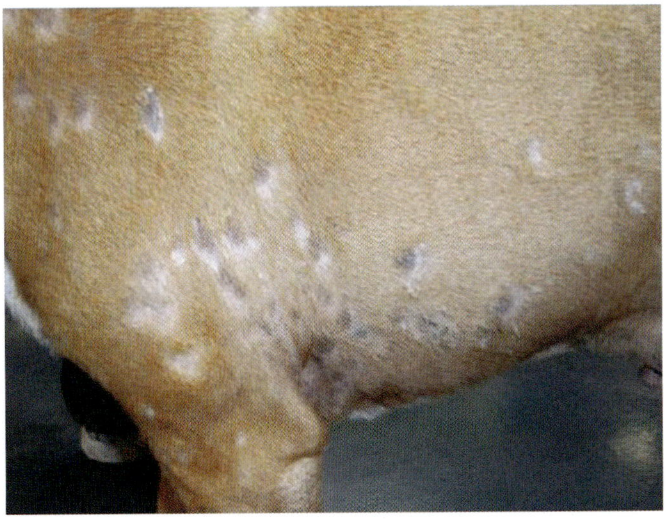

■ **Fig. 28.10.** Bacterial folliculitis secondary to hypothyroidism producing a "moth-eaten" appearance with punctate lesions of alopecia and scaling in a 4-year-old female-spayed pit bull mix.

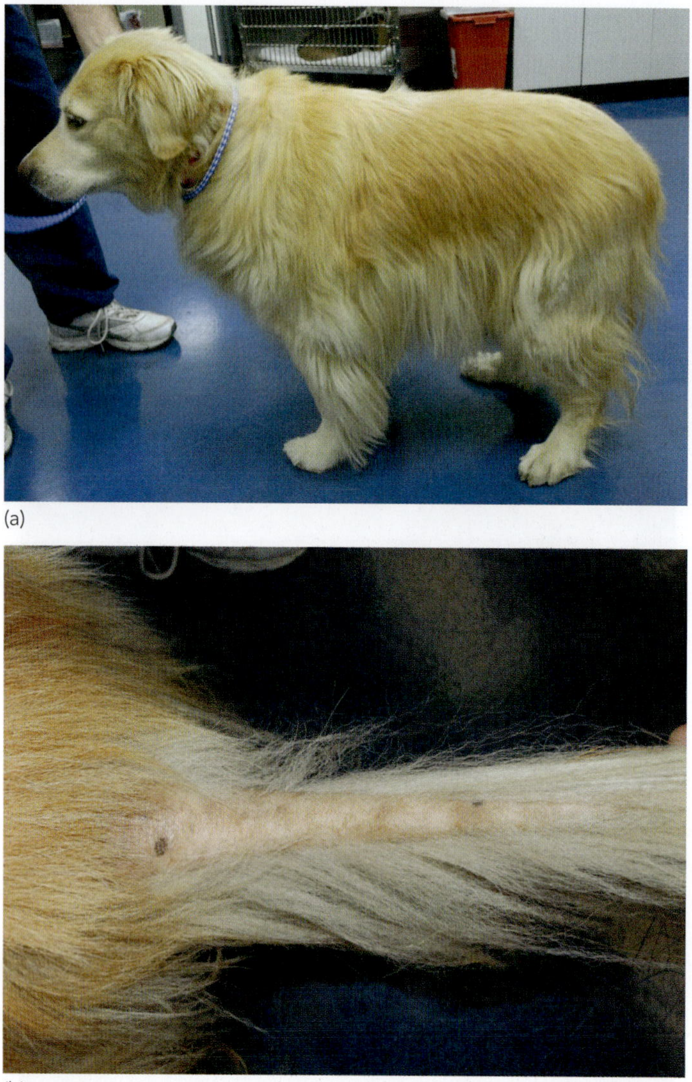

(a)

(b)

■ **Fig. 28.11.** Hypothyroidism in a 9-year-old female-spayed golden retriever before (a,b) and after (c,d) supplementation with L-thyroxine. Prior to treatment, the hair coat appeared thinner and lighter in color, with alopecia affecting the dorsum of the tail. After treatment, the hair coat has returned to a normal color and thickness, and hair regrowth on the tail is evident.

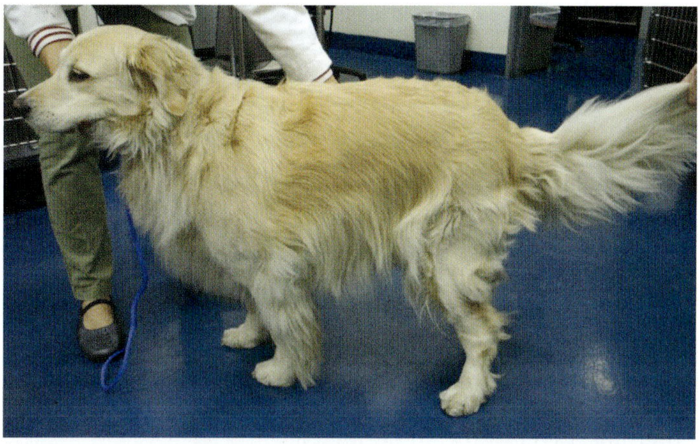

(c)

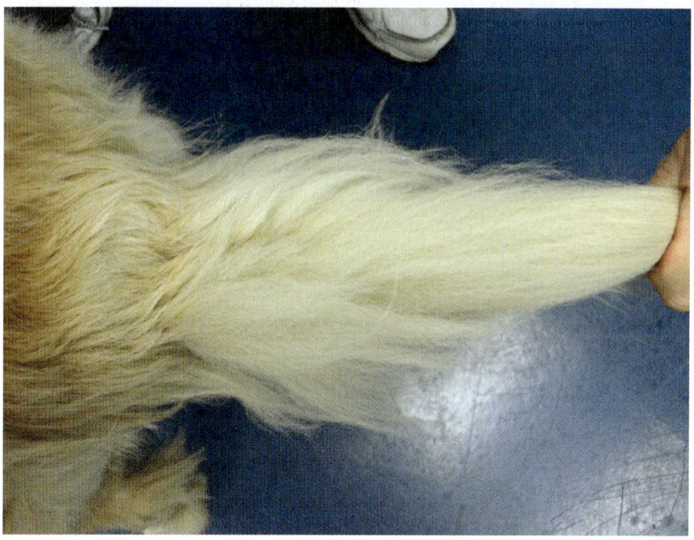

(d)

■ **Fig. 28.11.** (*Continued*)

chapter 29

Keratinization (Cornification) Disorders

DEFINITION/OVERVIEW

- Keratinization is the process by which the basal keratinocyte differentiates into the highly specialized corneocyte of the stratum corneum.
- Keratinization disorders occur when there is an inability to form a normal stratum corneum (outermost layer of the epidermis).
- Alterations in the formation, maturation, and desquamation of the epidermis result in visible abnormalities in the skin.
- Commonly referred to as *seborrhea*, a nonspecific term describing excessive scaling and crusting, with or without greasiness.
- Overall increased shedding (desquamation), as well as decreased shedding of individual epidermal cells, results in the clinical presentation of cutaneous scaling.
- The hydrophobic barrier of the stratum corneum is a fragile balance of phospholipid-derived free fatty acids, cholesterol, and ceramides; this outermost layer (epidermal lipid barrier) serves as the primary barrier between the body and the surrounding environment.
- Structural or physiologic abnormalities to the epidermal lipid barrier may cause excessive greasiness or dryness of the skin and encourage development of secondary infection.
- Keratinization disorders may be acquired (secondary to alterations induced by allergic skin disease, ectoparasitism, and/or endocrine/metabolic diseases) or inherited (ichthyotic and nonichthyotic).
- Treatment includes correction of the underlying etiology (if not primary), control of secondary infection, reduction in epidermal turnover, reduction of inflammation, restoration of epidermal barrier function, and removal of excessive epidermal accumulations.

ETIOLOGY/PATHOPHYSIOLOGY

- Keratinization disorders include a large number of syndromes and encompass dermatoses caused by a disruption in the normal and orderly process by which keratinocytes divide in the basal cell layer, mature, die, and are ultimately shed.

Blackwell's Five-Minute Veterinary Consult Clinical Companion: Small Animal Dermatology, Third Edition.
Karen Helton Rhodes and Alexander H. Werner.

- Increased production (epidermopoiesis), increased or decreased desquamation, and/or decrease in the cohesion of keratinocytes results in abnormal shedding of epidermal cells individually (fine scale) or in sheets (coarse scale).
- Normal epidermal turnover in the dog is approximately 21 days; this may decrease to as low as 7 days in primary seborrhea, resulting in a more rapid accumulation of scale.
- A flawed epidermal lipid barrier may allow transepidermal water loss (TEWL), resulting in decreased epidermal water content (loss of hydration) causing xerosis; normal skin hydration is 20–35%.
- An accelerated TEWL may be due to an inherent genetic defect in the epidermal lipid barrier (primary) or as a result of inflammatory or metabolic skin disease (secondary).
- In an attempt to heal the flawed barrier and restore normal hydrophobicity by making more lipid, the epidermis becomes hyperplastic and hyperkeratotic (thickened – seen clinically as excess scaling).
- Secondary infection (bacterial or yeast) produces inflammation and pruritus with excoriation and further epidermal damage.
- Abnormalities of sebaceous or apocrine gland function alter intercellular lipids and disrupt the epidermal barrier function.
- Primary disorders (ichthyotic and nonichthyotic): keratinization defects, in which the genetic control of epidermal cell proliferation and maturation and/or epidermal barrier formation is abnormal; known defects are related to mutations in genes that encode the structural proteins that form the corneocyte (cells of the stratum corneum) and/or enzymes responsible for lipid transport or formation.
- Secondary disorders: effects of disease alter the normal maturation and proliferation of epidermal cells; most keratinization disorders (over 80%) result from an underlying etiology.
- Assigning a specific category (primary versus secondary) for each of the discussed disorders is difficult and may be premature since the exact defect has yet to be identified.
- The nomenclature "seborrhea" is misused in the veterinary literature and may be more of an adaptive response to describe a defect in the keratinization (cornification) process; seborrhea sicca (dry scale) and seborrhea oleosa (greasy scale); seborrhea literally means "flow of sebum."

SIGNALMENT/HISTORY

- Primary: apparent by 2 years of age; characteristic in affected breeds; no sex predilection.
- Secondary: any age; any breed of dog or cat; any disorder affecting the skin can result in symptoms described as "seborrheic."
- Numerous syndromes have been identified; more frequent disorders listed below.

Primary Keratinization Disorders

- Ichthyosis:
  - Present at or near birth
  - Nonepidermolytic and epidermolytic; nonepidermolytic most common and associated with defects in various components of the epidermis; epidermolytic caused by a defect in keratin synthesis
  - Nonepidermolytic ichthyosis: autosomal recessive mutations affecting lipids and structural proteins; West Highland white terrier, golden retriever, doberman pinscher, Irish setter, collie, American bulldog, American Staffordshire terrier, Boston terrier, Labrador retriever, Jack Russell terrier, Manchester terrier, Australian terrier, cairn terrier, Norfolk terrier, Yorkshire terrier, soft-coated wheaten terrier (Figure 29.1)
  - Golden retriever ichthyosis (nonepidermolytic ichthyosis): mutation in the PNPLA1 gene that plays a role in lipid metabolism and organization in the epidermis; genetic testing available to assess for carrier status; characterized by large soft white adherent scale prominent on the trunk; diagnosed by 1 year of age (Figure 29.2)
  - American bulldog ichthyosis (nonepidermolytic ichthyosis): mutation in the NIPAL-4 gene that leads to decreased expression of the protein icthyin which is involved in epidermal lipid metabolism; genetic test available to assess carrier status; characterized by severe scruffy scaling haircoat, glabrous skin is erythematous with adherent light brown scale giving a wrinkled appearance; *Malassezia* dermatitis is a common severe secondary finding in adult dogs; clinical signs prior to weaning; may be clinically confused with canine atopic dermatitis (Figures 29.3, 29.4)
  - Keratoderma in dogue de Bordeaux: mutation in the keratin 16 gene (KRT16); hyperkeratosis of the footpad and planum nasale
  - Epidermolytic ichthyosis: mutation characterized by lysis of keratinocytes associated with hypergranulosis and hyperkeratosis corresponding with a defect in keratin formation; Rhodesian ridgeback, nasal parakeratosis of Labrador retriever, Norfolk terrier (epidermal keratin KRT10), cavalier King Charles spaniel (Figure 29.5)
  - Cavalier King Charles spaniel: keratoconjunctivitis sicca and ichthyosiform dermatosis; dry eye, curly coat, hyperkeratosis, footpad hyperkeratosis, nail dystrophy; mutation in the FAM83H gene; irregular keratin-14 labeling
  - Epidermolytic: lesions localized or generalized; large thick scales adhere to the epidermis and appear scale-like; underlying epidermis thickened with accentuated furrows and irregular texture (lichenification); erythema and exudation often present; fissures develop, especially with secondary infection; debris entrapped in the hair coat resulting in severe and generalized pigmented scaling; progressive alopecia may develop in severely affected areas; thick crusting of the footpads and nasal planum; keratin fronds produce horn-like projections (Figure 29.6)
  - Single case reported in an Abyssinian kitten.

- Primary "seborrhea" (primary keratinization disorder; idiopathic seborrhea and seborrheic dermatitis):
  - Accelerated epidermopoiesis and hyperproliferation of the epidermis, follicular infundibulum, and sebaceous gland due more likely to an adaptive response rather than to a true hereditary cellular defect
  - American cocker spaniel, English springer spaniel, West Highland white terrier, basset hound, English bulldog, German shepherd dog, doberman pinscher, Irish setter, Chinese shar-pei, miniature schnauzer, cavalier King Charles spaniel, dachshund, Labrador retriever
  - Mild to severe accumulations of scales, crusts, and greasiness; lesions discrete and focal with thickly crusted plaques and erythema, or diffuse and generalized (Figures 29.7, 29.8)
  - Ceruminous otitis externa
  - Alopecia and erythema, with lichenification, hyperpigmentation, and greasy exudation
  - Lesions predominantly truncal
  - Secondary bacterial folliculitis and *Malassezia* dermatitis common, especially in the folds of the ventral neck, axillae, and inguinum; treatment for infection reduces discomfort and malodor, but does not resolve lesions (Figure 29.9).
- Vitamin A-responsive dermatosis: rare; cocker spaniels, Labrador retrievers, miniature schnauzers, Gordon setters, French bulldogs; clinical signs similar to severe idiopathic seborrhea but usually adult onset; hyperkeratotic plaques with follicular plugging and predominant follicular casts; identified by cutaneous biopsy and response to oral vitamin A supplementation (Figure 29.10).
- Epidermal dysplasia (hyperplastic dermatosis) of West Highland white terrier: often associated with *Malassezia* infection and cutaneous hypersensitivity; may be a cause-and-effect and not a distinct syndrome; symptoms begin prior to 1 year of age; generalized and severe patches of alopecia, erythema, lichenification, and hyperpigmentation with greasiness, malodor, and pruritus; lesions begin on the trunk and skinfolds; otitis externa common (Figure 29.11).
- Generalized sebaceous gland hyperplasia in border collies and wire-haired terriers: greasy coat along the dorsum.
- Ear margin dermatosis: often secondary to hypothyroidism; primary disorder of dachshunds; thick and adherent crusts form on the medial and lateral edges of the pinnae; follicular casts; removal requires effort and produces erosions, pain, and fissuring; secondary bacterial folliculitis common (Figure 29.12).
- Acanthosis nigricans: dachshunds; less than 2 years of age; symmetric lesions of alopecia, striking hyperpigmentation and lichenification beginning in the axillae and often extending to the ventral neck and inguinum; lesions may generalize further; secondary bacterial folliculitis and *Malassezia* dermatitis common (Figure 29.13).
- Nasodigital hyperkeratosis: excessive accumulation of scale and crust on the nasal planum and footpad margins; possibly a senile change of the cocker spaniel, beagle, English bulldog, basset hound; lesions generally asymptomatic; cracking and secondary bacterial infection cause pain; similar in appearance but distinct from nasal

parakeratosis of Labrador retrievers (begins at less than 1 year of age; often more severe) (Figure 29.14).

- Footpad hyperkeratosis: severe keratin proliferations of all pads; fissuring results in secondary infection; Irish terrier, dogue de Bordeaux, Kerry blue terrier, Labrador retriever, golden retriever less than 6 months of age (Figure 29.15).
- Zinc-responsive dermatosis: supplement responsive; alopecia, dry scaling, crusting, and erythema around the eyes, ears, feet, lips, and other external orifices; two syndromes: syndrome 1 young adult dogs, primarily Siberian husky and Alaskan malamute; syndrome 2 rapidly growing, large-breed puppies (often fed an unbalanced diet) (Figures 29.16, 29.17).
- Color dilution alopecia: abnormal melanization of the hair shaft and structural hair growth; large melanosomes result in structural damage to the hair shaft and bulb; keratinization defect theorized as causative for several syndromes; blue and fawn doberman pinscher, Irish setter, dachshund, chow chow, Yorkshire terrier, poodle, Great Dane, whippet, saluki, Italian greyhound; failure to regrow blue or fawn hair with normal "point" hair growth, excessive scaliness, comedone formation, secondary pyoderma (Figures 29.18, 29.19).
- Sebaceous adenitis: autosomal recessive inheritance in the standard poodle and Akita; begins in the young adult dog; increased incidence in male dogs; caused by cell-mediated inflammation targeting the sebaceous gland and duct; may also be a response to abnormal lipid storage or keratinization; additional predisposed breeds include the samoyed, havanese, German shepherd, and vizsla; also occurs in their cross-breeds as well as in other breeds.
- Standard poodle, samoyed, and havanese: patchy or diffuse hair loss and excessive scaling; tightly adherent follicular casts ("keratin collaring"); commonly begins on the muzzle, dorsal head, and neck; most dogs are healthy and asymptomatic (Figures 29.20, 29.21).
- Akita: initial lesions similar to those of poodles but more generalized; significant alopecia; severe and deep bacterial pyoderma common as well as systemic signs of illness (Figures 29.22, 29.23).
- Vizsla: distinctly different and granulomatous; firm, coalescing plaques with fine adherent scales; lesions primarily on the trunk; also on the pinnae and face (Figure 29.24).
- Schnauzer comedo syndrome: miniature schnauzer; small comedones develop on the dorsal spine; lesions may coalesce and appear as large patches of hyperpigmentation; secondary bacterial folliculitis leads to alopecia and crusting (Figure 29.25).
- Psoriasiform-lichenoid dermatosis: predominantly in springer spaniel; also reported in English pointer, Irish setter, poodle; coalescing, crusted, erythematous papules form plaques with adherent debris; predilection for the pinnae and ventrum; may represent a staphylococcal hypersensitivity; similar pattern reported as an adverse reaction to cyclosporine (Figure 29.26).
- Acrodermatitis of bull terrier: rare; exclusively in white dogs; usually fatal; associated with decreased serum copper and zinc concentrations; lesions similar to but more severe than other metabolic and nutritional dermatoses (e.g., zinc-responsive dermatosis and superficial necrolytic dermatitis); thick crusts, papules, pustules,

erythema, and erosions on distal extremities and mucocutaneous junctions; associated with mental dullness, behavior abnormalities, diarrhea, bronchopneumonia, arched hard palate, secondary bacterial folliculitis, and *Malassezia* dermatitis; pinnal lesions and otitis externa.

- Facial dermatitis of Persian and Himalayan cats: greasy, adherent debris accumulates in facial and nasal folds; ceruminous otitis externa, secondary bacterial folliculitis, and *Malassezia* dermatitis, significant pruritus; begins between 10 months and 6 years of age (Figure 29.27).
- Primary seborrhea in newborn Persian kittens.

Secondary Keratinization Disorders

- Cutaneous hypersensitivity: atopy, flea allergic dermatitis, food allergy, and contact dermatitis; pruritus, secondary skin trauma and irritation.
- Ectoparasitism: scabies, demodicosis, and cheyletiellosis; inflammation and exfoliation (Figure 29.28).
- Bacterial folliculitis: bacterial enzymatic disadhesion and increased exfoliation of corneocytes in the attempt to shed pathogenic organisms (Figure 29.29).
- Dermatophytosis: usually exfoliative; increased shedding of infected corneocytes as primary skin mechanism in resolving fungal infection (Figure 29.30).
- Endocrinopathy:
  - Hypothyroidism: abnormal keratinization resulting in accumulation of scales, symmetric patches of alopecia, excessive sebum production; hyperpigmentation; secondary bacterial folliculitis and *Malassezia* dermatitis (Figure 29.31)
  - Hyperadrenocorticism: abnormal keratinization and decreased follicular activity; excessive scaling and secondary bacterial folliculitis; calcinosis cutis initially seen as firm, white plaques with scale (Figure 29.32)
  - Other hormonal abnormalities (e.g., sex hormone abnormalities, hyperthyroidism, and diabetes mellitus) associated with excessive scaling from metabolic abnormalities.
- Age: geriatric animals may have a dull, brittle, and scaly hair coat; alterations caused by natural changes in epidermal metabolism associated with age; no specific defect identified.
- Nutritional disorders: malnutrition and generic dog food dermatosis; scaling from abnormalities in keratinization (Figure 29.33).
- Autoimmune dermatoses: pemphigus complex – may appear exfoliative: vesicles become scaly and crusty; lupus erythematosus – cutaneous signs often appear as areas of alopecia and scaling (Figure 29.34).
- Neoplasia: primary epidermal neoplasia (epitheliotropic lymphoma); alopecia and scaling from epidermal structures damaged by infiltrating lymphocytes; preneoplastic conditions (actinic keratosis) initially appear exfoliative (Figure 29.35).
- Miscellaneous: any disease process may result in excessive scale formation owing to metabolic dyscrasia or cutaneous inflammation.
- Exfoliative disorders: rare in cats: tail gland hyperplasia, thymoma-associated exfoliative dermatitis (Figure 29.36).

CLINICAL FEATURES

- Syndromes may be visually distinctive or appear very similar.
- Focal or generalized, visible accumulations of epidermal debris.
- Small scales or large rafts of keratin.
- Excessive greasiness.
- Lichenification and hyperpigmentation with chronicity.
- Thickening of the footpads or nasal planum.
- Erosions beneath adherent keratinaceous debris.
- Fissures within thick crusts.
- Ceruminous otitis externa.
- Follicular casts.
- Comedones.
- Malodor.
- Variable pruritus leading to excoriation.
- Secondary bacterial folliculitis or *Malassezia* dermatitis.
- Nondermatologic symptoms dependent on etiology.

DIFFERENTIAL DIAGNOSIS

- Often based on the following criteria:
    - Signalment and history: paramount in distinguishing the possible causes of keratinization defect
    - Presence or absence of pruritus: noted with cutaneous hypersensitivity; primary keratinization defects often not pruritic unless secondary bacterial folliculitis or *Malassezia* dermatitis develops
    - Concurrent signs: lethargy, weight gain, polyuria/polydipsia, reproductive failure, change in body conformation, lack of hair regrowth
    - Response to therapy: antibiotics, antiyeast medication, thyroid supplementation.
- Differentiation between primary and secondary keratinization disorders based on exclusion of underlying etiology and dermatohistopathology results.

DIAGNOSTICS

- CBC/biochemistries/urinalysis: usually normal with primary keratinization disorders; mild, nonregenerative anemia and hypercholesterolemia (hypothyroidism); neutrophilia, monocytosis, eosinopenia, lymphopenia, elevated serum alkaline phosphatase, hypercholesterolemia, and hyposthenuria (hyperadrenocorticism).
- Thyroid hormone levels and adrenal function tests: see specific chapters for test recommendations.
- Skin scraping: ectoparasitism.
- Intradermal allergy test: atopy.
- Restricted-ingredient food trial: cutaneous adverse food reaction.

- Cytology of skin surface: bacteria folliculitis and/or *Malassezia* dermatitis.
- Examination of plucked hairs: macromelanosomes and structural abnormalities in follicular dysplasia and color dilution alopecia.
- Dermatohistopathology required for diagnosis.
- Genetic testing available for select disorders; Antagene-Lyon, France; Medical Genetics Department at The University of Pennsylvania School of Veterinary Medicine, USA.

THERAPEUTICS

- These disorders are characterized by damage to the integrity of the epidermal lipid barrier which results in accelerated TEWL; the skin attempts to heal the flawed barrier and produce more lipid by becoming hyperplastic and hyperkeratotic; harsh topicals may alter the "healing response" of the epidermis.
- Therapeutic focus is on identification and correction of the specific defect when possible as a means to restore the damaged epidermal lipid barrier.
- Frequent and adequate topical therapy is the cornerstone of proper treatment.
- Underbathing, rather than overbathing, is a common error.
- Diagnose and control all treatable primary and secondary diseases.
- Recurrence of secondary infections may require repeated therapy and further diagnostics.
- Maintaining control is often life-long.
- Recent treatment emphasizes restoring epidermal barrier integrity and function.

Topical Therapy

- Shampoos:
    - Contact time: 5–15 minutes; greater than 15 minutes discouraged: may result in epidermal maceration, loss of barrier function, and excessive epidermal drying and irritation
    - Hypoallergenic: useful only in mild cases of dry scale and to maintain secondary exfoliation after the primary disease has been controlled
    - Sulfur/salicylic acid: salicylic acid is keratolytic (aids desquamation by decreasing skin pH which subsequently increases water absorption in the stratum corneum); sulfur is keratolytic, keratoplastic, and bacteriostatic; moderately scaly patient; not overly drying
    - Benzoyl peroxide: strongly keratolytic and antimicrobial; may cause irritation and severe dryness; best for recurrent bacterial infection and/or greasiness
    - Ethyl lactate: antimicrobial; not as irritating or drying as benzoyl peroxide; most useful for moderate bacterial folliculitis and dry scale
    - Chlorhexidine: antimicrobial; mildly drying; useful for moderate bacterial folliculitis and *Malassezia* dermatitis; often combined with antifungal agents (e.g., miconazole, ketoconazole)

- Alpha-hydroxy acids (e.g., glycolic acid): enhances desmosomal breakdown only within the stratum corneum, promoting desquamation without loss of barrier function
- Sodium hypochlorite; useful for secondary bacterial and *Malassezia* overgrowth; best when combined with ceramides or moisturizers.

■ Moisturizers:
- Excellent for restoring skin hydration and increasing effectiveness of subsequent bathings
- Humectants: enhance hydration of the stratum corneum by attracting water from the dermis; high concentrations may be keratolytic
- Propylene glycol spray (50–75% dilution with water) applied frequently
- Emollients: coat the skin; smooth the roughened surfaces produced by excessive scaling; usually combined with occlusive compounds to encourage hydration of the epidermis.

■ Ceramides, phytosphingosines, and fatty acids: topical "repair products" can mimic the composition of epidermal lipids (free fatty acids, ceramides, cholesterol, phytosphingosines, etc.); phytosphingosines are proceramides that play a key role in the natural defense mechanisms of the skin; ceramides comprise 40–50% of epidermal lipids and function in the cohesion of the stratum corneum, control local flora, and balance hydration; ceramides also have an antiinflammatory effect by inhibiting protein kinase-C via anti-IL-1 activity and decreasing PGE_2; components of normal epidermal intracellular matrix; antimicrobial; necessary to maintain stratum corneum hydration; abnormal levels reported in multiple conditions; application helps restore epidermal barrier function; these components are available as "spot-on" topicals, moisturizers and shampoo ingredients.

Systemic Therapy

- Specific causes require specific treatments (e.g., L-thyroxine for hypothyroidism; zinc supplements for zinc-responsive dermatosis).
- Systemic antibiotics: secondary bacterial folliculitis.
- Ketoconazole 5–10 mg/kg PO q24h: *Malassezia* dermatitis.
- Prednisolone 0.5 mg/kg PO q24h tapered and discontinued when possible): inflammatory or hypersensitivity causes.
- Vitamin A in therapeutic dosages: 600–1200 IU/kg PO q24h.
- Retinoid drugs: varied success for idiopathic or primary seborrhea; reports of individual response to retinoids in refractory cases: isotretinoin (1 mg/kg PO BID to q24h); if response is seen, taper dosage (1 mg/kg q48h or 0.5 mg/kg q24h).
- Cyclosporine 5 mg/kg PO q24h until controlled, and then decreased to minimal effective maintenance dosage: keratinization disorder associated with hypersensitivity, sebaceous adenitis, epidermal dysplasia, ichthyosis and/or *Malassezia* dermatitis; cyclosporine has been shown to inhibit keratinocyte hyperproliferation in psoriatic human patients; some of the beneficial properties may be due to antiinflammatory effects of the drug.
- Essential fatty acid supplementation: may be helpful in replacing abnormal lipid levels in the skin.

COMMENTS

- Corticosteroids: may be used judiciously to control inflammation; mask signs of bacterial folliculitis and prevent accurate diagnosis of primary disease.
- Vitamins A and D analogs: side effects can be severe; patients should be referred to a dermatologist for treatment.
- Antibiotics and topical therapy: monitor response every 3 weeks; patients may respond differently to various topical therapies.
- Seasonal changes, development of additional diseases (e.g., cutaneous hypersensitivity), and recurrence of bacterial folliculitis: may cause previously controlled patients to worsen; reevaluation critical for determining whether new factors are involved and whether changes in therapy are necessary.
- Endocrinopathy: routine treatment monitoring; see specific chapters.
- Selective autoimmune disorders: reevaluate frequently during the initial phase of induction; less often after remission; clinical evaluation and laboratory data required; see specific chapters.
- Immunosuppressive therapy: monitor hemograms, serum chemistries, and urinalysis with culture.
- Retinoid drugs: monitor serum chemistries, including triglycerides, and tear production.
- Ketoconazole: monitor serum chemistries.
- Skin aging may worsen keratinization disorders or increase frequency of relapses.
- Dermatophytosis and several ectoparasites have either zoonotic potential or the ability to produce lesions in human beings.
- Systemic retinoids: extreme teratogen; do not use in intact females because of severe and predictable teratogenicity and the extremely long withdrawal period; women of child-bearing age should not handle this medication.

Synonyms

- Keratinization disorders = cornification disorders, seborrhea, idiopathic seborrhea, keratinization defect, dyskeratinization, and incorrect human terms (eczema, psoriasis, dander, dandruff); sebopsoriasis: appropriate term to describe the similarities between some human and canine keratinization defects.

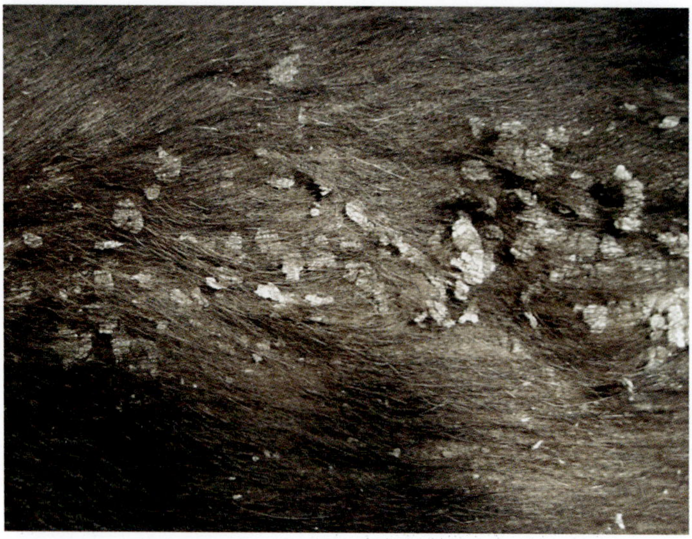

■ **Fig. 29.1.** Nonepidermolytic icthyosis seen as large rafts of scale on the dorsum of a 4-year-old Labrador retriever.

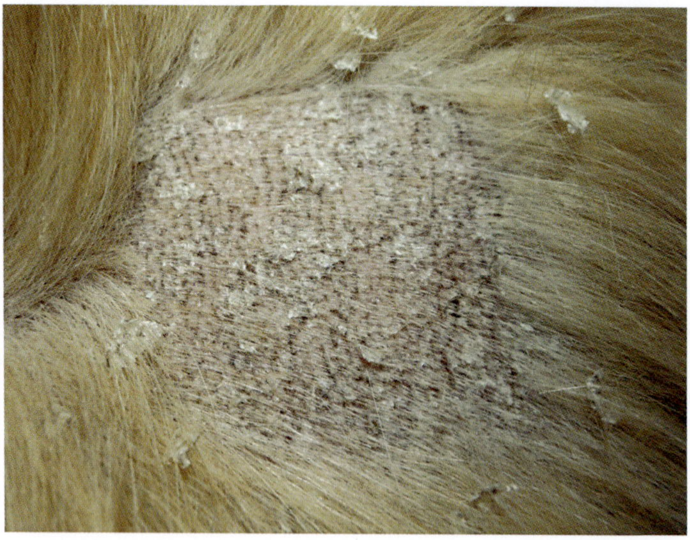

■ **Fig. 29.2.** Golden retriever icthyosis with large exfoliating scales over a skin with adherent fish scale-like crusts on the lateral thorax of a 7-year-old female-spayed dog.

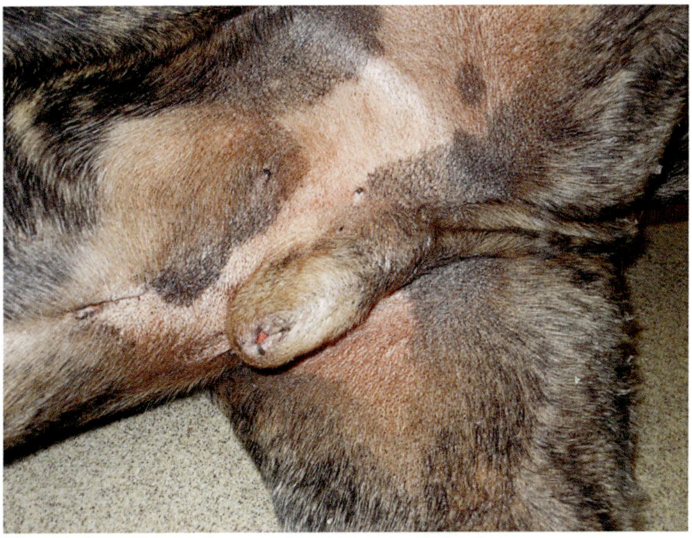

■ **Fig. 29.3.** Icthyosis in a 5-year-old male-castrate American bulldog. Lesions consist of tightly adherent scales with erythroderma on glabrous skin.

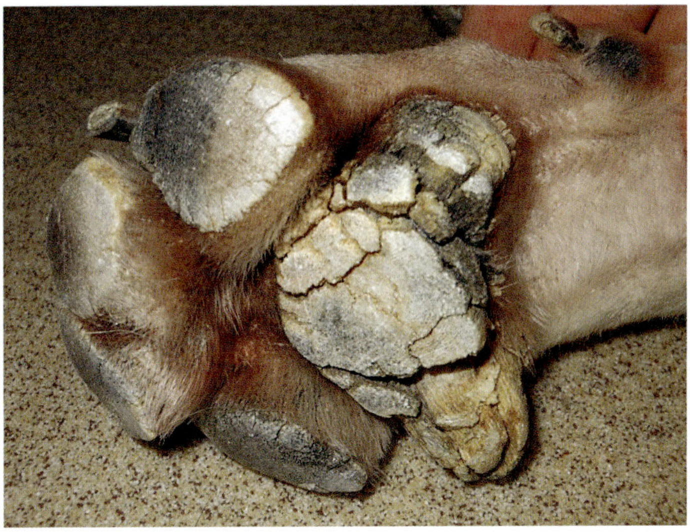

■ **Fig. 29.4.** Thickly-crusted footpads with fissures of the American bulldog in Figure 29.3.

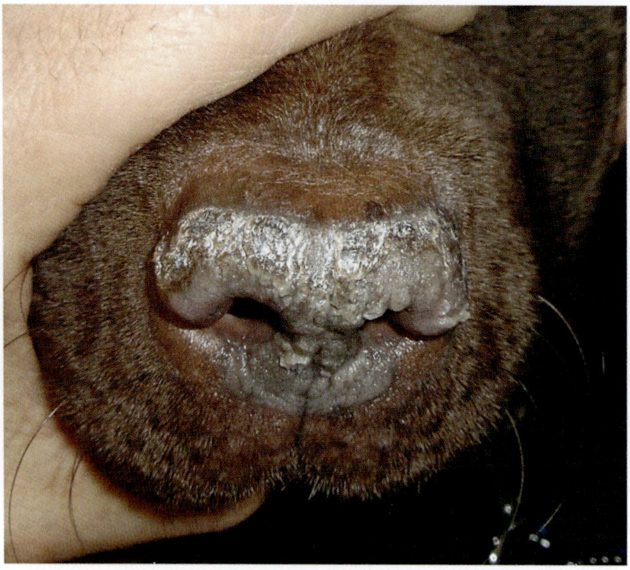

Fig. 29.5. Nasal parakeratosis: the nasal planum is hypopigmented with tightly adherent crusts over erosions in a 3-year-old female-spayed Labrador retriever.

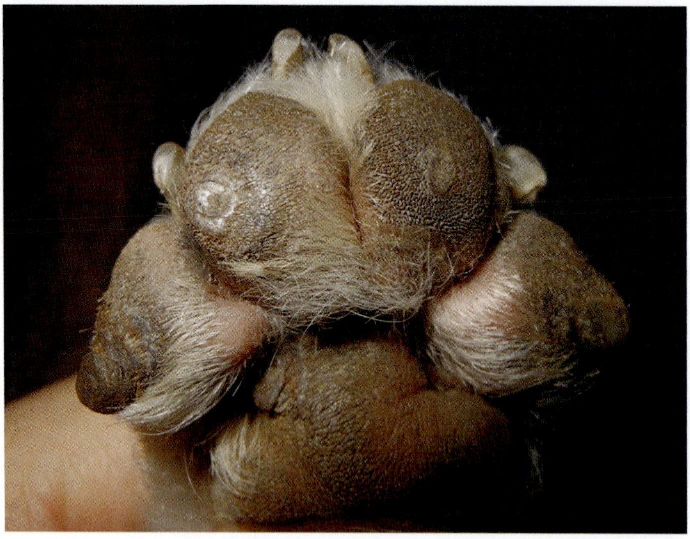

Fig. 29.6. Thickened footpads with horn-like projections with epidermolytic ichthyosis affecting a 7-month-old male-castrate chihuahua mix.

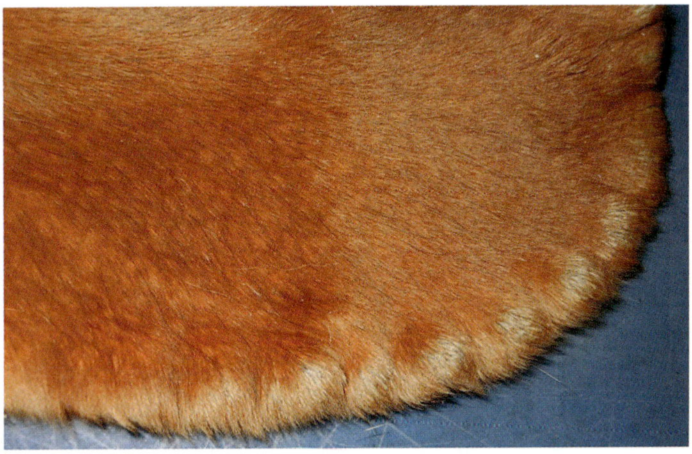

■ **Fig. 29.7.** Multiple patches of thick and adherent scale on the pinnal margin of a 5-year-old male-castrate basset hound with primary seborrhea.

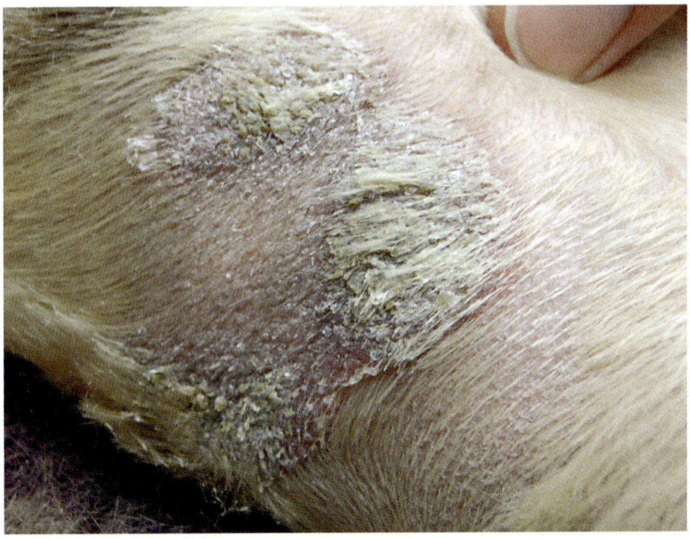

■ **Fig. 29.8.** Discrete patches of adherent crusts on the ventrum of a 2-year-old male-castrate cocker spaniel with primary seborrhea.

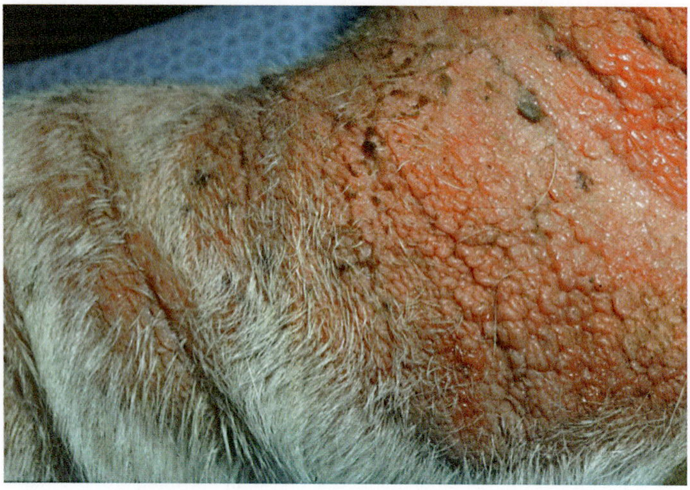

■ **Fig. 29.9.** Lichenification, erythema, and exudation in the axilla and medial foreleg due to *Malassezia* dermatitis in a basset hound with primary seborrhea.

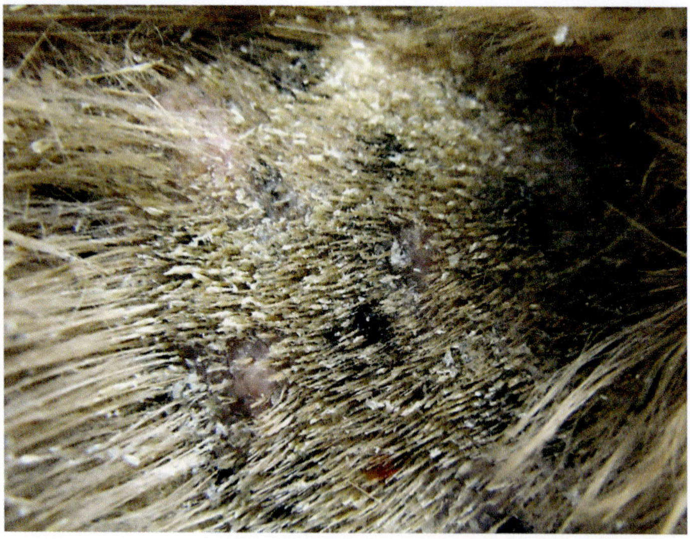

■ **Fig. 29.10.** Adherent, "candlewax" accumulations of keratinaceous debris on the hair shafts of a cocker spaniel with vitamin-A responsive seborrhea.

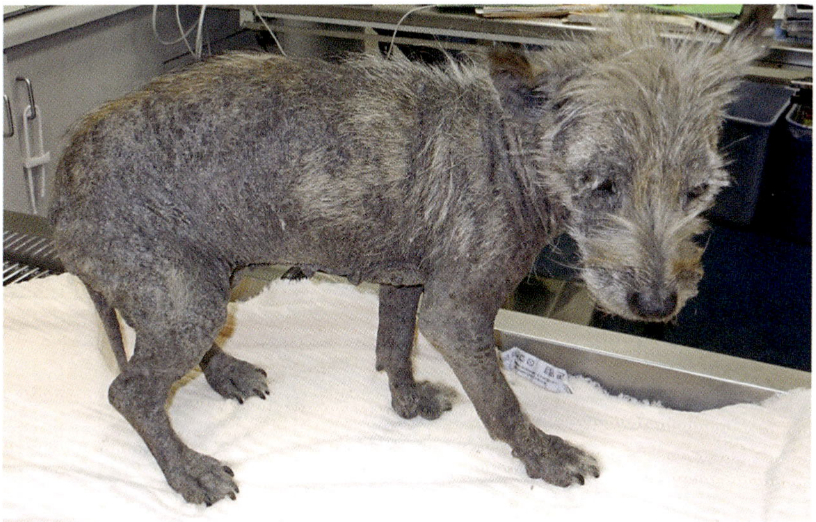

■ **Fig. 29.11.** Severe and generalized epidermal dysplasia in a 10-year-old female-spayed cairn terrier with chronic secondary bacterial folliculitis and *Malassezia* dermatitis.

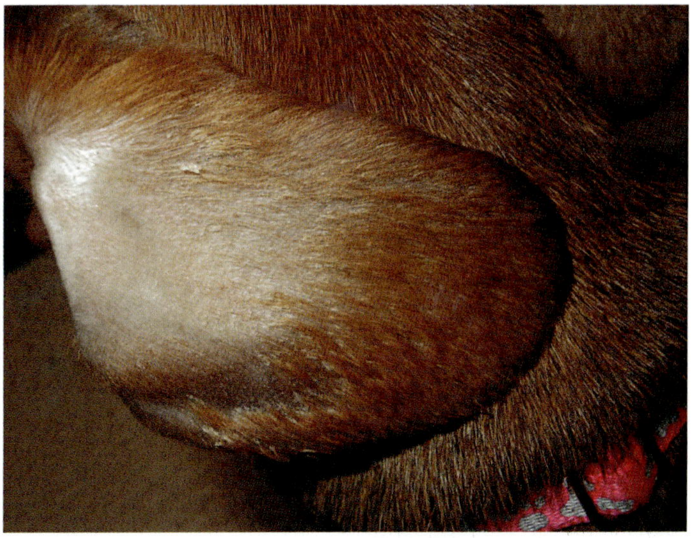

■ **Fig. 29.12.** Accumulations of crusts on hair shafts resulting in eventual loss of hair from the pinna of a 2-year-old female-spayed dachshund with pinnal margin seborrhea.

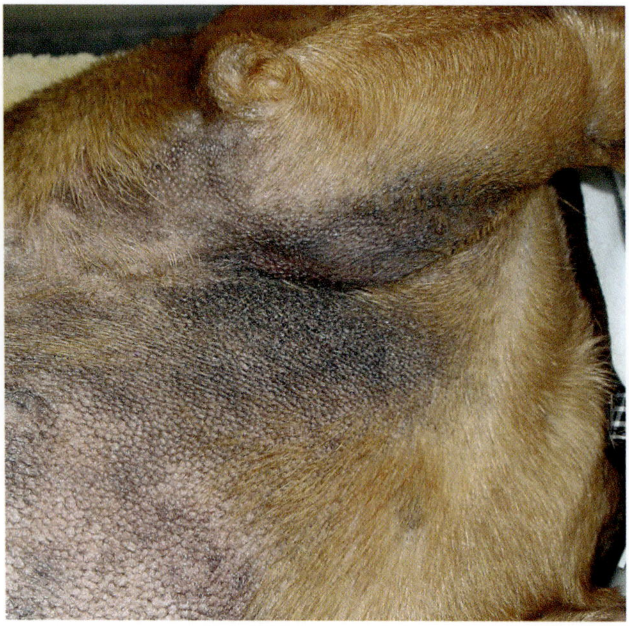

■ **Fig. 29.13.** Hyperpigmentation, lichenification, and exudation consistent with acanthosis nigricans affecting a 4-year-old male-castrate dachshund.

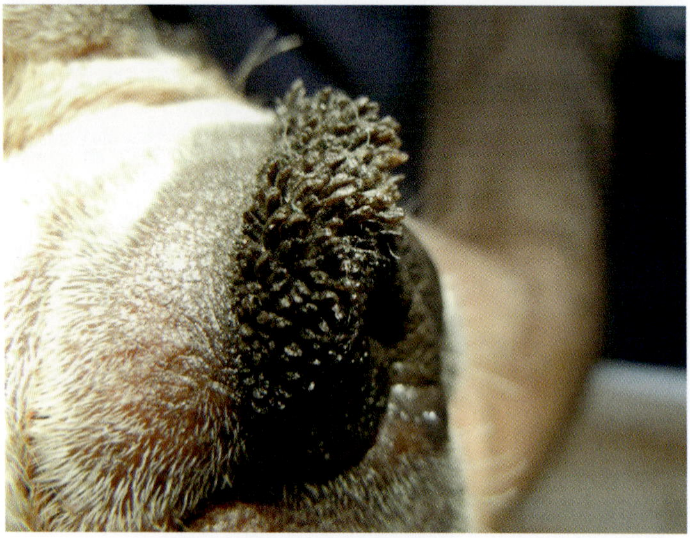

■ **Fig. 29.14.** Fronds of nasal hyperkeratosis on a 9-year-old female-spayed Boston terrier.

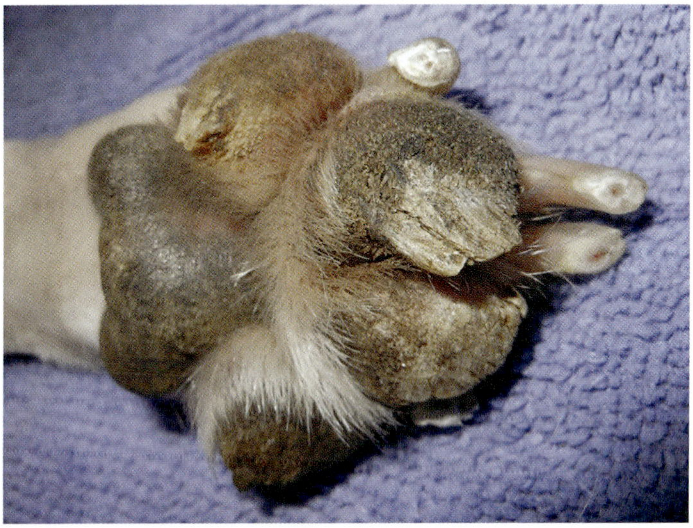

■ **Fig. 29.15.** Thickened footpads with accumulations of keratin into "horns" as well as painful fissures in a 6-year-old female-spayed Jack Russell terrier with digital hyperkeratosis.

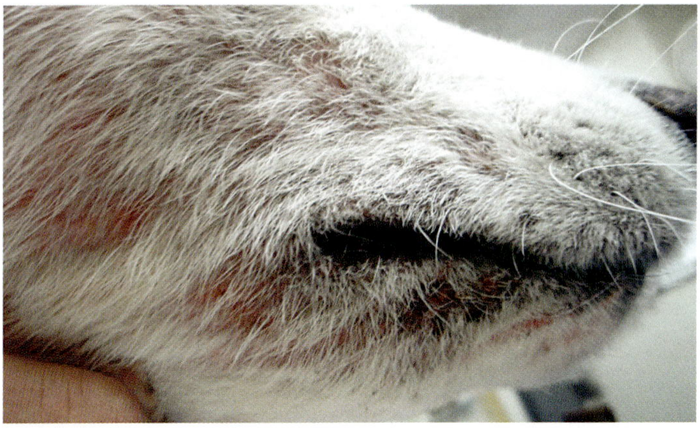

■ **Fig. 29.16.** Adherent crusts, alopecia, and erythema affecting the face and perioral areas of a 7-month-old male-intact Siberian husky with zinc-responsive dermatosis.

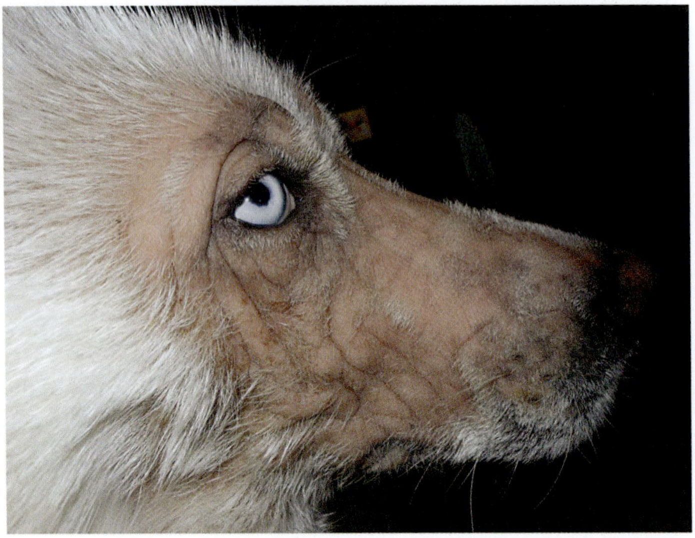

■ **Fig. 29.17.** Severe zinc-responsive dermatitis and secondary *Malassezia* dermatitis in a 2-year-old female-spayed Siberian husky fed a nutritionally deficient diet.

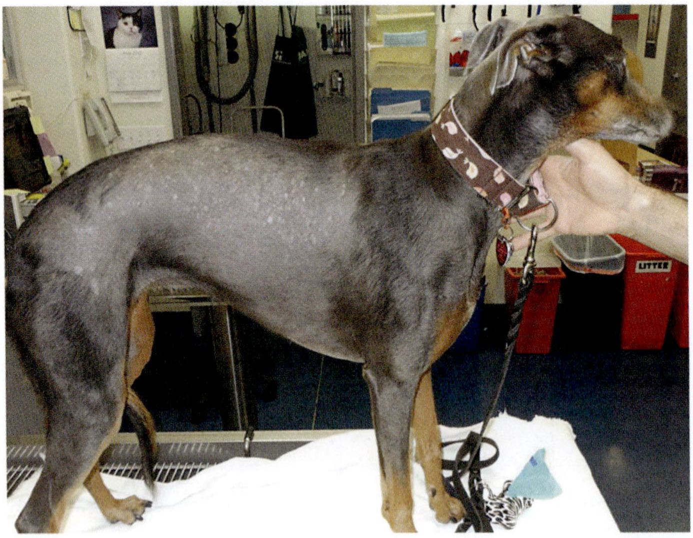

■ **Fig. 29.18.** Color dilution alopecia producing loss of the "blue" hair coat on the body of a 5-year-old female-spayed Italian greyhound.

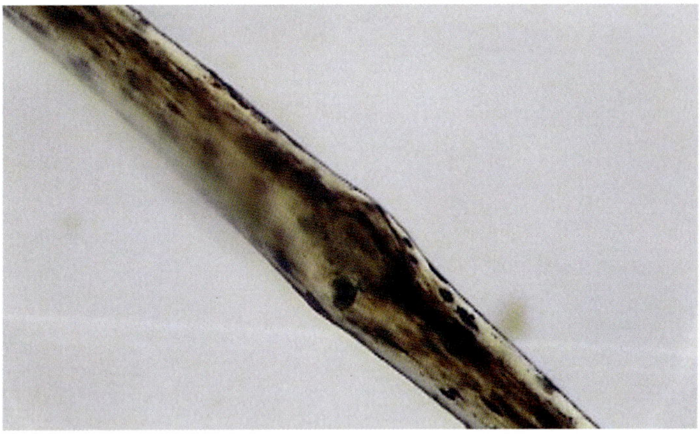

■ **Fig. 29.19.** Hair shaft from a dog with color dilution alopecia. Melanosomes are large and irregular in shape, producing a bulge and damage to the hair cuticle.

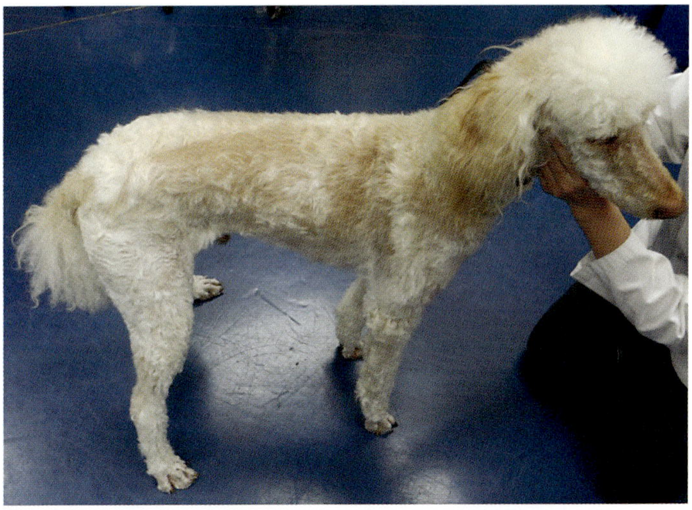

■ **Fig. 29.20.** Sebaceous adenitis in a 9-year-old male-castrate standard poodle. Affected areas of skin are noted as patches of darkened hair coat on the body, pinnae, and muzzle.

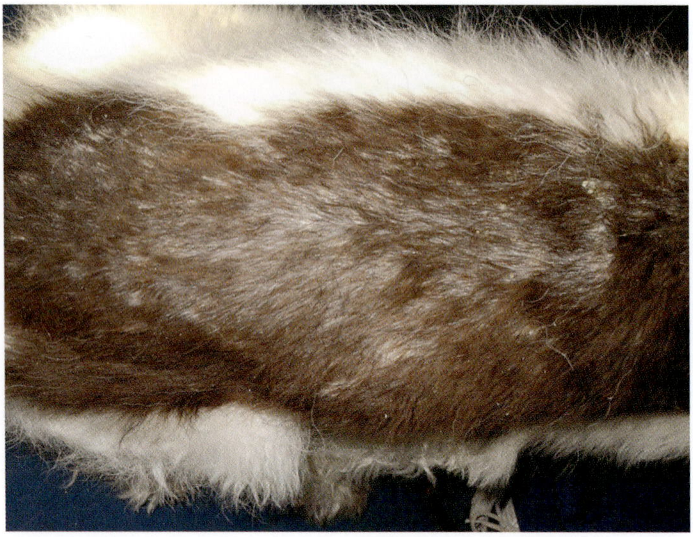

■ **Fig. 29.21.** Sebaceous adenitis producing alopecia and adherent crusts on the dorsum of an 18-month-old female-spayed standard poodle.

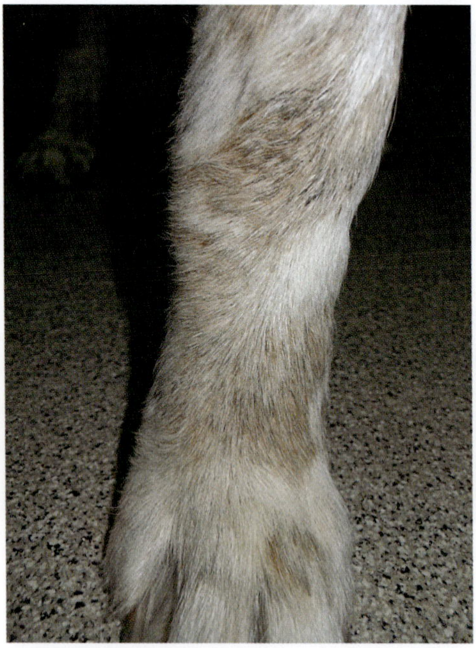

■ **Fig. 29.22.** Tightly adherent crusts on hair shafts with thinning of the hair coat discoloration of the hair and skin typical of sebaceous adenitis in 9-year-old female-spayed Akita.

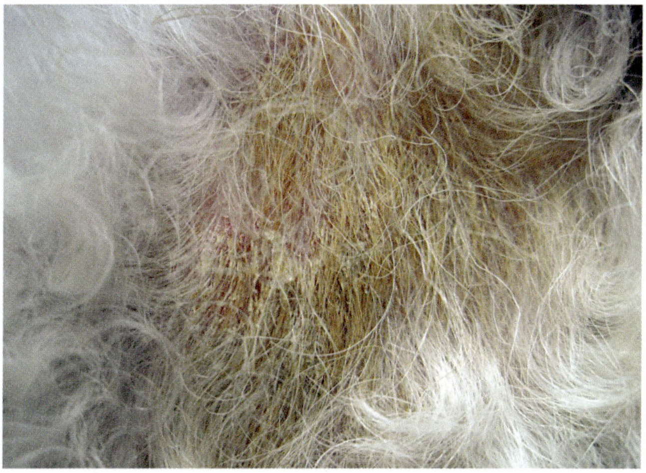

■ **Fig. 29.23.** Tightly adherent crusts surrounding hair shafts termed "keratin collaring" as seen in sebaceous adenitis.

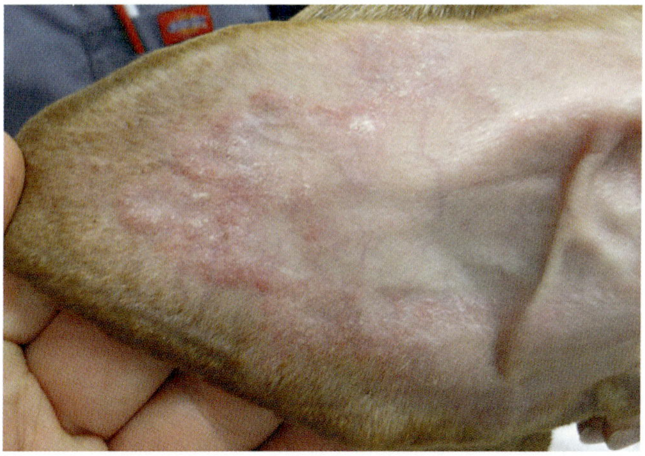

(a)

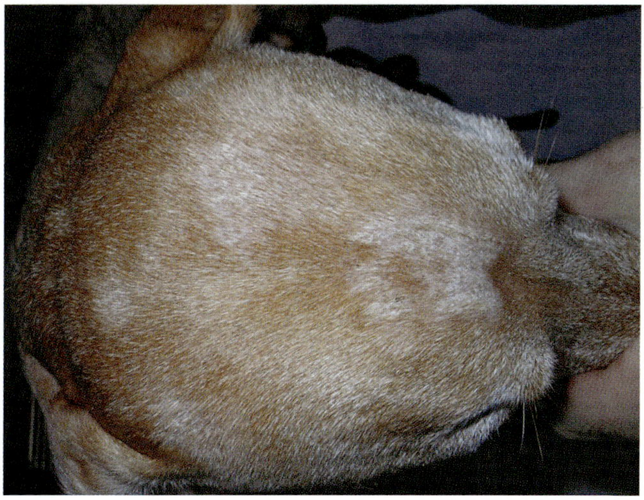

(b)

■ **Fig. 29.24.** Eight-year-old female-spayed vizsla with sebaceous adenitis. Lesions appear as irregularly shaped patches of alopecia, erythema, and fine scaling on the pinna (a) and head (b).

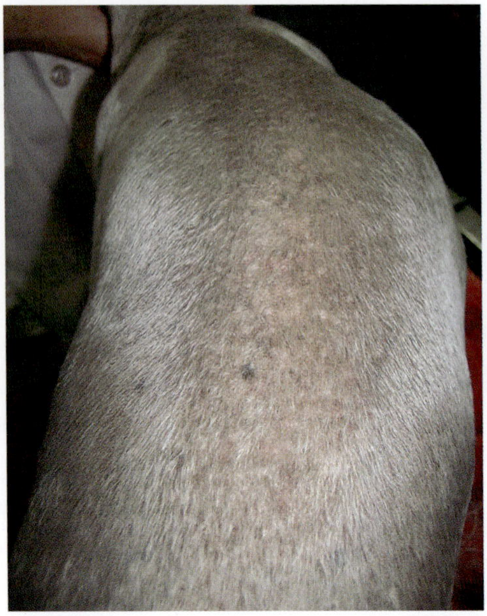

■ **Fig. 29.25.** Numerous adherent crusts protruding from follicles in a 5-year-old male-castrate miniature schnauzer with comedo syndrome.

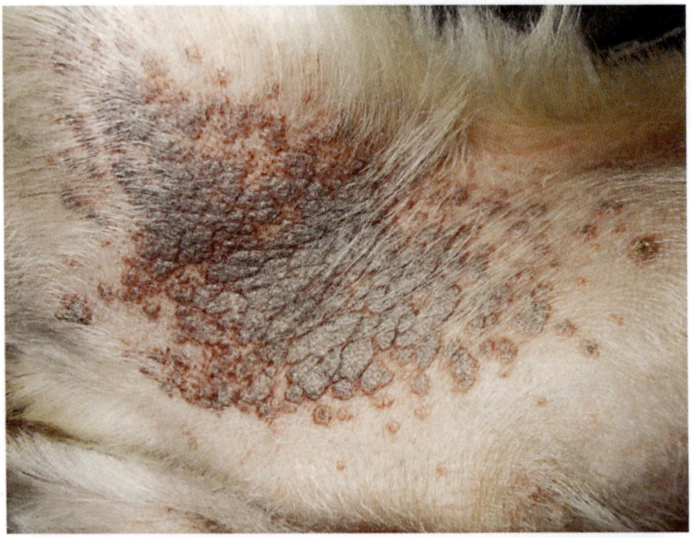

■ **Fig. 29.26.** Multiple flat-topped, lichenified, erythematous, and lightly crusted coalescing plaques in the flank fold region of a 7-year-old male-castrate mixed breed dog with cyclosporine-induced psoriasiform-lichenoid dermatitis.

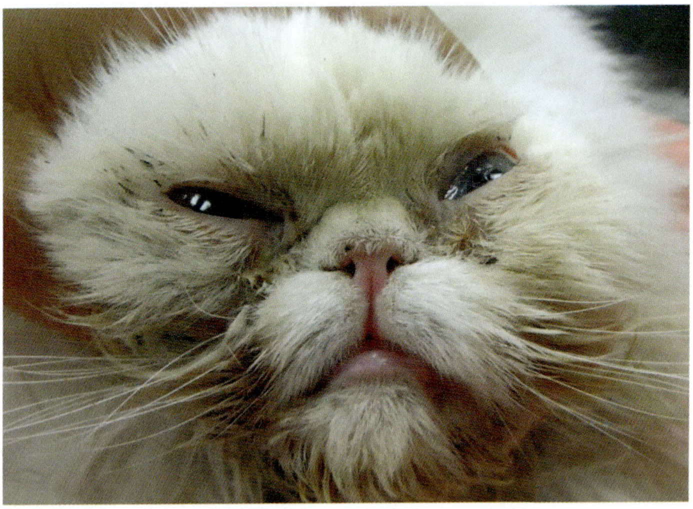

■ **Fig. 29.27.** Facial dermatitis in a 7-year-old female-spayed Persian. The facial and nasal folds, perioral region, and chin are exudative and inflamed.

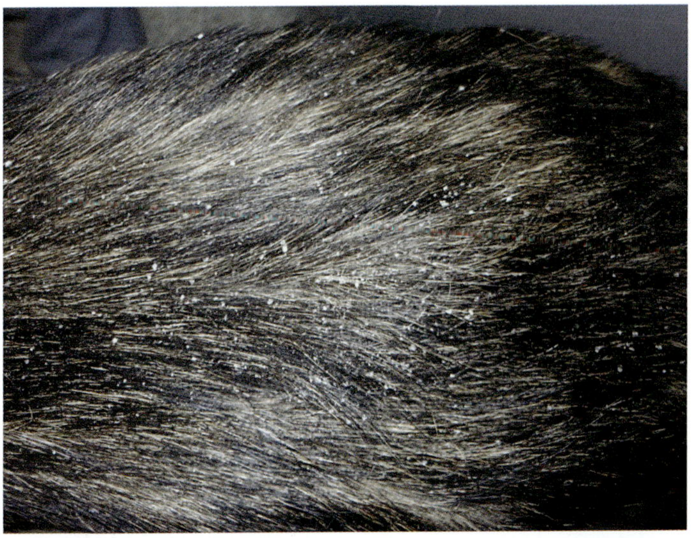

■ **Fig. 29.28.** Excessive scaling with large white flakes characteristic of cheyletiellosis affecting an 8-year-old male-castrate shepherd mix.

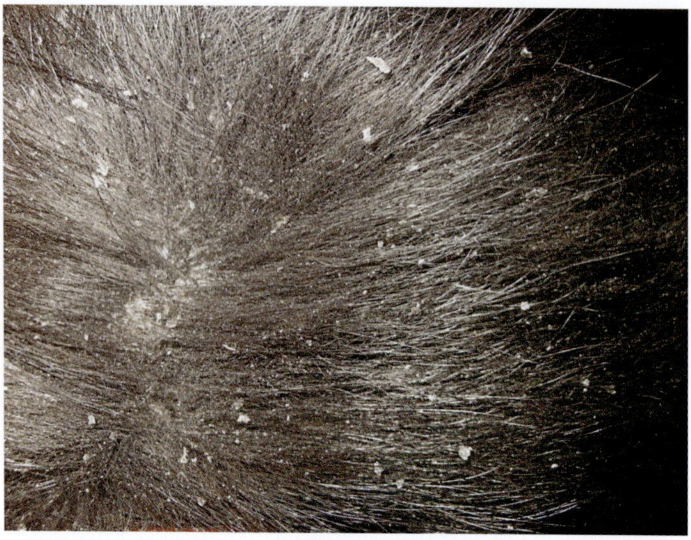

■ **Fig. 29.29.** Scaling dermatitis with resolving bacterial folliculitis secondary to atopic dermatitis in an 8-year-old male-castrate shepherd mix.

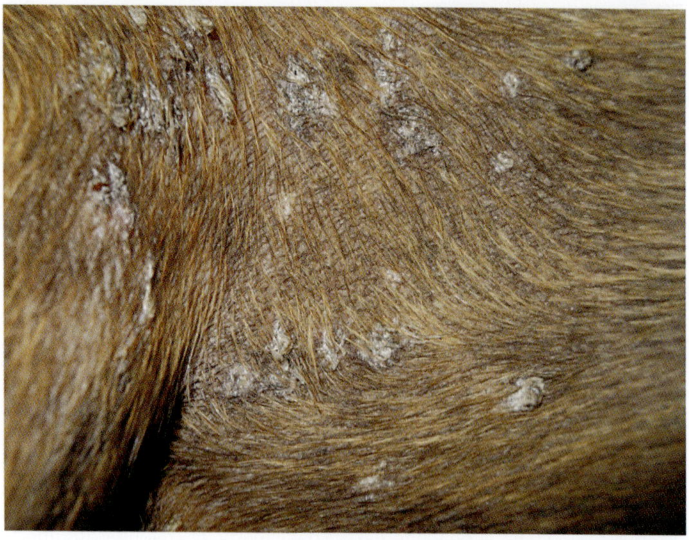

■ **Fig. 29.30.** Nine-year-old male-castrate boxer with multiple crusted lesions of dermatophytosis.

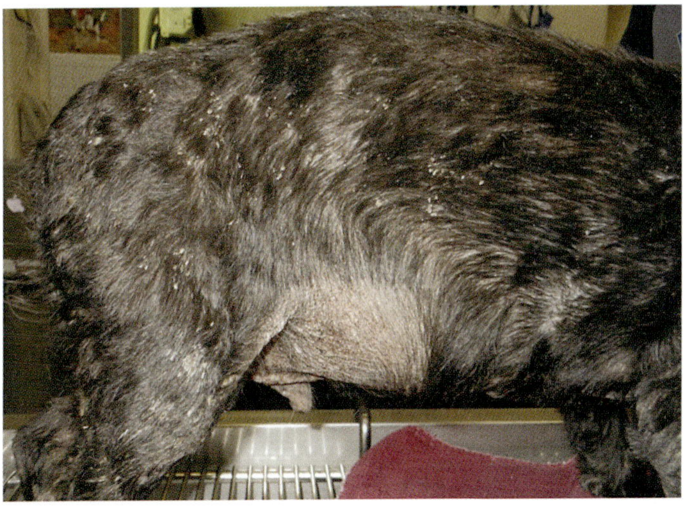

■ **Fig. 29.31.** Generalized crusts and moderate alopecia in a 12-year-old male-castrate cocker spaniel with hypothyroidism.

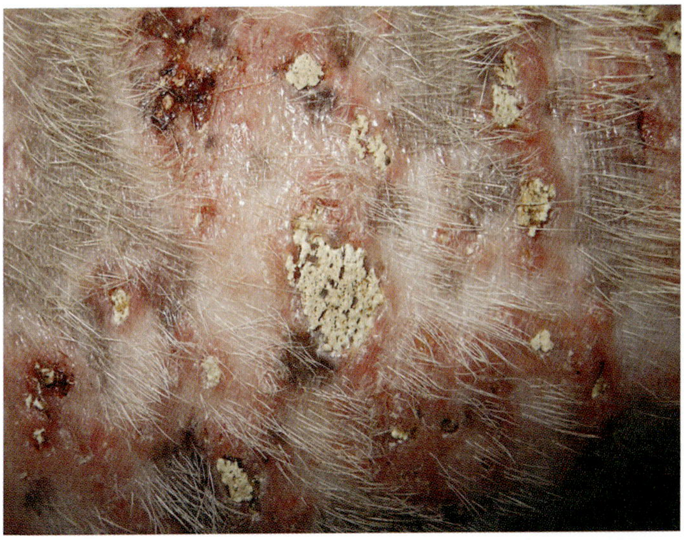

■ **Fig. 29.32.** Multiple erythematous plaques with accumulations of chalky-white adherent debris consistent with calcinosis cutis caused by hyperadrenocorticism in a 9-year-old female-spayed French bulldog.

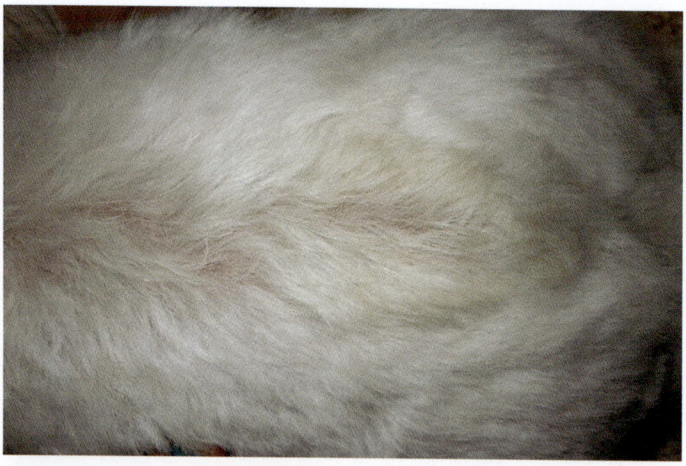

■ **Fig. 29.33.** Subtle changes in color with scaling and a brittle hair coat on the dorsum of a 6-year-old female-spayed Maltese with severe dietary fatty acid deficiency.

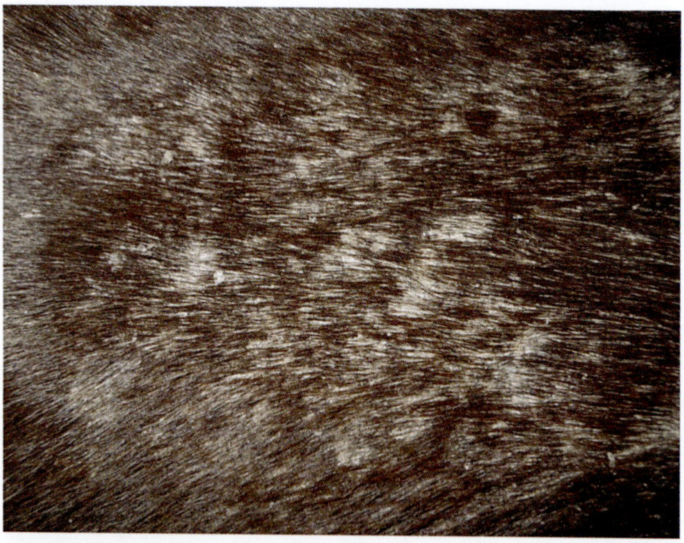

■ **Fig. 29.34.** Adherent crusts and scales on the dorsum of a 6-year-old female-spayed German short-haired pointer with exfoliative cutaneous lupus erythematosus.

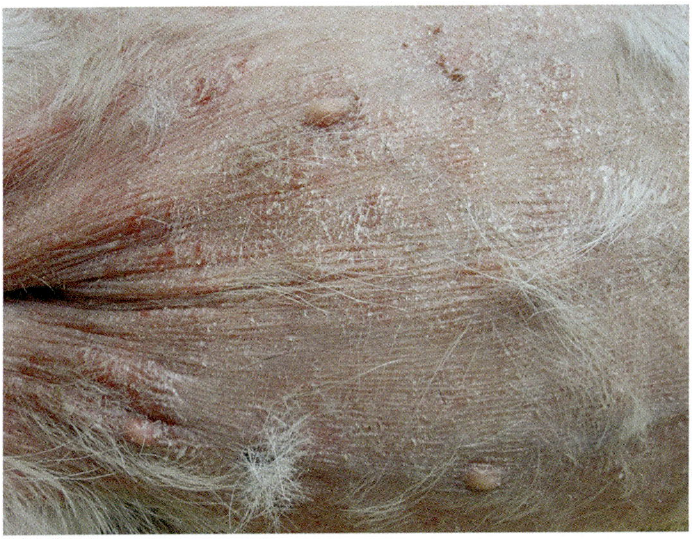

■ **Fig. 29.35.** Mycosis fungoides (epitheliotropic T cell lymphoma) producing erythroderma and scaling on the ventral abdomen of a 14-year-old female-spayed beagle.

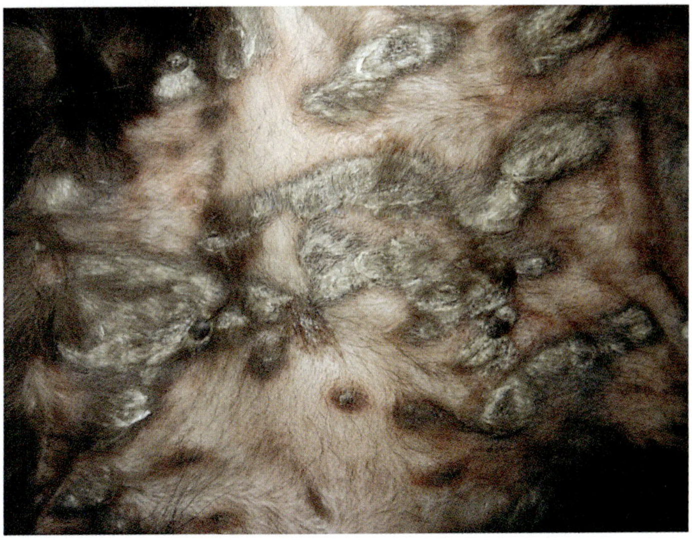

■ **Fig. 29.36.** Multiple crusted plaques of thymoma-associated exfoliative dermatitis in a 12-year-old female-spayed DSH.

chapter 30

Leishmaniasis: Protozoan Dermatitis

DEFINITION/OVERVIEW

- Flagellate protozoal infection causing cutaneous and visceral disease.
- Affects dogs, cats, rodents, horses, cattle, and human beings; canids are important reservoirs for human disease.
- Public health concern; zoonotic potential for fatal disease.
- Prevalence varies by geographic location.
- Dermatologic lesions caused by protozoa other than *Leishmania* (e.g., babesiosis, toxoplasmosis) are extremely rare and are not discussed in this chapter.

ETIOLOGY/PATHOPHYSIOLOGY

- Over 30 species identified; 8–10 considered pathogenic for dogs.
- *L. infantum*: most significant cause of leishmaniasis worldwide; Mediterranean basin, Portugal, and Spain; sporadic cases in Switzerland, northern France, West Africa, South Asia, Latin America, and the Netherlands; endemic populations recognized in the United States.
- Canine cases reported in Texas, Maryland, Oklahoma, Ohio, Alabama, Michigan, and North Carolina.
- *L. donovani* complex or *L. braziliensis*: endemic areas of South and Central America and southern Mexico.
- Different *Leishmania* species can produce different symptoms (e.g., *L. infantum* causing disseminated disease and *L. braziliensis* causing cutaneous/mucocutaneous disease); specific host incompetence in cellular immunity and compensatory humoral response leads to eventual tissue damage and the individual's unique clinical signs.
- Two-host flagellated parasite: vertebrate (including canids, rodents, human beings) and insect; transferred into the dermis of a host by sandfly vectors (*Phlebotomus* – Old World; *Lutzomyia* – New World); a competent insect vector in the United States has not been definitively identified.
- During feeding, female sand flies acquire amastigotes from the dermis and later deposit metacyclic promastigotes; organisms are entirely intracellular in monocytes/macrophages within the skin, bone marrow, and visceral organs.

Blackwell's Five-Minute Veterinary Consult Clinical Companion: Small Animal Dermatology, Third Edition.
Karen Helton Rhodes and Alexander H. Werner.

- Following inoculation, infection may be eliminated, sequestered in skin and lymph nodes, or distributed throughout tissues in the body; dogs may be asymptomatic or symptomatic; estimated 1–5 infected dogs will develop clinical disease.
- Dogs in endemic areas are continuously exposed; development of disease depends on the intensity of exposure, parasite virulence, host genetic factors, and the immune system's ability or inability to prevent organism replication.
- Cats: often localizes in skin.
- Dogs: invariably spreads throughout the body to most organs; nephrotic syndrome/chronic renal failure is the most common cause of death.
- Clinical symptoms are due to granulomatous/pyogranulomatous inflammation, deposition of immune complexes, and autoimmunity.
- Depletion of infected T cells in symptomatic dogs causes an exuberant B cell compensatory response and leads to detrimental hyperglobulinemia with circulating immune complexes producing indirect damage (e.g., arthritis, uveitis, nephritis, myositis, vasculitis) or autoantibodies producing direct damage (e.g., immune-mediated thrombocytopenia and glomerulonephritis).
- Migration of infected macrophages to areas of trauma may encourage localization of lesions (e.g., pressure points).
- Asymptomatic but infected dogs may be inapparent vectors of disease.
- Cell-mediated suppression in dogs with leishmaniasis may increase susceptibility to concurrent infections or disease (including other vector-borne organisms); the reverse may also be true, producing the increased incidence of disease in older dogs.
- Incubation period: 3 months to more than 7 years.

SIGNALMENT/HISTORY

- Travel to endemic regions inside or outside the United States.
- Breed predilection: boxer, German shepherd, rottweiler, cocker spaniel; Ibizan hound more resistant to symptomatic progression.
- Endemic in foxhound kennels in areas of the United States.
- Dogs usually less than 3 years of age or greater than 8 years.
- Resistance or susceptibility to infection and/or development of clinical symptoms may depend on *Leishmania*-specific cell-mediated immunity.
- Infection through transfusions of contaminated blood, secretions, venereally, and transplacental transmission (dog to dog may be the route of transmission in North America due to lack of a competent insect host).
- Almost all dogs develop visceral, or systemic, disease; 67–89% have cutaneous involvement.

CLINICAL FEATURES

- Visceral:
  - Peripheral lymphadenopathy (may be absent in advanced symptomatic cases as lymphoid tissue is depleted)

- Exercise intolerance
- Severe weight loss and anorexia
- Emaciation/chronic wasting
- Polymyositis and muscle atrophy
- Diarrhea, vomiting
- Epistaxis and melena
- Renal failure (polyuria, polydipsia, vomiting)
- Neuralgia
- Lameness due to polyarthritis, osteolytic lesions, and proliferative periostitis
- Pyrexia
- Splenomegaly
- Ocular disease (blepharitis, conjunctivitis, anterior uveitis, retinitis, keratoconjunctivitis sicca).

- Cutaneous:
  - Exfoliative dermatitis: may be localized, regional, generalized; symmetric or asymmetric; may be similar to pemphigus foliaceus (Figures 30.1, 30.2)
  - Ulcerative dermatitis: erosions leading to indolent ulcers; solitary or multiple; pinnae, nasal planum, mucocutaneous junctions, pressure points, and footpads (Figure 30.3)
  - Nodular dermatitis: solitary or multiple; often nonulcerated; more common in boxers; nodules located at areas of parasite inoculation may be painful (Figure 30.4)
  - Pustular dermatitis, often pruritic: small pustules leading to collarettes; most often on glabrous skin
  - Papular dermatitis: nonpainful and nonpruritic, discrete to coalescing papules; most often on glabrous skin
  - Regional (especially facial) alopecia
  - Cutaneous depigmentation
  - Nasodigital hyperkeratosis
  - Onychogryphosis: hypertrophy and abnormal curvature of claws
  - Lesions are typically nonpruritic unless secondarily infected
  - Secondary dermatoses including bacterial folliculitis and demodicosis may develop.

DIFFERENTIAL DIAGNOSIS

- Visceral:
  - Mycoses (blastomycosis, histoplasmosis)
  - Systemic lupus erythematosus
  - Ehrlichiosis
  - Anaplasmosis
  - Rickettsiosis
  - Bartonellosis
  - Babesiosis

  - Dirofilariasis
  - Hepatozoonosis
  - Multiple myeloma
  - Metastatic neoplasia
  - Distemper virus
  - Systemic vasculitis.
- Cutaneous:
  - Systemic or cutaneous lupus erythematosus
  - Keratinization disorder
  - Idiopathic sebaceous adenitis
  - Demodicosis
  - Dermatophytosis
  - Bacterial pyoderma
  - Sterile pustular dermatoses (e.g., subcorneal or eosinophilic)
  - Vasculitis
  - Nutritional dermatoses (e.g., vitamin A responsive, zinc responsive)
  - Idiopathic nasodigital hyperkeratosis
  - Superficial necrolytic dermatitis
  - Cutaneous adverse drug reaction
  - Lichenoid-psoriasiform-like dermatosis
  - Reactive histiocytosis
  - Leproid granuloma
  - Pemphigus foliaceus
  - Epitheliotropic lymphoma
  - Sterile granulomatous/pyogranulomatous dermatitis
  - Lupoid onychodystrophy (symptoms isolated to claws).

DIAGNOSTICS

- Diagnosis made by compatible clinical symptoms and positive serologic testing along with confirmation of the presence of organisms in sampled tissues by immunohistochemistry or polymerase chain reaction (especially lymph node and skin; bone marrow should be sampled if other sites fail to demonstrate organisms).
- Asymptomatic leishmanial dogs my exhibit symptoms due to coinfections and not *Leishmania*, leading to treatment failures from inappropriately directed therapy.
- CBC/biochemistries: thrombocytopenia, lymphocytosis, nonregenerative anemia; hyperproteinemia with hyperglobulinemia and hypoalbuminemia; elevated liver enzymes; azotemia; hyperamylasemia; elevated creatinine phosphokinase.
- Anemia and thrombocytopenia are partly produced by the high number of amastigotes in bone marrow.
- Parasite numbers in blood smears are typically low.
- Urinalysis: proteinuria.
- Coombs, ANA, LE cell tests: rare positive.
- Intradermal leishmanin injection (Montenegro test): positive skin reaction.

- Interferon-gamma production via ELISA from whole blood.
- Quantitative PCR: highly sensitive test; proves infection but not necessarily that infection has caused clinical symptoms; use in conjunction with other diagnostics.
- Serologic diagnosis: IFAT titer of 1:64 – recombinant antigen immunoassay (where available); false negatives estimated at 10%; false positives due to cross-reactivity to *Trypanosoma cruzi*; ELISA testing – positive in cases with active disease; used to monitor response to therapy.
- Cytology: identification of organism from aspirates of skin, spleen, bone marrow, lymph node, while diagnostic, can be difficult; aspirates from nodular lesions (especially skin) are most rewarding (Figure 30.5).
- Histopathology from mucosal ulcerations (endoscopy/surgical biopsy of stomach, intestine, and colon): histiocytic infiltrate with intracellular amastigotes.
- Renal histopathology: glomerulonephritis and tubulointerstitial nephritis.
- Dermatohistopathology from biopsy:
    - Macrophage infiltrate with intracellular amastigote forms in tissues from skin, lymph nodes, liver, spleen, and kidney (Figure 30.6)
    - Orthokeratosis, hyperkeratosis, and follicular keratosis
    - Dermal granulomatous or pyogranulomatous nodular inflammation
    - Sebaceous adenitis
    - Ulceration with epidermal hyperplasia and neutrophil exocytosis; histiocytic, lymphocytic, neutrophilic dermatitis
    - Predominance of macrophages and multinucleated giant cells containing organisms in nodular dermatitis
    - Subcorneal neutrophilic pustules with or without acantholytic keratinocytes
    - Nodular to diffuse pyogranulomatous dermatitis without multinucleated giant cells
    - Histopathologic changes may occur in "normal-looking" skin of infected dogs demonstrating systemic disease
    - Amastigote load tends to be highest in preferential feeding areas of the vector.

THERAPEUTICS

- Treatment aimed at reducing parasite load and resolving secondary clinical disease; inform client that organisms will never be eliminated; relapse is inevitable.
- Treatment controversial due to potential zoonotic transmission of organism to human beings from persistently infected dogs; documented cases reportable to the CDC.
- Prognosis very poor in emaciated, chronically infected animals.
- Pentavalent antimonial therapy provides increased quality of life but rarely cures.
- Cats: surgical excision of individual dermal nodules.
- Begin pentavalent antimonial drugs at lower doses in seriously ill patients.
- Prognosis depends on degree of renal insufficiency at the onset of treatment.
- Monitor therapy with frequent CBC, serum albumin, globulin, and creatinine, and urine protein:creatinine.

- Base continued treatment on clinical improvement, identification of organisms in repeat biopsies, and normalization of serum titers.
- Relapses occur often within months to a year; recheck at least every 2 months after completion of treatment.

Drugs of Choice

- Meglumine antimoniate (100 mg/kg intravenously or subcutaneously q24h or divided BID for 3–4 weeks).
- Allopurinol (10 mg/kg PO BID): administered with pentavalent antimonials and for long-term maintenance (Figure 30.7).
- Miltefosine (2 mg/kg PO q24h).
- Sodium stibogluconate (30–50 mg/kg intravenously or subcutaneously q24h for 3–4 weeks): available in the United States through the Centers for Disease Control.
- Alternative drugs include gamma-interferon, amphotericin-B, enrofloxacin, marbofloxacin, metronidazole, and spiramycin.

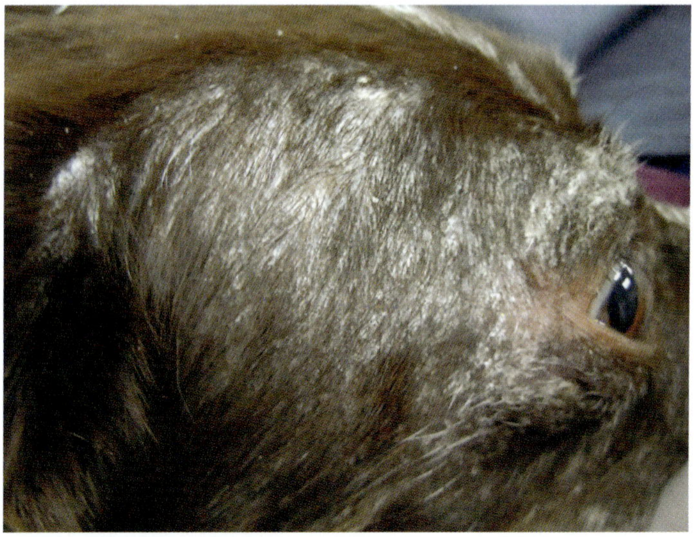

Fig. 30.1. Exfoliative dermatitis of leishmaniasis: characteristic fine, silvery, and adherent scales on the head of a 5-year-old female-spayed English pointer.

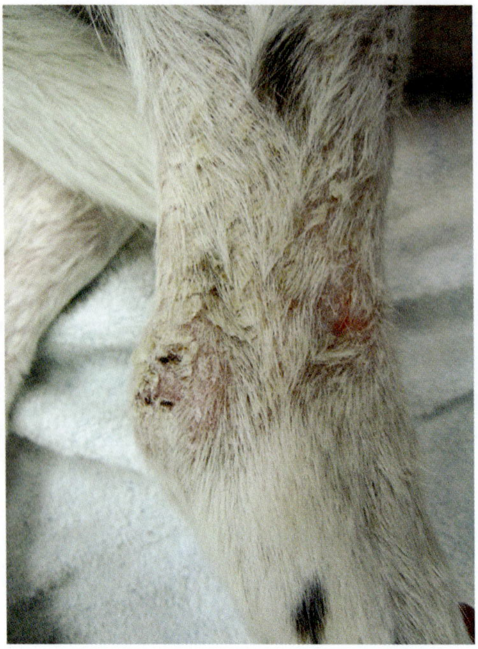

■ **Fig. 30.2.** Adherent scales with erythema and alopecia over a pressure point of the patient in Figure 30.1.

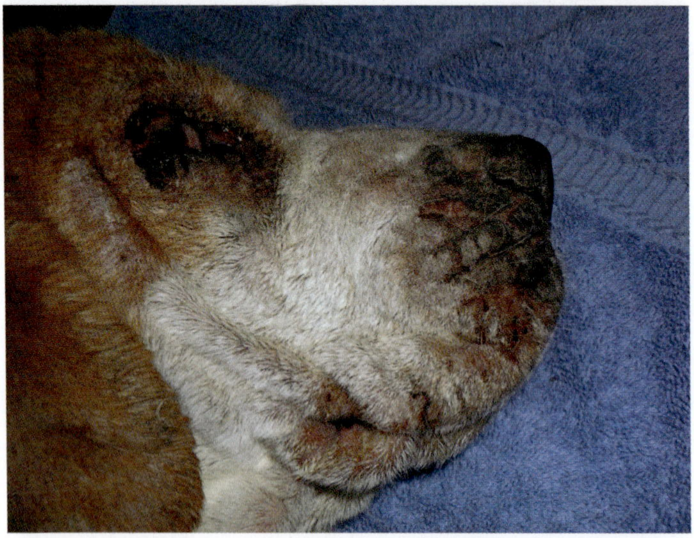

■ **Fig. 30.3.** Exudative and eroded lesions of leishmaniasis with secondary bacterial infection on the face of a 5-year-old male-castrate beagle. This patient had concurrent symptoms of lameness, keratoconjunctivitis sicca, and renal failure, and had been imported to the United States from Spain 6 months prior to development of lesions.

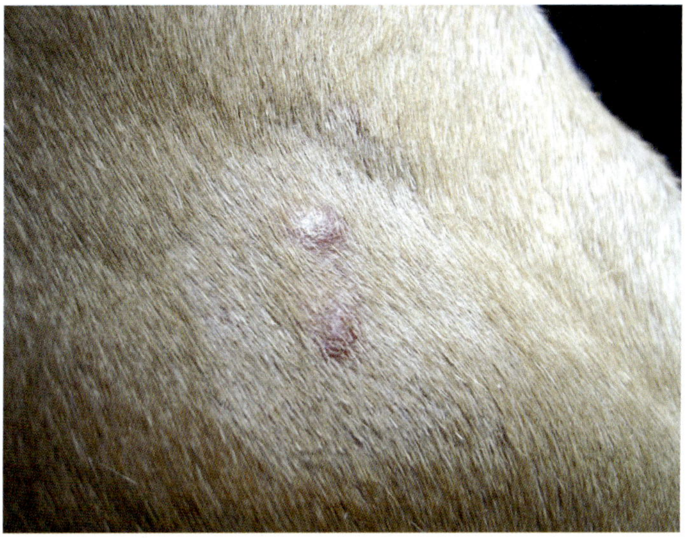

Fig. 30.4. Erythematous nodules of leishmaniasis on the lateral hock of an 8-year-old male-castrate Italian greyhound.

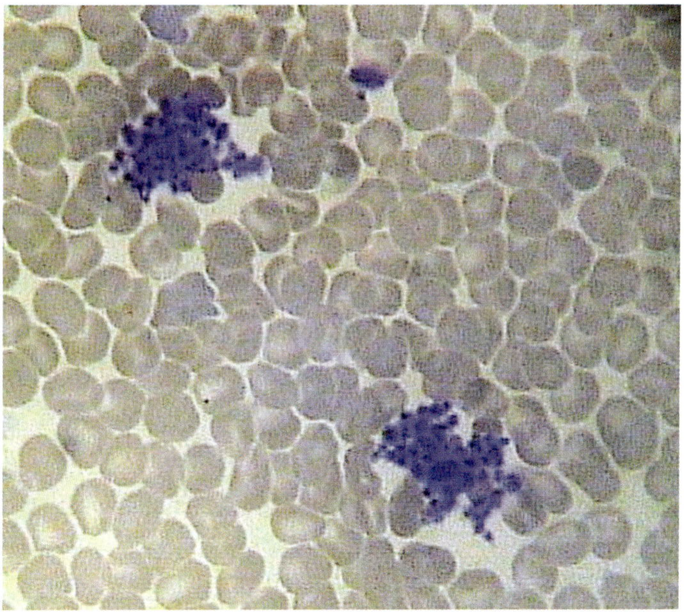

Fig. 30.5. Cytological preparation demonstrating macrophages filled with amastigotes.

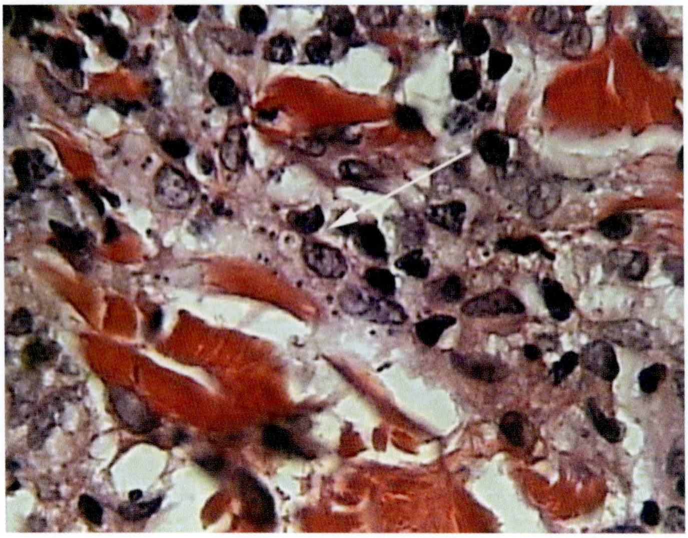

■ **Fig. 30.6.** Hematoxylin and eosin preparation of biopsy tissue revealing macrophages with multiple intracellular *Leishmania* amastigotes (*arrow*).

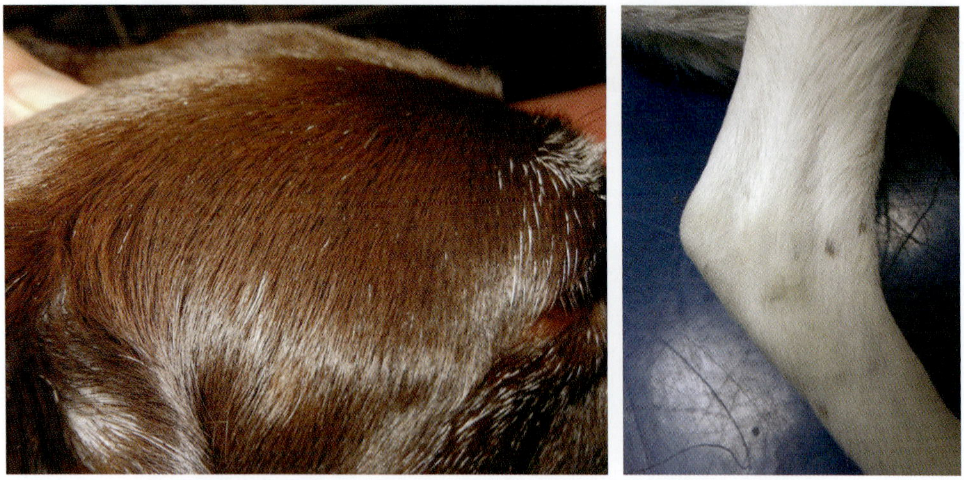

(a) (b)

■ **Fig. 30.7.** Images of patient in Figures 30.1 and 30.2 3 years after initial diagnosis of leishmaniasis. Excessive scales and crusts have resolved.

chapter 31

Lupus Erythematosus

DEFINITION/OVERVIEW

- Classification of lupus erythematosus (LE) in dogs and cats is evolving.
- "Lupus-specific" cutaneous disease (CLE) includes those with lymphocyte-rich interface dermatitis and basal keratinocyte damage.
- Further subdivision describes acute, subacute, and chronic CLE: most canine disease is considered to be a variant of chronic CLE (with the exception of vesicular CLE).
- Current recognized CLE diseases include:
    - Facial-predominant discoid lupus erythematosus (DLE)
    - Generalized discoid lupus erythematosus (GDLE)
    - Mucous membrane cutaneous lupus erythematosus (MCLE)
    - Vesicular cutaneous lupus erythematosus (VCLE)
    - Exfoliative cutaneous lupus erythematosus (ECLE)
    - Systemic lupus erythematosus (SLE).

ETIOLOGY/PATHOPHYSIOLOGY

- Exact mechanism undetermined but includes:
    - Genetic factors: forms of CLE more common in German shepherd
    - Hormonal factors: females possibly higher risk (unclear)
    - Environmental factors: drug reactions, viral initiation, and UV light exposure
    - T cell dysfunction
    - Polyclonal B cell activation
    - Cytokine production
    - Antigen/antibody complexes: deposited at the dermal-epidermal junction, glomerular basement membrane, blood vessels, and synovial membranes
    - Tissue injury: direct result of activation of complement by immune complexes and infiltration of inflammatory cells as well as by direct cytotoxic effect of autoantibodies against membrane-bound antigens.

Blackwell's Five-Minute Veterinary Consult Clinical Companion: Small Animal Dermatology, Third Edition.
Karen Helton Rhodes and Alexander H. Werner.

SIGNALMENT/HISTORY

Facial-Predominant Discoid Lupus Erythematosus (DLE)

- Dogs: age range reported as middle-aged to older; rare in cats.
- Most common immune-mediated skin disease in dogs.
- Also termed cutaneous lupus erythematosus (CLE).
- Predominant breeds affected: collie, German shepherd, Siberian husky, Shetland sheepdog, Alaskan malamute, chow chow, and their crosses.
- Predominantly involves the planum nasale and dorsal muzzle; pinnae and mucous membranes of the head (lips, eyelid) less commonly affected.
- Characterized primarily by depigmentation followed by erosion/ulceration of the planum nasale.
- Lack of systemic symptoms.

Generalized discoid lupus erythematosus (GDLE)

- Dogs: age range reported as 5–12 years (median 9 years).
- No sex or breed predilection.
- Generalized lesions similar in appearance to DLE develop on the body and extremities.
- Characterized by plaques of dyspigmentation with erosion/ulceration followed by scarring.
- Lack of systemic symptoms.

Mucous membrane cutaneous lupus erythematosus (MCLE)

- Dogs: age range reported as 3–13 years (median 6 years).
- No sex predilection.
- Predominant breed affected: German shepherd.
- Lesions noted at genital/perigenital, anal/perianal, perioral, and periocular regions.
- Characterized by well-demarcated erosions/ulcerations with peripheral hyperpigmentation.
- Lack of systemic symptoms.

Vesicular cutaneous lupus erythematosus (VCLE)

- Dogs: age range reported as middle-aged to older.
- Exacerbated by UV light.
- Breeds affected: Collie and Shetland sheepdog.
- Characterized by confluent patches of ulceration on the ventrum and mucocutaneous junctions.
- Lack of systemic symptoms.

Exfoliative cutaneous lupus erythematosus (ECLE)

- Dogs: reported as young adult at onset.
- Breed affected: German short-haired pointer.
- Characterized by large patches of adherent scales and alopecia beginning on head and dorsum but progressing to become generalized.
- Systemic symptoms may include lymphadenopathy, joint pain, pyrexia.

Systemic lupus erythematosus (SLE)

- Young adult dogs; rare in cats.
- Predominant breeds affected: collie, German shepherd, Siberian husky, Shetland sheepdog, Alaskan malamute, chow chow, and their crosses.
- Multisystem autoimmune disease characterized by the formation of autoantibodies and circulating antigen-antibody complexes.
- Clinical signs are dependent on target organ systems and may be quite severe; vasculitis is often a predominant clinical feature.
- May wax and wane.
- Systemic symptoms often include lethargy, anorexia, shifting leg lameness, fever, ulcerative dermatosis.

CLINICAL FEATURES

DLE

- Depigmentation of planum nasale and/or lip margins (Figures 31.1, 31.2).
- Loss of cobblestone appearance of the planum nasale.
- Depigmentation presents prior to crusting (Figure 31.3).
- Progresses to erosions and ulcerations (Figure 31.4).
- Tissue loss and scarring can occur (Figure 31.5).
- May involve pinnae and periocular region.

GDLE

- Erythematous macules, patches, and plaques.
- Progresses to erosions and ulcerations (Figure 31.6).
- Initial lesions on neck, thorax, dorsum (Figure 31.7).
- Progresses to involve ventrum and proximal limbs.
- May involve mucocutaneous junctions.
- Lesions often develop central scarring and peripheral dyspigmentation.

MCLE

- Symmetric, well-demarcated lesions of erosion and ulceration.
- Genital/perigenital and anal/perianal areas most frequently affected.

- Perioral and periocular skin often affected (Figure 31.8).
- Perinasal region, nasal planum, and oral mucosae may be affected.
- Hyperpigmentation at periphery of lesions.

VCLE

- Formerly considered a variant of dermatomyositis or hidradenitis suppurativa.
- Involves medial thigh, groin, axillae, and ventral abdomen.
- Mucocutaneous junctions often affected.
- Lesions seen as serpiginous or polycyclic ulcerations.

ECLE

- Fine adherent scales and alopecia starting on the muzzle and pinnae (Figures 31.9, 31.10).
- Lesions generalize to include entire body and extremities (Figure 31.11).
- Lymphadenopathy and pyrexia common.
- Often associated with lameness, stiffness, and pain.

SLE

- Cutaneous lesions characterized by erythema, erosion, and ulceration (Figures 31.12–31.14).
- Mucocutaneous and oral lesions common.
- Ulcerations of the lateral aspect of the tongue.
- Joints often swollen and painful.
- Fever, lymphadenopathy, hepatosplenomegaly, muscle wasting, myocarditis, pericarditis, pleuritis.

DIFFERENTIAL DIAGNOSIS

- Other immune-mediated diseases: pemphigus foliaceus, pemphigus erythematosus, mucous membrane pemphigoid, and uveodermatologic syndrome.
- Drug reactions, erythema multiforme, and toxic epidermal necrolysis: nasal and facial lesions.
- Mucocutaneous pyoderma; differentiated from LE by complete response to antibiotics.
- Dermatomyositis: affects some of the same predisposed breeds (collies and Shetland sheepdogs).
- Nasal pyoderma and nasal dermatophytosis: infectious conditions; can mimic DLE.
- Insect hypersensitivity (eosinophilic furunculosis).
- Contact allergy.
- Zinc-responsive dermatosis.
- Superficial necrolytic dermatitis.

- Dermatophytosis.
- Metabolic epidermal necrosis.
- Epitheliotropic lymphoma: may start on the planum and rostral aspect of the muzzle and lips.
- Squamous cell carcinoma: may affect the planum; may occur at a slightly higher incidence in chronic discoid lupus lesions.
- Idiopathic leukoderma leukotrichia (vitiligo): may cause depigmentation of the tissue and hair without concurrent inflammation.
- Neoplasia-induced vasculitis.
- Infectious diseases must be differentiated from SLE.

DIAGNOSTICS

- CBC/biochemistries: usually normal; thrombocytopenia in 25% of cases of ECLE.
- ANA, LE preparation, and Coombs tests: usually normal or negative except with SLE.
- SLE: nonerosive polyarthritis, proteinuria from glomerulonephritis, hemolytic anemia, leukopenia, thrombocytopenia, polymyositis, high concentration of beta and gamma globulins on serum electrophoresis.
- Dermatohistopathology from biopsy:
  - DLE: lymphocytic interface lichenoid dermatitis with pigmentary incontinence, prominent basal cell apoptosis, variable degrees of dermal mucin and epidermal atrophy
  - GDLE: more severe (than DLE) lymphocytic interface dermatitis with basal cell degeneration; suprabasal and lymphocytic satellitosis of apoptotic basal cells; pigmentary incontinence, basement membrane thickening
  - MCLE: lymphocytic interface lichenoid dermatitis with pigmentary incontinence, prominent basal cell apoptosis; basement membrane thickening; erosions and ulcerations without blistering; changes most prominent at ulcer margins
  - VCLE: lymphocytic interface dermatitis with dermoepidermal junction vesiculation; basal cell apoptosis
  - ECLE: lymphocytic interface dermatitis extending into follicular infundibulum and sebaceous glands; mural folliculitis; basal cell apoptosis
  - SLE: lymphocytic interface dermatitis with pigmentary incontinence and basal cell apoptosis; subepidermal vesiculation; leukocytoclastic vasculitis; panniculitis.
- Direct immunofluorescence or immunohistochemistry staining may reveal immunoglobulin and complement deposition at the dermoepidermal junction.

THERAPEUTICS

Drugs of Choice

- Cycline antibiotics: tetracycline (250 mg PO TID for dogs <10 kg; 500 mg PO TID dogs >10 kg); doxycycline (10 mg/kg PO q24h); minocycline (5 mg/kg PO BID); often administered with niacinamide 250 mg PO for dogs <10 kg and 500 mg PO for dogs >10 kg.

- Topical corticosteroids – betamethasone diproprionate 0.05% or fluocinolone 0.1%: apply sparingly q24h for 14 days; then EOD or twice weekly; if in remission, switch to less potent product (e.g., 0.5% or 2.5% hydrocortisone).
- Topical tacrolimus 0.1%: apply sparingly q24h for 14 days; then EOD or twice weekly.
- Prednisolone: 1–2 mg/kg PO BID initially tapered to EOD or twice weekly either solely or in combination with cytotoxic immunosuppressive drugs.
- Azathioprine: 2 mg/kg or 50 mg/m^2 PO daily until remission; then EOD or twice weekly; not for use in cats.
- Chlorambucil: 0.1–0.2 mg/kg q24h until remission; then EOD or twice weekly.
- Cyclosporine, microemulsion: 5–10 mg/kg q24h until remission; then EOD or twice weekly.
- Leflunomide: 2–4 mg/kg q24h or divided BID.
- Mycophenolate mofetil: 10 mg/kg PO BID.
- Vitamin E: 10–20 IU/kg PO q12h; may help reduce inflammation.

COMMENTS

- CBC and biochemistry: day 7; every 2–4 weeks until remission; then every 3–6 months when on oral medications.
- Avoid using affected animals for breeding.
- May be disfiguring; often scarring.
- Tissue loss of the nasal planum may create a source of trauma-induced bleeding.
- Avoid sunlight/apply sunblock.
- Monitor for development of secondary bacterial folliculitis.

Expected Course and Prognosis

- DLE is progressive but not usually life-threatening.
- DLE/GDLE/MCLE/VCLE: fair to good prognosis with treatment.
- ECLE: guarded to poor prognosis.
- SLE: guarded to poor prognosis especially with development of hemolytic anemia, glomerulonephritis or secondary bacterial infection.

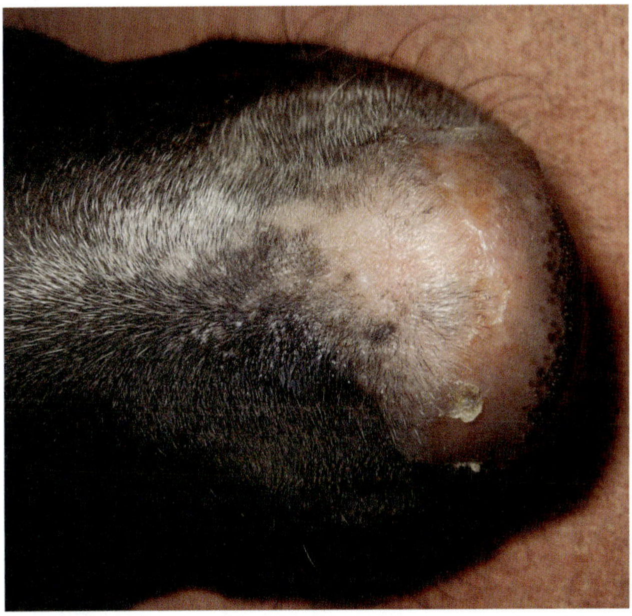

■ **Fig. 31.1.** DLE in a 3-year-old male-castrate pointer mix. The nasal planum and adjacent dorsal muzzle are depigmented, with mild erosions and scales. There is a loss of the normal cobblestone appearance of the nasal planum due to swelling.

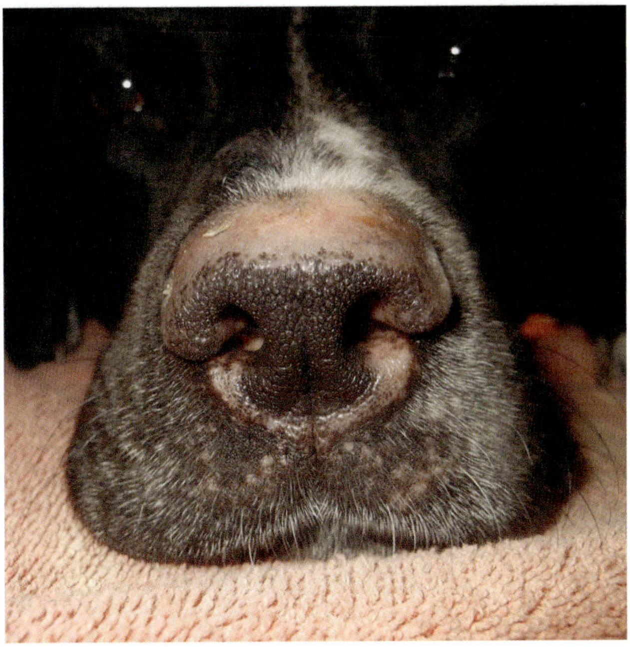

■ **Fig. 31.2.** Rostral aspect of the nasal planum of the patient in Figure 31.1. Loss of pigmentation occurring prior to development of scales or erosions in DLE.

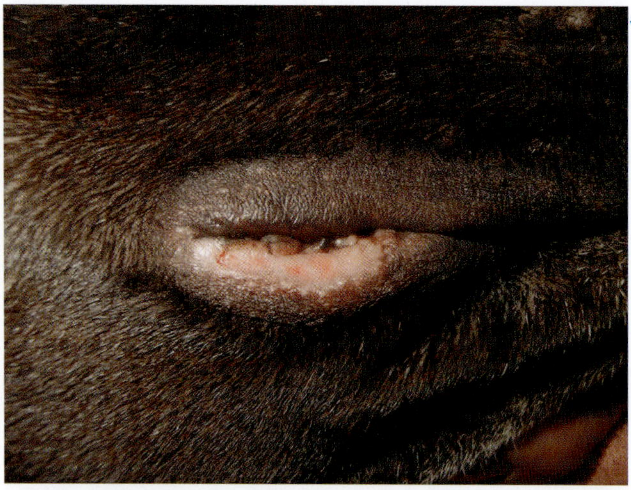

■ **Fig. 31.3.** Depigmentation and erosions on the lip margin of the patient in Figures 31.1 and 31.2.

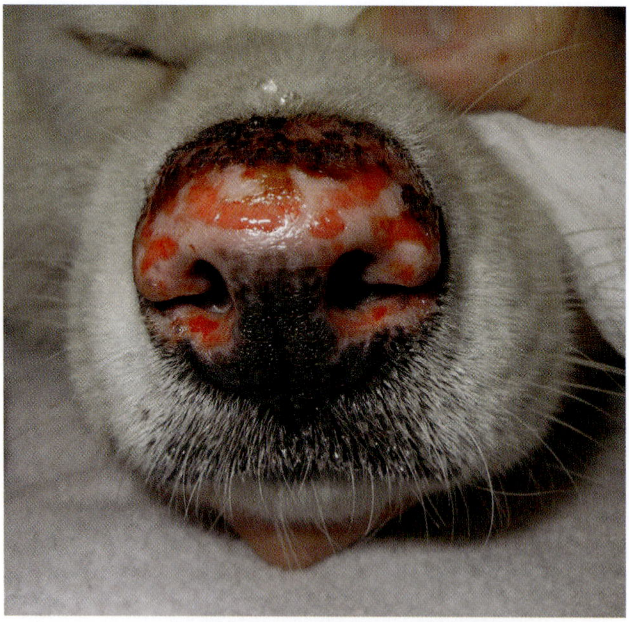

■ **Fig. 31.4.** Erosions and ulcerations developing within lesions of depigmentation on the nasal planum of a 3-year-old male-castrate Akita with DLE.

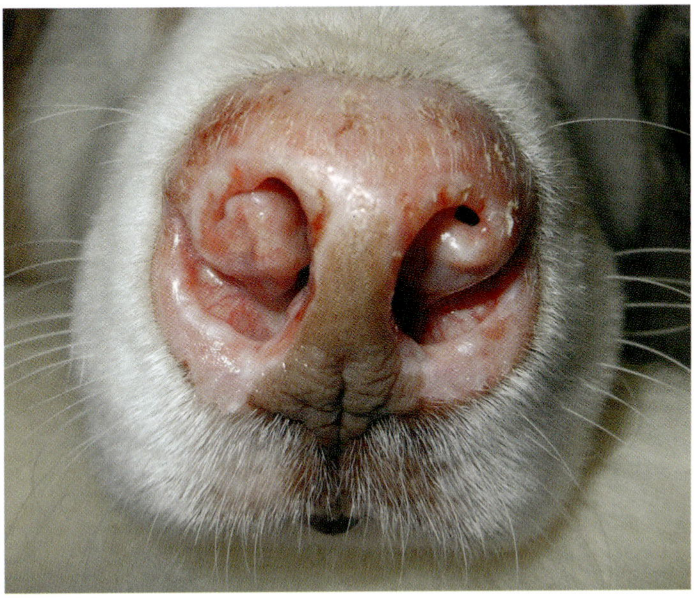

■ **Fig. 31.5.** Significant loss of tissue from chronic DLE in a 5-year-old male-castrate Australian shepherd.

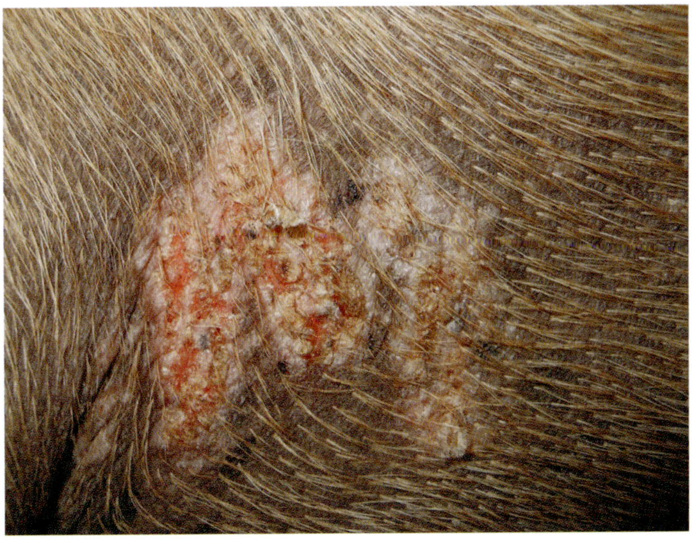

■ **Fig. 31.6.** Well-demarcated lesions of dyspigmentation with central erosion and peripheral hyperpigmentation in the axillae of a 4-year-old male-castrate boxer with GDLE.

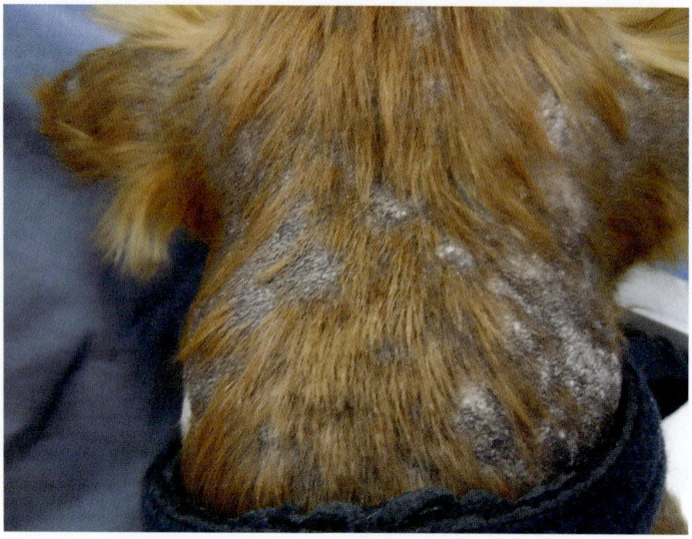

■ **Fig. 31.7.** More diffuse lesions developing initially on the head and neck of an 8-year-old male-castrate chow chow with GDLE. Lesions resulted in scarred coalescing patches with scales.

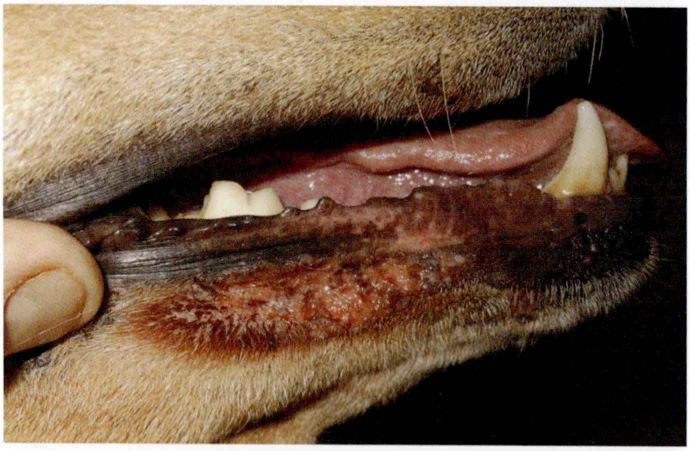

■ **Fig. 31.8.** Erosions and ulcerations at the margin of the lips with MCLE in a 6-year-old male-castrate Labrador retriever.

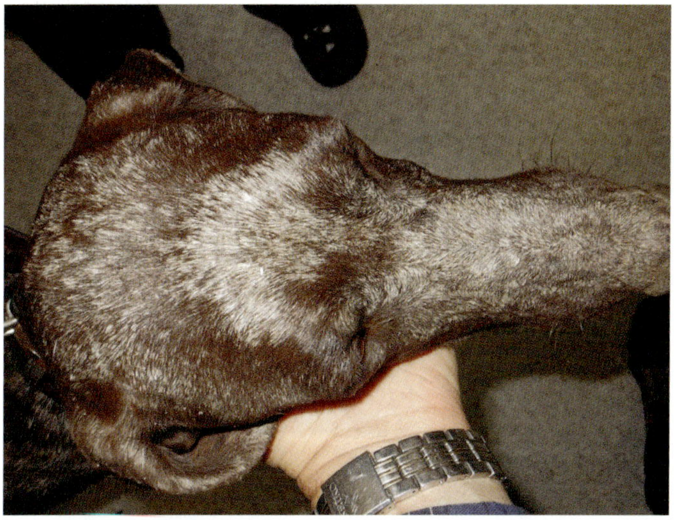

■ **Fig. 31.9.** ECLE in a 4-year-old female-spayed German short-haired pointer with fine adherent scales and alopecia starting on the muzzle and pinnae.

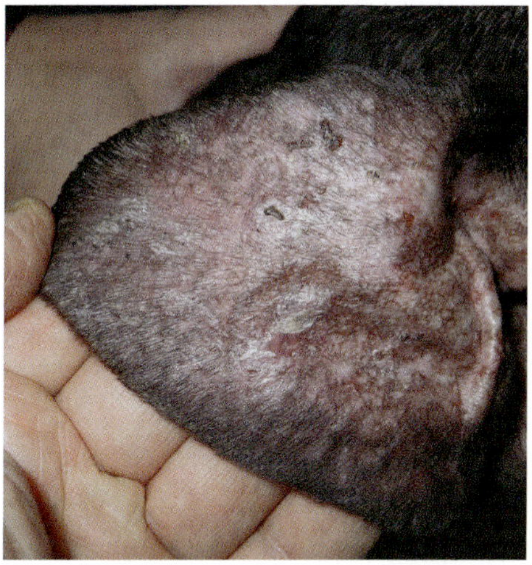

(a)

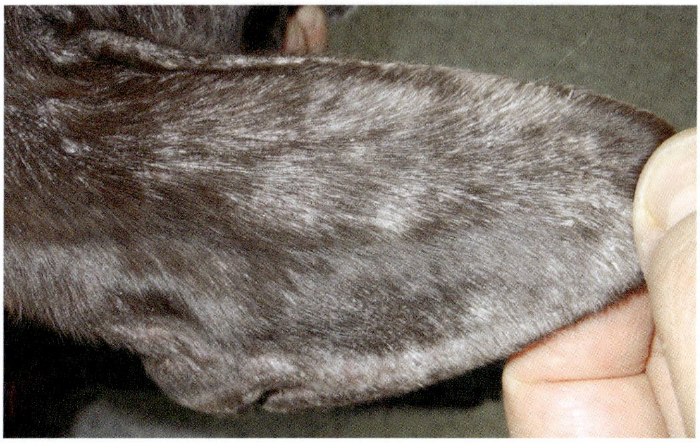

(b)

■ **Fig. 31.10.** Erythema, alopecia, and fine scaling affecting the pinna of a 6-year-old female-spayed German short-haired pointer with ECLE.

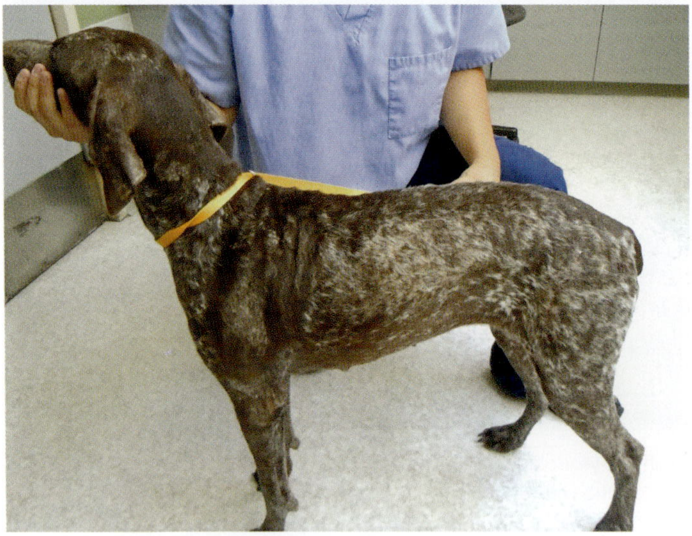

■ **Fig. 31.11.** Generalized lesions of the patient in Figure 31.9.

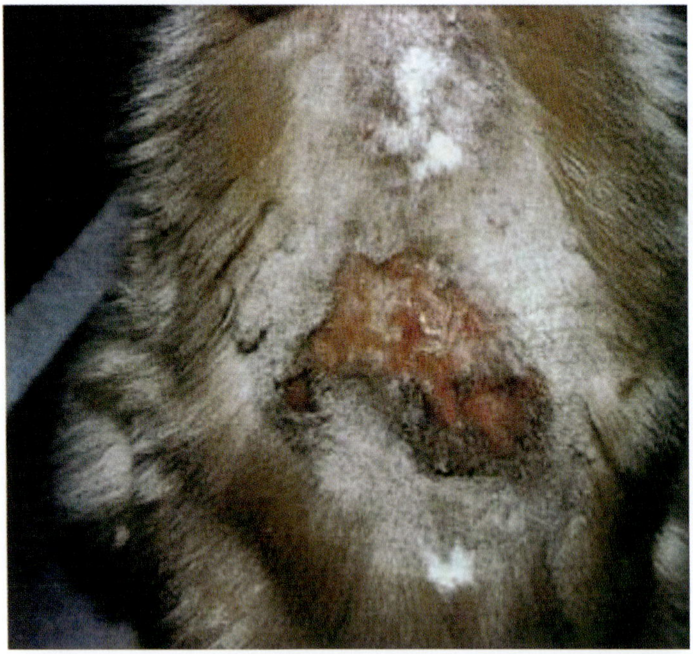

■ **Fig. 31.12.** Focal area of ulceration on the dorsum of a DLH with SLE. This patient also had intermittent fevers greater than 104 °F.

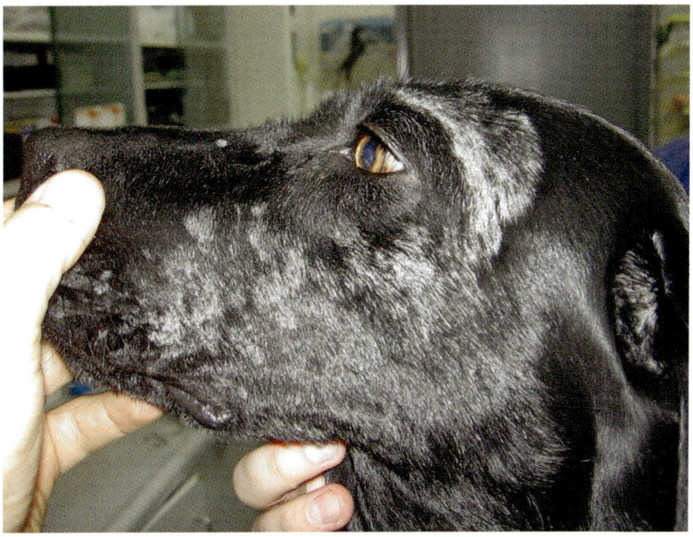

■ **Fig. 31.13.** Alopecia with fine scales similar in appearance to ECLE in a 4-year-old female Labrador retriever with SLE.

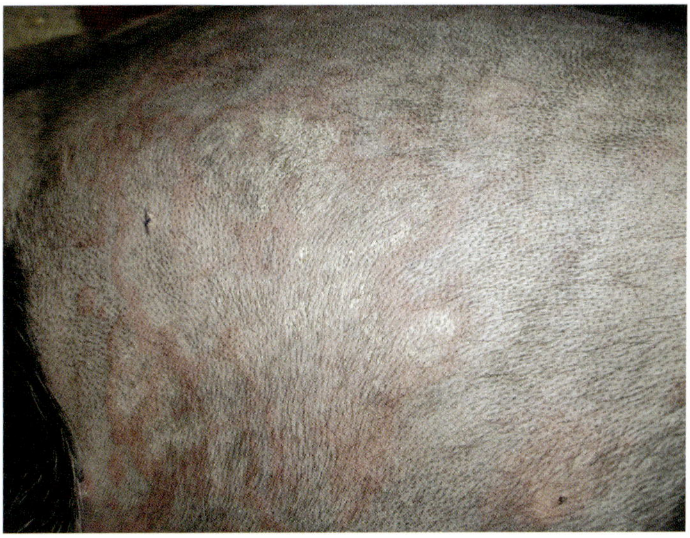

■ **Fig. 31.14.** Coalescing plaques with erythematous margins and central scales in a 12-year-old male-castrate Labrador mix with vasculitis secondary to SLE.

chapter 32

Malassezia Dermatitis

DEFINITION/OVERVIEW

- *Malassezia pachydermatis* (syn. *Malassezia canis*, *Pityrosporum canis*, and *Pityrosporum pachydermatis*): normal yeast commensal of the skin, ears, and mucocutaneous areas.
- *Malassezia* overgrowth syndrome (MOG)/*Malassezia* dermatitis – clinical disease due to overgrowth and colonization of a commensal organism causing dermatitis, cheilitis, paronychia, and otitis in dogs and cats.

ETIOLOGY/PATHOPHYSIOLOGY

- *M. pachydermatis* is nonlipid dependent; several species isolated from the cat and dog are lipid dependent (*M. sympodialis*, *M. globosa*, *M. nana*, *M. slooffiae*, *M. restricta*, and *M. furfur*).
- *Malassezia* species do not invade the skin beneath the stratum corneum.
- *Malassezia* may have a symbiotic relationship with commensal staphylococci; both yeast and bacterial numbers in diseased areas are typically excessive.
- Dermatitis likely results from inflammatory or hypersensitivity reactions to yeast products and antigens; the causes of the transformation from harmless commensal to pathogen are poorly understood but seem related to allergy, seborrheic conditions, and possibly congenital and hormonal factors.
- *Malassezia* produce many enzymes (e.g., lipases and proteases) which contribute to cutaneous inflammation by altering the lipidic cutaneous protective barrier (epidermal lipid barrier), changing cutaneous pH, and causing eicosanoid release and complement activation.
- *Malassezia* may be a primary allergen initiating a type I (immediate) hypersensitivity; skin testing with *Malassezia* extract results in an immediate hypersensitivity reaction in sensitized individuals; a delayed hypersensitivity pathway is also proposed.
- *Malassezia*-specific IgG and IgE are higher in atopic dogs compared to normal dogs; yeast may play a role in the pathogenesis of atopic dermatitis.
- *Malassezia* dermatitis is usually secondary to an underlying cause (e.g., allergy).

Blackwell's Five-Minute Veterinary Consult Clinical Companion: Small Animal Dermatology, Third Edition.
Karen Helton Rhodes and Alexander H. Werner.

SIGNALMENT/HISTORY

- Breeds predisposed:
  - Dogs: West Highland white terrier, miniature and toy poodle, basset hound, shih tzu, American cocker and cavalier King Charles spaniel, German shepherd, English setter, Australian and silky terriers, dachshund
  - Cats: Devon rex and sphynx.
- No gender predilection.

Risk Factors

- High humidity and elevated temperature.
- Anatomic factors: skinfolds, ear canals.
- Concurrent hypersensitivity disease (canine atopic dermatitis, flea allergy, cutaneous adverse reaction to food, contact dermatitis); causes mechanical disruption of the epidermal lipid barrier.
- Defects of keratinization/cornification increasing yeast nutrients.
- Endocrinopathy: hypothyroidism, hyperadrenocorticism, diabetes mellitus; causes changes in sebum production and immune dysfunction.
- Genetic factors: predisposed dog and cat breeds.
- Superficial staphylococcal folliculitis: yeast overgrowth is common with concurrent increase in cutaneous *Staphylococcus pseudintermedius* population; canine "seborrheic" dermatitis is proposed to be a result of this combination of pathogen overgrowth; treatment of one alone does not result in resolution of all signs, but just unmasks the other.
- Immunosuppression (e.g., neoplasia, viral disease including FIV).
- Medications: glucocorticoids or antibiotics without addressing the present yeast component.
- Ectoparasitic skin disease: demodicosis, scabies, etc.

CLINICAL FEATURES

- Pruritus (Figure 32.1).
- Erythema, alopecia, scale, and greasy, malodorous exudation (Figures 32.2–32.4).
- Hyperpigmentation and lichenification with chronicity (Figures 32.5, 32.6).
- Ceruminous otitis externa (Figure 32.7).
- Site predilection: lips, ear canals, axillae, inguinal area, perianal region, interdigital region, skinfolds, and ventral neck (Figures 32.8, 32.9).
- Facial pruritus and chin acne frequent in cats (Figure 32.10).
- Concurrent bacterial folliculitis.
- Paronychia/claw fold: red-brown discoloration of claws (Figure 32.11).
- Generalized erythematous scaly to waxy dermatitis (Figures 32.12, 32.13).

DIFFERENTIAL DIAGNOSIS

- Hypersensitivity dermatitis: canine atopic dermatitis, flea allergy, cutaneous adverse reaction to food, contact dermatitis.
- Superficial bacterial folliculitis.
- Primary and secondary seborrhea/keratinization disorders.
- Drug reaction.
- Epitheliotropic lymphoma.
- Dermatophytosis.
- Demodicosis.
- Scabies.

DIAGNOSTICS

- Diagnosis is made by demonstrating excessive numbers of the organism on diseased skin, and by a significant improvement in clinical signs following removal of the yeast.
- Skin cytology:
  - Direct impression, cotton swab, cellophane tape preparation, or "toothpick" for claw folds
  - Stained with modified Wright stain (Diff-Quik®)
  - Apply stain as a drop directly onto the slide; pass a flame under the slide to improve stain penetration and visualization
  - Greasy and/or scaly areas are most likely to produce positive results
  - Yeast are best visualized at 40× or 100× magnification
  - Seen as 3–8 μm in diameter, round to oval shaped with or without monopolar budding (described as "peanut" or "footprint" shape) (Figure 32.14)
  - There is no specific number of yeast organisms defined as abnormal; there is often overlap between normal and increased numbers based on anatomic location; few organisms may incite a hypersensitivity reaction.
- Intradermal skin test reactivity: *Malassezia* allergen-specific intradermal testing is a viable tool in determining immediate type hypersensitivity; should be included in immunotherapy vaccine (allergen-specific immunotherapy – ASIT).
- IgE serologic testing: enzyme-linked immunosorbent assay for *Malassezia* allergen-specific IgE; substantial agreement between IDST and ELISA for *Malassezia* allergen-specific IgE.
- IDST and ELISA: negative testing does not rule out a pathologic role for this organism; delayed type hypersensitivity may be clinically relative.
- Fungal culture:
  - Minimal value since *Malassezia* spp. are commensal organisms
  - Contact plates: Sabouraud agar or modified Dixon agar
  - Press plates onto the affected skin surface
  - Incubate at 32–37 °C for 3–7 days
  - *Malassezia* grows as distinctive yellow or buff, round, domed colonies (1–1.5 mm) (Figure 32.15).

- CBC/biochemistry to detect underlying diseases (e.g., hypothyroidism, hyperadrenocorticism).
- Ultrasonography and radiography to investigate possible internal malignancy.
- Histopathology:
  - Less sensitive method of diagnosis than cytology due to loss of superficial yeast during processing
  - Considered significant if yeast organisms are found within the infundibulum and interspersed within the stratum corneum
  - Superficial perivascular to interstitial dermatitis, accumulation of mast cells at the dermal-epidermal junction, lymphocytic exocytosis, and parakeratosis
  - Concurrent bacterial folliculitis.

THERAPEUTICS

- Identify and treat any predisposing factors or underlying diseases.

Topical Therapy

- Necessary component of the treatment since yeast organisms are located in the stratum corneum.
- Recommended twice weekly during active treatment; weekly maintenance in chronic cases.
- Antiseptic shampoo treatment: removes scale, exudation, and malodor; kills yeast and bacterial organisms.
- Active ingredients in creams/ointments/wipes: miconazole, clotrimazole, climbazole, ketoconazole, terbinafine.
- Active ingredients in shampoo/rinse therapy: sodium hypochlorite, chlorhexidine, ketoconazole, miconazole, selenium sulfide, enilconazole, lime sulfur, acetic and boric acids.

Systemic Therapy

- Ketoconazole: 5–10 mg/kg PO q24h for 2–4 weeks; discontinue or taper to the lowest possible or pulse dose; dogs only.
- Fluconazole: 5 mg/kg PO BID for 2–4 weeks; discontinue or taper to the lowest possible or pulse dose (dogs and cats).
- Itraconazole: 5 mg/kg PO q24h for 2 consecutive days and repeated weekly for 3–4 weeks (small dogs and cats).
- Terbinafine: 30–40 mg/kg PO q24h for 3 weeks; discontinue or taper to the lowest possible or pulse dose (dogs and cats).

Precautions/Interactions

- Ketoconazole: may cause gastrointestinal upset; masks signs of hyperadrenocorticism and interferes with adrenal function tests by blocking cortisol production; strong inhibitor of cytochrome p450 enzymes; avoid concurrent use with ivermectin – may exacerbate ivermectin toxicity; contraindicated in cats due to impaired metabolism of the drug; patients should be monitored with routine blood work for hepatotoxicity.

- Fluconazole: minimal side effects, safe option; moderate inhibitor cytochrome p450 enzymes.
- Itraconazole: often well tolerated; specific for fungal cytochrome p450 enzymes; mild inhibitor of mammalian cytochrome p450 enzymes; dose with food for best absorption; concurrent use with oral antacids will decrease oral absorption; monitor for hepatotoxicity; specific has little effect on hormone synthesis and will not produce endocrine effects; adverse effects – vasculitis and ulcerative skin lesions.
- Terbinafine: hepatotoxicity not reported from use in animals; facial pruritus has been reported in cats; no contraindications or drug interactions; vomiting most common side effect.

COMMENTS

Facts for Pet Owners about *Malassezia*

FACT Normal commensal yeast organism on the surface of the skin. *Malassezia pachydermatis* can be found on normal dogs primarily around the nose, ears, mouth, anus, axillae, anal sacs, skin folds, claw folds, and interdigital regions. Often seen as a red-brown discoloration at the base of the nails and interdigital webs. Yeasts love moist, dark crevices. Humidity is yeast's friend. Seborrheic skin and allergic skin are prone to yeast overgrowth.

FACT Yeasts create a rancid, pungent, musty odor (described as "corn chip" or "Frito-feet").

FACT *Malassezia* has a symbiotic relationship with staphylococcal bacteria. More bacteria on the skin = more yeast on the skin. Staphylococcal bacteria and *Malassezia* yeast produce mutually beneficial growth factors and alterations in their microenvironment. It is common for dogs with a yeast overgrowth to also have a bacterial folliculitis. Yeasts produce proteins and glycoproteins that allow staphylococcal bacteria to adhere to skin cells. Yeast organisms do not invade the skin beyond the outer layer (stratum corneum). Yeast "dermatitis" results from an inflammatory or hypersensitivity reaction to yeast products and antigens.

FACT *Malassezia pachydermatis* produces a number of inflammatory products that cause the skin to become moist, red, thickened with chronicity, and very itchy. These products alter the skin's pH and activate the inflammatory cascade in the skin that results in a hypersensitivity reaction. Chronic exposure to these products causes the skin to become thickened and lichenified (elephant skin). Constant scratching, licking or rubbing of the skin will also contribute to skin thickening … it is the "perfect storm."

FACT intradermal skin testing for environmental allergies (trees, grasses, weeds, pollens, molds, dust mites, etc.) can also identify an allergy to yeast.

Common Misconceptions Held by Pet Owners

Misconception	Fact
Antibiotic therapy in dogs causes yeast infections	*Malassezia* and staphylococci are synergistic on the skin; There is no evidence that antibiotics cause an overgrowth of yeast. Yeast numbers are enhanced when the skin is co-colonized with bacteria
Oatmeal shampoos "feed" yeast infections	Shampoos have too limited a contact time to encourage yeast overgrowth; carbohydrates do not "feed" yeast organisms
Coconut oil is anti-yeast	Topical coconut oil *encourages* yeast overgrowth by providing more lipids
Brewer's yeast induces yeast infections	No supporting scientific data; brewer's yeast is *Saccharomyces cerevisiae* (not *Malassezia* sp.); may increase salivary IgA in humans
Most important way to manage yeast infections is with diet	Most important way to manage yeast infections is identification and control of the underlying cause (e.g., allergy). The diet is not relevant *unless* the underlying etiology is a cutaneous adverse food reaction
Carbohydrates, sugars, and starch in the diet encourage yeast overgrowth Dietary supplements that reduce yeast organisms include garlic, thyme, oregano, parsley, apple cider vinegar, coconut oil, and fermented vegetables; probiotics, goldenseal, and caprylic acid can restore normal cutaneous yeast populations	No scientific support. Dietary carbohydrates have no direct link to *Malassezia* dermatitis. The quantity of these ingredients in the diet has no effect on yeast populations; these dietary ingredients do not directly reach the skin; hypersensitivity to dietary carbohydrates is uncommon
Antifungal rinses or sprays should be composed of apple cider vinegar, "essential oils," lemon juice, peppermint or lavender oil mixed with water	ASPCA reports that essential oils can be toxic if ingested. Vinegar (any type) applied as a 1:10 dilution is acidic and lowers skin pH – can help reduce yeast populations
Immune testing for IgG, IgA, and IgM will tell you if your dog is immunodeficient; these levels are low in a dog with chronic yeast infection	Tests are not specific; increased, rather than low, IgA and IgG levels have been detected in serum of dogs with yeast overgrowth; however, these immunoglobulins are not considered protective; immune deficiency may actually decrease *Malassezia* dermatitis by preventing a hypersensitivity reaction; intradermal allergy testing can detect hypersensitivity to *Malassezia*

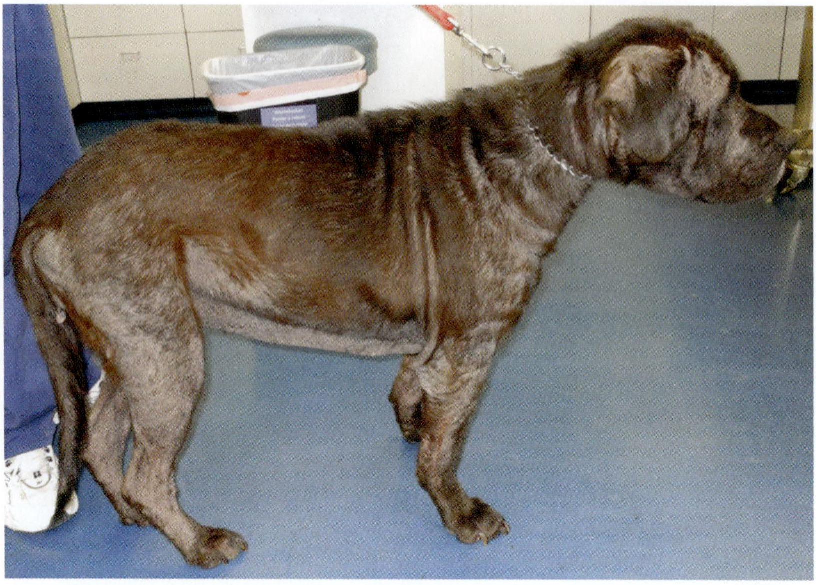

■ **Fig. 32.1.** Alopecia, hyperpigmentation, and lichenification resulting from pruritus and secondary *Malassezia* dermatitis in a 10-year-old female-spayed Labrador retriever mix.

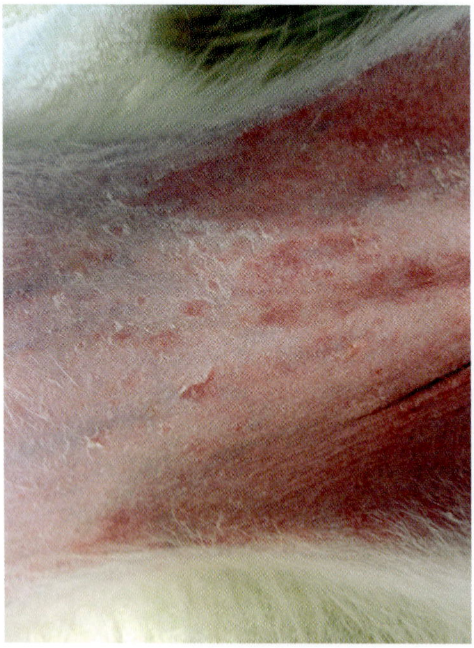

■ **Fig. 32.2.** Intense erythroderma with superficial scaling on the flank folds in a terrier mix with *Malassezia* hypersensitivity.

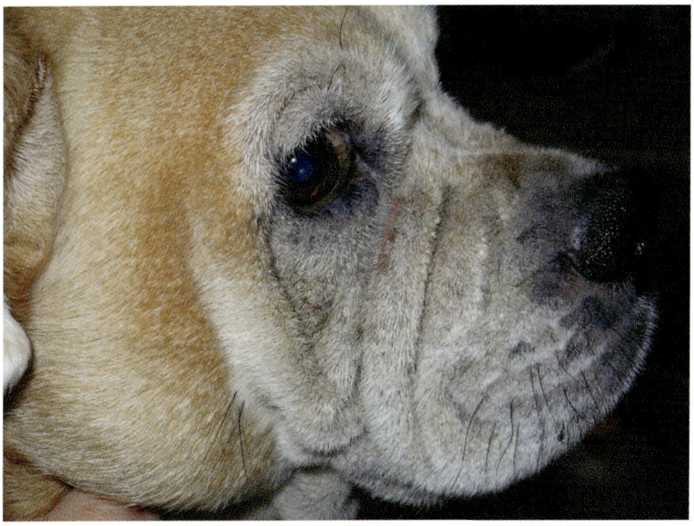

■ **Fig. 32.3.** Lichenification with crusts affecting the periocular region and facial folds in a 9-year-old female-spayed puggle with atopic dermatitis and secondary *Malassezia* dermatitis.

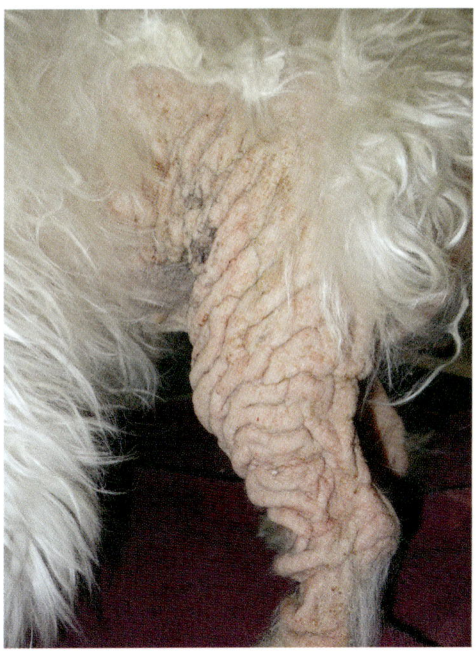

■ **Fig. 32.4.** Severe lichenification with crusting affecting the rear leg of a 2-year-old male-castrate Maltese with secondary *Malassezia* dermatitis.

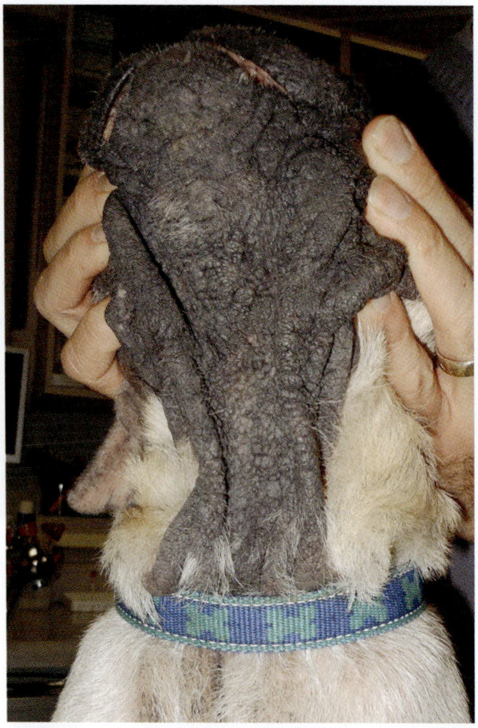

■ **Fig. 32.5.** Hyperpigmentation with lichenification and greasy exudate on the ventral neck and chin of a 13-year-old male-castrate pug with chronic *Malassezia* dermatitis secondary to atopic dermatitis.

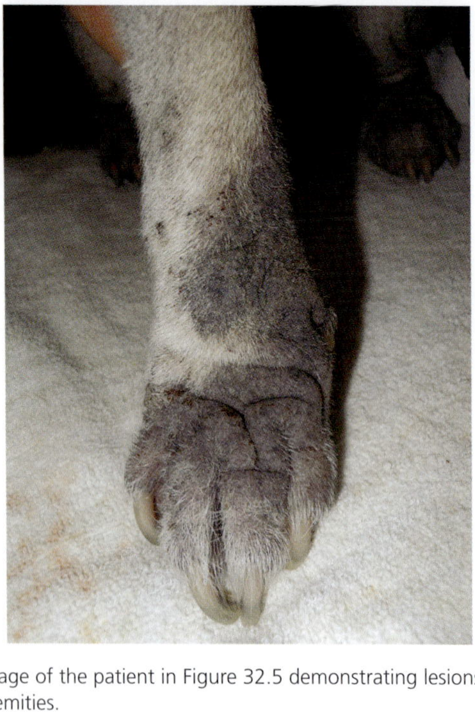

■ **Fig. 32.6.** Additional image of the patient in Figure 32.5 demonstrating lesions characteristic of *Malassezia* dermatitis on the distal extremities.

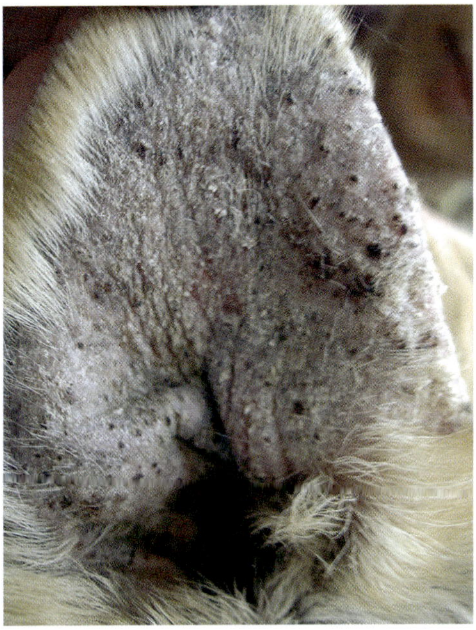

Fig. 32.7. *Malassezia* dermatitis affecting both the pinna and external ear canal in a dog with a cutaneous adverse reaction to food.

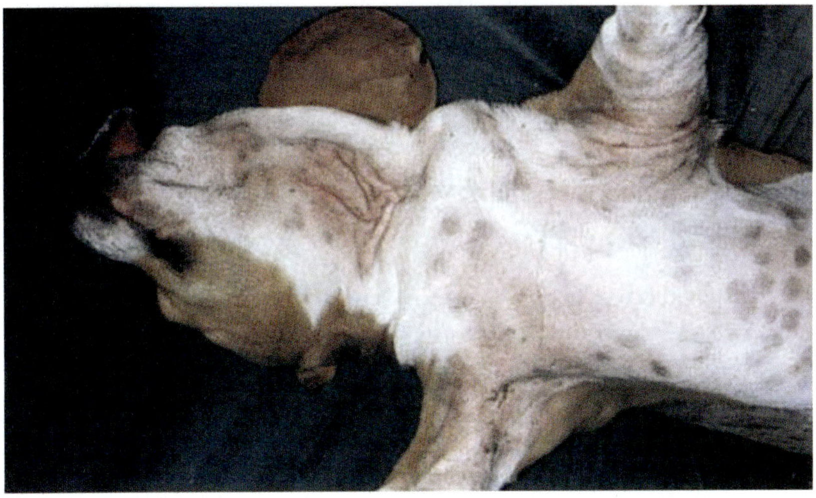

Fig. 32.8. Basset hound with *Malassezia* and "seborrheic" dermatitis in the fold regions of the ventral neck and axillae.

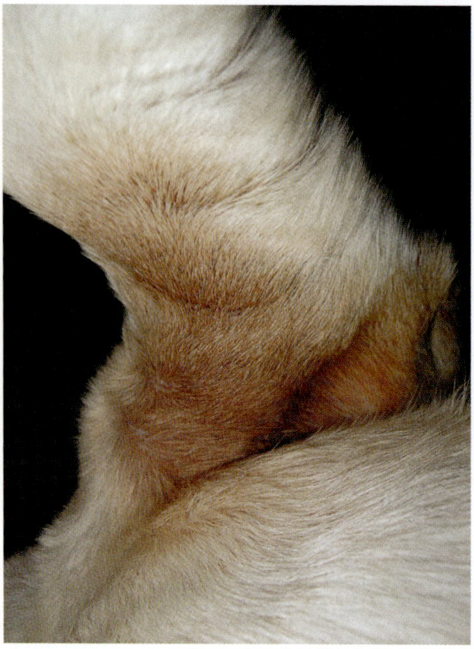

■ **Fig. 32.9.** Stained hair coat with greasy exudate in the axilla of a 7-year-old female-spayed Labrador with *Malassezia* dermatitis.

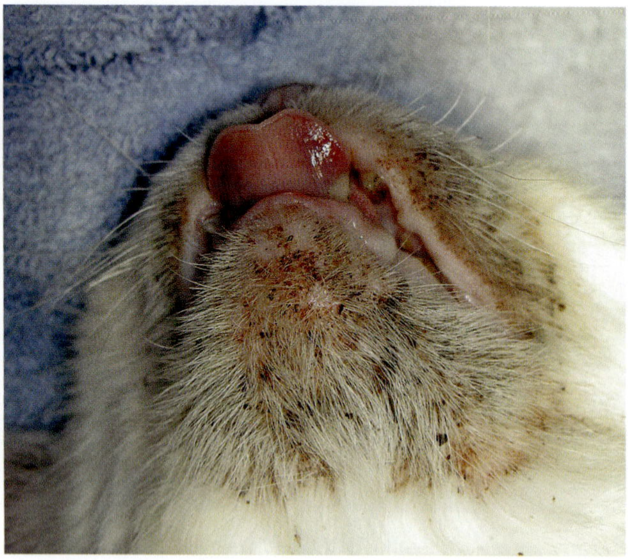

■ **Fig. 32.10.** Chin acne affecting a 13-year-old female-spayed Persian with *Malassezia* dermatitis and bacterial folliculitis secondary to pemphigus foliaceus.

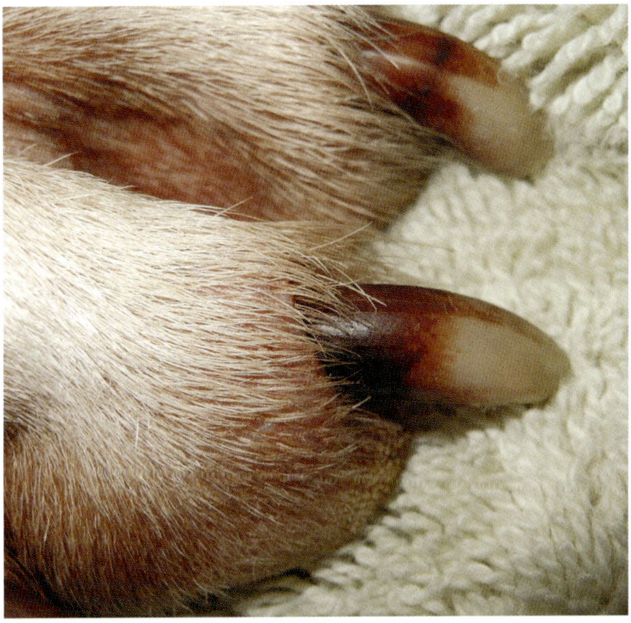

■ **Fig. 32.11.** Characteristic rust-brown staining of *Malassezia* on the proximal claw of a 5-year-old male-castrate pit bull terrier.

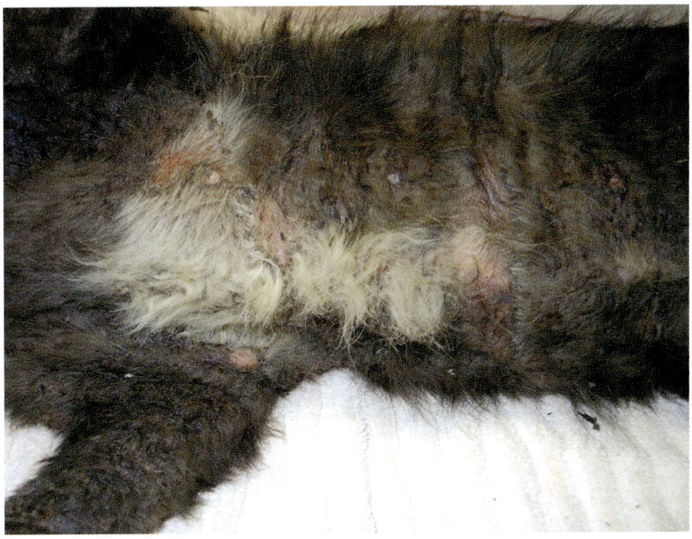

■ **Fig. 32.12.** Severe *Malassezia* dermatitis producing a generalized exfoliative and crusted dermatitis in a 6-month-old female-intact DSH.

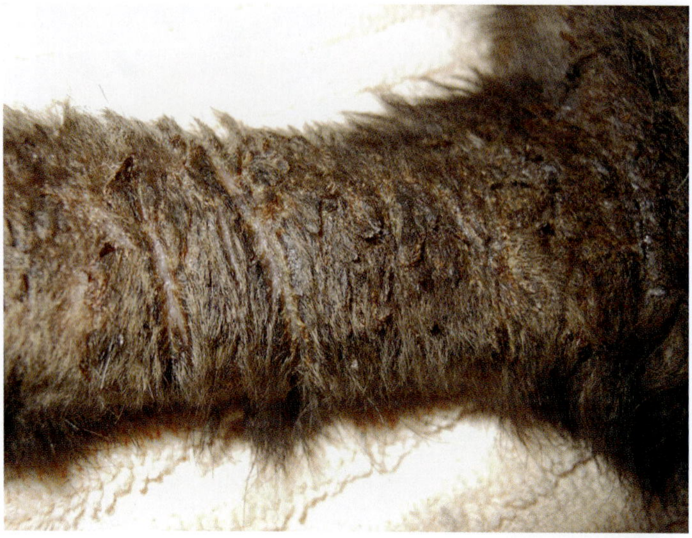

■ **Fig. 32.13.** Closer image of patient in Figure 32.12 demonstrating adherent crusts over exudative skin on the foreleg.

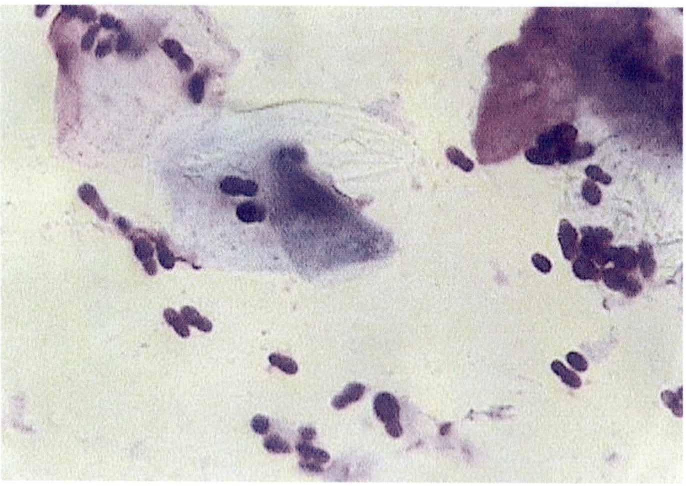

■ **Fig. 32.14.** Direct cytology of *Malassezia*: 3–8 μm in diameter, round to oval-shaped organisms with or without monopolar budding (described as "peanut" or "footprint" shape).

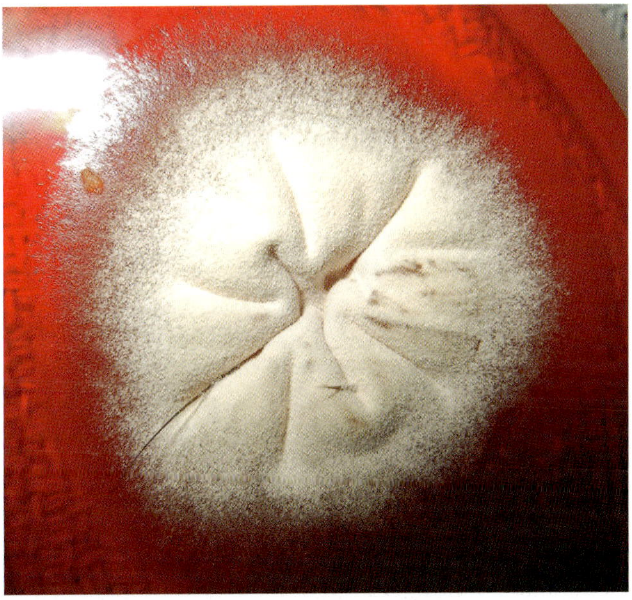

Fig. 32.15. *Malassezia* growth on dermatophyte test media (modified Sabouraud agar) forming a distinctive yellow or buff, round, domed colony (1–1.5 mm).

chapter 33

Mast Cell Tumors

DEFINITION/OVERVIEW

- Neoplasia arising from malignant round cells of hematopoietic origin.
- Mast cell granules contain many substances including histamine, heparin, platelet-activating factor, serine proteases, lysosomal enzymes, and cytokines.

ETIOLOGY/PATHOPHYSIOLOGY

- Histamine and other vasoactive substances released from mast cell tumors may cause erythema and edema; histamine may cause gastric and duodenal ulcers.
- Heparin release: increases likelihood of bleeding.
- Skin and subcutaneous tissue most common tumor sites in dogs.
- Hemic/lymphatic/immune-spleen: common primary location in cats (up to 50% of cases); rare in dogs; site of metastasis from the skin or subcutaneous tissue.
- Gastrointestinal: intestinal mast cell tumor uncommon in cats and rare in dogs; gastric and duodenal ulcers possible.
- Etiology unknown: viral etiology suspected by some investigators; current emphasis on genetic mutations of the tumor suppressor gene *p53* (13.75–44.6% of tumors) and c-KIT receptor tyrosine kinase.
- c-KIT mutations may result in increased recurrence and higher mortality; not all dogs with mast cell tumors have mutations (15%); often positive for mutation in higher grades of mast cell tumors (30–56%); measurement of c-KIT mutation by PCR may be a useful prognostic indicator.
- Histopathologic grading system valuable in the dog, not valuable in the cat; prognostication should rely on both histologic grading and clinical staging.

SIGNALMENT/HISTORY

- Most common skin tumor in the dog: 17–21% of skin and subcutaneous tumors; 11–14% of cases may develop multiple tumors synchronously or successively.
- Second most common skin tumor in cats (often benign in skin): 20% of skin tumors.

Blackwell's Five-Minute Veterinary Consult Clinical Companion: Small Animal Dermatology, Third Edition.
Karen Helton Rhodes and Alexander H. Werner.

- Predominant breeds: boxer, Staffordshire bull terrier, bulldog, English bulldog, dachshund, Boston terrier, shar pei, basset hound, weimaraner, fox terrier, beagle, pug, Labrador retriever, and golden retriever.
- Siamese cats: predisposed to histiocytic cutaneous mast cell tumors (young cats); may resolve spontaneously.
- Himalayan cats predisposed to urticaria pigmentosa (benign proliferative mast cell disorder seen in young cats).
- Dogs: mean age, 8 years; no sex predilection.
- Cats: mean age, 10 years except for urticaria pigmentosa and histiocytic cutaneous mast cell tumors; male predilection.
- Reported in animals <1 year old and in cats as old as 18 years.

Dogs

- Patient may have had skin or subcutaneous tumor for days to months at the time of examination.
- May have appeared to fluctuate in size.
- Recent rapid growth after months of quiescence common.
- Recent onset of erythema and edema most common with high-grade skin and subcutaneous tumors.

Cats

- Often no demonstration of systemic signs.
- Anorexia: most common complaint with splenic tumor.
- Vomiting: may occur secondary to both splenic and gastrointestinal tumors.

CLINICAL FEATURES

- Darier's sign: mechanical manipulation or extreme changes in temperature can lead to degranulation of mast cells with subsequent erythema and wheal formation and gastrointestinal ulceration causing anorexia, vomiting, and melena (Figures 33.1, 33.2).

Dogs

- Presentation extremely variable; may resemble any other type of skin or subcutaneous tumor (benign and malignant); may resemble an insect bite or allergic reaction, subcutaneous form may be mistaken clinically for a lipoma.
- Well-differentiated tumors: often slow growing; usually <3–4 cm in diameter; no ulceration of overlying skin; variably alopecic; commonly present for more than 6 months (Figures 33.3–33.5).
- Poorly differentiated mast cell tumors: rapidly growing; variably sized; variable ulceration of the overlying skin and inflammation/edema of the surrounding tissue; rarely present for more than 2–3 months prior to presentation (Figures 33.6, 33.7).
- Primarily a solitary skin or subcutaneous mass, but may be multifocal (Figure 33.8).

- Approximately 50% located on the trunk and perineum; 40% on extremities; 10% on the head and neck region; breed predilection for locations reported (especially hindlimb) (Figures 33.9, 33.10).
- Poorer prognosis associated with tumors on the perineum, prepuce, scrotum, groin, axillae, and digits (Figures 33.11–33.13).
- Regional lymphadenopathy: may develop when a high-grade tumor metastasizes to draining lymph nodes.
- Hepatomegaly and splenomegaly: features of disseminated mast cell neoplasia.

Cats

- Cutaneous: primarily found in the subcutaneous tissue or dermis; may be papular or nodular, solitary or multiple, and haired or alopecic or have an ulcerated surface; slight predilection for the head and neck regions (Figures 33.14, 33.15).
- Clusters of nodules that appear on the face and ears may regress spontaneously (histiocytic form especially in young Siamese) (Figure 33.16).
- Most feline tumors are well differentiated and benign.
- Urticaria pigmentosa appears as hyperpigmented and/or erythematous macules around the mouth, chin, neck, and eyes (spontaneous regression in some cases) (Figure 33.17).
- Intestinal mast cell tumor: firm, segmental thickenings of the small intestinal wall; measures 1–7 cm in diameter; metastases to the mesenteric lymph nodes, spleen, liver, and (rarely) lungs (Figure 33.18).

DIFFERENTIAL DIAGNOSIS

- Any other skin or subcutaneous tumor, benign or malignant, including lipoma.
- Insect bite or allergic reaction.

DIAGNOSTICS

- Cytologic examination of fine-needle aspirate:
    - Most important preliminary diagnostic test
    - Round cells with basophilic cytoplasmic granules that do not form sheets or clumps (Figure 33.19)
    - Malignant mast cells may be agranular; occurrence of a large eosinophilic infiltrate may suggest mast cell tumor
    - Granules may not stain well with Diff-Quick stain; may require methanol fixative for at least 2 minutes prior to routine staining
    - Cytology not useful to determine grade or prognosis.
- Use of buffy coat cytology and liver/spleen fine-needle aspirate is controversial and often not considered important in staging of disease.
- Tissue biopsy: necessary for definitive diagnosis and grading.

- Administer diphenhydramine 1 mg/kg SQ prior to biopsy of suspected mast cell tumor.
- Use caution when obtaining a biopsy sample from a mast cell tumor; sites may bleed excessively.
- Canine grading systems:
  - Patnaik: based on cellularity, cell morphology, mitotic index, extent of tissue involvement, and stromal reaction (survival greater than 1500 days reported):
    - Grade 1: well differentiated; located in the dermis and interfollicular spaces; low potential for metastasis; (93%)
    - Grade 2: intermediate with rare mitotic figures; infiltrate to the deep dermis and subcutaneous tissue; potential for local invasion and moderate potential for metastasis (47%)
    - Grade 3: undifferentiated or anaplastic with 3–6 mitotic figures; infiltrate into/beyond subcutaneous tissue; high potential for metastasis (6%)
  - Kiupel: low grade or high grade:
    - High grade: characterized by any one of these criteria (per 10 hpf):
      - At least 7 mitotic figures
      - At least 3 multinucleated cells
      - At least 3 bizarre nuclei
      - Karyomegaly
    - Median survival time greater than 2 years for low grade and less than 4 months for high grade.
- Cats: grading system not beneficial; no correlation between histopathologic appearance of cutaneous tumor and prognosis.
- Staging to determine the extent of disease and appropriate treatment:
  - Full physical exam
  - Bloodwork/urinalysis
  - Fine-needle aspirate of local lymph nodes even if they are not palpable
  - Abdominal ultrasound.
- Additional tests to achieve complete staging: cytologic examination or biopsy of local draining lymph node; cytologic examination of bone marrow aspirate is controversial; thoracic radiography and abdominal ultrasonography.
- Negative clinical prognostic factors include advanced stage, caudal half of body location, high tumor growth rate, aneuploidy, presence of systemic signs.
- Negative molecular-based prognostic factors include increased AgNOR (silver nucleolar organizing regions), increased PCNA/Ki67 immunohistochemistry expression (proliferation markers), increased vascularity and/or mitotic index, and increased c-KIT expression; the use of these panels is strongly recommended due to significant predictive ability for both development of metastasis and recurrence.

THERAPEUTICS

Dogs

- Aggressive surgical excision: treatment of choice.

- Histopathologic evaluation of the entire excised tissue: essential to determine surgical margins and to predict biologic behavior; recommend 2–3 cm lateral margins and one fascial plane deep to the mast cell tumor if possible; perform aggressive excision as soon as possible post diagnosis.
- Although incomplete excision may leave residual tumor, some reports indicate that incompletely excised grade 1 and 2 tumors may not regrow.
- Lymph node involvement but no systemic involvement: aggressive excision of the affected lymph node(s) and the primary tumor required; follow-up chemotherapy useful to prevent further metastasis.
- Primary tumor and/or affected lymph node cannot be excised: chemotherapy has minimal benefit.
- Systemic metastasis: excision of primary tumor and affected lymph nodes and follow-up chemotherapy have minimal effect on survival time.
- Radiotherapy: external beam radiation therapy: excellent adjuvant option for unresectable tumors; if possible, debulk tumor prior to radiotherapy; tumors on an extremity respond better than do tumors located on the trunk.

Cats

- Surgery: treatment of choice for cutaneous tumors.
- Some forms will spontaneously regress.
- Cats should be staged to insure that they do not have splenic primary mast cell tumor that is metastasizing to cutaneous locations as well as other sites.

Drugs of Choice

- Chemotherapy is typically less effective than surgery and radiation therapy; regardless of response rate, median time to progression 77–141 days.
- Prednisolone: induced remission and prolonged survival time in 20% of patients with grade 2 or 3 tumors; only one of the five responding patients had documented lymph node metastasis when initiated.
- Chlorambucil/prednisolone: overall response rate 38%.
- Lomustine: overall response rate 42%.
- Vinblastine/prednisolone: overall response rate 47%.
- Vinblastine/lomustine/prednisolone: overall response rate 65%.
- Vincristine alone: partial remission in 21% of patients.
- Studies suggest that lomustine, vinblastine, and cyclophosphamide have limited activity against mast cell tumors; may lengthen time of remission with prednisone-sensitive tumors.
- Dogs:
  - Prednisolone: 1 mg/kg PO q24h; taper slowly after 4 months; discontinue after 7 months
  - Vinblastine alone: 3.5 mg/m^2 IV q14 days; partial remission 21%
  - Vinblastine 2 mg/kg/m^2 IV q7 days for four treatments; then q14 days with prednisolone 1 mg/kg PO q24h

- Cyclophosphamide: 250–300 mg/m^2 PO divided over 4 days; administer on days 8, 9, 10, and 11 of each 21-day cycle; initiate at 250 mg/m^2 for two cycles; increase to 300 mg/m^2 for cycle 3 if well tolerated; continue for 6 months
- Lomustine (CCNU): 50–70 mg/m^2 PO q21 days
- Toceranib phosphate: 2.75 mg/kg PO M/W/F; tyrosine kinase inhibitor; also targets vascular endothelial growth factor receptor 2, and PDGFR-beta 42.8% response rate; median time to progression 126 days
- Mastinib 12.5 mg/kg PO q24h; tyrosine kinase inhibitor; also targets platelet-derived growth factors alpha and beta, and fibroblast growth factor 3; overall response 82.1%; median time to progression 79 days.

- Cats:
  - Lomustine 32–60 mg/m^2 PO q4–6 weeks
  - Vinblastine 2 mg/kg/m^2 IV q7 days for four treatments; then q14 days with prednisolone 1 mg/kg PO q21h.
- Histamine-blocking agents (e.g., cimetidine): helpful for systemic mastocytosis or when massive histamine release is of concern; helps to prevent gastric ulceration and counteract negative effects of histamine on fibroplasia in wound healing.
- Sucralfate helpful if gastrointestinal ulceration present: binds to ulcer site.
- Prednisolone-resistant tumor: chemotherapy does not appear to be beneficial.
- Intestinal tumor and systemic mastocytosis after splenectomy (cats): prednisolone and chemotherapy indicated.
- Vinblastine and lomustine: myelosuppressive; use with caution in patients with liver disease.
- Toceranib and mastinib: use with caution with other drugs that may induce gastric ulceration.

COMMENTS

Client Education/Patient Monitoring

- Warn client that a patient that has had more than one cutaneous tumor is predisposed to developing new mast cell tumors.
- Advise client that fine-needle aspiration and cytologic examination should be performed as soon as possible on any new mass.
- Inform client that appropriate surgical excision should be done as soon as possible.
- Evaluate any new masses cytologically or histologically.
- Evaluate regional lymph nodes at regular intervals to detect metastasis of grade 2 or 3 tumor.

Expected Course and Prognosis

- Dogs:
  - Tumors in the inguinal region: tend to be more aggressive than similarly graded tumors in other locations; always considered to have the potential to metastasize

- Survival times 6 months after surgery (Bostock): grade I, 77% alive; grade 2, 45% alive; grade 3, 13% alive
- Lymph node metastasis: survival may be prolonged if prednisolone and chemotherapy are given after the primary tumor and affected lymph node(s) are aggressively excised.

■ Cats:

- Solitary cutaneous tumor: prognosis excellent; rate of recurrence low (16–36%) despite incomplete excision; <20% of patients develop metastasis
- Survival after splenectomy for splenic tumor: reports of >1 year
- Concurrent development of mastocythemia: prognosis poor; prednisone and chemotherapy may achieve short-term remission
- Intestinal tumor: prognosis poor; survival times rarely >4 months after surgery.

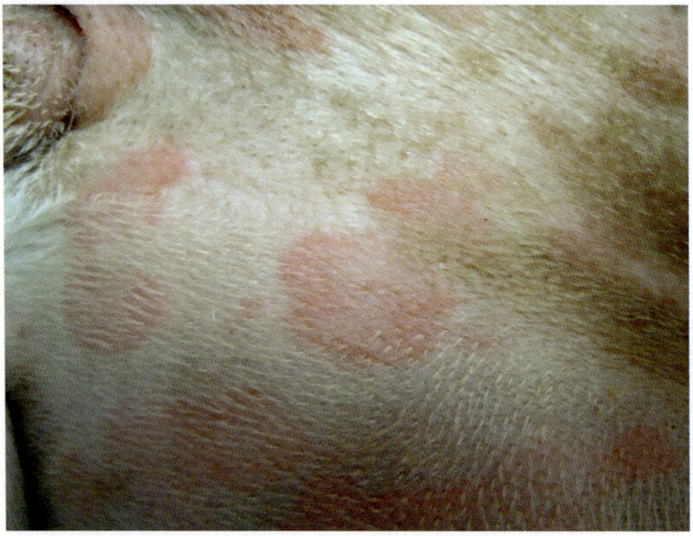

■ **Fig. 33.1.** Urticarial reaction from manipulation of a mast cell tumor on an 11-year-old female-spayed pit bull terrier.

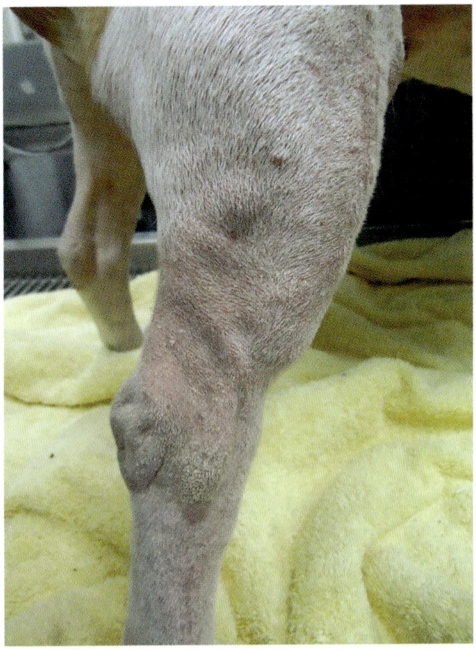

■ **Fig. 33.2.** Darier's sign: manipulation of the mast cell tumor produced erythroderma in the patient in Figure 33.1.

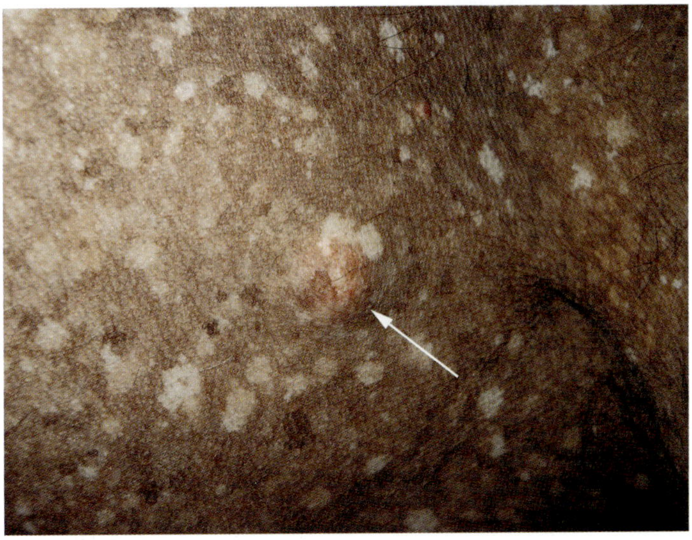

■ **Fig. 33.3.** Erythematous nodule (*arrow*) representing a grade 1 mast cell tumor on the lateral thorax of a 7-year-old male-castrate doberman pinscher.

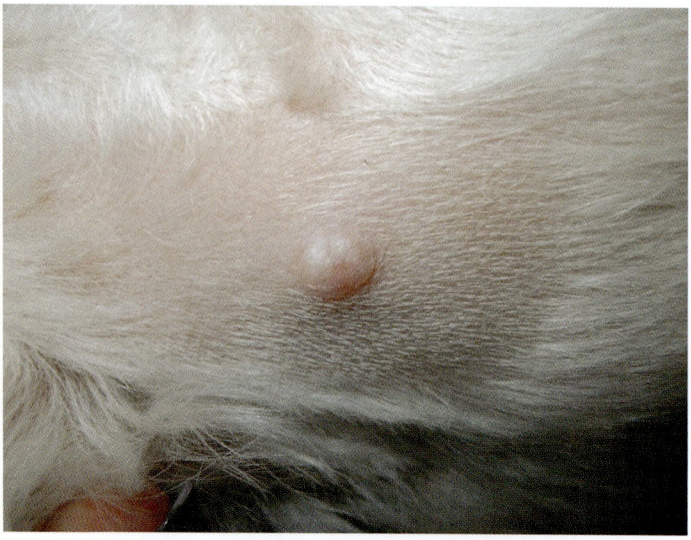

■ **Fig. 33.4.** Grade 1 mast cell tumor on the sternum of a $7\frac{1}{2}$-year-old male-castrate Maltese.

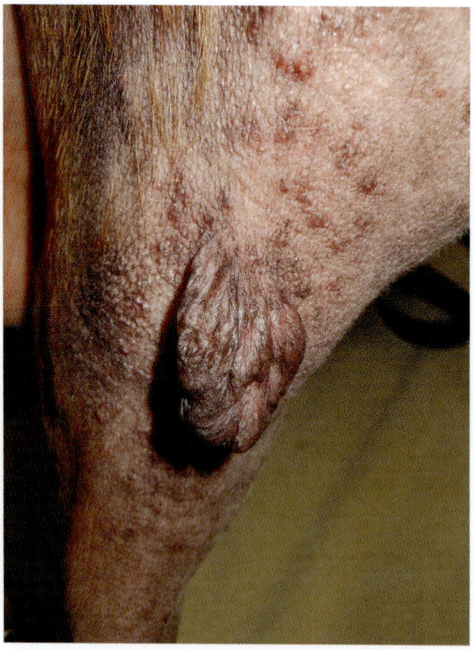

■ **Fig. 33.5.** Pedunculated grade 1 mast cell tumor on the hindlimb of a 5-year-old male-castrate boxer.

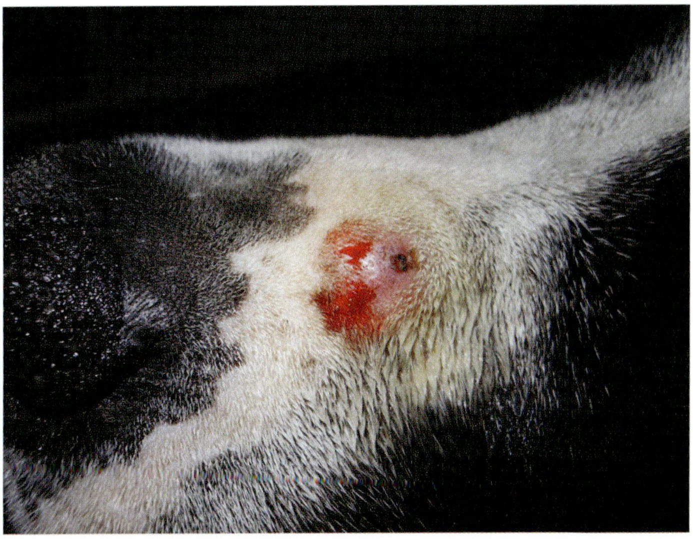

■ **Fig. 33.6.** Grade 1 mast cell tumor on the muzzle of a 3-year-old male-castrate pit bull mix.

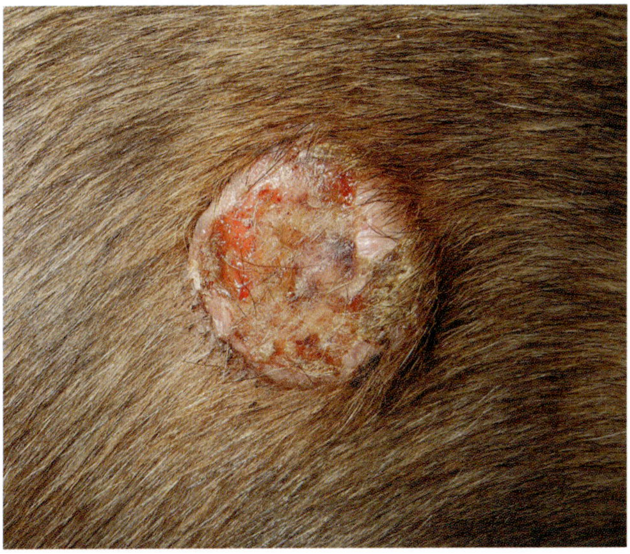

■ **Fig. 33.7.** Eroded and inflamed mast cell tumor on the lateral thorax of a 13-year-old female-spayed pit bull.

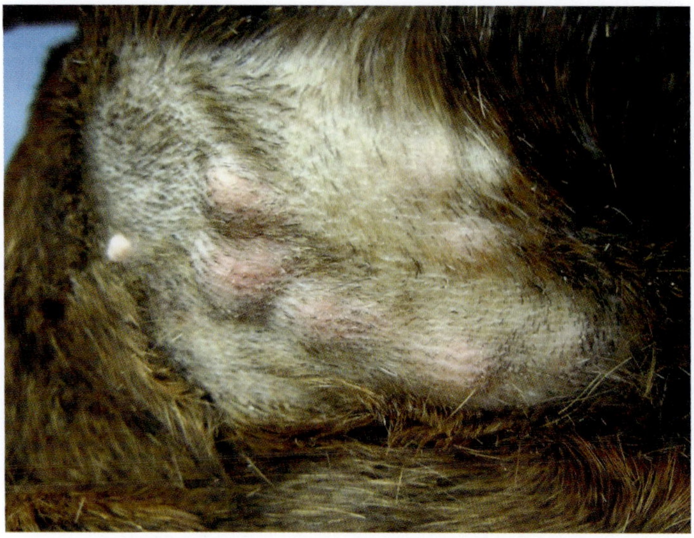

■ **Fig. 33.8.** Multiple mast cell tumors on the medial thigh of an 8-year-old male-castrate boxer.

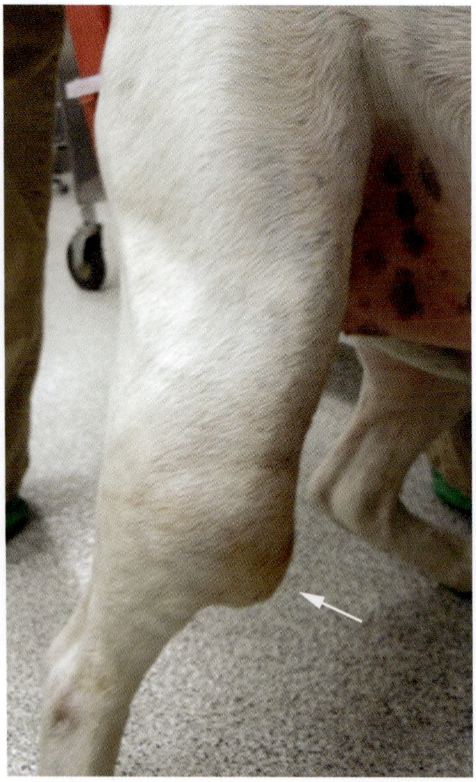

■ **Fig. 33.9.** Large mast cell tumor (*arrow*) on the stifle of a 10-year-old female-spayed American bull dog.

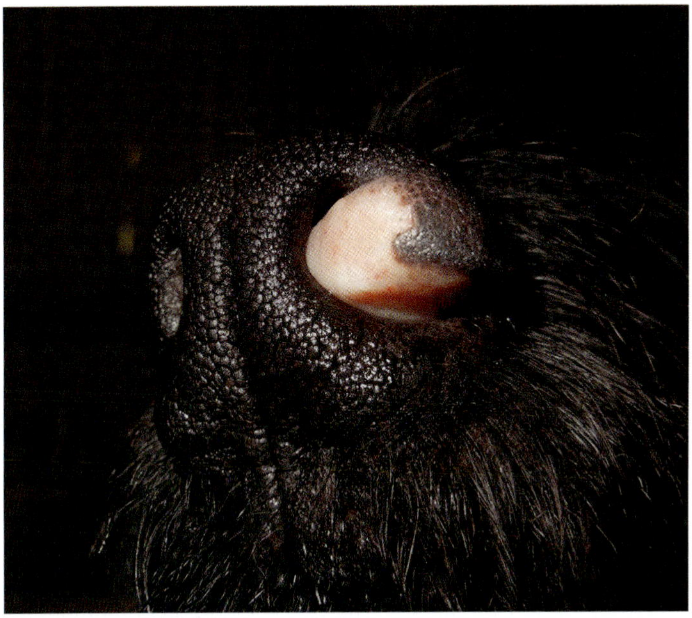

■ **Fig. 33.10.** Mast tumor causing swelling and depigmentation of the alar fold of a 10-year-old male-castrate Scottish terrier.

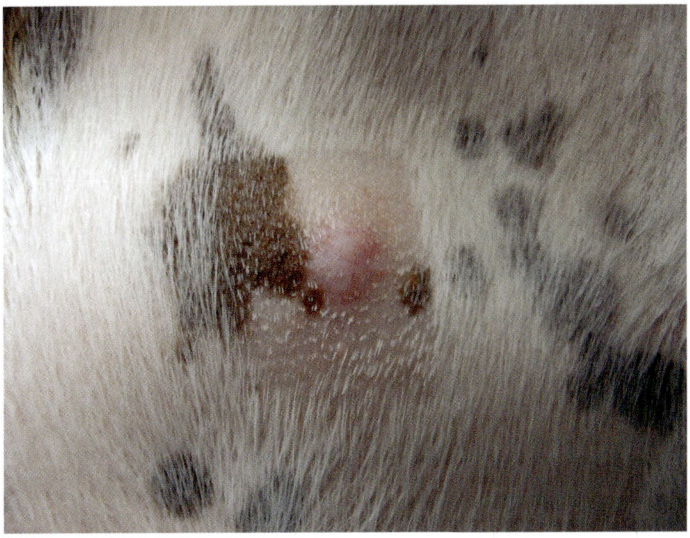

■ **Fig. 33.11.** Grade 2 mast cell tumor on the lateral thorax of a 7-year-old female-spayed boxer.

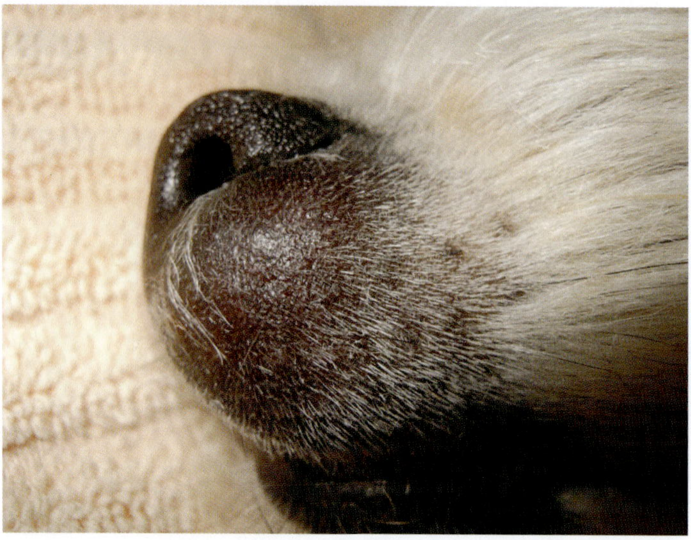

■ **Fig. 33.12.** Grade 2 mast cell tumor on the muzzle of an 18-month-old female pomeranian.

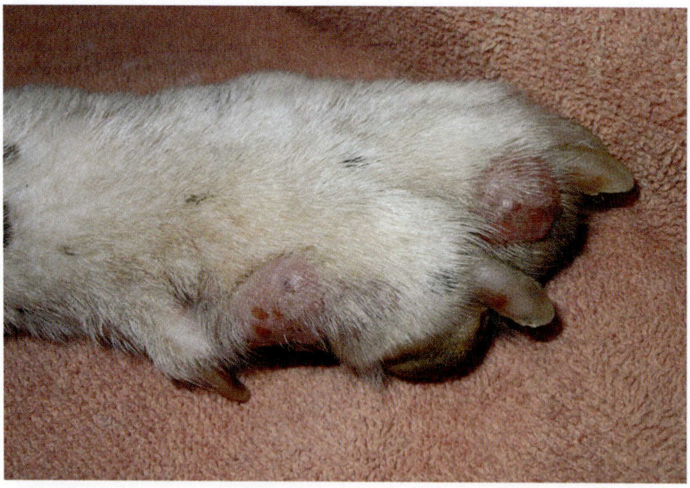

■ **Fig. 33.13.** Multicentric grade 3 mast cell tumors on the digits of a 5-year-old female-spayed English bulldog.

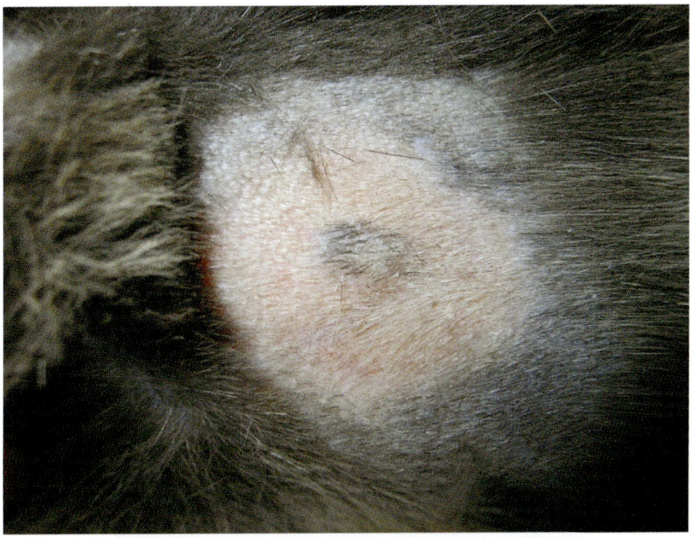

■ **Fig. 33.14.** Grade 1 mast cell tumor on the dorsum of a $10\frac{1}{2}$-year-old male-castrate Maine coon with the appearance of an erythematous plaque.

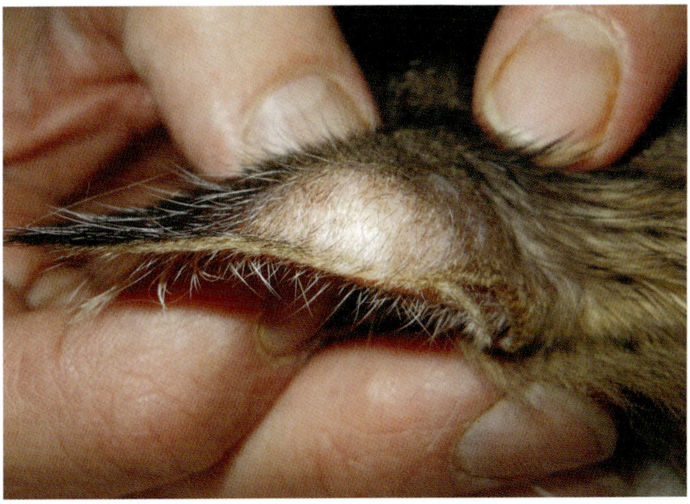

■ **Fig. 33.15.** Erythematous nodule of mast cell tumor on the pinnal margin of a 14-year-old female-spayed DLH.

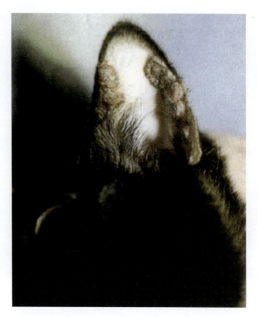

■ **Fig. 33.16.** Multifocal mast cell tumors on the pinna of a cat; these lesions were benign in nature.

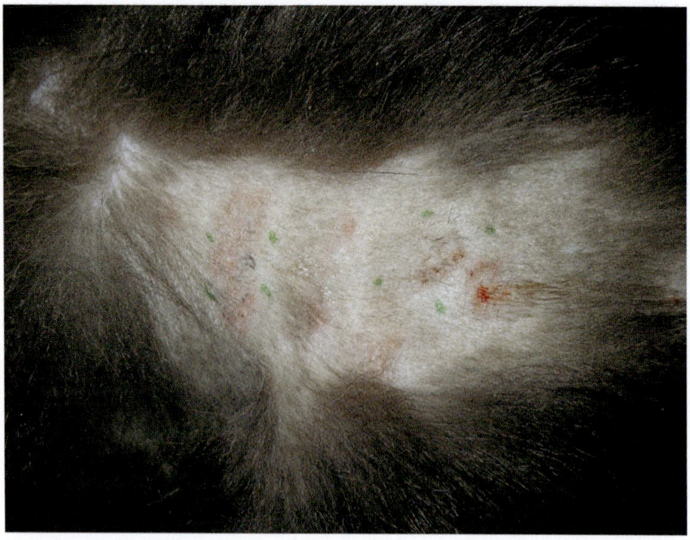

■ **Fig. 33.17.** Lesions of urticaria pigmentosa and mastocytosis on the ventrum of a 6-year-old female-spayed DSH.

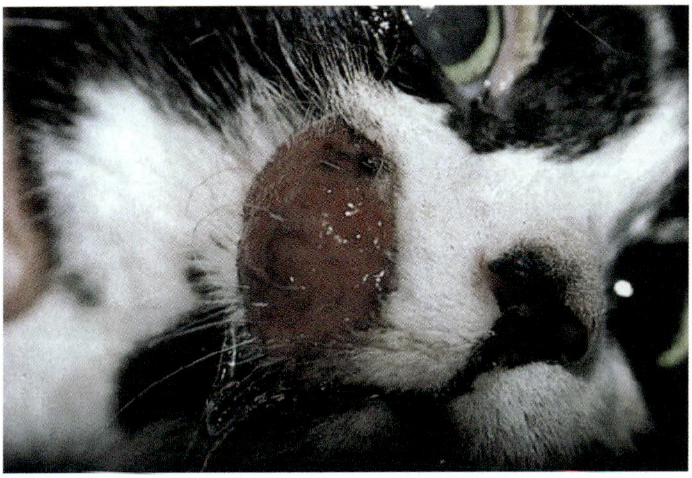

■ **Fig. 33.18.** Ulcerative mast cell tumor on the face of a cat. This was a metastatic lesion from primary gastrointestinal MCT.

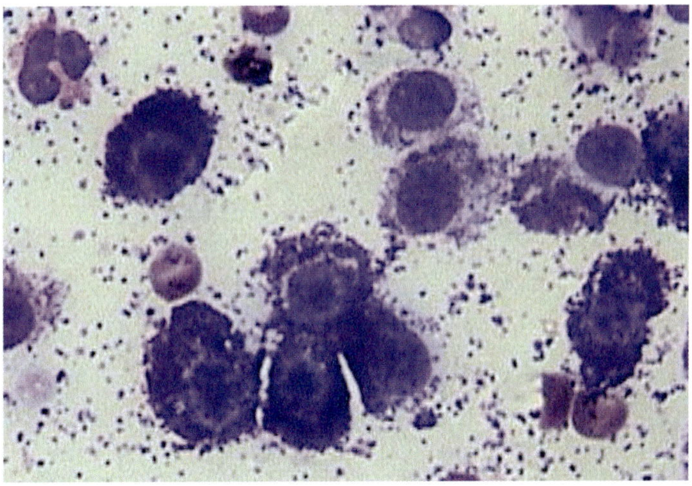

■ **Fig. 33.19.** Aspirate from a mast cell tumor demonstrating multiple round cells with basophilic cytoplasmic (and free) granules.

chapter 34

Mycobacterial Infections

DEFINITION/OVERVIEW

- Mycobacteria: genus of gram-positive, aerobic, acid-fast bacteria (genus *Mycobacterium*).
- Obligate or sporadic pathogens in humans and animals.
- Saprophytic pathogens may cause localized (immunocompetent host) or disseminated (immunodeficient host) disease.
- Relatively uncommon cause of nodular dermatoses in dogs and cats.

ETIOLOGY/PATHOPHYSIOLOGY

- Tuberculosis:
  - *Mycobacterium tuberculosis* (humans); uncommon infection in dogs and cats
  - *M. bovis* (cattle and some wild mammals); higher incidence in cats than in dogs
  - *M. microti* (voles); dogs and cats exposed to infected primary hosts sporadically infected
  - *M. avium* complex: consists of *M. avium* subspecies *avium*, *hominissus*, and *paratuberculosis*.
- Feline leprosy syndrome:
  - *M. lepraemurium*
  - *M. visibile*
  - *M. ulcerans*
  - *M. kansasii*
  - *M. szulgai*
  - *M. leprae*
  - *M. haemophilum*
  - *M. malmoense*
  - Additional unnamed species reported; *Mycobacterium* sp. strain Tarwin.
- Canine leproid granuloma syndrome:
  - Caused by unnamed slow-growing *Mycobacterium* sp. identified by DNA sequencing.

Blackwell's Five-Minute Veterinary Consult Clinical Companion: Small Animal Dermatology, Third Edition.
Karen Helton Rhodes and Alexander H. Werner.

- Systemic nontuberculous mycobacteriosis – nontuberculosis saprophytic mycobacteria: cutaneous/subcutaneous infections due to rapidly growing mycobacteria: also seen as mycobacterial panniculitis:
  - *M. chelonae-abscessus* group
  - *M. fortuitum group*
  - *M. perigrinum*
  - *M. phlei*
  - *M. terrae* complex
  - *M. genavense*
  - *M. massiliense*
  - *M. simiae*
  - *M. smegmatis* group
  - *M. thermoresistibile*
  - *M. xenopi*.

SIGNALMENT/HISTORY

- Tuberculosis:
  - Source of exposure: always an infected typical host
  - Dogs: usually exposed from an infected person in the household (*M. tuberculosis*); route is ingestion of expectorated infectious material; aerosol exposure possible; patients most often found in urban areas
  - Cats: classically exposed by drinking unpasteurized milk of infected cattle (*M. bovis*); much less common now than in the past; may be exposed by predation on infected small mammals (*M. bovis*, undefined tuberculosis species)
  - *M. microti:* natural infection common in voles; cats may act as a sentinel species; can infect human beings and other mammals
  - Cats and dogs of any age
  - *M. avium* complex: localized infections in immunocompetent hosts and disseminated disease in immunodeficient hosts; Abyssinian, Siamese, Somali cats; basset hounds, miniature schnauzers.
- Feline leprosy syndrome:
  - Adult free-roaming cats and kittens
  - Exposure to rodents postulated; lesions develop at locations of penetrating injury
  - Syndrome 1: young cats; males predisposed; localized nodular disease, affecting limbs with sparse to moderate numbers of acid-fast bacilli present in lesions (*M. lepraemurium*); cases reported from temperate coastal areas and port cities where cats are in contact with rats; cool climate may facilitate growth of the organism in extremities
  - Syndrome 2: older cats with generalized skin lesions and large numbers of acid-fast bacilli in lesions – *M. visibile* (United States); additional unnamed species reported (Australia, New Zealand); *Mycobacterium* sp. strain Tarwin (Australia); rural or semi-rural environments; risk factors of old age or immunodeficiency.

- Canine leproid granuloma:
  - Cases have been associated with fly bites and may seasonally fluctuate; short coat may predispose
  - Likely worldwide; most cases reported from Australasia and Brazil; United States reported in California, Hawaii, and Florida
  - Most often seen in short-haired outdoor-housed large-breed dogs, especially boxers (and their crosses), Staffordshire bull terriers, foxhounds, doberman pinschers, and German shepherds.
- Systemic nontuberculous mycobacteriosis:
  - Also known as opportunistic or atypical mycobacteriosis
  - Sporadic disease that can affect dogs and cats of any age
  - Most patients are immunosuppressed or have concurrent systemic diseases
  - Exposure: routes of exposure in pulmonary and systemic disease are unknown
  - Pleuritis; localized or disseminated granulomas; disseminated disease, neuritis; bronchopneumonia
  - Mycobacterial panniculitis; adult cats and dogs; infections follow trauma or bite wound, resulting in inoculation of the subcutaneous fat; risk factor with obesity.

CLINICAL FEATURES

- Tuberculosis:
  - Correlated with the route of exposure; major sites of involvement: oropharyngeal lymph nodes, cutaneous and subcutaneous tissues of the head and extremities; pulmonary system; gastrointestinal system
  - Dogs: respiratory, especially coughing; dyspnea uncommon
  - Cats: from contaminated milk: weight loss, chronic diarrhea, and thickened intestines; from predation: cutaneous nodules, ulcers, and draining tracts
  - Dogs and cats: pharyngeal and cervical lymphadenopathy; unproductive effort to vomit, ptyalism; tonsillar abscess; lymph nodes are visible or palpably firm, fixed, tender; may ulcerate and drain
  - Cutaneous ulcers, nodules, plaques; yellow foul-smelling discharge
  - Pyrexia
  - Depression
  - Partial anorexia and weight loss
  - Hypertrophic osteopathy or hypercalcemia may occur
  - Disseminated disease: body cavity effusion; visceral masses; bone or joint lesions; dermal and subcutaneous masses and ulcers; lymphadenopathy and/or abscesses; CNS signs; sudden death
  - *M. avium:* failure to regrow hair after clipping in Abyssinian cats.
- Feline leprosy syndrome:
  - Syndrome 1: initial localized nodules on limbs; progress rapidly, may ulcerate and drain; aggressive clinical course; recurrence after surgical excision; widespread lesions develop in several weeks; lack of systemic illness

- Syndrome 2: initial localized or generalized skin nodules that do not ulcerate, slowly progressive over months to years
- Feline multisystemic granulomatous mycobacteriosis: diffuse cutaneous thickening and multiple organ system involvement; caused by *M. visibile*
- Syndromes may overlap in cats of all ages.

■ Canine leproid granuloma:
- One or more well-circumscribed painless nodules (2 mm–5 cm) in dermis or subcutis; often on head or pinnae (especially dorsal fold), but may be anywhere on the body; only very large lesions ulcerate (Figures 34.1–34.4)
- Lack of systemic illness.

■ Systemic nontuberculous mycobacteriosis:
- Pulmonary and systemic infections reported rarely in dogs; may appear similar to tuberculosis
- Mycobacterial panniculitis: cutaneous: traumatic lesion that fails to heal with appropriate therapy; most often ventral abdominal and inguinal regions; spreads locally in the subcutaneous tissue (panniculitis); original lesion enlarges, forming a deep ulcer or fistula that drains greasy hemorrhagic exudate; surrounding tissue becomes firm; may form irregular ribbons or coalescing plaques; satellite pinpoint ulcerations open and drain (Figures 34.5–34.7)
- Wound dehiscence at surgery sites
- Lack of systemic illness when localized; pyrexia and anorexia when disseminated (immunodeficient host).

DIFFERENTIAL DIAGNOSIS

■ Mycobacterial infections have different prognoses, treatment recommendations, and public health consequences but may initially have similar signs, especially cutaneous lesions.
■ Focal or disseminated fungal infections (including dermatophytosis).
■ Actinomycosis.
■ Actinobacillosis.
■ Nocardiosis (can be clinically identical to mycobacterial panniculitis).
■ Bacterial pseudomycetoma.
■ Leishmaniosis.
■ Sterile pyogranulomatous dermatitis.
■ Cryptococcosis.
■ Neoplasia.

DIAGNOSTICS

Intradermal Skin Testing

■ Tuberculosis (dogs only): intradermal skin testing with PPD or BCG on inner pinna.
■ Test read at 48–72 hours post injection.

- May produce false-positive results owing to cross-reactions with nontuberculous mycobacteria.

Radiography

- Thoracic, abdominal, or skeletal lesions: suggest granulomatous infectious disease.
- No specific lesions for the mycobacterioses.
- Pulmonary tuberculosis lesions: may become calcified or cavitated.

Cytology/Histopathology

- Based on histopathologic and microbiologic evaluation of biopsy material from affected tissue.
- Aspiration of purulent material from any site after disinfection of overlying skin may be used for microbiological identification; ultrasound-guided aspiration techniques may be warranted.
- Biopsy specimens should incorporate the center of a granulomatous focus:
    - Tuberculosis: nodular to diffuse pyogranulomatous dermatitis with acid-fast bacilli
    - Feline leprosy syndrome: lepromatous form – epithelioid macrophages with large numbers of acid-fast bacilli; tuberculoid form – inflammatory cells surrounding necrotic foci with few acid-fast bacilli
    - Canine leproid granuloma: pyogranulomatous dermatitis with epithelioid macrophages; highly variable number of organisms
    - Systemic nontuberculous mycobacteriosis: nodular to diffuse pyogranulomatous dermatitis and panniculitis with a paucity of organisms.
- Cytology from infected tissues: with routine stains, negatively stained bacilli appear as "ghost rods" within macrophages; in positive stains including Ziehl–Neelson: acid-fast bacilli take up carbolfuchsin to appear pink; swabs or aspirations of draining cutaneous lesions or lymph nodes, transtracheal wash; endoscopic brushings; rectal cytology; impressions taken at surgical biopsy; heat-fixed samples should be submitted along with tissue for culture.

Culture

- Culture: special media and techniques required; referral to specialized laboratories may be required for no-tuberculous organisms (Mycobacterium.Mycology Referral, University of Texas Health Center at Tyler, Microbiology Section).

Special Testing (PCR)

- PCR methodologies: useful for any of the mycobacterial infections using tissue specimens or fluids; for canine leproid granuloma and the two feline leprosy syndromes the primers are not commercially available, but can be used to identify the suspect organisms.

THERAPEUTICS

- Tuberculosis:
  - Permission of local health authorities should be obtained in cases of *M. tuberculosis* and *M. bovis* infection due to their zoonotic potential
  - Multiple-agent chemotherapy with drugs used to treat human tuberculosis has been successful
  - *M. avium* complex infections are difficult to treat.
- Feline leprosy syndrome:
  - Before widespread dissemination, individual lesions may be excised with aggressive margins, which may be curative
  - Surgical treatment should be preceded by systemic therapy.
- Canine leproid granuloma:
  - Excision is curative
  - Lesions may self-cure within 1–3 months
  - Antimicrobial therapy may assist healing.
- Systemic nontuberculous mycobacteriosis:
  - Treatment should be based on organism identification and antibiotic sensitivity testing
  - Multiple drug therapy is often warranted
  - Aggressive surgical debulking may aid resolution; antimicrobial therapy pre- and intraoperatively is recommended.

Drugs of Choice

- Tuberculosis:
  - Multiple drug oral therapy required; never attempt single-drug therapy
  - Current recommendation: fluoroquinolone with clarithromycin and rifampin for 6–9 months:
    - Fluoroquinolone: marbofloxacin 2.75 mg/kg PO q24h; pradofloxacin 3–4.5 mg/kg PO q24h
    - Rifampin: 10–20 mg/kg PO q24h or divided BID (maximum 600 mg/day)
    - Clarithromycin: 7.5–15 mg/kg PO BID
  - Isoniazid and rifampin: combinations have been used; little is known about their use in cats; one recent report of treatment (cat) with isoniazid, rifampin, and dihydrostreptomycin for 3 months noted weight loss but eventual successful outcome
  - Isoniazid: 10–20 mg/kg PO (up to 300 mg total) q24h
  - Ethambutol: 10–25 mg/kg PO q24h
  - Pyrazinamide: instead of ethambutol; 15–40 mg/kg PO q24h
  - Dihydrostreptomycin: 15 mg/kg IM q24h
  - Clofazimine: 4–10 mg/kg PO q24h
  - Doxycycline: 10 mg/kg PO q24h or divided BID.

- Feline leprosy syndrome:
  - Multiple drug oral therapy recommended
  - Clofazamine: 25–50 mg/cat PO q24h or rifampin 10–15 mg/kg PO q24h or clarithromycin 62.5–125 mg/cat PO q24h with pradofloxacin 3 mg/kg PO q24h
  - Doxycycline: 5–7.5 mg/kg PO q24h
  - Amikacin: 10–15 mg/kg subcutaneously q24h.
- Canine leproid granuloma:
  - Doxycycline: 5 mg/kg PO BID
  - Rifampin: 10–15 mg/kg PO q24h with clarithromycin 7.5–12.5 mg/kg PO BID to TID.
- Systemic nontuberculous mycobacteriosis:
  - *In vitro* sensitivity testing may be used to choose chemotherapy for these cases; antibiotics reported to be effective against various isolates are macrolides, sulfonamides, tetracyclines, aminoglycosides, and fluoroquinolones
  - Anti-TB drugs are not generally effective
  - Multiple drug oral therapy recommended
  - Fluoroquinolone antibiotics, trimethoprim-sulfonamides, aminoglycosides, tetracyclines, and clarithromycin are useful for some individual isolates; long-term therapy should be based on sensitivity testing
  - Treatment should be continued for 2–6 months
  - Relapses upon cessation of treatment or during the course of treatment are common.

COMMENTS

Client Education/Prognosis

- Tuberculosis: guarded but in reality, currently undefined because experience with modern drugs that are better tolerated for long courses is limited.
- Feline leprosy: guarded to poor for syndrome 1; fair for syndrome 2, especially if lesions are amenable to surgical excision.
- Canine leproid granuloma: prognosis is good.
- Subcutaneous and systemic nontuberculous infections: relapses are common, but aggressive surgical approaches and multiple drug therapy may improve the outlook over what is reported in the literature.

Patient Monitoring

- Antituberculosis and antileprosy drugs: examine at least monthly; monitor for anorexia and weight loss.
- Hepatotoxicity: rifampin, clarithromycin, clofazamine; monitor liver enzymes monthly.
- Nephrotoxicity: amikacin; monitor urinalysis and renal chemistries weekly.
- Gastrointestinal adverse effects: clofazamine, doxycycline.
- Instruct owners to report cutaneous lesions immediately.

Zoonotic Potential

- Tuberculosis: affected domestic pets are potentially serious zoonotic threats to owners; public health authorities should be notified of any antemortem or postmortem diagnosis (may be required by law); do not attempt treatment without agreement of public health authorities.
- *M. tuberculosis*: greatest potential for zoonosis, especially with draining cutaneous lesions.
- Disease transmission from dogs and cats to humans: very rarely recorded; in recent outbreaks of tuberculosis in cats, no such case was documented.
- Clinicians aware of human tuberculosis in the household with dogs and cats should counsel owners about the risk of reverse zoonosis.

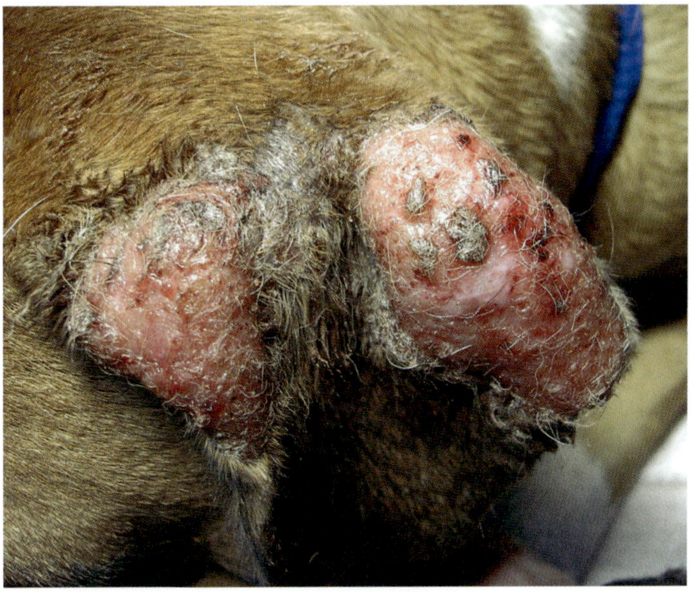

■ **Fig. 34.1.** Eroded and inflamed lesions of canine leproid granuloma on the pinna of a 1-year-old male-castrate boxer. Lesions were nonpainful.

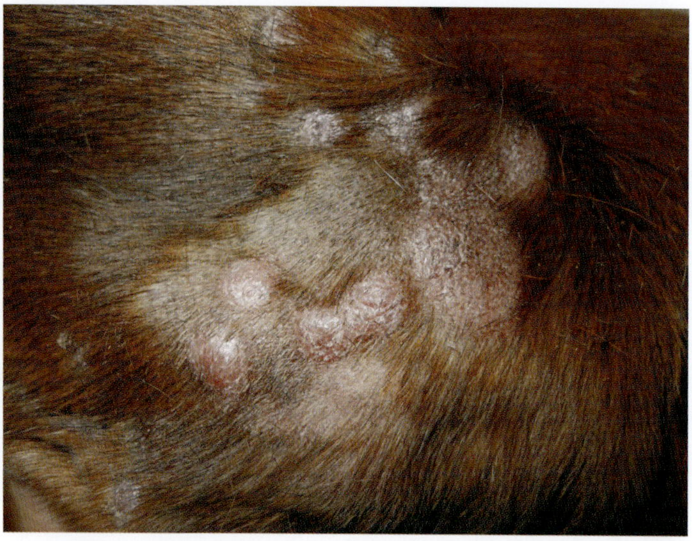

■ **Fig. 34.2.** Multiple erythematous and alopecic plaques with mild scaling on the pinna of a 10-year-old male-castrate boxer mix with canine leproid granuloma.

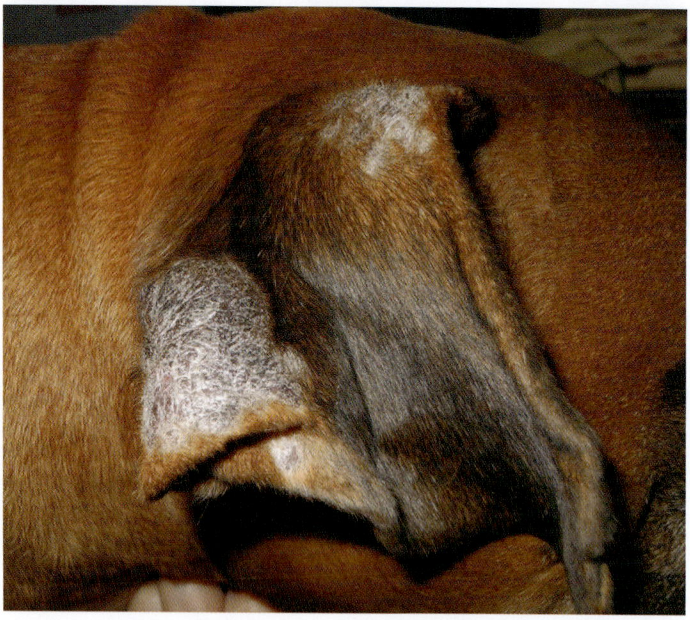

■ **Fig. 34.3.** Older, scarred lesions of canine leproid granuloma on the pinna of a 6-year-old male-castrate boxer. Patches are palpably thickened, nonpainful, alopecic, and lichenified.

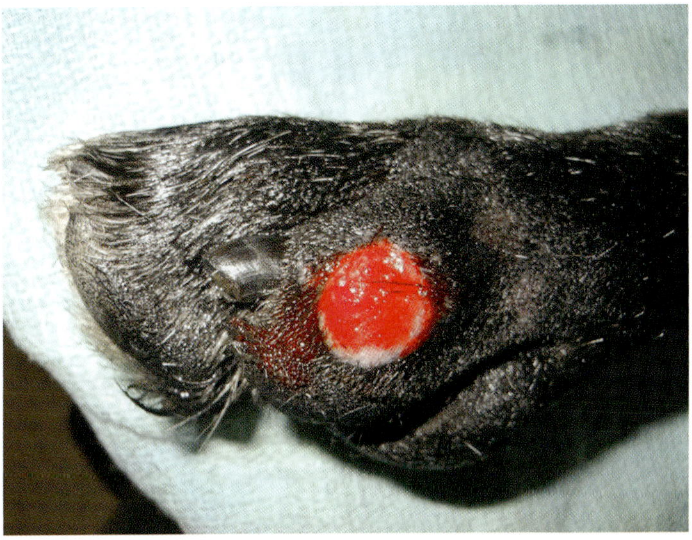

■ **Fig. 34.4.** Lesion of canine leproid granuloma on the foot of a 10-year-old male-castrate Labrador retriever.

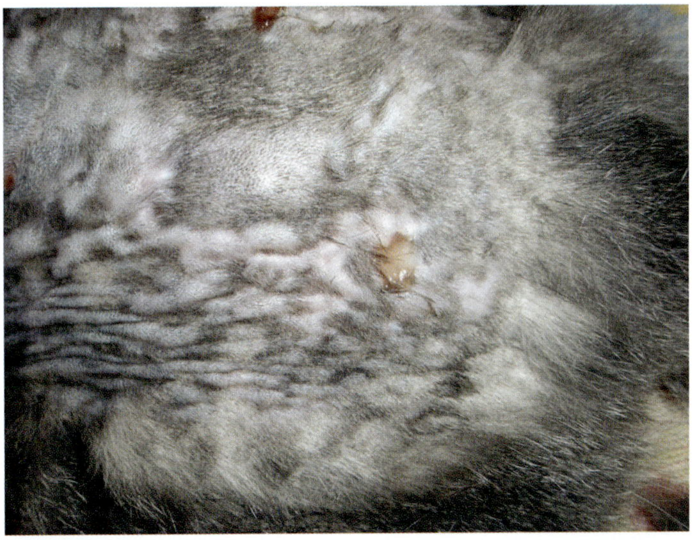

■ **Fig. 34.5.** *M. fortuitum* infection in an 11-year-old female-spayed DSH. Lesions on the ventrum palpated as thickened irregular ribbons of tissue with occasional draining tracts.

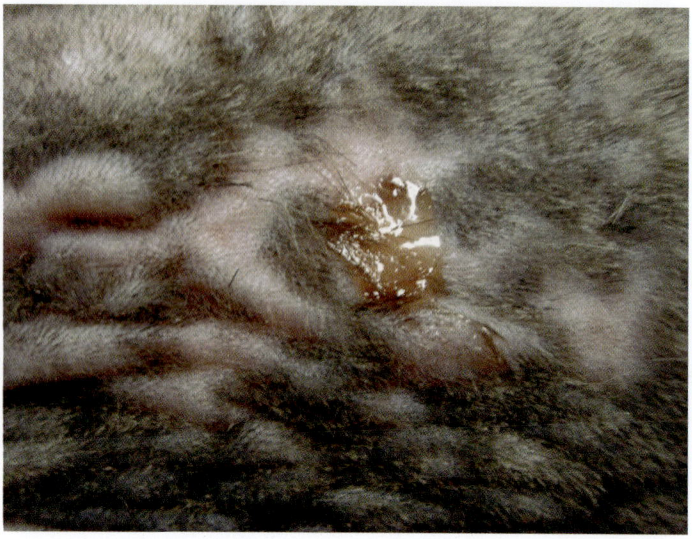

■ **Fig. 34.6.** Additional image of the patient in Figure 34.1 demonstrating irregular ribbons of tissue. Discharge is a yellow-oily foul-smelling exudate.

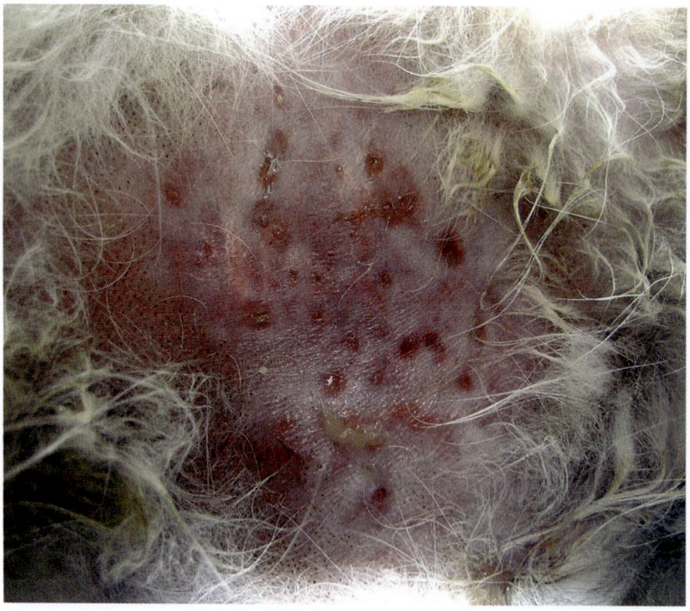

■ **Fig. 34.7.** Lesions in an adult DLH with an unidentified nontuberculous mycobacterial panniculitis. A large and firm plaque with punctate draining tracts was present on the ventral abdomen.

chapter 35

Mycoses, Deep

DEFINITION/OVERVIEW

- Cryptococcosis, coccidioidomycosis, blastomycosis: localized or disseminated systemic fungal infections.
- Clinical signs vary with the organ system involved.

ETIOLOGY/PATHOPHYSIOLOGY

- *Cryptococcus neoformans* and *C. gattii:* ubiquitous yeast-like organism; *C. neoformans* associated with bird droppings and decaying vegetation; *C. gattii* endemic in the environment as well as in humans and small ruminants.
- *Coccidioides immitis*: dimorphic saprophytic fungus; prefers warm and dry environments with alkaline soil (southwestern US).
- *Blastomyces dermatitidis* (Mississippi, Ohio, Tennessee river basins, and parts of Wisconsin) are soil-borne fungal organisms.

CLINICAL FEATURES

Cryptococcosis

- Most common systemic fungal infection in cats; seven times more common in cats; rare in dogs.
- Inhalation of the yeast organisms causes focal infection in the nasal passages; infection rarely caused by inoculation of organism through a wound; primary entry via the gastrointestinal tract may occur.
- Disseminated form spreads hematogenously from the nasal passages to the brain, eyes, lungs, and other tissues or by extension to the skin of the nose, eye, retroorbital tissue, and draining lymph nodes (lymphadenopathy).
- Immunosuppression (especially resulting from glucocorticoid administration) is a risk factor for development of disseminated disease (Figures 35.1, 35.2).
- Associated with fever, anorexia, nasal discharge, skin nodules/ulceration, lethargy, neurologic signs (seizures, ataxia, paresis, blindness).

Blackwell's Five-Minute Veterinary Consult Clinical Companion: Small Animal Dermatology, Third Edition.
Karen Helton Rhodes and Alexander H. Werner.

- Dogs:
  - Young adult, large-breed dogs
  - Doberman pinscher, German shepherd, Great Dane, boxer, American cocker spaniel predisposed
  - Rhinosinusitis, neurologic signs, and ocular signs most common; occasional lungs and abdominal organs.
- Cats:
  - Young adult cats
  - Possible increased incidence in male cats and Siamese cats
  - Upper respiratory signs and sinusitis most common (Figures 35.3, 35.4)
  - Subcutaneous lesions present in 40% of cases consisting of papules and nodules as well as abscesses, ulcers, and draining tracts (Figures 35.5–35.7)
  - Nasal lesions extremely common; present as a firm to boggy swelling of the bridge of the nose causing facial asymmetry (Figure 35.8).

Coccidioidomycosis

- Most dogs living in endemic areas have been infected; majority of cases are subclinical or present with mild respiratory symptoms.
- Dogs more susceptible than cats: rare disease in both species.
- Young adults; Boxer and doberman pinscher predisposed.
- Inhalation of infective arthroconidia is the primary route of infection: once inhaled, immature spherules mature and release hundreds of endospores.
- Clinical signs manifest 1–3 weeks post exposure; asymptomatic infections result in the development of immunity without clinical disease; dissemination, including to skin, may occur within 10 days.
- Clinical signs dependent on the organ system affected: lethargy, fever, anorexia, productive or dry cough/dyspnea, joint pain, seizures, uveitis/keratitis, ataxia, paraparesis, neck or back pain, bone swelling, cardiovascular symptoms, renal failure, lymphadenopathy.
- Cutaneous lesions characterized by nodules with draining tracts most often over sites of infected bone.

Blastomycosis

- Young adults; coonhound, walker hound, pointer, weimaraner, doberman pinscher predisposed; higher risk in males.
- Proximity to water increases risk of exposure.
- Inhalation of infective arthroconidia is the primary route of infection: once inhaled, yeast form initiates infection (mycotic pneumonia).
- Hematogenous dissemination results in a pyogranulomatous response.
- Clinical signs:
  - Dogs: 85% develop lung disease (harsh, dry cough); 50% develop fever; 40% develop cutaneous disease (granulomatous); 40% develop uveitis/glaucoma/visual impairment; 30% develop lameness (fungal osteomyelitis); additional

symptoms include anorexia, lymphadenopathy, endocarditis and myocarditis, testicular enlargement, and prostatomegaly (Figures 35.9–35.11)
- Cats: respiratory symptoms, ocular inflammation, weight loss.

- Cutaneous lesions consist of ulcerated nodules or plaques, subcutaneous abscesses, draining tracts, or large firm papules

DIFFERENTIAL DIAGNOSIS

- Pneumonia/respiratory disease
- Neoplasia (bone, respiratory)
- Cardiac disease
- Other systemic mycosis (e.g., coccidioidomycosis, histoplasmosis, blastomycosis)
- Bacterial infection (including osteomyelitis)
- Neurologic disease (e.g., rickettsial, granulomatous meningoencephalitis, bacterial meningoencephalitis, neoplasia)
- Distemper
- Immune-mediated disease

DIAGNOSTICS

- Complete blood count and serum chemistry: mild nonregenerative anemia, eosinophilia, neutrophilic leukocytosis, hyperglobulinemia, hypoalbuminemia, azotemia, hypercalcemia secondary to granuloma formation.
- Urinalysis: low specific gravity and proteinuria with inflammatory glomerulonephritis in *C. immitis*; blastomyces yeasts may be found in the urine of dogs with prostatic involvement.
- Imaging:
  - Cryptococcosis: tissue density (granuloma) behind the soft palate in cats or dense material filling the nasal passage with bone destruction on radiographs; CT or MRI for brain and nasal lesions
  - Coccidioidomycosis: pulmonary interstitial infiltrates, bone osteolysis on radiographs; CT or MRI for brain or CNS granulomas
  - Blastomycosis: pulmonary generalized interstitial to nodular infiltrate with nonuniform distribution (differentiates from pneumonia), tracheobronchial lymphadenopathy, lytic and proliferative focal bone lesions on radiographs.
- CSF culture and measurement of capsular antigen (cryptococcosis).
- Serology:
  - Cryptococcosis: latex agglutination or ELISA for capsular antigen in serum or CSF; highly sensitive (90–100%) and specific (97–100%); magnitude correlates with severity of infection; may be positive with colonization; titers greater than 1:32 diagnostic for infection
  - Coccidioidomycosis: serologic tests by ELISA or agar gel immunodiffusion (AGID) for antibody to *C. immitis*

- Blastomycosis: urine or serum antigen testing highly sensitive; agar gel immunodiffusion less sensitive but highly specific.

- Cytology: aspirates of mucoid material from nasal passages, lymph node aspirates, impression smears from skin lesions or draining exudates or even tracheal wash fluid may demonstrate organisms:
  - Cryptococcosis: pleopmorphic round 2–20 mm yeast-like organisms with mucinous capsules (Figure 35.12)
  - Coccidioidomycosis: 20–80 mm double-walled spherules with endospores
  - Blastomycosis: 5–20 mm round to oval, double-walled with broad-based budding (Figure 35.13).
- Histopathology:
  - Cryptococcosis: skin, bone, enucleated eye, lymph node: most diagnostic test along with cytology; scant pyogranulomatous inflammation with encapsulated organisms creates a "foamy" appearance
  - Coccidioidomycosis: discrete granulomas and pyogranulomas with organisms free in tissues; number of organisms varies from scarce to moderate
  - Blastomycosis: discrete granulomas and pyogranulomas with organisms in macrophages and free in tissues; number of organisms varies from scarce to moderate.
- Culture/sensitivity: caution when culturing *C. immitis* – mycelial form is highly contagious; infection has been reported in humans exposed to cultures (*C. immitis* and *Blastomyces dermatitidis*) and infected tissues (*C. immitis*) (Figure 35.14).

THERAPEUTICS

- Generally treated as outpatients; treatment with amphotericin B will require hospitalization several times a week during the treatment period.
- Concurrent clinical symptoms (e.g., seizures, pain, coughing) should be treated appropriately.
- Restrict activity until clinical signs begin to subside.
- Feed a high-quality palatable diet to maintain body weight.
- Review with client the necessity and expense of long-term therapy of a serious illness and the possibility of treatment failure.
- Surgical removal of the affected organ may be indicated in cases of focal granulomatous organ involvement (e.g., consolidated pulmonary lung lobe, eye, kidney).
- Cryptococcal pyogranulomatous lesions in the nasopharynx may require surgical removal to reduce respiratory difficulty.
- Coccidioidomycosis is considered the most severe and life-threatening of the systemic mycoses; treatment of disseminated disease requires at least 1 year of aggressive antifungal therapy.

Drugs of Choice

- Imidazole and triazole antifungals:

- Dogs:
  - Itraconazole 5–10 mg/kg PO q24h or divided BID: side effects (uncommon) include hepatotoxicity (elevated ALT), vasculitis
  - Fluconazole 5 mg/kg PO BID: side effects (mild) include anorexia, vomiting
  - Ketoconazole 5–15 mg/kg PO BID: side effects (mild) include anorexia, vomiting
  - Posaconazole 5–10 mg/kg PO q24h or divided BID: side effects include anorexia, vomiting, hepatotoxicity
- Cats:
  - Itraconazole 5–15 mg/kg PO q24h or divided BID or 25–50 mg total dose BID: side effects (uncommon) include anorexia, vomiting, depression, hepatotoxicity
  - Fluconazole 50 mg PO q24h to BID: side effects (uncommon) include anorexia, vomiting, depression, hepatotoxicity
  - Ketoconazole 5–10 mg/kg PO q24h or 50 mg total dose BID: side effects (common) include anorexia, vomiting, depression, fever, hepatotoxicity, neurologic disturbances
  - Posaconazole 5–7.5 mg/kg PO q24h or divided BID: side effects include anorexia, vomiting, hepatotoxicity, facial pruritus
- If side effects noted, discontinue until signs abate and restart at a lower dose; slowly increase to the recommended dose if possible
- Monitor serum ALT during treatment
- Treatment continued for at least 30 days after resolution of the clinical lesions; typical treatment length 3 months.

■ Amphotericin B:
- AMB/desoxycholate or L-AMB/lipid formulations
- Dogs: AMB 0.5 mg/kg IV over 4–6 h or L-AMB 1–3 mg/kg IV over 2 h; 3 times/week; fluid diuresis recommended
- Cats: AMB 0.25 mg/kg IV over 4–6 h or L-AMB 1 mg/kg IV over 2 h; 3 times/week; fluid diuresis recommended
- AMB may be administered subcutaneously with 300–500 mL sodium chloride 0.45%/dextrose 2.5%
- Side effects of AMB therapy can be severe and include cumulative nephrotoxicity, fever, inappetence, vomiting, and phlebitis
- Serum creatinine and BUN should be monitored during treatment; elevation in creatinine >20 of baseline or BUN greater than 50 mg/dL warrants discontinuation
- Urinalysis: discontinue treatment if granular casts are noted.

■ Combination of AMB and ketoconazole may be used in dogs that have not responded to either drug alone or have exhibited significant toxicity:
- Combination therapy may not be more effective than single-drug therapy in the treatment of coccidioidomycoses
- Administer AMB as described to a total cumulative dosage of 4–6 mg/kg, together with ketoconazole at 10 mg/kg PO divided daily for at least 8–12 months

  - AMB administered by rapid IV bolus at a dosage of 0.25 mg/kg, three times a week, for a total cumulative dosage of 4 mg/kg followed by long-term ketoconazole therapy, depending on the clinical response.
- Flucytosine 100 mg/kg PO divided TID to QID in addition to triazoles may be considered for resistant infections: associated with drug eruptions manifesting as depigmenting lesions of the skin, lips, and nose, as well as bone marrow suppression.

Precautions/Interactions

- Avoid use of antacids with imidazole and triazole medications.
- Drugs metabolized primarily by the liver should not be administered along with ketoconazole.
- Drugs metabolized primarily by the kidneys should not be administered along with AMB.
- Pulmonary disease resulting in severe coughing may temporarily worsen after therapy has begun due to inflammation in the lungs; low-dose short-term prednisone and cough suppressants may be required to alleviate the respiratory signs.

COMMENTS

Patient Monitoring

- Serologic titers (cryptococcosis, coccidioidomycosis) should be monitored every 1–3 months after initial 2-month treatment.
- Treatment is continued 60 days after antigen titers reach zero (cryptococcosis – may take >2 years) or less than 1:4 (coccidioidomycosis).
- Serum drug levels 2–4 h post administration may be considered in patients displaying poor response to assure adequate absorption.
- Blastomycosis: monitor thoracic radiographs at 90 days; continue treatment with repeat radiographs at 30-day intervals until lungs are normal or stable (indicating residual scarring).

Expected Course and Prognosis

- Cryptococcosis:
  - Chronic disease: requires months of therapy; patients with CNS disease may require life-long maintenance therapy
  - Not considered a zoonotic disease but may be transmitted via bite wounds, especially to an immunocompromised human
  - Capsular antigen titers determine response to therapy; if titers do not substantially decrease with 2 months of treatment, protocol may need to be changed
  - Poorer prognosis in cats with concurrent FeLV or FIV infection.
- Coccidioidomycosis:
  - Prognosis is guarded in disseminated disease

- Most dogs will improve following oral therapy; relapses may be seen, especially if therapy is shortened
- Overall recovery rate estimated at 60%; some report a 90% response to fluconazole therapy
- Prognosis for cats is not well documented; rapid dissemination requiring long-term therapy should be anticipated
- Serologic testing every 3–4 months after completion of therapy is recommended to monitor for possibility of relapse
- Spontaneous recovery from disseminated coccidioidomycosis without treatment is extremely rare
- Zoonosis:
  - Spherule form of the fungus, as found in animal tissues, is not directly transmissible to people or other animals
  - In rare circumstances, reversion to growth of the infective mold form of the fungus may occur on or within bandages placed over a draining lesion or in contaminated bedding
  - Draining lesions can lead to contamination of the environment with arthrospores
  - Care should be exercised whenever handling an infected draining lesion
  - Special precautions should be recommended with immunocompromised humans in the household.

■ Blastomycosis:
- 25% of dogs worsen or die within the first week of therapy due to inflammatory response to organism death
- Recurrence may occur in >20% of cases, necessitating retreatment
- Severity of lung and CNS involvement affects prognosis
- Thoracic radiographs are often the best monitor of therapeutic duration; continue treatment for at least 30 days after clinical/radiographic resolution
- Not considered a zoonotic threat unless transmitted via a bite wound
- Zoonosis:
  - Acquired from an environmental source
  - Human exposure at the same time as the dog/cat possible
  - Dogs may act as sentinels for exposure
  - Common source exposure has been documented in hunters
  - Incidence 10 times greater in dogs than in humans.

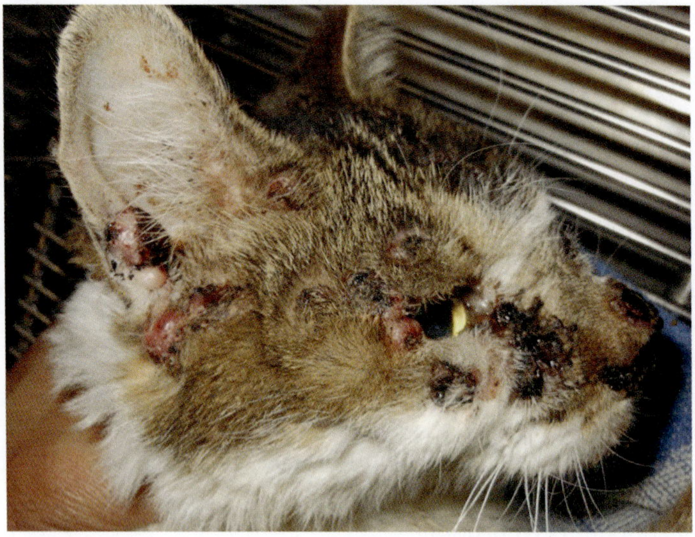

■ **Fig. 35.1.** Multiple ulcerated and exudative nodules of cryptococcosis in a 9-year-old male-castrate DLH treated with immunosuppressive dosages of corticosteroids for presumptive eosinophilic granuloma.

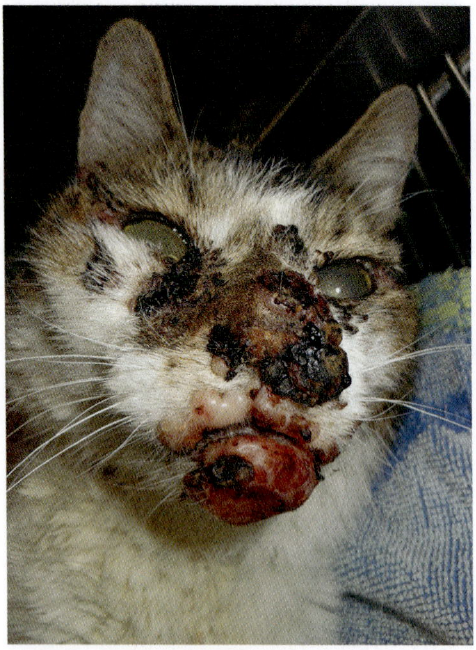

■ **Fig. 35.2.** Additional image of the patient in Figure 35.1.

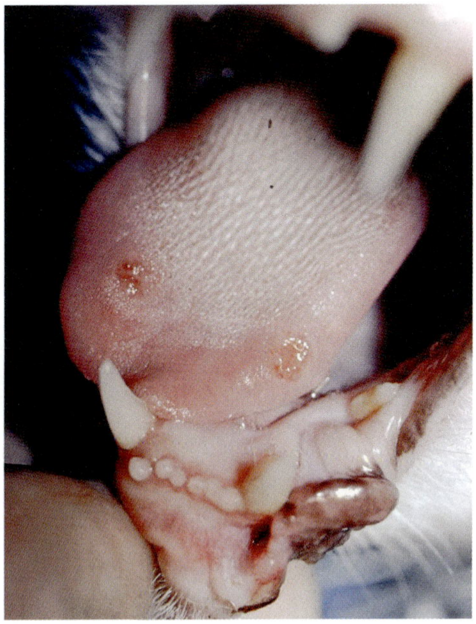

■ **Fig. 35.3.** Oral ulcerations in an adult cat with a diagnosis of cryptococcosis.

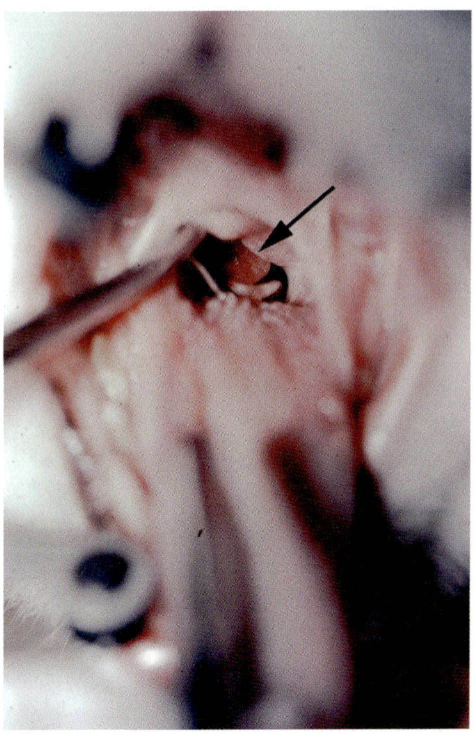

■ **Fig. 35.4.** Nasopharyngeal polyp (*arrow*) affecting the patient in Figure 35.3.

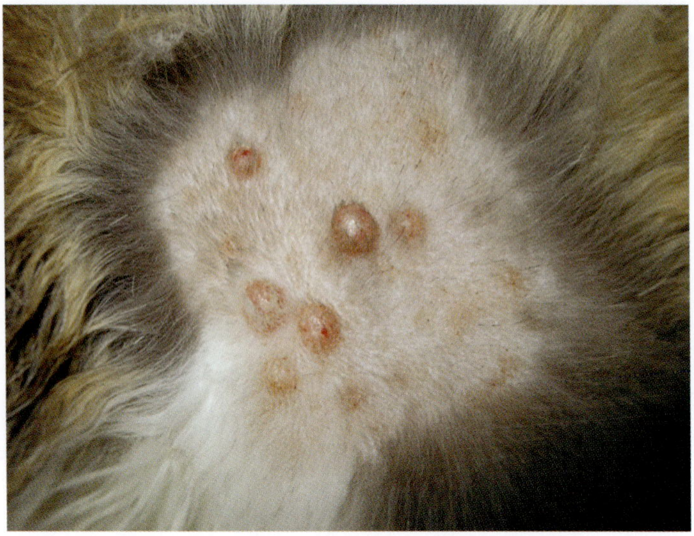

■ **Fig. 35.5.** Generalized erythematous cutaneous nodules of cryptococcosis affecting the patient in Figures 35.1 and 35.2.

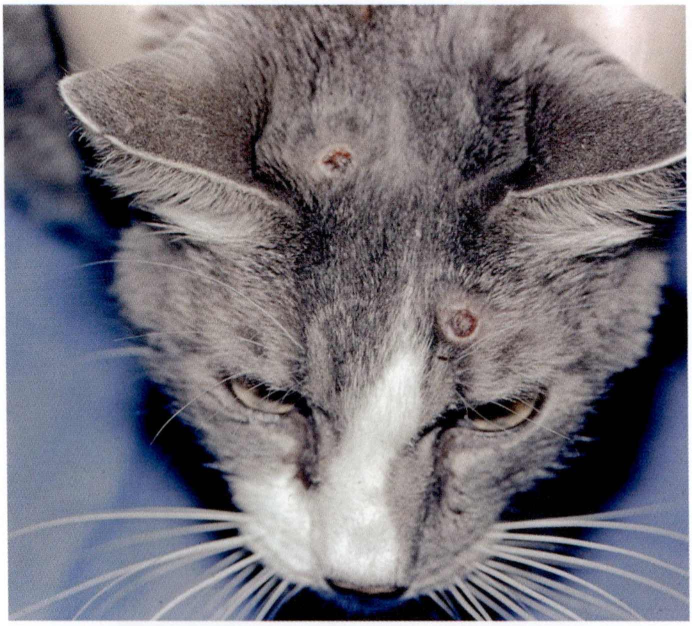

■ **Fig. 35.6.** Multiple ulcerated nodules characteristic of cryptococcosis in an adult DSH.

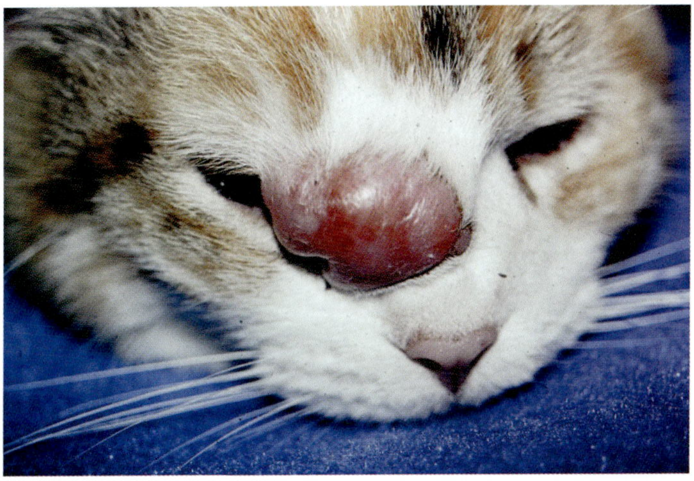

■ **Fig. 35.7.** Single large erythematous mass over the dorsal muzzle and right side of the face in a DSH with cryptococcosis.

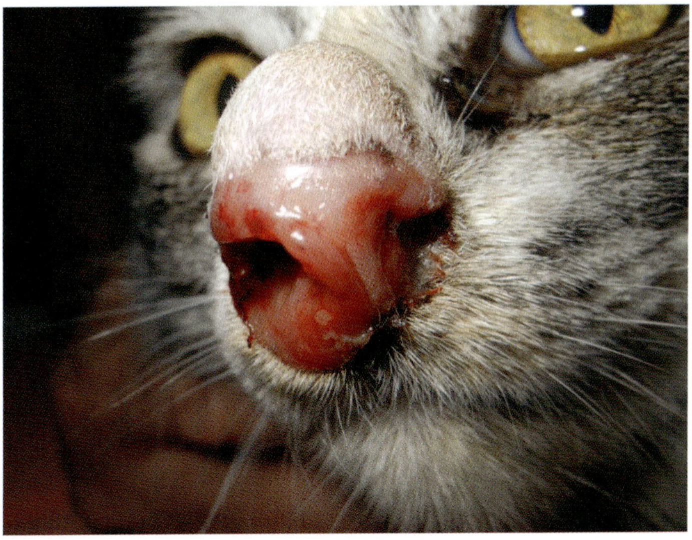

■ **Fig. 35.8.** Characteristic asymmetric swelling of the nasal planum and dorsal muzzle in a 7-year-old female-spayed DLH with cryptococcosis.

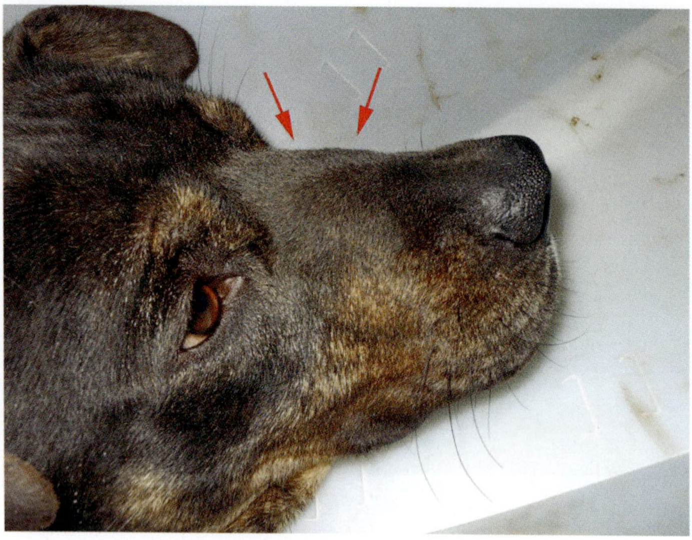

■ **Fig. 35.9.** Swelling of the dorsal muzzle (*arrows*) in a 2-year-old male-castrate pit bull mix with blastomycosis.

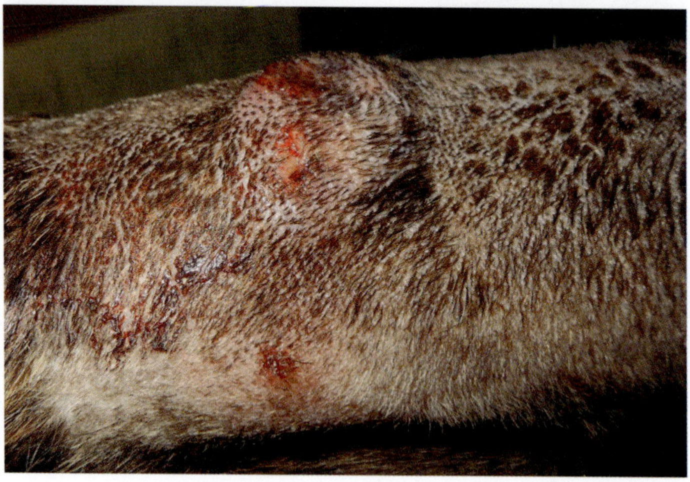

■ **Fig. 35.10.** Ulcerative and draining plaque of blastomycosis on the foreleg of the patient in Figure 35.9.

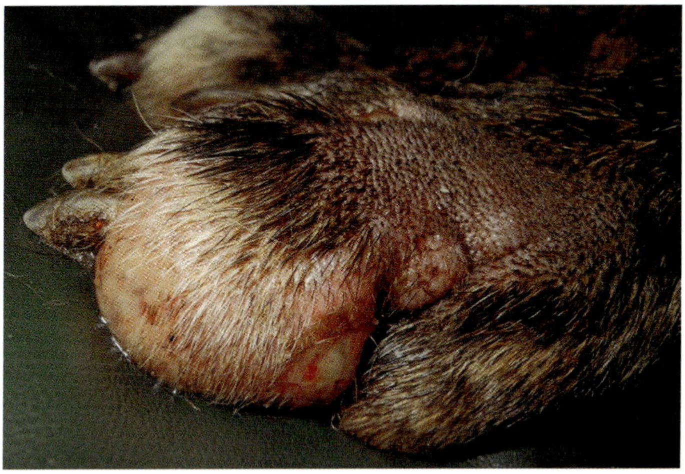

■ **Fig. 35.11.** Swollen and firm digit due to blastomycosis of the patient in Figures 35.9 and 35.10.

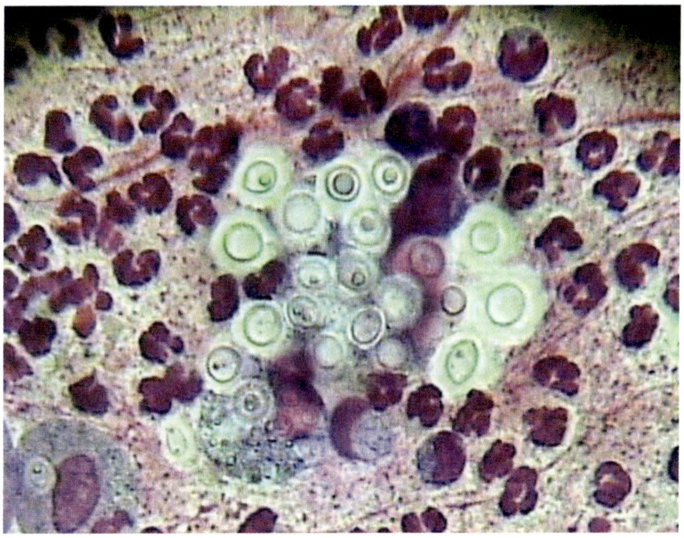

■ **Fig. 35.12.** Pyogranulomatous infiltrate with multiple pleomorphic organisms surrounded by distinctive capsules characteristic of *Cryptococcus neoformans* from exudates of the patient in Figure 35.1.

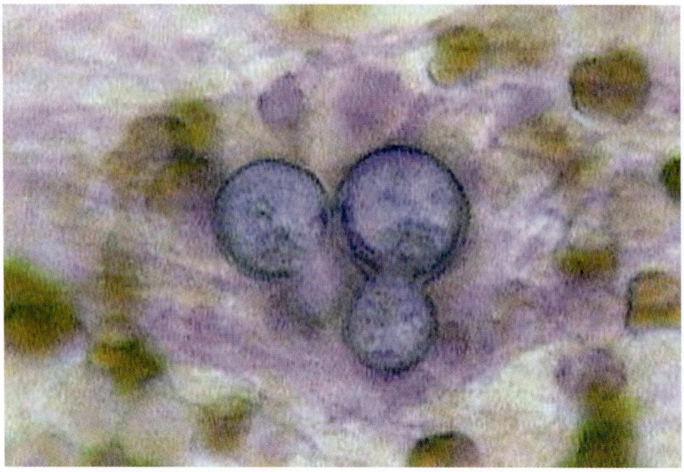

■ **Fig. 35.13.** Broad-based budding of a double-walled organism characteristic of *Blastomyces dermatitidis* in exudates from the patient in Figure 35.9.

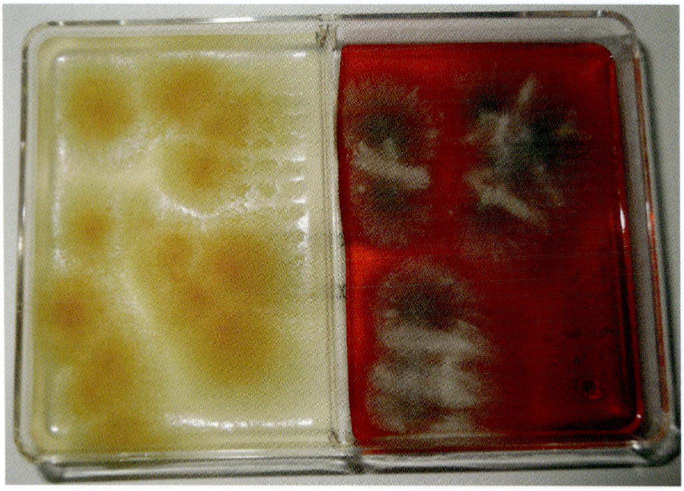

■ **Fig. 35.14.** Positive fungal culture of exudate from a 4-year-old male-castrate DMH. The organism was identified at the reference laboratory as *Coccidioides immitis*.

chapter 36

Nocardiosis and Actinomycosis

DEFINITION/OVERVIEW

- *Nocardia* spp. and *Actinomyces* spp.: uncommon pyogranulomatous and suppurative infection; dogs and cats.
- Opportunistic organism; enters body through contamination of wounds, respiratory inhalation, or ingestion.

ETIOLOGY/PATHOPHYSIOLOGY

Nocardia

- *Nocardia* spp. are aerobic, filamentous, gram-positive, partially acid-fast, branching soil saprophytes.
- Immunocompromise appears to be a significant predisposing factor for development of *Nocardia* infection.
- Causes three syndromes: localized cutaneous/subcutaneous; pulmonary; systemic/ disseminated.
- Systems affected: respiratory, skin/exocrine, lymphatic, musculoskeletal, nervous.
- *Nocardia asteroides* complex.
- *N. brasiliensis*.
- *N. nova* (main species affecting cats).
- *N. farcinica*.
- *N. otitidiscaviarum*.

Actinomyces

- *Actinomyces* spp. are anaerobic, filamentous, gram-positive, nonacid-fast, branching commensals in the oral cavity and bowel.
- Infection may have a latency period up to 2 years post exposure or trauma.
- Most often causes a subcutaneous swelling; less commonly causes osteomyelitis or pulmonary/pleural infection.

Blackwell's Five-Minute Veterinary Consult Clinical Companion: Small Animal Dermatology, Third Edition.
Karen Helton Rhodes and Alexander H. Werner.

SIGNALMENT/HISTORY

- Dogs and cats of any breed.
- Lesions may initially develop in the area of previous injury.
- Geographic distribution is worldwide.

CLINICAL FEATURES

- Nocardiosis:
    - Cutaneous/subcutaneous: cellulitis, ulcerated nodules, abscesses that develop draining sinuses; chronic, nonhealing wounds; often accompanied by fistulous tracts; if extended, may result in lymphadenopathy, draining lymph nodes, panniculitis, and osteomyelitis (Figures 36.1–36.3)
    - Pulmonary: pyothorax resulting in dyspnea, anorexia and emaciation, fever
    - Systemic/disseminated: most common in young dogs; usually begins in the respiratory tract; lethargy, fever, and weight loss; cyclic fever may be characteristic; CNS may be affected; pleural and/or abdominal effusion may occur.
- Actinomycosis:
    - Subcutaneous swelling or abscess on the head, neck, thorax, or flank
    - May have draining tracts or remain closed (Figure 36.4)
    - May discharge a malodorous exudate with or without sulfur granules.

DIFFERENTIAL DIAGNOSIS

- Nocardiosis:
    - Cutaneous/subcutaneous:
        - Actinomycosis
        - Atypical mycobacteriosis
        - Leprosy
        - Bite wound abscesses
        - Draining tracts resulting from foreign bodies
    - Pulmonary:
        - Thoracic neoplasia
        - Bacterial pyothorax
        - Chronic diaphragmatic hernia
    - Systemic/disseminated:
        - Feline infectious peritonitis
        - Systemic fungal infections.
- Actinomycosis:
    - Nocardiosis
    - Atypical mycobacteriosis
    - Leprosy

- Bite wound abscesses
- Draining tracts resulting from foreign bodies.

DIAGNOSTICS

- Nocardiosis:
  - Neutrophilic leukocytosis
  - Nonregenerative anemia with long-standing infections (anemia of chronic disease)
  - Chemistries: usually normal; hypergammaglobulinemia may be seen with long-standing infections; hypercalcemia with renal dysfunction
  - Radiographs: may reveal pleural or peritoneal effusion, pleuropneumonia, or osteomyelitis
  - Cytology: fine-needle aspirate; thoracentesis or abdominocentesis for samples; stain these or other exudates with Romanowsky, Gram or Brown-Brenn, and modified acid-fast stains for rapid diagnosis; may reveal gram-positive branching filamentous rods and cocci
  - Tissue culture: diagnostic; aerobic culturing on Sabouraud medium
  - Tissue PCR testing of 16S ribosomal DNA to permit speciation: assists in selection of antimicrobial therapy
  - *N. asteroides:* more suppurative pyogranulomatous reaction than with *Actinomyces* spp.
  - *N. brasiliensis:* granulomatous reaction with extensive fibrosis
  - Histopathology: nodular to diffuse dermatitis; panniculitis; with or without tissue grains
  - Although the organism is usually present, it cannot be distinguished in cytology or histopathologically from *Actinomyces* spp.
  - Hypercalcemia may be present and impair renal function.
- Actinomycosis:
  - Tissue culture; anaerobic culture may take several weeks
  - Histopathology: nodular to diffuse pyogranulomatous dermatitis and panniculitis
  - Sulfur granules noted in approximately 50% of cases
  - Stain with Gram, Brown-Brenn, or Gomori methanamine silver.

THERAPEUTICS

- Pleural or peritoneal effusions and disseminated form: inpatient until clinically stable and effusion removed; fluid therapy for rehydration and maintenance often needed.
- Long-term antibiotic therapy and draining fistulous tracts: outpatient.
- Diet: encourage consumption by offering foods with appealing tastes and smells; forced enteral feeding for anorectic inpatients essential; orogastric tube feeding preferred.

- Surgery: surgical drainage should accompany medical therapy; thoracotomy tube for pleural effusion; debridement of draining tracts and lymph nodes.

Drugs of Choice

- Culture organism and perform antibiotic sensitivity testing.
- Nocardiosis: empirical choices (or pending culture results):
  - Sulfadiazine-trimethoprim combinations (15–30 mg/kg PO q24h)
  - Aminoglycosides: gentamicin 9–12 mg/kg (dogs) or 5–8 mg/kg (cats) IV, IM, SC q24h; amikacin 15–30 mg/kg (dogs) or 10–15 mg/kg (cats) IV, IM, SC q24h
  - Cycline antibiotics: tetracycline 15–20 mg/kg PO TID; doxycycline 10 mg/kg PO q24h; minocycline 5–12.5 mg/kg PO BID
  - Erythromycin: 10–20 mg/kg PO q8h; or combined with ampicillin 20–40 mg/kg PO q8h or amoxicillin 6–20 mg/kg PO BID to TID; or clarithromycin 7.5 mg/kg PO BID
  - Amoxicillin plus an aminoglycoside: synergistic combination; consider in any serious infection when culturing is not possible or is pending
  - Chloramphenicol: 40–50 mg/kg PO TID (dogs); 12.5–20 mg/kg PO BID (cats)
  - Fluoroquinolones (third or fourth generation) may be effective.
- Actinomycosis: empirical choices (or pending culture results):
  - Amoxicillin 6–20 mg/kg PO BID to TID
  - Erythromycin: 10–20 mg/kg PO TID; or combined with ampicillin 20–40 mg/kg PO TID.
- Average treatment period is 6 weeks; however, medical treatment should extend several weeks past apparent remission of the disease.

COMMENTS

- Prognosis is guarded.
- Aggressive early therapy when lesions are localized improves outcome.
- Tetracyclines (cats): may cause fever up to 41.5 °C (107 °F); discontinue and replace if fever increases during therapy.
- Monitor carefully for fever, weight loss, seizures, dyspnea, and lameness the first year after apparently successful therapy because of the potential for bone and CNS involvement.
- Treatment should be continued for at least 1 month after clinical remission.

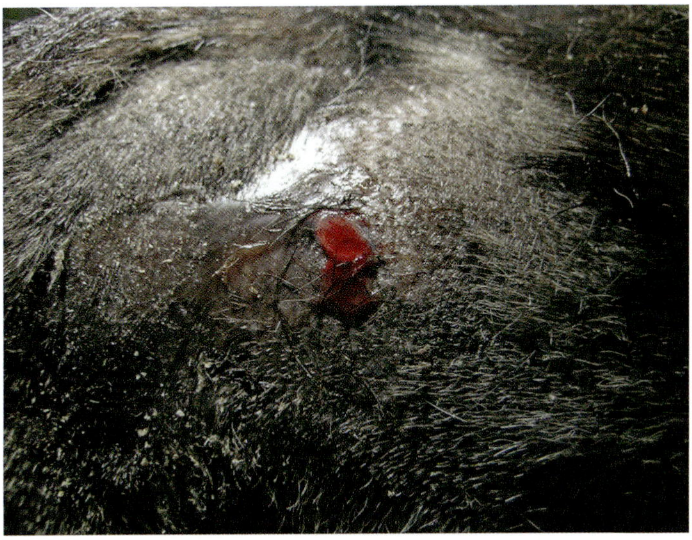

■ **Fig. 36.1.** Exudative and nonhealing wound characteristic of nocardiosis in a DSH.

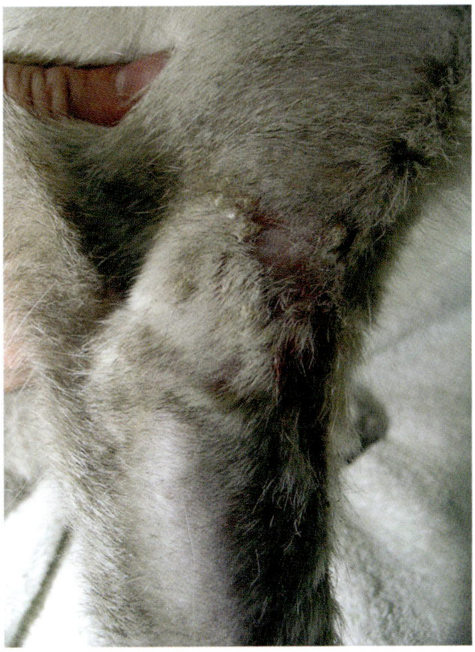

■ **Fig. 36.2.** Patch of dried exudation over exudative wound on the lateral elbow.

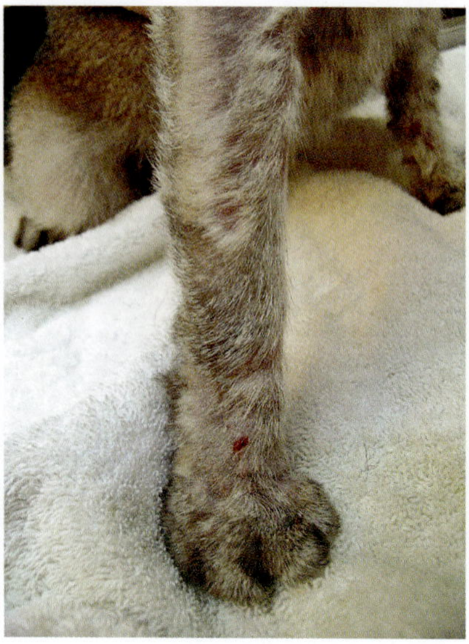

■ **Fig. 36.3.** Persistent draining lesions on the foot of the cat in Figure 36.2.

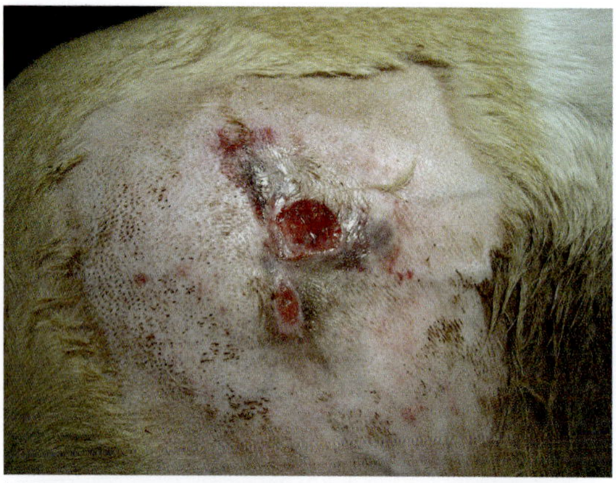

(a)

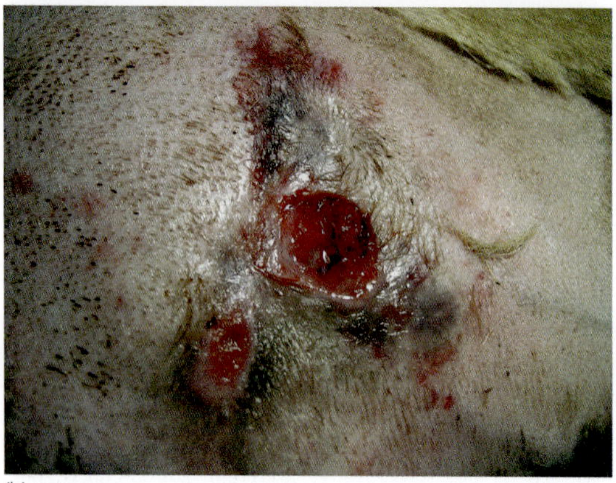

(b)

■ **Fig. 36.4.** Lesions of *Actinomyces* in a Labrador mix. Subcutaneous and draining nodules are very similar in appearance to nocardiosis.

chapter 37

Otitis Externa, Media, and Interna

DEFINITION/OVERVIEW

- Otitis externa: inflammation of the external ear canal; includes anatomic structures of the pinna, horizontal and vertical canals, and the external wall of the tympanic membrane.
- Otitis media: inflammation of the middle ear; includes anatomic structures of the medial wall of the tympanic membrane, bulla (tympanic cavity), auditory ossicles, and auditory tube.
- Otitis interna: inflammation of the inner ear; includes anatomic structures of the cochlea, semicircular canals, and associated nerves (cranial nerves VII and VIII).
- Terms are descriptions of clinical signs, not diagnoses.
- Ototoxicity: impairment or damage of the inner ear and/or eighth cranial nerve; neurotoxicity (specifically during treatment of otitis externa/media) damage of the eight cranial nerve.

ETIOLOGY/PATHOLOGY

- External ear canal:
    - Auricular cartilage: funnel-shaped structure that creates the pinna and the proximal section of the vertical canal
    - Annular cartilage overlaps with the auricular cartilage and extends to the external wall of the tympanum
    - Auricular projection: a fold of cartilage in the vertical canal near the junction with the horizontal canal; must be displaced dorsally to gain access to the horizontal canal
    - Sebaceous glands and modified apocrine glands (cerumen glands) line the canal and produce a secretion with varying amounts of lipid (higher levels in dogs with otitis externa); increased density of cerumen glands associated with predisposition to otitis externa

Blackwell's Five-Minute Veterinary Consult Clinical Companion: Small Animal Dermatology, Third Edition.
Karen Helton Rhodes and Alexander H. Werner.

- Epithelial migration moves epithelial cells, cerumen, and canal contents up and out of the external canal
- Tufts of hair may be present on the ventral surface of the external ear canal proximal to the opening of the acoustic meatus near the ventral attachment of the tympanic membrane.

■ Tympanum (Figures 37.1, 37.2):
- Pars flaccida: alternatively called the dorsal membrane; small portion dorsal to the osseous ring of the external acoustic meatus; may swell with inflammation or increased pressure in the middle ear
- Pars tensa: thin firm structure attached to the osseous ring of the external acoustic meatus; manubrium of the malleus on the medial surface curves rostrally.

■ Middle ear canal: medial surface of the tympanic membrane, bulla (tympanic cavity – normally air filled) and auditory ossicles and associated structures; dog – incomplete septum (bulla ridge) and promontory (contains cochlea and communicates with the bulla through the oval and round windows); cat – bulla divided by a nearly intact septum (associated with postganglionic sympathetic nerves); three auditory ossicles transfer movement from the tympanum to the inner ear; bulla connected to the nasopharynx by the auditory tube.

■ Inner ear: anatomic structures of the cochlea, semicircular canals, and associated nerves (cranial nerves VII and VIII).

■ Otitis externa:
- Common disease in dogs; frequent in cats
- Chronic inflammation results in alterations of the normal environment of the canal
- With inflammation, glands enlarge and produce excessive wax
- Epidermis and dermis thicken and become fibrotic
- Thickened canal folds effectively reduce canal width
- End-stage calcification of the auricular cartilage results in permanent changes.

■ Causes of otitis externa are frequently classified as primary, secondary, predisposing, or perpetuating:
- Primary causes directly initiate or cause inflammation in a normal ear canal (e.g., parasites, hypersensitivity, endocrinopathy)
- Secondary causes initiate or cause inflammation in an abnormal ear canal (e.g., bacterial or yeast infection, medication reaction)
- Predisposing causes change the environment of the normal ear canal, facilitating inflammation and encouraging secondary infection
- Perpetuating causes result from changes in the external ear canal from inflammation that prevent resolution of the inflammation and/or infection of the ear canal.

■ Otitis media: most often an extension of otitis externa through a ruptured tympanum; may occur without membrane rupture; may occur from polyps or neoplasia within the middle ear or auditory tube.

■ Otitis interna: extension of otitis media or hematogenous spread of infection; extension of neoplasia from surrounding tissue.

SIGNALMENT/HISTORY

Breed Predilections

- Pendulous-eared dogs: spaniels, retrievers, and hounds.
- Hirsute canals: terriers and poodles.
- Stenotic canals: Chinese shar pei.
- Primary secretory otitis media: cavalier King Charles spaniel and boxer.

Historical Findings

- Pain (shying from touching of the head or refusing to open the mouth).
- Head shaking (if both ear canals are severely affected, the patient may not shake the head as vigorously as expected due to pain).
- Scratching at the pinnae.
- Malodor.
- Peripheral vestibular deficits.
- Loss of hearing acuity.
- Facial nerve deficits and/or Horner's syndrome.
- Unilateral (i.e., foreign body, polyp, tumor) versus bilateral (i.e., hypersensitivity, endocrinopathy).
- Otitis externa was reported as being more disturbing to clients than to patients in one study.

Risk Factors

- Abnormal or breed-related conformation of the external canal (e.g., stenosis, hirsutism, and pendulous pinnae) restricts proper airflow into the canal.
- Excessive moisture (e.g., swimming, environmental humidity, or frequent cleanings) can lead to infection; overzealous client compliance with recommendations for ear cleanings and/or use of inappropriate solutions.
- Topical drug reaction and irritation or trauma from abrasive cleaning techniques.
- Underlying systemic diseases producing abnormalities in the microenvironment of the ear canal environment and in the immune response.
- Otitis media is a frequent sequela of chronic otitis externa.
- Nasopharyngeal polyps, and inner, middle, or external ear canal neoplasia.
- Inhalant anesthesia may change middle ear pressure.

CLINICAL FEATURES

Otitis Externa

- Deafness.
- Erythroceruminous: ceruminous discharge with erythema; often associated with secondary *Malassezia* or staphylococcal infection; pruritic (Figure 37.3).

- Suppurative: purulent and malodorous exudates; erosion and ulceration of the epithelial lining; frequently associated with *Pseudomonas aeruginosa* infection; painful (Figure 37.4).
- Inflammation, pain, pruritus, and erythema of the pinnae and external canals.
- Aural hematoma.
- Swelling of the canal leading to stenosis.
- Cerumen gland hyperplasia (Figure 37.5).
- Fibrosis and ossification of the auricular cartilage; canals palpate as firm and thickened.
- Holding of the pinnae down and/or head tilt toward affected side (if unilateral).
- Chronic otitis externa in dogs results in tympanic membrane rupture (71%) and otitis media (82%) (one study).
- Allergic dermatitis: most common cause of otitis externa in dogs.
- Polyps and ectoparasites: most common cause of recurrent otitis externa in cats.

Otitis Media

- Intact tympanic membrane: bulging tissue with evidence of fluid and/or gas caudally; membrane may be opaque; fluid may be purulent or hemorrhagic (Figure 37.6).
- Swelling of the pars flaccida: may indicate increased pressure in the middle ear; commonly seen with primary secretory otitis media in the cavalier King Charles spaniel (Figures 37.7–37.9).
- Ruptured tympanic membrane: discharge into canal or bullae filled with debris (Figure 37.10).
- Deafness.
- Pain on palpation of bullae or opening of the mouth.
- Pharyngitis, tonsillitis, or discharge through auditory tube (Figure 37.11).
- Lymphandenopathy if severe or chronic.

Otitis Interna

- Deafness.
- Neurologic findings:
    - Vestibular (cranial nerve VIII) deficits: nystagmus, head tilt (ipsilateral), ataxia, anorexia or vomiting, and reluctance to move the head (Figure 37.12)
    - Facial nerve (cranial nerve VII) deficits: paresis/paralysis of eyelids, lips, tongue, nares; reduced tear production; miosis, ptosis, protrusion of the nictitans, and enophthalmos (Horner's syndrome) (Figure 37.13).

DIFFERENTIAL DIAGNOSIS

Otitis Externa and Media

- Primary causes:
    - Parasite: *Otodectes cynotis*, *Demodex* spp., *Sarcoptes scabiei*, *Notoedres cati*, and *Otobius megnini* (Figure 37.14).

- Hypersensitivity: atopy, cutaneous adverse reaction to food, contact allergy, and systemic or local drug reaction; most common cause of chronic otitis externa; present in over 50% of cases of cutaneous adverse reaction to food (Figure 37.15).
- Foreign body: plant material, accumulation of hair, medication.
- Keratinization disorder: increased cerumen production resulting in functional obstruction of the canal.
- Endocrinopathy: causes immunosuppression and changes in cerumen production.
- Autoimmune disease: frequently affects the pinnae and less often the external ear canal.

- Secondary causes:
  - Bacterial infection: *Staphylococcus pseudintermedius*, *Pseudomonas aeruginosa*, *Enterococcus* spp., *Proteus mirabilis*, *Streptococcus* spp., *Corynebacterium* spp., and *Escherichia coli*
  - *Pseudomonas aeruginosa* most commonly cultured in otitis media
  - Fungal infection: *Malassezia pachydermatis*, *Candida albicans*, and rarely other fungi (*Sporothrix schenckii*, *Cryptococcus neoformans*).
- Perpetuating causes:
  - Chronic changes: stenosis of the canal due to cerumen gland hyperplasia and polyp formation, swelling from inflammation, scarring and calcification
  - Chronic change increases retention of debris in the ear by increased cerumen production and decreased removal by epidermal migration and by physical obstruction.
- Predisposing causes:
  - Obstruction: neoplasia, inflammatory polyp, cerumen gland hyperplasia, accumulation of hair (Figures 37.16–37.19)
  - Ceruminous cystomatosis: multiple dark nodules on the concave portion of the pinna and proximal horizontal canal of middle-aged cats (Figure 37.20).
- Otitis media:
  - Most often caused by descending otitis externa
  - May develop secondary to upper respiratory infection by ascension of infection through the auditory tube or by hematogenous spread
  - Otitis media may perpetuate otitis externa
  - Patency of tympanic membrane may be difficult to assess; careful cleaning may reveal a small defect (Figures 37.21, 37.22)
  - Primary secretory otitis media: associated with accumulation of mucoid viscous exudate in the middle ear causing discomfort and intermittent otitis externa following rupture of the tympanic membrane; may be unilateral or bilateral; possibly due to abnormality in the structure or function of the auditory tube; exudate is often aseptic.

Otitis Interna

- Extension of infection from otitis externa/media.

- Central vestibular disease: differentiated by brainstem signs such as stupor and lethargy.
- Neoplasia: diagnosed by imaging studies.
- Endocrinopathy: polyneuropathy and Horner's syndrome associated with hypothyroidism.
- Metronidazole toxicity.
- Thiamine deficiency (cats).
- Trauma.
- Idiopathic vestibular disease (older dogs and middle-aged cats): diagnosis made by exclusion of other causes.

DIAGNOSTICS

- CBC/biochemistry/urinalysis: usually normal; may indicate a primary underlying disease (e.g., hypothyroidism, hematogenous spread of infection).
- Allergy testing: restricted-ingredient food trial for cutaneous adverse reaction to food; intradermal and/or serum allergy testing for atopy.
- Neurologic examination: may indicate otitis interna.
- Direct otoscopy: visualization of the external canal, tympanic membrane, and dorsal and middle portions of the bulla (if tympanum ruptured).
- Video-otoscopy:
  - Provides a magnified view of the canal
  - Improved visualization for diagnosis of otitis media
  - Permits more controlled sample collection
  - Allows direct visualization during cleaning, myringotomy, and surgical procedures (including laser ablation and mass biopsy or removal) (Figure 37.23).
- Imaging:
  - Radiographs: not highly sensitive for diagnosis of otitis media; useful for evaluating chronic changes; bullae should appear thin-walled and air-filled; bullae may appear cloudy if filled with exudate; stenosis of external ear canal; thickening of bullae and petrous temporal bones with mineralization; presence of bone lysis with osteomyelitis or neoplastic disease
  - Ultrasound: poor sensitivity in detecting otitis media compared with CT, MRI or video-otoscopy
  - CT or MRI:
    - Detailed evidence of fluid or tissue density (e.g., polyp) in the bulla, adjacent tissues, or auditory tube
    - CT: useful for bony changes; stenosis or calcification of the canals; contrast used to differentiate debris from soft tissues
    - MRI: useful for evaluation of the tympanic membrane and soft tissues; helpful to differentiate central versus peripheral vestibular disease.
- Skin scrapings from pinnae: ectoparasites.
- Dermatohistopathology: autoimmune disease, neoplasia, cerumen gland hyperplasia; pinnae difficult to biopsy; avoid damaging auricular cartilage.

- Myringotomy: spinal needle or sterile catheter is inserted through the ventral aspect of the pars tensa caudal to the manubrium of the malleolus to sample fluid within the bulla for cytologic examination, culture and sensitivity testing; frequent contamination of samples from the external ear canal occurs during sampling (Figure 37.24).
- Histopathologic examination of tissue obtained by biopsy forceps from the external ear canal or middle ear.
- Brainstem auditory evoked responses: only way to detect bilateral or (especially) unilateral hearing loss; can differentiate deficits originating in the middle ear, cochlea, or central auditory pathways.
- CSF analysis: detect CNS involvement.
- Culture of exudates for identification and sensitivity: may be useful with persistent/nonresponsive infection; most indicated when rod bacteria found in exudate samples or systemic antibiotics are prescribed; concentration of antibiotics instilled into the ear are often significantly higher than used to determine sensitivity *in vitro*.

Cytology

- Microscopic evaluation of exudates: single most important diagnostic tool after complete examination of the ear canal.
- Appearance of the exudates (guidelines – not definitive):
  - Yeast infections: yellow-tan and adherent (especially in proximal horizontal canal) to brown or gray and waxy in deeper canal
  - Bacterial infections: yellow-green, purulent (especially *Pseudomonas*) to brown-black thin exudate (especially staphylococcal)
  - Mucoid or viscous: associated with biofilm production.
- Gross appearance of exudates does not allow an accurate diagnosis of the type of infection; microscopic examination is necessary.
- Samples obtained from the proximal and distal external ear canal, as well as from the middle ear, are frequently different; cytological examination and submission of samples from each location may be necessary for accurate assessment of otitis externa and otitis media.
- Exudates and infection within each canal can differ; samples should be examined from each canal; separate samples may need to be submitted for culture and sensitivity if cytology results demonstrate disparate populations of organisms.
- Infections within the canal can change with prolonged or recurrent therapy; repeat examination of exudates is required in chronic cases.
- Response to therapy also monitored by repeat cytological examination.
- Preparations: made from both canals: contents of each canal may differ; spread samples thinly on a glass microscope slide; examine both unstained and Romanowsky (Diff-Quik®) stained samples: stain chambers should be changed regularly.
- Heat fixing may help with waxy debris but is not required for most samples.
- Mites: presumptive diagnosis.
- Type(s) of bacteria or yeast: assist in the choice of therapy as well as determine whether culture is needed.

- Note findings (e.g., type of organisms; cells present) in the record; rank the number of organisms and cell types present on a standardized scale (e.g., 0 to 4) to allow treatment monitoring:
    - Bacteria: cocci – *Staphylococcus* (clusters or pairs), *Streptococcus* or *Enterococcus* (small, chains); rods – *Pseudomonas* (long, narrow) or *Proteus* (short, bipolar)
    - Yeast: *Malassezia* (broad-based budding, "peanut-shaped") or *Candida* (narrow-based budding)
    - Neutrophils: absence associated with colonization of the canal with bacteria or yeast or mild infection; increased numbers especially with degenerate changes and intracellular organisms indicates active response to infection
    - Red blood cells: associated with ulceration of the epithelial lining; often associated with *Pseudomonas* spp.

THERAPEUTICS

- Diet: no restrictions unless a cutaneous adverse reaction to food is suspected.
- Client education: instruct clients, by demonstration, in the proper method for cleaning and medicating ears (especially the volume of medication to instill; average external ear canal volume is 2.7 mL; there are 15–20 drops/mL).
- Surgical considerations:
    - Indicated when the canal is severely stenotic or obstructed, or when neoplasia or a polyp is diagnosed
    - Severe, unresponsive otitis media may require a bullae osteotomy
    - Lateral ear resection or total ear ablation required with obstructed canals or neoplasia.
- Chronic otitis externa frequently leads to ruptured tympanae and otitis media.
- Complications following external ear flushing in cats (vestibular signs) are not uncommon; clients should be warned of possible residual effects.
- Corticosteroid use is controversial with otitis media/interna.
- Avoid vigorous flushing of the ear with otitis media/interna.
- Osteomyelitis of petrous temporal bone and bulla may require 6–8 weeks of antibiotics.
- Uncontrolled otitis externa and media, as well as treatment complications, can lead to deafness, vestibular disease, cellulitis, facial nerve paralysis, progression to otitis interna, and, rarely, meningoencephalitis.
- Vestibular signs usually improve within 2–6 weeks.
- Tympanum integrity should be assessed prior to introduction of solutions and/or medications into the external ear canal.
- Ear cleanser ingredients:
    - Tympanum not intact:
        - Saline solution
        - 2.5% acetic acid (1:1 vinegar/water) rinses; acetic acid solutions may be irritating if not buffered
        - 2% N-acetyl-L-cysteine (NAC) solutions when biofilms suspected

- Intact tympanum:
  - Ceruminolytic: dioctyl sodium sulfosuccinate, squaline, carbamide peroxide, propylene glycol (mild cleanser); most often used for in-hospital cleaning; irritating if not removed from ear canal
  - Antiseptics: acetic acid or 0.2% chlorhexidine gluconate; parachlorometaxylenol (PCMX); monosaccharide complex; trisaminomethane ethylenediaminetetraacetic acid (tris-EDTA) has antibacterial and synergistic properties with certain antibiotics
  - Astringents: isopropyl alcohol, boric acid, salicylic acid
  - Antiinfective/parasiticide agents: specific to identified organism(s).

- Ear flushing:
  - Antiinflammatory therapy may be necessary prior to flushing to reduce swelling
  - Sedation may be required in painful cases and to prevent further trauma to the canal
  - Gentle solutions should be used initially
  - A bulb syringe or properly trimmed French red rubber catheter is used to flush in solution and remove debris
  - A catheter can be introduced into the bullae to permit flushing of the middle ear; intubation is recommended if heavy sedation or general anesthesia is administered
  - Repeat cleansing at a tapering frequency during therapy
  - Primary secretory otitis media treated by complete flushing of the middle ear; repeat flushing may be required.

Drugs of Choice

- Topical medication:
  - Antibiotic: based on cytologic evaluation, culture and sensitivity testing, and/or empiric choice; common commercial formulations contain gentamicin, neomycin, marbofloxacin, enrofloxacin, orbifloxacin, florfenicol, polymyxin B, or silver sulfadiazine
  - Additional antibiotics used topically (based on culture/sensitivity testing): amikacin, ticarcillin disodium/clavulanate potassium, and tobramycin
  - Antifungal: imidazoles – lotrimazole, ketoconazole, miconazole, posaconazole, thiabendazole; also nystatin, terbinafine
  - Antiinflammatory: corticosteroids: dexamethasone, fluocinolone, betamethasone, triamcinolone, hydrocortisone, and mometasone; also dimethyl sulfoxide (DMSO); adrenal suppression occurs with topically applied corticosteroids
  - Combination antibiotic/antifungal/corticosteroid combination products are widely used
  - Formulated products with excipients to permit longer exposure times for infecting organisms with antimicrobials and longer contact time of the canal epithelium with corticosteroids are available; particularly effective in acute otitis when compliance with daily instillation of products is challenging
  - Caution when patency of the tympanic membrane is not known

- Standard ointments and lotions may be occlusive and perpetuate disease unless used judiciously
- NAC: 2% solution used to disrupt biofilm formation to increase antibiotic efficacy; administered systemically to reduce chemotherapy-induced ototoxicity
- Antiparasite: ivermectin, amitraz, pyrethrins, milbemycin, and thiabendazole.

■ Systemic medication:
- May be required if topical therapy is ineffective or cannot be administered due to patient temperament or pain
- Cytological examination of exudates helps determine the type of systemic medication needed
- Inflammation perpetuates disease; high-dose corticosteroids may be required initially to reduce swelling of the canal epithelium so that medications can be instilled effectively
- Otitis interna, otitis media, and chronic/severe otitis externa may require systemic medication for at least 4–6 weeks
- Antibiotic choice should be based on culture/sensitivity with recurrent infections; should be performed when initial treatment is ineffective
- Staphylococcal bacteria: cephalexin 22 mg/kg PO BID, amoxicillin trihydrate-clavulanate potassium 10–15 mg/kg PO BID; clindamycin 11 mg/kg PO q24h to BID for bone involvement; mupirocin topical solution, and chloramphenicol 40 mg/kg PO BID to TID – reserve unless indicated by culture and sensitivity testing
- Mixed or rod bacteria: fluoroquinolone: trimethoprim-sulfadiazine 10–15 mg/kg PO BID, ormetoprim-sulfadimethoxine 55 mg/kg PO first day then 27.5 mg/kg PO q24h, enrofloxacin 10–20 mg/kg PO q24h (dogs) maximum 5 mg/kg PO q24h (cats) – dose may be divided and administered BID, ciprofloxacin 20–25 mg/kg PO q24h, orbifloxacin 2.5–7.5 mg/kg PO q24h, marbofloxacin 2.75–5.5 mg/kg PO q24h – higher-range dosage recommended for *Pseudomonas* spp. infection
- Subcutaneously: amikacin 20 mg/kg by subcutaneous injection q24h; beta-lactam: ticarcillin disodium/clavulanate potassium 10–25 mg/kg by intramuscular injection, imipenem 5 mg/kg by subcutaneous or intramuscular injection TID to QID, meropenem 8.5 mg/kg BID (dogs), 10 mg/kg BID (cats), ceftazidime 30 mg/kg by subcutaneous injection TID to QID
- Antifungal: may be prescribed along with topical therapy for otitis media; ketoconazole 5 mg/kg PO q24h to BID, fluconazole 5 mg/kg PO q24h to BID, itraconazole 5 mg/kg PO q24h; usefulness of oral antifungal medications in otitis externa is controversial
- Antiinflammatory: prednisolone 1–2 mg/kg PO q24h, dexamethasone 0.1–0.2 mg/kg PO q24h, triamcinolone 0.1–0.2 mg/kg PO q24h – tapering dosages; intralesional triamcinolone (0.1 mg/kg total dosage placed in multiple sites)
- Parasiticide: ivermectin 200–400 μg/kg by subcutaneous injection every 2 weeks for three treatments or PO weekly for four treatments, selamectin – as labeled, moxidectin – as labeled, isoxazolines (afoxolaner, fluralaner, sarolaner) – as labeled.

Maintenance Therapy Goals

- Keep canals clear of debris with routine cleanings weekly to every other week; balance overcleaning/overwetting with undercleaning.
- Reduce bacterial and yeast colonization of the ear canal environment with cleansing solutions or judicious use of topical medications.
- Reduce inflammation and wax production with topical corticosteroids and treatment of underlying causes of ear canal disease.
- Examine ear canals at routine intervals to detect changes prior to the onset of clinical symptoms.

COMMENTS

- Do not use ivermectin in heartworm-positive dogs, or in collies, Shetland sheepdogs, Old English sheepdogs, Australian shepherds, and their cross-breeds; there is increased risk of ivermectin toxicity in herding breeds; prevent ingestion of topical ivermectins in herding dogs and their cross-breeds (due to possible ABCB1Δ [MDR1] gene mutation).
- Ototoxicity has been reported with a large number of topical medications and ingredients; avoidance (if possible) is recommended if the tympanae are not intact (or cannot be properly assessed); commonly reported ototoxic medications include aminoglycoside and macrolide antibiotics, antineoplastic (platinum-based) agents, and loop diuretics.

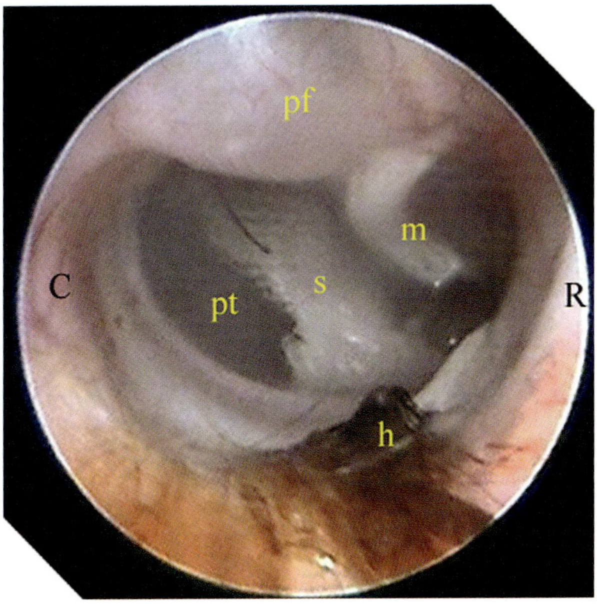

■ **Fig. 37.1.** Normal tympanum in a 2-year-old male-castrate golden retriever. C, caudal; R, rostral; pf, pars flaccida; pt, pars tensa; S, septum bulla (as visualized through intact tympanum); m, manubrium of the malleus; h, tufts of hair on ventrum of canal proximal to tympanum.

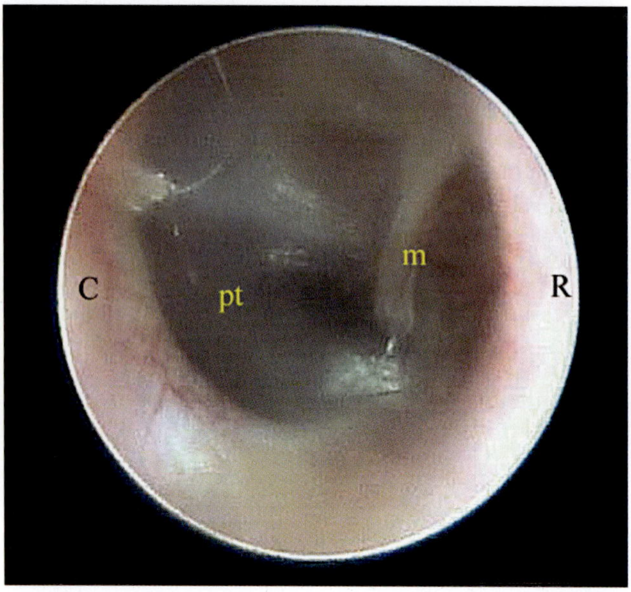

■ **Fig. 37.2.** Normal tympanum in a 9-year-old male-castrate DSH. The manubrium of the malleus in the cat appears straighter than in the dog. C, caudal; R, rostral; pt, pars tensa; m, manubrium of the malleus.

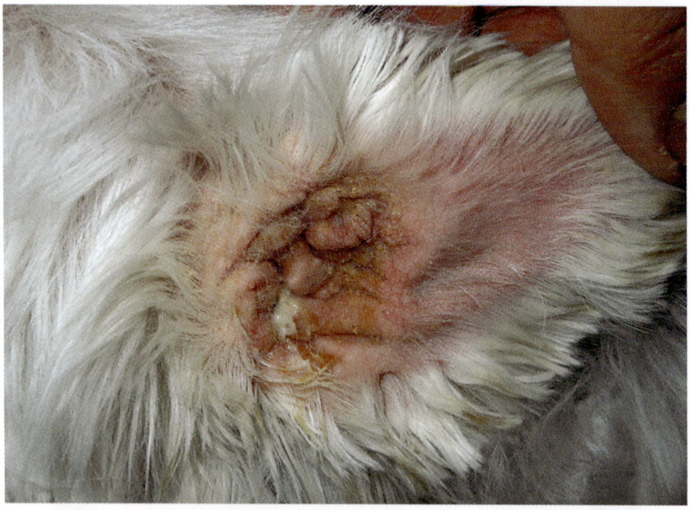

■ **Fig. 37.3.** Erythroceruminous otitis externa as a result of chronic atopic dermatitis in an 11-year-old male-castrate Maltese. The pinna is thickened and erythematous, with accumulations of waxy to purulent exudate.

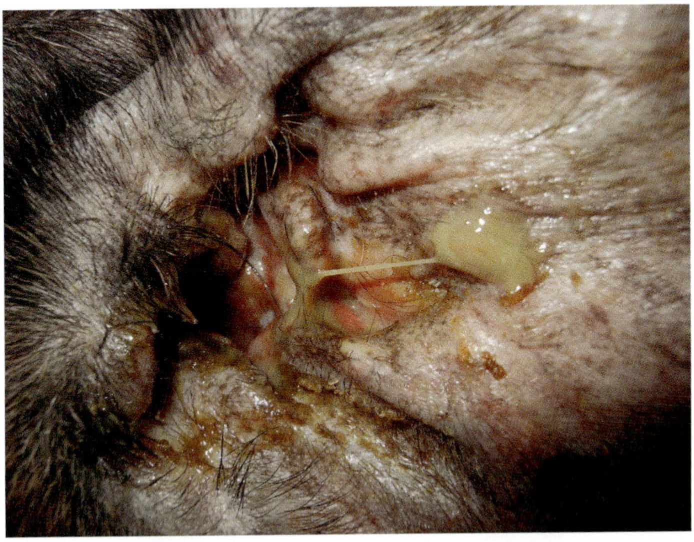

■ **Fig. 37.4.** Suppurative otitis externa with secondary *Pseudomonas aeruginosa* infection in an adult male-castrate mix-breed dog. *Pseudomonas* spp. infection often causes a foul-smelling, yellow-green exudate with erosion and ulceration of the epithelial lining of the canal. Mucoid appearance to the discharge may indicate biofilm production.

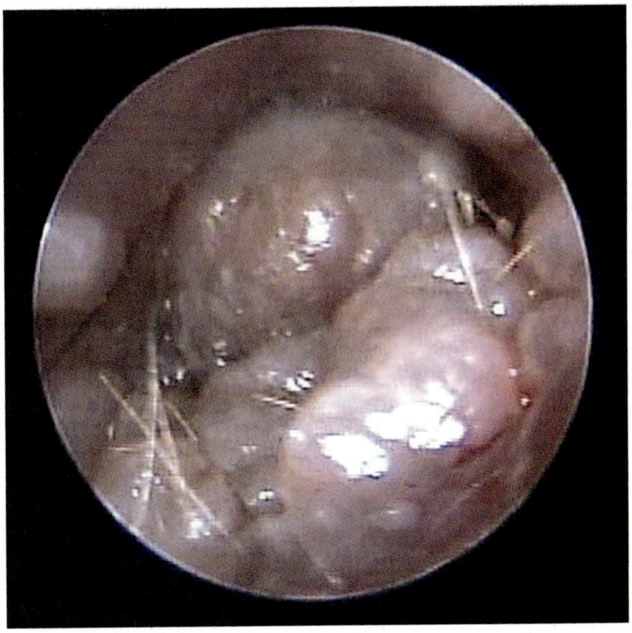

■ **Fig. 37.5.** Polypoid cerumen gland hyperplasia causing functional obstruction of the external ear canal in an 11-year-old male-castrate cocker spaniel.

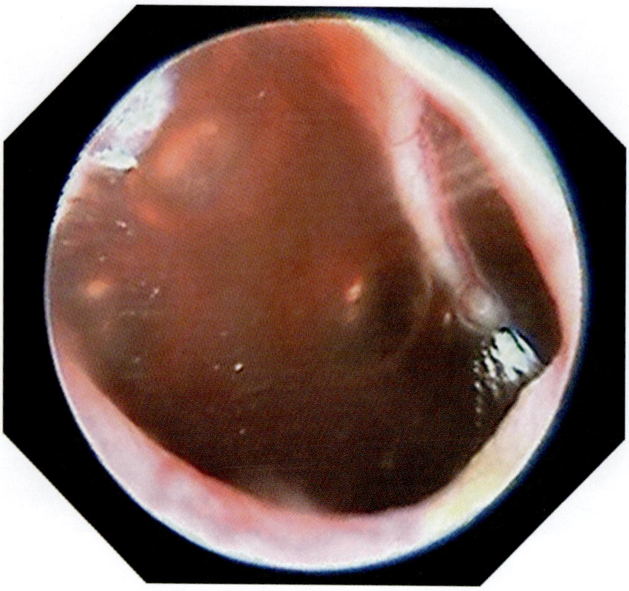

■ **Fig. 37.6.** Otitis media with blood-tinged fluid behind the tympanum in an adult DLH. Note the gas bubble adjacent to the manubrium of the malleus.

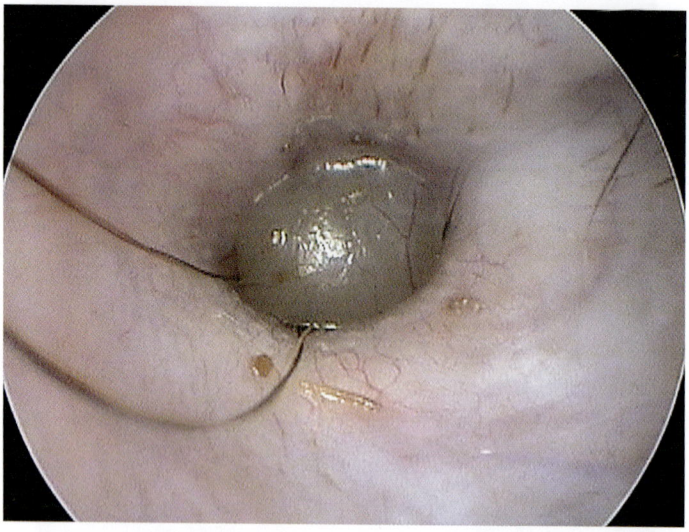

■ **Fig. 37.7.** Primary secretory otitis media in a 7-year-old female-spayed cavalier King Charles spaniel. A pale-yellow mucoid exudate has caused the pars flaccida of the tympanum to swell into the external ear canal.

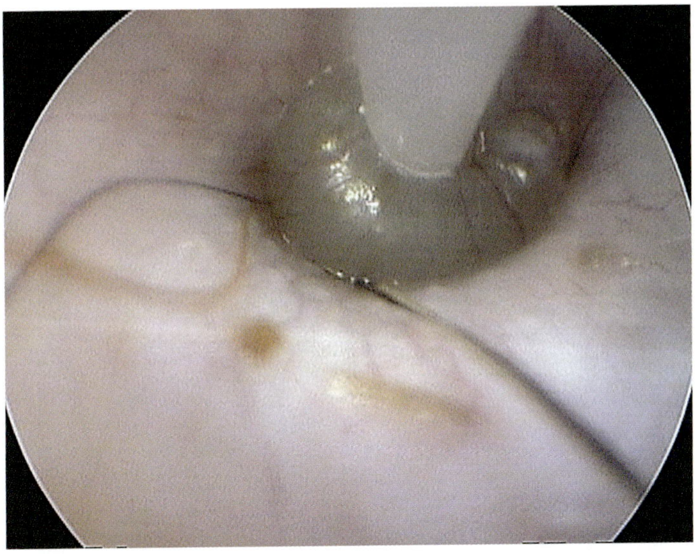

■ **Fig. 37.8.** Pressure from a myringotomy catheter demonstrates the accumulation of fluid behind the tympanum in the patient in Figure 37.7.

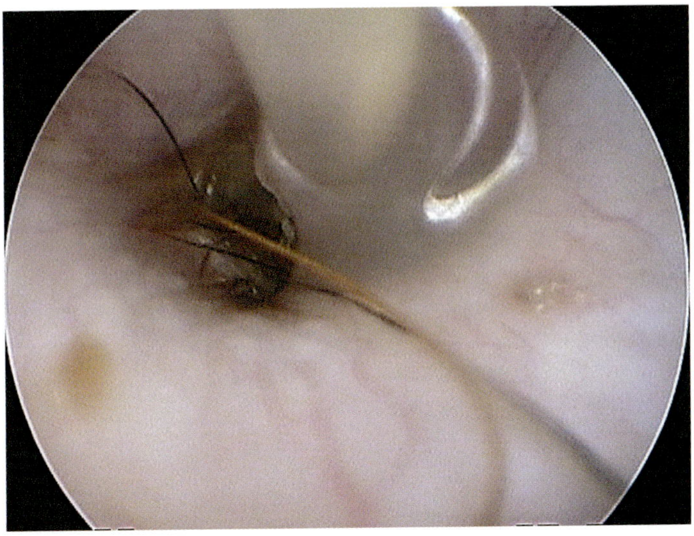

■ **Fig. 37.9.** Postmyringotomy image of the patient in Figure 37.7. Surrounding the myringotomy tube is mucoid exudate from the middle ear.

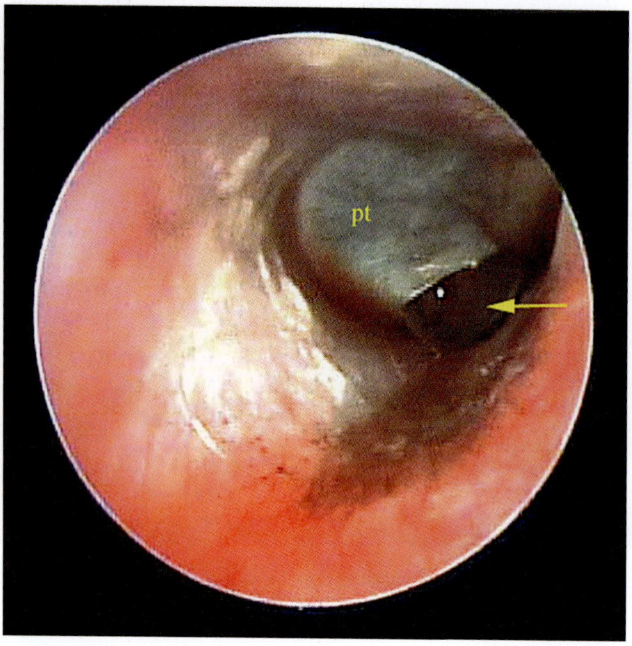

■ **Fig. 37.10.** Otitis externa leading to rupture of the tympanum in an 11-year-old male-castrate cocker spaniel. pt, pars tensa; yellow arrow, defect in tympanum.

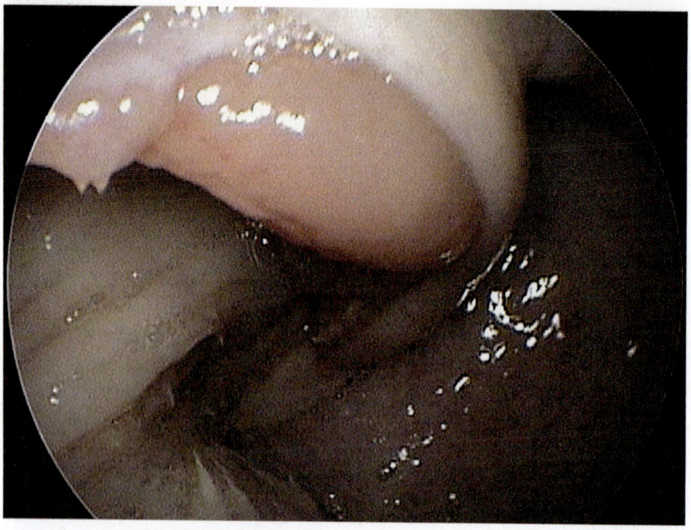

■ **Fig. 37.11.** Enlarged tonsil due to chronic otitis media in a 10-year-old male-castrate rottweiler.

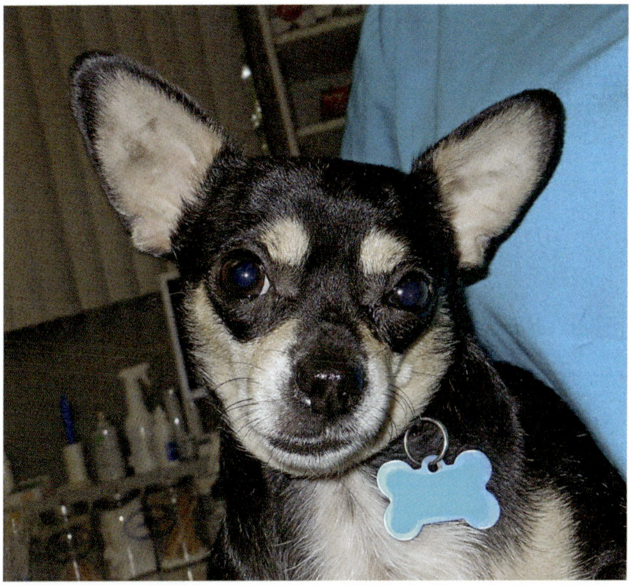

■ **Fig. 37.12.** Head tilt as a result of otitis media in a 1-year-old male-castrate chihuahua. External ear canals appeared normal on examination.

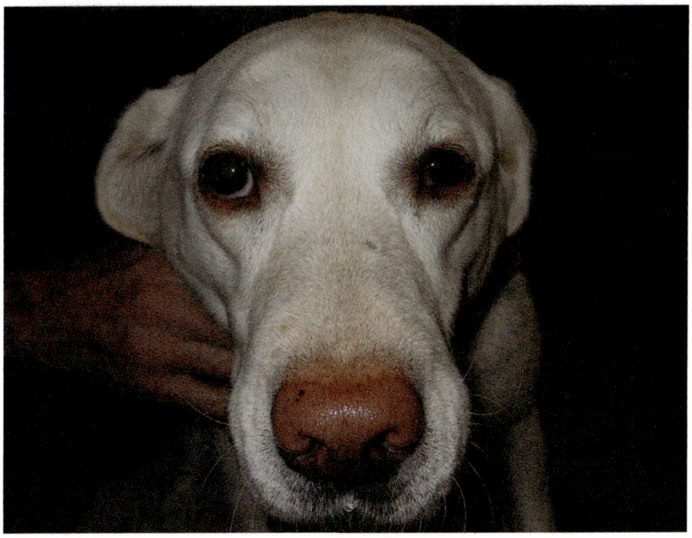

■ **Fig. 37.13.** Horner's syndrome as a result of otitis externa and media in a 2-year-old male-castrate Labrador retriever. Facial nerve (cranial nerve VII) deficits in this case include miosis, ptosis, protrusion of the nictitans, and enophthalmos.

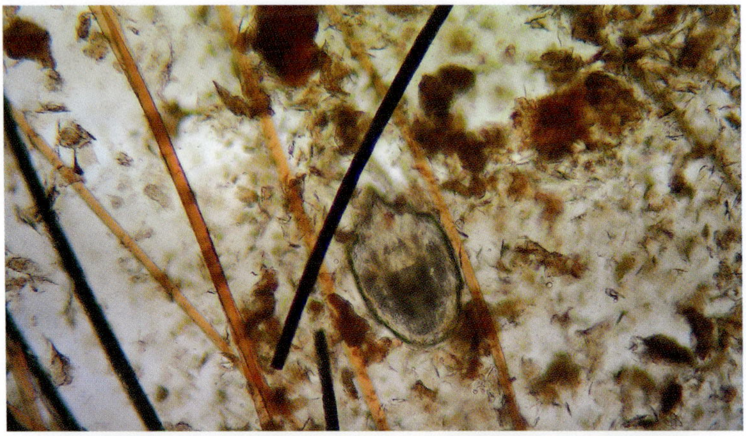

■ **Fig. 37.14.** *Otodectes cynotis* mite in otic exudate from a 10-month-old female-spayed Kerry blue terrier.

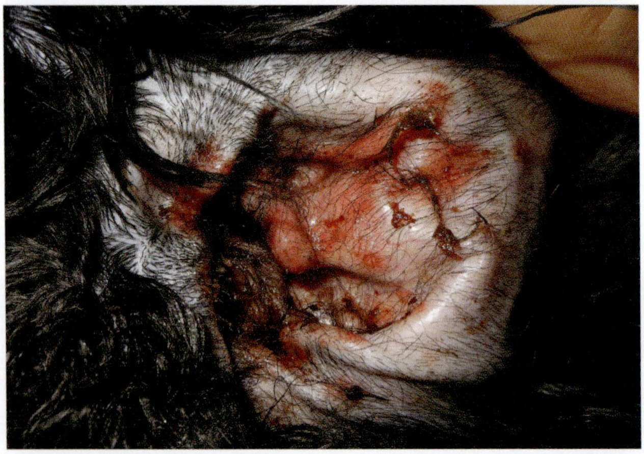

■ **Fig. 37.15.** Erythema and exudation caused by reaction to a common ear medication in a 5-month-old male-intact standard poodle.

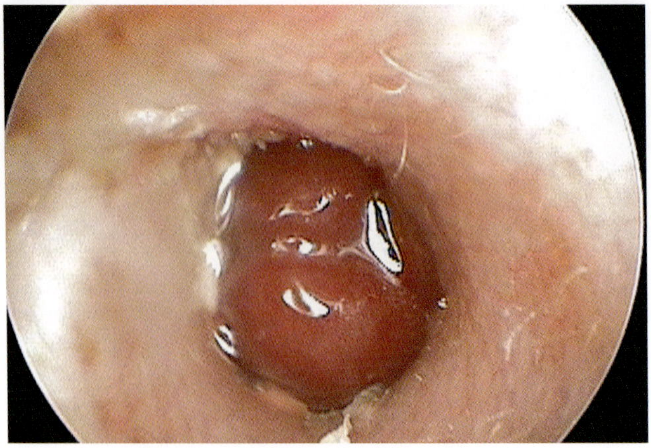

■ **Fig. 37.16.** Feline inflammatory polyp from the middle ear protruding through the tympanum and into the external ear canal in a 1-year-old male-castrate DMH.

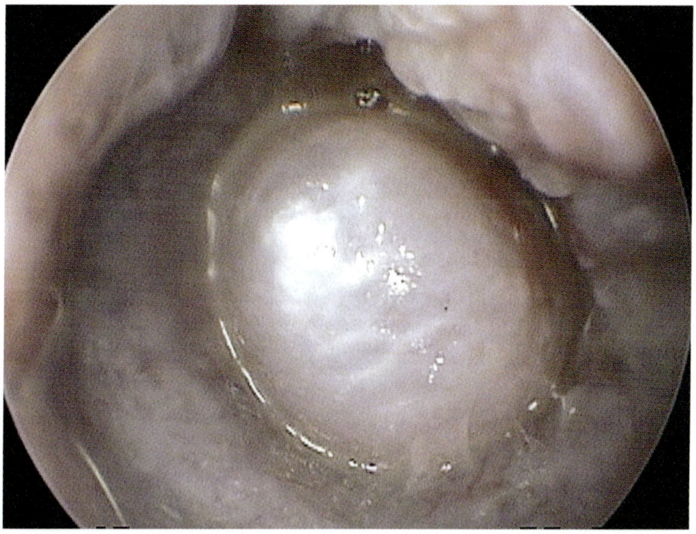

■ **Fig. 37.17.** Presence of a large polyp causing the tympanum to bulge into the horizontal ear canal of a 7-year-old male-castrate French bulldog.

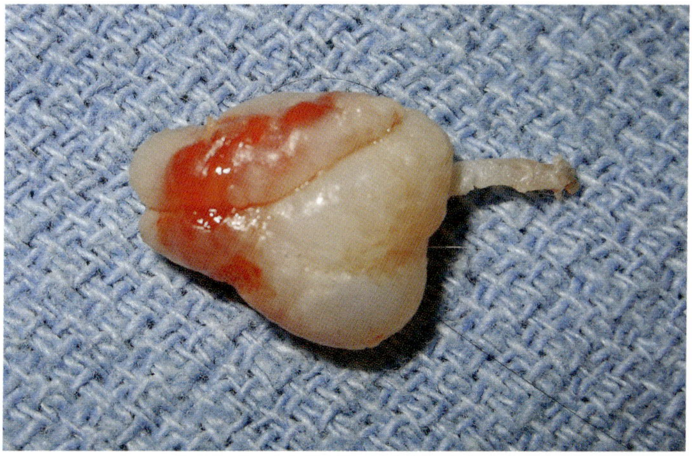

■ **Fig. 37.18.** Polyp after removal from the ear canal of the patient in Figure 37.17. Note the stalk attached at the base; polyps often develop from the lining of the middle ear.

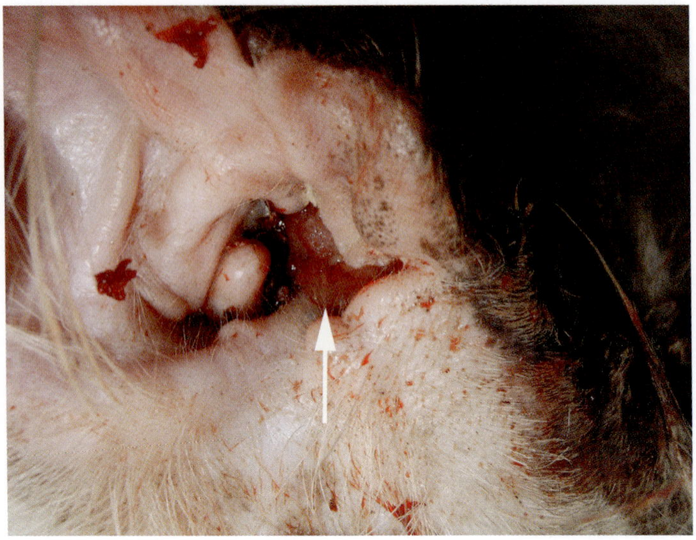

■ **Fig. 37.19.** Cerumen gland adenocarcinoma (*white arrow*) in the anthelix portion of the external ear canal in a 12-year-old male-castrate Persian cat.

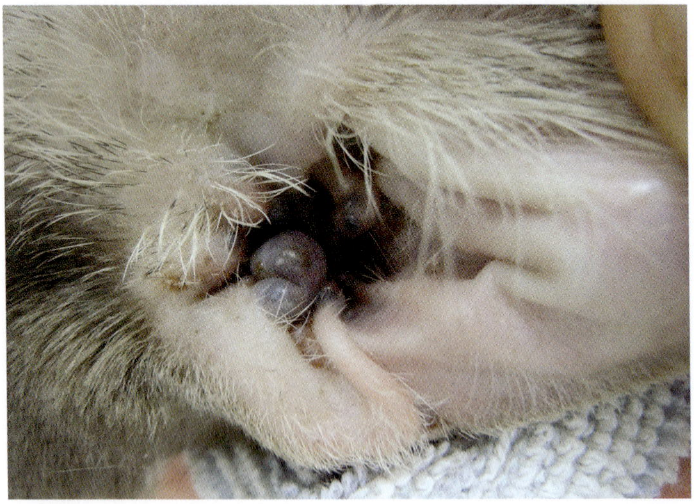

■ **Fig. 37.20.** Ceruminous cystomatosis affecting the concave pinna and proximal vertical ear canal of a 9-year-old male-castrate DSH.

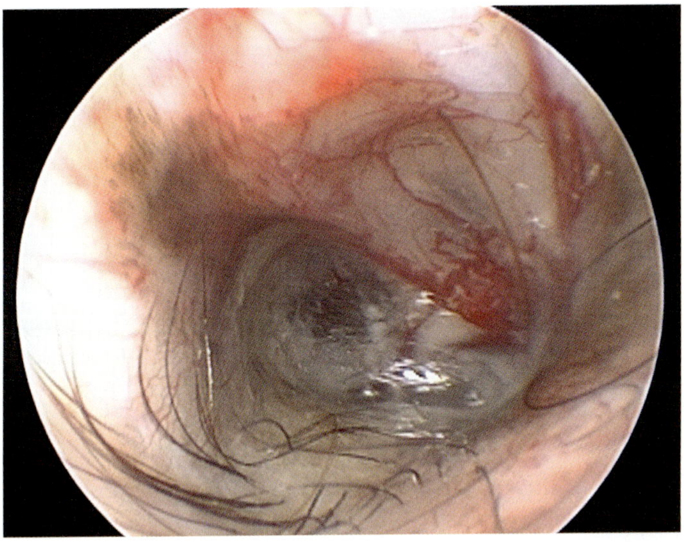

■ **Fig. 37.21.** Tympanic membrane in a 5-year-old male-castrate wheaten terrier appears intact prior to gentle cleaning. Note prominent vasculature of the pars flaccida and debris that appears caudal to the tympanum.

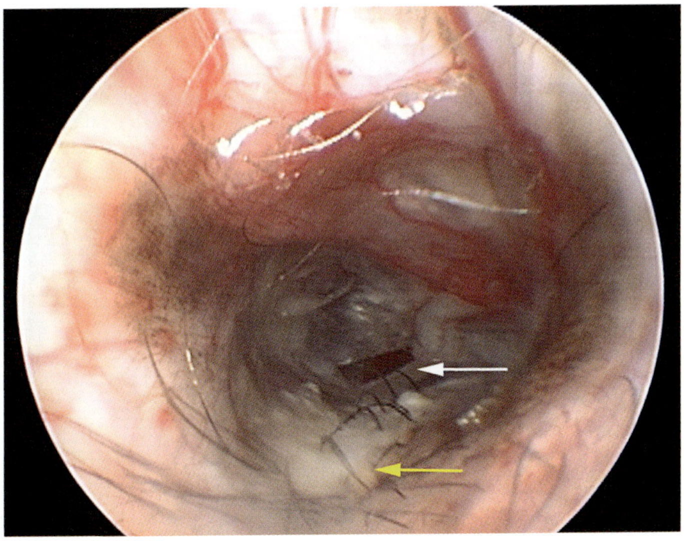

■ **Fig. 37.22.** Gentle cleaning of the ear seen in Figure 37.21 reduced pressure within the bulla, revealing a defect in the tympanic membrane (*white arrow*) that was not apparent until debris was removed from the surface (*yellow arrow*).

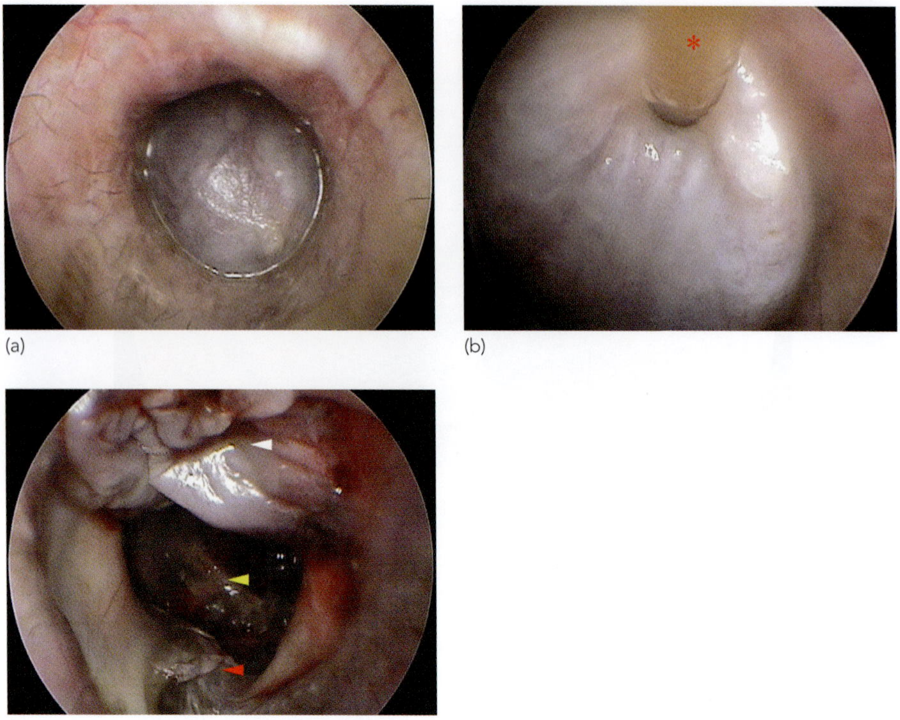

■ **Fig. 37.23.** (a) Cerumen cyst occupying the external ear canal of a 5-year-old male-castrate mix breed dog. (b) Under visualization with video-otoscopy, the cerumen cyst is punctured and drained of tan-yellow fluid by rigid catheter (*asterisk*). (c) Following drainage, the wall of the cerumen cyst has retracted towards the dorsal aspect of the external ear canal (*white arrowhead*). Remnants of the tympanum are visualized on the ventral aspect of canal (*red arrowhead*). The ruptured tympanic membrane allows visualization of the tympanic bulla (*yellow arrowhead*).

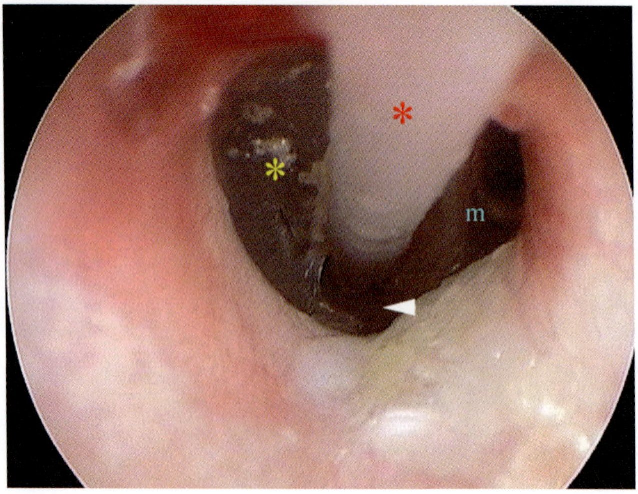

■ **Fig. 37.24.** Myringotomy procedure in a 12-year-old male-castrate DSH. The myringotomy tube (*red asterisk*) is inserted through the tympanic membrane (*yellow asterisk*) ventral and caudal to the manubrium of the malleus (m) to produce a defect in the tympanum (*white arrowhead*), permitting sample collection and cleaning of the tympanic bulla.

chapter 38

Panniculitis

DEFINITION/OVERVIEW

- Inflammation of the subcutaneous fat tissue; variety of etiologies; infectious versus idiopathic; uncommon in dogs and cats.

ETIOLOGY/PATHOPHYSIOLOGY

- Lipocyte (adipocyte, fat cell) is susceptible to trauma, ischemic disease, and inflammation from adjacent tissues.
- Damage to lipocytes results in lipid hydrolysis into glycerol and fatty acids.
- Fatty acids incite an inflammatory response leading to granulomatous tissue reaction.
- Causes:
  - Infectious: parasites, bacteria, mycosis, atypical *Mycobacteria*, *Nocardia*, *Bartonella*, poxvirus
  - Immune mediated: lupus panniculitis, erythema nodosum, drug reaction, vasculitis, rheumatoid arthritis, lymphoplasmacytic colitis
  - Idiopathic form: sterile nodular panniculitis (SNP)
  - Puncture wounds, blunt trauma, foreign body
  - Neoplastic: multicentric mast cell tumors, cutaneous lymphosarcoma, pancreatic tumors
  - Arthropod bite
  - Nutritional (vitamin E deficiency: steatitis in cats)
  - Post injection: corticosteroids, vaccines (rabies, etc.), other subcutaneous injections
  - Inflammatory: pancreatitis
  - Drug eruption
  - Thermal burns: heating pad injuries.

SIGNALMENT/HISTORY

- Sterile nodular panniculitis: Australian shepherd, Brittany spaniel, chihuahua, dalmatian, dachshund and pomeranian are predisposed; collies and miniature poodles are at risk.
- Age of onset: 3–6 years (dogs).

Blackwell's Five-Minute Veterinary Consult Clinical Companion: Small Animal Dermatology, Third Edition.
Karen Helton Rhodes and Alexander H. Werner.

CLINICAL FEATURES

- Single or multiple discrete subcutaneous nodules or draining tracts; more often multiple in dogs (Figures 38.1, 38.2).
- Dogs (SNP): primarily dorsal trunk and neck.
- Cats (panniculitis): primarily ventral abdomen and ventrolateral thorax; most often single nodule.
- Early cases of single or multifocal disease: nodules are freely movable underneath the skin; skin overlying the nodule is usually normal but may become erythematous or purpuric (Figure 38.3).
- Nodules may become cystic, ulcerate, and develop draining tracts (Figures 38.4, 38.5).
- Often painful before and just after rupturing.
- Ulcerations heal with crusting and scarring (Figures 38.6, 38.7).
- Nodules vary from a few millimeters to several centimeters in diameter; may be firm and well circumscribed or soft and poorly defined; may affix to the deep dermis with enlargement (Figure 38.8).
- Involved fat may necrose.
- Exudate: small amount of oily discharge; yellow-brown to bloody.
- Multiple lesions (dogs and cats): systemic signs common (e.g., anorexia, pyrexia, lethargy, and depression).
- Occasionally associated with arthropathies in dogs.

DIFFERENTIAL DIAGNOSIS

Deep Pyoderma

- More common than panniculitis.
- More likely over pressure points, often more generalized.
- May have associated superficial pyoderma (e.g., papules, pustules, and epidermal collarettes).
- Aspirates and impression smears: marked numbers of neutrophils with variable numbers of mononuclear cells and bacteria; culture/sensitivity and biopsies: confirm diagnosis.

Cutaneous Cysts

- Usually nonpainful.
- Well demarcated and usually not characterized as "melting," as is often noted with panniculitis.
- Minimal inflammation.
- Aspirates: amorphous debris; no inflammatory cells, not characterized as fat necrosis but rather a thick sebaceous secretion.
- Biopsies: confirm diagnosis.

Cutaneous Neoplasia

- Lipomas: soft; usually well demarcated.
- No inflammation or draining tracts.
- Aspirates: lipocytes; no inflammatory cells.
- Biopsies: confirm diagnosis.

Mast Cell Tumors/Cutaneous Lymphosarcoma/Pancreatic Panniculitis

- Multifocal.
- May affect the head, legs, and mucous membranes.
- Often erythematous.
- Variable presentations.
- Aspirates: often suggestive.
- Biopsies: confirm diagnosis.

Sterile Nodular Panniculitis

- Diagnosis made by ruling out other causes of panniculitis.
- Tissue cultures negative.
- Special stains on histopathologic samples are negative.

DIAGNOSTICS

- Occasional regenerative left shift or eosinophilia.
- Mild leukocytosis.
- Mild normochromic, normocytic nonregenerative anemia.
- Antinuclear antibody.
- Direct immunofluorescence testing.
- Serum protein electrophoresis.
- Serum lipase/amylase levels.
- Ultrasound: pancreatitis may be a contributing factor (rare).
- Bacterial culture and sensitivity testing: necessary for identifying primary or secondary bacteria.
- Fungal and atypical mycobacteria culture.
- Aspirates from fluctuant nodules may appear oily, with examination revealing large numbers of adipocytes in addition to pyogranulomatous inflammation (Figures 38.9, 38.10).
- Biopsies: negative tissue cultures support diagnosis of sterile nodular panniculitis.
- Histopathology divided into four forms: nodular inflammatory aggregates, lobular (within fat lobules), septal (interlobular connective tissue), and diffuse (involves both lobular and interlobular septa).
- Diffuse form most common in dogs.
- Septal form most common in cats.

- Special stains of histopathologic samples: help identify causative agent.
- Surgical excisional biopsies: much more accurate than punch biopsy specimens in most cases; punch biopsies do not provide a sample deep enough to make the diagnosis.
- Histopathologic lesions: required to make a diagnosis of panniculitis; determine septal, lobular, or diffuse inflammatory infiltrate by neutrophils, histiocytes, plasma cells, lymphocytes, eosinophils, or multinucleated giant cells; identify necrosis, fibrosis, or vasculitis (Figures 38.11–38.13).

THERAPEUTICS

- Single lesions: cured with surgical excision.
- Multiple lesions: require systemic medications.
- Positive culture results require appropriate antifungal, antibacterial, or antimycobacterial treatment.
- Sterile nodular panniculitis: systemic treatment with steroids; prednisolone (2.2 mg/kg daily) until lesions completely regress (3–6 weeks); after remission, gradually taper dosage over 2 weeks; may need slower taper to minimize chance of recurrence; many patients cured; some patients require low-dose alternate-day treatment to maintain remission.
- Oral vitamin E: may control mild cases.
- Oral azathioprine 1 mg/kg or 50 mg/m^2 PO q24h then tapered: alternative when steroids are contraindicated.
- Cyclosporine 5–10 mg/kg PO q24h: alternative for sterile idiopathic panniculitis.
- Cycline antibiotics: tetracycline 250 mg PO TID for dogs <10 kg; 500 mg PO TID dogs >10 kg; doxycycline 10 mg/kg PO q24h; minocycline 5 mg/kg PO BID; often administered with niacinamide 250 mg PO for dogs <10 kg and 500 mg PO for dogs >10 kg.

COMMENTS

- Monitor CBC, platelet count, chemistry profile, and urinalysis if immunosuppressive agents or long-term glucocorticosteroids are used.
- Infectious cases may require long-term therapy with high doses of medications.
- Sterile idiopathic nodular panniculitis often responds rapidly to high doses of corticosteroids.
- Young animals have a more rapid and complete recovery than older animals; older patients may require a maintenance protocol.

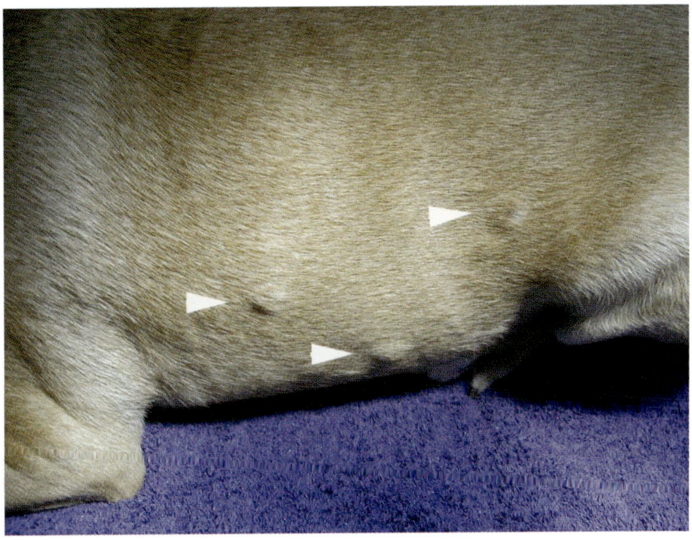

■ **Fig. 38.1.** Multiple subdermal nodules (*arrowheads*) of panniculitis in a 3-year-old female-spayed pit bull mix.

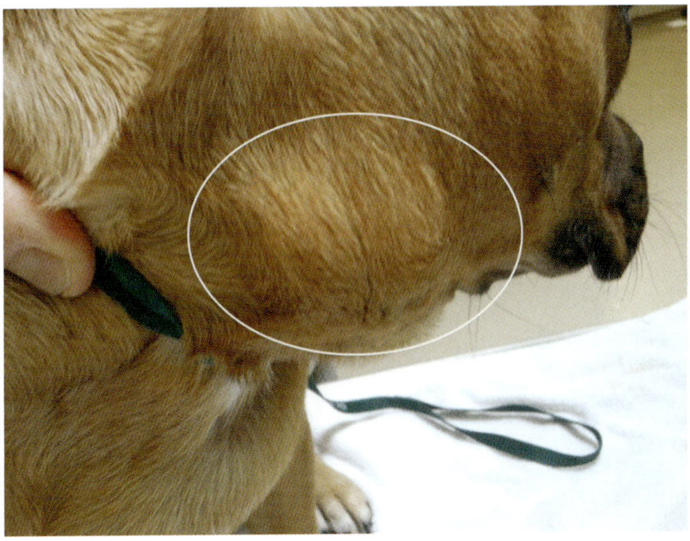

■ **Fig. 38.2.** Large submandibular mass-like panniculitis in a 4-year-old male-castrate puggle. This patient developed generalized and multiple lesions.

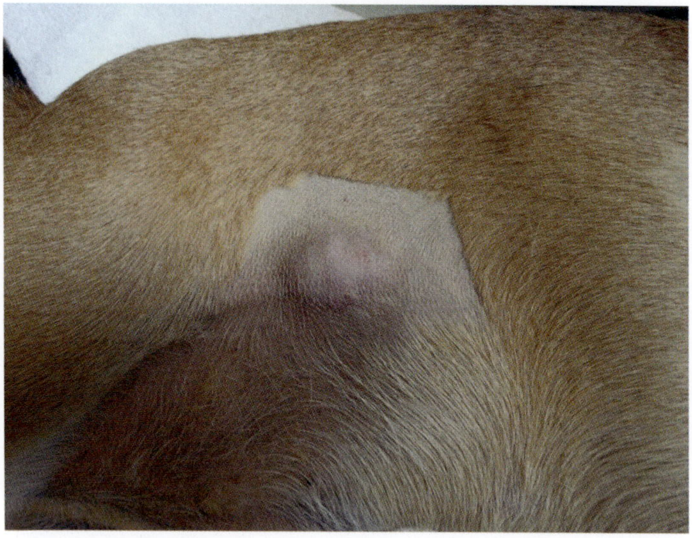

■ **Fig. 38.3.** Nodules of panniculitis may become erythematous and tender prior to rupturing, as noted in the flank region of the patient in Figure 38.2.

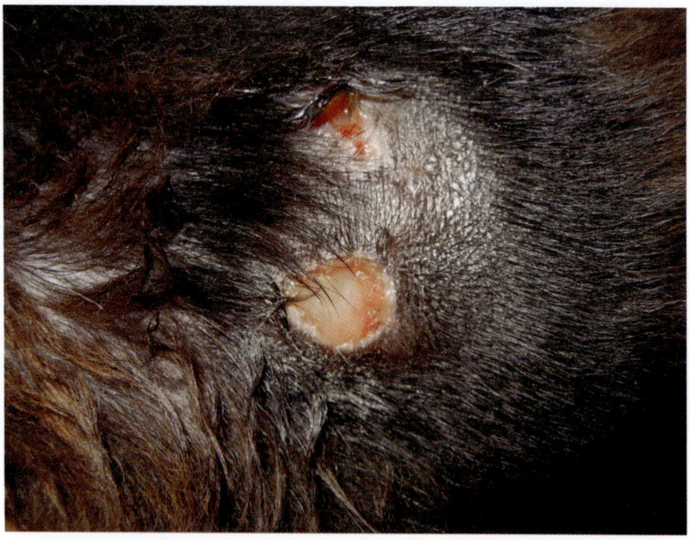

■ **Fig. 38.4.** Older lesions of panniculitis may rupture and discharge an oily exudate; lesions on a 4-year-old male-castrate Australian shepherd.

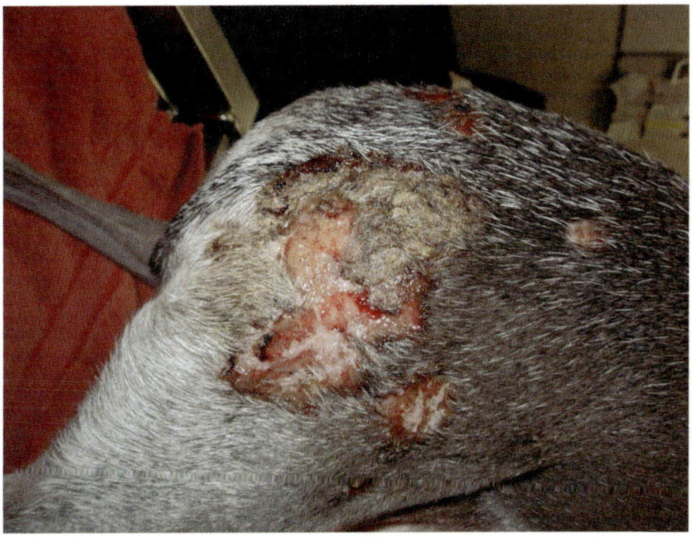

■ **Fig. 38.5.** Large exudative lesions on the lateral thighs and pelvic region of panniculitis secondary to sepsis in a 9-year-old male-castrate Italian greyhound.

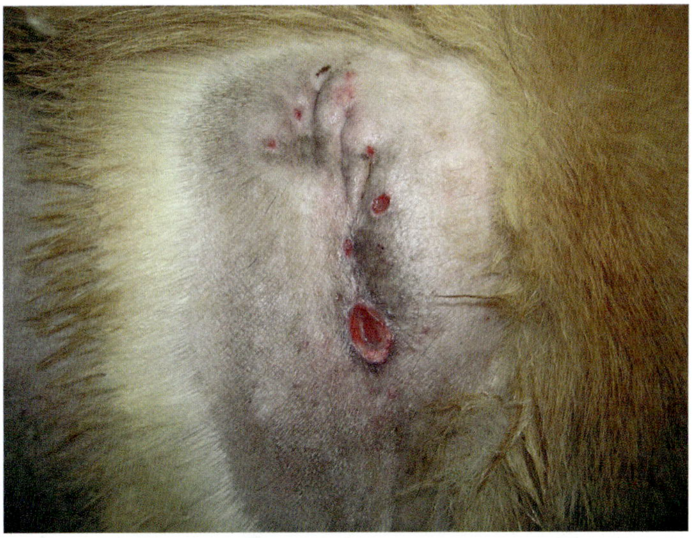

■ **Fig. 38.6.** Chronic lesions of panniculitis developing fistulae between scars on the flank of an 8-year-old female-spayed chow mix.

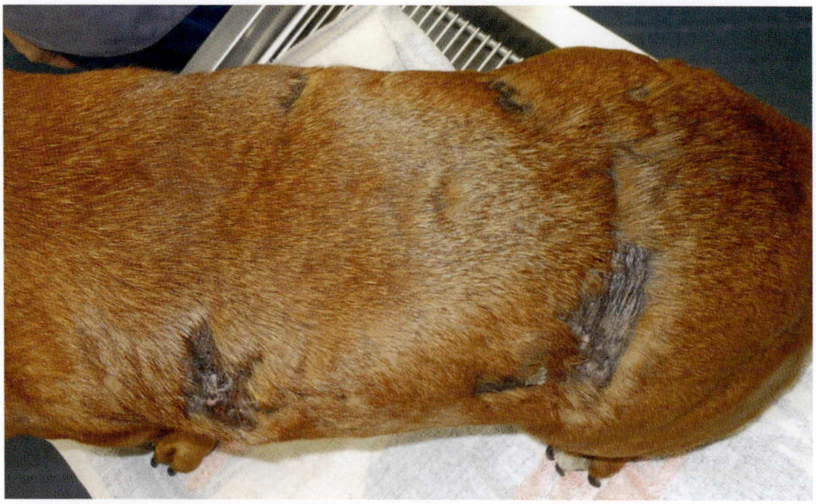

■ **Fig. 38.7.** Multiple scarred and depressed lesions of panniculitis secondary to vaccination in a 6-year-old male-castrate corgi mix.

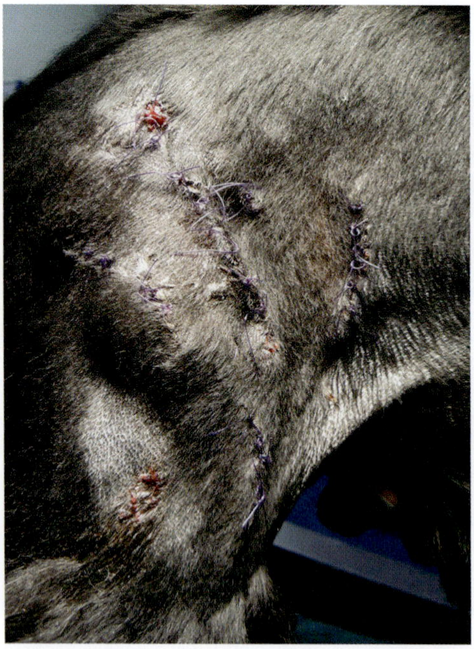

■ **Fig. 38.8.** Multiple lesions of varying size on the flanks and lateral abdomen of a 9-year-old female-spayed cocker spaniel mix. This patient underwent multiple surgical procedures to remove developing nodules (most recent evidenced by remaining sutures) prior to referral and diagnosis.

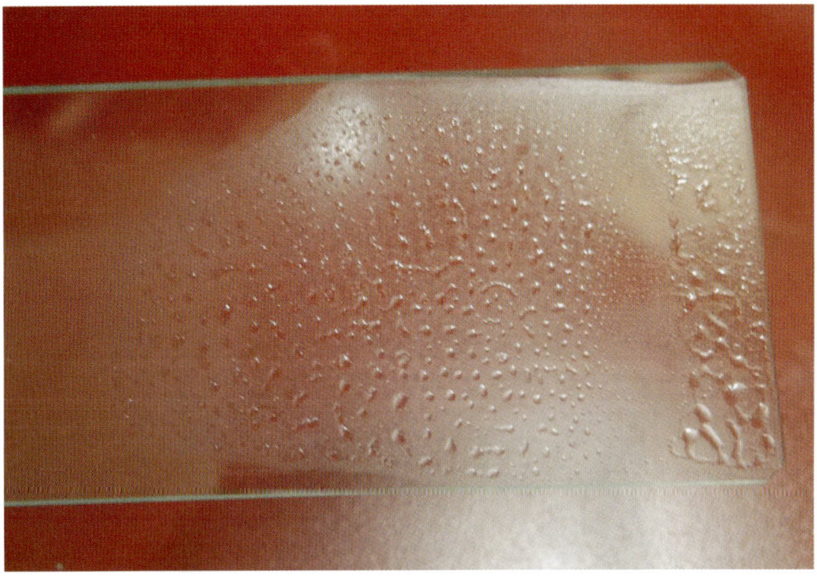

■ **Fig. 38.9.** Aspirated fluid from the patient in Figures 38.2 and 38.3 appears oily or fat-like.

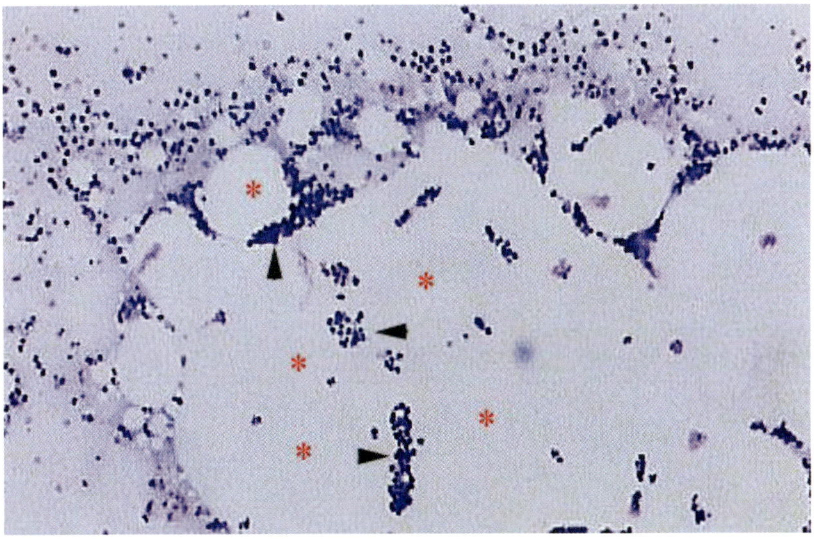

■ **Fig. 38.10.** Cytological examination of the fluid in Figure 38.9 reveals inflammatory cells within septae (*dark arrowheads*) surrounding lipocytes (*red asterisks*).

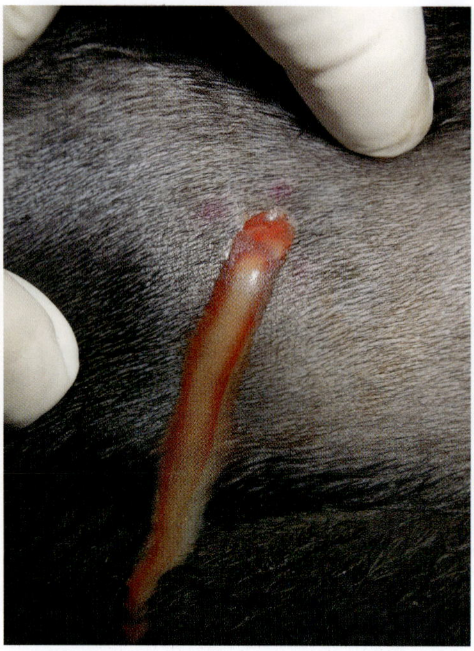

■ **Fig. 38.11.** Tissue collection using a biopsy punch from one of the nodules present in the patient of Figure 38.4 resulted in drainage of characteristic blood-tinged creamy-oily exudate of panniculitis.

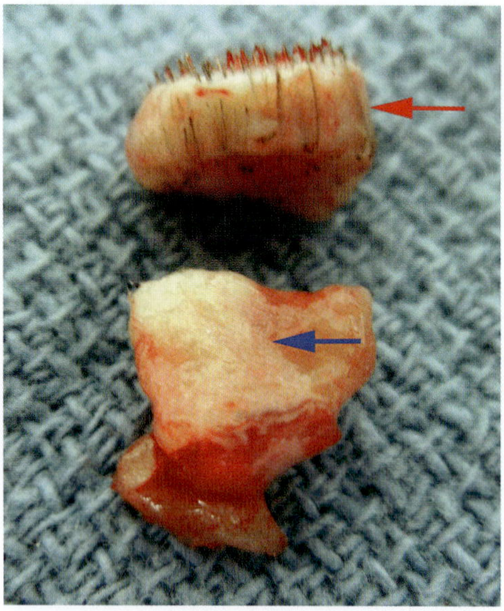

■ **Fig. 38.12.** A small nodule excised by biopsy punch and transected reveals a creamy-white accumulation of tissue within the panniculus (*blue arrow*) – beneath the epidermis and dermis (*red arrow*).

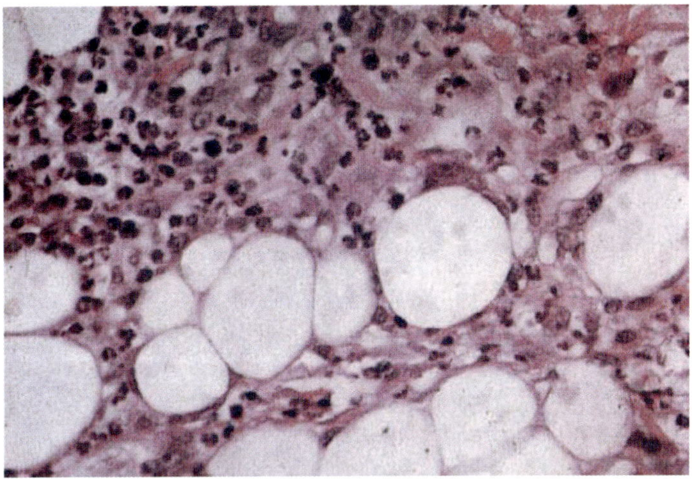

■ **Fig. 38.13.** Histopathologic example of panniculitis. Note the influx of inflammatory cells around the fat lobules.

chapter 39

Photodermatoses

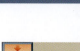

DEFINITION/OVERVIEW

- Electromagnetic radiation, primarily ultraviolet light (UVL), is absorbed by and directly damages keratinocytes, and alters the epithelial environment.
- Nonpigmented and/or glabrous areas of both dogs and cats are most affected.
- Photodermatoses include solar dermatitis, actinic keratoses (AK), actinic comedones and furunculosis, hemangioma (HA), hemangiosarcoma (HSA), and squamous cell carcinoma (SCC).

ETIOLOGY/PATHOPHYSIOLOGY

- Both UVA and UVB cause photodermatitis by:
  - Direct phototoxicity (sunburn)
  - Alteration of cell markers (seen with discoid lupus erythematosus and pemphigus erythematosus)
  - Damage by photoactive compounds (photosensitivity)
  - Cellular hyperproliferation and mutagenesis (actinic keratosis and solar-induced neoplasia).
- Natural barriers to UVL (e.g., melanin) are overcome by chronic and prolonged exposure to sunlight.
- UVL causes DNA damage directly and indirectly by free radicals; specific UVL-induced mutations have been documented in the tumor suppressor gene *p53*, leading to expansion of mutated keratinocytes.
- Patients often develop a spectrum of UVL-caused disorders concurrently, including nonneoplastic (actinic comedones and furunculosis), preneoplastic (actinic keratoses), and neoplastic (hemangioma, hemangiosarcoma, and squamous cell carcinoma).

SIGNALMENT/HISTORY

- Most affected dogs and cats are known sunbathers; dogs may preferentially expose one side when sunbathing, resulting in asymmetric lesions.

Blackwell's Five-Minute Veterinary Consult Clinical Companion: Small Animal Dermatology, Third Edition.
Karen Helton Rhodes and Alexander H. Werner.

- Lesions develop in sun-exposed, lightly pigmented or unpigmented skin (naturally or scarred) in areas not sufficiently protected by hair and in junctions between haired and nonhaired skin.
- Dogs: nasal planum, dorsal muzzle, axillae, and glabrous areas of the ventral abdomen and medial thigh.
- Cats: pinnal margins and nasal planum.
- No sex predilection.
- Age: usually older animals; reported as young as 2 years.
- Geographic distribution: higher elevations; animals housed outdoors in tropical, desert, or mountainous regions.
- Breed predilections: dalmatian, whippet, Italian greyhound, greyhound, American Staffordshire and bull terrier, beagle, German short-haired pointer, boxer, basset hound.

CLINICAL FEATURES

- Solar dermatitis (Figures 39.1–39.3):
  - Extent of damage directly related to duration and intensity of sun exposure
  - Erythema, swelling, crusting, erosion, ulceration, and exudation
  - Pruritus variable; develops more in chronic lesions
  - Vasculopathy may be underrecognized
  - Lesions may expand as adjacent skin becomes inflamed, depigmented, and alopecic
  - Severe cases develop secondary bacterial folliculitis and scarring
  - Cats: erythema, scaling, scabbing, and thickening of pinnal margins, eyelid margins, nasal planum, dorsal muzzle, lip margins; white cats; pinnal margins may curl.
- Actinic comedones and furunculosis (Figures 39.4–39.6):
  - Seen in conjunction with other chronic actinic dermatoses
  - Inflamed and dilated follicles with caseous debris result from dermal fibrosis
  - Nonfolliculocentric dermal cysts and nodules
  - Ruptured comedones and cysts lead to furunculosis (bacterial)
  - Scabbing, hemorrhage, and scarring are common sequelae
  - Large, hemorrhagic bullae develop with chronicity.
- Actinic keratoses (Figures 39.7, 39.8):
  - Actinic keratoses (AK) may represent a premalignant condition; there is a close association of and genetic similarities between AK and squamous cell carcinoma (SCC). Actinic carcinoma *in situ* denotes SCC that has not penetrated to the dermis
  - Early erythematous patches appear slightly lichenified or roughened
  - Epithelial plaques may be palpable as firm thickenings prior to becoming visible and may be distinguishable from nonthickened (normal) adjacent pigmented skin
  - Crusted, indurated, and exfoliating plaques
  - Severe hyperkeratosis may be seen as cutaneous horns

- Individual plaques and nodules (often with actinic comedones) coalesce to form larger lesions
- Affected areas become extensive; inflammation and exudation develop with secondary furunculosis
- Axillae, ventral abdomen, and medial thigh primary sites; less often dorsal muzzle and eyelid margin
- Cats: preauricular regions, as well as pinnal margins, nasal planum, and eyelid margins; lesions often traumatized, resulting in scabbing and crusting.

■ Solar-induced hemangioma (HA) and hemangiosarcoma (HAS) (Figures 39.9–39.12):
- UVL-induced HA and HSA are superficial and dermal in location; behavior differs from non-UVL-induced tumors
- HA is more common than HSA
- Early lesions may appear as erythematous or purpuric plaques (mimicking telangiectasia); vasoproliferative plaque
- Lesions may be discrete and well demarcated or poorly circumscribed, reddened, or dark-appearing nodules to masses
- Often multiple
- UVL-induced HA and HSA often associated with other forms of photodermatosis
- HA: behaviorally benign
- HSA: metastasis in fewer than 20% of superficial (solar-induced) cases.

■ Squamous cell carcinoma (SCC) (Figures 39.13–39.18):
- 80% of cases arise in association with AK
- SCC may also develop secondary to chronic inflammation or viral infection
- Most common cutaneous malignant neoplasm in cats (15–49%); second most common in dogs (3–20%)
- Single or multiple
- Initial lesions: shallow, crusted ulcerations with peripheral alopecia and erythema
- Intermediate lesions: eroded and exudative plaques; scabbed surface
- Late lesions: deep, crateriform and indurated patches or plaques
- Cutaneous horns (rare)
- Cats: external nares may be proliferative and scabbed or ulcerative; pinnal lesions often traumatized
- Locally highly invasive and destructive with significant tissue loss; neoplastic tissue may extend beyond visible boundaries
- Hemorrhage may be severe from erosion through local blood vessels
- Metastasis is rare
- Secondary bacterial infection results in pain and systemic symptoms.

DIFFERENTIAL DIAGNOSIS

■ Solar dermatitis: lupus erythematosus (discoid, cutaneous, systemic), pemphigus erythematosus, dermatomyositis, vasculitis, thermal burn, neoplasia, and bacterial folliculitis.

- Actinic comedones and furunculosis: deep bacterial, fungal, or mycobacterial furunculosis, demodicosis, schnauzer comedo syndrome, endocrinopathy, and neoplasia.
- Actinic keratoses: bacterial furunculosis, lichenoid keratosis, squamous cell carcinoma, topical drug eruption, and severe contact dermatitis.
- Hemangioma and hemangiosarcoma: bacterial furunculosis, other vascular abnormalities, and nonsolar-induced vascular neoplasia.
- Squamous cell carcinoma: other neoplasia, deep vessel thrombosis, vasculitis, sterile granulomatous disease, deep bacterial, fungal, or mycobacterial furunculosis.

DIAGNOSTICS

- Cytologic examination of aspirated samples: demonstrates infectious organisms.
- Bacterial culture and sensitivity from draining tracts (recurrent infections).
- Dermatohistopathology of representative tissues necessary to establish diagnosis:
    - Solar elastosis: replacement of collagen of the superficial dermis by basophilic fibers; characteristic of UVL damage; may be associated with laminar fibrosis
    - Solar dermatitis: decreased melanocytes, epidermal hyperplasia, intraepidermal edema, apoptotic keratinocytes, thickening or obscuring of the dermal-epidermal junction, vascular dilation, and solar elastosis
    - Actinic comedones and furunculosis: epidermal hyperplasia, plugging of follicular ostea and intrafollicular accumulation of keratin debris, perifollicular fibrosis, solar elastosis; ruptured comedones produce furunculosis with accompanying dermal inflammation and infiltration with neutrophils (similar to bacterial furunculosis); should be associated with other photodermatoses
    - Actinic keratoses: epidermal hyperplasia and dysplasia with severe hyperkeratosis and/or "stacked" parakeratosis; keratinocytes appear distorted and/or apoptotic; perivascular to lichenoid dermal infiltrate with solar elastosis and fibrosis; absence of invasion through the dermal-epidermal junction
    - Hemangioma: blood-filled vascular ectasia lined by endothelial cells; endothelial cells may show varying degrees of atypia representing a continuum from HA to HSA; less well circumscribed than non-UVL-induced HA; associated with dermal solar elastosis and fibrosis
    - Hemangiosarcoma: invasive vascular ectasia not uniformly confined by endothelial cells; endothelial cells demonstrate marked cellular and nuclear pleomorphism and mitotic activity; associated with dermal solar elastosis and fibrosis
    - Squamous cell carcinoma: trabeculae of squamous cells invade into the dermis; neoplastic cell aggregates; keratin pearls (accumulations of compact keratin); keratinocyte cellular and nuclear pleomorphism; mitotic activity higher in dogs than cats; associated with dermal solar elastosis and fibrosis.

THERAPEUTICS

- Avoid exposure to UVL by keeping patients indoors and by applying sunblock.
- Use protective clothing.

- Individual tumors should be surgically excised; large areas may require extensive procedures.
- Vitamin E 200 mg BID less than 10 kg body weight; 400 mg BID greater than 10 kg body weight; vitamin C 500 mg BID; beta-carotene 30 mg BID to q24h; vitamin A 400 IU/kg q24h; may have a protective effect.
- Topical corticosteroids may reduce localized areas of inflammation.
- Firocoxib 5 mg/kg PO q24h; overexpression of cyclooxygenase (COX-2) documented in actinic keratoses in humans and dogs; improvement noted with use of COX-2 selective inhibitor.
- Prednisolone 0.5 mg/kg PO q24h then tapered dosage: reduces significant inflammation.
- Cephalexin 22 mg/kg PO BID: secondary bacterial furunculosis; alternative antibiotics selected by culture and sensitivity testing results.
- Tretinoin 0.1%: apply daily to individual lesions for 14 days; then 2–3 times weekly; may cause irritation.
- Isotretinoin 1 mg/kg PO q24h for 30 days; then alternate days or as needed to control lesions.

COMMENTS

- Routinely screen for the development of suspicious lesions; remove individual tumors as soon as identified.
- Prognosis is fair to guarded in cases with extensive disease.
- Patients with severe disease may have affected areas reduced in size with medications to permit more effective surgical intervention.
- Euthanasia is due to secondary complications of open lesions and neoplasia, not due to metastasis.
- Isotretinoin: oral synthetic retinoids have become difficult to dispense due to very strict prescription procedures; may cause keratoconjunctivitis sicca; extreme teratogen; do not use in intact females because of severe and predictable teratogenicity and the extremely long withdrawal period; women of child-bearing age should not handle this medication; monitor serum chemistries including triglycerides, and tear production.

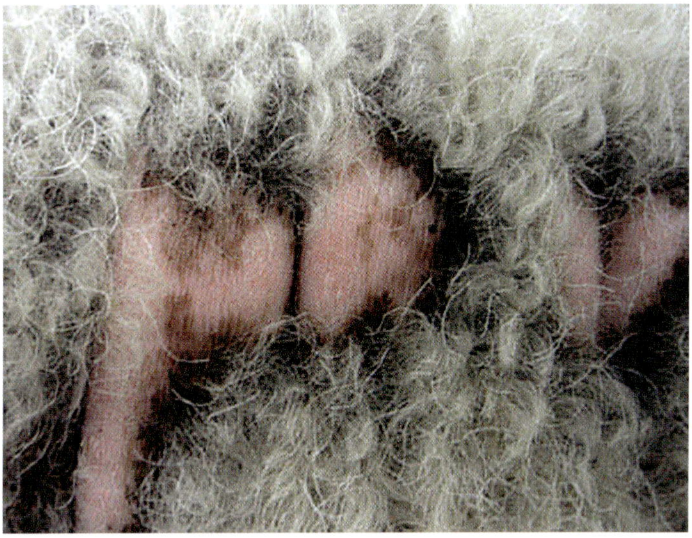

■ **Fig. 39.1.** Scarred and depigmented plaques of chronic solar dermatitis.

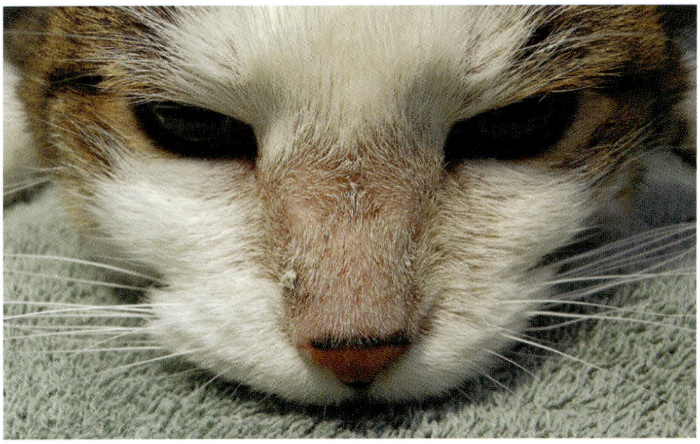

■ **Fig. 39.2.** Feline solar dermatitis. Note erythema and crusting on the dorsal muzzle and nasal planum.

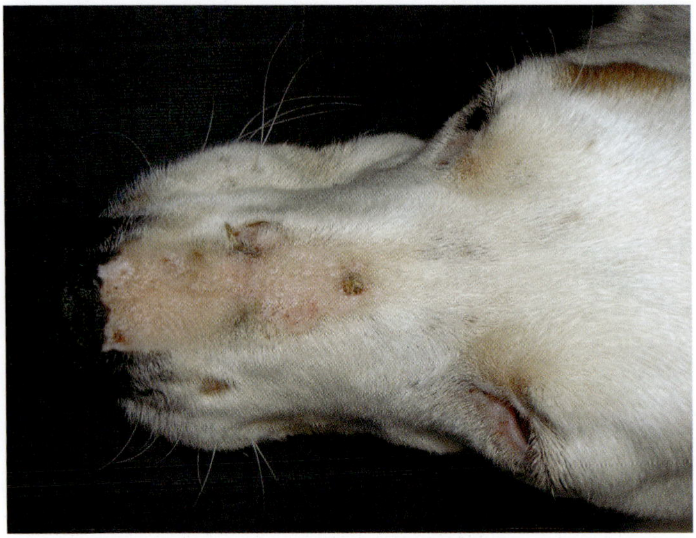

■ **Fig. 39.3.** Canine solar dermatitis. Similar lesions as for the cat in Figure 39.2. Note additional lesions on the nonpigmented margins of the eyelids.

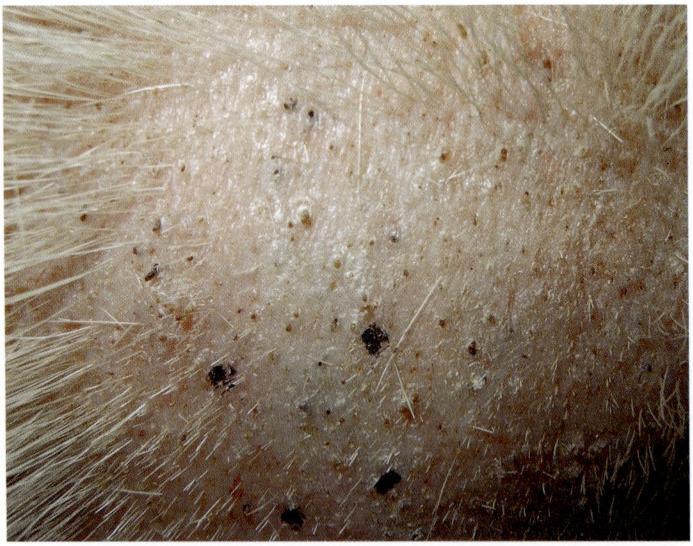

■ **Fig. 39.4.** Actinic comedones seen as inflamed and dilated, debris-filled follicles.

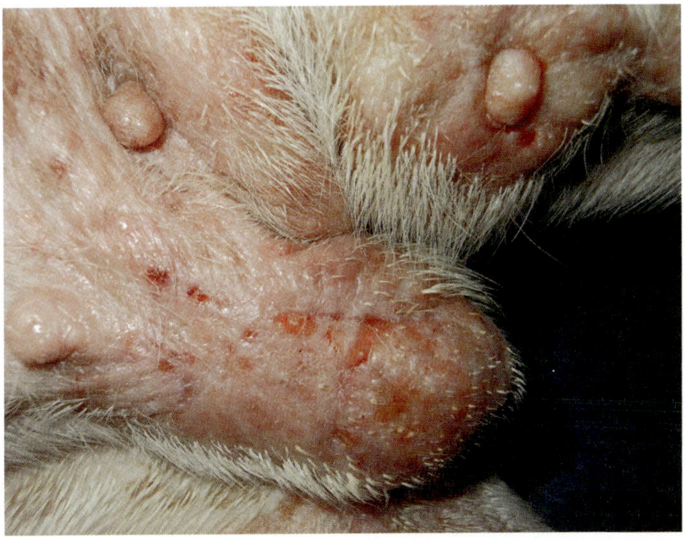

■ **Fig. 39.5.** Exudative and thickened skin associated with actinic comedones and furunculosis on the prepuce and ventrum. This 10-year-old male-castrate pit bull also has sun-induced squamous cell carcinoma.

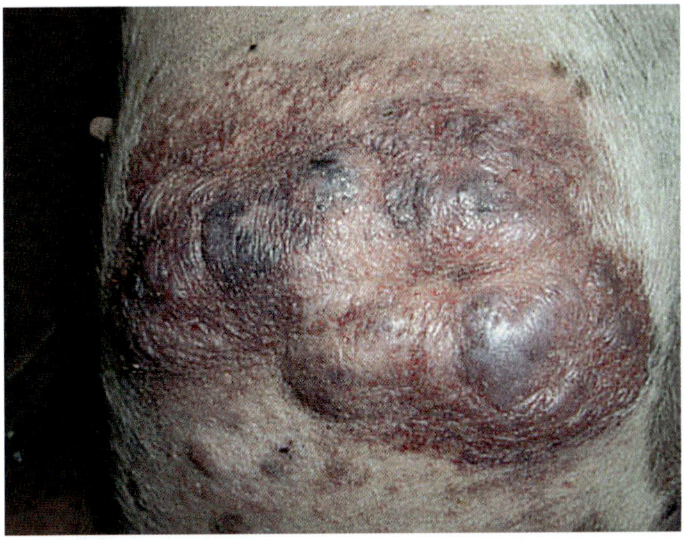

■ **Fig. 39.6.** Ruptured actinic comedones leading to furuncles and bullae.

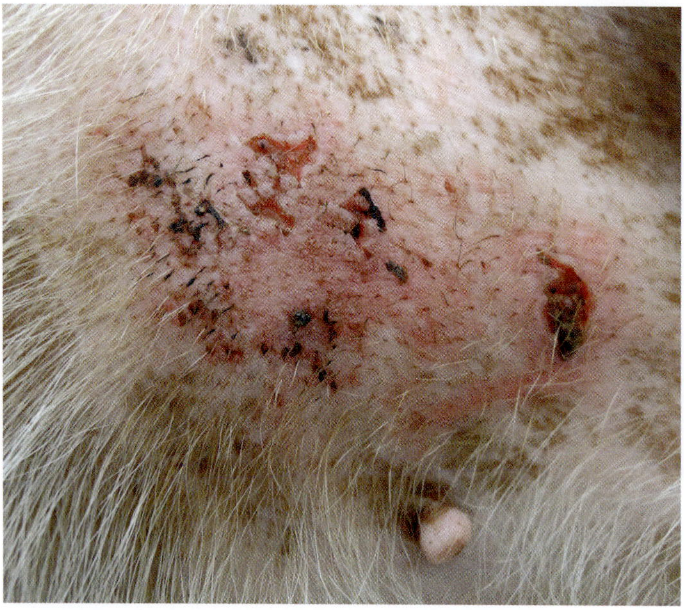

Fig. 39.7. Actinic keratoses with crusted, indurated, and exfoliating plaques on the ventrum of a 9-year-old pointer mix.

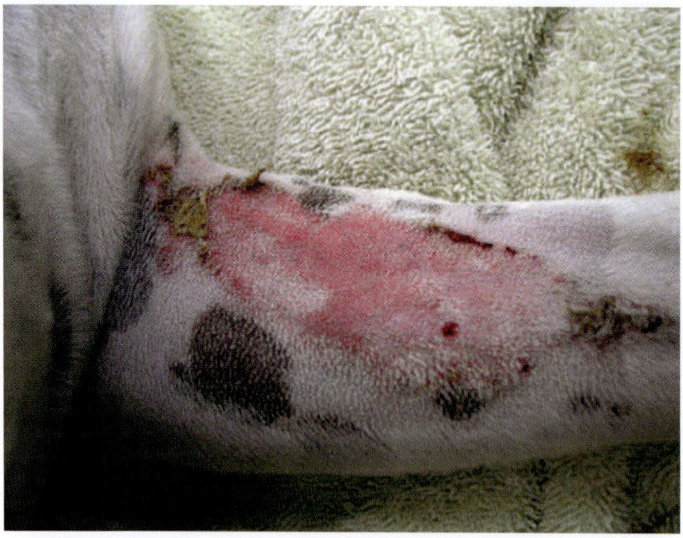

Fig. 39.8. Actinic keratoses on the medial aspect of the foreleg in a dalmatian.

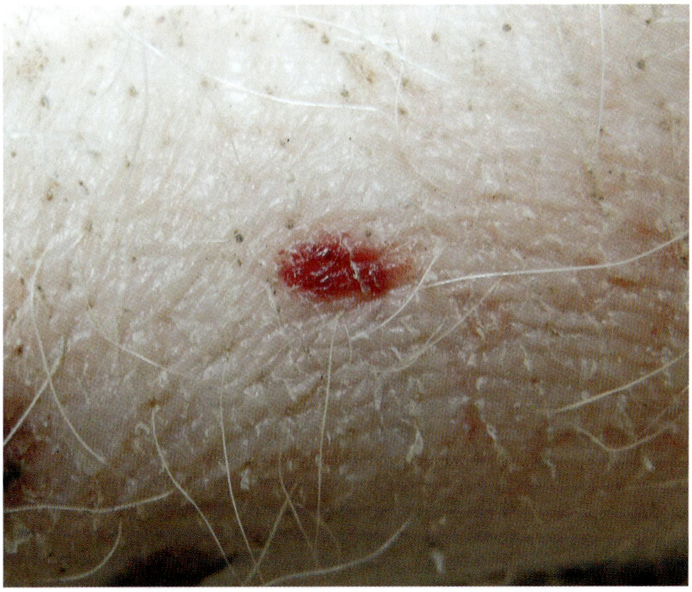

Fig. 39.9. Vasoproliferative plaque – this lesion may be a precursor to HA or HSA.

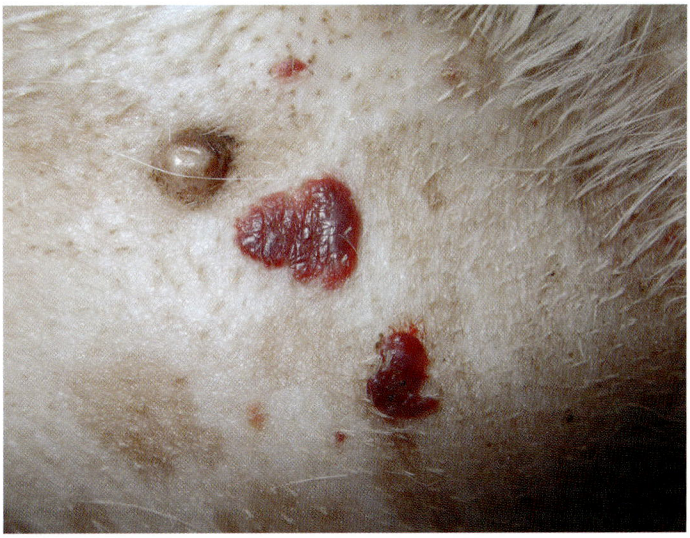

Fig. 39.10. Multiple sun-induced hemangiomas seen as purpuric plaques on the ventrum.

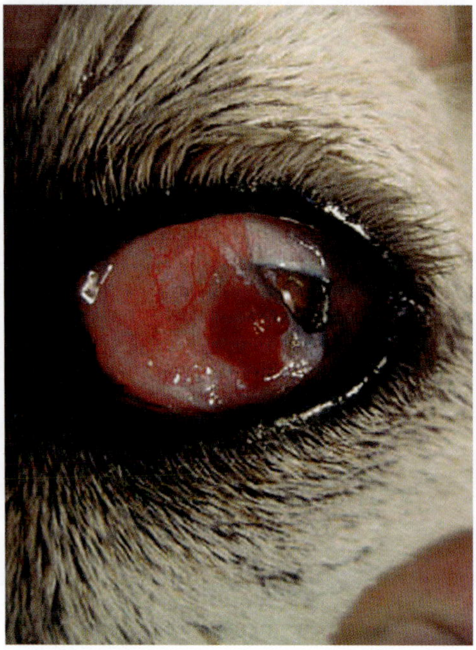

■ **Fig. 39.11.** Solar-induced hemangiosarcoma on the nictitans of an adult female-spayed basset hound.

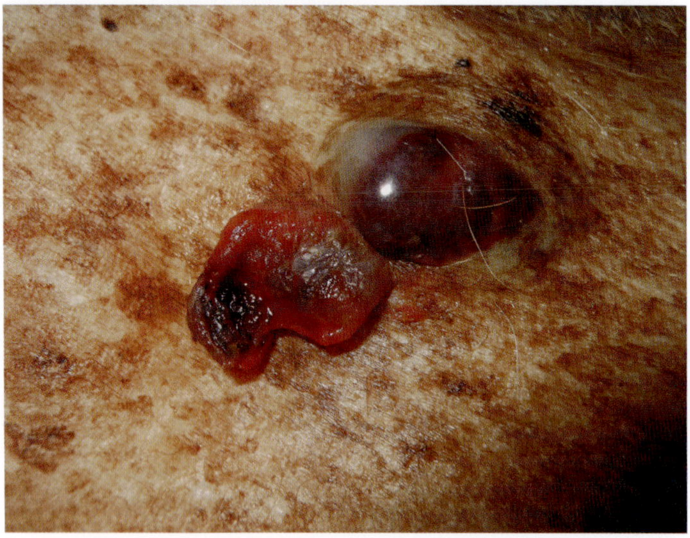

■ **Fig. 39.12.** Eroded and non-eroded HSAs on the flank seen as well-demarcated reddened and/or blood-filled nodules.

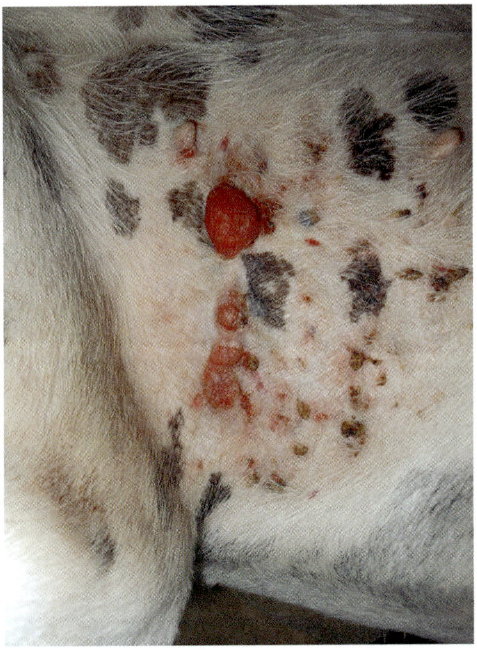

■ **Fig. 39.13.** Multiple eroded and noneroded plaques of squamous cell carcinoma associated with AKs.

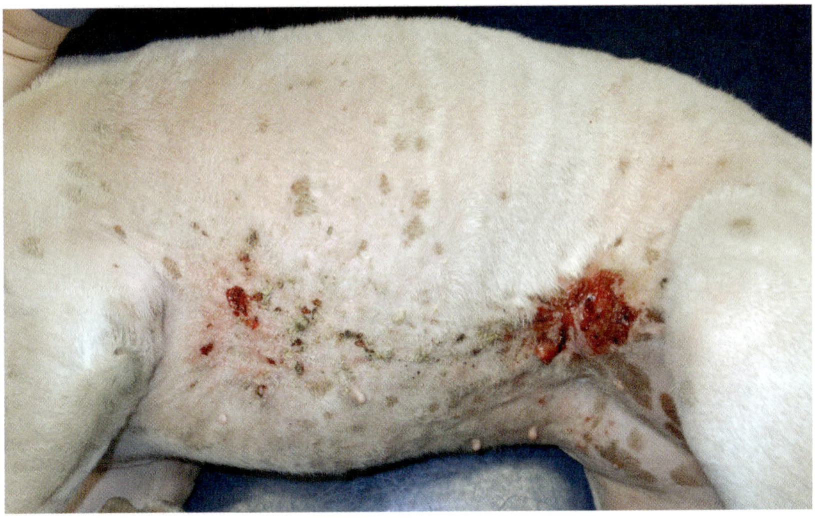

■ **Fig. 39.14.** Actinic keratoses and squamous cell on the left lateral aspect of the body from axilla to flank in a 9-year-old female-spayed pit bull.

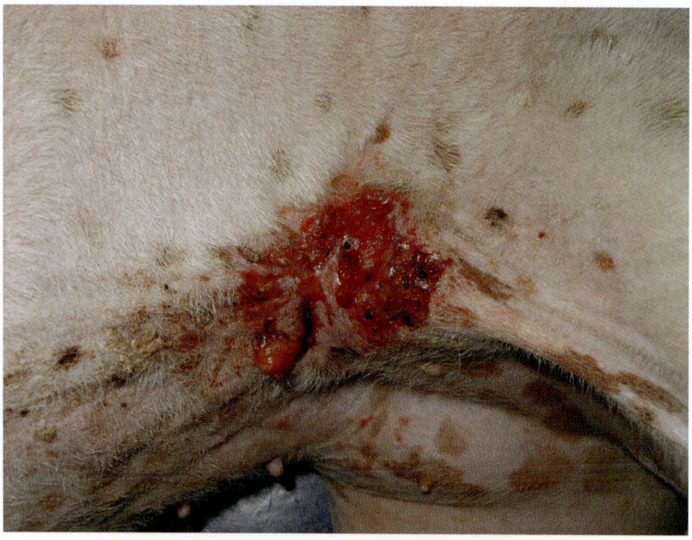

■ **Fig. 39.15.** Additional image of the patient in Figure 39.14. Large exudative squamous cell carcinoma in the flank fold restricting movement.

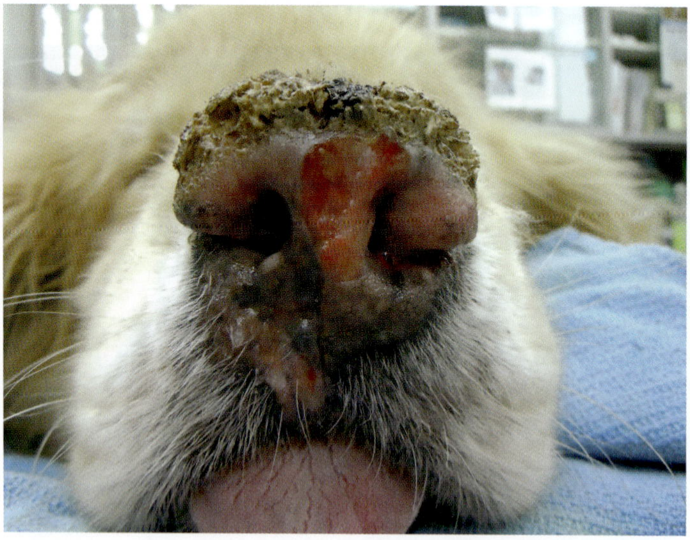

■ **Fig. 39.16.** Squamous cell carcinoma on the nasal planum of an adult golden retriever.

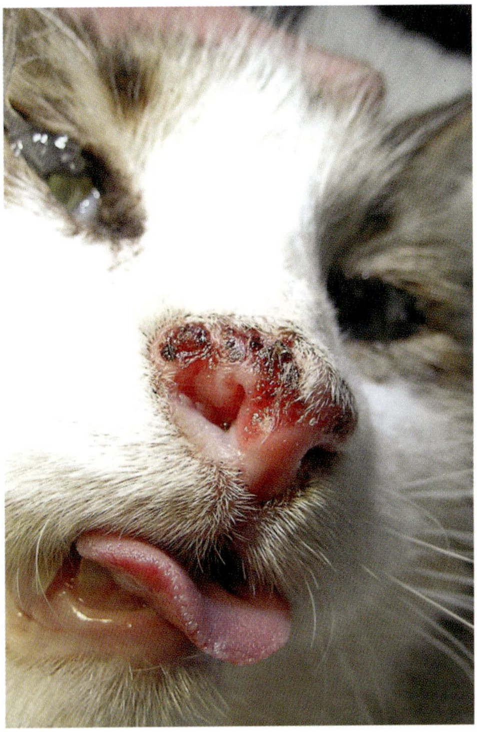

■ **Fig. 39.17.** Squamous cell carcinoma in a DSH. Note punctate scabs on the external nares and philtrum.

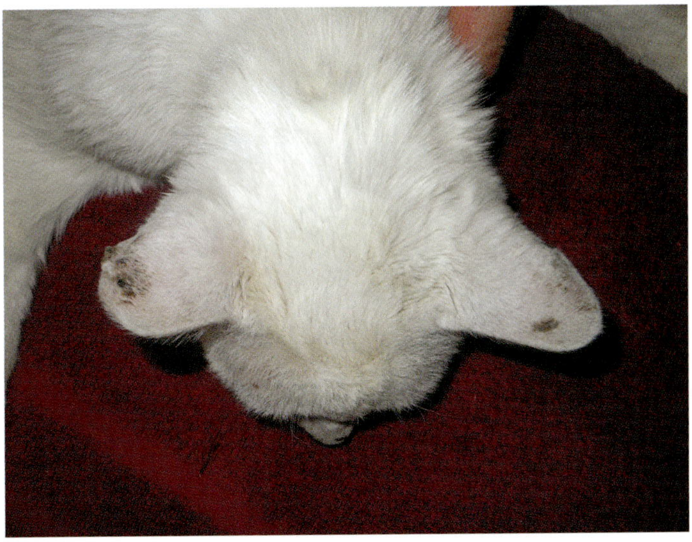

■ **Fig. 39.18.** Erythema, thickening, and scabbing on the pinnal margins of a white 13-year-old male-castrate DSH with solar dermatitis, actinic keratoses, and squamous cell carcinoma.

chapter 40

Pododermatitis and Claw Disorders

DEFINITION/OVERVIEW

Pododermatitis: descriptive term for dermatoses affecting the pedal region; not a final diagnosis.

Claw Anatomy

- Ungual fold: crescent-shaped tissue that surrounds the proximal claw.
- Coronary band and dorsal ridge (dorsal surface of the ungual crest): produce most of the claw; contribute to curvature of the claw.

Claw Terminology

- Onychopathy: disease of claws.
- Paronychia: inflammation of soft tissue around the claw.
- Pachyonychia: thickening of the claw.
- Onychitis: inflammation of the claw (all inclusive).
- Pyonychia: purulent exudates from the claw.
- Onychomycosis: fungal infection of the claw.
- Onychorrhexis: brittle claws that tend to split or break.
- Onychoschizia: splitting and/or lamination of the claw, usually beginning distally.
- Onychomadesis: sloughing of the claws.
- Onychodystrophy: deformity caused by abnormal growth.
- Onychomalacia: softening of the claws.
- Onychoclasis: breaking of the claw.
- Onychocryptosis: ingrown claw.
- Anonychia: absence of claws.
- Brachyonychia: shortened claws.
- Leukonychia: claw whitening.
- Macronychia: unusually large claws.
- Micronychia: unusually small claws.
- Onychalgia: claw pain.
- Onychatrophia: atrophy of claws.
- Onychauxis: hypertrophy of claws.

Blackwell's Five-Minute Veterinary Consult Clinical Companion: Small Animal Dermatology, Third Edition.
Karen Helton Rhodes and Alexander H. Werner.

- Onychogryphosis: abnormal curvature of the claw.
- Onycholysis: separation of claw at proximal attachment.

ETIOLOGY/PATHOPHYSIOLOGY

- Claw, claw/ungual folds, footpads: subject to trauma, infection, vascular insufficiency, immune-mediated disease, parasites, neoplasia, defects in keratinization, and congenital abnormalities.
- A particular claw deformity may be caused by a variety of diseases; claw disease is most often associated with other dermatoses – rarely the only epithelial structure affected.
- A single disease can present with various claw lesions.
- Pododermatitis is a multifaceted disease complex.
- One foot affected: top differentials include foreign body, neoplasia, trauma, fungal infection, bacterial infection.
- Multiple feet affected: allergy, endocrine, secondary infections, demodicosis, immune-mediated disorders, epidermolysis bullosa, symmetric lupoid onychodystrophy, plasma cell pododermatitis, superficial necrolytic dermatitis, nutritional deficiencies, psychogenic dermatoses, idiopathic.

SIGNALMENT/HISTORY

- Claw and claw fold diseases: 1.3% dogs and 2.2% cats.
- Collie and Shetland sheepdog: dermatomyositis (Figure 40.1).
- Dachshund: onychorrhexis (Figures 40.2, 40.3).
- German shepherd dog, rottweiler, giant schnauzer and doberman pinscher: symmetric lupoid onychodystrophy (Figures 40.4–40.6).
- Siberian husky, dachshund, Rhodesian ridgeback, rottweiler, cocker spaniel: idiopathic onychodystrophy; keratinization defects.
- Bull terrier: acrodermatitis, footpad hyperkeratosis.
- Irish terrier, French mastiff, Kerry blue terrier, Labrador retriever, golden retriever: familial footpad hyperkeratosis.
- English bulldog, Great Dane, dachshund: idiopathic sterile granuloma (Figures 40.7, 40.8).
- German shepherd dog, whippet, English springer spaniel: idiopathic onychomadesis.
- Devon rex cats: *Malassezia* paronychia.
- German shepherd dog: nodular dermatofibroma.
- Gordon setter: genetic predisposition for symmetric lupoid onychitis.

Risk Factors

- Claw and claw fold are carrier sites for *Malassezia pachydermatis* and *Bartonella henselae*.

- Clipping too closely can lead to embedded debris and secondary infections, including onychomadesis; trauma to P3 may cause onychodystrophy (Figure 40.9).
- Paronychia (infectious): immunosuppression (endogenous or exogenous), FeLV or FIV infection (may be associated with plasma cell pododermatitis), trauma, and diabetes mellitus.
- Dogs that dig or hunting dogs.
- Dogs with conformational disorders and obesity are at risk due to abnormal weight distribution and increased friction.
- Concurrent diseases increase risk: allergy, immune-mediated diseases, keratinization disorders, parasites (e.g., *Demodex*, *Leishmania*, hookworms), metabolic disease (hepatocutaneous syndrome), neoplasia (epitheliotropic lymphoma, metastatic bronchogenic adenocarcinoma, squamous cell carcinoma, keratoacanthoma, inverted papilloma, melanoma, mast cell tumor) (Figures 40.10–40.12).

CLINICAL FEATURES

- Licking at the feet and/or claw/ungual folds; nail biting.
- Lameness.
- Pain.
- Pruritus.
- Swelling, erythema, or exudate within the claw.
- Swelling, erythema, or exudate affecting the ungual fold.
- Swelling, erythema, or exudate affecting the interdigital region.
- Swelling, or erythema affecting the footpad.
- Hyperkeratosis, crusting, or ulceration of the ungual fold.
- Hyperkeratosis, crusting, or ulceration of the footpad.
- Deformity or sloughing of claw.
- Deformity or sloughing of the footpad.
- Discoloration of the claw (red-brown discoloration associated with *Malassezia*).
- Hemorrhage from the claw or following the loss of a claw.
- Previous description of being "tender-footed."
- Malodor.

Paronychia

- Infection: bacteria, dermatophyte, yeast, viral (*Candida, Malassezia*) (Figures 40.13–40.15).
- Parasites: *Demodex*, *Leishmania*.
- Immune mediated: pemphigus, bullous pemphigoid, lupus erythematosus, drug eruption, symmetric lupoid onychodystrophy (Figures 40.16, 40.17).
- Neoplasia: subungual squamous cell carcinoma, melanoma, eccrine carcinoma, osteosarcoma, subungual keratoacanthoma, inverted squamous papilloma (Figures 40.18–40.20).
- Arteriovenous fistula.

Onychomycosis

- Dogs: *Trichophyton mentagrophytes* – usually generalized (Figure 40.21).
- Cats: *Microsporum canis*.

Onychorrhexis

- Idiopathic: especially in dachshunds; multiple nails.
- Trauma.
- Infection: dermatophytosis.
- Parasites: *Leishmania*.

Onychomadesis

- Trauma.
- Infection.
- Immune mediated: pemphigus, bullous pemphigoid, lupus erythematosus, drug eruption, symmetric lupoid onychodystrophy.
- Vascular insufficiency: vasculitis, cold agglutinin disease.
- Neoplasia: subungual squamous cell carcinoma, melanoma, eccrine carcinoma, osteosarcoma, subungual keratoacanthoma, inverted squamous papilloma (Figure 40.22).
- Idiopathic.

Claw Dystrophy

- Acromegaly.
- Feline hyperthyroidism.
- Zinc-responsive dermatosis.
- Congenital malformations.

DIFFERENTIAL DIAGNOSIS

- Classification based on clinical presentation.
- Interdigital erythema with pruritus:
    - Atopic dermatitis
    - Food hypersensitivity
    - Demodicosis
    - Bacterial overgrowth.
- Nonpruritic alopecia of the foot:
    - Demodicosis
    - Bacterial overgrowth
    - Dermatophytosis (Figure 40.23)
    - Ischemic folliculopathy (dermatomyositis, postvaccination).

- Crusted/hyperkeratotic/fissured footpads:
  - Pemphigus foliaceus (Figures 40.24–40.26)
  - Zinc-responsive dermatosis
  - Superficial necrolytic dermatitis (hepatocutaneous syndrome) (Figure 40.27)
  - Erythema multiforme (Figure 40.28)
  - Feline paraneoplastic pancreatic adenocarcinoma
  - Feline thymoma-associated exfoliative dermatitis (Figure 40.29)
  - Idiopathic/hereditary hyperkeratosis (Figure 40.30)
  - Dermatophytosis
  - Drug eruption
  - Feline plasma cell pododermatitis (Figure 40.31)
  - Eosinophilic granuloma complex (Figure 40.32)
  - Viral (distemper).
- Sloughing/ulcerative footpads:
  - Trauma (Figures 40.33, 40.34)
  - Epitheliotropic lymphoma (Figure 40.35)
  - Ischemic vasculopathy
  - Erythema multiforme
  - Drug eruption
  - Feline plasma cell pododermatitis.
- Nodular disorders of the foot:
  - Sterile granuloma syndrome
  - Pyoderma
  - Demodicosis
  - Dermatophytosis (kerion)
  - Nodular dermatofibroma in German shepherd dogs
  - Calcinosis cutis/circumscripta (Figure 40.36)
  - Xanthomatosis (Figure 40.37)
  - Neoplasia (Figures 40.38–40.40).
- Asymmetrical claw disorders:
  - Bacterial paronychia/pyonychia
  - Onychomycosis
  - Trauma: physical, chemical, pedicure
  - Ungual polyp (see Figure 40.19)
  - Arteriovenous fistula (postsurgical declaw or trauma)
  - Neoplasia: squamous cell carcinoma, melanoma, mast cell tumor, metastatic bronchogenic adenocarcinoma, keratoacanthoma.
- Symmetrical claw disorders:
  - Bacterial infection
  - Metabolic disease
  - Symmetric lupoid onchodystrophy
  - Autoimmune disorders (especially pemphigus foliaceus in the cat)
  - Keratinization disorders
  - Viral diseases
  - Leishmaniasis

  - Severe ascarid infestation, hookworms
  - Nutritional deficiencies (zinc)
  - Toxins (thallium)
  - Idiopathic (breed-related and senile changes).

DIAGNOSTICS

- Antinuclear antibody (ANA): systemic lupus erythematosus.
- Complete blood count and urinalysis.
- Serum chemistry to evaluate for diabetes mellitus, thyroid function, liver function, other systemic illness.
- FeLV and FIV antibody titers.
- Radiographs: osteomyelitis of third phalanx, neoplastic change.
- Biopsy: often involves a third phalanx amputation; inclusion of the coronary band required for diagnosis of most diseases.
- Cytology of exudate from the nail and/or fold.
- Peripheral lymph node aspirates of affected limbs.
- Skin scraping.
- Bacterial and/or fungal culture.
- Fecal examination.
- Limited allergen diet trial.
- Intradermal allergy testing/serologic allergy testing.
- Ultrasonography: renal or uterine tumors with dermatofibroma; cystic with renal adenoma/adenocarcinoma syndrome.

THERAPEUTICS

- Paronychia:
  - Surgical removal of nail plate (shell)
  - Antimicrobial soaks
  - Identify underlying condition and treat specifically.
- Onychomycosis:
  - Antifungal soaks: chlorhexidine, povidone-iodine, lime sulfur
  - Surgical removal of nail plate: may improve response to systemic medication
  - Amputation of third phalanx.
- Onychorrhexis:
  - Repair with fingernail glue (the type used to attach false nails in humans)
  - Remove splintered pieces
  - Amputate third phalanx
  - Treat underlying cause.
- Onychomadesis:
  - Antimicrobial soaks
  - Treat underlying cause.
- Neoplasia:
  - Determined by biologic behavior of specific tumor

    - Surgical excision
    - Amputation of digit or leg
    - Chemotherapy and/or radiation therapy.
- Nail dystrophy:
    - Treat underlying cause.

Drugs of Choice

- Bacterial paronychia: systemic antibiotics based on culture and sensitivity.
- Yeast (*Candida* or *Malassezia*) paronychia: ketoconazole 5–10 mg/kg PO BID to q24h (dogs) or fluconazole 5 mg/kg PO BID (dogs and cats) for 2–4 weeks; topical nystatin, miconazole, terbinafine.
- Onychomycosis: ketoconazole 5–10 mg/kg PO BID for 6–12 months until negative cultures; itraconazole 5–10 mg/kg PO q24h for 3 weeks and then pulse therapy twice a week until resolved.
- Onychomadesis: determined by cause; immunomodulation therapy for immune-mediated diseases; medication options include essential fatty acid supplementation; cycline antibiotics: tetracycline 250 mg PO TID for dogs <10 kg; 500 mg PO TID dogs >10 kg); doxycycline 10 mg/kg PO q24h; minocycline 5 mg/kg PO BID; often administered with niacinamide 250 mg PO for dogs <10 kg and 500 mg PO for dogs >10 kg; pentoxifylline 10–15 mg/kg PO BID to TID; corticosteroids, and cyclosporine 5 mg/kg PO q24h; vitamin E; appropriate chemotherapeutic agents (e.g., azathioprine, chlorambucil).
- Symmetric lupoid onychodystrophy; options include essential fatty acid supplementation; cycline antibiotics: tetracycline 250 mg PO TID for dogs <10 kg; 500 mg PO TID dogs >10 kg; doxycycline 10 mg/kg PO q24h; minocycline 5 mg/kg PO BID; often administered with niacinamide 250 mg PO for dogs <10 kg and 500 mg PO for dogs >10 kg; pentoxifylline 10–15 mg/kg PO BID to TID; corticosteroids, and cyclosporine 5 mg/kg PO q24h.

COMMENTS

Expected Course and Prognosis

- Slow claw growth cycle may require 6–8 months of therapy to fully correct an abnormality; improvement may be noted after 6–8 weeks of appropriate treatment.
- Bacterial or yeast paronychia and onychomycosis: treatment may be prolonged and response may be influenced by underlying factors.
- Onychorrhexis: may require amputation of the third phalanx for resolution.
- Onychomadesis: prognosis determined by underlying cause; immune-mediated diseases and vascular problems carry a more guarded prognosis than do trauma or infectious causes.
- Nail dystrophy: prognosis is good when underlying cause can be controlled.
- Neoplasia: excised by amputation of the digit; malignant tumors may have metastasized by the time of diagnosis.

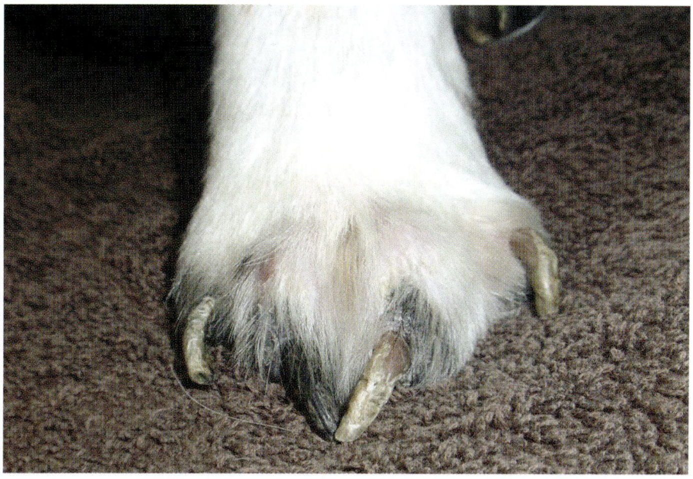

■ **Fig. 40.1.** Onychodystrophy with misshapen and flaking layers of the claws secondary to dermatomyositis.

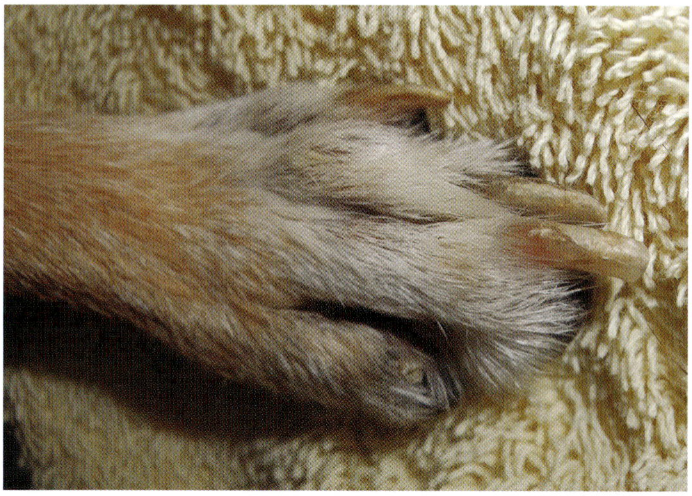

■ **Fig. 40.2.** Onychorrhexis with onychomadesis affecting multiple claws in a 6-year-old female-spayed dachshund mix.

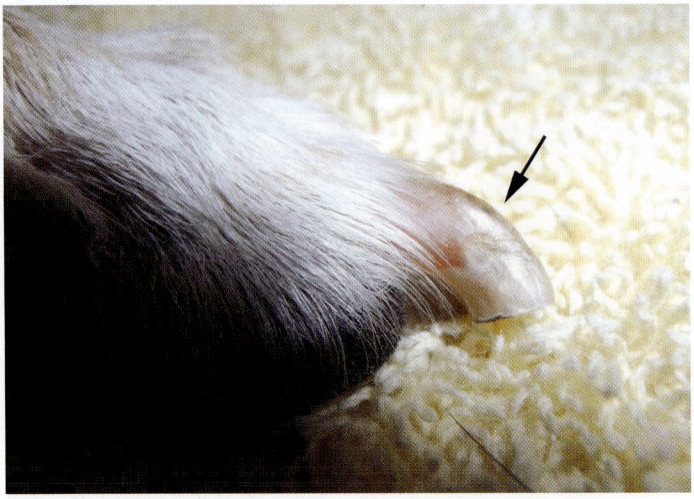

■ **Fig. 40.3.** Additional image of the patient in Figure 40.2 demonstrating horizontal fracturing of the dorsal aspect of a claw (*arrow*) due to onychorrhexis.

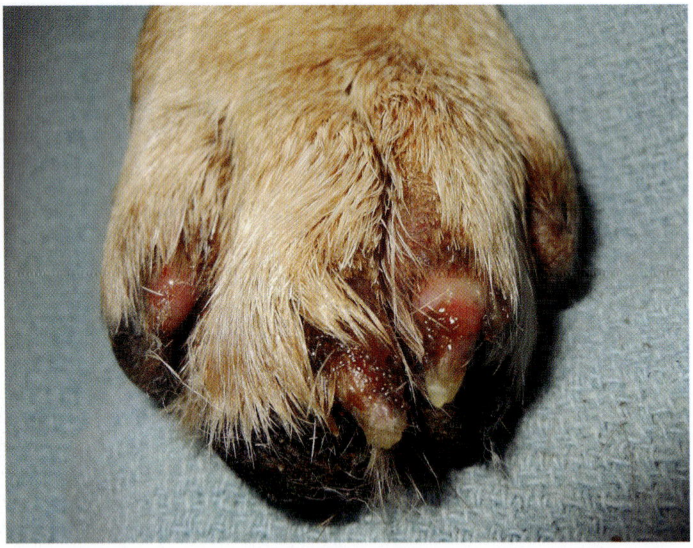

■ **Fig. 40.4.** Onycholysis leading to onychomadesis and paronychia with hemorrhagic to purulent exudation in a 10-year-old male-castrate puggle with symmetric lupoid onychodystrophy.

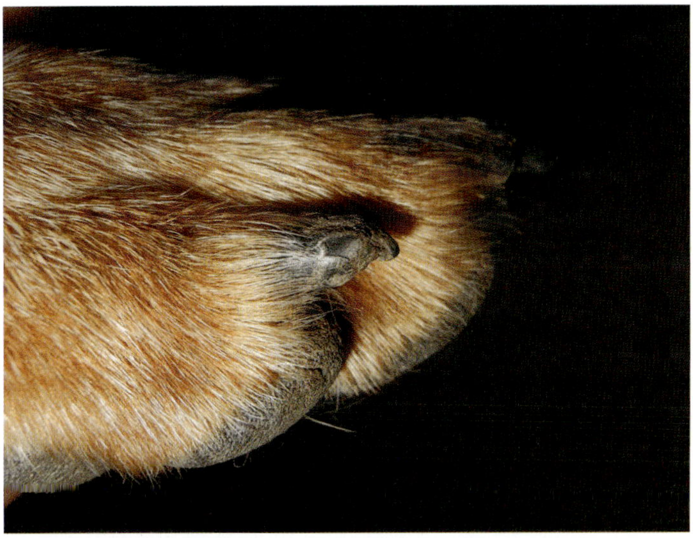

■ **Fig. 40.5.** Symmetric lupoid onychodystrophy in a 6-year-old female-spayed German shepherd. Following onychomadesis, regrowth resulted in brittle, misshapen, and shortened claws.

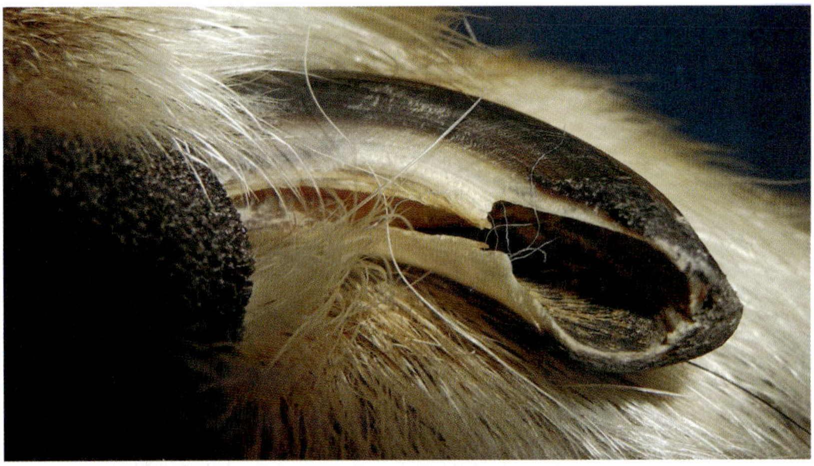

■ **Fig. 40.6.** Symmetric lupoid onychodystrophy in an 11-year-old male-castrate German shepherd. Onycholysis has caused separation of the claw proximally from the coronary band and lateral and medial walls, resulting in a hollowed-out appearance to the claw prior to sloughing.

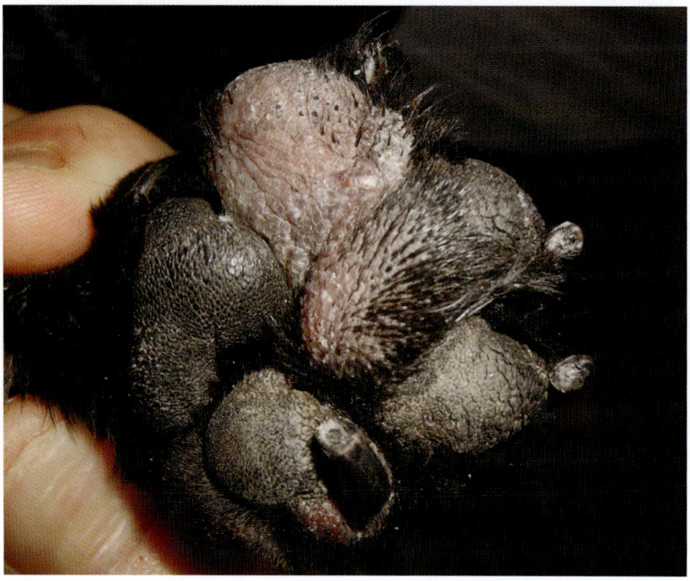

■ **Fig. 40.7.** Erythematous thickening of interdigital tissue on the palmar surface of a 4-year-old female-spayed dachshund with idiopathic sterile granuloma. Resulting unprotected (nonfootpad) tissue contact with the ground causes lameness.

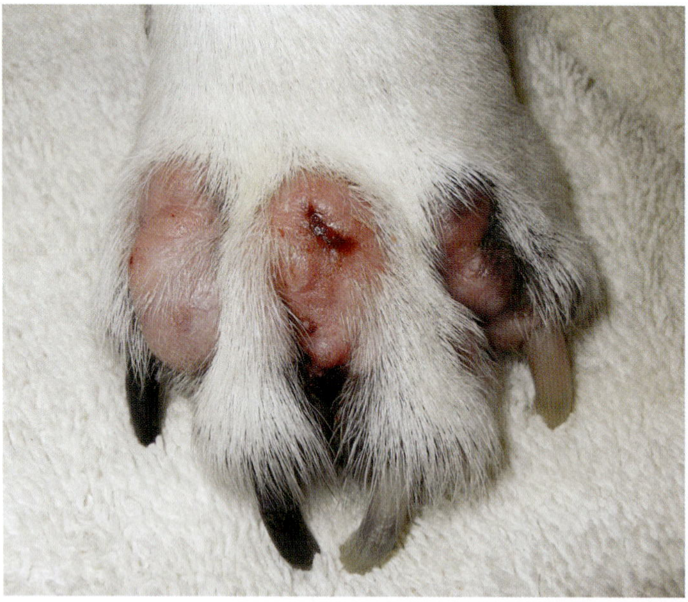

■ **Fig. 40.8.** Sterile idiopathic interdigital granulomas in a 9-year-old female-spayed French bulldog. Secondary bacterial folliculitis and furunculosis is a common sequelae to tissue trauma, often leading to permanent scarring.

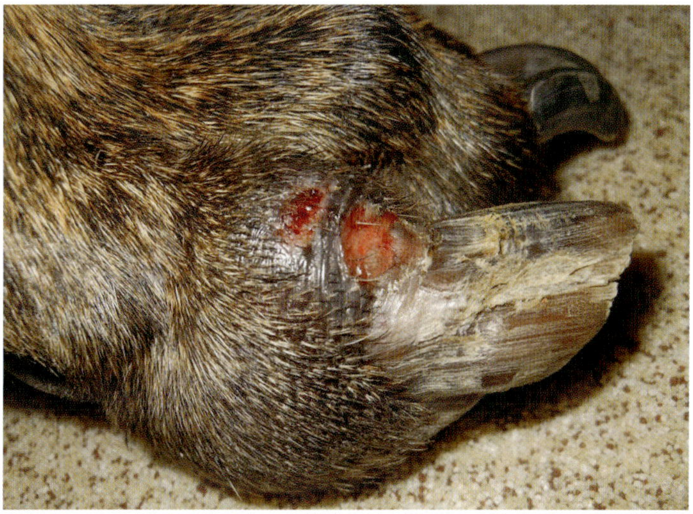

■ **Fig. 40.9.** Physical trauma to the toe has caused damage to the coronary band in this 11-year-old female-spayed plott hound, leading to macronychia and onychodystrophy (note adjacent claw for comparison).

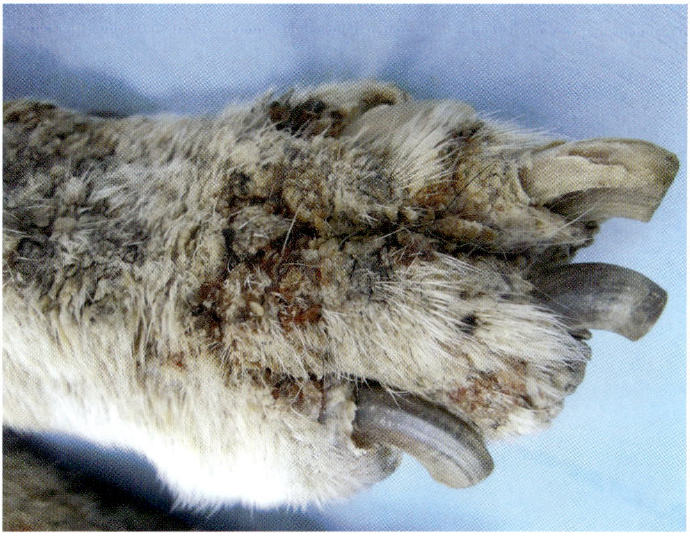

■ **Fig. 40.10.** Inflammation and infection from demodicosis causing crusts and lichenification on the paw and onychorrhexis of a claw of a 12-year-old male-castrate terrier mix.

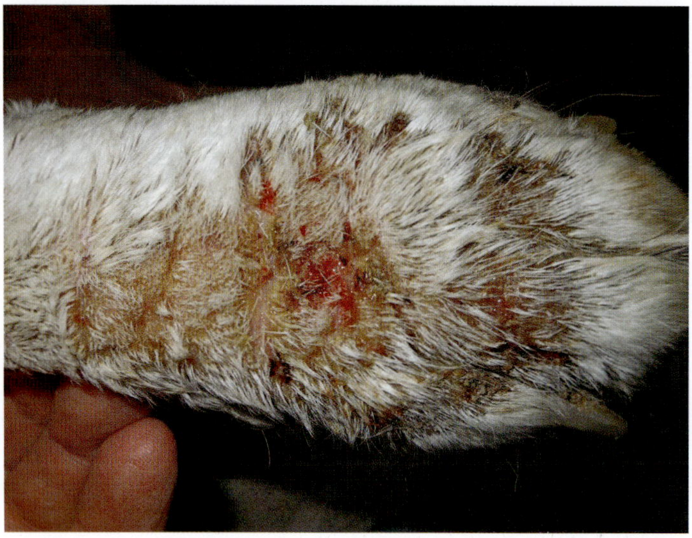

■ **Fig. 40.11.** Exudation and swelling of the carpus of a 5-year-old male-castrate beagle with leishmaniasis.

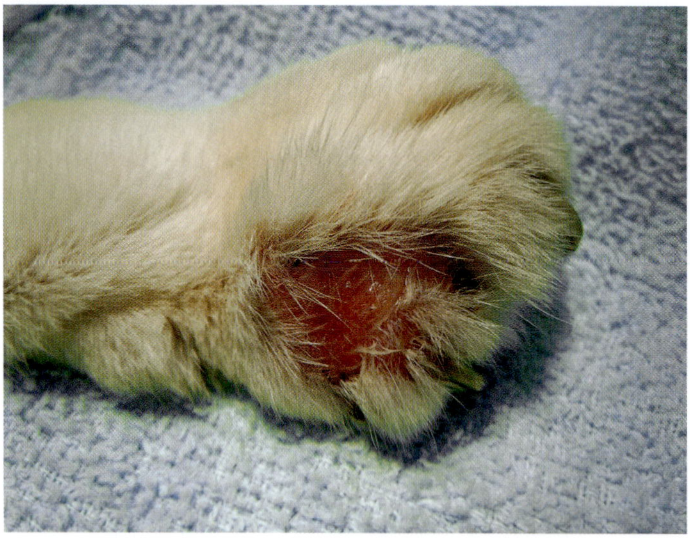

■ **Fig. 40.12.** Exudative and eroded lesion of pulmonary metastatic adenocarcinoma (lung-digit) on the carpus of a 16-year-old female-spayed DSH.

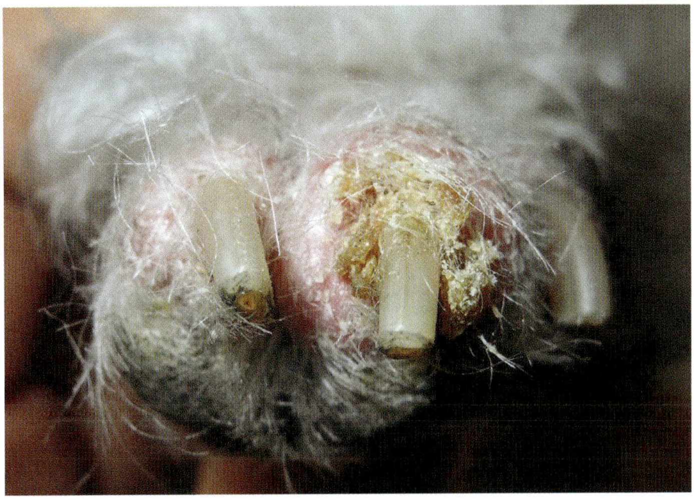

Fig. 40.13. Swelling and exudation due to bacterial paronychia in an 8-year-old male-castrate Maltese.

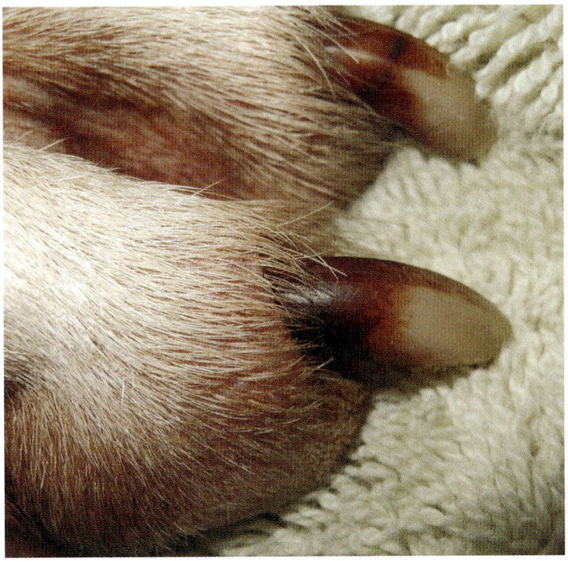

Fig. 40.14. Adherent brown debris staining of proximal claws in a 5-year-old male-castrate pit bull terrier characteristic of *Malassezia* dermatitis.

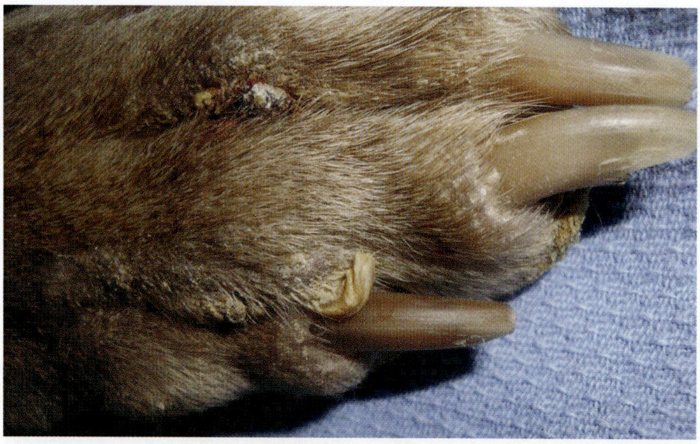

■ **Fig. 40.15.** Cutaneous horn secondary to papilloma virus infection at the ungual fold of a 9-year-old male-castrate weimaraner.

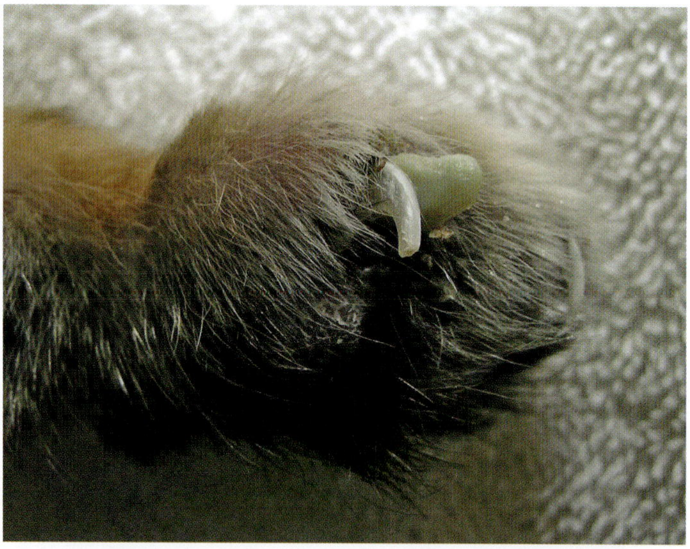

■ **Fig. 40.16.** Caseous to purulent exudate from the ungual fold of a DSH with pemphigus foliaceus.

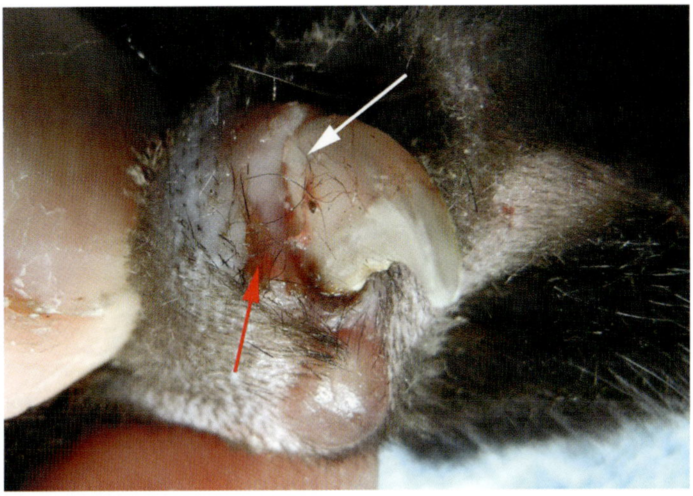

■ **Fig. 40.17.** Pemphigus foliaceus causing exudation at the base of the claw (*white arrow*) and erosions in the ungual fold (*red arrow*) of a 1-year-old male-castrate DSH.

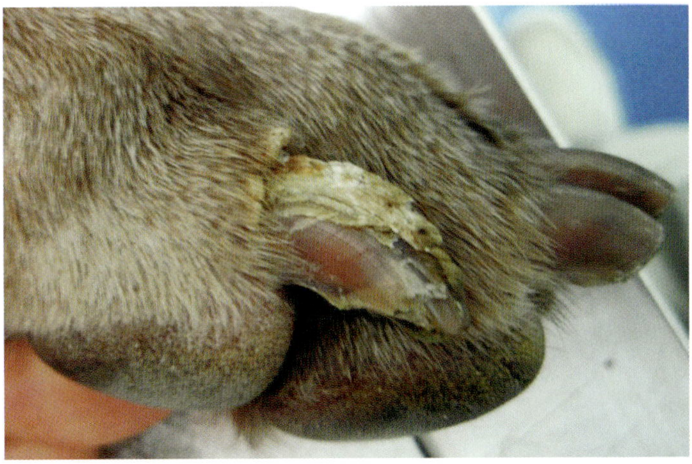

■ **Fig. 40.18.** Accumulation of crusts with onychodystrophy affecting the external coronary horn portion of the claw of a 4-year-old female-spayed weimaraner due to a subungual keratoacanthoma.

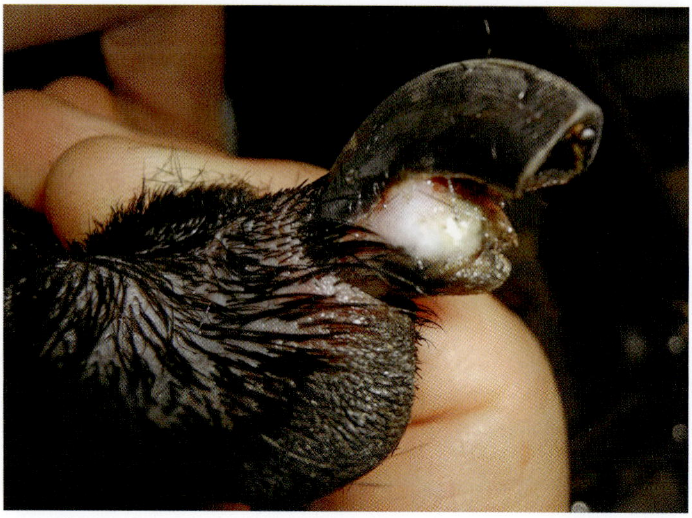

■ **Fig. 40.19.** Benign polyp developing at the base of a claw in a 4-year-old female-spayed German shepherd with symmetric lupoid onychodystrophy. Polyps develop in areas of trauma to the coronary horn, causing pain and onycholysis.

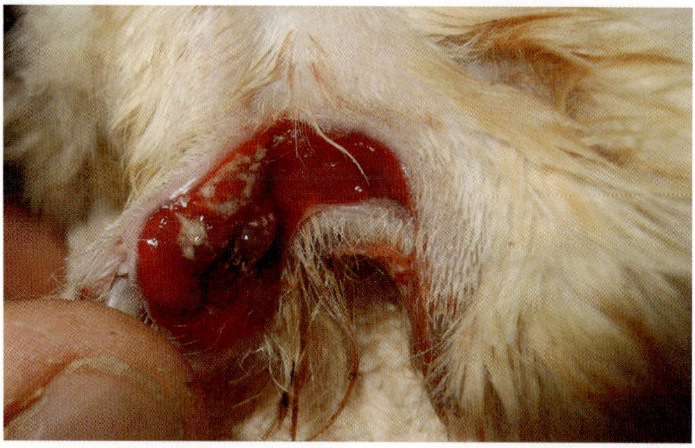

■ **Fig. 40.20.** Lymphosarcoma affecting the interdigital region and ungual fold in a 15-year-old female-spayed DMH.

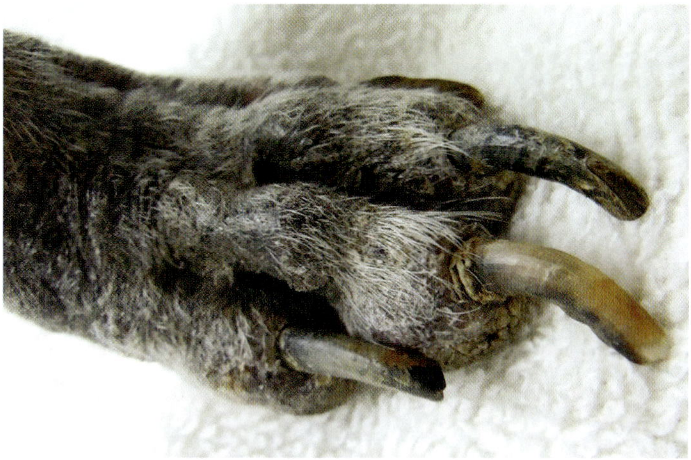

■ **Fig. 40.21.** Alopecia with crusting of the paw and onychodystrophy of adjacent claws secondary to *Trichophyton mentagrophytes* infection in a 14-year-old male chihuahua mix.

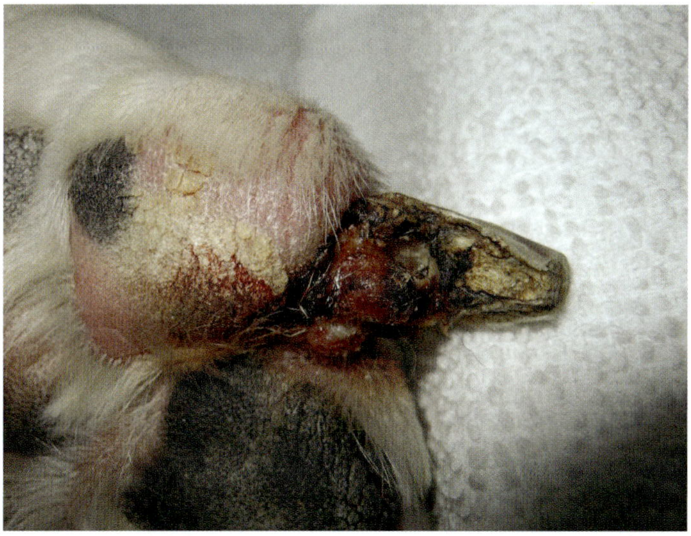

■ **Fig. 40.22.** Osteosarcoma of P3 causing onycholysis and onychodystrophy of one toe in a 9-year-old male-castrate English bulldog.

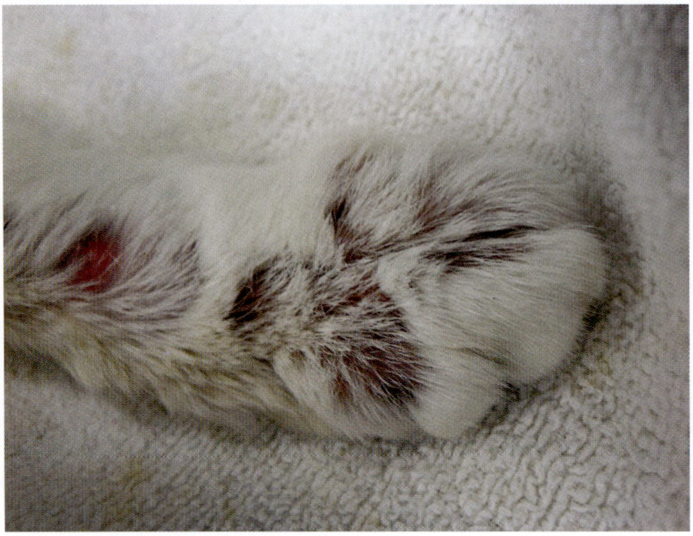

■ **Fig. 40.23.** Alopecia with erythema on the dorsal paw due to *Microsporum canis* infection in a 4-year-old male-castrate DSH.

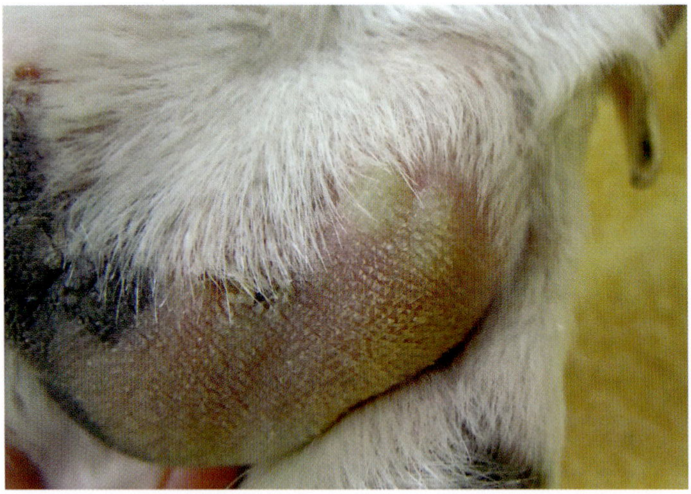

■ **Fig. 40.24.** Pustules due to pemphigus foliaceus forming at the footpad margin of a 2-year-old female-spayed American bulldog. These superficial pustules are fragile and rapidly rupture to form crusts.

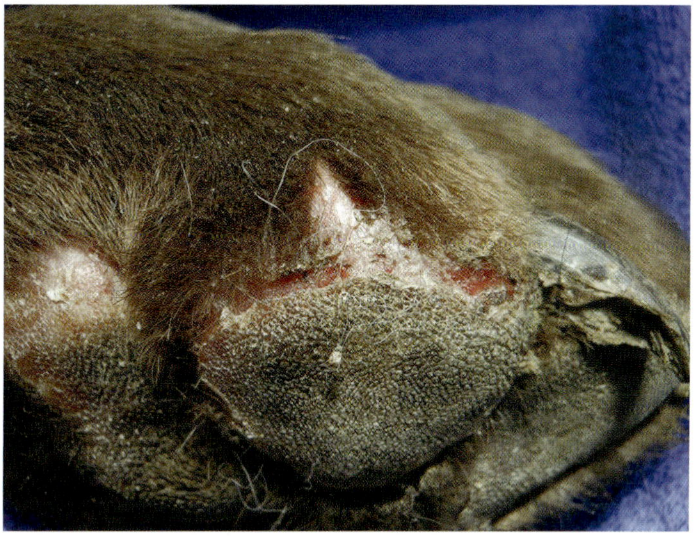

■ **Fig. 40.25.** Erythema and erosions with crusting at the footpad margins in a 10-year-old male-castrate Labrador retriever with pemphigus foliaceus. Note onychodystrophy affecting the claw of this toe.

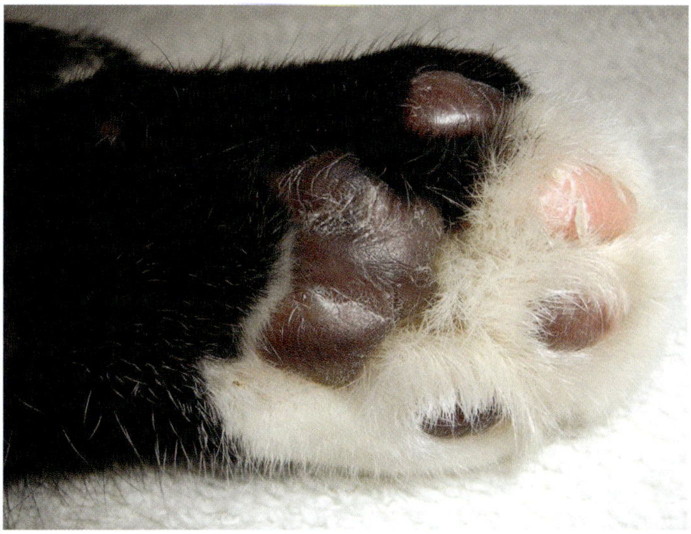

■ **Fig. 40.26.** Thin sheets of peeling epidermis can be seen on the footpads of a 1-year-old male-castrate DSH with pemphigus foliaceus.

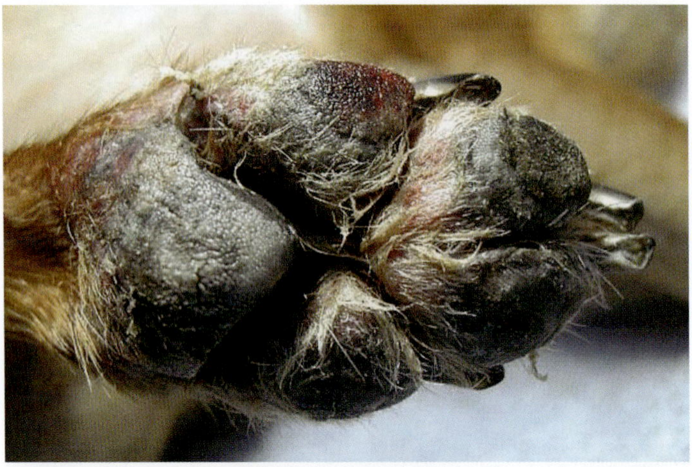

■ **Fig. 40.27.** Crusting and erosion of the footpads with interdigital exudation in a 12-year-old male-castrate terrier mix with superficial necrolytic dermatitis.

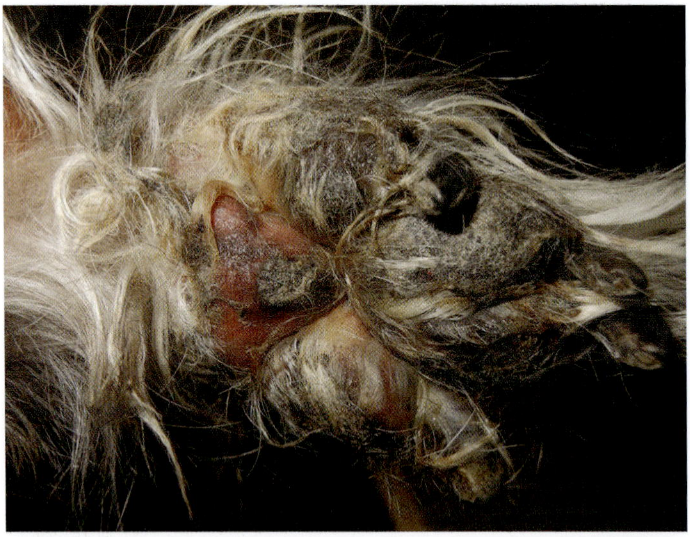

■ **Fig. 40.28.** Full-thickness necrosis and sloughing of the footpads associated with erythema multiforme major in a 7-year-old female-spayed terrier mix.

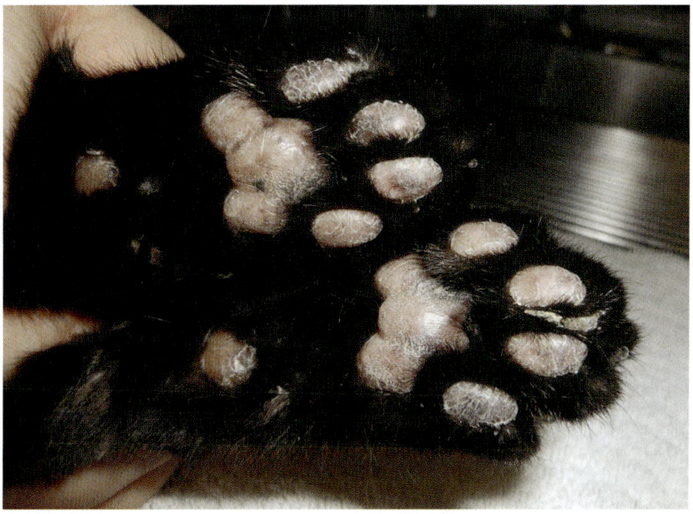

■ **Fig. 40.29.** Erythema and fine crusting affecting all the footpads in a 12-year-old female-spayed DSH with feline thymoma-associated exfoliative dermatitis.

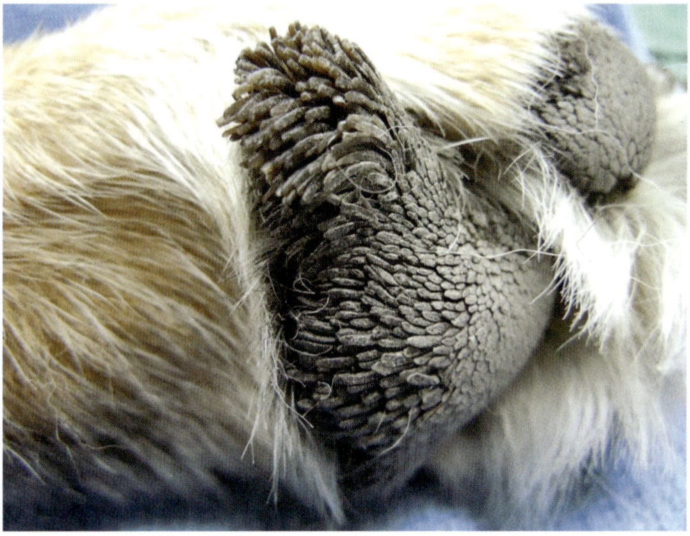

■ **Fig. 40.30.** Digital hyperkeratosis seen as verrucous accumulations of keratin, particularly at the edge of footpads, in a 15-year-old female-spayed cattle dog mix.

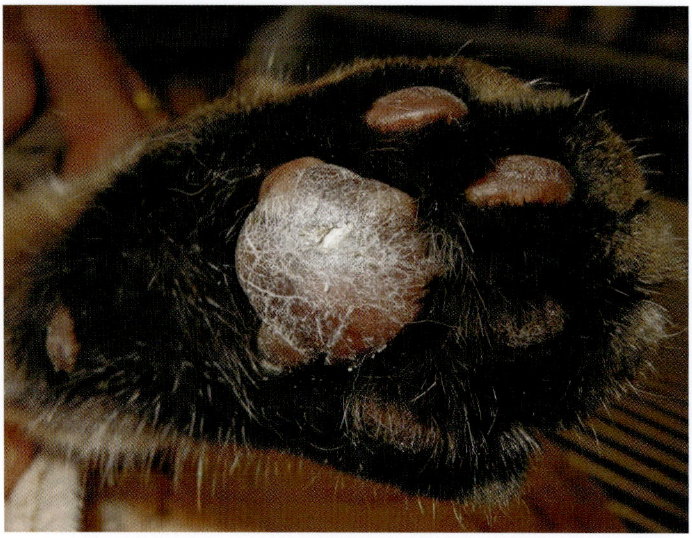

■ **Fig. 40.31.** Plasma cell pododermatitis in a 7-year-old female-spayed DSH demonstrating a characteristic "pillow" soft swelling of the metacarpal pad.

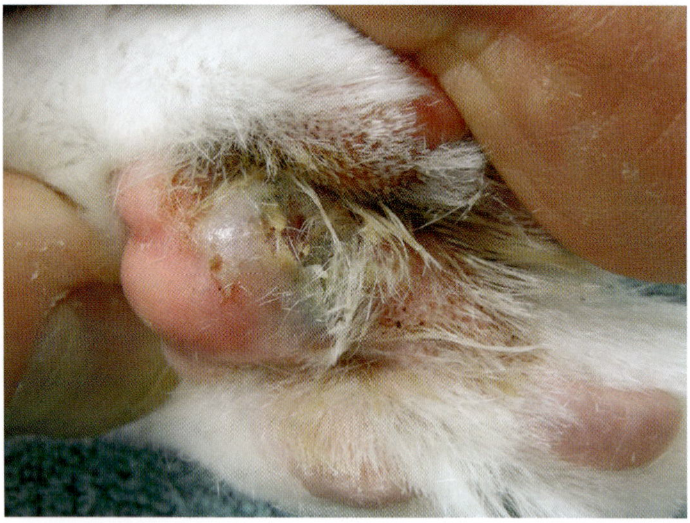

■ **Fig. 40.32.** Eroded and exudative lesion of eosinophilic granuloma on the metacarpal pad of a DSH.

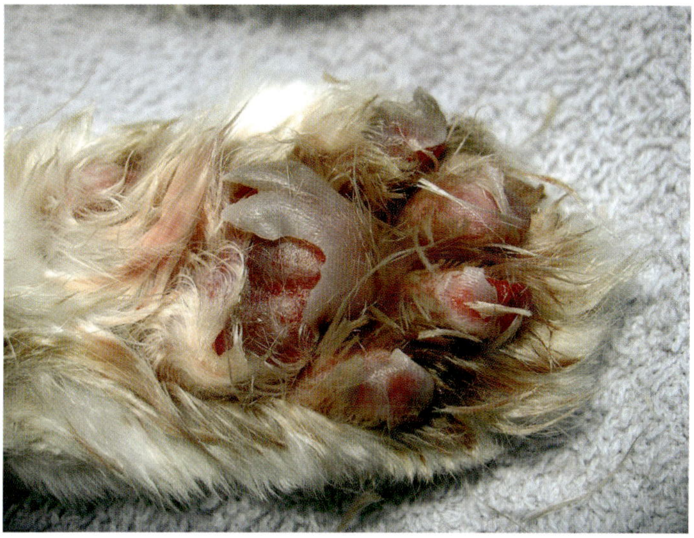

■ **Fig. 40.33.** Severe and full-thickness sloughing of the footpads due to electrical shock in a 3-year-old female-spayed ragdoll.

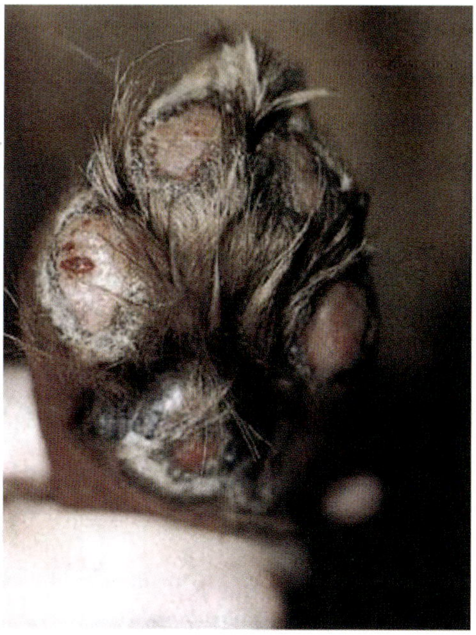

■ **Fig. 40.34.** Footpad erosion and ulceration secondary to rock salt exposure along the streets of New York City after a snowstorm.

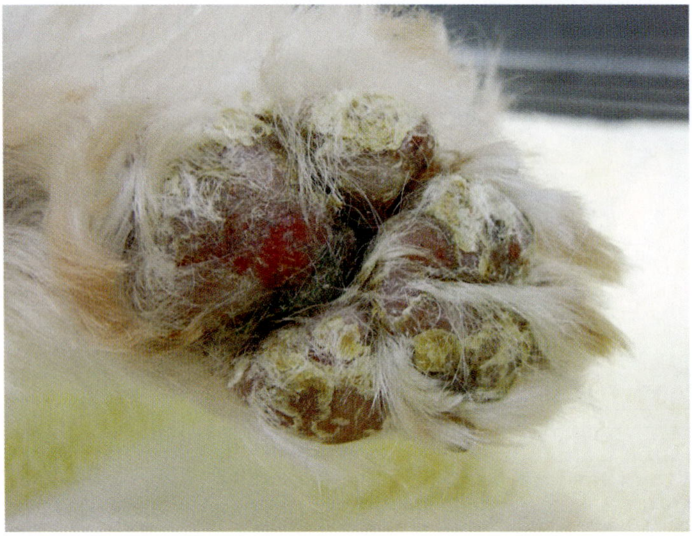

■ **Fig. 40.35.** Depigmentation, swelling, erythema, and crusting seen with epitheliotropic lymphoma in a 9-year-old female-spayed Maltese.

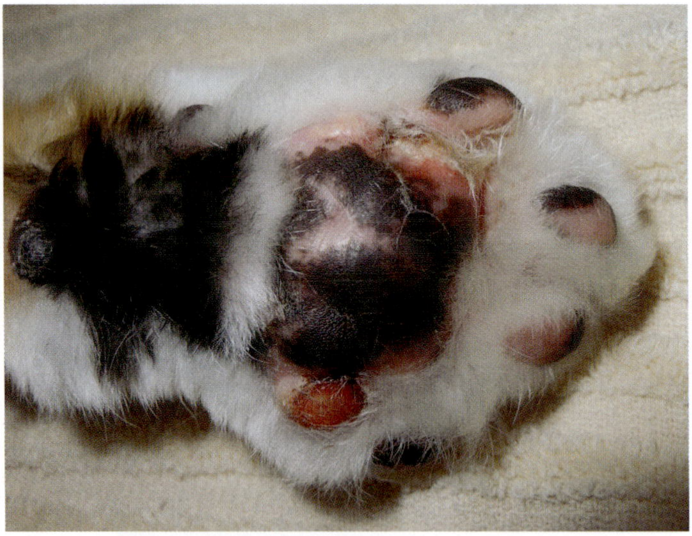

■ **Fig. 40.36.** Firm swelling of the metacarpal pad in a 1-year-old female-spayed DSH. The tissues contained a white, crumbling material identified as calcium with calcinosis circumscripta caused by severe renal failure.

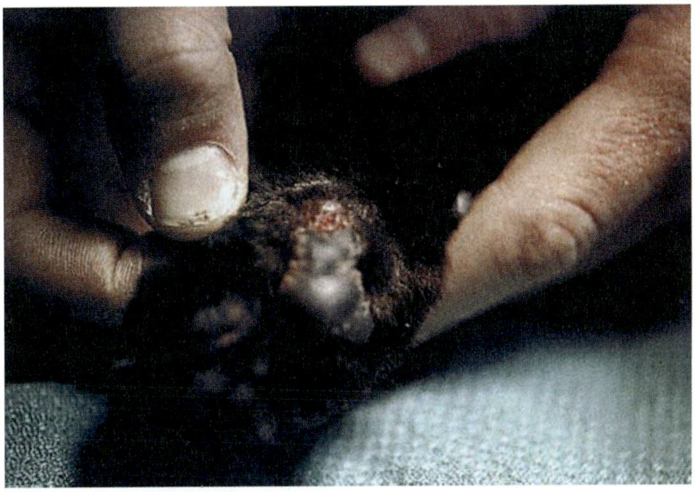

■ **Fig. 40.37.** Cutaneous xanthomatosis of the footpads in a cat associated with idiopathic hyperlipidemia. Note the yellow-pink plaques along the margins of the footpads.

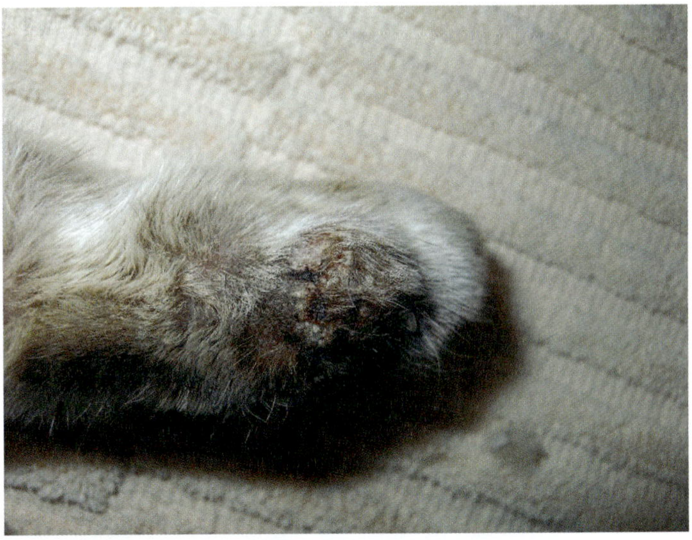

■ **Fig. 40.38.** Cutaneous large T cell lymphoma causing a nodular and crusted lesion on the extremity of a 12-year-old female-spayed DSH.

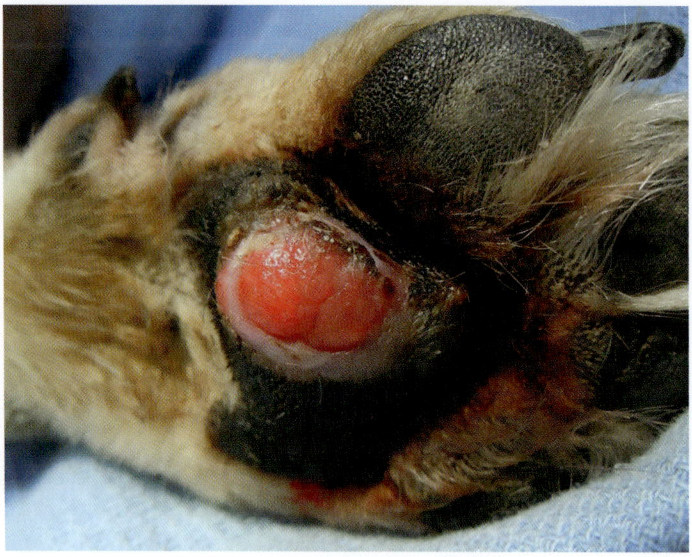

■ **Fig. 40.39.** Tumor tissue erupting through the footpad in this 15-year-old female-spayed cattle dog with malignant melanoma.

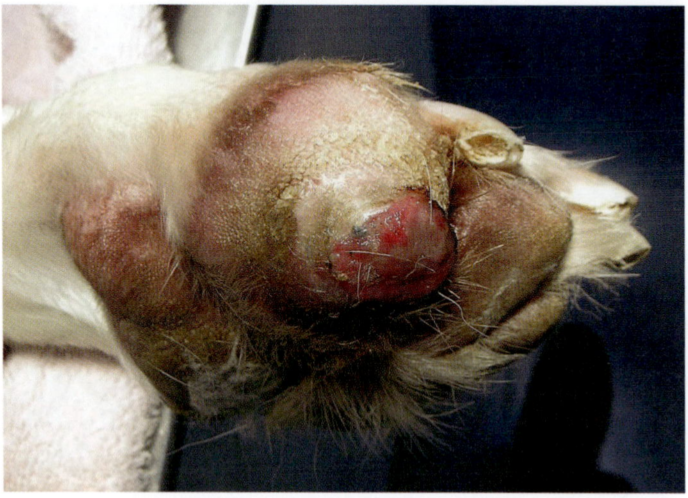

■ **Fig. 40.40.** Squamous cell carcinoma of the footpad; the lesion has a similar appearance to that seen in Figure 40.39.

chapter 41

Pre- and Paraneoplastic Syndromes

DEFINITION/OVERVIEW

- Preneoplastic dermatoses: lesions with a malignant predisposition; a *tendency* to become tumors (not consistent).
- Paraneoplastic dermatoses: lesions resulting from the metabolic effects of internal malignancy; often a marker for specific cancer.
- Categorizing preneoplastic versus paraneoplastic dermatoses: difficult in some syndromes – progression from a reactive pattern to overt neoplasia may be inconsistent.

ETIOLOGY/PATHOPHYSIOLOGY

- Canine preneoplastic dermatoses:
  - Actinic keratoses: ultraviolet light (UVL) causes DNA damage directly and indirectly by free radicals; specific UVL-induced mutations have been documented in the tumor suppressor gene p53, leading to expansion of mutated keratinocytes; may represent a premalignant condition; close association of and genetic similarities between AK and squamous cell carcinoma (SCC); actinic carcinoma *in situ* denotes SCC that has not penetrated to the dermis (see relevant chapter)
  - Cutaneous lymphocytosis: expansion of T cells in response to persistent antigenic stimulation such as drugs or vaccines; clonal rearrangement may result in overt lymphoma
  - Cutaneous mastocytosis: a specific mutation in mast cells leading to systemic mastocytosis has not been identified; associated with mutations of the *c-kit* oncogene in human beings
  - Nodular fasciitis: benign reactive lesion, possibly due to trauma; occasionally used to describe proliferative inflammatory processes, including reactive histiocytosis.
- Canine paraneoplastic dermatoses:
  - Cutaneous (primary nodular) amyloidosis: increased production of amyloidogenic immunoglobulin light chains by proliferating plasma cells; associated with multiple myeloma and extramedullary plasmacytoma; associated with chronic inflammatory conditions
  - Cutaneous mucinosis (secondary): excessive accumulation of mucin in the dermis rarely associated with mast cell tumors

Blackwell's Five-Minute Veterinary Consult Clinical Companion: Small Animal Dermatology, Third Edition.
Karen Helton Rhodes and Alexander H. Werner.

- Paraneoplastic pemphigus: multiple epidermal plakin family proteins and desmogleins targeted; T cell-mediated keratinocyte apoptosis may contribute to lesion development
- Multiple collagenous nevi: potential increase in local production of TGF-alpha and beta-1 cytokine resulting in proliferation of fibroblasts and excess collagen
- Renal cystadenocarcinoma and nodular dermatofibrosis: result of autosomal dominant genetic defect; a missense mutation of the *FLCN*(folliculin)/*BHD* gene on chromosome 5 may contribute to renal or uterine muscle tumors in German shepherd dogs
- Superficial necrolytic dermatitis (hepatocutaneous syndrome, necrolytic migratory erythema, metabolic epidermal necrosis): most often associated with hepatopathy; rare association with glucagon-secreting pancreatic or extrapancreatic neoplasia; glucagonemia-induced glycogenesis results in hypoaminoacidemia, causing keratinocyte degeneration
- Cutaneous changes due to hyperadrenocorticism (see relevant chapter).

- Feline preneoplastic dermatoses:
  - Actinic keratoses: similar to canine (see relevant chapter)
  - Cutaneous lymphocytosis: expansion of T cells in response to persistent antigenic stimulation such as drugs or vaccines; clonal rearrangement may result in overt lymphoma.
- Feline paraneoplastic dermatoses:
  - Pancreatic/hepatic paraneoplastic alopecia:
    - Majority of cases are associated with an underlying pancreatic adenocarcinoma
    - Other internal carcinomas, such as bile duct and hepatocellular carcinomas, may be involved
    - Most affected cats with pancreatic adenocarcinomas have metastases to liver, lungs, pleura, and/or peritoneum; reports of bile duct and hepatocellular carcinomas
    - Clinical symptoms may involve cytokines producing atrophy of the hair follicles
  - Feline thymoma-associated exfoliative dermatitis:
    - Elevated numbers of CD3+ lymphocytes within the dermis
    - Proposed induction of autoreactive T lymphocyte attack on follicles.

SIGNALMENT/HISTORY

- Canine preneoplastic dermatoses:
  - Actinic keratoses:
    - No sex predilection
    - Age: usually older animals; reported as young as 2 years
    - Breed predilections: dalmatian, whippet, Italian greyhound, greyhound, American Staffordshire and bull terrier, beagle, German short-haired pointer, boxer, basset hound

- Cutaneous lymphocytosis:
  - □ Very rare; older dogs; median 8 years; range 5–14 years
  - □ Female predilection
  - □ Possible breed predilection: golden retriever, Shetland sheepdog, Chinese crested, Welsh corgi
- Cutaneous mastocytosis:
  - □ Rare; reported primarily in dogs under 1 year of age
  - □ Newfoundland, cocker spaniel, Labrador retriever, Jack Russell terrier, other breeds
- Nodular fasciitis:
  - □ No age, breed, or sex predilection.

■ Canine paraneoplastic dermatoses:
- Cutaneous (primary nodular) amyloidosis
  - □ Very rare; older dogs
  - □ Chinese shar-pei, cocker spaniels and beagles may be predisposed
- Cutaneous mucinosis (secondary):
  - □ Rare; may be associated with mast cell tumors
- Multiple collagenous nevi: nodular dermatofibrosis:
  - □ Rare; middle-aged dogs; range 3–7 years
  - □ German shepherd dog (autosomal dominant inheritance); golden retriever, boxer, other breeds
  - □ Associated with renal cysts, cystadenomas, cystadenocarcinomas, and uterine leiomyomas
- Paraneoplastic pemphigus:
  - □ Very rare; too few reports to characterize
- Superficial necrolytic dermatitis:
  - □ Rare; primarily old dogs (mean age 10 years)
  - □ Males possibly overrepresented
  - □ May have a heritable component in some breeds (shih tzu)
  - □ Predilection for medium and small breeds: West Highland white terrier, Scottish terrier, American cocker spaniel, Shetland sheepdog, Lhasa apso, border collie; syndrome also identified in large breeds
  - □ Lesions often precede systemic symptoms.

■ Feline preneoplastic dermatoses:
- Actinic keratoses:
  - □ No sex predilection
  - □ Age: usually older animals
- Cutaneous lymphocytosis:
  - □ Rare: older cats – median age 13 years; range 6–15 years
  - □ Female predilection (61%).

■ Feline paraneoplastic dermatoses:
- Pancreatic/hepatic paraneoplastic alopecia
  - □ Domestic shorthair cats
  - □ Older cats – median age: 13 years; range 7–16 years

- Feline thymoma-associated exfoliative dermatitis:
  - Middle-aged to older cats
  - No breed or sex predilection.

CLINICAL FEATURES

- Canine preneoplastic dermatoses:
  - Actinic keratoses:
    - Lesions develop in sun-exposed lightly pigmented or unpigmented skin (naturally or scarred) in areas not sufficiently protected by hair, and in junctions between haired and nonhaired skin.
    - Nasal planum, dorsal muzzle, axillae, and glabrous areas of the ventral abdomen and medial thigh
    - Early erythematous patches appear slightly lichenified or roughened
    - Epithelial plaques may be palpable as firm thickenings before becoming visible and may be distinguishable from nonthickened (normal) adjacent pigmented skin
    - Crusted, indurated, and exfoliating plaques (Figure 41.1)
    - Severe hyperkeratosis may be seen as cutaneous horns
    - Individual plaques and nodules (often with actinic comedones) coalesce to larger lesions
    - Affected areas become extensive; inflammation and exudation develop with secondary furunculosis
    - Axillae, ventral abdomen, and medial thigh primary sites; less often dorsal muzzle and eyelid margin
  - Cutaneous lymphocytosis:
    - Patches of erythema or erythematous plaques on head, neck, thorax, and axillae (Figure 41.2)
    - Multiple lesions
    - Slow progression without regression; potential to progress to high-grade lymphoma
    - Rarely pruritic
  - Cutaneous mastocytosis:
    - Cutaneous lesions in dogs similar to urticaria pigmentosa of human beings
    - Small erythematous macules, papules or plaques, wheals, and hemorrhagic bullae on the head, neck, trunk, and legs
    - Manipulation induces erythema and induration
    - Nonmalignant conditions are more likely to have multiple lesions as opposed to a single, discrete neoplasm
  - Nodular fasciitis:
    - Solitary, subcutaneous mass often less than 2 cm in diameter
    - Predilection for the head, face, and eyelids.

- Canine paraneoplastic dermatoses:
  - Cutaneous (primary nodular) amyloidosis: solitary or grouped, firm, dermal, or subcutaneous nodules on the pinnae, oral mucosa, digits, legs, and trunk; cutaneous hemorrhage (Figure 41.3)
  - Cutaneous mucinosis (secondary):
    - Excessive dermal accumulation of mucin, often asymptomatic
    - Rare reports of papular mucinosis seen as puffy, thickened, nonpitting patches with vesicles or bullae (Figure 41.4)
  - Multiple collagenous nevi: nodular dermatofibrosis: multiple, firm, well-demarcated nodules varying in size from very small to large on the head, legs, and ears; may be alopecic and ulcerated in areas of trauma or friction (Figures 41.5–41.7)
  - Paraneoplastic pemphigus:
    - Blistering disease affecting the mucosa and mucocutaneous junctions (Figures 41.8, 41.9)
    - Systemic signs associated with both neoplasia and cutaneous lesions (weight loss, lethargy, purulent discharge)
  - Superficial necrolytic dermatitis:
    - Progressive development of erythema, hyperkeratosis, and exudation at the margins of the footpads (Figure 41.10)
    - Crusting, ulcerative, and painful dermatitis
    - Lesions affect the mucocutaneous junctions of lips, eyes, and anus; develop at the same time or immediately following footpad lesions (Figure 41.11)
    - Skin lesions also pronounced in areas of trauma: muzzle, distal limbs, elbows, footpads
    - Fissuring and severe crusting of footpads result in pruritus and pain
    - Hyperpigmentation and lichenification common with chronicity
    - Secondary bacterial folliculitis and *Malassezia* dermatitis common
    - Lesions develop on pressure points, pinnae, and external genitalia
    - Dermatitis often precedes systemic symptoms by weeks
    - Systemic signs include lethargy, polyuria, polydipsia (when associated with diabetes mellitus), anorexia, and weight loss
    - Poor to grave prognosis.
- Feline preneoplastic dermatoses:
  - Actinic keratoses: preauricular regions, as well as pinnal margins, nasal planum, and eyelid margins; lesions often traumatized, resulting in scabbing
  - Cutaneous lymphocytosis:
    - Alopecia with or without erythema, scaling, crusting, excoriation (70%)
    - Erythematous plaques (30%)
    - Solitary lesions (60%)
    - Slow, progressive disorder.
- Feline paraneoplastic dermatoses:
  - Pancreatic/hepatic paraneoplastic alopecia:
    - Decrease in appetite followed by rapid 2–5-week history of anorexia, weight loss, lethargy, and excessive shedding

- Most cases euthanized within 8 weeks of developing dermatitis
- Hair loss: rapidly progressive with sudden onset leading to total loss in affected region; primarily ventral distribution (ventral trunk, medial aspect of limbs) (Figure 41.12)
- Some affected cats may be reluctant to walk, owing to painful fissuring of the footpads
- Hairs epilate easily
- Severe alopecia: ventral neck, abdomen, and medial thighs
- The stratum corneum may "peel," leading to a glistening appearance to the skin (Figure 41.13)
- Alopecic skin is shiny, inelastic and thin, but not fragile
- Pruritus: variable; sometimes with excessive grooming
- Gray lentigines may develop in alopecic areas
- Footpads may be fissured and/or scaly, often painful
- May have secondary *Malassezia* overgrowth

- Exfoliative dermatitis associated with thymoma:
  - Slowly progressive scaling dermatitis
  - Cats present with skin lesions and no evidence of neoplasia
  - Systemic signs develop late in the course of disease; coughing, dyspnea, anorexia, lethargy
  - Lesions often begin on the head and neck; become generalized (Figure 41.14)
  - Large, nonadherent, white scales and crusts (Figure 41.15)
  - Erythema mild initially and then becomes severe
  - Brown waxy deposits adhere around the eyes and lips as well as the ear canal
  - Usually nonpruritic unless associated with secondary *Malassezia* overgrowth
  - Rare associated myasthenia gravis and megaesophagus.

DIFFERENTIAL DIAGNOSIS

- Canine preneoplastic dermatoses:
  - Actinic keratoses: bacterial furunculosis, lichenoid keratosis, squamous cell carcinoma, topical drug eruption, severe contact dermatitis
  - Cutaneous lymphocytosis: epitheliotropic lymphoma, lymphocytic leukemia with cutaneous involvement, hypersensitivity reaction, drug eruption, bacterial folliculitis
  - Cutaneous mastocytosis: hypersensitivity reaction, drug eruption, bacterial folliculitis, mast cell tumor
  - Nodular fasciitis: infectious granuloma, sterile granuloma, local trauma, dermal neoplasia, fibroma, fibrosarcoma, spindle cell lipoma.
- Canine paraneoplastic dermatoses:
  - Cutaneous (primary nodular) amyloidosis:dermal neoplasia or cyst, infectious granuloma, sterile granuloma, pyogranulomatous dermatitis

- Cutaneous mucinosis (secondary): causes of diffuse dermal edema, vesicular or bullous dermatitis
- Nodular dermatofibrosis: dermal neoplasia, infectious granuloma, sterile granuloma, pyogranulomatous dermatitis, fibroma, hematoma, nodular scar
- Paraneoplastic pemphigus: pemphigus vulgaris, bullous pemphigoid, erythema multiforme
- Superficial necrolytic dermatitis: pemphigus foliaceus, zinc-responsive dermatosis, systemic lupus erythematosus, erythema multiforme, drug eruption, generic dog food dermatosis, irritant contact dermatitis, demodicosis, dermatophytosis, vasculitis, epitheliotropic lymphoma, toxic epidermal necrolysis.

- Feline preneoplastic dermatoses:
  - Actinic keratoses: squamous cell carcinoma, topical drug eruption, severe contact dermatitis
  - Cutaneous lymphocytosis: epitheliotropic lymphoma, hypersensitivity reaction, drug eruption, bacterial folliculitis, dermatophytosis.
- Feline paraneoplastic dermatoses:
  - Pancreatic/hepatic paraneoplastic alopecia: hyperadrenocorticism, hyperthyroidism, feline symmetric alopecia, demodicosis, dermatophytosis, alopecia areata, telogen effluvium/defluvium, skin fragility syndrome, alopecia mucinosa, epitheliotropic lymphoma, erythema multiforme (idiopathic and herpes virus associated), sebaceous adenitis
  - Exfoliative dermatitis associated with thymoma: demodicosis, dermatophytosis, hyperadrenocorticism, epitheliotropic lymphoma, erythema multiforme (idiopathic and herpes virus associated), drug reaction, hypersensitivity reaction, systemic lupus erythematosus, FeLV or FIV-related dermatitis.

DIAGNOSTICS

- CBC/biochemistry/urinalysis: depends upon specific condition and involvement of other organ systems.
- Elevated plasma glucagon levels: consistently noted with glucagon-secreting pancreatic or extrapancreatic neoplasia and hypoaminoacidemia (notably glutamine, proline, cysteine, hydroxyproline) in superficial necrolytic dermatitis.
- Cytology of lesions: rarely definitive; pattern of cellular aggregation significant to determination of cause.
- Imaging: depends upon specific condition and involvement of other organ systems.
- Dermatohistopathology required for diagnosis; immunohistochemical studies from tissues may be required to distinguish nonmalignant from malignant cell populations.
- Ultrasonography: pathognomonic "Swiss cheese" hepatic appearance with superficial necrolytic dermatitis; pancreatic mass and/or nodular lesions in the liver or peritoneal cavity with pancreatic/hepatic paraneoplastic alopecia; mediastinal mass in exfoliative dermatitis associated with thymoma.
- Thoracic radiographs: metastatic lesions in the lungs or pleural cavity in pancreatic/hepatic cases.
- CT scans.
- Laparoscopy or exploratory laparotomy: identify primary and metastatic tumors.

Dermatohistopathology

- Canine preneoplastic dermatoses:
  - Actinic keratoses: epidermal hyperplasia and dysplasia with severe hyperkeratosis and/or "stacked" parakeratosis; keratinocytes appear distorted and/or apoptotic; perivascular to lichenoid dermal infiltrate with solar elastosis and fibrosis; absence of invasion through the dermal-epidermal junction
  - Cutaneous lymphocytosis: perivascular to diffuse infiltration of small lymphocytes in the superficial dermis with a zone of acellularity (Grenz zone); nonepitheliotrophic; immunohistochemistry demonstrates $CD3^+$ T cells; clonality supports the potential for neoplastic cell population
  - Cutaneous mastocytosis: perivascular to diffuse infiltration with well-differentiated mast cells
  - Nodular fasciitis: poorly demarcated and disorganized accumulation of spindle cells attached to fascia; highly vascular; immunohistochemistry consistent with fibroblasts.
- Canine paraneoplastic dermatoses:
  - Cutaneous (primary nodular) amyloidosis: accumulations of amorphous-appearing eosinophilic deposits in beta-pleated configuration (electron microscopy); associated with plasma cells; deposits may be surrounded by macrophages and giant cells; immunohistochemistry demonstrates amyloid derived from light-chain immunoglobulin
  - Cutaneous mucinosis (secondary): epidermal hyperplasia; accumulations of pale substance (mucin) between collagen fibers in the superficial dermis with scattered focal, large accumulations; minimal inflammation unless associated with concurrent dermatitis
  - Multiple collagenous nevi: nodular dermatofibrosis: increased and thickened collagen bundles (nodular collagen hyperplasia); subcutaneous lesions may be well demarcated as opposed to less distinct dermal lesions; collagen bundles surround adnexal structures
  - Paraneoplastic pemphigus: transepidermal pustulation with suprabasilar and superficial acantholysis; prominent apoptotic keratinocytes; dermal or submucosal infiltrate of lymphocytes, macrophages, and plasma cells; variable numbers of neutrophils
  - Superficial necrolytic dermatitis: parakeratosis and neutrophilic crusting; pallor of epidermis above the basal layer due to intracellular and intercellular edema; hyperplastic basal cell layer producing a distinctive "red/white/blue" pattern; clefting within the epidermis; mild neutrophilic superficial to perivascular dermal infiltrate; marked parakeratosis with absence of epidermal pallor noted in chronic cases.
- Feline preneoplastic dermatoses:
  - Actinic keratoses: similar to canine
  - Cutaneous lymphocytosis: moderate to marked perivascular to diffuse, superficial and deep, round cell infiltrate consisting primarily of T cells; small aggregates of B cells; mild epitheliotrophism; occasional excoriation noted.

- Feline paraneoplastic dermatoses:
  - Pancreatic/hepatic paraneoplastic alopecia: severe atrophy of hair follicles and adnexa; miniaturization of hair bulbs; mild acanthosis; variable absence of stratum corneum; variable mixed superficial perivascular infiltrates of neutrophils, eosinophils, and mononuclear cells; some have secondary *Malassezia* infections/primary tumor – usually pancreatic adenocarcinoma, rarely primary bile duct or hepatocellular carcinomas/metastatic nodules – common in the liver, lungs, pleura, and peritoneum
  - Exfoliative dermatitis associated with thymoma: cell-poor hydropic interface dermatitis with apoptosis of basal keratinocytes, pockets of satellitosis, and lymphocytic dermal infiltrate.

THERAPEUTICS

- Canine preneoplastic dermatoses:
  - Actinic keratoses:
    - Avoid exposure to UVL by keeping patients indoors and by applying sunblock
    - Vitamin E 200 mg PO BID less than 10 kg body weight; 400 mg PO BID greater than 10 kg body weight; vitamin C 500 mg PO BID; beta-carotene 30 mg PO BID to q24h; vitamin A 400–600 IU/kg PO q24h – may have a protective effect
    - Topical corticosteroids: reduce localized areas of inflammation
    - Prednisolone 0.5 mg/kg PO q24h then tapered dosage: reduce significant inflammation
    - Cephalexin 22 mg/kg PO BID: secondary bacterial furunculosis; alternative antibiotics selected by culture and sensitivity test results
    - Tretinoin 0.1% (Retin-A): apply daily to individual lesions for 14 days; then 2–3 times weekly; may cause irritation
    - Isotretinoin 1 mg/kg PO q24h for 30 days; then alternate days or as needed to control lesions
    - Firocoxib 5 mg/kg PO q24h: overexpression of cyclooxygenase (COX-2) documented in actinic keratoses in humans and dogs; improvement noted with use of COX-2 selective inhibitor
  - Cutaneous lymphocytosis: undetermined; too few cases documented; poor response to corticosteroids
  - Cutaneous mastocytosis:
    - Spontaneous resolution
    - Antihistamines: hydroxyzine 1 mg/kg PO BID; chlorpheniramine 0.2–0.5 mg/kg PO BID
    - Corticosteroids: prednisolone 0.5 mg/kg PO q24h then tapered dosage
  - Nodular fasciitis: surgical excision curative.
- Canine paraneoplastic dermatoses:
  - Cutaneous (primary nodular) amyloidosis:

    - Surgical excision of individual lesions
    - Application of DMSO may inhibit amyloid synthesis
  - Cutaneous mucinosis (secondary):
    - Antihistamines: diphenhydramine 1 mg/kg PO BID; hydroxyzine 1 mg/kg PO BID
    - Corticosteroids: prednisolone 0.5 mg/kg PO q24h then tapered dosage
  - Nodular dermatofibrosis:
    - Surgical excision of internal neoplasia
    - Surgical excision of individual lesions
  - Paraneoplastic pemphigus:
    - Surgical excision of internal neoplasia
    - Treatment similar to pemphigus foliaceus
    - Prednisolone: 1.1–2.2 mg/kg PO divided BID to initiate control, tapering to maintenance at 0.5 mg/kg PO q48–72h
    - More than half of patients require the addition of other immunomodulating drugs
    - Azathioprine: 2.2 mg/kg PO q24h, then EOD
  - Superficial necrolytic dermatitis:
    - Surgical excision of tumor
    - Patient survival: 6 months without tumor excision; euthanasia most often due to diabetic crisis or hepatic failure
    - Treatment of secondary bacterial folliculitis and/or *Malassezia* dermatitis with appropriate antimicrobials
    - Prednisolone 0.5 mg/kg q24h; taper dosage and discontinue as soon as possible: temporary relief of pruritus and inflammation; may exacerbate diabetes mellitus; may aggravate hepatopathy
    - Octreotide 2–3.2 μg/kg by subcutaneous injection BID to QID: somatostatin analog; nonresected glucagon-producing pancreatic tumor
    - Amino acid infusion: intravenous administration of amino acids to replenish serum levels from excessive hepatic catabolism
    - 10% crystalline amino acid solution; 25 mL/kg over 8 h
    - 3% amino acid and electrolyte solutions; 25 mL/kg over 8 h
    - Initial replacement therapy twice weekly until symptoms improve
    - Maintenance infusions every 7–14 days as indicated by patient response.
- Feline preneoplastic dermatoses:
  - Actinic keratoses:
    - Avoid exposure to UVL by keeping patients indoors and by applying sunblock
    - Topical corticosteroids: reduce localized areas of inflammation
    - Prednisolone (0.5 mg/kg PO tapered dosage): reduce significant inflammation
    - Cephalexin (22 mg/kg PO BID): secondary bacterial furunculosis; alternative antibiotics selected by culture and sensitivity test results
    - Tretinoin 0.1% (Retin-A): apply daily to individual lesions for 14 days; then 2–3 times weekly; may cause irritation
    - Surgical excision of affected tissue

- Cutaneous lymphocytosis:
  - Prednisolone: 0.5 mg/kg PO q24h until remission; then EOD or twice weekly
  - Chlorambucil: 0.1–0.2 mg/kg PO q24h until remission; then EOD or twice weekly
  - Lomustine: 40–60 mg/m^2 PO every 3–6 weeks; or 10 mg PO every 3 weeks.

- Feline paraneoplastic dermatoses:
  - Pancreatic/hepatic paraneoplastic alopecia:
    - Removal of tumor by partial pancreatectomy may be curative; prognosis is grave; majority of cases have metastatic disease; ultrasonography and thoracic radiographs may demonstrate progression
    - Chemotherapy or other medications: no reported response
    - Affected animals rapidly deteriorate; euthanasia should be suggested as humane intervention
    - Supportive care: only if owners refuse to consider euthanasia; feed highly palatable, nutrient-dense foods and/or tube feed
    - Progressive deterioration; death most often occurs within 2–20 weeks after onset of skin lesions
  - Exfoliative dermatitis with thymoma:
    - Prognosis guarded
    - Complete surgical removal of the thymoma and sternal lymph nodes produces resolution of clinical signs within months (average 4–5 months)
    - Radiation therapy recommended for unresectable tumors.

COMMENTS

- Preneoplastic dermatoses require regular monitoring for early detection of developing neoplasia.
- Paraneoplastic dermatoses require treatment of underlying etiology (if identified) to prevent recurrences of symptoms.
- Corticosteroids: may cause polyuria, polydipsia, polyphagia, temperament changes, diabetes mellitus, pancreatitis, and hepatotoxicity.
- Azathioprine: may cause pancreatitis.
- Chlorambucil: monitor CBC weekly until remission; then every 3–6 months.
- Lomustine: monitor CBC 1 week after and just prior to next dosage; serum chemistries prior to next dosage.
- Isotretinoin: may cause keratoconjunctivitis sicca; extreme teratogen; do not use in intact females because of severe and predictable teratogenicity and the extremely long withdrawal period; women of child-bearing age should not handle this medication; monitor serum chemistries including triglycerides, and tear production.

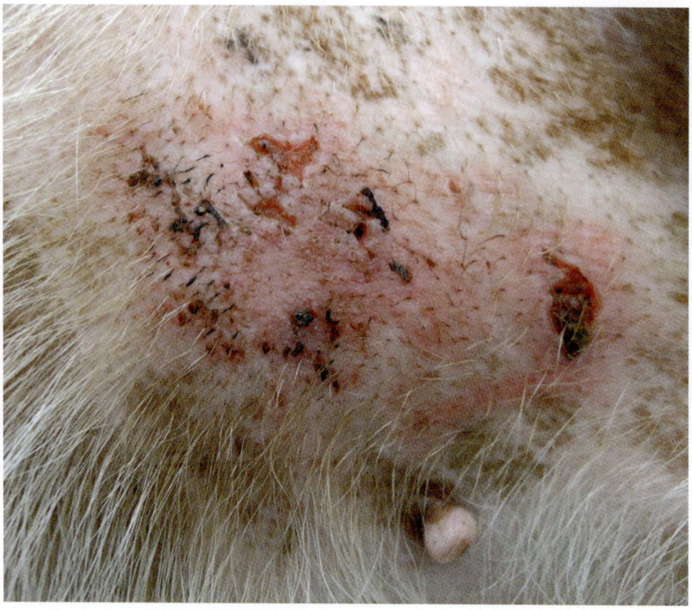

■ **Fig. 41.1.** Crusted, indurated, and erythematous plaque characteristic of actinic keratosis on the ventral abdomen of a 9-year-old female-spayed pointer mix.

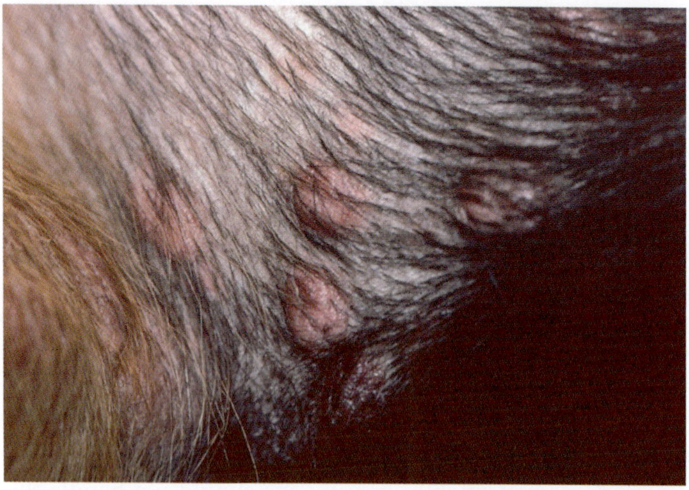

■ **Fig. 41.2.** Multiple erythematous plaques on the ventrum of a mix-breed dog with cutaneous lymphocytosis.

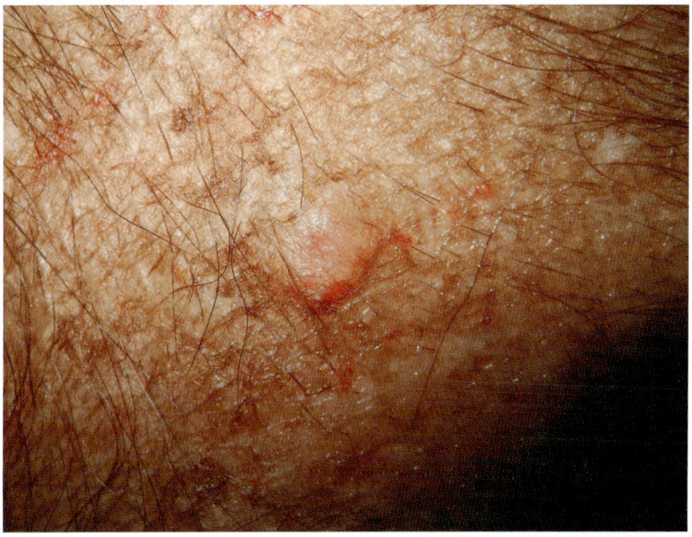

■ **Fig. 41.3.** Single firm and excoriated plaque of amyloidosis on the ventrum of an 11-year-old male-castrate Labrador retriever with pemphigus erythematosus.

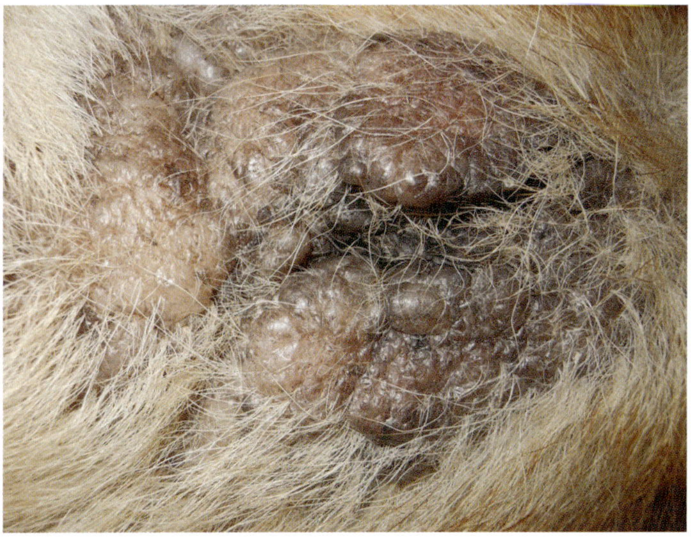

■ **Fig. 41.4.** Irregularly surfaced plaque consisting of multiple fluid-filled bubbles on the ventrum of an adult female-spayed Chinese shar-pei with cutaneous mucinosis.

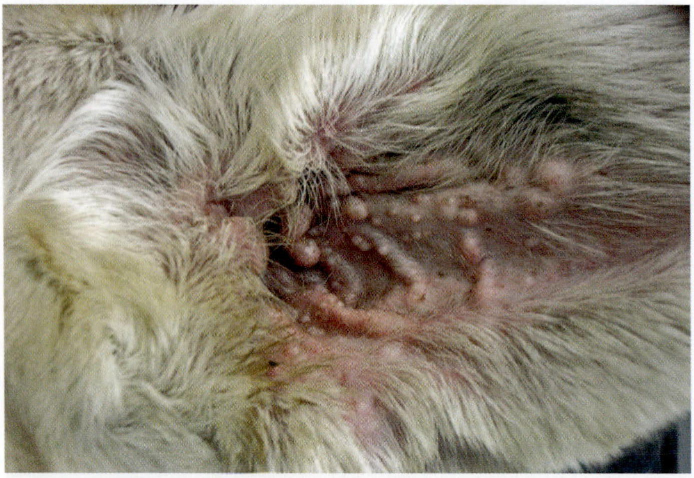

■ **Fig. 41.5.** Multiple firm nodular on the concave surface of the pinna of an 8-year-old male-castrate Labrador retriever with multiple collagenous nevi (nodule dermatofibrosis).

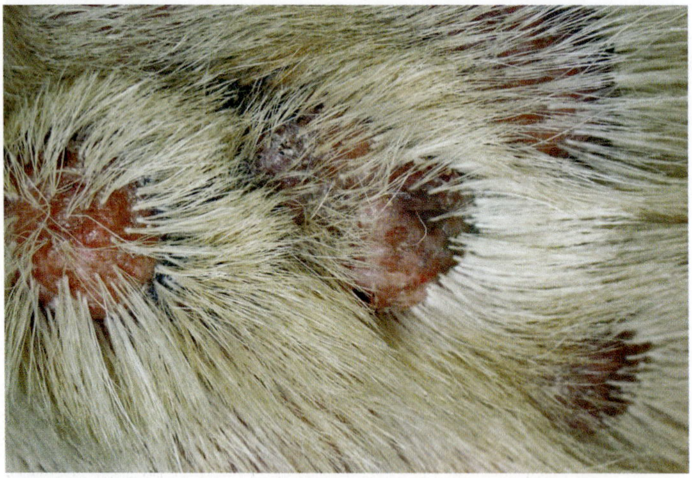

■ **Fig. 41.6.** Additional example of firm nodules affecting the patient in Figure 41.5.

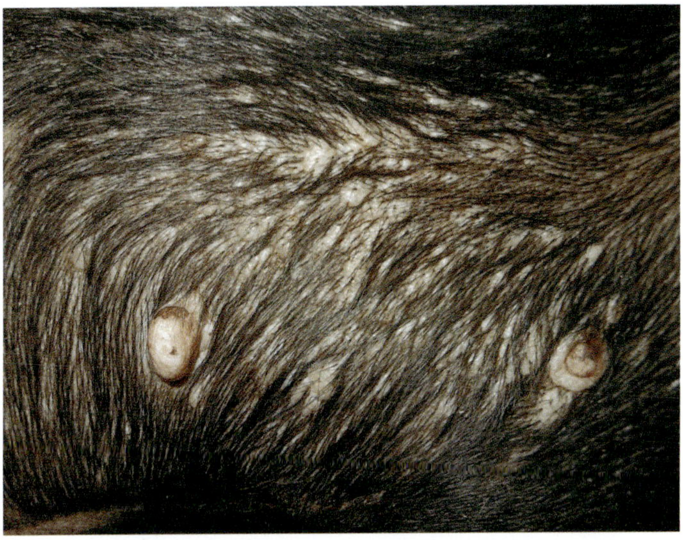

■ **Fig. 41.7.** Multiple firm nodules of collagenous nevi on the ventrum of a 4-year-old female-spayed dachshund.

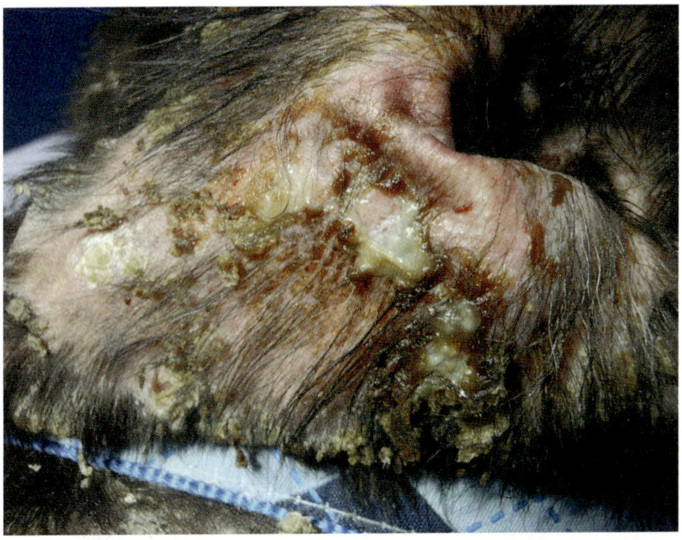

■ **Fig. 41.8.** Thickly crusted, exudative lesions on the pinna of an 11-year-old male-castrate Newfoundland-labrador retriever mix with paraneoplastic pemphigus. The patient was diagnosed with a splenic hemangiosarcoma.

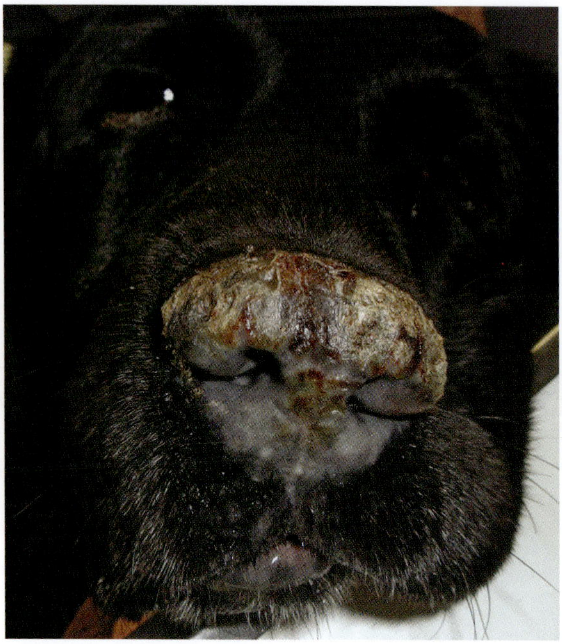

■ **Fig. 41.9.** Depigmented nasal planum with adherent crusts over erosions due to paraneoplastic pemphigus. An undetermined thoracic tumor was identified in this patient on radiographs.

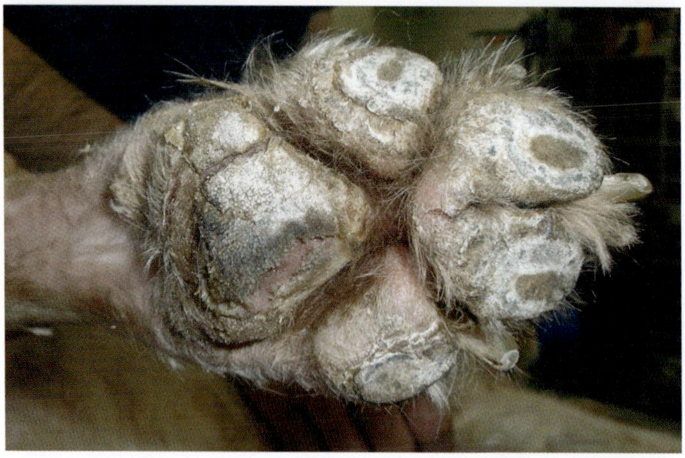

■ **Fig. 41.10.** Superficial necrolytic dermatitis producing thickly crusted footpads with fissures affecting a 6-year-old female-spayed mix-breed dog.

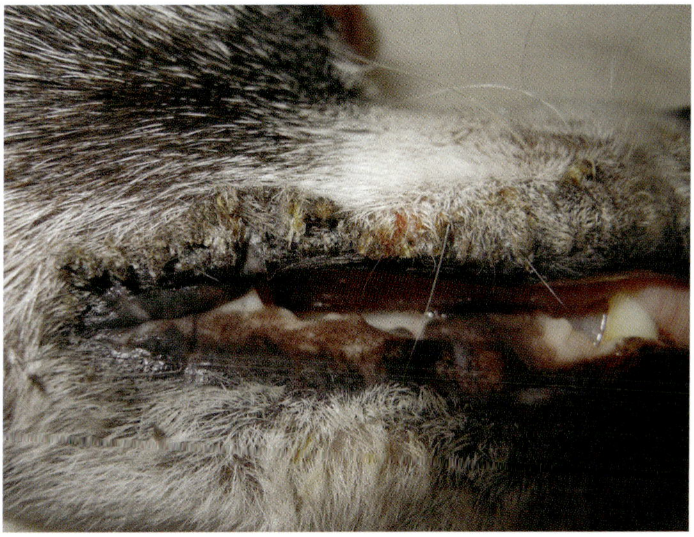

Fig. 41.11. Crusted and inflamed lip margins of an adult male-castrate chihuahua mix dog with superficial necrolytic dermatitis and hyperadrenocortisolism.

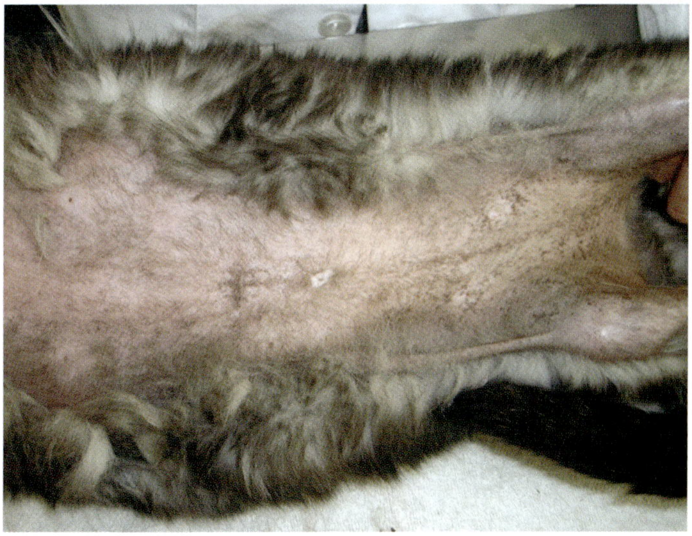

Fig. 41.12. Severe alopecia with accumulations of brown exudate on the entire ventrum and medial thighs of an 11-year-old male-castrate DLH with paraneoplastic alopecia.

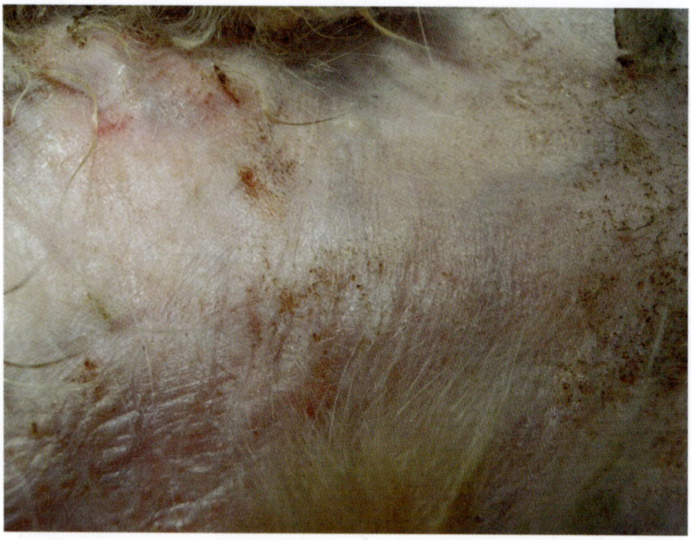

■ **Fig. 41.13.** Alopecia with thin and "glistening" skin on the ventral abdomen due to paraneoplastic alopecia in an 11-year-old female-spayed DSH.

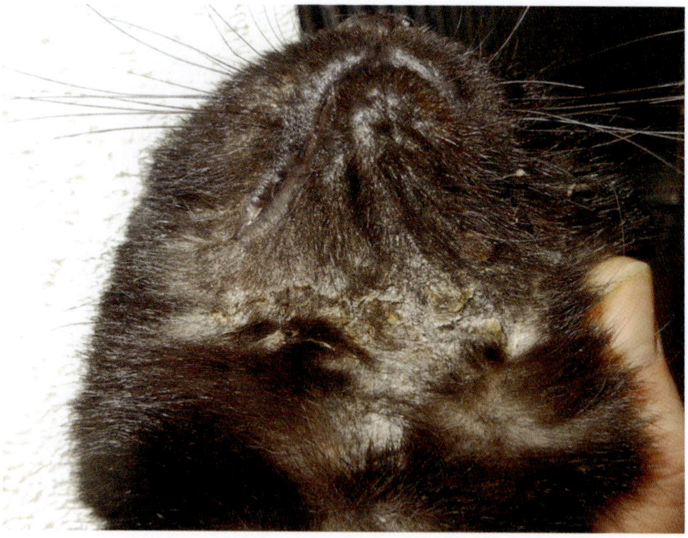

■ **Fig. 41.14.** Accumulations of brown adherent crusts on the chin and lip margins of a 12-year-old female-spayed DSH with exfoliative dermatitis associated with thymoma.

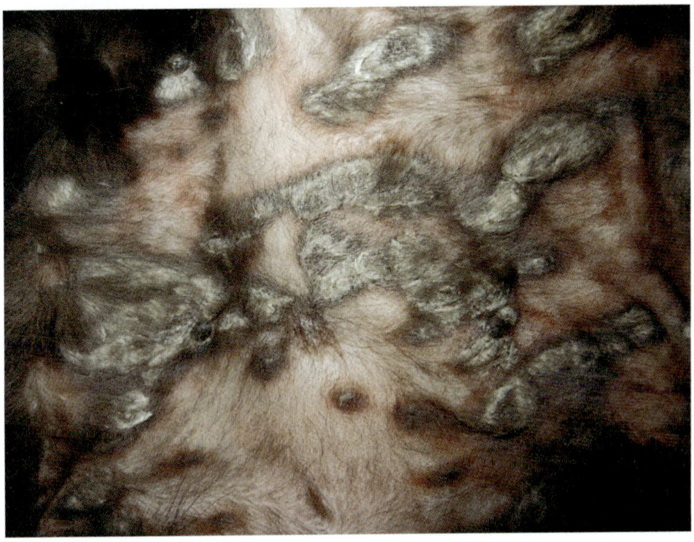

Fig. 41.15. Examples of lesions on the ventrum of the patient in Figure 41.14. There are marked thickly crusted and erythematous patches and plaques affecting most of the body.

chapter 42

Sarcoptid Mites

DEFINITION/OVERVIEW

- Nonseasonal, intensely pruritic, highly contagious parasitic skin diseases of dogs and cats caused by infestation with sarcoptid mites.

ETIOLOGY/PATHOPHYSIOLOGY

- *Sarcoptes scabiei* var. *canis*: dogs – sarcoptic mange/scabies (Figures 42.1, 42.2).
- *Notoedres cati:* cats – notoedric mange (Figures 42.3, 42.4).
- *Cheyletiella yasguri*: dogs – "walking dandruff" (Figure 42.5).
- *Cheyletiella blakei:* cats – "walking dandruff."
- *Otodectes cynotis*: dogs and cats – ear mites (Figure 42.6).
- *Sarcoptes scabiei* and *Notoedres cati*: mites burrow through the stratum corneum and cause intense pruritus by mechanical irritation, production of irritating by-products, and secretion of allergenic substances that produce both antibody- and cell-mediated immune reactions.
- *Cheyletiella* spp.: live in the upper epidermis between follicles; piercing mouthparts cause mechanical irritation; pruritus significantly increases with development of hypersensitivity.
- *Otodectes cynotis:* do not burrow; entire life cycle occurs within the external ear canal; feed on epidermal debris; irritation and later development of hypersensitivity cause accumulation of cerumen and blood within the ear canal; can produce "ectopic" symptoms at other body sites; associated with 50–80% of otitis externa in cats.
- Life cycle for all mites may be completed in as few as 21 days.
- Mites can transiently affect species other than the host species (dog, cat, fox, rabbit, human) via direct contact; lack of host specificity may affect treatment requirements.
- Considered highly contagious within the host species.
- Zoonosis: mites can burrow and survive for limited periods on humans.

SIGNALMENT/HISTORY

- Animals of all ages and breeds; most often seen in younger animals.
- Exposure to a carrier often 2–6 weeks before development of symptoms.

Blackwell's Five-Minute Veterinary Consult Clinical Companion: Small Animal Dermatology, Third Edition.
Karen Helton Rhodes and Alexander H. Werner.

- Nonseasonal extremely intense pruritus.
- Zoonosis: pruritic papular dermatitis affecting in-contact humans.
- Sources of exposure:
    - Catteries and multiple cat households
    - Living outside
    - Kennels
    - Veterinary offices
    - Groomers
    - Animal shelters.

CLINICAL FEATURES

- *Sarcoptes scabiei* infestation:
    - Alopecia and erythematous rash: pinnal margins, elbows, hocks, ventral abdomen, and chest (Figures 42.7–42.9).
    - Lesions on pinnal margins and elbows: vary from barely perceptible scaling to alopecia or thick crusts; ear canals not affected.
    - Chronic: periocular and truncal alopecia; thick secondary crusts, excoriations, and secondary bacterial folliculitis; diffuse papular eruption.
    - Possible peripheral lymphadenopathy.
    - Frequently bathed dogs will often have chronic pruritus with minimal skin lesions ("scabies incognito").
    - Often minimal or no response to antiinflammatory doses of steroids.
    - Multiple dog households: more than one dog typically pruritic; asymptomatic carriers rare.
- *Notoedres cati* infestation:
    - Intense pruritus with thick adherent crusting dermatitis
    - Areas most affected include the pinnae, head, face, neck and forelegs; may generalize from grooming behavior (Figures 42.10–42.12)
    - Peripheral lymphadenopathy is common
    - Cats may become anorexic and emaciated if left untreated.
- *Cheyletiella* spp. infestation:
    - Characterized by excessive scaling and variable pruritus (Figures 42.13, 42.14)
    - "Walking dandruff" due to large mite size: mites may be visible without magnification
    - Cocker spaniels, poodles, long-haired cats, and rabbits may be asymptomatic carriers
    - Young animals most at risk
    - Dorsal orientation of scale with minimal erythema is a common initial symptom
    - Some cats may exhibit bilateral and symmetric alopecia.
- *Otodectes cynotis* infestation:
    - Pruritus and resultant excoriation usually located around the ears, head, and neck; may generalize
    - Thick, red-brown or black crusts within and around the ear canal (Figure 42.15).

DIFFERENTIAL DIAGNOSIS

- Cutaneous adverse reaction to food
- Atopic dermatitis
- *Malassezia* dermatitis
- Flea-allergic dermatitis
- Dermatophytosis
- Pyoderma
- Demodicosis
- Contact allergy
- Pelodera dermatitis
- Pruritic impetigo
- Otitis externa/media
- Pediculosis
- Seborrhea

DIAGNOSTICS

- ELISA technique: identify *Sarcoptes* mite-infested dogs; detection of circulating IgG antibodies against *Sarcoptes* antigens; seroconversion 2–5 weeks after exposure; high false-positive results in dogs previously treated for scabies mites and false-negative results in young dogs and those receiving corticosteroids; not widely used.
- Positive pinnal-pedal reflex: rubbing the ear margin between the thumb and forefinger induces scratching with the ipsilateral hindleg; occurs in 75–90% of cases of scabies, notoedres, and otodectes; not diagnostic.
- Superficial skin scrapings:
    - Technique (also see Chapter 5):
        - ☐ Apply a small amount of mineral oil directly onto the selected lesional skin
        - ☐ Scrape the area in the direction of hair growth and transfer accumulated material to the glass slide
        - ☐ Select several sites for sampling and sample a large surface area; preferred sites include pinnal margins and lateral forelegs just proximal to the elbow
        - ☐ Finding mite eggs or feces is diagnostic of infestation
    - *Sarcoptes scabiei:* may be difficult to demonstrate; positive in less than 50% of scrapings
    - *Notoedres cati:* large number of mites easily demonstrated in scrapings.
- Touch tape prep and "flea combing" for collection of epidermal debris: *Cheyletiella* spp. (Figure 42.16).
- Ear swab in mineral oil: *Otodectes cynotis.*
- Fecal flotation: occasionally reveals mites or ova.
- Diagnosis inferred by favorable response to a "therapeutic trial" for suspect cases with negative skin scrapings.
- Dogs with nonseasonal pruritus that respond poorly to steroids should be treated with a scabicide (even if skin scrape results are negative) to definitively rule out sarcoptic mange.

THERAPEUTICS

- Scabicidal rinses: the entire dog must be treated; treatment failures often linked to owner's reluctance to apply rinse to the patient's face and ears; swimming and bathing are prohibited between treatments.
- *Cheyletiella* spp. and *Otodectes cynotis*: all in-contact dogs, cats, rabbits should be treated, even those with no clinical signs; asymptomatic carriers possible.
- *Sarcoptes scabiei* and *Notoedres cati*: all in-contact dogs or cats (respectively) should be treated, even those with no clinical signs; asymptomatic carriers possible.
- Thoroughly clean and treat the environment; mites can survive for up to 3 weeks off a host animal (depending on species, temperature, and humidity).
- Corticosteroids may be used concurrently with miticidal therapy; immunomodulatory drugs administered without miticidal therapy (prior to diagnosis) may cause increased pruritus and be associated with a higher rate of positive skin scrapings.

Therapeutic Options

- Avermectins:
    - Macrocyclic lactone with GABA agonist activity
    - Ivermectin: 0.2–0.4 mg/kg PO or by subcutaneous injection every 1–2 weeks for 4 treatments:
        - Systemic use contraindicated in collies, Shetland sheepdogs, Australian shepherds, Old English sheepdogs, white German shepherds, long-haired whippets, greyhounds, silken windhound, other herding breeds, and crosses with these breeds; sensitivity derived from a deletion mutation of the multidrug-resistant gene (*ABCB1*); see demodicosis treatment
        - Toxicity seen as hypersalivation, mydriasis, tremors, depression, ataxia, blindness
        - Intravenous lipid emulsion therapy has shown success in the treatment of ivermectin toxicosis
        - Do not use with Spinosad-containing flea control products; enhances toxicity of ivermectin
    - Ivermectin topical: *Otodectes cynotis*
    - Selamectin: 6–12 mg/kg applied topically every 2 weeks for 3–4 treatments (dogs and cats)
    - Moxidectin: 200 mg/kg PO or by subcutaneous injection every 2 weeks for two treatments
    - Imidacloprid 10% with moxidectin 1% topical: applied monthly for two treatments; *Otodectes cynotis*
    - Milbemycin: 0.75 mg/kg PO q24h or 2 mg/kg PO weekly for 3–4 treatments (dogs)
    - Milbemycin 0.1% topical: *Otodectes cynotis*
    - Doramectin: 0.2–25 mg/kg PO or by subcutaneous injection weekly for two treatments.

- Isoxazolines:
  - Selective inhibitor of arthropod GABA and L-glutamate-gated chloride channels
  - Off-label use; number of treatments required undetermined
  - Well tolerated; adverse effects include transient vomiting or diarrhea, and anorexia
  - Afoxalaner 2.5 mg/kg every 4 weeks; approved for use in dogs over 1.8 kg and over 8 weeks of age for flea/tick control; use with caution in patients with a history of seizures
  - Fluralaner 25 mg/kg every 12 weeks; approved for use in dogs over 2 kg and over 6 months of age for flea/tick control
  - Sarolaner 2 mg/kg every 4 weeks; approved for use in dogs over 1.4 kg and over 6 months of age for flea/tick control
- Fipronil spray or spot-on: applied monthly for 1–2 treatments; *Cheyletiella* spp.
- Amitraz (Mitaban) dip: 250 ppm; every 1–2 weeks for three treatments; treat entire body including the face and ears (dogs).
- Lime sulfur: 2–4% solution of lime sulfur; apply weekly for 4–6 weeks; treat entire body including face and ears (dogs and cats).
- Topical antiseborrheic shampoo therapy in conjunction with scabicidal agent helps speed clinical resolution.
- Systemic antibiotics: may be needed for 21 days or longer to resolve any secondary bacterial folliculitis.
- Low-dose glucocorticoids: prednisolone 0.5 mg/kg BID for first week of treatment then tapered dosage in conjunction with miticidal therapy; beneficial in resolving pruritus.

COMMENTS

- Bedding should be disposed of and the environment thoroughly cleaned and treated with parasiticidal sprays/foggers/bombs (flea insecticides for the environment are often effective).
- Intense pruritus and clinical signs should resolve within 4–6 weeks after initiation of treatment.
- Reinfection can occur if contact with infected animals continues.
- Sarcoptid mite infestation should be considered for pruritus of unknown origin as well as in previously controlled allergic patients with sudden and poorly responsive flaring of symptoms.
- Approximately 30% of dogs with sarcoptid mite infestations will also react to house dust mite antigens on intradermal skin testing.
- Humans in close contact with an affected animal may develop a pruritic, papular rash on their arms, chest, or abdomen; human lesions are usually transient and should resolve spontaneously after the affected animal has been treated; if lesions persist, clients should seek advice from their physician for appropriate therapy (Figure 42.17).

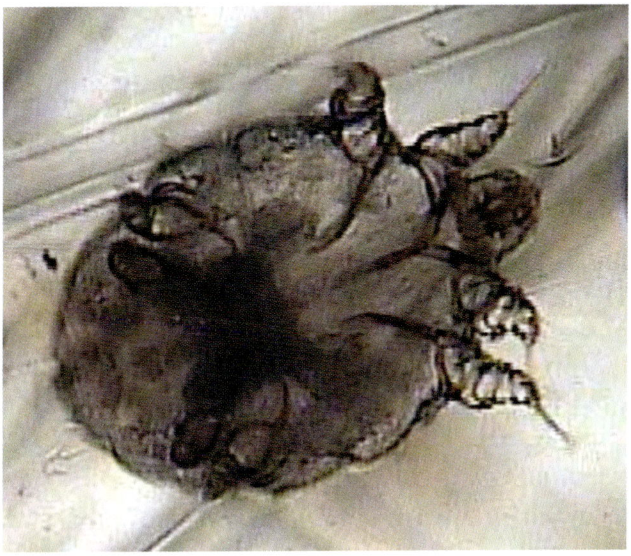

■ **Fig. 42.1.** *Sarcoptes scabiei* var. *canis* from scrapings of an infested dog.

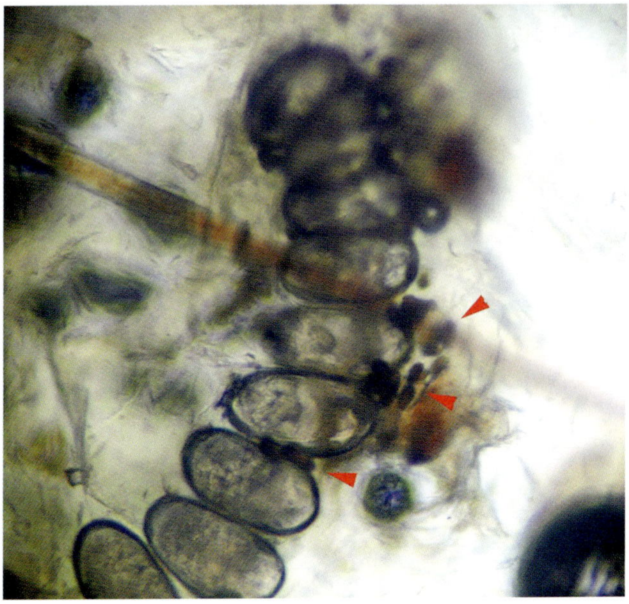

■ **Fig. 42.2.** *Sarcoptes scabiei* eggs are produced in a linear pattern as the female mite burrows through the epidermis. Arrowheads indicate mite feces.

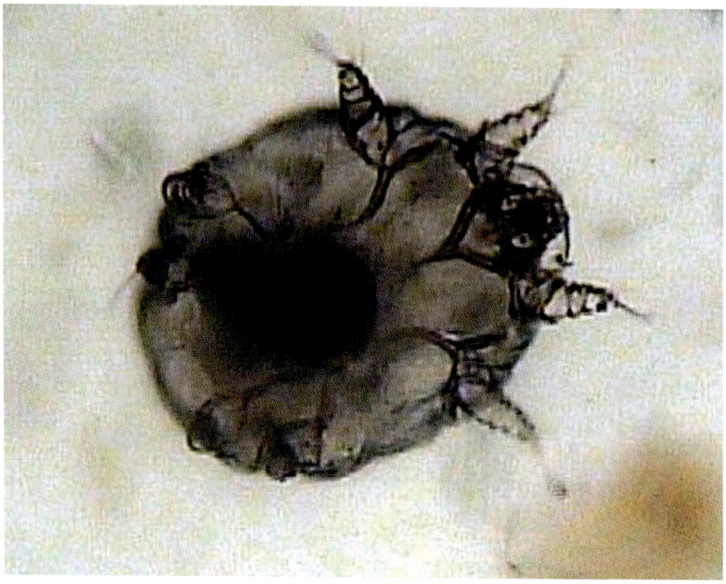

■ **Fig. 42.3.** *Notoedres cati* mite from scrapings of the cat in Figure 42.11.

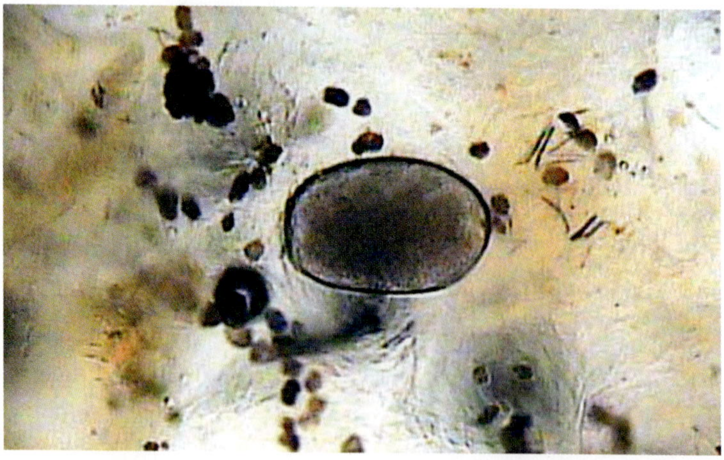

■ **Fig. 42.4.** Eggs and feces of *Notoedres cati* from the patient in Figure 42.11.

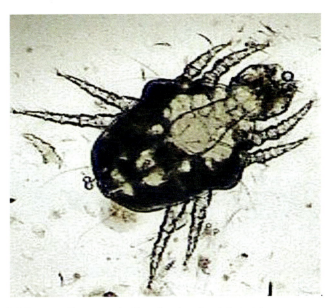

■ **Fig. 42.5.** *Cheyletiella yasguri* from examination of scales of an infested dog.

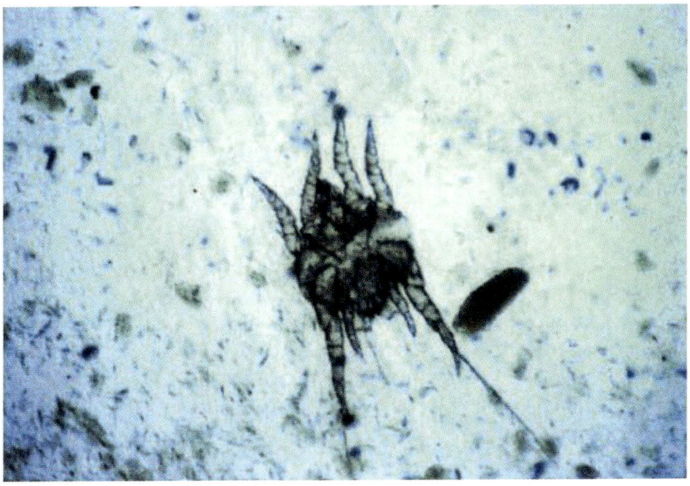

■ **Fig. 42.6.** *Otodectes cynotis* mite from the external ear canal.

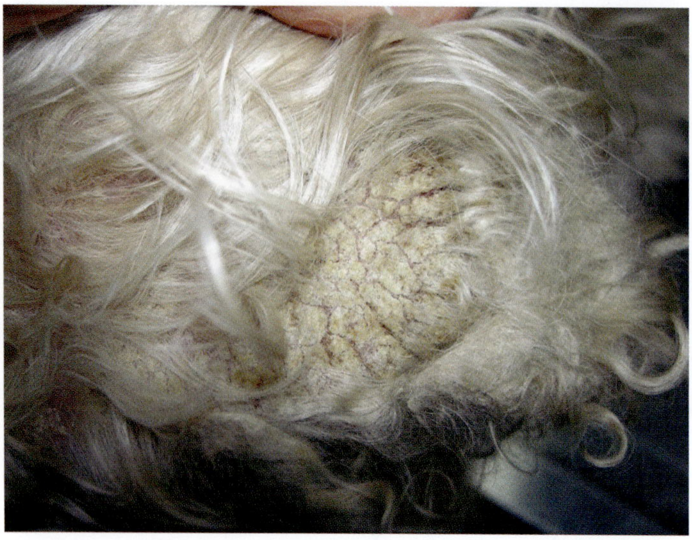

■ **Fig. 42.7.** Accumulations of thick crusts on the pinnal margin of an 8-year-old female-spayed cocker spaniel with severe and chronic scabies.

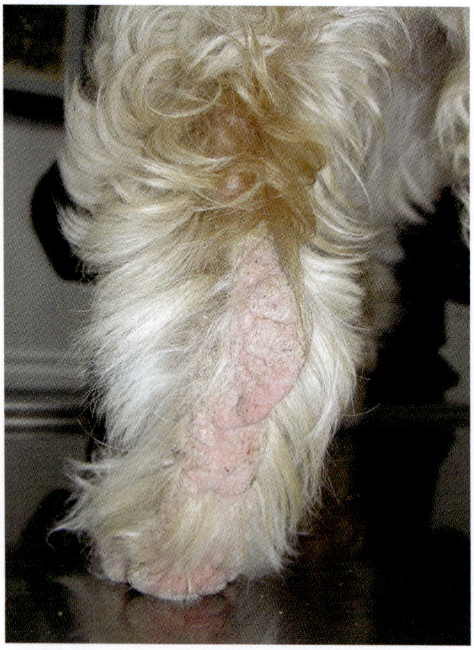

■ **Fig. 42.8.** Caudal aspect of left rear leg of the patient in Figure 42.7. Pruritus and chronic inflammation have caused lichenification and accumulations of crusts in alopecic areas.

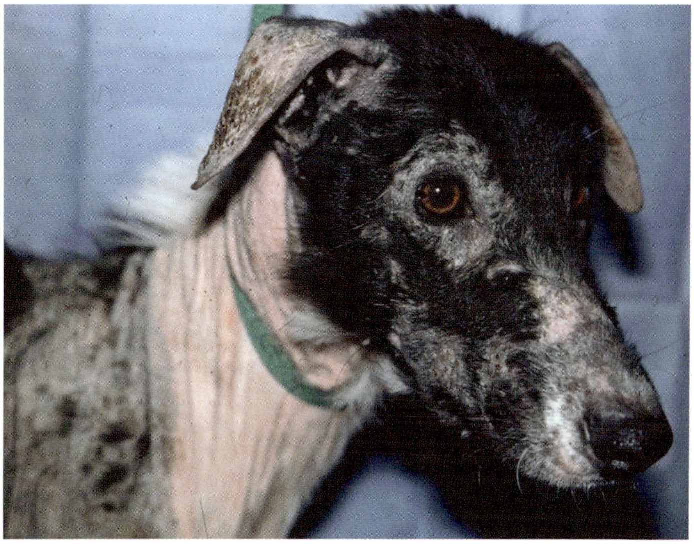

■ **Fig. 42.9.** Generalized alopecia with lichenification and crusting in a young dog with scabies.

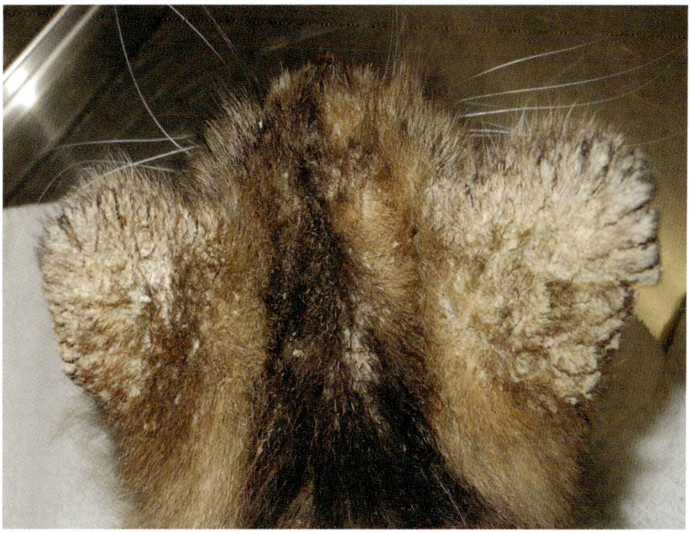

■ **Fig. 42.10.** Accumulations of crusts on the pinnae and head of an 8-year-old female-spayed DLH with *Notoedres cati* infestation.

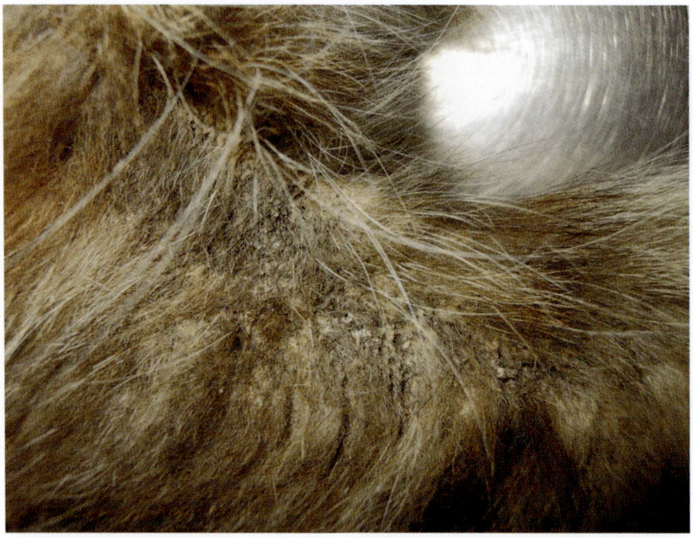

■ **Fig. 42.11.** Patient in Figure 42.10 with accumulations of thick crusts on the foreleg.

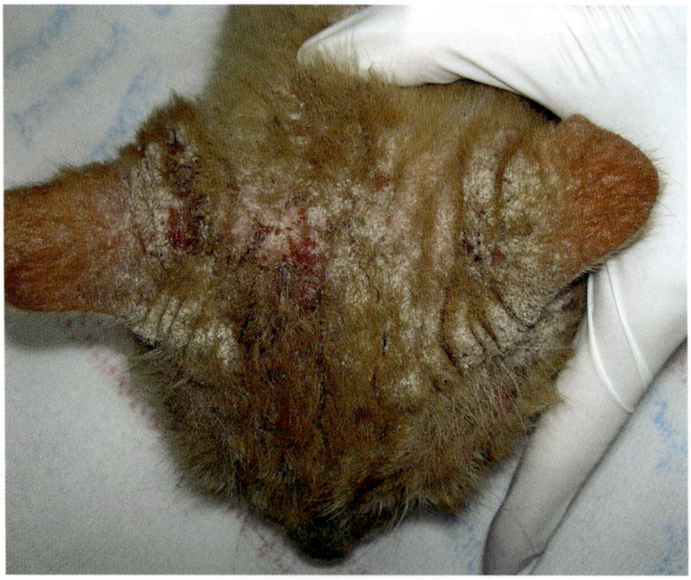

■ **Fig. 42.12.** Accumulations of crusts on the head and pinnae of an adult DSH with severe *Notoedres cati* infestation. Note lichenification and excoriations from severe pruritus.

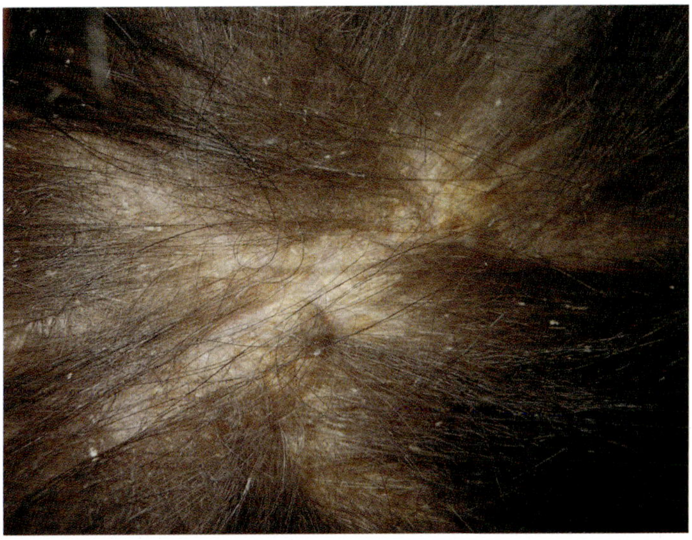

■ **Fig. 42.13.** Cheyletiellosis in a 6-year-old female-spayed Australian shepherd. Thick yellow crusts and scales are noted attached to the epidermis through the parted hair coat.

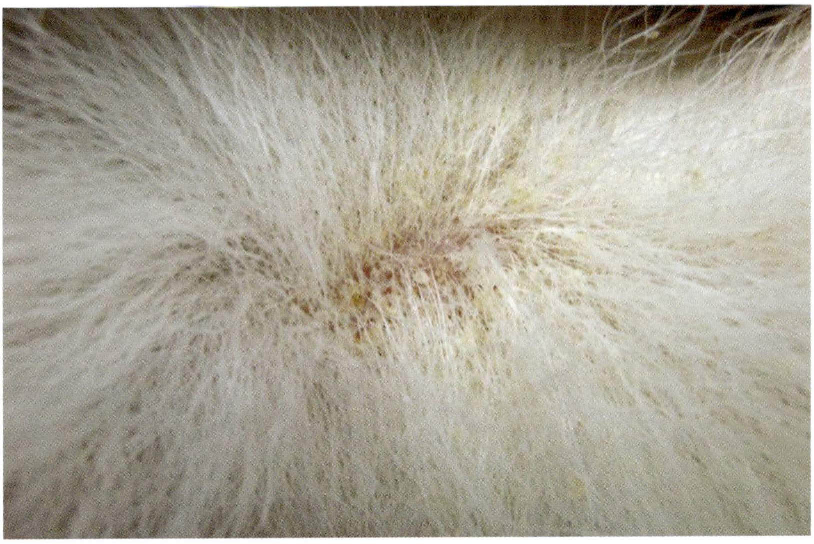

■ **Fig. 42.14.** Adherent yellow crusts deep in the hair coat attached to the skin in a 14-year-old female-spayed pug with cheyletiellosis.

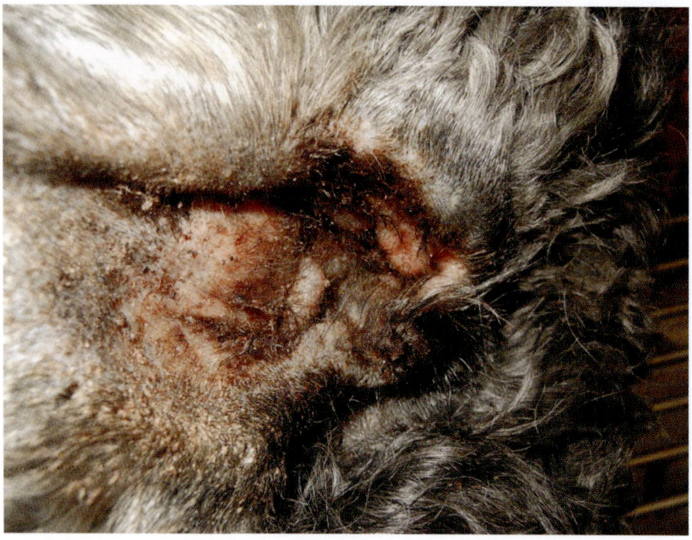

■ **Fig. 42.15.** Coffee-ground, dark brown, crumbling exudate characteristic of *Otodectes cynotis* infestation in the external ear canal of a 2-year-old female-spayed Kerry blue terrier.

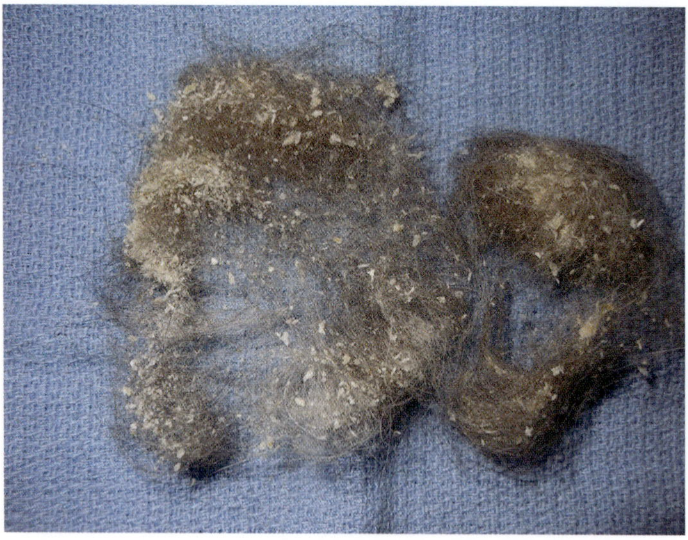

■ **Fig. 42.16.** Example of the scales removed for examination by combing through the hair coat of the patient in Figure 42.13 with cheyletiellosis.

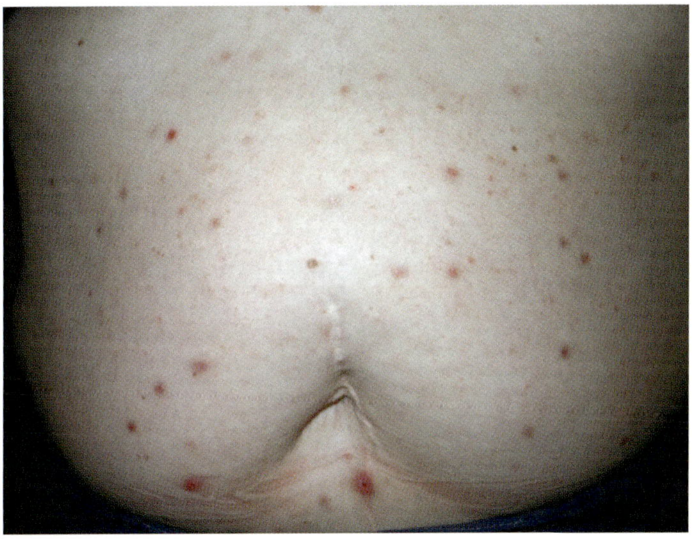

■ **Fig. 42.17.** Pruritic and erythematous papular rash on the abdomen of a human caused by contact with a *Sarcoptes scabiei*-infested dog.

chapter 43

Sebaceous Adenitis, Granulomatous

DEFINITION/OVERVIEW

- An inflammatory disease process directed against the sebaceous glands (cutaneous holocrine adnexal structures).

ETIOLOGY/PATHOPHYSIOLOGY

- Idiopathic.
- Genetic: inherited/congenital sebaceous gland destruction: autosomal recessive mode of inheritance in standard poodle and Akita.
- Immune mediated: cell-mediated reaction to a component of the sebaceous gland.
- Metabolic: initial defect may be a keratinization disorder or an abnormality in lipid metabolism leading to accumulation of toxic intermediate metabolites and sebaceous gland destruction.

SIGNALMENT/HISTORY

- Young adult to middle-aged dogs.
- Male predilection possible.
- Two forms (predisposed breeds):
    - Long-coated: standard poodle, samoyed, Akita, German shepherd, hovawart, havanese, Lhasa apsos,
    - Short-coated: vizsla, beagle, miniature pinscher.
- Seen in many purebreds as well as cross-bred dogs.
- Rare in cats.

CLINICAL FEATURES

Long-Coated Dog Breeds

- Lesions first observed along dorsal midline and dorsum of the head.
- Change in hair color (especially poodles or due to adherent scales) (Figures 43.1, 43.2).

Blackwell's Five-Minute Veterinary Consult Clinical Companion: Small Animal Dermatology, Third Edition.
Karen Helton Rhodes and Alexander H. Werner.

- Change in hair from wavy to straight (Figure 43.3).
- Symmetric, partial to diffuse alopecia (Figures 43.4–43.6).
- Dull brittle hair.
- Follicular casts: hairs with tightly adherent silver-white scale (keratin collaring) (Figures 43.7, 43.8); often first observed along dorsal midline and head.
- Tufts of matted hair; loss of hair and matted hair with scale on the tail give the appearance of a rat tail.
- Secondary bacterial folliculitis, pruritus, and malodor (Figure 43.9).

Short-Coated Dog Breeds

- Alopecia: "moth-eaten" pattern of coalescing circular to serpiginous lesions.
- Lesions may be erythematous.
- Scaling: fine and adherent.
- Affects the trunk, head, and pinnae (Figures 43.10–43.14).
- Secondary bacterial folliculitis rare.

Cats

- Initial lesions on the head and pinnae; may become generalized.
- Hypotrichosis progressing to alopecia and scaling.
- Black waxy debris noted along the eyelid margins, nasal folds, perioral.
- Secondary bacterial folliculitis.

DIFFERENTIAL DIAGNOSIS

- Primary keratinization disorder
- Bacterial folliculitis
- Demodicosis
- Dermatophytosis
- Endocrine skin disease
- Ichthyosis
- Follicular dysplasia
- Epitheliotropic lymphoma
- Feline specific differentials: mural infiltrative folliculitis, feline exfoliative dermatitis, pseudopelade, paraneoplastic syndrome (thymoma-associated exfoliative dermatitis).

DIAGNOSTICS

- Skin scrapings: normal.
- Dermatophyte culture: negative.
- Endocrine function tests: normal.
- Skin biopsies are diagnostic.

Pathologic Findings

- Nodular granulomatous to pyogranulomatous inflammatory reaction at the level of the sebaceous glands (isthmus region of hair follicles).
- Orthokeratotic hyperkeratosis and follicular cast formation; more prominent in long-coated breeds.
- Advanced: complete loss of sebaceous glands; perifollicular granulomas and fibrosis.
- Destruction of entire hair follicle and adnexal unit rare.

THERAPEUTICS

- Clinical signs may wax and wane irrespective of treatment.
- Response may depend on severity of disease at the time of diagnosis; early diagnosis and initiation of treatment prevents complete loss of sebaceous glands.
- Akita: often more refractory to treatment; develop more severe secondary bacterial folliculitis.

Drugs of Choice: Topical Therapy

- Antibacterial and/or keratolytic shampoo: bathe once to twice weekly; follow with conditioner or propylene glycol spray.
- Propylene glycol: (1:1 with water); humectant; attracts water into the stratum corneum: apply lightly daily or as a prebathing treatment to soften scale.
- Baby oil: occlusive emollient; prevents transepidermal water loss; apply as a prebathing aid in removal of adherent scale.
- Topical fatty acid spot-on containing essential oils, smoothing and purifying agents, vitamin E, and a bio-diffusing vector (Dermoscent Essential-6 spot-on, LCDA, France).
- Topical products containing novasomes, spherulites, and/or phytosphingosine: slow release augments emollients to increase epidermal hydration.

Drugs of Choice: Systemic Therapy

- Cyclosporine 5 mg/kg PO BID: often best therapeutic option, may cause vomiting, diarrhea, gingival hyperplasia, hirsutism, papillomatous skin lesions, increased incidence of infections, nephrotoxicity (rare), and hepatotoxicity (infrequent).
- Cycline antibiotics: tetracycline 250 mg PO TID for dogs <10 kg; 500 mg PO TID dogs >10 kg); doxycycline 10 mg/kg PO q24h; minocycline 5 mg/kg PO BID; often administered with niacinamide 250 mg PO for dogs <10 kg and 500 mg PO for dogs >10 kg.
- Isotretinoin 1–3 mg/kg PO BID initial dose: reduce to 1 mg/kg q24h after 1 month and taper further and maintain as needed; teratogenic, may cause keratoconjunctivitis, gastrointestinal signs, hepatotoxicity.
- Pentoxifylline 10 mg/kg PO BID to TID.
- Essential fatty acid supplementation: reduces transepidermal water loss; may be supplemented directly or by feeding diets formulated for joint mobility.

- Vitamin A: 1000 IU/kg q24h; do not use with retinoids.
- Bactericidal antibiotics (e.g., cephalexin 22 mg/kg PO BID).

COMMENTS

- Urge owners to register affected dogs so that mode of inheritance can be determined.
- Sebaceous glands are not able to regenerate after complete destruction; lifelong therapy is necessary to help remove excess scaling and replace lost sebum.
- Hair regrowth is variable and is frequently a different texture from the original hair coat (i.e., loss of curl in poodles).

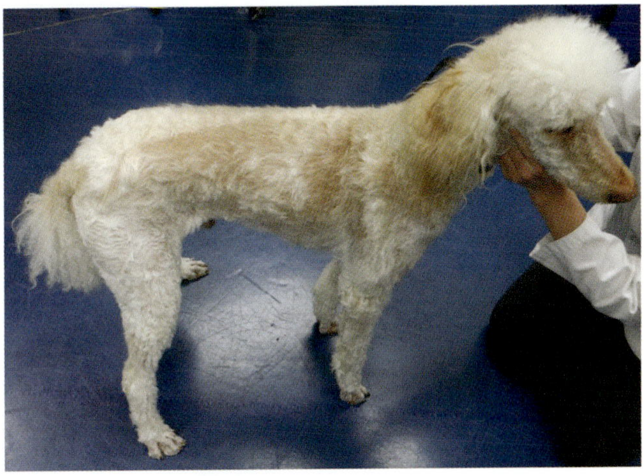

Fig. 43.1. Initial signs of sebaceous adenitis in a 9-year-old male-castrate standard poodle seen as darkening of the hair coat on the body and pinnae.

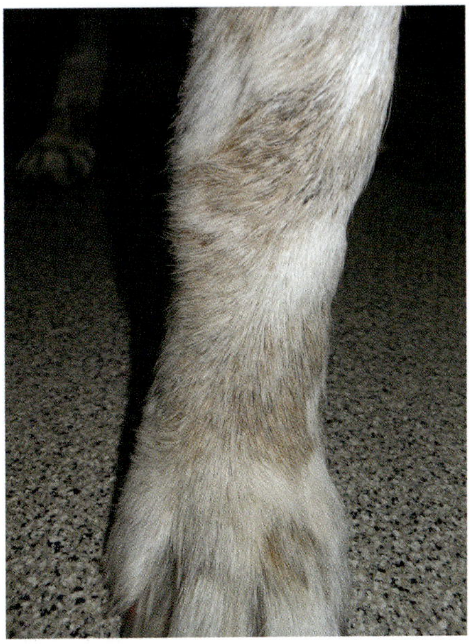

Fig. 43.2. Adherent scales causing a darkened appearance of the hair coat on the foreleg of a 9-year-old female-spayed Akita with sebaceous adenitis.

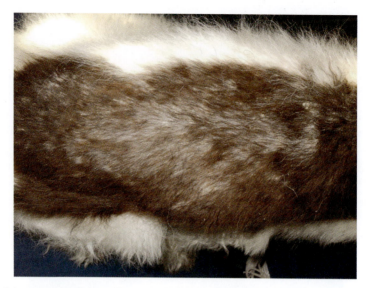

■ **Fig. 43.3.** Sebaceous adenitis in an 18-month-old female-spayed standard poodle causing the normally curly hair coat to become straightened, thin, and scaly.

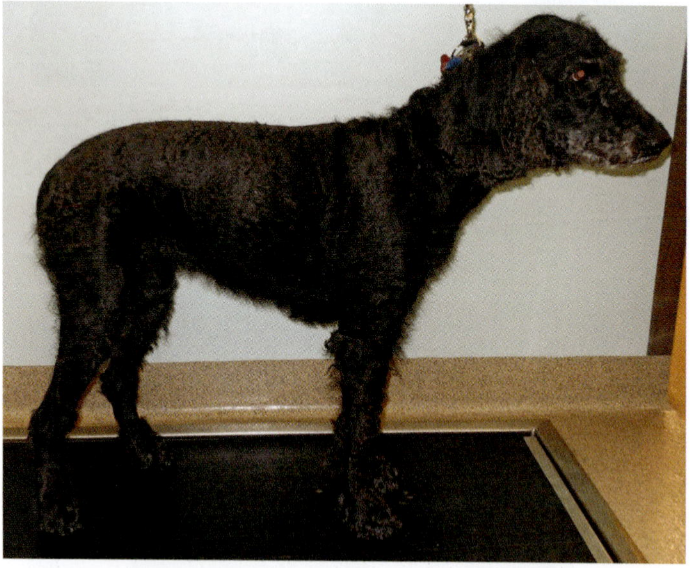

■ **Fig. 43.4.** Generalized thinning and straightening of the hair coat with sebaceous adenitis. Changes in this 9-year-old female-spayed standard poodle are most evident on the pinnae and truncal region (hair coat has not been clipped).

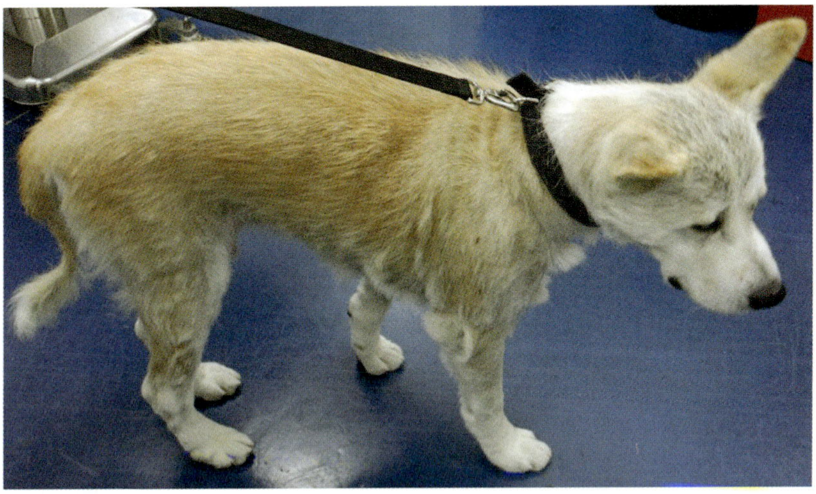

■ **Fig. 43.5.** Sebaceous adenitis in a 7-year-old male-castrate Akita the hair coat is thin and excessively brittle.

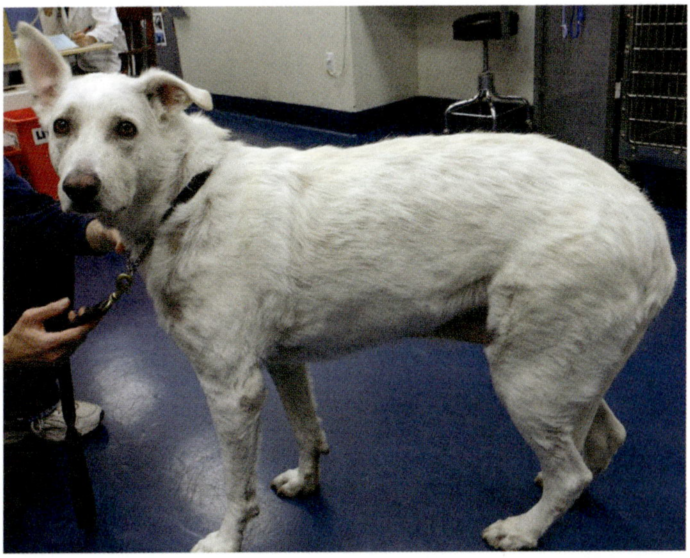

■ **Fig. 43.6.** Generalized thinning of the hair coat with patches of crusts in a 3-year-old male-castrate German shepherd with sebaceous adenitis.

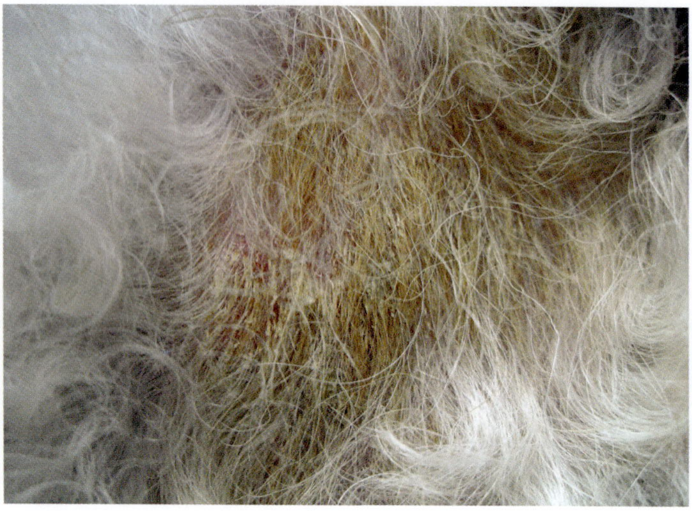

■ **Fig. 43.7.** Keratin collaring: the hairs of this 18-month-old female-spayed standard poodle appear "glued together" by keratin adherence.

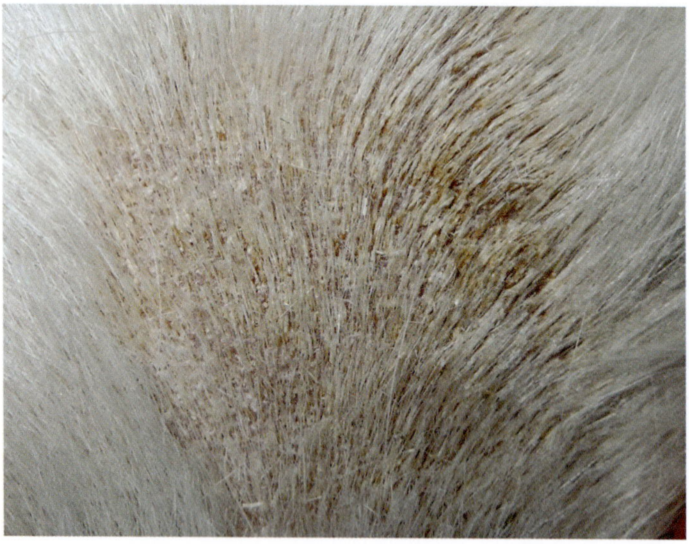

■ **Fig. 43.8.** Keratin collaring: shortened hairs have firm and adherent follicular casts in this 4-year-old male-castrate maltipoo with sebaceous adenitis.

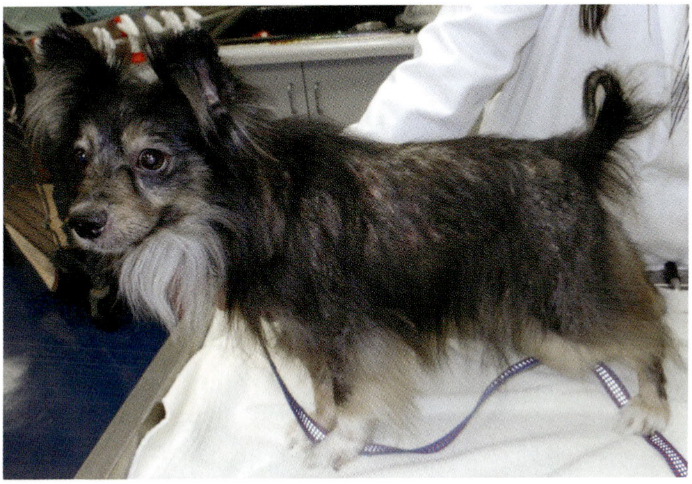

■ **Fig. 43.9.** Bacterial folliculitis secondary to sebaceous adenitis seen as truncal and head alopecia with erythema and crusting in a 4-year-old male-castrate pomeranian mix with sebaceous adenitis.

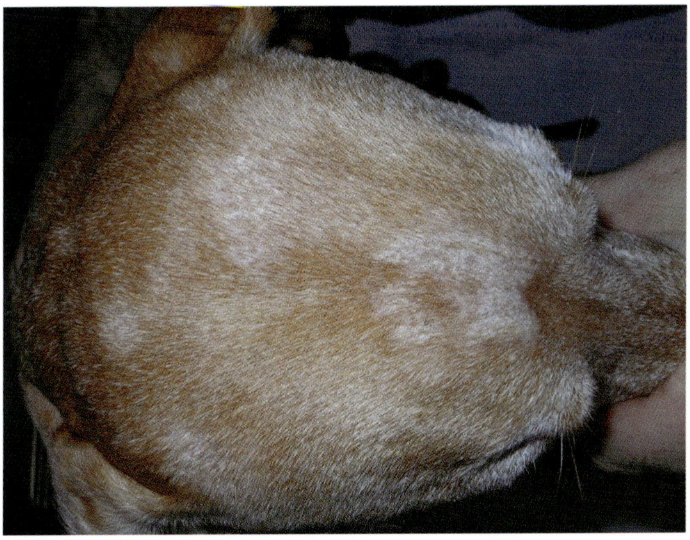

■ **Fig. 43.10.** Erythematous, coalescing, and circular lesions with alopecia and fine scales characteristic of sebaceous adenitis on the head of an 8-year-old male-castrate vizsla.

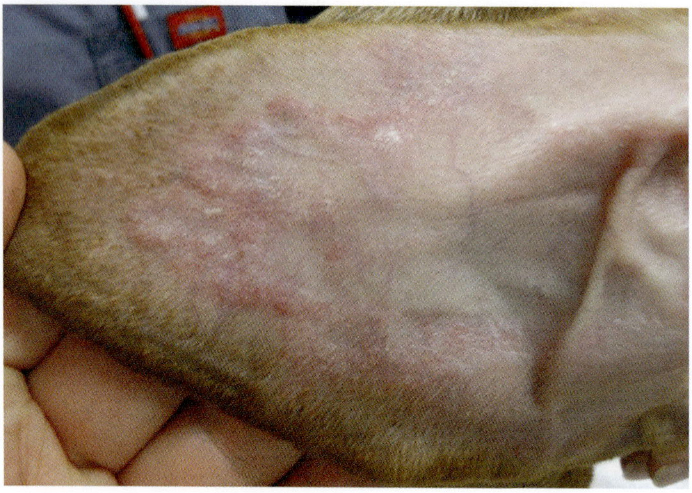

■ **Fig. 43.11.** Concave aspect of the pinna of the patient in Figure 43.10 with multiple coalescing papules and fine adherent scale.

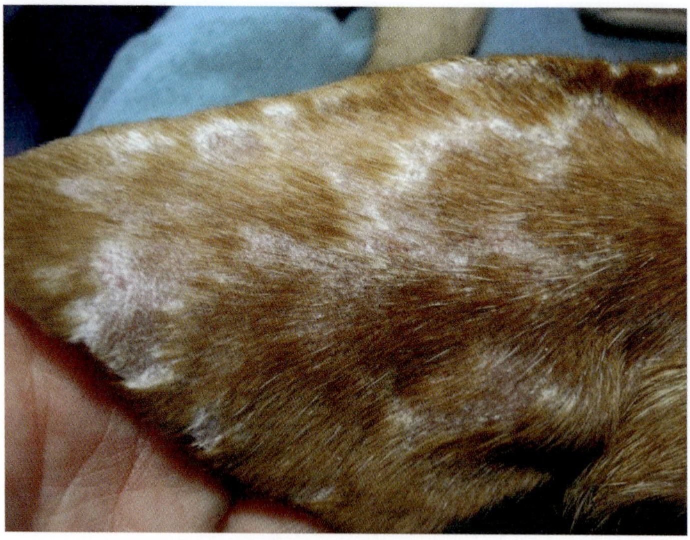

■ **Fig. 43.12.** Characteristic lesions of sebaceous adenitis in short-coated breeds, with alopecic and coalescing patches of dermatitis affecting the pinna of a 9-year-old male-castrate vizsla.

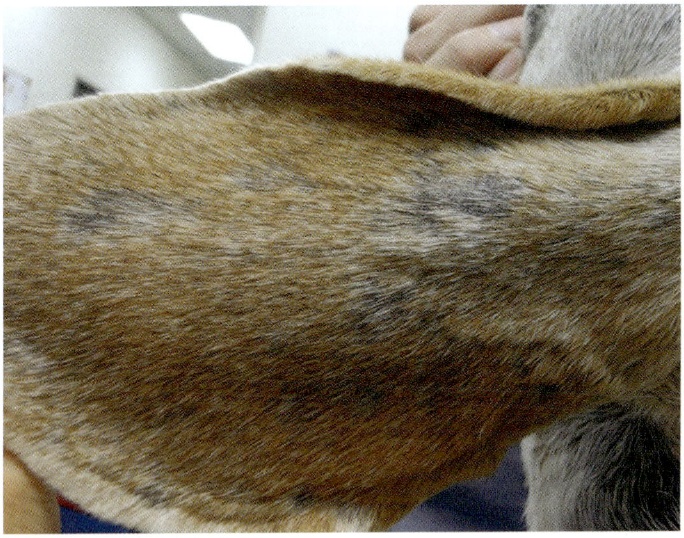

Fig. 43.13. Sebaceous adenitis causing lesions on the pinna of a 9-year-old female-spayed beagle similar to those of the patient in Figure 43.12.

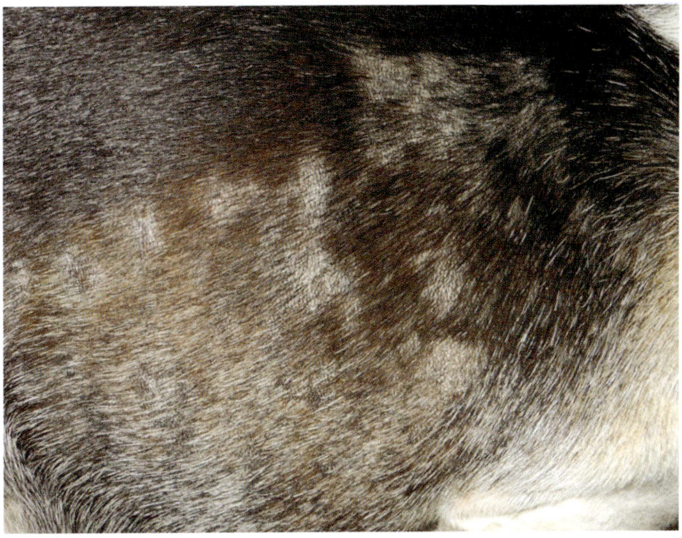

Fig. 43.14. Truncal lesions of sebaceous adenitis on the patient in Figure 43.13.

chapter 44

Sporotrichosis

DEFINITION/OVERVIEW

- Zoonotic fungal disease affecting the skin and lymphatics; may become systemic.

ETIOLOGY/PATHOPHYSIOLOGY

- *Sporothrix* spp. are saprophytes in soil, decomposing plants, peat moss, rose thorns, and wood.
- Disease caused by direct inoculation into subcutaneous tissues of the thermally dimorphic fungus with conversion from mycelial form to yeast form in mammalian tissues.
- Described on all continents: most prevalent serotype differs by geographic location.
- *S. schenckii* is a cryptic species with a high level of intraspecific DNA variability, leading to two or more species having been originally classified as a single species.
- Pathogenic serotypes within the *Sporothrix* complex include *S. brasiliensis*, *S. schenckii sensu stricto*, *S. globosa*, *S. mexicana*, and *S. luriei*.
- Lesions in cats typically contain high fungal loads: yeast forms scarce in human and canine lesions.
- Cats may be subclinical carriers as well as being the main zoonotic disseminators of *Sporothrix* infection.
- Cellular immunity is involved in disease resolution – severe systemic disease and high fungal load are associated with increased expression of $CD8^+$ cells; localized, organized control of disease and low fungal load are associated with increased expression of $CD4^+$ cells (cats); recent studies correlate $CD8^+$ release and subsequent activation (by inflammasomes/caspase-1) of IL-1-beta with severity of lesions.
- Disease manifestation is dependent on species virulence; independent of coinfection with feline retroviruses.

SIGNALMENT/HISTORY

Causes and Risk Factors

- Dogs: hunting dogs from puncture wounds associated with thorns or splinters.

Blackwell's Five-Minute Veterinary Consult Clinical Companion: Small Animal Dermatology, Third Edition.
Karen Helton Rhodes and Alexander H. Werner.

- Cats: male-intact outdoor or stray cats innoculated from claws and teeth during fights.
- Exposure to soil rich in decaying organic debris; increased prevalence in tropical and subtropical zones.
- Exposure to infected animals or clinically healthy cats sharing a household with an affected cat.
- Immunosuppression is a risk factor for development of disseminated disease.
- *CAUTION* – zoonotic disease: proper precautions should be taken to prevent infection; a break in the skin is not required for transmission; disease has become endemic in some areas.

CLINICAL FEATURES

- Cutaneous form – dogs: multiple firm nodules or plaques that may crust or ulcerate and drain; typically affecting the head or trunk.
- Cutaneous form – cats: multiple ulcerating nodules to lesions that appear initially as nonhealing wounds or abscesses mimicking wounds associated with fighting; typically affecting the head, lumbar region, or distal limbs (Figures 44.1–44.3).
- Cutaneolymphatic form: extension of the cutaneous form through the lymphatics resulting in the formation of new nodules that frequently ulcerate to form draining tracts or crusts; lymphadenopathy is common.
- Disseminated form: systemic signs of malaise and fever.

DIFFERENTIAL DIAGNOSIS

- Infectious: bacterial and fungal diseases presenting with nodules and draining tracts (e.g., cryptococcosis, blastomycosis, feline leprosy, histoplasmosis).
- Other causes of granulomatous to pyogranulomatous dermatitis (e.g., foreign body, panniculitis).
- Neoplasia.
- Deep bacterial infection.

DIAGNOSTICS

- Cytology of exudates: cigar- to round-shaped yeast found intracellularly or free in the exudate; organisms are generally plentiful in cat lesions but scarce in dogs (Figures 44.4, 44.5).
- Biopsy: organisms usually numerous, especially in cats; fungal stains (PAS or GMS) may aid in the diagnosis; the absence of demonstrable organisms in tissues from dogs does not preclude diagnosis (Figures 44.6, 44.7).
- Cultures: samples obtained from deep within draining tracts.
- *CAUTION* – zoonotic disease; laboratory personnel must be warned of the potential differential diagnosis; cultures should not be attempted until other differential diagnoses have been eliminated.

THERAPEUTICS

- The zoonotic nature of sporotrichosis must be considered when treating an animal with this disease; outpatient therapy increases the potential for human exposure; human infection has been reported without history of an injury or wound.
- Sensitivity testing is particularly difficult due to the dimorphic nature of *Sporothrix* spp. as well as a lack of standardization for testing methods; geographic differences in sensitivity have been reported; the broth microdilution assay is most often utilized.

Drugs of Choice

- Supersaturated solution of potassium iodide (SSKI: potassium iodide oral solution):
  - Dogs: 40 mg/kg PO BID with food
  - Cats: initial dosage 2.5 mg/kg PO q24h with food, increasing every 5 days until clinical remission or toxicity is noted; final dosage typically 10–20 mg/kg
  - Treatment continued for at least 30 days after resolution of the clinical lesions; typical treatment length 2 months
  - Discontinue treatment for 1 week if signs of iodism are noted; reinstitute at a lower dosage and increase in increments of 2.5 mg/kg to the highest dosage that does not cause signs of iodism
  - Signs of iodism:
    - Dogs: dry or scaly hair coat, nasal or ocular discharge, inappetance or vomiting, depression or collapse; if symptoms are severe or recurrent, other drugs should be considered
    - Cat: depression, vomiting, anorexia, twitching, hypothermia, or cardiovascular collapse.
- Imidazole and triazole antifungals:
  - Dogs:
    - Ketoconazole 5–15 mg/kg PO BID: side effects (mild) include anorexia, vomiting
    - Itraconazole 5–10 mg/kg PO q24h or divided BID: side effects (uncommon) include hepatotoxicity (elevated ALT), vasculitis
    - Posaconazole 5–10 mg/kg PO q24h or divided BID: side effects include anorexia, vomiting, hepatotoxicity
  - Cats:
    - Ketoconazole 5–10 mg/kg PO q24h: side effects (common) include anorexia, vomiting, depression, fever, hepatotoxicity, neurologic disturbances
    - Itraconazole 5–15 mg/kg PO q24h or divided BID: side effects (uncommon) include anorexia, vomiting, depression, hepatotoxicity
    - Posaconazole 5–7.5 mg/kg PO q24h or divided BID: side effects include anorexia, vomiting, hepatotoxicity, facial pruritus
  - Treatment continued for at least 30 days after resolution of the clinical lesions; typical treatment length 3 months.

- Terbinafine:
  - Dogs 30 mg/kg PO BID to TID: side effects include anorexia, vomiting, diarrhea, hepatopathy
  - Cats 30 mg/kg PO q24h: side effects include lethargy, facial pruritus; may be combined with itraconazole.
- Cryotherapy: treatment of individual cutaneous lesions in conjunction with oral antifungal therapy.
- Amphotericin B:
  - AMB/desoxycholate or L-AMB/lipid formulations
  - Dogs: AMB 0.5 mg/kg IV over 4–6h or L-AMB 1–3 mg/kg IV over 2h; three times/week; fluid diuresis recommended
  - Cats: AMB 0.25 mg/kg IV over 4–6h or L-AMB 1 mg/kg IV over 2h; three times/week; fluid diuresis recommended
  - AMB may be administered subcutaneously with 300–500 mL sodium chloride 0.45%/dextrose 2.5%.

COMMENTS

Patient Monitoring/Prognosis

- Reevaluations, including serum chemistries, are recommended every 2–4 weeks to monitor clinical signs and side effects associated with treatment.
- Guarded prognosis: clinical cure reported in 28.6–47.9% of patients.

Zoonotic Potential

- *CAUTION*: this is a zoonotic disease and proper precautions should be taken to prevent infection.
- Client education is of paramount importance.
- An absence of a break in the skin does not protect against the disease.
- Zoonotic transmission from bites and scratches from rodents, parrots, cats, dogs, horses, and armadillos has been reported.
- Clinically healthy cats sharing a household with an infected cat may be a source of infection.

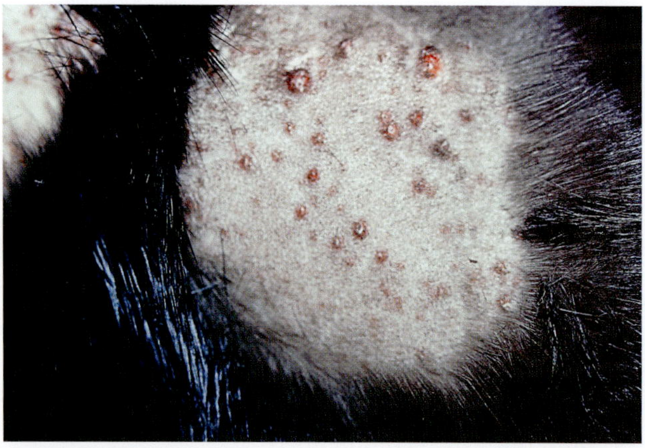

■ **Fig. 44.1.** Multiple firm and ulcerated nodules of sporotrichosis affecting a 5-year-old female-spayed DSH.

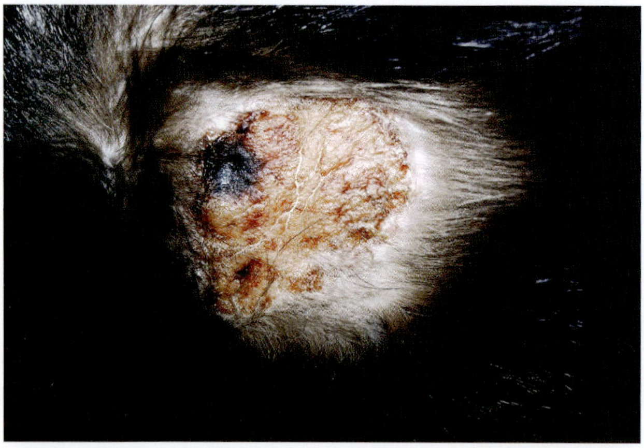

■ **Fig. 44.2.** Large ulcerated plaque on the lateral thorax of the patient in Figure 44.1.

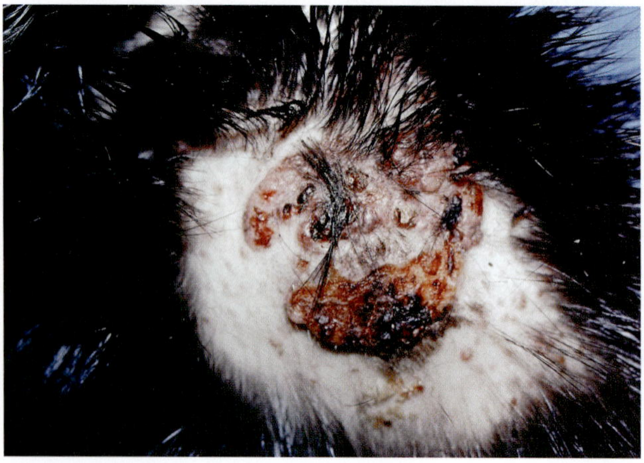

■ **Fig. 44.3.** Eroded plaques on the dorsum of the patient in Figure 44.1.

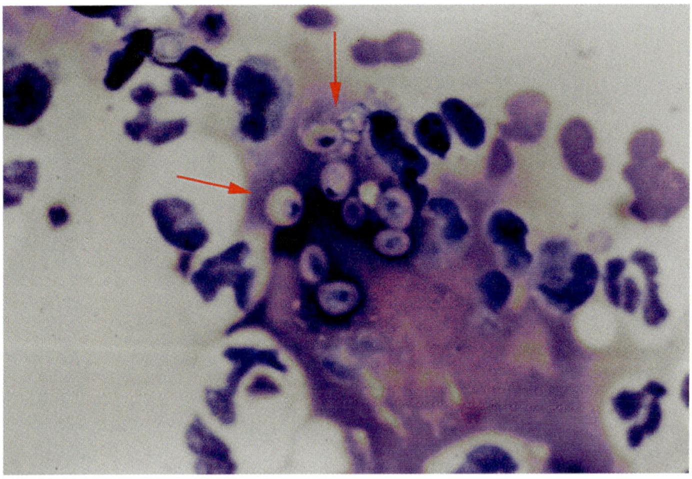

Fig. 44.4. Exudate from lesions of sporotrichosis demonstrating pleomorphic yeast (*red arrows*) and neutrophils.

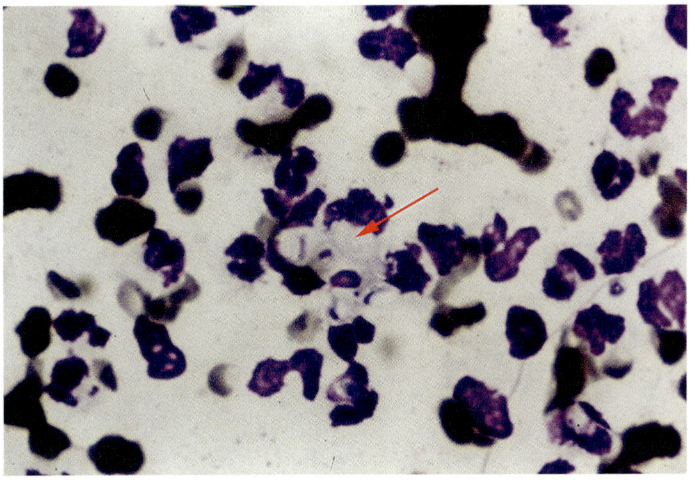

Fig. 44.5. Additional image of cytology from a lesion of sporotrichosis demonstrating the pleomorphic nature of the yeast (*red arrow*).

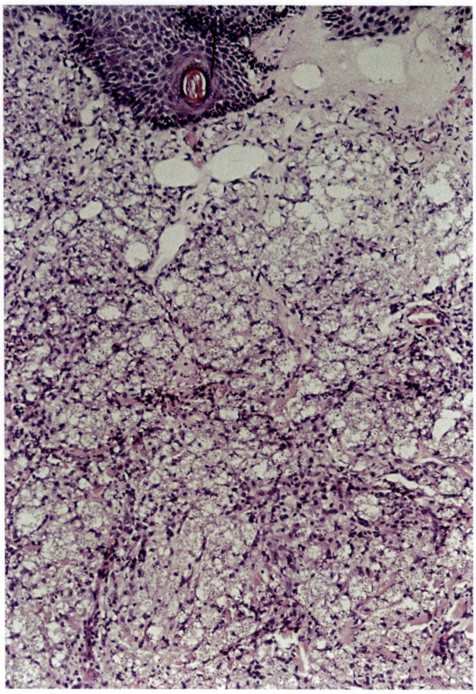

■ **Fig. 44.6.** Histologic image (hematoxylin and eosin) obtained from lesion biopsy of sporotrichosis. Epidermis is located at the top of the image; there is a diffuse granulomatous and suppurative dermatitis with numerous fungal organisms.

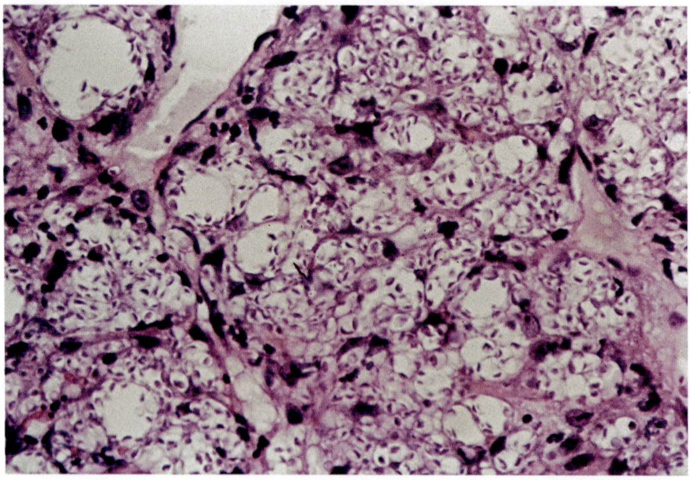

■ **Fig. 44.7.** Higher magnification image of the histologic tissue in Figure 44.6. Numerous pleomorphic yeast organisms are present within the dermis.

chapter 45

Superficial Necrolytic Dermatitis

DEFINITION/OVERVIEW

- Synonyms: hepatocutaneous syndrome; necrolytic migratory erythema; metabolic epidermal necrosis.
- Complex, progressive, and usually fatal disorder affecting the skin and liver (and rarely pancreas).
- Necrotizing dermatitis resulting from cutaneous nutritional deprivation.
- Predominantly associated with hepatic disorder; rarely with glucagonoma.

ETIOLOGY/PATHOPHYSIOLOGY

- Hypoaminoacidemia: amino acids involved in the urea cycle and synthesis of glutathione or collagen are those predominantly measured as low.
- Metabolic hepatopathy (not cirrhosis) resulting in increased hepatic catabolism of amino acids proposed; variable high serum bile acids concentrations.
- Predominantly associated with severe vacuolar hepatopathy:
  - Rarely associated with phenobarbital or phenytoin administration
  - Rarely associated with severe hepatic insult; mycotoxin
  - Rarely associated with glucagon-secreting pancreatic or extrapancreatic neoplasia; these cases do not exhibit signs of hepatopathy.
- Occurs with or without diabetes mellitus; development of diabetes mellitus may be an indicator of disease progression and worsening prognosis.
- Hypoaminoacidemia, with or without deficiencies in zinc, essential fatty acids, or other nutrients.
- Clinical symptoms produced by keratinocyte degeneration from cellular starvation or nutritional imbalance.
- Resolution by excision of a glucagon-secreting pancreatic tumor reported.
- Symptoms temporarily relieved by intravenous infusions of amino acid solutions.
- Associated with secondary bacterial follicultis and *Malassezia* dermatitis.
- Feline cases very rare; most often associated with neoplasia (pancreatic carcinoma, intestinal lymphoma) and hepatopathy.

Blackwell's Five-Minute Veterinary Consult Clinical Companion: Small Animal Dermatology, Third Edition.
Karen Helton Rhodes and Alexander H. Werner.

SIGNALMENT/HISTORY

- Primarily old dogs; mean age 10 years; rare in cats.
- Males overrepresented.
- May have a heritable component in some breeds (shih tzu).
- Predilection for medium and small breeds: West Highland white terrier, Scottish terrier, American cocker spaniel, Shetland sheepdog, Lhasa apso, border collie; syndrome also identified in large breeds.
- Cutaneous lesions often precede systemic symptoms.

CLINICAL FEATURES

- Progressive development of erythema, hyperkeratosis, and exudation at the margins of the footpads (Figure 45.1).
- Crusting, ulcerative, and painful dermatitis (Figures 45.2, 45.3).
- Lesions affect the mucocutaneous junctions of lips, eyes, and anus; develop at the same time as or immediately following footpad lesions (Figure 45.4).
- Skin lesions also pronounced in areas of trauma: muzzle, distal limbs, elbows, footpads (Figure 45.5).
- Fissuring and severe crusting of footpads result in pruritus and pain.
- Hyperpigmentation and lichenification common with chronicity.
- Secondary bacterial folliculitis and *Malassezia* dermatitis common.
- Lesions develop on pressure points, pinnae, and external genitalia.
- Dermatitis often precedes systemic symptoms by weeks.
- Systemic signs include lethargy, polyuria, polydipsia (when associated with diabetes mellitus), anorexia, and weight loss.
- Poor to grave prognosis.

DIFFERENTIAL DIAGNOSIS

- Pemphigus foliaceus
- Zinc-responsive dermatosis
- Systemic lupus erythematosus
- Erythema multiforme
- Drug eruption
- Generic dog food dermatosis
- Irritant contact dermatitis
- Demodicosis
- Dermatophytosis
- Vasculitis
- Epitheliotropic lymphoma

- Toxic epidermal necrolysis
- Cats: exfoliative dermatitis (thymoma associated), pancreatic paraneoplastic alopecia, epitheliotropic lymphoma, erythema multiforme, pemphigus foliaceus, FeLV- and FIV-associated dermatoses

DIAGNOSTICS

- CBC: inconsistent findings: microcytosis (40–67%), low PCV, monocytosis, thrombocytosis.
- Biochemistries:
  - Hepatic: elevated serum alkaline phosphatase, alanine aminotransferase, aspartate aminotransferase
  - Hyperglycemia
  - Elevated total bilirubin and bile acids
  - Hypoalbuminemia variable.
- Elevated plasma glucagon levels: consistently noted with glucagon-secreting pancreatic or extrapancreatic neoplasia; rarely observed with hepatopathy.
- Hypoaminoacidemia: notably glutamine, proline, cysteine, hydroxyproline.
- Urinalysis: rare ammonium biurate crystalluria; aminoaciduria – notably lysinuria, prolinuria.
- Abdominal ultrasound:
  - Pathogonomic "honeycomb" or "Swiss cheese" hepatic appearance
  - Variably sized, hypoechoic regions measuring 0.5–1.5 cm in diameter surrounded by highly echogenic borders
  - Hypoechoic regions correspond to distinct regenerative nodules (nodular hyperplasia) bounded by regions of severe parenchymal collapse.
- Lesions lack extensive fibrosis and reduced liver size usually associated with chronic cirrhosis.
- Rare pancreatic or extrapancreatic neoplasia (Figures 45.6, 45.7).
- Dermatohistopathology:
  - Distinctive "red/white/blue" pattern:
    - Parakeratosis and neutrophilic crusting
    - Pallor of epidermis above the basal layer due to intracellular and intercellular edema
    - Hyperplastic basal cell layer
  - Clefting within the epidermis
  - Mild neutrophilic superficial to perivascular dermal infiltrate
  - Marked parakeratosis with absence of epidermal pallor noted in chronic cases.
- Hepatic histopathology:
  - Vacuolar hepatopathy (not seen with pancreatic tumor)
  - Hepatocyte degeneration
  - Parenchymal collapse
  - Nodular hyperplasia.

THERAPEUTICS

- Excision of pancreatic or extrapancreatic neoplasia.
- Supportive care for systemic symptoms: appropriate management of diabetes mellitus (if present).
- Nutritional support: high-quality protein supplement; cooked whole eggs or yolks.
- Dietary supplementation of zinc 1 mg/kg PO q24h (of elemental zinc), essential fatty acids, and vitamin E 200–400 IU PO BID.
- S-adenosylmethionine 18–22 mg/kg PO q24h.
- Silymarin 1–2 mg/kg PO q24h.
- Frequent bathing and hydrotherapy to remove crusts and reduce pruritus.

Drugs of Choice

- Treatment of secondary bacterial folliculitis and/or *Malassezia* dermatitis with appropriate antimicrobials.
- Prednisolone 0.5 mg/kg q24h then taper dosage and discontinue as soon as possible: temporary relief of pruritus and inflammation; may exacerbate diabetes mellitus; may aggravate hepatopathy.
- Octreotide 2–3.2 μg/kg by subcutaneous injection BID to QID: somatostatin analog; nonresected glucagon-producing pancreatic or extrapancreatic neoplasia.
- Amino acid infusion: intravenous administration of amino acids to replenish serum levels from excessive hepatic catabolism:
    - 10% crystalline amino acid solution or 3% amino acid-electrolyte solution: 25 mL/kg over 8h
    - Initial replacement therapy twice weekly until symptoms improve
    - Maintenance infusions every 7–14 days as indicated by patient response.

COMMENTS

- Frequent monitoring of serum chemistries needed to monitor for hepatic failure and/or development of diabetes mellitus.
- Repeated treatment for secondary infection.
- Poor prognosis;
    - Worsening prognosis associated with the development of diabetes mellitus
    - Survival time typically less than 6 months post development of cutaneous lesions
    - 18% survival more than 12 months
    - Euthanasia most often due to diabetic crisis or hepatic failure.

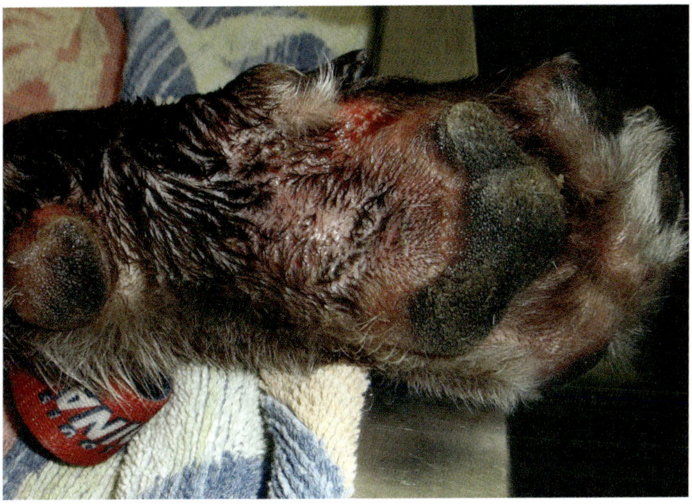

■ **Fig. 45.1.** Superficial necrolytic dermatitis-induced erythema and crusting at footpad margins of a 13-year-old female-spayed Labrador retriever mix.

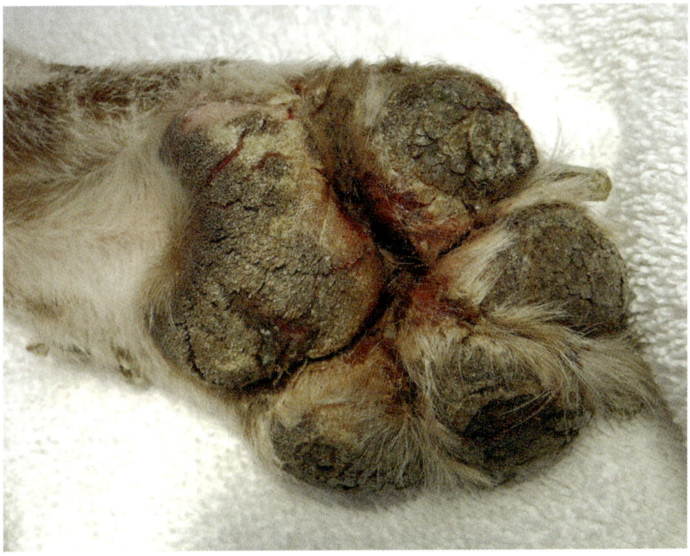

■ **Fig. 45.2.** Characteristic accumulations of crusts and interdigital inflammation of SND in an 11-year-old male-castrate beagle mix.

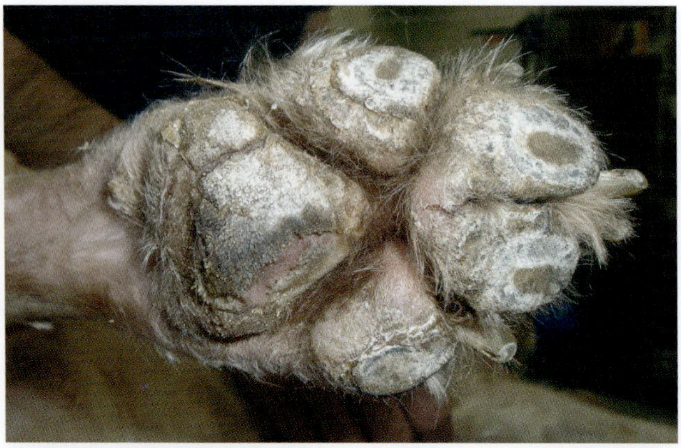

■ **Fig. 45.3.** Thick crusting of footpads similar to pemphigus foliaceus seen with superficial necrolytic dermatitis in a 6-year-old female-spayed terrier mix.

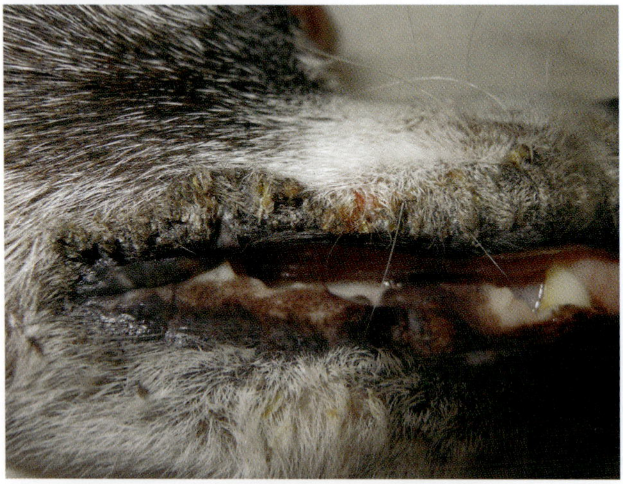

■ **Fig. 45.4.** Lip margin crusting and exudation with SND in an adult male-castrate chihuahua.

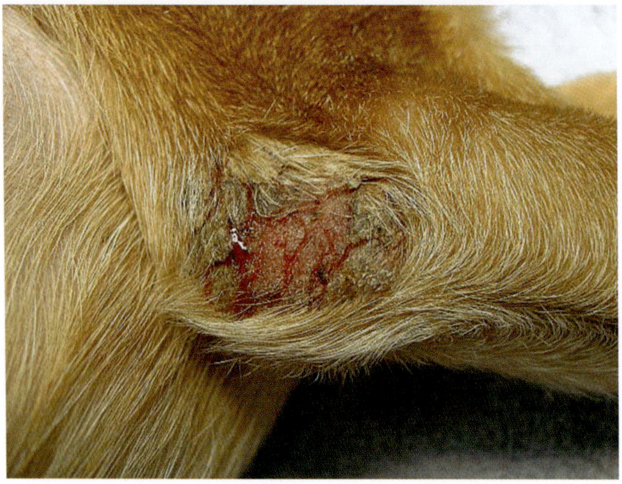

■ **Fig. 45.5.** SND in a 12-year-old male-castrate terrier mix. Note pressure point (lateral elbow) crusting, erosions, and erythema.

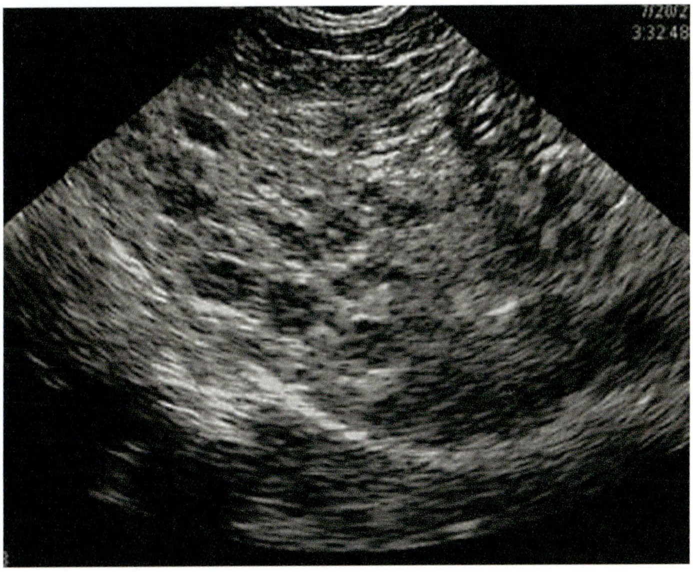

■ **Fig. 45.6.** Honeycomb hepatic appearance with SND on ultrasound.

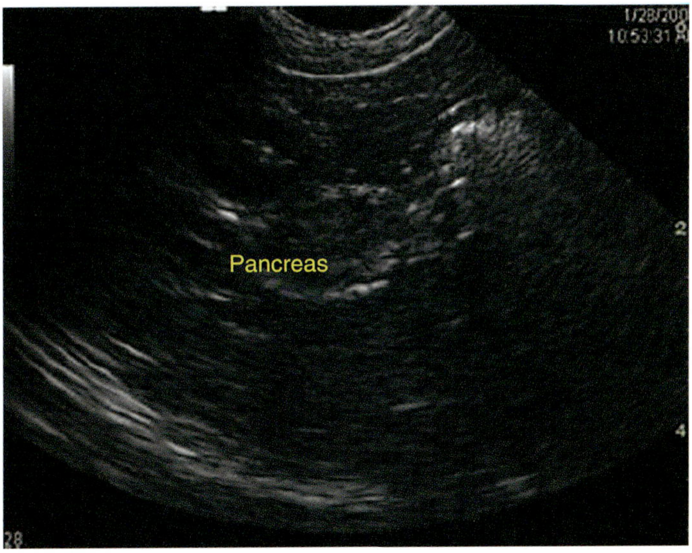

■ **Fig. 45.7.** Pancreatic nodule with SND on ultrasound.

chapter 46

Tumors, Common Skin and Hair Follicle

DEFINITION/OVERVIEW

- Skin and hair tumors are common in dogs; less common in cats.
- These neoplasms involve the epidermis, dermis, hair follicles, and adnexal structures.
- This chapter is intended as a list of the more frequent tumors arising from the skin and adnexa.

ETIOLOGY/PATHOPHYSIOLOGY

- Squamous cell carcinoma:
  - Neoplasia consisting of differentiating keratinocytes
  - May be well, moderately, or poorly differentiated; aggressiveness varies
  - Bowen's disease (Bowenoid *in situ* carcinoma, multicentric SCC *in situ*):
    - More benign form
    - Most common in the cat; occurs in dogs as pigmented epidermal plaques
    - SCC "*in situ*" histopathology (dysplastic cells do not extend past the epidermal basement membrane)
    - Potential viral etiology: papillomavirus (cat – FcaPV2, FcaPV3, FdPV2; dog – novel viruses identified)
    - May progress to multicentric squamous cell carcinoma in situ
  - Solar induced:
    - Ultraviolet light causes mutation of tumor suppressor gene (*p53*); this gene encodes a protein that prevents mutations by arresting the cell cycle when DNA damage is detected, giving the damaged cell time to repair
    - Mutant form of *p53* has been detected in 82% of feline pinnal SCC
  - SCC may also develop secondary to chronic inflammation or viral infection
  - Metastasis is rare; often related to tumor depth
  - Secondary bacterial infection results in pain and systemic symptoms.
- Melanocytic tumors (skin/digit):
  - Benign or malignant neoplasm arising from melanocytes and melanoblasts
  - Most melanomas arise from haired skin
  - Ultraviolet light exposure does not appear to play a role in the etiology
  - Genetic susceptibility may be a factor because breed and familial clustering is noted

Blackwell's Five-Minute Veterinary Consult Clinical Companion: Small Animal Dermatology, Third Edition.
Karen Helton Rhodes and Alexander H. Werner.

- MAB IBF9: cell surface antigen (protein) present during all phases of the cell cycle in malignant canine melanoma cell lines; may be helpful in studying melanoma etiology as well as aiding in immunotherapeutic options.

■ Basal cell tumors:
- Umbrella term for a heterogenous group of tumors arising from basal cells of the epidermis, hair follicle epithelium, sebaceous gland, or sweat glands
- Basal cell tumors may be benign or malignant
- May be triggered by papilloma virus
- Majority of these tumors are benign, solitary, and slow growing.

■ Sebaceous gland tumors:
- Primarily benign (rarely malignant) tumors of the sebocytes
- Forms: nodular sebaceous hyperplasia, sebaceous adenoma, sebaceous epithelioma, sebaceous gland adenocarcinoma.

■ Hair follicle tumors:
- Tumors, typically benign, that arise from germinal hair follicle cells
- Classified according to adnexal differentiation
- Trichoepitheliomas, pilomatrixoma, trichoblastoma, tricholemmoma, trichofolliculoma, dilated pore of Winer.

SIGNALMENT/HISTORY

Breed/Coat Color Predilection

■ Squamous cell carcinoma:
- Cats: no breed predisposition; black cats may be predisposed to Bowen's disease; more aggressive disease in Devon rex
- Dogs: giant schnauzer, Scottish terrier, pekingese, boxer, poodle, Norwegian elkhound, dalmatian, beagle, whippet, and white English bull terrier may be predisposed; large breeds with black skin and hair coats may be predisposed to multiple squamous cell carcinoma involving the digits
- Solar-induced breed predilections: dogs – dalmatian, whippet, Italian greyhound, greyhound, American Staffordshire and bull terrier, beagle, German short-haired pointer, boxer, basset hound; cats – light or unpigmented skin in thinly haired regions.

■ Melanocytic tumors:
- Dogs: dark-skinned individuals predisposed
- Airedale terriers, Boston terrier, boxer, chow chow, chihuahua, cocker spaniel, doberman pinscher, Irish setter, springer spaniel.

■ Basal cell tumors:
- Cats: Siamese, Himalayan, and Persian
- Dogs: cocker spaniel, poodles, sheltie, Kerry blue terrier, Siberian husky.

■ Sebaceous gland tumors:
- Cats: uncommon; Persians predisposed
- Dogs: adenomas/hyperplasia: poodle, cocker spaniel, miniature schnauzer, terrier, shih tzu, Lhasa apso, Siberian husky, wheaten terrier, beagle, dachshund

- Sebaceous epitheliomas: Irish setter, malamute, shih tzu
- Sebaceous adenocarcinomas: rare; cocker spaniel, cavalier King Charles spaniel, Scottish terrier, husky.

- Hair follicle tumors:
  - Trichoepithelioma: cats – Persian; dogs – basset hound, golden retriever, German shepherd, miniature schnauzer, standard poodle, spaniel
  - Pilomatrixoma: Kerry blue terrier, poodle, Old English sheepdog
  - Trichoblastoma: poodle, cocker spaniel
  - Tricholemmoma: Afghan
  - Trichofolliculoma: none
  - Dilated pore of Winer: older cats, no breed predisposition.

Mean Age and Range

- Squamous cell carcinoma:
  - Cats 9–12.4 years
  - Dogs 9 years.
- Melanocytic tumors:
  - Cats 8–14 years (rare)
  - Dogs average age 9 years (common).
- Basal cell tumors:
  - Older cats predisposed
  - Uncommon in dogs.
- Sebaceous gland tumors:
  - Uncommon in older cats; 10–13 years
  - Common in older dogs; 8–11 years
  - Adenocarcinomas – rare in both dogs and cats.
- Hair follicle tumors:
  - 5–13 years of age; dogs and cats.

Historical Findings

- Squamous cell carcinoma:
  - Most common cutaneous malignant neoplasm in cats (15–49%); second most common in dogs (3–20%)
  - Feline SCC more prevalent in sunny climates and high altitudes (high ultraviolet light exposure)
  - Crusts, ulcer, or mass present for months and unresponsive to conservative treatment
  - Bowen's disease (cats): skin becomes pigmented; ulcer/crust may develop with or without progressive pigmented hyperkeratosis
  - Lips, nose, eyelids, and pinnae: may start as shallow crusting lesion that progresses to a deep ulcer
  - Facial skin involvement (cats)
  - Claw fold involvement (dogs)

- Solar induced: dogs – nasal planum, dorsal muzzle, axillae, and glabrous areas of the ventral abdomen and medial thigh; cats – pinnal margins and nasal planum.

- Melanocytic tumors:
  - 1–7% of all skin tumors in cats
  - 4–20% of all skin tumors in dogs
  - Slow or rapidly growing mass
  - Patient may be lame if a digit is involved.
- Basal cell tumors:
  - 15–26% of all skin tumors in the cat
  - 6% of skin tumors in dogs.
- Sebaceous gland tumors:
  - 6–21% of skin tumors in dogs; rare in cats
  - Often considered incidental finding in certain breeds; cocker spaniel and poodle.
- Hair follicle tumors:
  - Trichoepithelioma: common in dogs, uncommon in cats
  - Pilomatrixoma: uncommon in dogs, rare in cats
  - Trichoblastoma: uncommon in middle-aged dogs and cats
  - Tricholemmoma: rare in dogs and cats
  - Trichofolliculoma: rare in dogs and cats
  - Dilated pore of Winer: uncommon in older cats.

CLINICAL FEATURES

- Squamous cell carcinoma:
  - Bowen's disease:
    - Solitary or multiple lesions on head, digits, neck, thorax, shoulders, and ventral abdomen
    - Hair associated with lesions epilates easily
    - Crusts cling to the epilated hair shaft
    - Characterized by hyperpigmented and hyperkeratotic plaques of primarily the face, shoulders, and extremities (Figures 46.1, 46.2)
  - Solar induced:
    - Initial lesions: shallow, crusted ulcerations with peripheral alopecia and erythema
    - Intermediate lesions: eroded and exudative plaques; scabbed surface
    - Late lesions: deep, crateriform, and indurated patches or plaques
    - Cutaneous horns (rare)
    - Locally highly invasive and destructive with significant tissue loss; neoplastic tissue may extend beyond visible boundaries
    - Hemorrhage may be severe from erosion through local blood vessels.
    - Ulcerative tumors appear shallow and erosive; rapidly progress to deep craters with tissue remodeling (Figure 46.3)
    - Cats: external nares may be proliferative and scabbed or ulcerative; pinnal lesions often traumatized (Figures 46.4, 46.5)

  - Single or multiple, proliferative tumors have a cauliflower appearance that is friable and bleeds easily (Figures 46.6, 46.7)
  - Most common sites: cats – nasal planum, eyelids, lips, and pinnae; dogs – digits, scrotum, nose, legs, and anus
  - Digital lesions are typically swollen and painful and have a misshapen or absent claw
  - Lesions may also be found in the oral cavity, cornea, lungs, esophagus, and urinary bladder.
- Melanocytic tumors:
  - 85% of melanomas are benign
  - Benign, locally invasive, or metastatic (bone, lung, regional lymph nodes)
  - Pigmented or nonpigmented
  - Benign tumors are typically brown macules, plaques, or dome-shaped nodules that are well circumscribed and less than 2 cm diameter (Figure 46.8)
  - Malignant melanomas are rapidly growing, nonpigmented to black, ulcerated or pedunculated masses or nodules that are usually greater than 2 cm in diameter (Figure 46.9, 46.10)
  - Most common on the head, trunk, and digits but may occur anywhere on the body (most common on the head of cats)
  - More common in male dogs.
- Basal cell tumors:
  - Typically manifest as a solitary, well-circumscribed firm to fluctuant nodule; 1–10 cm diameter (Figure 46.11)
  - Often alopecic, may be pigmented, and may be ulcerative (Figure 46.12)
  - Lesions most commonly found on the head (lip, cheek, pinnae, periocular), neck, thorax, dorsal trunk
  - Feline basal cell carcinomas are highly metastatic
  - Canine malignant forms are rare; locally invasive; rarely metastasize.
- Sebaceous gland tumors:
  - Adenoma/hyperplasia: distinctive wart-like or cauliflower appearance in most cases (Figures 46.13–46.16)
  - Adenocarcinomas: firm raised nodules that ulcerate; may have metastasized from a primary bronchogenic site to the digits; in cats, swelling of multiple digits may occur due to multicentric ungual metastasis, solitary metastasis is more common than multicentric in dogs (Figures 46.17, 46.18)
  - Most common sites: cats – head, eyelids, extremities; dogs – head, neck, trunk, legs, and eyelids
  - Few millimeters to several centimeters in diameter, typically multiple in number
  - Yellow in color, alopecic, oily, may ulcerate; may become traumatized
  - Adenocarcinomas are usually solitary, alopecic, ulcerated, or erythematous intradermal nodules.
- Hair follicle tumors:
  - Single to multiple, alopecic, firm, white to gray multilobulated nodules that may ulcerate; typically well circumscribed (Figures 46.19–46.23)
  - Location: head, tail, trunk, limbs

- Some tumors (trichofolliculoma and dilated pore of Winer) have a central depression or opening that contains keratin, hair, or sebaceous material (Figure 46.24)
- Dilated pore of Winer may appear to form a cutaneous horn.

DIFFERENTIAL DIAGNOSIS

- Squamous cell carcinoma:
  - Draining abscesses or infected wounds
  - Claw bed infection/osteomyelitis
  - Other neoplasia (lymphoma, mast cell tumor)
  - Melanoma (may mimic Bowen's disease)
  - Eosinophilic plaque.
- Melanocytic tumors:
  - Amelanotic melanomas may look similar to undifferentiated sarcomas
  - Other neoplasms as well as infection.
- Basal cell tumors:
  - Other neoplasms: mast cell tumors, melanoma, hemangioma, hemangiosarcoma
  - Epidermal or follicular cyst.
- Sebaceous adenomas:
  - Other neoplasms
  - Cellulitis
  - Nevus
  - Apocrine adenomas, adenocarcinomas.
- Hair follicle tumors: cysts, other neoplasms.

DIAGNOSTICS

- Routine blood work: hemogram and serum chemistry.
- Urinalysis.
- Thoracic radiography: detects lung metastasis (3 view).
- Abdominal radiography: evaluates and monitors sublumbar lymph nodes, if clinically relevant (3 view).
- Radiography of extremities: with digital tumor; determines extent of underlying bone involvement.
- Ultrasonography and CT/MRI may be helpful (especially tumors invading the ear canal, oral cavity, sinonasal cavity).
- Cytologic examination: fine-needle aspirate of the mass; evaluate regional and/or large lymph nodes for metastasis.
- Biopsy: needed to confirm diagnosis.

Histopathology

- Squamous cell carcinoma: cords or irregular masses of dysplastic epidermal cells infiltrating into the dermis and subcutis, keratin pearls (accumulations of compact keratin) in well-differentiated tumors, desmosomes and mitotic figures common; *Bowen's disease* – dysplastic, highly ordered keratinocytes proliferate, replacing normal epidermis, but do not penetrate the basement membrane into the surrounding dermis (*in situ*): *solar induced* – trabeculae of squamous cells invade into the dermis; neoplastic cell aggregates; keratin pearls; keratinocyte cellular and nuclear pleomorphism; mitotic activity higher in dogs than cats; associated with dermal solar elastosis and fibrosis.

- Melanocytic tumors: neoplastic melanocytes that may be spindle, epithelial, or round in appearance with variable degrees of pigmentation; cells arranged in clusters, cords, or whorls; infiltration of pigment-laden macrophages; variable mitotic figures and pleomorphism related to the degree of malignancy; mitotic index most reliable way to predict tumor behavior; 10% of histologically benign tumors may behave in a malignant manner.
- Basal cell tumor: nonencapsulated dermal to subcutaneous mass composed of cords or nests of neoplastic basal cells; may be pigmented or cystic; central areas of squamous differentiation; nuclear hyperchromasia; frequent mitotic figures.
- Sebaceous gland tumors:
  - Hyperplasia: multiple enlarged mature sebaceous lobules with single peripheral layer of basaloid epithelial cells clustered around dilated sebaceous ducts; no mitotic activity
  - Sebaceous adenoma: mature sebaceous lobules with increased numbers of basaloid epithelial cells; sebaceous ducts not prominent; cystic degeneration; low mitotic activity
  - Epithelioma: irregular islands and lobules of basaloid epithelial cells with reactive collagen; higher mitotic activity
  - Adenocarcinoma: poorly defined lobules of large epithelial cells with varying degrees of differentiation; high mitotic activity.
- Hair follicle tumors:
  - Trichoepithelioma: germinal hair follicle cells differentiate toward hair follicles and shaft structures
  - Pilomatrixoma: germinal cells tend to differentiate toward hair bulb/matrix
  - Trichoblastoma: germinal cells differentiate toward hair bulb
  - Trichofolliculoma: may actually be a follicular or pilosebaceous hamartoma rather than a true neoplasm
  - Dilated pore of Winer: benign hair follicle tumor or cyst.

THERAPEUTICS

- Invasive tumors: inpatient; require aggressive surgical excision or radiotherapy.
- Superficial tumors: surgery, cryosurgery, photodynamic therapy, or irradiation.
- Plesiotherapy (topical radiation, strontium-90).
- Photodynamic therapy.
- Topical synthetic retinoids or imiquimod: early superficial lesions.
- Wide surgical excision.

- Digit involvement: amputation.
- Pinna involvement: may require partial or total resection.
- Invasive tumors of the nares: removal of the nasal planum recommended.
- Radiotherapy: recommended for inoperable tumors or as adjunct to surgery.
- Adjunctive chemotherapy: recommended with incomplete surgical excision, nonresectable mass, and metastasis.
- Cisplatin (dogs, do not use in cats), carboplatin, and mitoxantrone: reported to induce partial and complete remission; generally of short duration; small number of patients; do not use with concurrent renal disease.
- Intralesional sustained-release chemotherapeutic gel implants (dogs): contain either 5-fluorouracil or cisplatin.
- Firocoxib 5 mg/kg PO q24h: overexpression of cyclooxygenase (COX-2) documented in actinic keratoses in humans and dogs; improvement noted with use of COX-2 selective inhibitor; may be helpful in conjunction with chemotherapeutic agents.
- Vitamin E: stabilize cell membranes: 400–600 IU PO BID.
- Cimetidine: reported to have some benefit as a biologic response modifier in malignant melanoma by reversing suppressor T cell-mediated immune suppression.

COMMENTS

Client Education/Prognosis

- Squamous cell carcinoma:
  - Discuss risk factors associated with the development of the tumor (ultraviolet light exposure)
  - Monitor patient with physical examination and radiography 1, 3, 6, 9, 12, 18, and 24 months after treatment or if the owner thinks the tumor is recurring
  - Thoracic and abdominal radiography: at each recheck examination, if the lesion is on the caudal portion of the patient
  - Limit sun exposure, especially between the hours of 10.00 a.m. and 2.00 p.m.
  - Sunscreens: may help in some areas (e.g., pinnae)
  - Prognosis: good with superficial lesions that receive appropriate treatment; guarded with invasive lesions and those involving the claw fold or digit.
- Melanocytic tumors:
  - Breed may be prognostic: 85% of miniature poodle melanomas are behaviorally malignant, >75% of melanomas in dobermans and schnauzers are benign
  - Location may be prognostic: most oral, scrotal, and mucocutaneous (except the eyelid) melanomas are malignant, 50% of claw fold melanomas are malignant
  - 35–50% of melanomas in cats are reported to be malignant.
- Basal cell tumors:
  - Most are benign and easily cured with excision
  - Malignant tumors are typically slow growing and of low-grade malignancy; complete staging, including regional lymph node aspiration, chest radiography, and abdominal ultrasonography are advised.

- Sebaceous gland tumors:
  - Prognosis is good
  - Malignant form (adenocarcinoma) rarely metastasizes and is locally infiltrative involving regional lymph nodes.
- Hair follicle tumors:
  - Prognosis is good; surgical or laser excision is curative
  - Rare report of metastatic pilomatrixoma with neurologic complications.

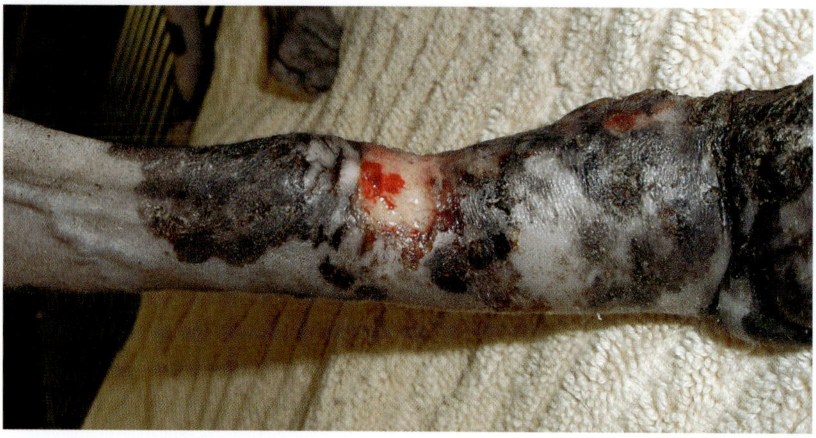

■ **Fig. 46.1.** Multiple hyperpigmented plaques with areas of ulceration on an extremity with Bowen's disease caused by papillomavirus in a 12-year-old female-spayed sphynx.

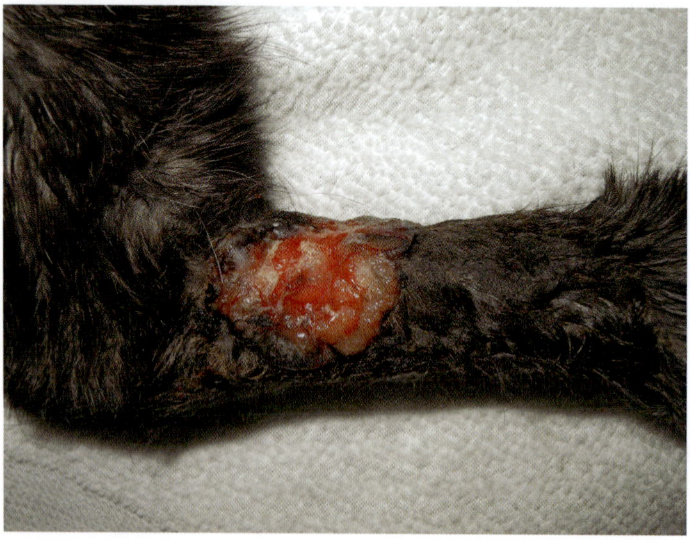

■ **Fig. 46.2.** Squamous cell carcinoma *in situ* of Bowen's disease on the tarsus of a 19-year-old male-castrate DSH.

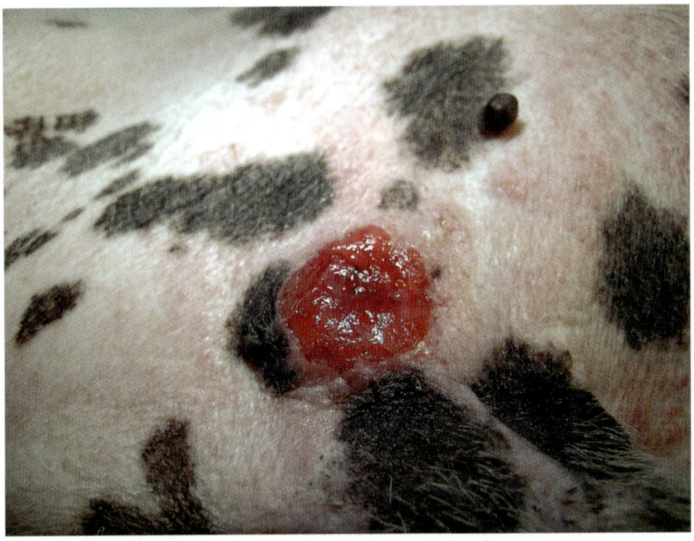

■ **Fig. 46.3.** Ulcerated plaque of squamous cell carcinoma surrounded by erythema typical of actinic dermatitis on the ventrum of a 6-year-old male-castrate pit bull terrier mix.

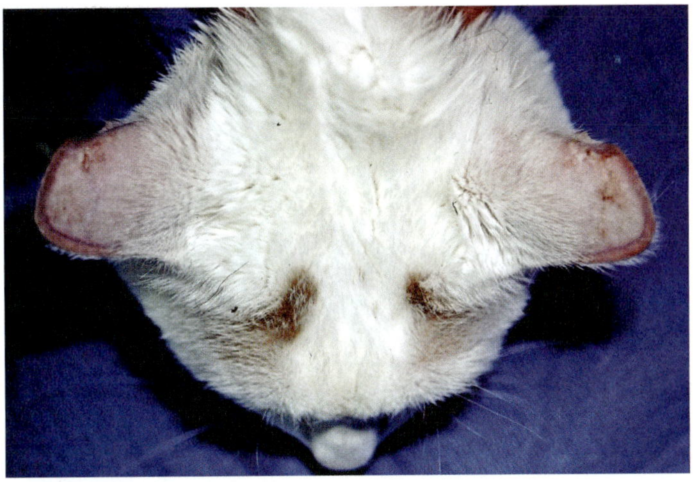

■ **Fig. 46.4.** Solar-induced squamous cell carcinoma affecting the pinnae of an adult DSH. Neoplastic tissue is located on the caudal aspects of the pinnae with actinic dermatitis present on pinnal margins.

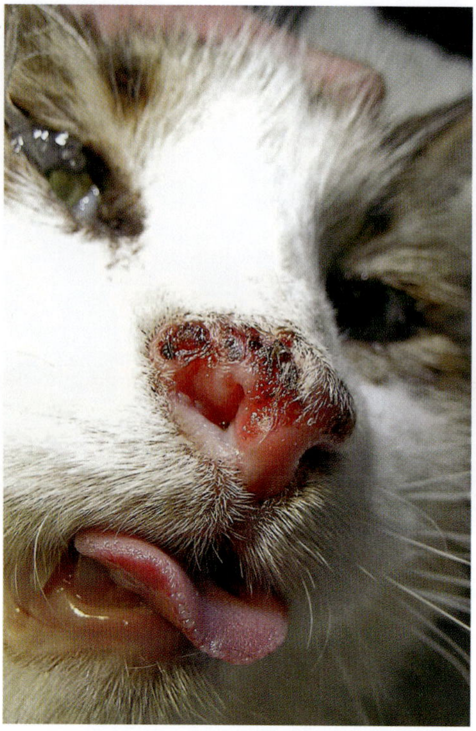

■ **Fig. 46.5.** Solar-induced squamous cell carcinoma affecting the nasal planum of a 14-year-old female-spayed DSH.

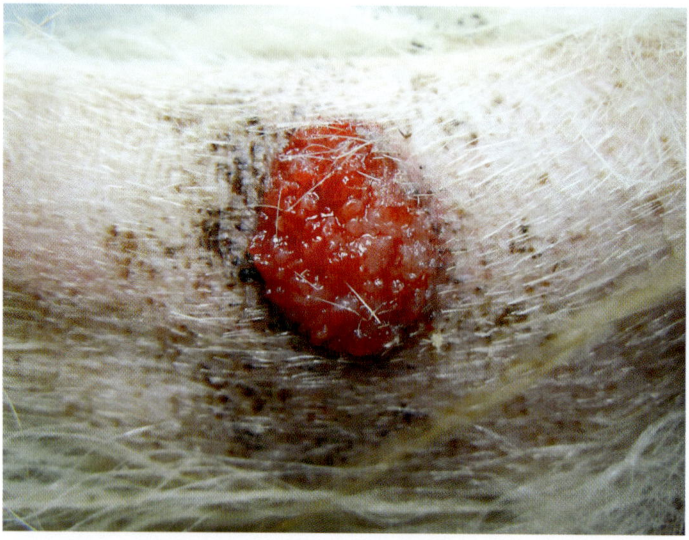

■ **Fig. 46.6.** Squamous cell carcinoma *in situ* on the ventral aspect of the tail of a 12-year-old male-castrate chow chow. Tissue is friable and bleeds easily.

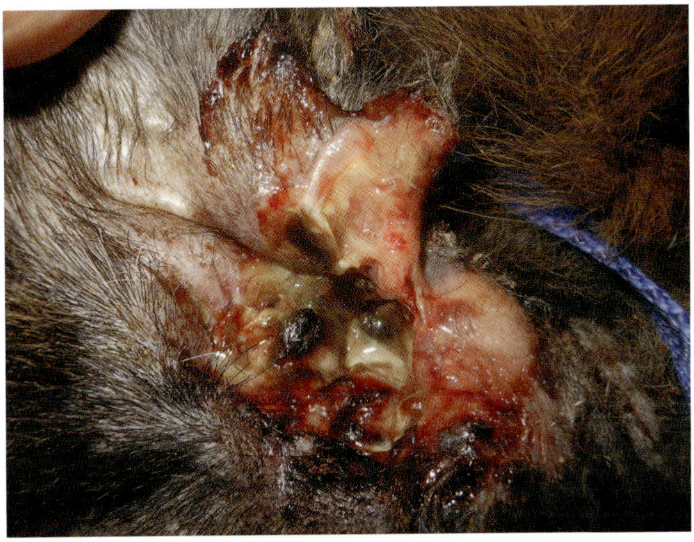

Fig. 46.7. Necrotic tissue resulting from an aggressive squamous cell carcinoma at the base of the pinna of a 12-year-old male-castrate shepherd mix.

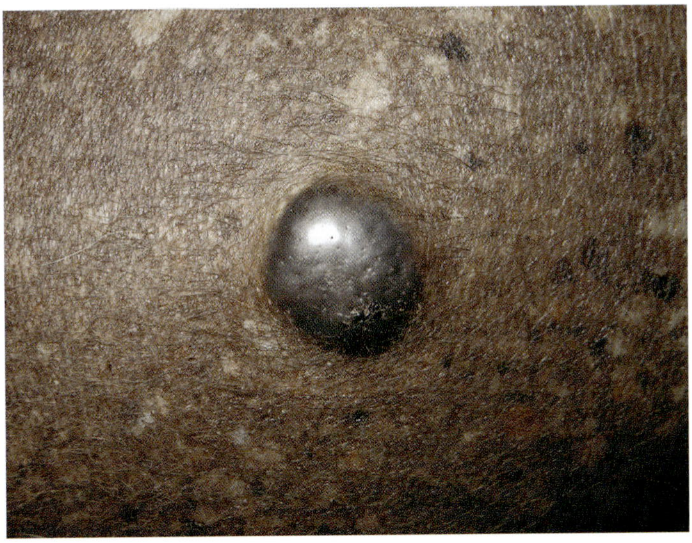

Fig. 46.8. Pigmented, dome-shaped melanocytoma on the ventrum of an 8-year-old male-castrate doberman pinscher.

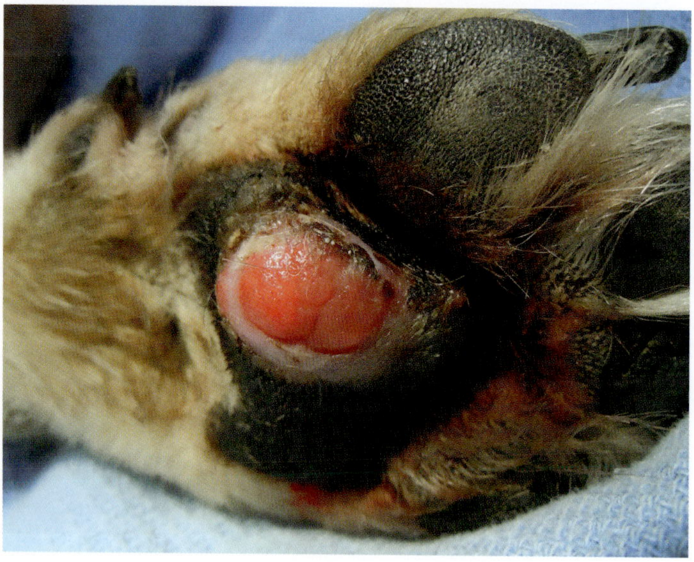

■ **Fig. 46.9.** Malignant melanoma affecting the footpad of a 15-year-old female-spayed cattle dog. This tumor is not pigmented and caused significant lameness.

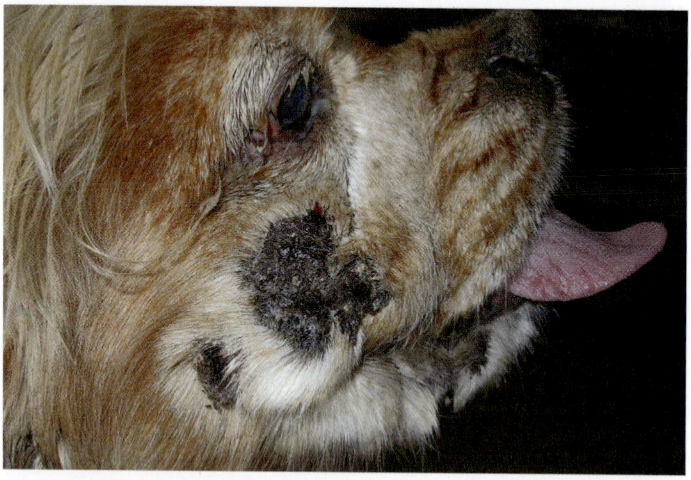

■ **Fig. 46.10.** Multiple pigmented plaques of malignant melanoma on the face of a 12-year-old female-spayed cocker spaniel. Secondary infection caused pain and malodor.

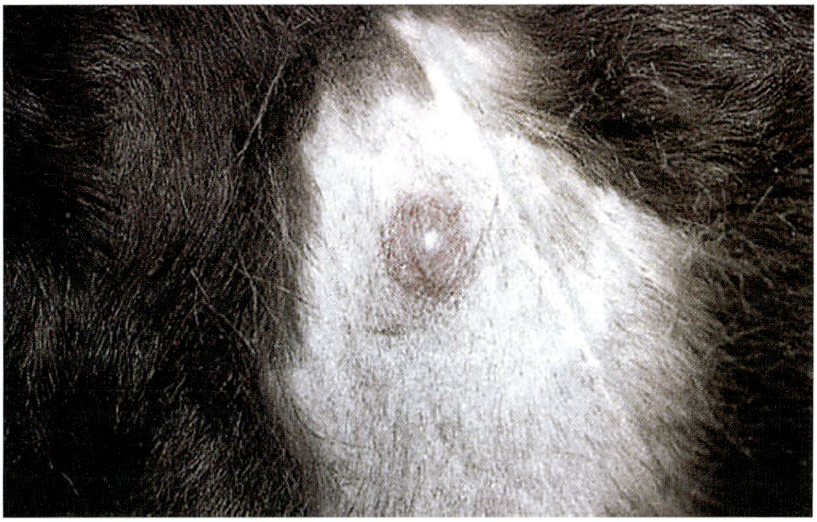

■ **Fig. 46.11.** Small solitary firm dermal nodule of basal cell tumor located on the neck of a dog.

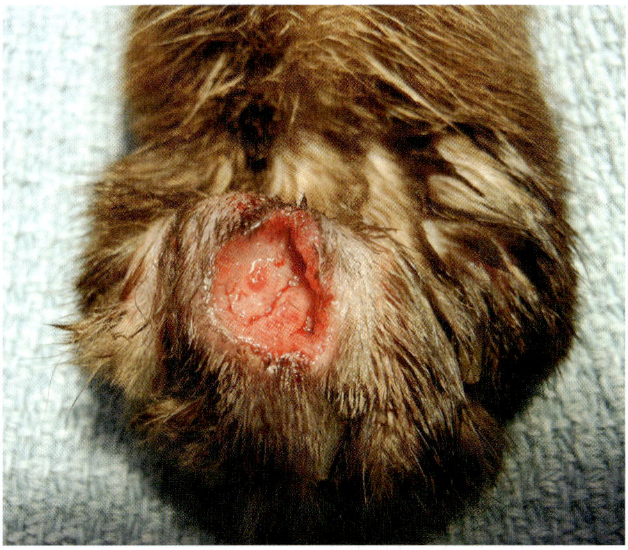

■ **Fig. 46.12.** Ulcerated aggressive basal cell carcinoma on the digit of an 18-year-old male-castrate DMH.

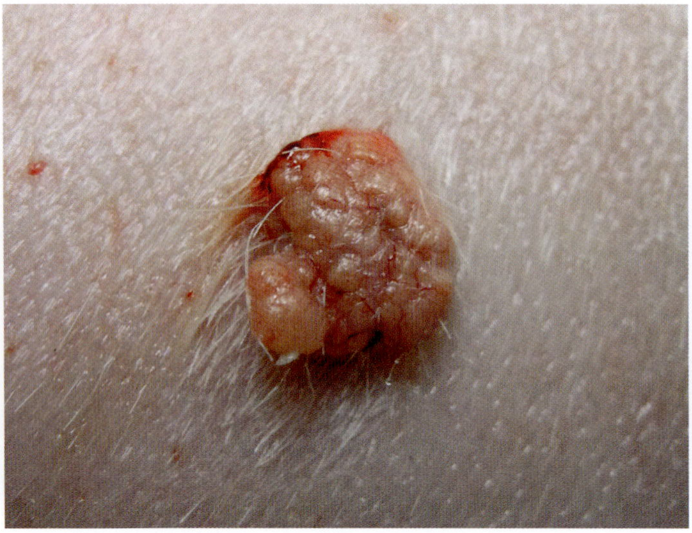

■ **Fig. 46.13.** Cauliflower-appearance of the surface of a nodule characteristic of sebaceous gland hyperplasia on a 7-year-old male-castrate bichon frise mix.

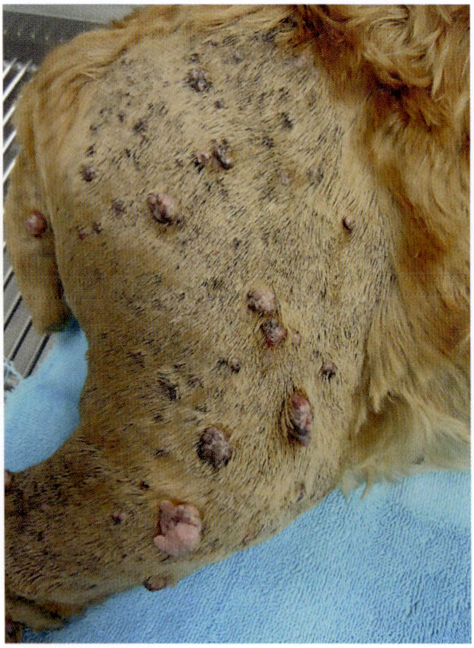

■ **Fig. 46.14.** Multiple sebaceous gland adenomas affecting a 10-year-old male-castrate cocker spaniel. Hair coat has been clipped.

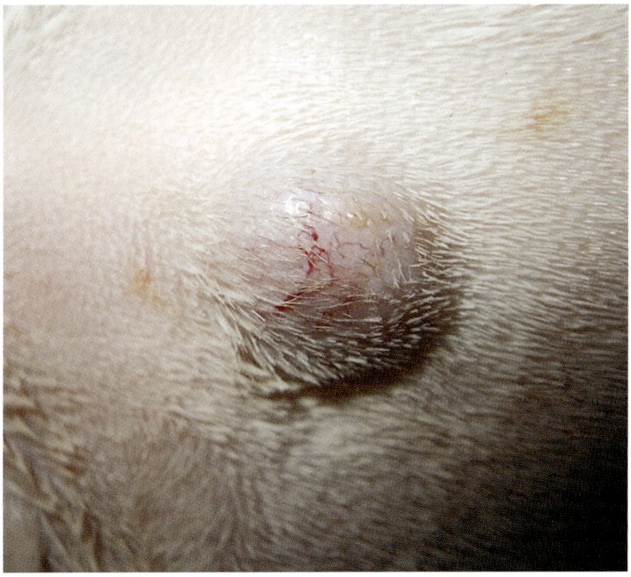

Fig. 46.15. Sebaceous gland adenoma on a 6-year-old male-castrate ragdoll cat.

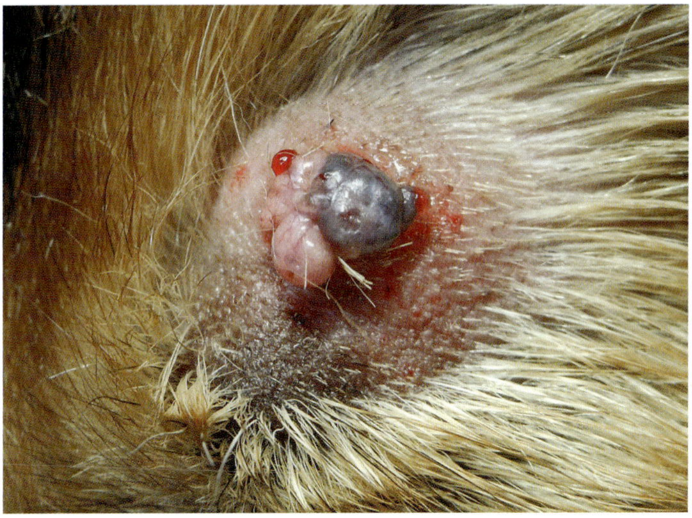

Fig. 46.16. Compound sebaceous gland adenoma on the head of a 13-year-old female-spayed chow chow.

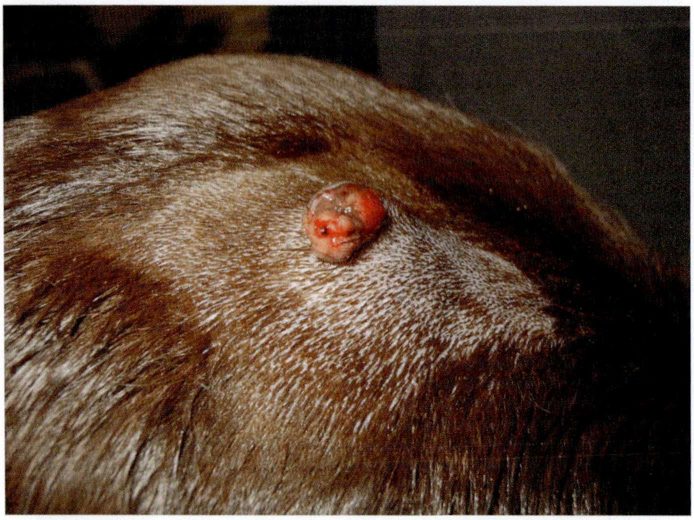

■ **Fig. 46.17.** Epitheliomatous sebaceous gland adenocarcinoma on the forehead of an 11-year-old female spayed Labrador retriever.

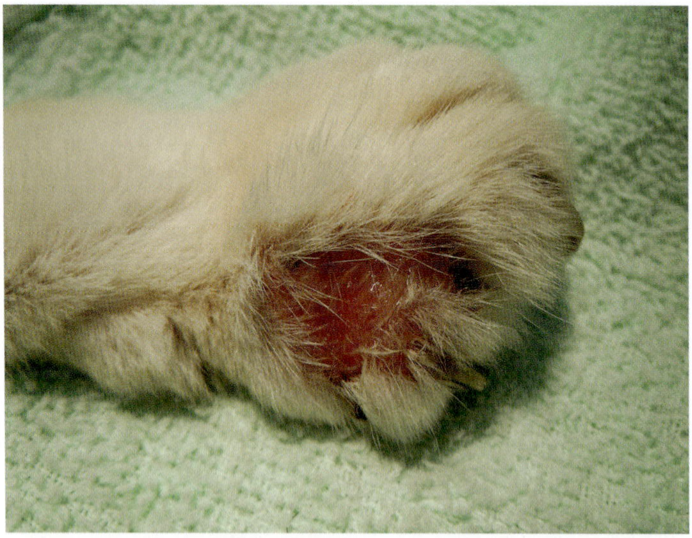

■ **Fig. 46.18.** Pulmonary metastatic adenocarcinoma on the foot of a 16-year-old female-spayed DSH. This lesion is representative of lung-digit syndrome.

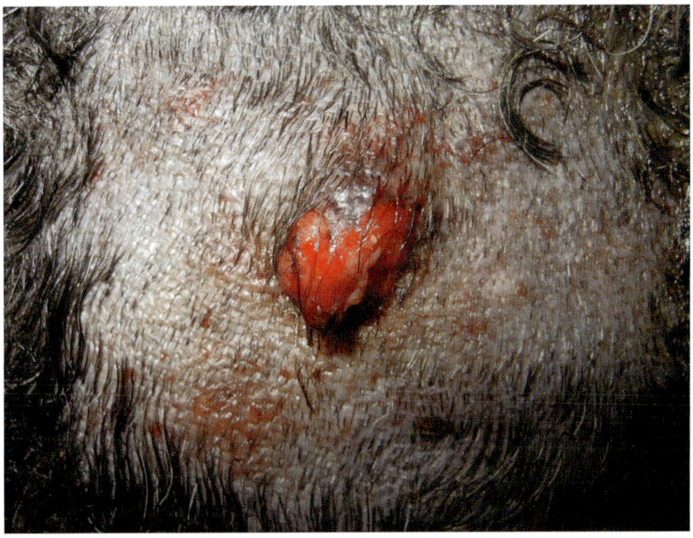

■ **Fig. 46.19.** Infiltrative trichoepithelioma in a 12-year-old male-castrate standard poodle.

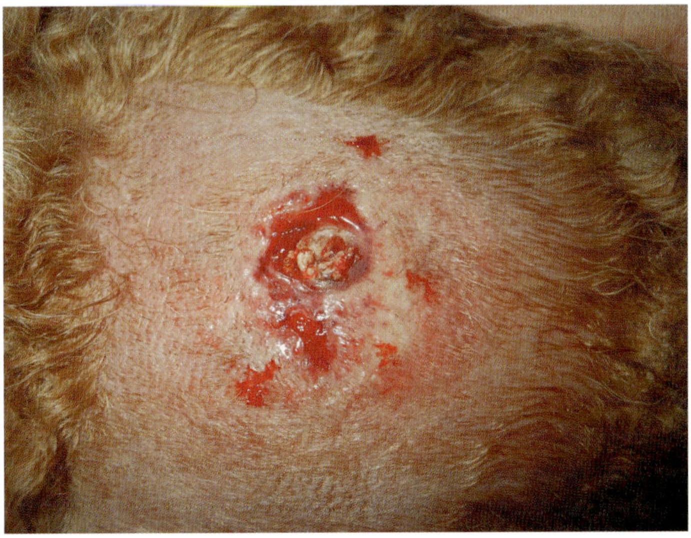

■ **Fig. 46.20.** Ulcerated trichoepithelioma on a 7-year-old female-spayed labradoodle.

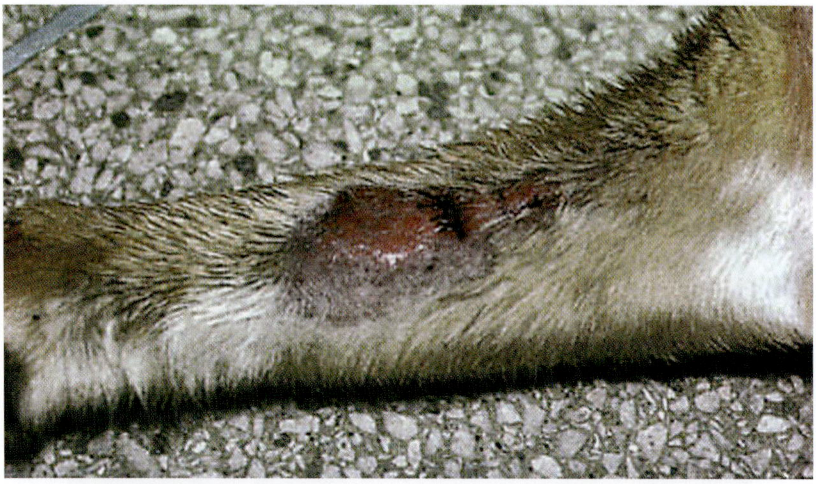

■ **Fig. 46.21.** Solitary raised mass of the medial aspect of the forelimb of a DSH diagnosed as pilomatrixoma.

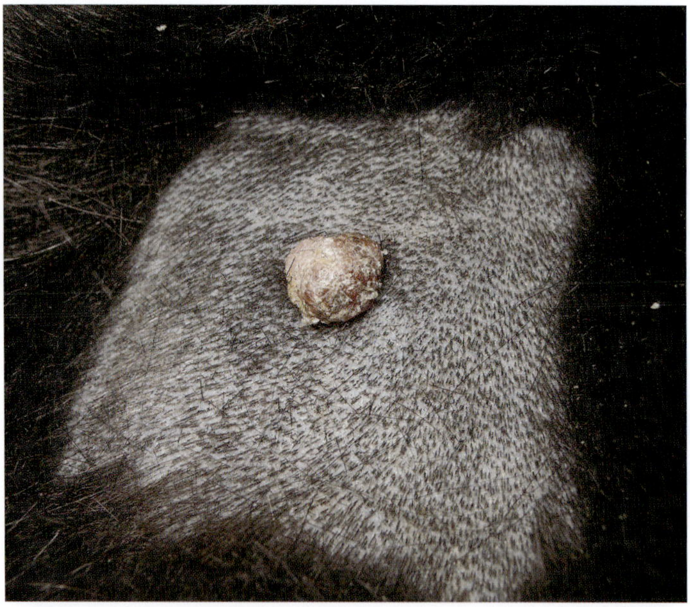

■ **Fig. 46.22.** Mildly crusted nodule diagnosed as isthmus tricholemmoma on an 8-year-old male-castrate border collie.

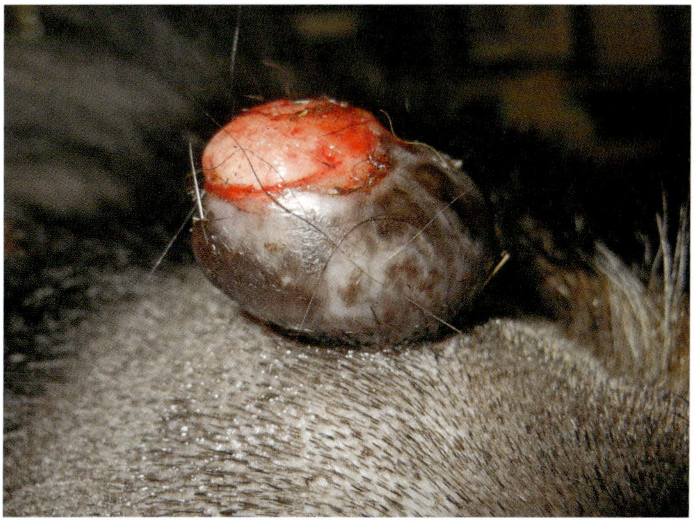

■ **Fig. 46.23.** Ribbon trichoblastoma on an 11-year-old male-castrate chow mix.

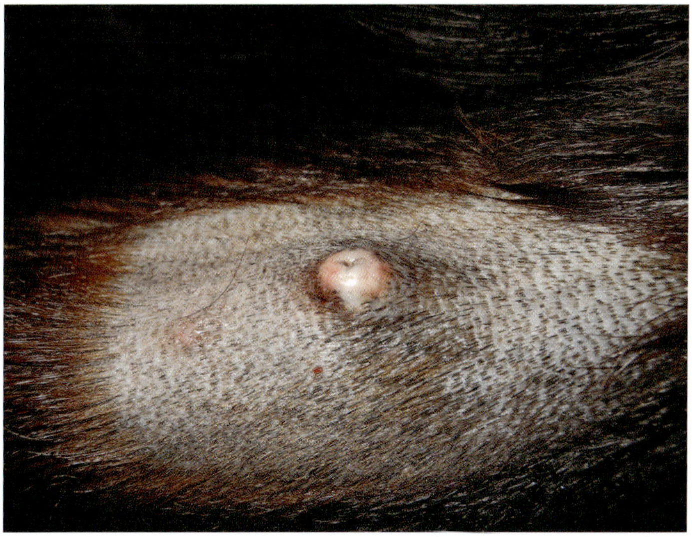

■ **Fig. 46.24.** Erythematous nodule with a central indentation characteristic of a trichofolliculoma on a 5-year-old male-castrate Labrador retriever.

chapter 47

Uveodermatologic Syndrome

DEFINITION/OVERVIEW

- Rare syndrome similar to Vogt–Koyanagi–Harada syndrome in humans.
- Considered to be an autoimmune disorder resulting in concurrent granulomatous uveitis and depigmenting dermatitis (skin and hair) and rare meningoencephalitis.
- Multisystem autoimmune disease affecting pigmented tissue of the eye, ear, nervous system, skin, and hair.

ETIOLOGY/PATHOPHYSIOLOGY

- Autoimmune disease with genetic factors; autoantibodies against melanocytes result in panuveitis, leukoderma, and leukotrichia.
- Antiretinal antibodies have been found in affected dogs.
- T_H1 cytokines involved in skin pathology; T_H2 cytokines may be more involved with ocular pathology.
- Exposure to sunlight exacerbates symptoms.

SIGNALMENT/HISTORY

- Predominant breeds: akitas, samoyeds, and Siberian huskies.
- Young adult and middle-aged dogs.
- No sex predilection reported.
- Rarely reported in other breeds: chow chow, Alaskan malamute, Australian shepherd, basset hound, Irish setter, fox terrier, dachshund, Shetland sheepdog, St Bernard, old English sheepdog, Brazilian fila, German shepherd dog, shiba inu.

CLINICAL FEATURES

- Sudden-onset bilateral uveitis: may be painful and progress to blindness.
- Concurrent or subsequent leukoderma of the nose, lips, and eyelids.
- Footpads, scrotum, anus, and hard palate may also become depigmented.

Blackwell's Five-Minute Veterinary Consult Clinical Companion: Small Animal Dermatology, Third Edition.
Karen Helton Rhodes and Alexander H. Werner.

- Ophthalmic signs: photophobia, diminished or absent papillary light reflexes, blepharospasm, anterior uveitis, hyphema, chorioretinitis, conjunctivitis, retinal detachment, iris bombe, glaucoma, blindness.
- Dermatologic signs: symmetric (often striking) depigmentation of the planum nasale, perioral/oral (lips and oral mucosa), and periocular tissue; less frequently, scrotum, vulva, anus, and footpads may be depigmented (Figures 47.1–47.4).
- Rarely, leukoderma and leukotrichia may become generalized.
- Skin lesions may ulcerate and become crusted.
- Meningoencephalitis is reported rarely.

DIFFERENTIAL DIAGNOSIS

- Immune-mediated diseases: pemphigus complex, systemic lupus erythematosus, cutaneous lupus erythematosus, bullous pemphigoid, vitiligo (idiopathic leukoderma/leukotrichia), vasculitis.
- Neoplasia (cutaneous lymphoma) and numerous other inflammatory and infectious skin diseases that can cause depigmentation.

DIAGNOSTICS

- Biopsy: lichenoid interface granulomatous pattern with large histiocytes and pronounced pigmentary incontinence; hydropic degeneration of the epidermal basal cell layer rare.
- Evaluate the retina; often the first abnormal clinical feature (granulomatous panuveitis).

THERAPEUTICS

- Aggressive and rapid initiation of immunosuppressive therapy is recommended to prevent formation of posterior synechiae and secondary glaucoma, cataracts, or blindness.
- Subconjunctival or topical glucocorticoids (i.e., 0.1% dexamethasone ophthalmic solution q4h, dexamethasone 1–2 mg subconjunctivally) until the uveitis has resolved.
- Cycloplegics: 1% atropine ophthalmic solution q6–24h.
- Retinal examinations: most important means of monitoring progress; improvement in dermatologic lesions may not reflect the retinal pathology.
- Enucleation: sometimes recommended because of pain.

Drugs of Choice

- Corticosteroids: initial high doses of prednisolone 1.1–2.2 mg/kg PO BID to q24h.
- Azathioprine 1–2 mg/kg or 50 mg/m2 PO q24h.

- Cyclosporine 5–10 mg/kg PO q24h.
- Dosage and frequency of medications tapered with response.
- Long-term therapy necessary.
- Topical or subconjunctival steroids and atropine may be indicated with anterior uveitis.

COMMENTS

- CBC and biochemistry: day 7; every 2–4 weeks until remission; then every 3–6 months when on azathioprine; routine monitoring with use of prednisolone and cyclosporine.
- Avoid using affected animals for breeding.
- Referral to a veterinary ophthalmologist recommended for management of ocular disease.
- Weekly or biweekly examinations including retinal evaluations: recommended initially for monitoring side effects associated with therapeutics.
- Retinal examinations are required; improvement in dermatologic lesions may not reflect improvement in retinal lesions.
- Azathioprine may be discontinued after a few months of therapy; prednisolone may be necessary indefinitely.
- Iatrogenic hyperadrenocorticism: often a result of the steroid therapy.
- Cyclosporine may be used as a steroid-sparing protocol.
- Prognosis is fair to guarded.
- Blindness is a common sequela.
- Depigmentation of the skin/hair is often permanent; may improve in some cases.

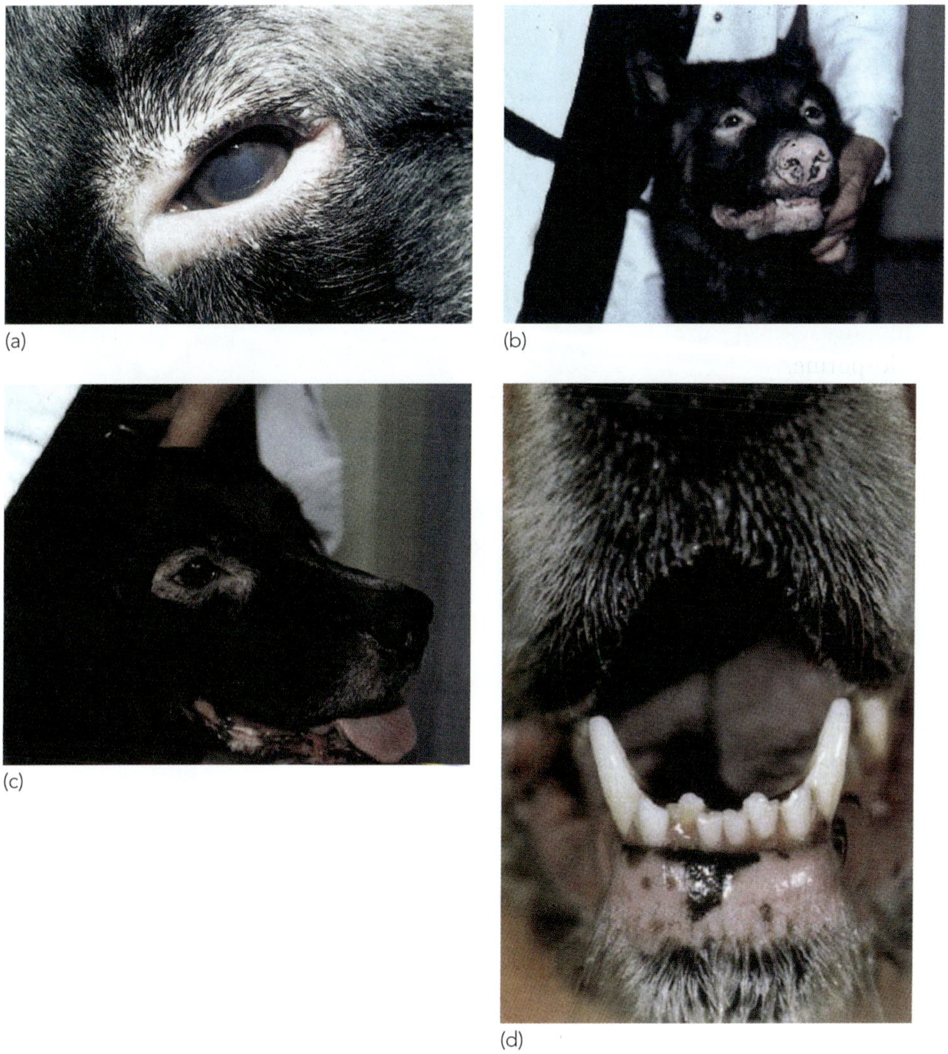

■ **Fig. 47.1.** Uveodermatologic syndrome in an adult Akita. (a) Note the early evidence of uveitis, which is often the initial clinical feature recognized. (b) Characteristic striking depigmentation of the planum nasale and periocular mucocutaneous junctions. (c) Depigmentation of the periocular region. (d) Depigmentation affecting the mucous membranes.

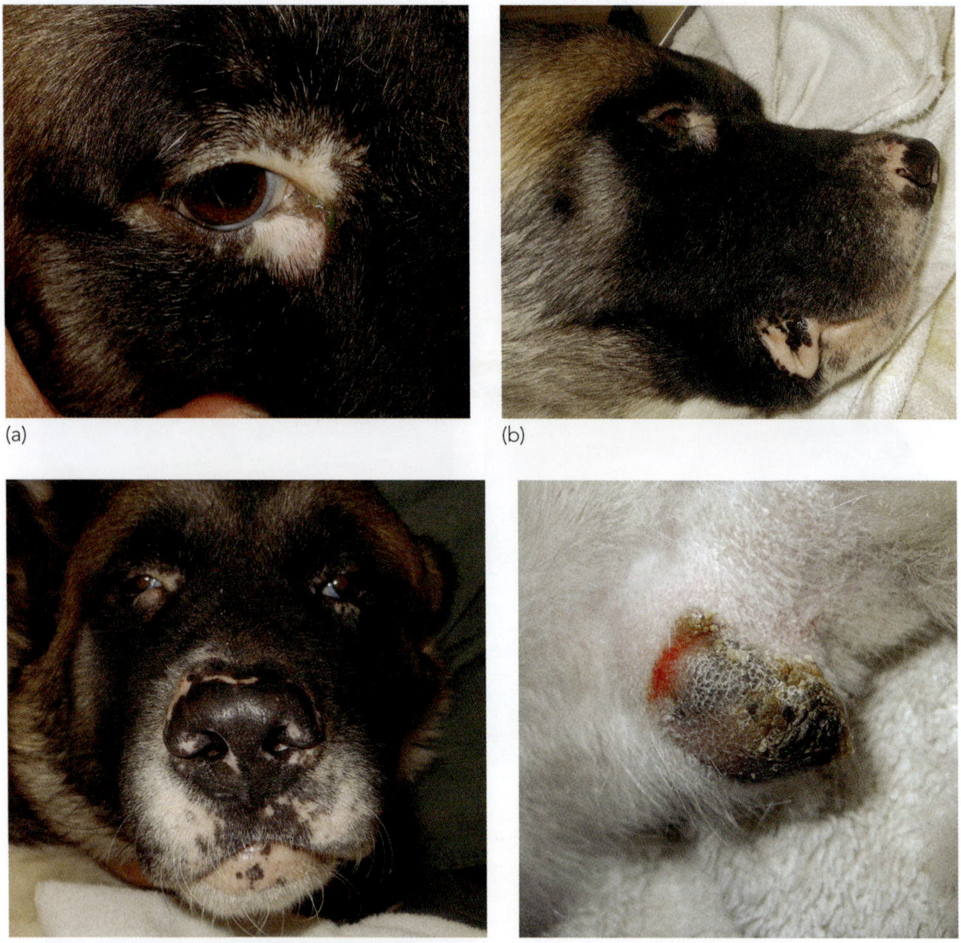

(a) (b) (c) (d)

Fig. 47.2. Uveodermatologic syndrome in a 2-year-old male-castrate Akita. (a) Depigmentation affecting the eyelid margin. (b) Characteristic pattern of depigmentation of the periocular skin, planum nasale, and lip margins. (c) Depigmentation of the muzzle region. (d) Depigmentation and mild crusting affecting a footpad.

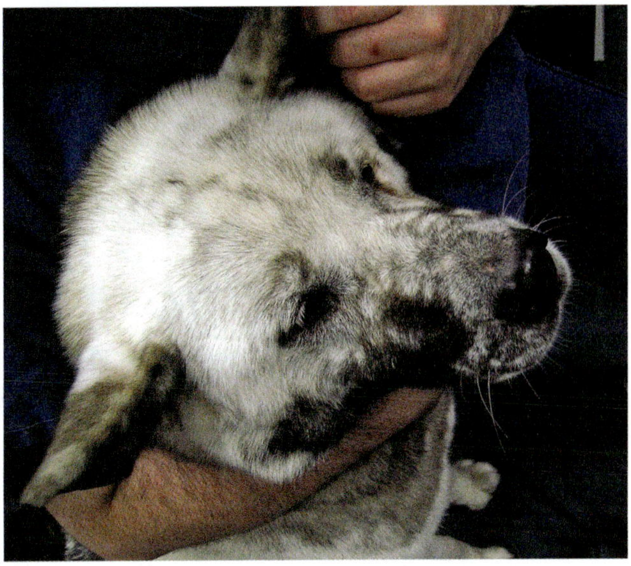

■ **Fig. 47.3.** An 11-year-old female-spayed Akita during treatment for uveodermatologic syndrome: repigmentation of the mucous membranes is evident but there is persistent patchy leukotrichia.

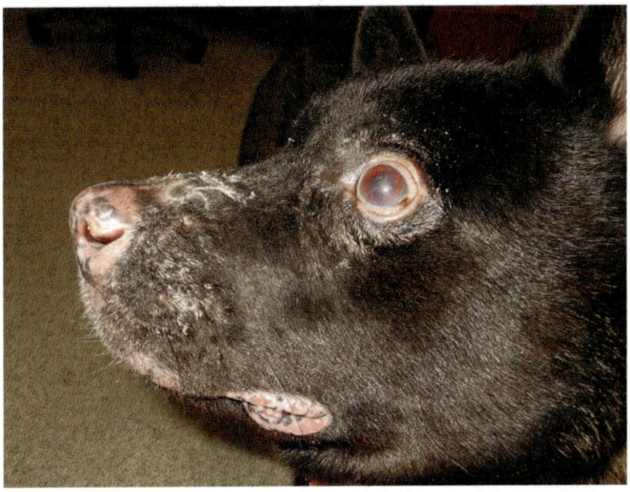

■ **Fig. 47.4.** Uveodermatologic syndrome in a 1-year-old male-castrate Akita. Note the striking depigmentation with crusting along the lip margins and nasal planum/dorsal muzzle. Uveitis is evident in the image and progressed to permanent blindness prior to referral for treatment.

chapter 48

Vasculitis

DEFINITION/OVERVIEW

- Specifically denotes the targeted damage of blood vessels by inflammation; often inferred from tissue changes consistent with a disruption in blood flow.
- Inflammation may be neutrophilic (leukocytoclastic or nonleukocytoclastic), lymphocytic, eosinophilic, granulomatous, or of mixed cell type.
- Leukocytoclastic vasculitis is the inflammation of small blood vessels seen as perivascular nuclear fragments; may be a major feature seen histologically.
- Clinical signs related to type or size, location, and cause of vessel(s) affected.
- May be associated with additional or underlying conditions, a drug reaction, or idiopathic.
- Cutaneous adverse reaction to food associated with urticarial vasculitis.
- Pathomechanisms: type III (immune complex) and type I (immediate) reactions:
  - Endothelial damage caused by infectious agent, parasite infestation, endotoxin, or immune complex deposition along the vessel wall
  - Initiation of local inflammation, neutrophil accumulation, and complement activation
  - Neutrophils release lysosomal enzymes leading to necrosis of vessel wall, fibrinoid change, endothelial swelling, thrombosis, and hemorrhage
  - Polyarteritis nodosa: systemic vasculitis with intimal (vascular smooth muscle cell) proliferation and vessel wall degeneration and necrosis; leads to microaneurysm, hemorrhage, thrombosis, and necrosis of involved vessels and adjacent tissues.
- Nondermal vasculitis (e.g., renal, hepatic, and serosal surfaces of body cavities) may be the mechanism leading to development of clinically apparent signs of systemic disease (e.g., polyarthritis and proteinuria) without causing obvious external lesions.

SIGNALMENT/HISTORY

- Any age, breed, or sex may be affected.
- Predisposed breeds: dachshund, rottweiler, Chinese shar-pei, greyhound, German shepherd, Scottish terrier, Jack Russell terrier, St Bernard.

Blackwell's Five-Minute Veterinary Consult Clinical Companion: Small Animal Dermatology, Third Edition.
Karen Helton Rhodes and Alexander H. Werner.

- Vaccination associated: poodle, Maltese, silky terrier, Yorkshire terrier.
- Varies depending on cause.
- Provocative drug exposure (e.g., penicillin, sulfonamides, streptomycin, and hydralazine) given to sensitized animal.
- Exposure to ticks.
- Dirofilariasis.
- Skin lesions may be the only symptom, or precede or follow systemic symptoms.

CLINICAL FEATURES

- Alopecia.
- Palpable purpura.
- Hemorrhagic bullae.
- Crusting and scarring.
- Mottled pigmentary changes (hyper- or hypopigmentation).
- Necrosis and "punched-out" ulcers.
- Affects extremities, pinnae, lips, tail, and oral mucosa, especially "dependent" or distant regions (tail tip, pinnal tip, claws) and areas of pressure (elbows, footpads) (Figures 48.1–48.5).
- May be painful or pruritic.
- Anorexia, depression, pyrexia, pitting edema of the extremities, arthropathy or polyarthropathy, hepatopathy, neuropathy, nephropathy, and myopathy – dependent on the underlying cause (Figures 48.6, 48.7).
- Systemic signs reflecting organ involvement (e.g., hepatic, renal, and CNS).
- Systemic signs of illness (e.g., lethargy, lymphadenopathy, pyrexia, vague signs of pain, and weight loss).
- Cutaneous lesions of polyarteritis nodosa (subcutaneous nodules: less common in dogs than in human beings).
- Signs associated with underlying infectious or immune-related disease (e.g., thrombocytopenia and polyarthropathy).
- Proliferative arteritis of the nasal philtrum: St Bernard (Figure 48.8).
- Juvenile polyarteritis syndrome of beagle dogs (JPS) – multisystemic necrotizing vasculitis of small vessels.
- Ear margin vasculitis/vasculopathy/seborrhea in dachshunds.
- Familial cutaneous vasculopathy of German shepherd dogs.
- Cutaneous and renal glomerular vasculopathy of greyhound dogs: verotoxin-induced (proposed) palpable purpura leading to multiple lesions of ulceration and necrosis; associated with renal compromise or failure.
- Solar vasculopathy: associated with other sun-aggravated or induced dermatoses (e.g., discoid lupus erythematosus).
- Proliferative thrombovascular necrosis: focal to multifocal areas of pinnal ulceration and crusting (Figure 48.9).
- Neutrophilic leukocytoclastic vasculitis of Jack Russell terriers.

- Ischemic dermatopathy:
  - Dermatomyositis in predisposed breeds – see Chapter 20 (Figures 48.10–48.12)
  - Vaccine induced: 2–6 months post vaccination (most often rabies); progressive, noninflamed alopecia beginning at the site of injection; may be associated with generalized symptoms (Figures 48.13, 48.14)
  - Idiopathic – not associated with vaccination.

Causes and Risk Factors

- Systemic lupus erythematosus
- Cold agglutinin disease
- Frostbite
- Disseminated intravascular coagulopathy
- Lymphoreticular neoplasia
- Drug reactions, e.g., itraconazole-induced necrotizing vasculitis
- Post vaccination
- Spider bites
- Immune-mediated disease
- Erythema nodosum-like panniculitis
- Rheumatoid arthritis
- Rocky Mountain spotted fever
- Staphylococcal hypersensitivity
- Food hypersensitivity causing urticarial vasculitis
- FeLV- and FIV-associated vasculitis in cats
- 50% of all cases are idiopathic

DIFFERENTIAL DIAGNOSIS

- Ear margin seborrhea
- Chemical or thermal burn
- Coagulopathy
- Toxic epidermal necrolysis
- Erythema multiforme
- Ulcerative dermatosis of collies and shelties
- Deep pyoderma
- Sepsis

DIAGNOSTICS

- Diascopy: erythema that does not blanch with pressure from a glass slide indicates hemorrhage into the skin (Figure 48.15).
- CBC: thrombocytopenia, anemia – dependent on the underlying cause.
- Immunodiagnostics: ANA titer, Coombs test, and cold agglutinin tests.

- Serologic tests may aid diagnosis of tick-related (i.e., rickettsial) disease.
- ANA titer positive in patient with SLE; may also be positive in patients with other systemic illnesses.
- Occult heartworm test positive in patients with dirofilariasis.
- *Angiostrongylus vasorum* infestation diagnosed by fecal examination and cytologic examination of tracheal wash.
- Radiographs: assist diagnosis of dirofilariasis and angiostronglyiasis.
- Skin scrapings: possible demodicosis (with secondary sepsis).
- Representative cultures (e.g., blood, urine, skin) if CBC, chemistry screen, or urinalysis reveals systemic disease.
- Biopsy representative lesions (wedge-type biopsy rather than "punch biopsy" sample):
    - Findings depend on the underlying cause
    - Subtle changes associated with tissue hypoxia (e.g., follicular atrophy, cell-poor interface dermatitis, pale-staining collagen)
    - Neutrophilic (leukocytoclastic/nonleukocytoclastic) vasculitis
    - Lymphocytic, eosinophilic, granulomatous, or mixed cellular inflammation in and around the vessels
    - Vascular necrosis and fibrin thrombi may be prominent
    - Perivascular hemorrhage and edema may occur
    - Ischemic dermatopathy
    - Direct immunofluorescence or immunohistochemistry staining – deposition of immunoglobulin in vessel walls.

THERAPEUTICS

- First priority: diagnose and treat the underlying disease.
- No systemic abnormalities: treat as outpatient.
- Systemic disease: inpatient care may be required.
- Topical therapy: antiseptic solutions to clean lesions and reduce secondary infection underneath accumulations of exudates.
- Systemic or severe cases: inform owner that the prognosis may be guarded unless a cause is found; prognosis is based on the etiology.

Drugs of Choice

- Broad-spectrum antibiotics: first line of therapy while awaiting histopathology results – cephalexin 22 mg/kg PO BID.
- Pentoxifylline 10–20 mg/kg PO BID to TID.
- Vitamin E 400 IU PO BID.
- Prednisolone 1–2 mg/kg PO BID then tapered to EOD or twice weekly either solely or in combination with cytotoxic immunosuppressive drugs.
- Cycline antibiotics: tetracycline 250 mg PO TID for dogs <10 kg; 500 mg PO TID dogs >10 kg); doxycycline 10 mg/kg PO q24h; minocycline 5 mg/kg PO BID; often

administered with niacinamide 250 mg PO for dogs <10 kg and 500 mg PO for dogs >10 kg.

- Dapsone:
    - Dogs only
    - Added to treatment when prednisolone alone is not sufficient and the primary cause is unknown
    - Tapering dosage schedule: 1 mg/kg PO TID for 2 weeks; then 1 mg/kg BID for 2 weeks; then 1 mg/kg q24h for 2 weeks; then 1 mg/kg EOD if sufficient to maintain control of symptoms.
- Sulfasalazine 20–40 mg/kg PO TID (maximum of 3 g/day); once remission is achieved, the dose is tapered by giving 10 mg/kg BID for 3 weeks, then 10 mg/kg q24h.
- Azathioprine: 2 mg/kg or 50 mg/m2 PO q24h until remission; then EOD or twice weekly; not for use in cats.
- Chlorambucil: 0.1–0.2 mg/kg q24h until remission; then EOD or twice weekly.
- Cyclosporine, microemulsion: 5–10 mg/kg q24h until remission; then EOD or twice weekly.

Precautions/Interactions

- Dapsone and sulfasalazine: not recommended with preexisting renal disease, hepatic disease, or blood dyscrasias.
- Sulfasalazine: not recommended with preexisting or borderline keratoconjunctivitis sicca; use with caution in cats; may displace highly protein-bound drugs (e.g., methotrexate, warfarin, phenylbutazone, thiazide diuretics, salicylates, probenecid, and phenytoin); bioavailability decreased by antacids; may decrease bioavailability of folic acid or digoxin; blood levels may be decreased if concurrently administering ferrous sulfate or other iron salts.
- Pentoxifylline: may increase prothrombin times; may decrease blood pressure.

COMMENTS

- Depending on medication(s) prescribed: CBC and biochemistry: day 7; every 2–4 weeks until remission; then every 3–6 months when on oral medications; monitor urinalysis with systemic vasculitis.
- Vasculitis may be difficult to treat and the prognosis is guarded if idiopathic.
- Immunosuppressive therapies should always be reduced to the lowest effective therapeutic dose.

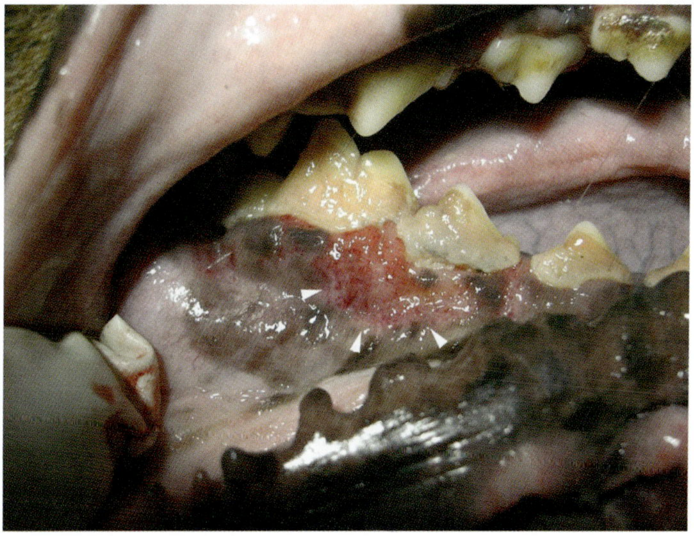

Fig. 48.1. Presumptive drug-induced vasculitis lesions in an 11-year-old male-intact rottweiler. Lesions were generalized as well as affecting the oral mucosae (*arrowheads*).

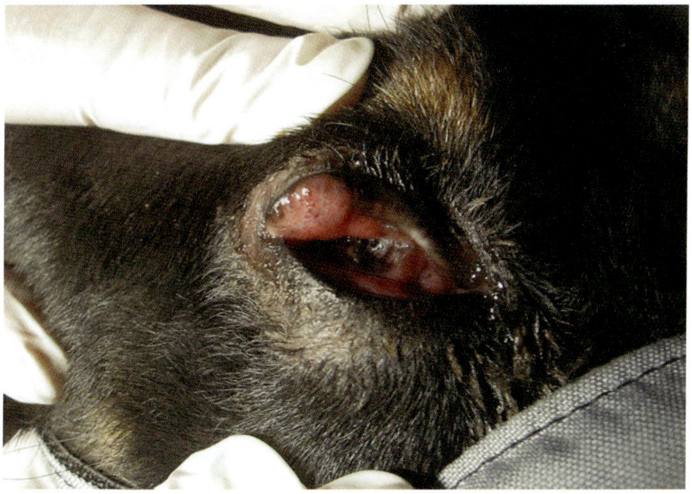

Fig. 48.2. Lesions affecting the conjunctiva of the patient in Figure 48.1.

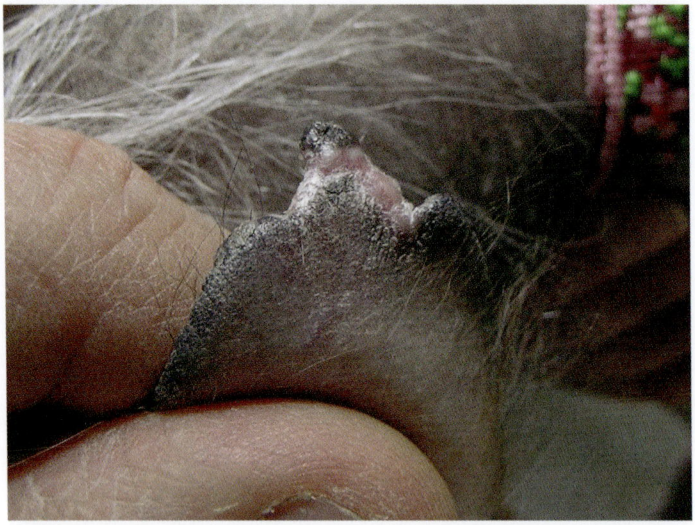

■ **Fig. 48.3.** Pinnal lesions of vasculitis in a 5-year-old male-castrate Chinese crested. Note the scalloped edges with scar tissue on either side of the pinnal tip.

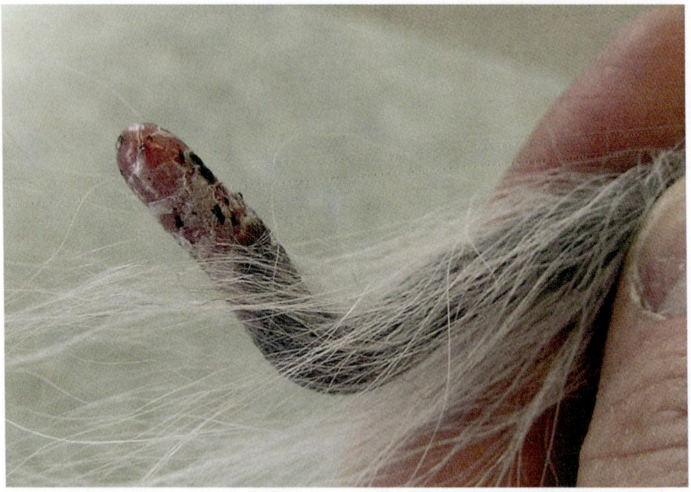

■ **Fig. 48.4.** Similarly affected tail tip of the patient in Figure 48.3.

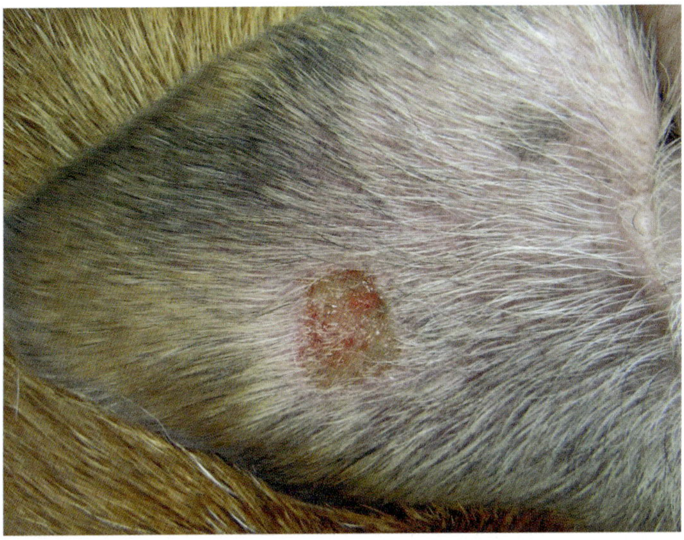

■ **Fig. 48.5.** Focal area of vasculitis consisting of loss of epidermis producing an erosion on the concave surface of the pinna in a 14-year-old female-spayed German shepherd.

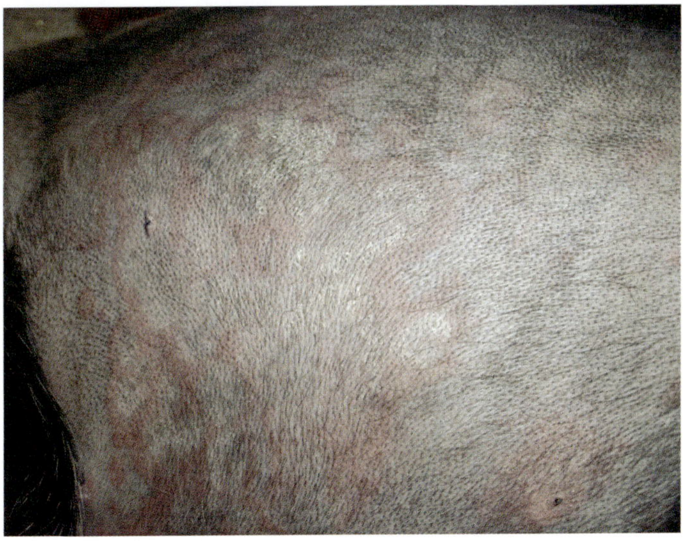

■ **Fig. 48.6.** Coalescing annular lesions producing a serpiginous pattern of erythema caused by systemic lupus erythematosus in a 12-year-old male-castrate Labrador retriever mix.

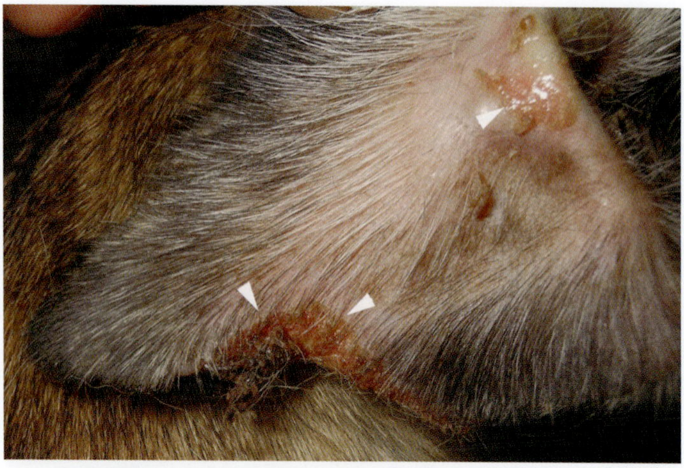

■ **Fig. 48.7.** Erosions and loss of tissue on the concave surface of the pinna at the fold and on the margin (*arrowheads*). Lesions were due to a generalized ischemic dermatopathy and vasculitis, with hepatitis and glomerulonephritis in a 6-year-old male-castrate Labrador retriever mix.

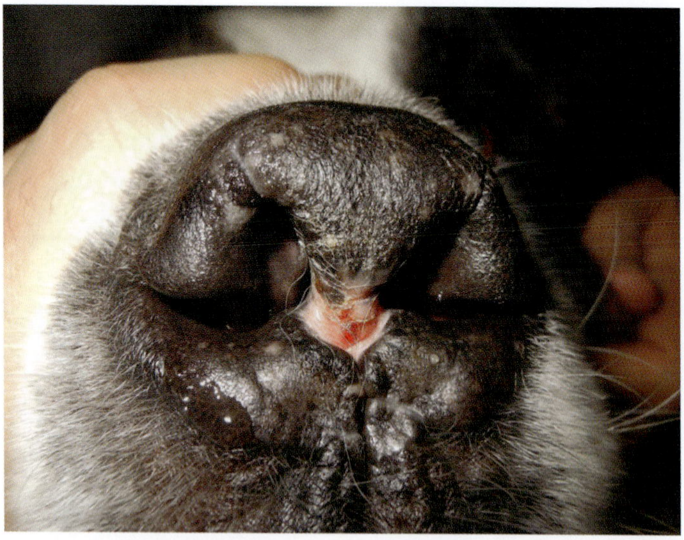

■ **Fig. 48.8.** Proliferative arteritis of the nasal philtrum in a 3-year-old female-spayed St Bernard. Note the significant loss of tissue and ulceration in a linear pattern across the nasal planum.

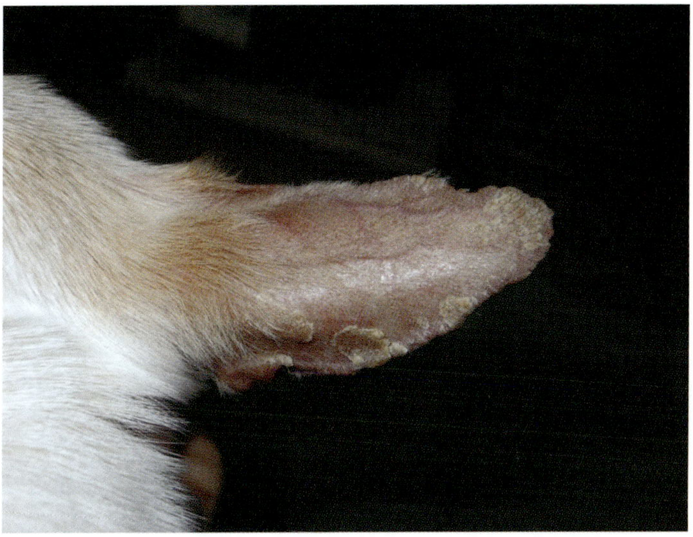

■ **Fig. 48.9.** Proliferative thrombovascular necrosis in a 3-year-old male-castrate chihuahua. The pinnae are alopecic and inflamed, with crusted margins and scalloped edges indicating tissue loss.

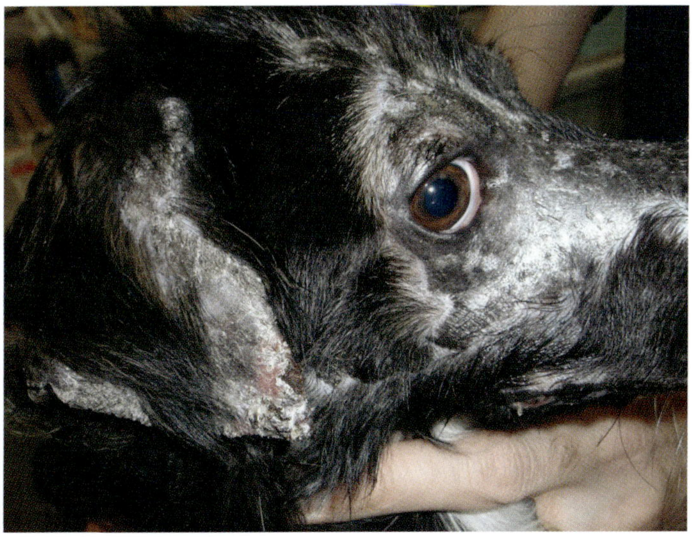

■ **Fig. 48.10.** Severe lesions of dermatomyositis in a 6-year-old male-castrate Shetland sheepdog mix. Chronic inflammation has resulted in alopecia with scarring on the face as well as the pinnae.

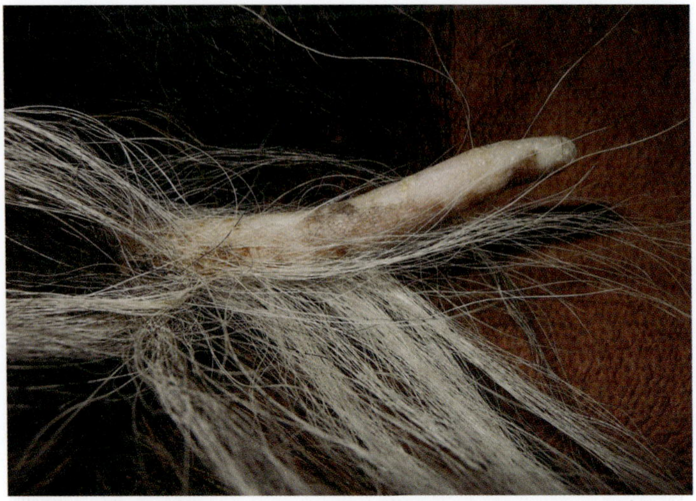

■ **Fig. 48.11.** Alopecia and scarring on the tail tip of the patient in Figure 48.10.

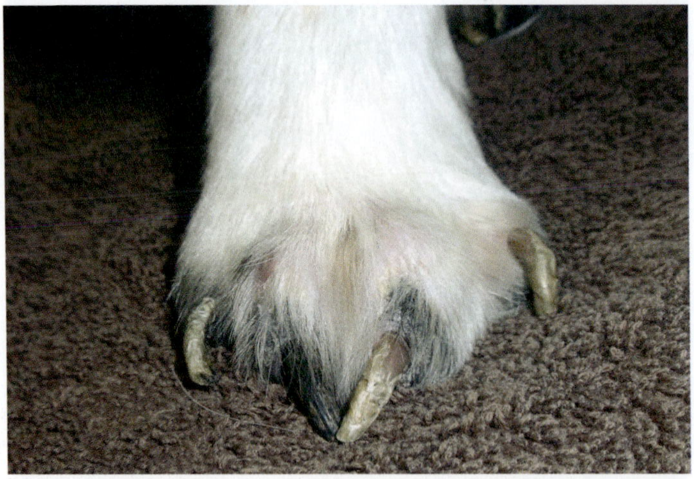

■ **Fig. 48.12.** Onychodystrophy caused by dermatomyositis affecting the patient in Figure 48.10.

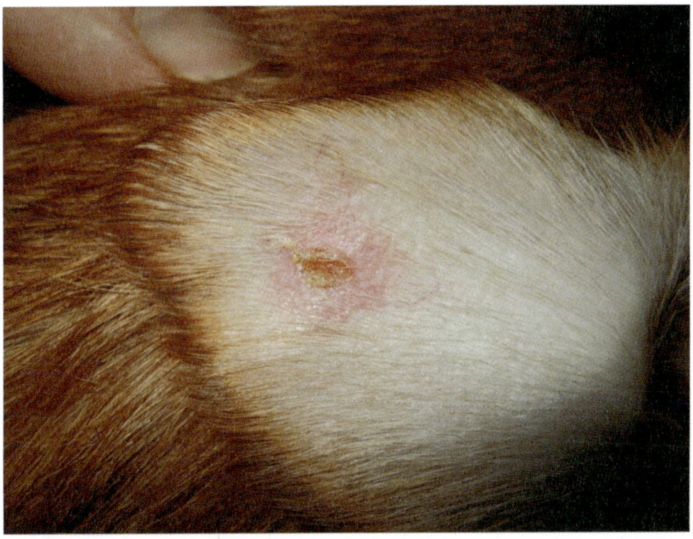

Fig. 48.13. Punctate lesion of erythema surrounding an erosion on the concave surface of the pinna of a 2-year-old male-castrate chihuahua mix dog secondary to rabies vaccination. Lesions may also develop at pinnal margins.

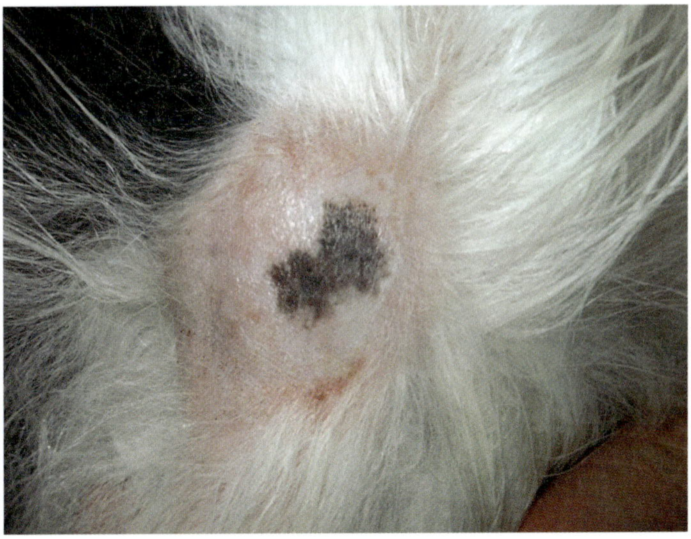

Fig. 48.14. Rabies vaccination-induced ischemic dermatopathy affecting the right lateral thigh of a 4-year-old female-spayed pomeranian mix. Quiescent alopecia with a central plaque (may be pigmented as present in this case) is typical of these lesions.

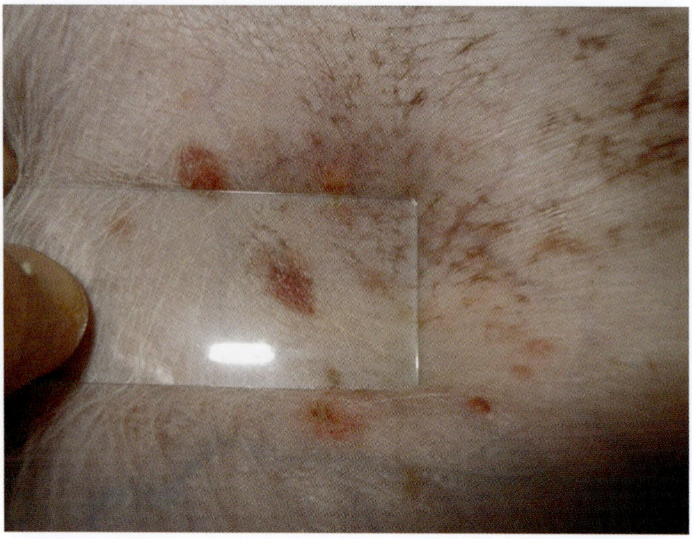

■ **Fig. 48.15.** Diascopy: pressing a glass slide against a lesion demonstrates whether or not there has been extravasation of red blood cells. Hemorrhagic lesions do not blanch as seen in the above image.

chapter 49

Viral Dermatoses

DEFINITION/OVERVIEW

- Dermatoses caused by viral infection within keratinized structures.
- Often underdiagnosed due to difficulty in identifying an exact causative viral agent.

ETIOLOGY/PATHOPHYSIOLOGY

- Viral replication within keratinized structures may cause cytosuppressive effects or upregulate keratinization, resulting in hyperplastic or crusted conditions.
- Most of the recognized viral dermatoses in veterinary medicine involve poxvirus-, coronavirus-, papillomavirus-, retrovirus-, herpesvirus-, and calicivirus-associated disease.
- Several widely recognized cutaneous syndromes in animals have not been proven to be a direct result of viral infection, but have a strong association suggestive of a causal effect.
- Papillomavirus: viral genome contains an oncogene that degrades p53 tumor suppressor protein; papillomavirus may be involved in the development of squamous cell carcinoma (SCC) in dogs and cats.

SIGNALMENT/HISTORY

- Head, neck, feet, and footpads common sites.
- Clinical dermatologic signs are variable with each specific virus; may involve other organ systems such as the respiratory, gastrointestinal, and/or nervous system.
- Risk factors for infection or development of viral dermatoses:
  - Fighting or hunting behavior
  - Exposure to an infected animal
  - Ingestion of infected materials
  - Immunosuppression – inherited or induced (corticosteroid or chemotherapy administration).

Blackwell's Five-Minute Veterinary Consult Clinical Companion: Small Animal Dermatology, Third Edition.
Karen Helton Rhodes and Alexander H. Werner.

Causes – Cat

- FeLV associated (retrovirus): vasculitis – seborrheic or ulcerative necrosis of the pinnae and tail tip; giant cell dermatosis – pruritic, ulcerative dermatosis of face, neck, pinnae; cutaneous horns – multicentric horns on the footpads and rarely nasal planum or eyelid margins; tumor – lymphoma, fibrosarcoma; immunosuppressive effects – produces secondary symptoms of gingivitis, recurrent bacterial folliculitis, dermatophytosis, malassezia dermatitis, and demodicosis (Figures 49.1, 49.2).
- FIV associated (retrovirus): plasma cell stomatitis: painful, proliferative lesion on palatoglossal folds and arches; plasma cell pododermatitis – spongy metacarpal and metatarsal pads ± painful and ulcerative; immunosuppressive effects – produces secondary symptoms of oral disease, recurrent bacterial folliculitis, dermatophytosis, *Malassezia* dermatitis, cryptococcosis, candidiasis, and demodicosis; generalized crusting dermatitis – head and limbs most affected (Figures 49.3–49.5).
- Plasma cell chondritis (retrovirus): symmetrical painful swelling of the pinnae, followed by shrinkage when healing, pyrexia, FeLV/FIV associated.
- Feline sarcoma virus (FeSV): multicentric fibrosarcoma.
- Feline cowpox virus infection (orthopoxvirus): initial small solitary "pock" lesion on the face or limbs that progresses to nodules, erosions, abscesses, and cellulitis; 20% of cases have oral lesions, depression, anorexia, pyrexia, respiratory signs or pneumonia; lesions usually resolve in 3–8 weeks; cat to cat, dog, and human reported; may be fatal in exotic felids.
- Feline infectious peritonitis (coronavirus FcoV): ascites, pleural effusion, hepatitis, uveitis, and, rarely, skin lesions characterized by vasculitis causing nodules or ulcers and focal necrosis affecting the head and neck.
- Feline papillomavirus (papillomavirus FcaPV2, FcaPV3, and FdPV2): hyperplastic multicentric scaly papules or plaques that may be hyperpigmented; implicated as precursory lesions of multicentric squamous cell carcinoma *in situ* (Bowen's disease, bowenoid *in situ* carcinoma – BISC) and characterized by hyperpigmented hyperkeratotic plaques of primarily the face, shoulders, and extremities (more aggressive disease seen in Devon rex); rare sarcoid lesions (facial nodules) caused by papillomavirus infection of dermal fibroblasts rather than epidermal keratinocytes; possible basal cell carcinoma (Figures 49.6–49.10).
- Feline rhinotracheitis (alpha-herpesvirus-1): vesicles, blisters, ulcerations of facial and nasal regions, often associated with URI; virus persists in the trigeminal nerve; may mimic allergic dermatitis (head and neck pruritus); herpes virus-associated erythema multiforme – skin lesions appear 10 days after infection causing respiratory signs and conjunctivitis; generalized erosive and exfoliative dermatosis that resolves within a few weeks (Figures 49.11–49.14).
- Feline calicivirus (calicivirus): conjunctivitis and stomatitis; vesicles that rapidly ulcerate, URI, pneumonia, acute death or spontaneously resolution; one syndrome involves only the skin presenting with fever, swollen feet and erosive lesions on the face (nose predominant) with spontaneous resolution in 2–3 days.

- Feline orofacial pain (FOP) syndrome (calicivirus): Burmese and Siamese cats predisposed, trigeminal neuralgia, unilateral intense pruritus, may be associated with oral disease.
- Pseudorabies (alpha-herpesvirus): intense self-mutilating pruritus; pigs are main reservoir; acute and fatal.

Causes – Dog

- Canine papillomavirus (seven canine subtypes identified); oral or mucocutaneous junction viral papillomas – young dogs or immunologically naive patients, associated with cyclosporine drug use; exophytic horns – footpads of older dogs; multiple cutaneous papillomas – cocker spaniel and Kerry blue terrier predisposed; pigmented viral plaques (chipapillomavirus) — multiple deeply pigmented small plaques on ventrum and medial forelegs (pugs and miniature schnauzer predisposed); cutaneous inverted papillomas – small, firm nodules with central indentation (Figures 49.15–49.22).
- Canine distemper (morbillivirus/paramyxovirus): nasodigital hyperkeratosis, "hard-pad disease," pustular dermatitis, fever, anorexia, oculonasal discharge, pneumonia, diarrhea, neurologic disorders.
- Contagious viral pustular dermatitis (parapoxvirus): sheep and goat reservoir; pustules, ulceration and crusts typically on the head; both dogs and cats affected; transmission to humans possible.
- Pseudorabies (alpha-herpesvirus): intense self-mutilating pruritus; pigs are main reservoir; acute and fatal.
- Canine herpesvirus (herpesvirus): petechial hemorrhages on mucous membranes, acute death in puppies, keratitis and conjunctivitis in adult dogs.

CLINICAL FEATURES

- Crusts
- Associated superficial bacterial folliculitis
- Abscess
- Paronychia
- Poor wound healing
- Seborrhea
- Exfoliative dermatitis
- Cutaneous horns
- Exophytic papillomas
- Gingivitis/stomatitis
- Cutaneous or oral (MCJ) ulceration
- Nasodigital hyperkeratosis
- Pigmented macules or plaques
- Progression to bowenoid *in situ* carcinoma (papillomavirus)

DIFFERENTIAL DIAGNOSIS

- Crusting diseases: if crust formation precedes other symptoms – drug eruption, pemphigus foliaceus, systemic lupus erythematosus additional causes for exfoliative dermatitis.
- Allergic disorders: if pruritus is the initial clinical sign – flea-allergic dermatitis, cutaneous adverse reaction to food, atopic dermatitis, *Malassezia* overgrowth/hypersensitivity.
- Parasitic diseases: canine and/or feline scabies, demodicosis, cheyletiellosis.
- Infectious diseases: superficial and deep bacterial and fungal infections, leishmaniasis.
- Keratinization disorders: nasodigital hyperkeratosis, zinc-responsive dermatoses.
- Neoplasia: mast cell tumors and epitheliotropic lymphoma.
- Metabolic disorders: hepatocutaneous syndrome (superficial necrolytic dermatitis).

DIAGNOSTICS

CBC/Biochemistry/Urinalysis

- Often normal; abnormalities present may reflect severity of other systemic disease processes.

Cytology/Serology/Virus Isolation

- Rule out other differentials with skin scrapings and trichograms, dermatophyte culture, epidermal cytology.
- Viral serology: FeLV and FIV; hemagglutination inhibition, virus neutralizing, complement fixation, Western blot (immunoblot), or ELISA; demonstrate rising titers indicative of active infection on paired serum samples.
- Virus isolation from crusted material is often diagnostic (90% positive in poxvirus infection).
- Polymerase chain reaction (PCR) or reverse transcriptase PCR (RT-PCR).
- Cerebrospinal spinal fluid analysis, bone marrow aspirate.

Histopathologic Findings

- Light microscopy:
  - Hyperplasia
  - Ballooning degeneration
  - Hydropic interface dermatitis
  - Syncytial-type giant cell formation within the epidermis and/or outer root sheath of the hair follicle
  - Keratinocyte inclusion bodies

- Immunohistochemistry: immunofluorescent or avidin-biotin complex method often employed for detection of papillomavirus group-related antigens; requires active viral replication for detection, leading to possible false-negative results.
- Electron microscopy:
    - Highly selective and diagnostic
    - May be performed on crust, biopsy specimen, or exudate.

THERAPEUTICS

- Usually outpatient, except for systemically ill patients.
- Systemically ill: may require IV fluids, parenteral antibiotics; supportive care and treatment of secondary infections.
- Azithromycin 10 mg/kg PO q24h for 10–14 days; papillomavirus (questionable efficacy).
- L-lysine 200–500 mg/cat PO BID (questionable efficacy).
- Famcyclovir 62.5–125 mg/cat PO TID for 3 weeks (lower dose for kittens).
- Zidovudine (Retrovir or Retrovis – Glaxo SmithKline): direct antiviral agent, most effective against acute FIV infections, monitor for bone marrow suppression; 5–15 mg/kg PO BID (primarily FIV, FeLV).
- Interferon-alpha: 1000–2000 units q24h orally (immunomodulating dose) or 1–2 million units/m^2 by subcutaneous injection three times weekly.
- Topical imiquimod (Aldara): primarily used for Bowen's syndrome (SCC *in situ*); applied 2–3 consecutive days/week.
- Topical 5-fluorouracil (0.5%): contraindicated in cats due to neurotoxicity.
- Vaccinations as preventive for certain virus infections (e.g., distemper, FeLV).
- Immunomodulators with limited success: *Proprionibacterium acnes* (ImmunoRegulin – Neogen) and acemannan (Carrisyn – Carrington Labs).
- Ophthalmic antivirals: vidarabine (Vira-A – Parke-Davis); used for herpetic ulcers q2h.
- Surgical removal of papillomas; surgical excision, cryosurgery, laser surgery.

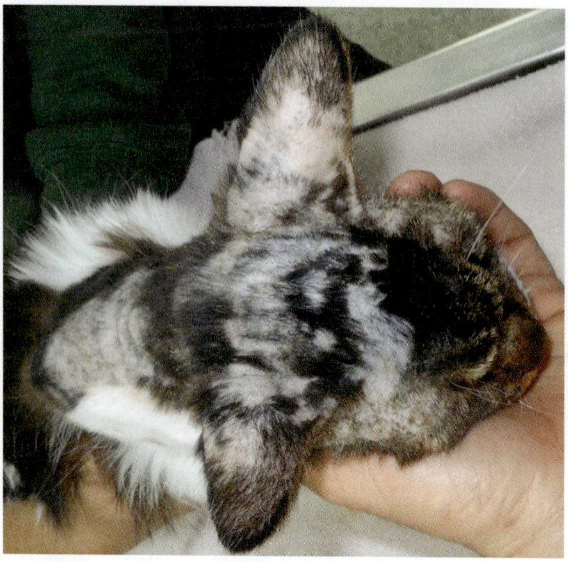

■ **Fig. 49.1.** Intense head and neck pruritus exacerbated by FeLV in a 13-year-old male-castrate DLH with cutaneous adverse reaction to food.

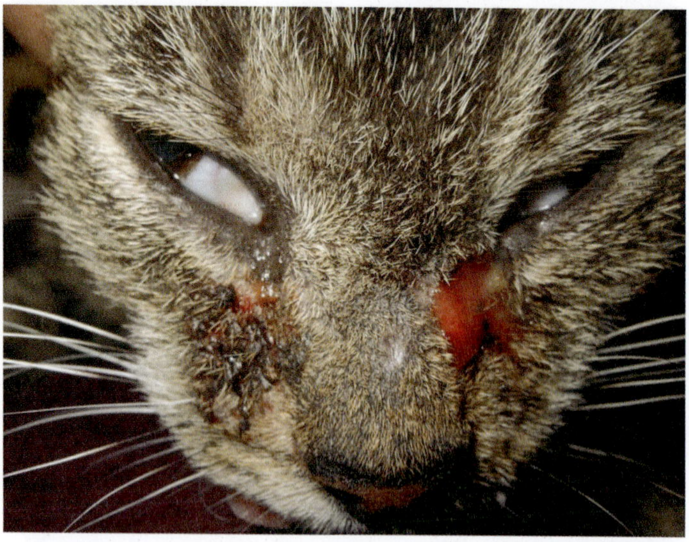

■ **Fig. 49.2.** FeLV-related facial pruritus and demodicosis in a 13-year-old female-spayed DSH.

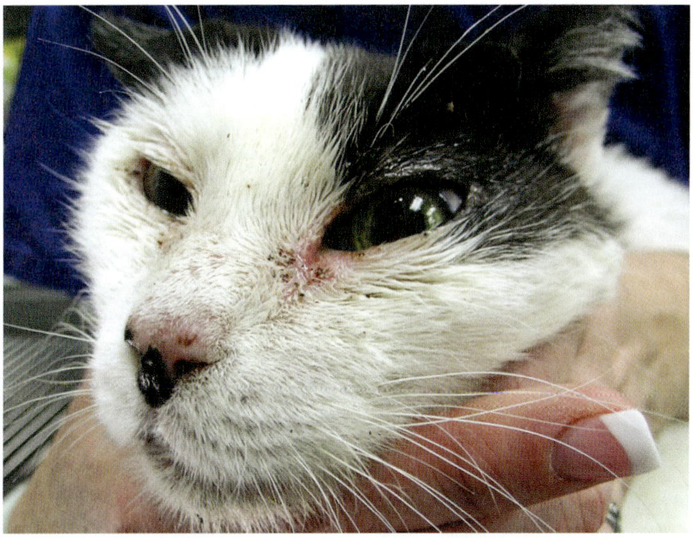

■ **Fig. 49.3.** Facial pruritus associated with FIV in an adult DSH.

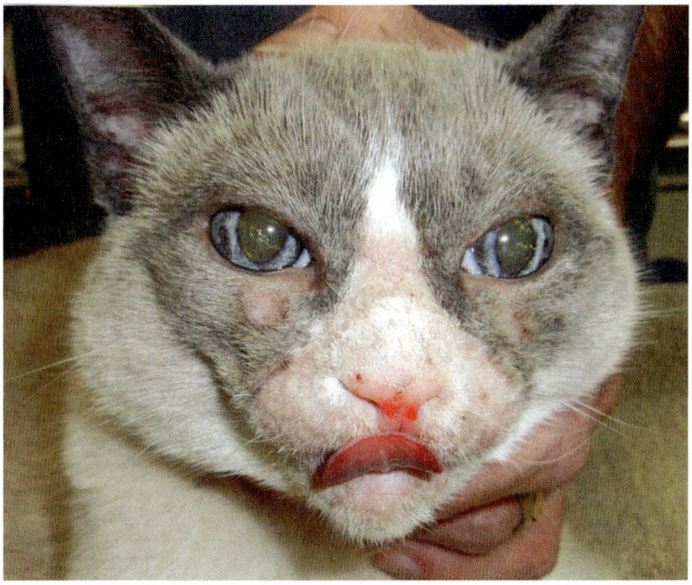

■ **Fig. 49.4.** Facial pruritus and erythema associated with FIV in a 5-year-old female-spayed Siamese mix.

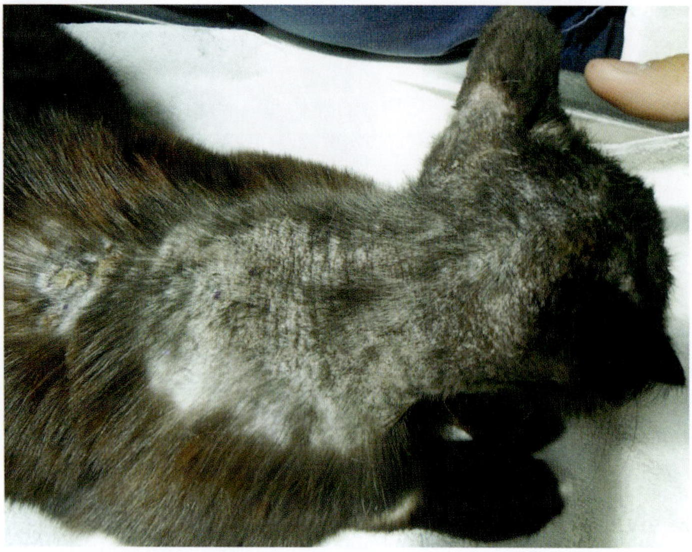

Fig. 49.5. Head and neck pruritus and exfoliative dermatitis associated with FIV in a 7-year-old male-castrate DMH.

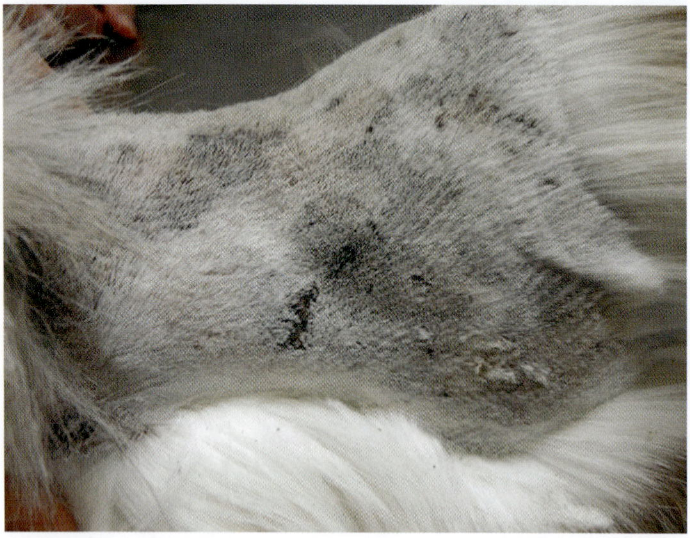

Fig. 49.6. Characteristic pigmented macules and plaques of multicentric squamous cell carcinoma *in situ* (Bowen's disease) on the dorsal and lateral aspects of the neck of a 12-year-old female-spayed DLH.

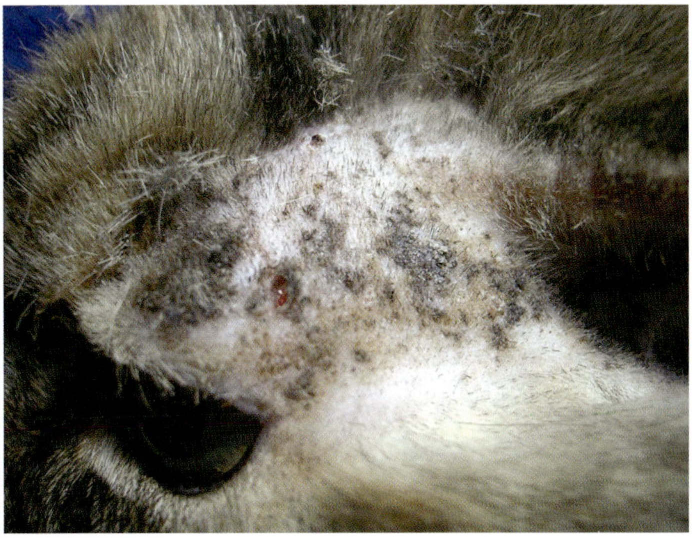

■ **Fig. 49.7.** Punctate pigmented plaques in the preauricular area of an adult DSH with Bowen's disease.

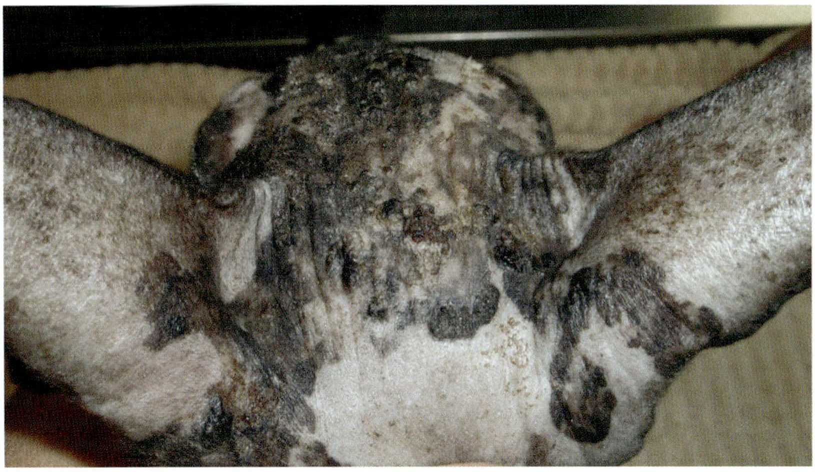

■ **Fig. 49.8.** Multiple, large, coalescing, and hyperpigmented plaques of Bowen's disease in a 12-year-old female-spayed sphynx.

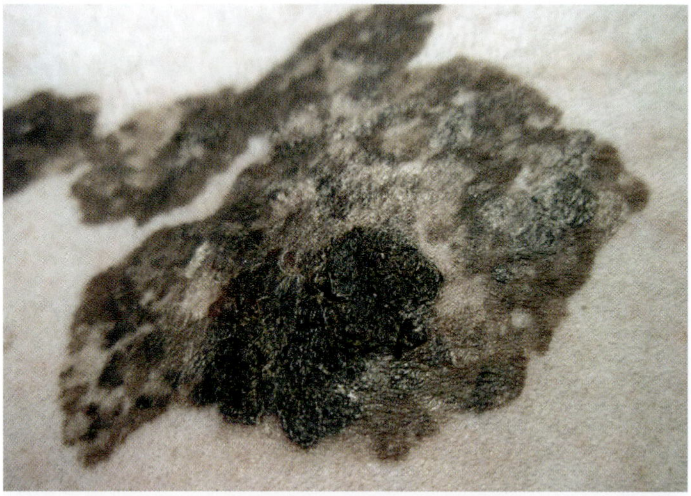

■ **Fig. 49.9.** Closer image of lesions from the patient in Figure 49.8. Note that pigmented plaques are irregular in both depth of pigmentation and thickness.

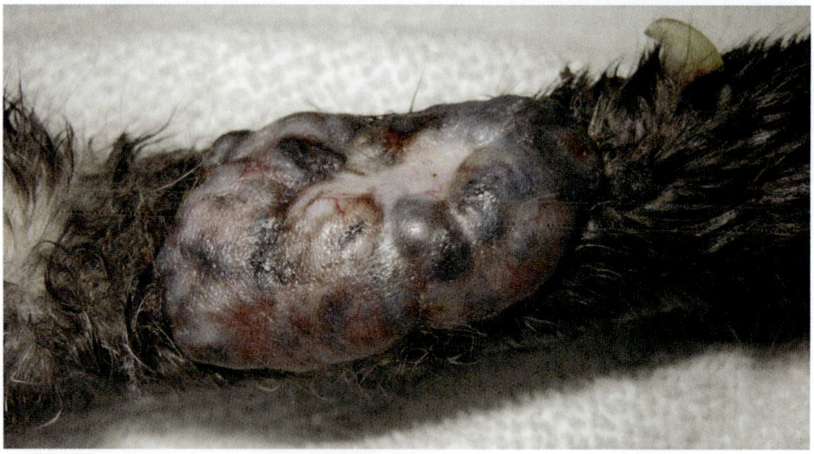

■ **Fig. 49.10.** Single large tumor on the foreleg of a 19-year-old male-castrate DSH with Bowen's disease.

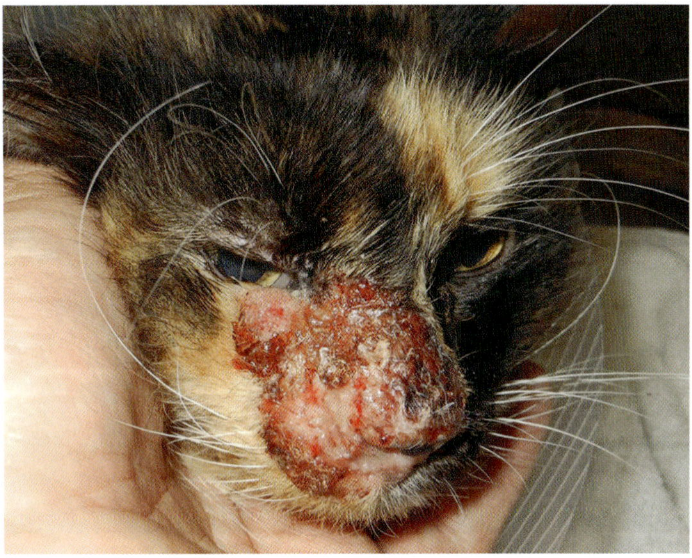

■ **Fig. 49.11.** Large eroded and ulcerated plaque associated with herpes virus infection in a 14-year-old female-spayed DLH.

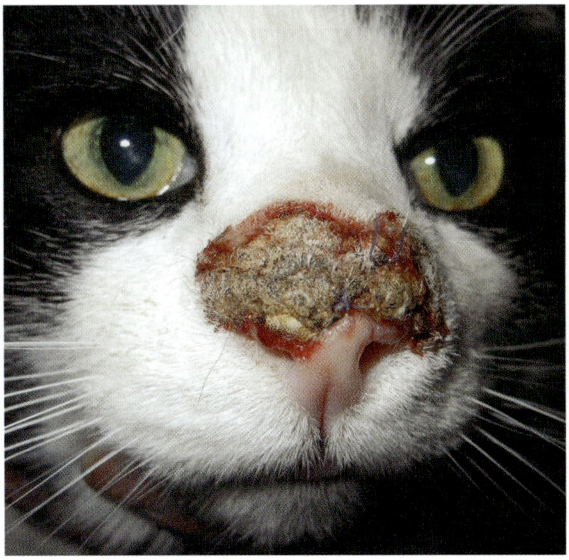

■ **Fig. 49.12.** Adherent crust over eroded and ulcerated patch on the dorsal muzzle and nasal planum of a 12-year-old male-castrate DSH with herpes virus dermatitis.

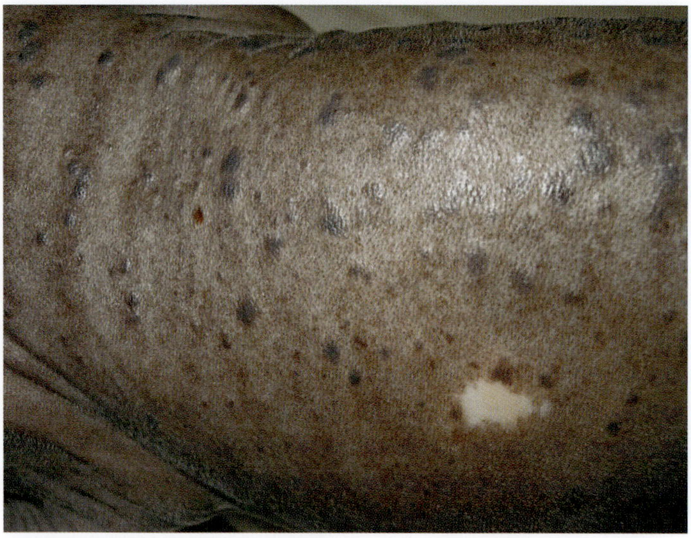

■ **Fig. 49.13.** Herpes virus-associated erythema multiforme in a 7-year-old female-spayed sphynx. Note generalized multiple hyperpigmented plaques. Patient experienced a flare-up of ocular disease prior to onset of skin lesions; lesions responded to oral antiviral therapy.

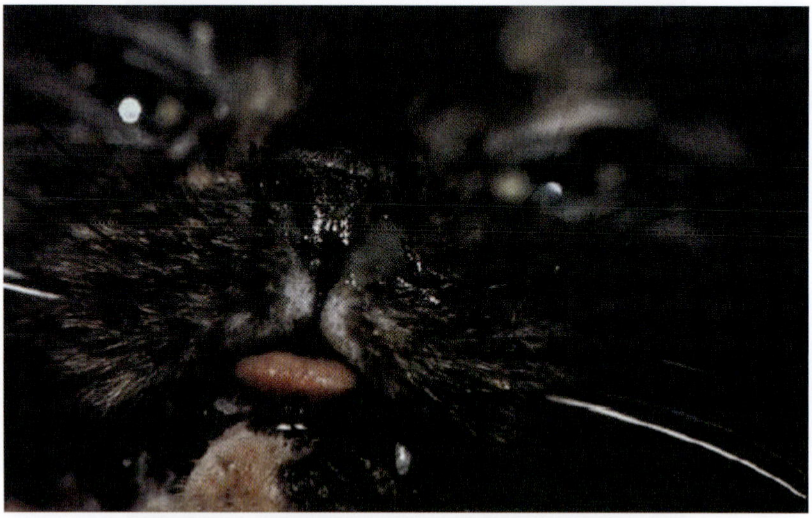

■ **Fig. 49.14.** Calicivirus infection in the cat. Note the erythema and erosions along the periocular and facial region. Source: Reproduced with permission of Dr J. Taboada.

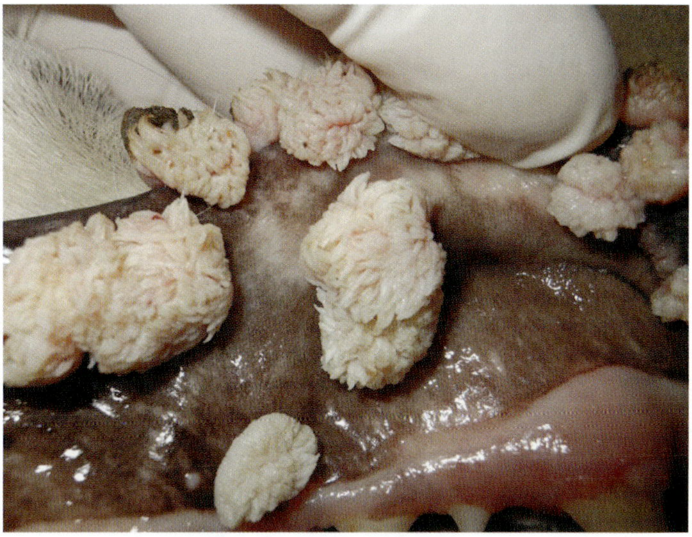

Fig. 49.15. Multiple irregularly surfaced and pedunculated nodules on the mucous membranes of a 2-year-old female-spayed Siberian husky with oral viral papillomatosis.

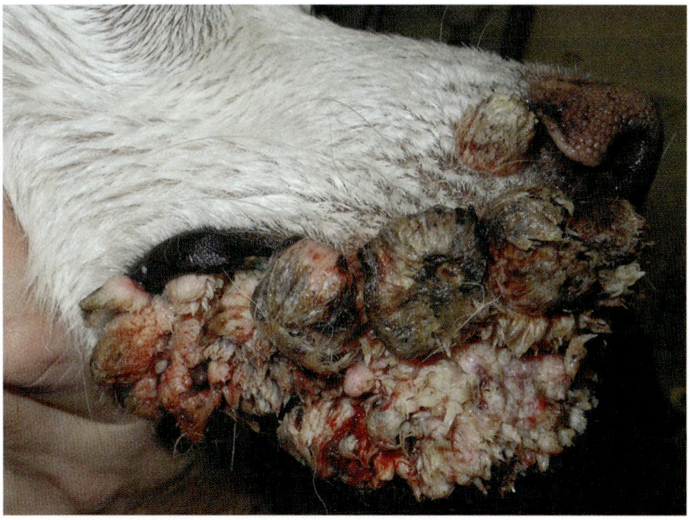

Fig. 49.16. Large, coalescing papillomavirus lesions on the muzzle and lip margins of the patient in Figure 49.15.

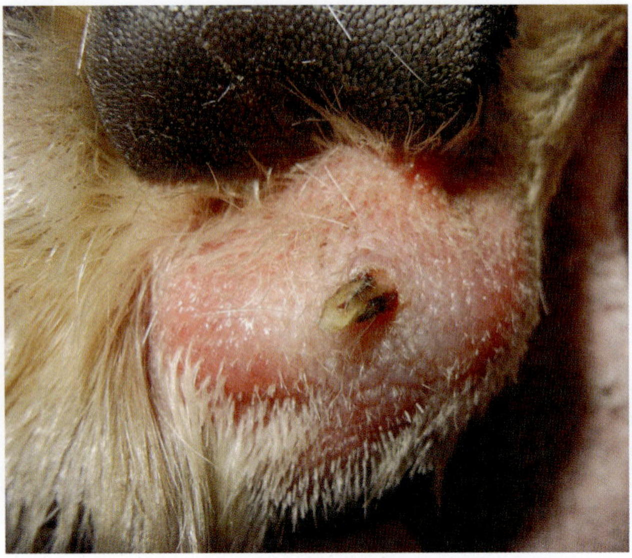

■ **Fig. 49.17.** Exophytic cutaneous horn on a footpad margin associated with papillomavirus in a 1-year-old female-spayed chihuahua.

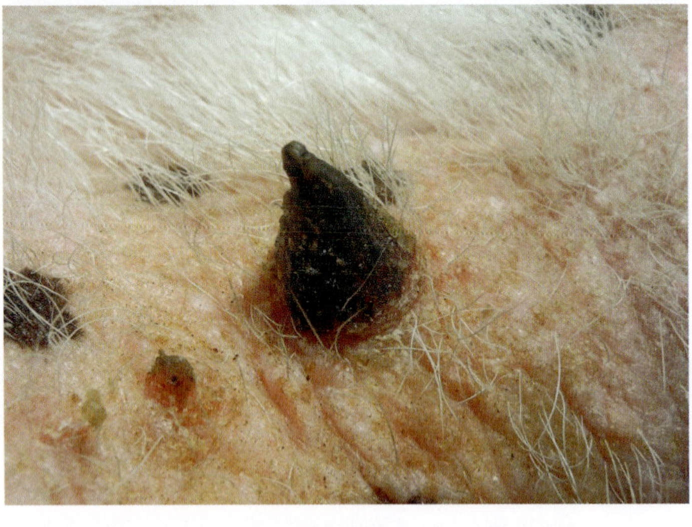

■ **Fig. 49.18.** Cutaneous horn associated with papillomavirus on the dorsum of a 4-year-old male-castrate pit bull. Lesions were also associated with generalized demodicosis.

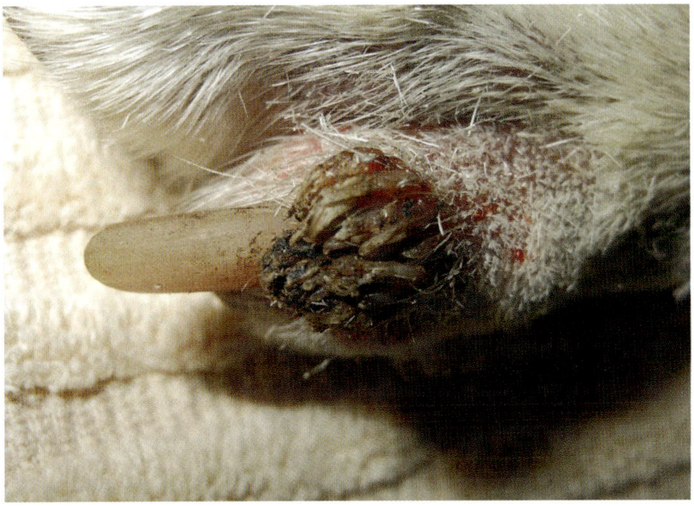

■ **Fig. 49.19.** Viral papilloma at the ungual fold of a 7-year-old male-castrate French bulldog. This nodule demonstrates the characteristic irregular "cauliflower-like" appearance.

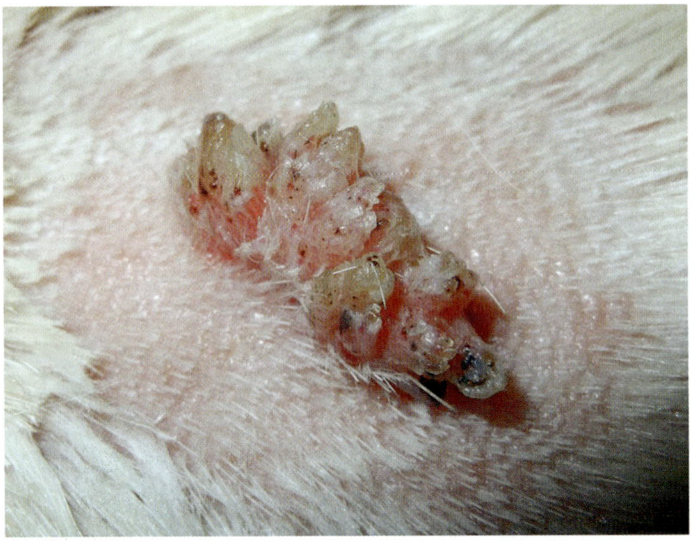

■ **Fig. 49.20.** Viral papilloma on a 2-year-old female-spayed French bulldog. There were multiple similar lesions noted in this patient.

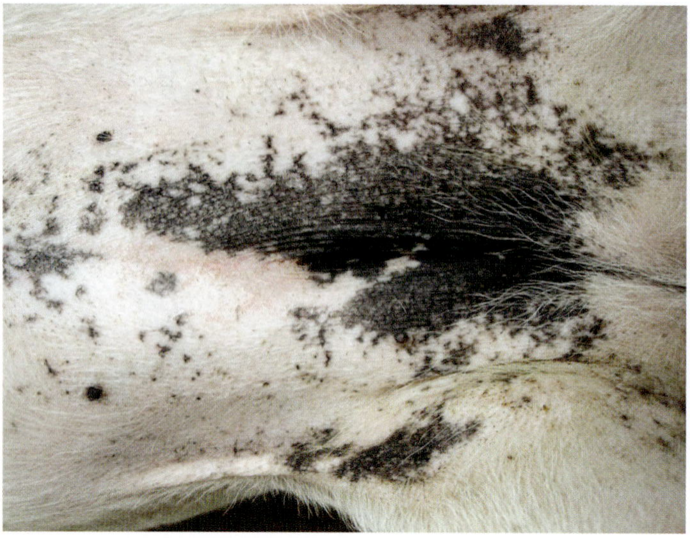

■ **Fig. 49.21.** Pigmented viral plaques associated with papillomavirus. Lesions were distributed on the ventrum of an 8-year-old female-spayed pug.

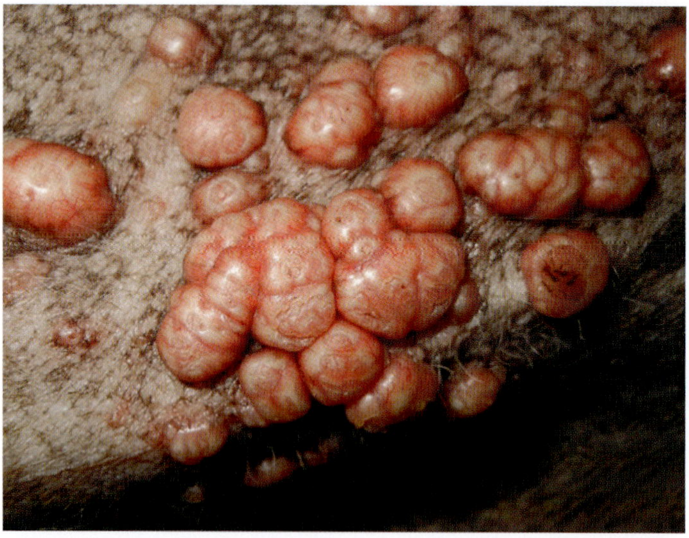

■ **Fig. 49.22.** Multiple inverted papillomas on the ventrum of a 10-year-old male-castrate golden retriever.

chapter 50

Zoonosis

DEFINITION/OVERVIEW

- Zoonosis can be defined broadly (any disease/organism shared by animals and humans) or narrowly (a disease/organism transmitted directly from animals to humans).
- Distinction can blur with diseases affecting the skin, especially if vectors (especially fleas and ticks) are included in this category.
- A further consideration is whether external parasites carried by companion animals that can irritate but not infest humans are included in this category.
- Recent discussions include the concept that genes coding for multidrug resistance may transfer from the bacterial populations on companion animals to humans, and vice versa.
- Similar drug resistance patterns have been found in bacterial populations residing on people and on animals in a household; this may be loosely considered as a zoonosis – the transfer of drug resistance directly from animal to human may affect (though not cause) disease in people.
- Zoonotic diseases and their vectors vary significantly geographically.
- The lists in the following sections are not meant to be exhaustive and list dermatologic diseases more commonly acquired directly from dogs and cats, diseases transmitted by their ectoparasites, or dermatitis caused by ectoparasites carried on dogs and cats (Figures 50.1–50.4).

PARASITES

- *Cheyletiella* spp.
- *Sarcoptes scabiei*
- *Otodectes cynotis*
- *Leishmania*
- *Notoedres cati*
- *Ctenocephalides felis* and *canis*
- *Pulex* spp.
- *Echnidnophaga gallinacea*
- *Dipylidium caninum*

Blackwell's Five-Minute Veterinary Consult Clinical Companion: Small Animal Dermatology, Third Edition.
Karen Helton Rhodes and Alexander H. Werner.

- Cutaneous larval migrans:
    - *Ancylostoma caninum*
    - *Ancylostoma brazilense*
    - *Uncinaria stenocephala*

BACTERIA

- Tuberculosis
- *Dermatophilus congolensis*
- *Streptococcus* spp.
- *Staphylococcus* spp.
- L-form/*Mycoplasma* spp.
- *Yersinia pestis*
- *Brucella canis*
- *Ehrlichia* spp.
- *Anaplasma phagocytophilum*
- *Rickettsia* spp.
- *Francisella tularensis*
- *Borrelia burgdorferi*

FUNGI

- Sporotrichosis
- Cryptococcosis
- Blastomycosis
- Histoplasmosis
- Rhinosporidiosis
- Aspergillosis
- Penicilliosis
- Protothecosis
- *Coccidioides immitis*
- *Malassezia pachydermatis*
- Dermatophytosis:
    - *Microsporum canis*
    - *Microsporum gypseum*
    - *Trichophyton mentagrophytes*
    - *Epidermophyton* spp.

VIRUSES

- Orthopoxvirus (feline cowpox virus)
- Parapoxvirus (contagious viral pustular dermatitis)

PROTOZOA

- *Babesia* spp.

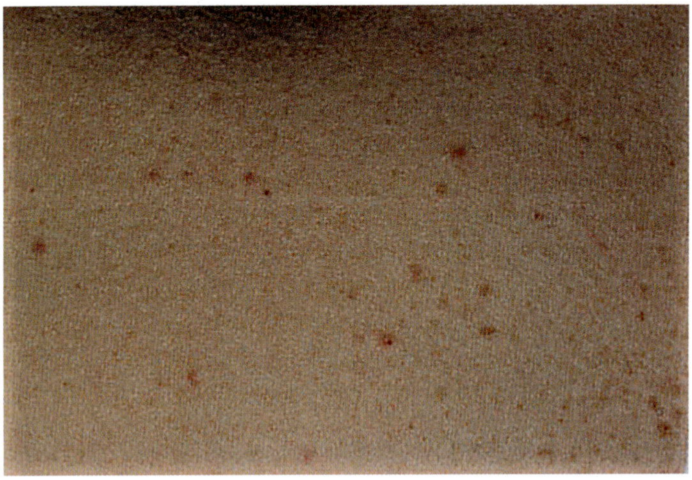

Fig. 50.1. Erythematous papules on the abdomen from cheyletiellosis.

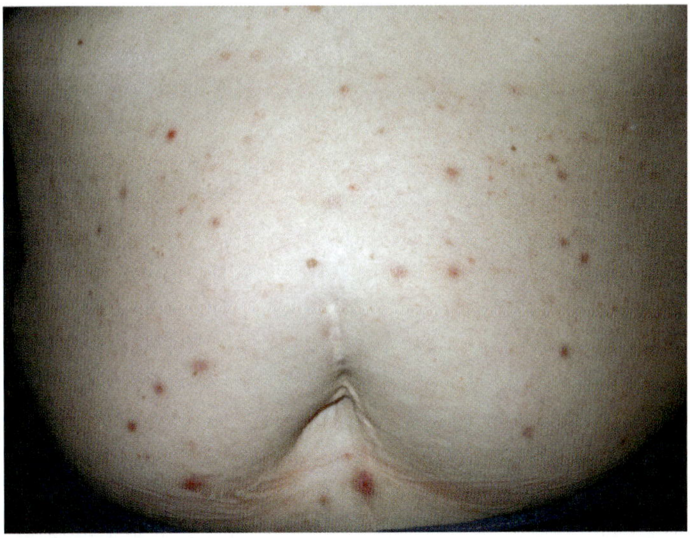

Fig. 50.2. Erythematous and excoriated papules on the abdomen caused by *Sarcoptes scabiei*.

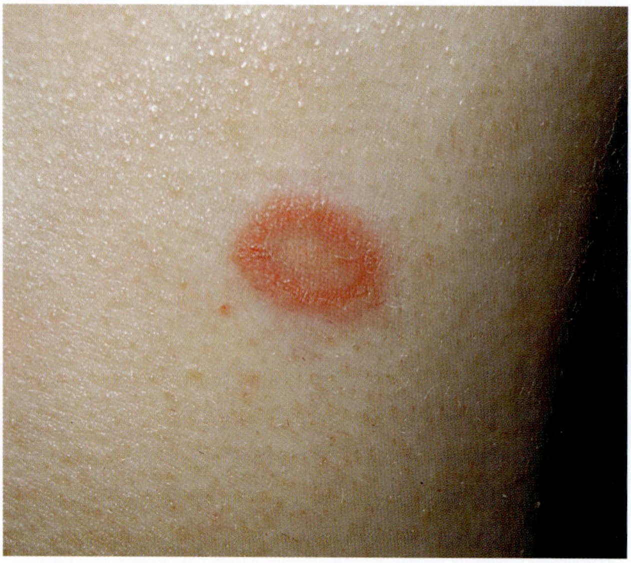

Fig. 50.3. Slowly expanding, annular lesion of erythema and scale forming the "classic" ringworm lesion seen in a human infected with *Microsporum canis*.

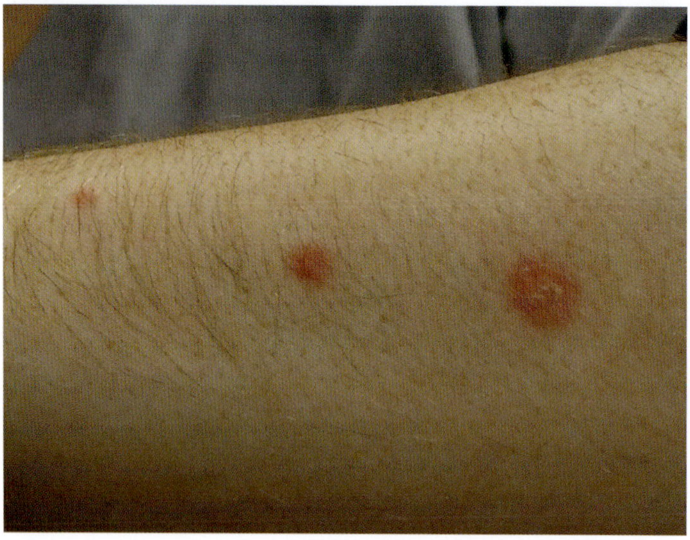

Fig. 50.4. Additional lesions on the forearm of a human due to *Microsporum canis*.

appendix A

Canine Genodermatoses

This list represents some of the more common canine dermatologic (or dermatologic-related) disorders recognized within certain breeds. Some of the diseases have a genetic etiology whereas others seem to have a breed predisposition. The exact etiologies/pathogenesis of many of the conditions are changing as canine dermatologic research progresses.

Affenpinscher	Hyperadrenocorticism
Afghan hound	Hypothyroidism
	Demodicosis
Airedale terrier	Lymphoma
	Hypothyroidism
	Demodicosis
	Flank alopecia
Akita	Juvenile-onset polyarthritis
	Uveodermatologic syndrome
	Pemphigus foliaceus
	Deafness
	Hypothyroidism
	Granulomatous sebaceous adenitis
Alaskan malamute	Anemia with chondrodysplasia
	Follicular (color) dysplasia (red)
	Follicular dysplasia (plush-coated breeds)
	Dwarfism
	Demodicosis
	Hypothyroidism
	Hyperadrenocorticism
	Zinc-responsive dermatosis
American foxhound	Deafness
	Microphthalmia
	Leishmaniasis
American Staffordshire terrier	Mast cell tumor
	Deafness
	Flank alopecia
American water spaniel	Hermaphroditism
	Pattern baldness

Blackwell's Five-Minute Veterinary Consult Clinical Companion: Small Animal Dermatology, Third Edition.
Karen Helton Rhodes and Alexander H. Werner.

Australian cattle dog	Deafness
	Keratinization disorders
Australian kelpie	Microphthalmia
	Cutaneous asthenia
Australian shepherd dog	Microphthalmia
	Deafness
	Dwarfism
	Discoid lupus erythematosus
	ABCB1 gene defect/drug sensitivity
Australian terrier	Diabetes mellitus
Basenji	Immunoproliferative enteropathy (alopecia, hyperkeratosis, pinnal necrosis)
Basset hound	Seborrhea
	Malassezia dermatitis
	Actinic/solar dermatitis
	Atopic dermatitis
	Otitis externa/media
	Achondrodysplasia
	Congenital hypotrichosis
	Black-hair follicular dysplasia
Beagle	Lymphocytic thyroiditis
	Cutaneous asthenia
	Congenital hypotrichosis
	Atopic dermatitis
	Amyloidosis
	Deafness
	Hypothyroidism
	Systemic necrotizing vasculitis
Bearded collie	Hypopigmentation
	Pemphigus foliaceus
	Black-hair follicular dysplasia
Beauceron	Epidermolysis imperfecta
	Dermatomyositis
	Systemic lupus erythematosus
Bedlington terrier	Lacrimal duct atresia
	Melanotrichia
	Senile perifollicular mineralization
Belgian sheepdog	Granulomatous sebaceous adenitis
Belgian tervuren	Idiopathic leukoderma/leukotrichia
	Hypothyroidism
Bernese mountain dog	Color dilution alopecia
	Histiocytosis: cutaneous, systemic, malignant
Bichon frise	Pemphigus foliaceus
	Congenital hypotrichosis

Bloodhound	*Malassezia* dermatitis
	Atopic dermatitis
	Otitis externa/media
Border collie	Deafness
	Black-hair follicular dysplasia
	ABCB1 gene defect/drug sensitivity
Border terrier	Mast cell tumors
	Pituitary tumors
Borzoi	Hygromas
	Calcinosis circumscripta
	Hypothyroidism
Boston terrier	Atopic dermatitis
	Mast cell tumor
	Hyperadrenocorticism
	Deafness
	Stenotic nares
	Intertrigo (facial/tail fold)
	Demodicosis
	Pattern baldness
	Color dilution alopecia
Bouvier des Flandres	Flank alopecia
	Lymphosarcoma
Boxer	Atopic dermatitis
	Cutaneous adverse reaction to food
	Acne/muzzle furunculosis
	Bacterial folliculitis
	Cutaneous asthenia
	Mast cell tumor
	Histiocytoma
	Gingival hyperplasia
	Dermoid cyst
	Interdigital pyogranulomatous dermatitis/furunculosis
	Vaginal hyperplasia
	Hyperadrenocorticism
	Hypothyroidism
	Actinic/solar dermatitis
	Deafness
	Fibrosarcoma
	Melanoma
	Flank alopecia
	Leishmaniasis
Briard	Hypothyroidism
Brittany spaniel	Lip fold dermatitis
	Cryptorchidism
	Discoid lupus erythematosus

Bull terrier	Deafness Lethal acrodermatitis Zinc-responsive dermatitis Actinic/solar dermatitis Interdigital pyogranulomatous dermatitis/furunculosis Nasal/muzzle furunculosis Demodicosis Waardenburg–Klein syndrome (amelanotic skin, blue eyes, deafness)
Bulldog	Muzzle furunculosis Ichthyosis Interdigital pyogranulomatous dermatitis/furunculosis Intertrigo (facial/tail fold) Demodicosis Blepharitis Atopic dermatitis Pemphigus foliaceus Lymphoma Mast cell tumor Hypothyroidism Deafness Flank alopecia Calcinosis cutis Lymphedema
Bullmastiff	Idiopathic leukoderma/leukotrichia Interdigital pyogranulomatous dermatitis/furunculosis
Cairn terrier	Atopic dermatitis Hyperadrenocorticism
Canaan dog	Diabetes mellitus Hypothyroidism
Cardigan Welsh corgi	Cutaneous asthenia
Cavalier King Charles spaniel	Diabetes mellitus Keratoconjunctivitis sicca and ichthyosiform dermatosis Primary secretory otitis media (PSOM) Syringomyelia Black-hair follicular dysplasia Ichthyosis Canine eosinophilic granuloma
Chesapeake Bay retriever	Entropion Atopic dermatitis Ectodermal dysplasia – skin fragility syndrome

Chihuahua	Color dilution alopecia
	Pattern baldness
	Demodicosis
Chinese crested	Atopic dermatitis
	Comedones
	Ectodermal dysplasia
Chinese shar-pei	Cutaneous mucinosis
	Hypothyroidism
	Renal amyloidosis (Mediterranean/periodic fever)
	Bacterial folliculitis
	Atopic dermatitis
	Cutaneous adverse reaction to food
	Cutaneous Langerhans cell histiocytosis
	Fold dermatitis
	Demodicosis
	Malassezia hypersensitivity
Chow chow	Pemphigus foliaceus
	Color dilution alopecia
	Follicular dysplasia (plush-coated breeds)
	Hypothyroidism
	Microphthalmia
	Uveodermatologic syndrome
	Postclipping alopecia
	Tyrosinase deficiency (depigmentation)
Collie	Dermatomyositis
	Vesicular cutaneous lupus erythematosus
	Discoid lupus erythematous
	Pemphigus erythematosus
	Bullous pemphigoid
	Deafness
	Systemic lupus erythematosus
	Autosomal recessive cyclic neutropenia
	Dwarfism
	Cyclic hematopoiesis (immunodeficiency)/gray haircoat
	Waardenburg–Klein syndrome (blue eyes, amelanotic skin, deaf)
	ABCB1 gene defect/drug sensitivity
Curly-coated retriever	Hyperadrenocorticism
	Hypothyroidism
	Pattern baldness
	Flank alopecia
Dachshund	Diabetes mellitus
	Hypothyroidism
	Hyperadrenocorticism

	Deafness
	Dermoid cyst
	Idiopathic sterile nodular panniculitis
	"Acanthosis nigricans"
	Color dilution alopecia
	Cutaneous asthenia
	Pattern baldness
	Sensory neuropathy
	Pemphigus foliaceus
	Linear IgA pustular dermatosis
	Vasculitis
	Alopecia areata
	Interdigital pyogranulomatous dermatitis/furunculosis
	Black-hair follicular dysplasia
	Juvenile cellulitis
	Bacterial folliculitis
	Malassezia hypersensitivity
	Ear margin dermatosis/pinnal seborrhea
	Pinnal vasculitis
	Idiopathic onchodystrophy
Dalmatian	Bacterial folliculitis
	Atopic dermatitis
	Cutaneous adverse reaction to food
	Actinic/solar dermatitis
	Deafness
	Globoid cell leukodystrophy
	Allergic dermatitis
	Waardeburg–Klein syndrome (amelanotic skin, blue eyes, deaf)
Dandie Dinmont terrier	Hyperadrenocorticism
	Lymphoma
Doberman pinscher	Hypothyroidism
	"Flank sucking"
	Immune complex disorders drug sensitivity (trimethoprim-sulfa antibiotics)
	Interdigital pyogranulomatous dermatitis/furunculosis
	Muzzle furunculosis
	Color dilution alopecia
	Follicular dysplasia
	Deafness
	Idiopathic leukoderma/leukotrichia
	Oculocutaneous albinism
	Granulocytopathy (immunodeficiency)

	Selective IgM deficiency
	Pemphigus foliaceus
	Canine benign familial chronic pemphigus
	Ichthyosis
Dogue de Bordeaux	Footpad hyperkeratosis
	Interdigital pyogranulomatous dermatitis/furunculosis
English foxhound	Deafness
English setter	Deafness
	Carcinoma and lymphoma of the oral and nasal cavity
	Canine benign familial chronic pemphigus
Finnish spitz	Pemphigus foliaceus
Flat-coated retriever	Histiosarcoma
	Symmetric lupoid onchodystrophy
Fox terrier	Deafness
	Atopic dermatitis
French bulldog	Atopic dermatitis
	Congenital hypotrichosis
	Intertrigo (facial/tail folds)
	Follicular dysplasia
	Flank alopecia
German shepherd dog	Symmetric lupoid onychodystrophy
	Discoid lupus erythematosus
	Systemic lupus erythematosus
	Pemphigus foliaceus
	Perineal fistula
	Metacarpal/metatarsal fistulae
	Atopic dermatitis
	Pituitary dwarfism
	Hypothyroidism
	Nodular dermatofibrosis with renal cystadenocarcinoma
	Calcinosis circumscripta
	Mucocutaneous pyoderma
	Granulomatous sebaceous adenitis
	Deafness
	Nasal furunculosis
	German Shepherd dog folliculitis/furunculosis
	Vasculitis
	Lymphedema
	ABCB1 gene defect/drug sensitivity (white German shepherds)
	Ectodermal dysplasia
	Leishmaniasis

Giant schnauzer	Keratinization disorder Hypothyroidism Vitamin A-responsive dermatosis
Golden retriever	Lymphoma Atopic dermatitis Otitis externa Hypothyroidism Ichthyosis Footpad hyperkeratosis Juvenile cellulitis Epidermolysis bullosa, dystrophic
Gordon setter	Hypothyroidism Black-hair follicular dysplasia Juvenile cellulitis
Great Dane	Acral lick dermatitis Interdigital pyogranulomatous dermatitis/furunculosis Muzzle furunculosis Demodicosis Deafness Ichthyosis Calcinosis circumscripta Color dilution alopecia Lymphedema Epidermolysis bullosa aquisita
Great Pyrenees	Deafness
Greyhound	Low normal thyroid values Pattern baldness/bald thigh syndrome Color dilution alopecia Cutaneous and renal glomerular vasculopathy Ventral comedone syndrome
Havanese	Granulomatous sebaceous adenitis
Irish setter	Atopic dermatitis Hypothyroidism Granulocytopathy (immunodeficiency)
Irish terrier	Footpad hyperkeratosis (digital hyperkeratosis)
Irish water spaniel	Follicular dysplasia Symmetric lupoid onchodystrophy
Jack Russell terrier	Familial vasculopathy Atopic dermatitis Black-hair follicular dysplasia Pinnal vaculitis Ichthyosis Dermatophytosis

Keeshond	Melanoma
	Hypothyroidism
	Sebaceous cyst
	Infundibular keratinizing acanthoma
Kerry blue terrier	Hair follicle tumor
	Spiculosis
	Footpad hyperkeratosis
Kuvasz	Deafness
Labrador retriever	Color dilution alopecia ("silver labs")
	Atopic dermatitis
	Cutaneous adverse reaction to food
	Otitis externa
	Hypothyroidism
	Diabetes
	Melanoma
	Idiopathic leukoderma/leukotrichia
	Mast cell tumor
	Congenital hypotrichosis
	Keratinization disorder
	Nasodigital hyperkeratosis
	Nasal parakeratosis
	Lymphedema
	Vitamin A-responsive dermatosis
	"Wells' syndrome" (eosinophilic dermatitis and edema)
Lakeland terrier	Dermatomyositis
Lhasa apso	Atopic dermatitis
	Malassezia hypersensitivity
	Hypotrichosis
	Vasculitis – vaccine induced
	Granulomatous sebaceous adenitis
Maltese	Deafness
	Allergic dermatitis
	Vasculitis – vaccine induced
Manchester terrier	Cutaneous asthenia
	Follicular dysplasia
	Pattern baldness
Mastiff	Bacterial folliculitis
	Interdigital pyogranulomatous dermatitis/furunculosis
	Muzzle furunculosis
	Vaginal hyperplasia
Miniature pinscher	Leukoderma/leukotrichia
	Pattern baldness
	Color dilution alopecia
	Idiopathic vitiligo

Miniature schnauzer	Schnauzer comedone syndrome
	Atopic dermatitis
	Hyperadrenocorticism
	Hypothyroidism
	Sertoli cell tumor
	Aurotrichia (hairs become gold in color)
	Subcorneal pustular dermatosis
	Pigmented viral plaques
Newfoundland	Pyotraumatic dermatitis
	Bacterial folliculitis
	Atopic dermatitis
	Pemphigus foliaceus
	Idiopathic leukoderma/leukotrichia
	Interdigital pyogranulomatous dermatitis/furunculosis
Norfolk terrier	Hyperkeratosis, epidermolytic
Norwegian elkhound	Subcutaneous cyst
	Keratinization disorder
	Follicular dysplasia (plush-coated breeds)
	Infundibular keratinizing acanthoma
Norwich terrier	Atopic dermatitis
Old English sheepdog	Immune-mediated hemolytic anemia
	ABCB1 gene defect/drug sensitivity
	Lymphedema
	Idiopathic leukoderma/leukotrichia
Otter hound	Sebaceous cyst
Papillon	Deafness
	Microphthalmia with lacrimal duct atresia
Pekingese	Vasculitis – vaccine induced
	Intertrigo (facial fold)
Pembroke Welsh corgi	Cutaneous asthenia
	Dermoid cyst
Pointer, English	Calcinosis circumscripta
	Deafness
	Dwarfism
	Nasolacrimal puncta atresia
	Sensory neuropathy (acral mutilation syndrome)
	Black-hair follicular dysplasia
Pointer, German short-haired	Lymphedema
	Exfoliative cutaneous lupus erythematosus
	Fibrosarcoma
	Melanoma
	Acral mutilation syndrome (sensory neuropathy)
	Epidermolysis bullosa, junctional

Pomeranian	Follicular dysplasia (plush-coated breeds)
	Cyclic hematopoiesis (immunodeficiency)
Poodle, miniature and toy	Vasculitis – vaccine induced
	Atopic dermatitis
	Cutaneous adverse reaction to food
	Deafness
	Lacrimal duct atresia
	Pattern baldness
	Follicular dysplasia (plush-coated breeds)
	Hyperadrenocorticism
	Lymphedema
	Senile perifollicular mineralization
	Congenital hypotrichosis
	Pseudoachondroplastic dysplasia
	Epidermolysis bullosa
Poodle, standard	Atopic dermatitis
	Cutaneous adverse reaction to food
	Otitis externa/media
	Granulomatous sebaceous adenitis
	Lacrimal duct atresia
	Microphthalmia
	Color dilution alopecia
	Hypothyroidism
Portuguese water dog	Follicular dysplasia
	Pattern baldness
Pug	Demodicosis
	Hypothyroidism
	Intertrigo (facial/tail fold)
	Atopic dermatitis
	Mast cell tumor
	Pigmented viral plaques
Puli	Deafness
Rhodesian ridgeback	Dermoid sinus
	Hypothyroidism
	Deafness
	Color dilution follicular dysplasia associated with cerebellar degeneration
	Idiopathic onychodystrophy
Rottweiler	Idiopathic leukoderma/leukotrichia
	Hypothyroidism
	Symmetric lupoid onychodystrophy
	Diabetes
	Vasculitis
	Interdigital pyogranulomatous dermatitis/furunculosis

	Muzzle furunculosis
	Idiopathic vitiligo
	Follicular lipidosis (hypotrichosis of red-colored points)
	Follicular parakeratosis
Saint Bernard	Vaginal hyperplasia
	Intertrigo (lip fold)
	Deafness
	Nasal arteritis
	Lymphoma
	Uveodermatologic syndrome
	Diabetes
	Acromegaly
	Elbow hygroma
Saluki	Color dilution alopecia
Samoyed	Uveodermatologic syndrome
	Sebaceous cyst
	Dwarfism
	Follicular dysplasia (plush-coated breeds)
	Diabetes
	Granulomatous sebaceous adenitis
Schipperke	Pemphigus foliaceus
	Hypothyroidism
Scottish terrier	Melanoma
	Deafness
	Atopic dermatitis
	Cutaneous adverse reaction to food
	Histiocytoma
	Hyperadrenocorticism
	Vasculitis
	Flank alopecia
	Familial vasculopathy
Sealyham terrier	Deafness
	Atopic dermatitis
	Waardenburg–Klein syndrome (deaf, blue eyes, amelanotic skin)
Shetland sheepdog	Dermatomyositis
	Vesicular cutaneous lupus erythematosus
	Discoid lupus erythematosus
	Systemic lupus erythematosus
	Epidermolysis bullosa
	Staphylococcal hypersensitivity
	Hypothyroidism
	ABCB1 gene defect/drug sensitivity

Shih tzu	Sebaceous adenoma
	Atopic dermatitis
	Malassezia hypersensitivity
Siberian husky	Uveodermatologic syndrome
	Zinc-responsive dermatosis
	Discoid lupus erythematosus
	Atopic dermatitis
	Postclipping alopecia
	Follicular (color) dysplasia (red)
	Follicular dysplasia (plush-coated breeds)
	Canine eosinophilic granuloma
	Idiopathic onychodystrophy
Silky terrier	Color dilution alopecia
	Diabetes mellitus
	Vasculitis – vaccine induced
	Short-hair syndrome —follicular dysplasia
Skye terrier	Hypothyroidism
Spinone	Hypothyroidism
Spaniel, cocker	Hermaphroditism
	Atopic dermatitis
	Proliferative otitis externa
	Seborrhea
	Malassezia hypersensitivity
	Fold dermatitis (lip)
	Sebaceous adenoma
	Idiopathic facial paralysis (may be related to otitis)
	Hypothyroidism
	Deafness
	Cyclic hematopoiesis (immunodeficiency)
	Pemphigus foliaceus
	Black-hair follicular dysplasia
	Vitamin A-responsive dermatosis
	Idiopathic onychodystrophy
Spaniel, English springer	Seborrhea
	Psoriasiform lichenoid dermatosis of springer spaniels
	Acral mutilation syndrome (sensory neuropathy)
	Hypothyroidism
	Granulomatous sebaceous adenitis
	Acral mutilation syndrome (sensory neuropathy)
	Cutaneous asthenia
	Otitis externa
	Malassezia hypersensitivity
	Atopic dermatitis

Staffordshire terrier	Atopic dermatitis
	Interdigital pyogranulomatous dermatitis/furunculosis
	Demodicosis
	Actinic/solar dermatitis
	Follicular dysplasia
	Flank alopecia
Standard schnauzer	Atresia of nasolacrimal puncta
	Perianal adenoma
	Hypothyroidism
Tibetan terrier	Hypothyroidism
Vizsla	Granulomatous sebaceous adenitis
	Facial nerve paralysis
	Atopic dermatitis
Weimaraner	Syringomyelia
	Melanoma
	Fibrosarcoma
	Mast cell tumor
	Dwarfism
	Granulocytopathy (immunodeficiency)
	Muzzle furunculosis
	Demodicosis
	Interdigital pyogranulomatous dermatitis/furunculosis
Welsh terrier	Idiopathic onychodystrophy
West Highland white terrier	Atopic dermatitis
	Cutaneous adverse reaction to food
	Malassezia hypersensitivity
	Epidermal dysplasia
	Ichthyosis
	Seborrhea
	Demodicosis – *Demodex canis*, *Demodex injai*
Wheaten terrier	Cutaneous asthenia
	Atopic dermatitis
	Ichthyosis
Whippet	Pattern baldness
	Color dilution alopecia
	Symmetric lupoid onychodystrophy
	ABCB1 gene defect/drug sensitivity (long-haired)
Yorkshire terrier	Melanoderma
	Pattern baldness
	Color dilution alopecia
	Dermatophytosis
	Vasculitis – vaccine induced
	Short-hair syndrome – follicular dysplasia

Sources for Information on DNA-Based Tests

Online Mendelian Inheritance in Animals (OMIA): http://omia.angis.org.au/home/
Inherited diseases in dogs (IDID): https://www.vet.cam.ac.uk/idid/
WSAVA Testing Laboratories: http://research.vet.upenn.edu/DNAGeneticsTesting LaboratorySearch/tabid/7620/Default.aspx

appendix B

Drug Formulary

Blackwell's Five-Minute Veterinary Consult Clinical Companion: Small Animal Dermatology, Third Edition.
Karen Helton Rhodes and Alexander H. Werner.

Drug name (trade or other names)	Pharmacology and indications	Adverse effects and precautions	Dosing information and comments	Formulations	Dosage (unless otherwise indicated, dose is the same for dogs and cat)
ACTH	See Corticotropin.				
Afoxalaner	Antiparasitic drug. Isoxazoline: selective inhibitor of arthropod GABA and L-glutamate-gated chloride channels.		Labeled use: flea and tick preventative. Off-label efficacy against sarcoptid mites and demodicosis.		Dog: 2.5 mg/kg every 4 weeks po.
Amikacin (Amiglyde-V [veterinary] and Amikin [human])	Aminoglycoside antibacterial drug (inhibits protein synthesis). Mechanism is similar to other aminoglycosides (see Gentamicin sulfate), but may be more active than gentamicin.	May cause nephrotoxicosis with high doses or prolonged therapy. May also cause ototoxicity and vestibulotoxicity. (See Gentamicin sulfate.)	Once-daily doses are designed to maximize peak minimum inhibitory concentration (MIC) ratio. Consider therapeutic drug monitoring for chronic therapy. (See also Gentamicin sulfate.)	50, 250 mg/mL injection.	Dog and cat: 6.5 mg/kg q8h IV, IM, SC; or Dog: 15–30 mg/kg q24h IV, IM, SC; Cat: 10–14 mg/kg q24h IV, IM, SC.
Amitraz (Mitaban)	Antiparasitic drug for ectoparasites. Used for treatment of mites, including *Demodex*. Inhibits monoamine oxidase in mites.	Causes sedation in dogs (α_2-agonist), which may be reversed by yohimbine or atipamezole. When high doses are used, other side effects reported include pruritus, polyuria and polydipsia (PU/PD), bradycardia, hypothermia, hyperglycemia, and (rarely) seizures.	Manufacturer's dose should be used initially. But for refractory cases, this dose has been exceeded to produce increased efficacy.	10.6 mL concentrated dip (19.9%).	10.6 mL per 7.5 L water (0.025% solution). Apply 3–6 topical treatments q14d. For refractory cases, this dose has been exceeded to produce increased efficacy. Doses that have been used include: 0.025, 0.05, and 0.1% concentration applied 2 × per week and 0.125% solution applied to one-half of the body every day for 4 weeks to 5 months.

Amitriptyline hydrochloride (Elavil)	Tricyclic antidepressant drug. Action is via inhibition of uptake of serotonin and other transmitters at presynaptic nerve terminals. Used in animals to treat variety of behavioral disorders, such as anxiety. Used in cats for chronic idiopathic cystitis.	Multiple side effects are associated with tricyclic antidepressants, such as antimuscarinic effects (dry mouth, rapid heart rate) and antihistamine effects (sedation). High doses can produce life-threatening cardiotoxicity. In cats, reduced grooming, weight gain, and sedation are possible.	Doses are primarily based on empiricism. There are no controlled efficacy trials available for animals. There is evidence for success treating idiopathic cystitis in cats. Clomipramine is preferred for behavior problems.	10, 25, 50, 75, 100, 150 mg tablets; 10 mg/mL injection.	Dog: 1–2 mg/kg po q12–24h. Cat: 2–4 mg per cat/day po; cystitis: 2 mg/kg/day (2.5–7.5 mg/cat/day).
Amoxicillin + clavulanate potassium (Clavamox)	β-lactam antibiotic + β-lactamase inhibitor. Inhibits bacterial cell wall synthesis. Generally broad-spectrum activity. Used for a variety of infections in all species (clavulanate/clavulanic acid).	Usually well tolerated. Allergic reactions are possible. Diarrhea is possible with oral doses.	Dose recommendations vary depending on the susceptibility of bacteria and location of infection. Generally, more frequent or higher doses needed for gram-negative infections.	62.5, 125, 250, 375 mg tablets and 62.5 mg/mL suspension.	Dog: 12.5–25 mg/kg q12h po. Cat: 62.5 mg/cat q12h po. Consider administering these doses q8h for gram-negative infections.
Amphotericin B (Fungizone)	Antifungal drug. Fungicidal for systemic fungi, by damaging fungal membranes.	Produces a dose-related nephrotoxicosis. Also produces fever, phlebitis, and tremors.	Administer IV via slow infusion diluted in fluids, and monitor renal function closely. When preparing IV solution, do not mix with electrolyte solutions (use D-5-W, for example); administer NaCl fluid loading before therapy.	50 mg injectable vial.	0.5 mg/kg IV (slow infusion) q48h to a cumulative dose of 4–8 mg/kg.

(continued)

Drug name (trade or other names)	Pharmacology and indications	Adverse effects and precautions	Dosing information and comments	Formulations	Dosage (unless otherwise indicated, dose is the same for dogs and cat)
Amphotericin B, liposomal formulation (ABLC, Abelcet)	Same indications as for conventional amphotericin B. Liposomal formulations may be used at higher doses, and safety margin is increased. Expense is much higher than for conventional formulations.	Renal toxicity is the most dose-limiting effect.	Higher doses can be used compared to conventional formulation of amphotericin B. Dilute in 5% dextrose in water to 1 mg/mL, and administer IV over 1–2 hours.	100 mg/20 mL in lipid formulation.	Dog: 2–3 mg/kg IV 3 times/week for 9–12 treatments to a cumulative dose of 24–27 mg/kg. Cat: 1 mg/kg IV 3 times/week for 12 treatments.
Ampicillin (Omnipen, Principen, others [human forms])	β-lactam antibiotic. Inhibits bacterial cell wall synthesis.	Use cautiously in animals allergic to penicillin-like drugs.	Dose requirements vary depending on susceptibility of bacteria. Absorbed approximately 50% less, compared with amoxicillin, when administered orally. Generally, more frequent or higher doses needed for gram-negative infections.	250, 500 mg capsules; 125, 250, 500 mg vials of ampicillin sodium. Ampicillin trihydrate: 10 and 25 g vials for injection.	Ampicillin sodium: 10–20 mg/kg q6–8h IV, IM, SC or 20–40 mg/kg q8h po. Ampicillin trihydrate: Dog: 10–50 mg/kg q12–24h IM, SC. Cat: 10–20 mg/kg q12–24h IM, SC.
Antacid drugs	See Aluminum hydroxide, Magnesium hydroxide, Calcium carbonate.				
Atipamezole (Antisedan)	α_2-antagonist. Used to reverse α_2-agonists, such as medetomidine and xylazine.	Safe. Can cause some initial excitement in some animals shortly after reversal.	When used to reverse medetomidine, inject same volume as used for medetomidine.	5 mg/mL injection	Inject same volume as used for medetomidine.

Atropine (many generic brands)	Anticholinergic agent (blocks acetylcholine effect at muscarinic receptor), parasympatholytic. Used primarily as adjunct to anesthesia or other procedures to increase heart rate and decrease respiratory and gastrointestinal secretion. Also used as antidote for organophosphate intoxication.	Potent anticholinergic agent. Do not use in patients with glaucoma, intestinal ileus, gastroparesis, or tachycardia. Side effects of therapy include xerostomia, ileus, constipation, tachycardia, urine retention.	Used ordinarily as adjunct with anesthesia or other procedures. Do not mix with alkaline solutions.	400, 500, 540 µg/mL injection; 15 mg/mL injection.	0.02–0.04 mg/kg q6–8h IV, IM, SC; 0.2–0.5 mg/kg (as needed) for organophosphate and carbamate toxicosis.
Auranofin (triethylphosphine gold) (Ridaura)	Used for gold therapy (chrysotherapy). Mechanism of action is unknown, but may relate to immunosuppressive effect on lymphocytes. Used primarily for immune-mediated diseases.	Adverse effects include dermatitis, nephrotoxicity, and blood dyscrasias.	Use of this drug has not been evaluated in veterinary medicine. No controlled clinical trials are available to determine efficacy in animals. It has been suggested that this product (oral) is not as effective as injectable products, such as aurothioglucose.	3 mg capsules.	0.1–0.2 mg/kg q12h po.

(continued)

Drug name (trade or other names)	Pharmacology and indications	Adverse effects and precautions	Dosing information and comments	Formulations	Dosage (unless otherwise indicated, dose is the same for dogs and cat)
Aurothioglucose (Solganol)	Used for gold therapy (chrysotherapy). Mechanism of action is unknown, but may relate to immunosuppressive effect on lymphocytes. Used primarily for immune-mediated diseases (such as dermatologic disease).	Adverse effects include dermatitis, nephrotoxicity, and blood dyscrasias.	Use of this drug has not been evaluated in veterinary medicine. No controlled clinical trials are available to determine efficacy in animals. This drug is often used in combination with other immunosuppressive drugs, such as corticosteroids.	50 mg/mL injection.	Dog < 10 kg: 1 mg IM first week, 2 mg IM second week, 1 mg/kg/week maintenance. Dog > 10 kg: 5 mg IM first week, 10 mg IM second week, 1 mg/kg/week maintenance. Cat: 0.5–1 mg/cat every 7 days IM.
Azathioprine (Imuran)	Thiopurine immunosuppressive drug. Acts to inhibit T cell lymphocyte function. This drug is metabolized to 6-mercaptopurine, which may account for immunosuppressive effects. Used to treat various immune-mediated diseases.	Bone marrow suppression is most serious concern. Cat particularly are susceptible. There has been some association with development of pancreatitis when administered with corticosteroids.	Usually used in combination with other immunosuppressive drugs (such as corticosteroids) to treat immune-mediated disease. Doses of 2.2 mg/kg in cats have produced toxicity.	50 mg tablets; 10 mg/mL for injection.	Dog: 2 mg/kg q24h po initially then 0.5–1 mg/kg q48h. Cat (use cautiously): 0.3 mg/kg q24h po initially, then q48h, with careful monitoring.
Azithromycin (Zithromax)	Azalide antibiotic. Similar mechanism of action as macrolides (erythromycin), which is to inhibit bacteria protein synthesis via inhibition of ribosome. Spectrum is primarily gram-positive.	Vomiting is likely with high doses. Diarrhea may occur in some patients.	Azithromycin may be better tolerated than erythromycin. Primary difference from other antibiotics is the high intracellular concentrations achieved.	250 mg capsules, 250 and 600 mg tablets, 100 or 200 mg/5 mL oral suspension, and 500 mg vials for injection.	Dog: 10 mg/kg po once every 5 days, or 3.3 mg/kg q24h for three days Cat: 5–10 mg/kg po q48h.

Bactrim (sulfamethoxazole + trimethoprim) (See Trimethoprim-sulfonamide combinations)					
Betamethasone (Celestone)	Potent, long-acting corticosteroid. Antiinflammatory and immunosuppressive effects are approximately 30 × more than cortisol. Antiinflammatory effects are via inhibition of inflammatory cells and suppression of expression of inflammatory mediators. Use is for treatment of inflammatory and immune-mediated disease.	Side effects from corticosteroids are many and include polyphagia, PU/PD, and hypothalamic pituitary adrenal (HPA) axis suppression. Adverse effects include GI ulceration, hepatopathy, diabetes, hyperlipidemia, decreased thyroid hormone, decreased protein synthesis and wound healing, and immunosuppression.	Antiinflammatory effects are seen at doses of 0.1–0.2 mg/kg, immunosuppressive effects at 0.2–0.5 mg/kg.	500 µg (0.6 mg) tablets; 3 mg/mL sodium phosphate injection.	Antiinflammatory effects: 0.1–0.2 mg/kg q12–24h po. Immunosuppressive effects: 0.2–0.5 mg/kg q12–24h po.
Budesonide (Enterocort)	Corticosteroid. Budesonide is a locally acting corticosteroid. It is designed to release locally – in the intestine – after oral administration. Only a small fraction is absorbed systemically. Budesonide is used to treat inflammatory bowel disease.	No serious adverse effects are reported. Systemic absorption may cause glucocorticoid effects in animals.	The capsules are designed for human use. When administering to animals, do not disrupt the coating on the drug or the intestinal release may be compromised.	3 mg capsule	0.125 mg/kg q6–8h po. Dose interval may be increased to every 12 hours when condition improves.

(*continued*)

Drug name (trade or other names)	Pharmacology and indications	Adverse effects and precautions	Dosing information and comments	Formulations	Dosage (unless otherwise indicated, dose is the same for dogs and cat)
Bupivacaine hydrochloride (Marcaine and generics)	Local anesthetic. Inhibits nerve conduction via sodium channel blockade. Longer acting and more potent than lidocaine or other local anesthetics.	Adverse effects rare with local infiltration. High doses absorbed systemically can cause nervous system signs (tremors and convulsions). After epidural administration, respiratory paralysis is possible with high doses.	Used for local infiltration or infusion into epidural space. One may admix 0.1 mEq sodium bicarbonate per 10 mL solution to increase pH, decrease pain from injection, and increase onset. Use immediately after mixing with bicarbonate.	2.5 and 5 mg/mL solution injection.	1 mL of 0.5% solution per 10 cm for an epidural.
Buprenorphine hydrochloride (Buprenex [Vetergesic in the UK])	Opioid analgesic. Partial (μ-receptor agonist, κ-receptor antagonist. 25–50 × more potent than morphine. Buprenorphine may cause less respiratory depression than other opiates.	Adverse effects are similar to other opiate agonists, except there may be less respiratory depression. Dependency from chronic use may be less than with pure agonists.	Used for analgesia, often in combination with other analgesics or in conjunction with general anesthesia. Longer acting than morphine. Only partially reversed by naloxone.	0.3 mg/mL solution	Dog: 0.006–0.02 mg/kg IV, IM, SC q4–8h. Cat: 0.005–0.01 mg/kg IV, IM, q4–8h. Buccal administration in cat: 0.01–0.02 mg/kg q12h.
Buspirone (BuSpar)	Antianxiety agent. Acts by binding to serotonin receptors. In veterinary medicine, has been primarily used for treatment of urine spraying in cats.	Some cats show increased aggression; some cats show increased affection to owners.	Some efficacy trials suggest effectiveness for treating urine spraying in cats. There may be a lower relapse rate compared to other drugs.	5, 10 mg tablets.	Dog: 2.5–10 mg/dog q12–24h po or 1 mg/kg q12h po. Cat: 2.5–5 mg/cat q24h po (may be increased to 5–7.5 mg per cat twice daily for some cat).

Carprofen (Rimadyl; Zenecarp in the UK) Novox (generic)	NSAID. Used for treatment of pain and inflammation, particularly pain and inflammation associated with osteoarthritis. Shown to be safe and effective for perioperative use for surgical pain either by injection or po. Carprofen's action may be via cyclooxygenase inhibition but is relatively COX-1 sparing. Other mechanisms also may explain its efficacy.	Most common adverse effects in clinical patients have been GI (vomiting, nausea, diarrhea). Other adverse effects are more rare and include idiosyncratic hepatotoxicosis. If they occur, signs of hepatotoxicosis appear 2–3 weeks after beginning therapy. Perioperative use has not adversely affected renal function or bleeding times. Avoid use with other NSAIDs or with corticosteroids.	Doses are based on manufacturer's field trials and US registration data. Clinical trials conducted with canine patients with osteoarthritis and surgical patients. There is not sufficient safety information available to recommend carprofen for use in cats. Injectable carprofen administered for surgery may be given 2 hours prior to the procedure.	25, 75, 100 mg tablets (regular and chewable); 50 mg/mL injectable solution.	Dog: 4.4 mg/kg/day po, administered either once a day or divided into 2.2 mg/kg q12h; 4.4 mg/kg/day SC, administered once daily or 2.2 mg/kg q12h. To control postoperative pain, administer prior to surgery. Cat: not recommended.
Cefadroxil (Cefa-Tabs, Cefa-Drops)	Cefadroxil is a first-generation cephalosporin antibiotic with broad-spectrum activity.	Cefadroxil has been known to cause vomiting after oral administration in dogs.	Spectrum of cefadroxil is similar to other first-generation cephalosporins. For susceptibility test, use cephalothin as test drug.	50 mg/mL oral suspension; 50, 100, 200, 1000 mg tablet. Availability of some oral formulations is questionable.	Dog: 22 mg/kg q12h, up to 30 mg/kg q12h po. Cat: 22 mg/kg q24h po.
Cefazolin sodium (Ancef, Kefzol, and generic)	Cefazolin is a first-generation cephalosporin.	For cefazolin, use cephalothin to test susceptibility.	Commonly used first-generation cephalosporin as injectable drug for prophylaxis for surgery as well as for acute therapy for serious infections.	50 and 100 mg/50 mL for injection.	20–35 mg/kg q8h IV, IM. For perisurgical use: 22 mg/kg q2h during surgery.

(continued)

Drug name (trade or other names)	Pharmacology and indications	Adverse effects and precautions	Dosing information and comments	Formulations	Dosage (unless otherwise indicated, dose is the same for dogs and cat)
Cefdinir (Omnicef)	Oral third-generation cephalosporin. Activity includes staphylococci and many gram-negative bacilli.	Similar to those of other cephalosporins.	Use in veterinary medicine has not been reported. Use and doses are extrapolated from human medicine.	300 mg capsules, 25 mg/mL oral suspension.	Dose not established. Human dose is 7 mg/kg q12h po.
Cefixime (Suprax)	Cefixime is a third-generation cephalosporin.	Similar to those of other cephalosporins.	Although not approved for veterinary use, pharmacokinetic studies in dogs have provided recommended dosages.	20 mg/mL oral suspension and 200 and 400 mg tablets.	10 mg/kg q12h po; for cystitis: 5 mg/kg q12–24h po.
Cefotaxime sodium (Claforan)	Cefotaxime is a third-generation cephalosporin. It is used when resistance is encountered to other antibiotics or when infection is in central nervous system.	Similar to those of other cephalosporins.	Third-generation cephalosporin used when resistance encountered to first- and second-generation cephalosporins.	500 mg; 1, 2, and 10 g vials for injection.	Dog: 50 mg/kg IV, IM, SC q12h. Cat: 20–80 mg/kg q6h IV, IM.
Cefotetan disodium (Cefotan)	Cefotetan is second-generation cephalosporin.	Similar to those of other cephalosporins.	Second-generation cephalosporin similar to cefoxitin, but may have longer half-life in dogs.	1, 2, and 10 g vials for injection.	30 mg/kg q8h IV, SC.
Cefoxitin sodium (Mefoxin)	Cefoxitin is a second-generation cephalosporin. May have increased activity against anaerobic bacteria.	Similar to those of other cephalosporins.	Second-generation cephalosporin, which is often used when activity against anaerobic bacteria is desired.	1, 2, and 10 g vials for injection.	30 mg/kg q6–8h IV.

Cefpodoxime proxetil (Simplicef)	Oral third-generation cephalosporin. Activity includes gram-negative bacilli and staphylococci.	Vomiting and diarrhea are the most common adverse effects.	Approved for skin and soft tissue infections in dogs.	100, 200 mg tablets.	Dog: 5–10 mg/kg po q24h. Cat: dose not established.
Ceftazidime (Fortaz, Ceptaz, Tazicef)	Third-generation cephalosporin. Ceftazidime has more activity than other cephalosporins against *Pseudomonas aeruginosa*.	Similar to those of other cephalosporins.	Third-generation cephalosporin. May be reconstituted with 1% lidocaine for IM injection.	Vials (0.5, 1, 2, 6 g) reconstituted to 280 mg/mL.	Dog and cat: 30 mg/kg q6h IV, IM. Dog: 30 mg/kg q4–6h SC.
Ceftiofur (Naxcel [ceftiofur sodium]; Excenel [ceftiofur HCl]).	Ceftiofur spectrum resembles many of the third-generation cephalosporins.	Similar to those of other cephalosporins.	Available as powder for reconstitution prior to injection. After reconstitution, stable for 7 days when refrigerated or 12h at room temperature, or frozen for 8 weeks.	50 mg/mL injection.	2.2–4.4 mg/kg SC q24h (for urinary tract infections).
Cephalexin (Keflex and generic forms)	Cephalexin is a first-generation cephalosporin.	Similar to those of other cephalosporins.	Although not approved for veterinary use, trials in dogs with pyoderma show efficacy.	250, 500 mg capsules; 250, 500 mg tablets; 100 mg/mL or 125, 250 mg/5 mL oral suspension.	10–30 mg/kg q6–12h po; for pyoderma, 22–35 mg/kg q12h po.

(continued)

Drug name (trade or other names)	Pharmacology and indications	Adverse effects and precautions	Dosing information and comments	Formulations	Dosage (unless otherwise indicated, dose is the same for dogs and cat)
Cetirizine (Zyrtec)	Antihistamine (H1 blocker). It acts by blocking the histamine type-1 receptor (H1) and suppressing inflammatory reactions caused by histamine. The H1 blockers have been used to control pruritus and skin inflammation, rhinorrhea, and airway inflammation. Cetirizine is considered a second-generation antihistamine, which may be associated with less sedation than older drugs.	No adverse effects have been reported in dogs or cats.	There are no studies published that demonstrate clinical efficacy in dogs and cats. Clinical use is based on experimental animals.	1 mg/mL oral syrup; 5 and 10 mg tablets.	2.5–5 mg per animal, once daily po.
Chlorambucil (Leukeran)	Cytotoxic agent. Acts in similar manner as cyclophosphamide as alkylating agent. Used for treatment of various tumors and immunosuppressive therapy.	Myelosuppression is possible. Cystitis does not occur with chlorambucil as with cyclophosphamide.	Consult anticancer drug protocol for specific regimens.	2 mg tablets.	Dog: 2–6 mg/m^2 q24h initially, then q48h po. Cat: 0.1–0.2 mg/kg q24h initially, then q48h po.

Chloramphenicol and chloramphenicol palmitate (Chloromycetin, generic forms)	Antibacterial drug. Mechanism of action is via inhibition of protein synthesis via binding to ribosome. Broad spectrum of activity.	Bone marrow suppression is possible with high doses or prolonged treatment (especially in cats). Avoid use in pregnant or neonatal animals. *Drug interactions* with other drugs (e.g., barbiturates) possible because chloramphenicol will inhibit hepatic microsomal enzymes.	Chloramphenicol palmitate requires active enzymes and should not be administered to fasted (or anorectic) animals. *Note:* Some forms of chloramphenicol are no longer available in the US.	30 mg/mL oral suspension (palmitate), 250 mg capsules, and 100, 250, and 500 mg tablets.	Dog: 40–50 mg/kg q8h po. Cat: 50 mg/cat q12h po or 12.5–20 mg/kg q12h po.
Chlorpheniramine maleate (Chlor-Trimeton, Phenetron, and others)	Antihistamine (H1 blocker). Blocks action of histamine on receptors. Also may have direct antiinflammatory action. Used most often to prevent allergic reactions. Used for pruritus therapy in dogs and cats.	Sedation is most common side effect. Antimuscarinic effects (atropine-like effects) also are common.	Chlorpheniramine is included as ingredient in many OTC cough/cold and allergy medications.	[illegible], 8 mg tablets.	Dog: 4–8 mg/dog q12h po (up to a maximum of 0.5 mg/kg q12h). Cat: 2 mg/cat q12h po.
Cimetidine (Tagamet [OTC and prescription])	Histamine-2 antagonist (H2 blocker). Blocks histamine stimulation of gastric parietal cells to decrease gastric acid secretion. Used to treat ulcers and gastritis.	Adverse effects usually seen only with decreased renal clearance. In people, CNS signs may occur with high doses. *Drug interactions:* May increase concentrations of other drugs used concurrently (e.g., theophylline) because of inhibition of hepatic enzymes.	Precise doses needed to treat ulcers have not been established.	100, 200, 300, 400, 800 mg tablets; 60 mg/mL oral solution; 6 mg/mL injection.	10 mg/kg q6–8h IV, IM, po (in renal failure, administer 2.5–5 mg/kg q12h IV, po).

(*continued*)

Drug name (trade or other names)	Pharmacology and indications	Adverse effects and precautions	Dosing information and comments	Formulations	Dosage (unless otherwise indicated, dose is the same for dogs and cat)
Ciprofloxacin (Cipro and generic forms)	Fluoroquinolone antibacterial. Acts to inhibit DNA gyrase and inhibit cell DNA and RNA synthesis. Bactericidal. Broad antimicrobial activity.	Avoid use in dogs 4 weeks to 7 months of age. High concentrations may cause CNS toxicity, especially in animals with renal failure. Use cautiously in epileptic patients. Causes occasional vomiting. IV solution should be given slowly (over 30 min).	Doses are based on plasma concentrations needed to achieve sufficient plasma concentration above MIC. Efficacy studies have not been performed in dogs or cats. Ciprofloxacin is not absorbed orally as well as enrofloxacin.	250, 500, 750 mg tablets; 2 mg/mL injection.	10–20 mg/kg q24h po, IV.
Clarithromycin (Biaxin)	Macrolide antibiotic with bacteriostatic activity. Spectrum includes primarily gram-positive bacteria. Resistance is expected for most gram-negative bacteria. Efficacy is not established for animals. Most common use in people is for treatment of *Helicobacter* gastritis and respiratory infections.	Well tolerated in animals. Most common side effects are vomiting, nausea, and diarrhea.	Doses are not established for animals due to lack of clinical trials. Dose recommendations are extrapolated from human or empirical use.	250, 500 mg tablets; 25 and 50 mg/mL oral suspension.	7.5 mg/kg q12h po.
Clavamox	See Amoxicillin/clavulanate potassium.				
Clavulanic acid	See Amoxicillin/clavulanate potassium.				

Clemastine (Tavist, Contac 12 Hour Allergy, and generic forms)	Antihistamine (H1 blocker). Blocks action of histamine on tissues. Used primarily for treatment of allergy. Some evidence suggests that clemastine is more effective than other antihistamines for pruritus in dogs.	Sedation is most common side effect.	Used for short-term treatment of pruritus in dogs. May be more efficacious when combined with other antiinflammatory drugs. Tavist syrup contains 5.5% alcohol.	1.34 mg tablets (OTC), 2.64 mg tablets (Rx), and 0.134 mg/mL syrup.	Dog: 0.05–0.1 mg/kg q12h po.
Clindamycin (Antirobe [veterinary], Cleocin [human])	Antibacterial drug of the lincosamide class (similar in action to macrolides). Inhibits bacterial protein synthesis via inhibition of bacterial ribosome. Primarily bacteriostatic, with spectrum of activity primarily against gram-positive bacteria and anaerobes.	Generally well tolerated in dogs and cats. Oral liquid product may be unpalatable to cats. Lincomycin and clindamycin may alter bacterial population in intestine and cause diarrhea; for this reason, do not administer to rodents or rabbits.	Most doses are based on manufacturer's drug approval data and efficacy trials. See dosing column for specific guidelines for different infections.	Oral liquid 25 mg/mL; 25, 75, 150 and 300 mg capsules, and 150 mg/mL injection (Cleocin).	Dog: 11–33 mg/kg q12h po; for periodontal and soft tissue infection, 5.5–33 mg/kg q12h po. Cat: 11–33 mg/kg q24h po; for skin and anaerobic infections, 11 mg/kg q12h po; for toxoplasmosis, 12.5–25 mg/kg po q12h.
Clofazimine (Lamprene)	Antimicrobial agent used to treat feline leprosy. Slow bactericidal effect on *Mycobacterium leprae*.	Adverse effects have not been reported in cats. In people, the most serious adverse effects are GI.	Doses based on empiricism or extrapolation of human studies.	50 and 100 mg capsules.	Cat: 1 mg/kg up to a maximum of 4 mg/kg/day po.

(continued)

Drug name (trade or other names)	Pharmacology and indications	Adverse effects and precautions	Dosing information and comments	Formulations	Dosage (unless otherwise indicated, dose is the same for dogs and cat)
Clomipramine (Clomicalm [veterinary]; Anafranil [human])	Tricyclic antidepressant (TCA) drug. Used in people to treat anxiety and depression. Used in animals to treat variety of behavioral disorders, including obsessive compulsive disorders and separation anxiety. Action is via inhibition of uptake of serotonin at presynaptic nerve terminals.	Reported adverse effects include sedation, reduced appetite. Other side effects associated with TCAs are antimuscarinic effects (dry mouth, rapid heart rate) and antihistamine effects (sedation). Overdoses can produce life-threatening cardiotoxicity.	When adjusting doses, one may initiate therapy with low dose and increase gradually. There may be a 2–4 week delay after initiation of therapy before beneficial effects are seen.	5, 20, 80 mg tablets (veterinary); 10, 25, 50 mg tablets (human).	Dog: 1–2 mg/kg q12h po. Cat: 1–5 mg per cat q12–24h po.
Cloxacillin sodium (Cloxapen, Ortoenin, Tegopen)	β-lactam antibiotic. Inhibits bacterial cell wall synthesis. Spectrum is limited to gram-positive bacteria, especially staphylococci.	Use cautiously in animals allergic to penicillin-like drugs.	Doses based on empiricism or extrapolation from human studies. No clinical efficacy studies available for dogs or cats. Oral absorption is poor; if possible, administer on empty stomach.	250, 500 mg capsules, 25 mg/mL oral solution.	20–40 mg/kg q8h po.
Colchicine (generic)	Antiinflammatory agent. Used primarily to treat gout. In animals, used to decrease fibrosis and development of hepatic failure (possibly by inhibiting formation of collagen).	Do not administer to pregnant animals. Adverse effects are not well documented in animals. Colchicine may cause dermatitis in people.	Doses based on empiricism. There are no well-controlled efficacy studies in veterinary species.	500, 600 µg tablets and 500 µg/mL ampule injection.	0.01–0.03 mg/kg q24h po.

Corticotropin (ACTH) (Acthar)	Used for diagnostic purposes to evaluate adrenal gland function. Stimulates normal synthesis of cortisol from adrenal gland.	Adverse effects unlikely when used as single injection for diagnostic purposes.	Doses established by measuring normal adrenal response in animals.	80 U/mL gel.	Response test: collect pre-ACTH sample and inject 2.2 IU/kg IM. Collect post-ACTH sample at 2h in dogs and at 1 and 2h in cats.
Cosyntropin (Cortrosyn)	Cosyntropin is a synthetic form of corticotropin (ACTH) used for diagnostic purposes only. In humans, it is preferred over corticotropin because it is less allergenic.	Same as for corticotropin.	Use for diagnostic purposes only; not intended for treatment of hypoadrenocorticism. Maximum dosage for dogs should be 250 µg.	250 µg per vial.	ACTH response test: collect pre-ACTH sample and inject 5 µg/kg IV or IM (dog) or 125 µg (0.125 mg) IM (cat). Cat: collect sample at 60 and 90 min after IV administration and 30 and 60 min after IM administration. Collect post sample at 30 and 60 min.
Cyclophosphamide (Cytoxan, Neosar)	Cytotoxic agent. Bifunctional alkylating agent. Disrupts base-pairing and inhibits DNA and RNA synthesis. Cytotoxic for tumor cells and other rapidly dividing cells. Used primarily as adjunct for cancer chemotherapy and as immunosuppressive therapy.	Bone marrow suppression is most common adverse effect. Can produce severe neutropenia (that usually is reversible). Vomiting and diarrhea may occur in some patients. Dogs are susceptible to bladder toxicity (sterile hemorrhagic cystitis). May cause hair loss when used in some chemotherapeutic protocols.	Cyclophosphamide is usually administered with other drugs (other cancer drugs in cancer protocols or corticosteroids) when used for immunosuppressive therapy. Consult specific anticancer protocols for specific regimens.	25 mg/mL injection; 25, 50 mg tablet.	Dog: anticancer: 50 mg/m^2 once daily 4 days/week po, or 150–300 mg/m^2 IV, and repeat in 21 days Immunosuppressive therapy: 50 mg/m^2 (approx. 2.2 mg/kg) q48h po, or 2.2 mg/kg once daily for 4 days/week. Cat: 6.25–12.5 mg/cat once daily 4 days/week.

(continued)

Drug name (trade or other names)	Pharmacology and indications	Adverse effects and precautions	Dosing information and comments	Formulations	Dosage (unless otherwise indicated, dose is the same for dogs and cat)
Cyclosporine (Neoral [human], Atopica® [veterinary], Optimmune [ophthalmic]. Also called cyclosporin A)	Immunosuppressive drug. Suppresses induction of T cell lymphocytes. Used in dogs for atopic dermatitis, and treatment of immune-mediated diseases.	Can cause vomiting, diarrhea, anorexia. In comparison to other immunosuppressive drugs, does not cause myelosuppression. *Drug interactions:* erythromycin or ketoconazole may increase cyclosporine concentrations when used concurrently.	Suggested trough blood concentration range (whole blood assay) is 300–400 ng/mL. Neoral oral products are the same formulation as Atopica®. Topical cyclosporine has been used successfully as treatment for keratoconjunctivitis sicca.	10, 25, 50 and 100 mg capsules.	Dog: 3–7 mg/kg/day po. Dose for atopic dermatitis may be changed to 5 mg/kg q48h in some patients. Cat: 3–5 mg/kg/day po.
Cyproheptadine hydrochloride (Periactin)	Phenothiazine with antihistamine and antiserotonin properties. Used as appetite stimulant (probably by altering serotonin activity in appetite center).	May cause increased appetite and weight gain.	Clinical studies have not been performed in veterinary medicine. Use is based primarily on empiricism and extrapolation from human results. Syrup contains 5% alcohol.	4 mg tablet; 2 mg/5 mL syrup.	Antihistamine: 0.5–1.1 mg/kg q8–12h po. Appetite stimulant: 2 mg/cat po. Feline asthma: 1–2 mg/cat q12h po.
Danazol (Danocrine)	Gonadotropin inhibitor. Suppresses luteinizing hormone (LH) and follicle-stimulating hormone (FSH) and estrogen synthesis. In humans, used for endometriosis. May reduce destruction of platelets or RBC in immune-mediated disease.	May cause signs similar to other androgenic drugs. Adverse effects have not been reported in animals. Gonadotropin inhibitor.	When used to treat autoimmune disease, usually used in conjunction with other drugs (e.g., corticosteroids).	50, 100, 200 mg capsules.	5–10 mg/kg q12h po.

Dantrolene sodium (Dantrium)	Muscle relaxant. Inhibits calcium leakage from sarcoplasmic reticulum. In addition to muscle relaxation, it has been used for malignant hyperthermia. Also has been used to relax urethral muscle in cats.	Muscle relaxants can cause weakness in some animals.	Doses have been primarily extrapolated from experimental studies or extrapolation of human studies. No clinical trials available in veterinary medicine. Studies in which dantrolene relaxed urethra in cats used 1 mg/kg IV.	100 mg capsule and 0.33 mg/mL injection.	For prevention of malignant hyperthermia: 2–3 mg/kg IV for muscle relaxation: dog: 1–5 mg/kg q8h po; cat: 0.5–2 mg/kg q12h po.
Dapsone (generic)	Antimicrobial drug used primarily for treatment of *Mycobacterium*. May have some immunosuppressive properties or inhibit function of inflammatory cells. Used primarily for dermatologic diseases in dogs and cats.	Hepatitis and blood dyscrasias may occur. Toxic dermatologic reactions have been seen in people. *Drug interactions:* Do not administer with trimethoprim (may increase blood concentrations). Do not administer to cats.	Doses are derived from extrapolation of human doses or empiricism. No well-controlled clinical studies have been performed in veterinary medicine.	25 and 100 mg tablets.	Dog: 1.1 mg/kg q8–12h po. Cat: do not use.
Deprenyl (L-deprenyl)	See Selegiline.				
Deracoxib (Deramaxx)	NSAID of the coxib class; high COX-1: COX-2 *in vitro* inhibitory ratio. Indicated for the control of postoperative pain and inflammation associated with orthopedic surgery and pain and inflammation associated with osteoarthritis.	Most common adverse effect from clinical trials has been GI (vomiting and diarrhea). In safety studies at doses above 25 kg/mg, reduced body weight, melena, and vomiting occurred.	Recommended doses are for dogs weighing > 1.8 kg (4 lb). Safety has not been established for dogs under 4 months of age, dogs used for breeding, pregnant or lactating dogs, or for cats.	25, 100 mg tablets; chewable tablets.	Dog (postoperative pain): 3.0–4.0 mg/kg q24h po as needed for 7 days. Dog (osteoarthritis): 1–2 mg/kg po q24h for long-term treatment over 7 days. Cat: safe dose not established.

(continued)

Drug name (trade or other names)	Pharmacology and indications	Adverse effects and precautions	Dosing information and comments	Formulations	Dosage (unless otherwise indicated, dose is the same for dogs and cat)
DES	See Diethylstilbestrol.				
Desoxycorticosterone pivalate (Percorten-V, DOCP, or DOCA pivalate)	Mineralocorticoid. Used for adrenocortical insufficiency (hypoadrenocorticism). No glucocorticoid activity.	Excessive mineralocorticoid effects with high doses.	Initial dose based on studies performed in clinical patients. Individual doses may be based on monitoring electrolytes in patients. Actual interval between doses may range from 14–35 days.	25 mg/mL injection.	1.5–2.2 mg/kg every 25 days IM.
Dexamethasone (dexamethasone solution and dexamethasone sodium phosphate) (Azium, Decaject SP, Dexavet, and Dexasone. Tablets include Decadron and generic)	Corticosteroid. Dexamethasone has approximately 30 × potency of cortisol. Multiple antiinflammatory effects.	Corticosteroids produce multiple systemic side effects and adverse effects from chronic therapy.	Doses based on severity of underlying disease. Dexamethasone is used for testing hyperadrenocorticism. Low-dose dexamethasone suppression test: dog 0.01 mg/kg IV, cat 0.1 mg/kg IV, and collect sample at 0, 4, and 8 hours. For high-dose dexamethasone suppression test: dog 0.1 mg/kg, cat 1.0 mg/kg.	Azium solution, 2 mg/mL. Sodium phosphate forms are 3.33 mg/mL 0.25, 0.5, 0.75, 1, 1.5, 2, 4, 6 mg tablets.	Antiinflammatory: 0.07–0.15 mg/kg q12–24h IV, IM po. Dexamethasone 21-isonicotinate 0.03–0.05 mg/kg IM.

Diazepam (Valium and generic)	Benzodiazepine. Central-acting CNS depressant. Mechanism of action appears to be via potentiation of GABA receptor-mediated effects in CNS. Used for sedation, anesthetic adjunct, anticonvulsant, and behavioral disorders. Diazepam metabolized to desmethyl diazepam (nordiazepam) and oxazepam.	Sedation is most common side effect. May cause paradoxical excitement in dogs. Causes polyphagia. In cats, idiopathic fatal hepatic necrosis has been reported.	Clearance in dogs is many times faster than in people (half-life in dogs less than 1h), requires frequent administration. For treatment of status epilepticus, may be administered IV or rectally. Avoid administration IM.	2, 5 mg tablets; 5 mg/mL solution for injection.	Preanesthetic: 0.5 mg/kg IV. Status epilepticus: 0.5 mg/kg IV, 1 mg/kg rectal; repeat if necessary. Appetite stimulant (cat): 0.2 mg/kg IV. For behavior treatment in cats: 1–4 mg per cat q12–24h po.
Dicloxacillin sodium (Dynapen)	β-lactam, antibiotic. Inhibits bacterial cell wall synthesis. Spectrum is limited to gram-positive bacteria, especially staphylococci.	Use cautiously in animals allergic to penicillin-like drugs.	No clinical efficacy studies available for dogs or cats. In dogs, oral absorption is very low and may not be suitable for therapy. Administer, if possible, on empty stomach.	125, 250, 500 mg capsules, 12.5 mg/mL oral suspension.	11–55 mg/kg q8h po.
Diethylstilbestrol (DES)	Synthetic estrogen compound. Used for estrogen replacement in animals. DES is most commonly used to treat estrogen-responsive incontinence in dogs. Also has been used to induce abortion in dogs.	Side effects may occur that are caused by excess estrogen. Estrogen therapy may increase risk of pyometra and estrogen-sensitive tumors.	Doses listed are for treating urinary incontinence and vary depending on response. Titrate dose to individual patients. Although used to induce abortion, it was not efficacious in one study that administered 75 µg/kg.	1, 5 mg tablets; 50 mg/mL injection (no longer manufactured in US but available from compounding pharmacist).	Dog: 0.1–1.0 mg/dog q24h po. Cat: 0.05–0.1 mg/cat q24h po.

(*continued*)

Drug name (trade or other names)	Pharmacology and indications	Adverse effects and precautions	Dosing information and comments	Formulations	Dosage (unless otherwise indicated, dose is the same for dogs and cat)
Difloxacin hydrochloride (Dicural)	Fluoroquinolone antibacterial drug. Acts via inhibition of DNA gyrase in bacteria to inhibit DNA and RNA synthesis. Bactericidal with broad spectrum of activity. Used for variety of infections, including skin infections, wound infections, and pneumonia.	Adverse effects include seizures in epileptic animals, arthropathy in young animals, vomiting at high doses. *Drug interactions:* May increase concentrations of theophylline if used concurrently. Coadministration with di- and trivalent cations (e.g., sucralfate) may decrease absorption. Ocular safety not established in cats.	Dose range can be used to adjust dose, depending on severity of infection and susceptibility of bacteria. Difloxacin is primarily eliminated in feces rather than urine (urine is < 5% of clearance). Sarafloxacin is an active desmethyl metabolite.	11.4, 45.4, and 136 mg tablets.	Dog: 5–10 mg/kg q24h po. Cat: safe dose not established.
Dimenhydrinate (Dramamine, [Gravol in Canada])	Antihistamine drug. Converted to active diphenhydramine. Used for antiemetic treatment.	Primary side effect is sedation.	There have been no clinical studies on the use of dimenhydrinate. It is primarily used empirically for treatment of vomiting.	50 mg tablets and 50 mg/mL injection.	Dog: 4–8 mg/kg q8h po, IM, IV. Cat: 12.5 mg/cat q8h IV, IM, po.
Diphenhydramine hydrochloride (Benadryl)	Antihistamine used for allergy treatment and antiemetic.	Primary side effect is sedation.	Antihistamine used primarily for allergic disease in animals.	Available OTC; 2.5 mg/mL elixir; 25, 50 mg capsules and tablets; 50 mg/mL injection.	Dog: 25–50 mg/dog q8h IV, IM, po. Cat: 2–4 mg/kg q6–8h po, or 1 mg/kg q6–8h IM, IV.

Diphenoxylate (Lomotil)	Opiate agonist. Stimulates smooth muscle segmentation in intestine, as well as electrolyte absorption. Used for acute treatment of nonspecific diarrhea.	Adverse effects have not been reported in veterinary medicine. Diphenoxylate is poorly absorbed systemically and produces few systemic side effects. Excessive use can cause constipation.	Doses are based primarily on empiricism or extrapolation of human dose. Clinical studies have not been performed in animals. Contains atropine, but dose is not high enough for significant systemic effects.	2.5 mg tablets.	Dog: 0.1–0.2 mg/kg q8–12h po. Cat: 0.05–0.1 mg/kg q12h po.
Doxycycline (Vibramycin and generic forms)	Tetracycline antibiotic. Mechanism of action of tetracyclines is to bind to 30S ribosomal subunit and inhibit protein synthesis. Usually bacteriostatic. Broad spectrum of activity including bacteria, some protozoa, *Rickettsia*, *Ehrlichia*.	Severe adverse reactions not reported with doxycycline. Tetracyclines in general may cause renal tubular necrosis at high doses. Tetracyclines can affect bone and teeth formation in young animals but this is less likely with doxycycline.	Many pharmacokinetic and experimental studies have been conducted in small animals, but no clinical studies. Ordinarily considered the drug of choice for *Rickettsia* and *Ehrlichia* infections in dogs. Doxycycline IV infusion is stable for only 12h at room temperature and 72h if refrigerated.	10 mg/mL oral suspension; 100 mg injection vial. Doxycycline hyclate 50, 100 mg tablets or capsules. Doxycycline monohydrate 50 or 100 mg tablets or capsules.	3–5 mg/kg q12h po IV or 10 mg/kg q24h po. For *Rickettsia* in dogs: 5 mg/kg q12h.
Enilconazole (Imaverol, Clinafarm EC)	Azole antifungal agent for topical use only. Like other azoles, inhibits membrane synthesis (ergosterol) in fungus. Highly effective for dermatophytes.	Administered topically. Adverse effects have not been reported.	Imaverol is available only in Canada as 10% emulsion. In the US, Clinafarm EC is available for use in poultry units as 13.8% solution. Dilute solution to at least 50:1, and apply topically every 3–4 days for 2–3 weeks. Enilconazole also has been instilled as 1:1 dilution into nasal sinus for nasal aspergillosis.	10% or 13.8% emulsion.	Nasal aspergillosis: 10 mg/kg q12h instilled into nasal sinus for 14 days (10% solution diluted 50/50 with water). Dermatophytes: dilute 10% solution to 0.2%, and wash lesion with solution 4 times at 3–4 day intervals.

(*continued*)

Drug name (trade or other names)	Pharmacology and indications	Adverse effects and precautions	Dosing information and comments	Formulations	Dosage (unless otherwise indicated, dose is the same for dogs and cat)
Enrofloxacin (Baytril)	Fluoroquinolone antibacterial drug. Acts via inhibition of DNA gyrase in bacteria to inhibit DNA and RNA synthesis. Bactericidal. broad spectrum of activity.	Adverse effects include seizures in epileptic animals, arthropathy in dogs 4–28 weeks of age, vomiting in dogs and cats at high doses. Blindness in cats has been reported. *Drug interactions*: May increase concentrations of theophylline if used concurrently. Coadministration with di- and trivalent cations (e.g., sucralfate) may decrease absorption.	Solution is not approved for IV use but has been administered via this route safely if given slowly. Do not mix IV solutions with cation-containing fluids (e.g., Mg^{++}, Ca^{++}).	22.7, and 68 mg tablets. Taste Tabs are 22.7, 68 and 136 mg. 22.7 mg/mL injection.	Dog: 5–20 mg/kg/q24h po, IV, IM. Cat: 5 mg/kg q24h po, IM. Do not administer to cats at doses higher than 5 mg/kg and do not administer to cats IV.
Ergocalciferol (vitamin D2) (Calciferol, Drisdol)	Vitamin D analogue. Used for vitamin D deficiency and as treatment of hypocalcemia, especially that associated with hypothyroidism. Vitamin D promotes absorption and utilization of calcium.	Overdose may cause hypercalcemia. Avoid use in pregnant animals because it may cause fetal abnormalities. Use cautiously with high doses of calcium-containing preparations.	Should not be used for renal hypoparathyroidism because of inability to convert to active compound. Available as oral solution, tablets, capsules, and injection. Doses for individual patients should be adjusted by monitoring serum calcium concentrations.	400 U tablets (OTC); 50 000 U tablets (1.25 mg); 500 000 U/mL (12.5 mg/mL) injection.	500–2000 U/kg/day po.

Erythromycin (many brands and generic)	Macrolide antibiotic. Inhibits bacteria by binding to SOS ribosome and inhibiting protein synthesis. Spectrum of activity limited primarily to gram-positive aerobic bacteria. Used for skin and respiratory infections.	Most common side effect is vomiting (probably caused by cholinergic-like effect or motilin-induced motility). May cause diarrhea in some animals. Do not administer po to rodents or rabbits.	There are several forms of erythromycin, including the ethylsuccinate and estolate esters, and stearate salt for oral administration. There is no convincing data to suggest that one form is absorbed better than another, and one dose is included for all.	250 or 500 mg capsules or tablets.	10–20 mg/kg q8–12h po; prokinetic effects at 0.5–1.0 mg/kg q8–12h po.
Estradiol cypionate (ECP, Depo-Estradiol Cypionate, generic)	Semi-synthetic estrogen compound. Used primarily to induce abortion in animals.	High risk of endometrial hyperplasia and pyometra. High doses can produce leukopenia, thrombocytopenia, and fatal aplastic anemia.	Ordinarily, 22 µg/kg is administered once IM during days 3–5 of estrus or within 3 days of mating. However, in one study, a dose of 44 µg/kg was more efficacious than 22 µg/kg when given during estrus or diestrus.	2 mg/mL injection.	Dog: 22–44 µg/kg IM (total dose not to exceed 1.0 mg). Cat: 250 µg/cat IM between 40h and 5 days of mating.
Etodolac (EtoGesic [veterinary]; Lodine [human])	An NSAID of the pyranocarboxylic acid group. Inhibits inflammatory prostaglandins.	NSAIDs may cause GI ulceration. Other adverse effects caused by NSAIDs include decreased platelet function and renal injury. Keratoconjunctivitis sicca has been reported in dogs. In clinical trials with etodolac, some dogs at recommended doses showed weight loss, loose stools, or diarrhea. At high doses, etodolac caused GI ulceration in dogs.	Studies in dogs showed etodolac to be more efficacious than placebo for treatment of arthritis	150 and 300 mg tablets.	Dog: 10–15 mg/kg q24h po. Cat: dose not established.

(continued)

Drug name (trade or other names)	Pharmacology and indications	Adverse effects and precautions	Dosing information and comments	Formulations	Dosage (unless otherwise indicated, dose is the same for dogs and cat)
Famcyclovir	Antiviral drug. Synthetic purine analogue (acyclic nucleoside analogue). Converted to penciclovir via deacetylation and oxidation. Used to treat feline herpesvirus infection.	Possible adverse effects: mild anemia, mild increase in WBC.	Response can be variable in some cats.	125, 250, and 500 mg tablets.	Cat: feline herpes: 62.5 mg/cat q8h po for 3 weeks. Higher dose of 125 mg/cat may be more effective. Kittens: 30–50 mg/kg q12h po.
Famotidine (Pepcid)	Histamine H2 receptor antagonist. Used to suppress acid secretion for treatment and prevention of ulcers.	None reported for animals.	Clinical studies for famotidine have not been performed, therefore optimal dose for ulcer prevention and healing is not known.	10 mg tablet; 10 mg/mL injection.	Dog: 0.1–0.2 mg/kg po, IV, SC, IM q12h. Cat: 0.2–0.25 mg/kg IM, IV, SC, po q12–24h.
Fentanyl citrate (Sublimaze, generic)	Synthetic opiate analgesic. Approximately 80–100 times more potent than morphine.	Adverse effects similar to morphine.	Doses are based on empiricism and experimental studies. No clinical studies have been reported. In addition to fentanyl injection, transdermal fentanyl is available (see below).	250 mg/5 mL injection.	Anesthetic use: 0.02–0.04 mg/kg IV q2h IM SC or 0.01 mg/kg IV, IM, SC (with acetylpromazine or diazepam). Analgesia: dog: 0.002–0.01 mg/kg, cat: 0.001–0.005 mg/kg q2h IV, IM, SC.

Fentanyl, transdermal (Duragesic)	Same as for fentanyl. Transdermal fentanyl incorporates fentanyl into adhesive patches applied to skin of dogs and cats. Studies have determined that patches release sustained levels of fentanyl for 72–108 hours in dogs and cats. One 100 µg/h patch is equivalent to 10 mg/kg of morphine q4h IM.	Adverse effects have not been reported. However, if adverse effects are observed (e.g., respiratory depression, excess sedation, excitement in cats), remove patch and, if necessary, administer naloxone.	Patches available in sizes of 25, 50, 75, and 100 µg/h. Patch size is related to release rate of fentanyl. Studies have determined that 25 µg/h patches are appropriate for cats; 50 µg/h patches are appropriate for dogs 10–20 kg. Follow manufacturer's recommendations carefully when applying patches.	25, 50, 75, and 100 µg/h patch.	Dog: 10–20 kg, 50 µg/h patch every 72h. Cat: 25 µg patch every 118h.
Firocoxib (Previcox)	Firocoxib is a nonsteroidal antiinflammatory drug (NSAID). Like other drugs in this class, firocoxib produces analgesic and antiinflammatory effects by inhibiting the synthesis of prostaglandins. Firocoxib is highly selective for COX-2.	GI problems are the most common adverse effects associated with NSAIDs and can include vomiting diarrhea, nausea, ulcers, and erosions of the GI tract.	Dose for cats has been reported from only one study. Not registered for cats.	Tablets 57 or 277 mg.	Dog: 5 mg/kg po, q24h. Cat: 1.5 mg/kg, once. Long-term safety in cats has not been determined.
Florfenicol (Nuflor)	Chloramphenicol derivative with same mechanism of action as chloramphenicol (inhibition of protein synthesis) and broad antibacterial spectrum. Use in small animals has been infrequent.	Use in dogs and cats has been limited; therefore adverse effects have not been reported. Chloramphenicol has been linked to dose-dependent bone marrow depression, and similar reactions may be possible with florfenicol. However, there does not appear to be a risk of aplastic anemia, as for chloramphenicol.	Dose form is approved for use only in cattle, and these doses have not been thoroughly evaluated in small animals. Doses listed are derived from pharmacokinetic studies.	300 mg/mL injectable solution.	Dog: 20 mg/kg q6h po, IM, q6h. Cat: 22 mg/kg q8h IM, po.

(continued)

Drug name (trade or other names)	Pharmacology and indications	Adverse effects and precautions	Dosing information and comments	Formulations	Dosage (unless otherwise indicated, dose is the same for dogs and cat)
Fluconazole (Diflucan)	Azole antifungal drug. Similar mechanism as other azole antifungal agents. Inhibits ergosterol synthesis in fungal cell membrane. Fungistatic. Active against dermatophytes and variety of systemic fungi, but not *Aspergillus* sp.	Adverse effects have not been reported from fluconazole administration. Compared to ketoconazole, has less effect on endocrine function. However, increased liver enzyme plasma concentrations and hepatopathy are possible. Compared to other oral azole antifungals, fluconazole is absorbed more predictably and completely, even on an empty stomach.	Doses for fluconazole are primarily based on studies performed in cats for treatment of cryptococcosis. Efficacy for other infections has not been reported. The primary difference between fluconazole and other azoles is that fluconazole attains higher concentrations in the CNS.	50, 100, 150 or 200 mg tablets; 10 or 40 mg/mL oral suspension; 2 mg/mL IV injection.	Dog: 10–12 mg/kg q24h po. For *Malassezia*, 5 mg/kg q12h po has been used. Cat: 50 mg/cat q12h–24h, po.
Flucytosine (Ancobon)	Antifungal drug. Used in combination with other antifungal drugs for treatment of cryptococcosis. Action is to penetrate fungal cells and is converted to fluorouracil, which acts as antimetabolite.	Anemia and thrombocytopenia are possible.	Flucytosine is used primarily to treat cryptococcosis in animals. Efficacy is based on flucytosine's ability to attain high concentrations in cerebrospinal fluid. Flucytosine may be synergistic with amphotericin B.	250 mg capsule; 75 mg/mL oral suspension.	25–50 mg/kg q6–8h po (up to a maximum dose of 100 mg/kg q12h po).

Fludrocortisone acetate (Florinef)	Mineralocorticoid. Used as replacement therapy in animals with adrenal atrophy/adrenocortical insufficiency. Has high potency of mineralocorticoid activity compared to glucocorticoid activity.	Adverse effects are primarily related to glucocorticoid effects with high doses. Long-term treatment for hypoadrenocorticism may result in glucocorticoid side effects.	Dose should be adjusted by monitoring patient response (i.e., monitoring electrolyte concentrations). In some patients, it is administered with a glucocorticoid and sodium supplementation.	100 μg (0.1 mg) tablets.	Dog: 0.2–0.8 mg per dog or 0.02 mg/kg q24h po (15–30 μg/kg). Cat: 0.1–0.2 mg per cat q24h po.
Flumethasone (Flucort)	Potent glucocorticoid antiinflammatory drug. Potency is approximately 15 × that of cortisol. Used to treat inflammatory disorders when a potent drug is needed.	Corticosteroids produce multiple systemic side effects. Adverse effects are common with chronic therapy.	Doses are based on severity of underlying disease.	0.5 mg/mL injection.	Antiinflammatory uses: 0.15–0.3 mg/kg q12–24h IV, IM, SC.
Fludrocortisone acetate (Florinef)	Mineralocorticoid. Used as replacement therapy in animals with adrenal atrophy/adrenocortical insufficiency. Has high potency of mineralocorticoid activity compared to glucocorticoid activity.	Adverse effects are primarily related to glucocorticoid effects with high doses. Long-term treatment for hypoadrenocorticism may result in glucocorticoid side effects.	Dose should be adjusted by monitoring patient response (i.e., monitoring electrolyte concentrations). In some patients, it is administered with a glucocorticoid and sodium supplementation.	100 μg (0.1 mg) tablets.	Dog: 0.2–0.8 mg per dog or 0.02 mg/kg q24h po (15–30 μg/kg). Cat: 0.1–0.2 mg per cat q24h po.
Flumethasone (Flucort)	Potent glucocorticoid antiinflammatory drug. Potency is approximately 15 × that of cortisol. Used to treat inflammatory disorders when a potent drug is needed.	Corticosteroids produce multiple systemic side effects. Adverse effects are common with chronic therapy.	Doses are based on severity of underlying disease.	0.5 mg/mL injection.	Antiinflammatory uses: 0.15–0.3 mg/kg q12–24h IV, IM, SC.

(continued)

Drug name (trade or other names)	Pharmacology and indications	Adverse effects and precautions	Dosing information and comments	Formulations	Dosage (unless otherwise indicated, dose is the same for dogs and cat)
Flunixin meglumine (Banamine)	NSAID. Acts to inhibit cyclooxygenase (COX) enzyme, which synthesizes prostaglandins. Other antiinflammatory effects may occur (such as effects on leukocytes), but have not been well characterized. Used primarily for short-term treatment of moderate pain and inflammation.	Most severe adverse effects related to GI system. Causes gastritis, GI ulceration with high doses or prolonged use. Renal ischemia has also been documented. Therapy in dogs should be limited to 4 consecutive days. Avoid use in pregnant animals near term. *Drug interactions*: Ulcerogenic effects are potentiated when administered with corticosteroids.	Not approved for small animals, but has been shown in experimental studies to be an effective prostaglandin synthesis inhibitor.	250 mg packet granules; 10, 50 mg/mL injection.	1.1 mg/kg once IV, IM, SC or 1.1 mg/kg/day 3 day/week po. Ophthalmic: 0.5 mg/kg once IV.
5-Fluorouracil (Fluorouracil)	Anticancer agent. Antimetabolite. Action is via inhibition with nucleic acid synthesis.	Causes mild leukopenia, thrombocytopenia. CNS toxicity. Do not use in cats.	Used in anticancer protocols. Consult anticancer treatment protocol for precise dosage and regimen.	50 mg/mL vial.	Dog: 150 mg/m^2 once/week IV. Cat: do not use.

Fluoxetine (Reconcile [veterinary], Prozac [human])	Antidepressant drug. Used to treat behavioral disorders, such as obsessive-compulsive disorders and dominance aggression. Mechanism of action via selective inhibition of serotonin reuptake and downregulation of 5-HT1 receptors.	Most common adverse effects during field trials were lethargy, reduced appetite, shaking, diarrhea, restlessness, aggression, and vocalization. In cats, nervousness and increased anxiousness have been observed.	Because of long half-life, accumulation in plasma may take several days to weeks.	Human formulations: 10 and 20 mg capsules; 4 mg/mL oral solution. Veterinary formulations: 8, 16, 32, 64 mg chewable tablets.	Dog: 1–2 mg/kg q24h po. Cat: 0.5–4 mg/cat q24h po.
Fluralaner (Bravecto)	Antiparasitic drug. Isoxazoline: selective inhibitor of arthropod GABA and L-glutamate-gated chloride channels.	Vomiting, diarrhea.	Labeled use: flea and tick preventative. Off-label efficacy against sarcoptid mites and demodicosis.	Dog chews and topical: 112.5, 250, 500, 1000, and 1400 mg/chew or tube. Cat topical: 112.5, 250, and 500 mg/tube.	Dog: 25 mg/kg q12 weeks po.
Gabapentin (Neurontin)	Anticonvulsant and analgesic. Gabapentin is an analogue of the inhibitory neurotransmitter GABA. The mechanism of anticonvulsant action and analgesic effects are not known.	Warning: oral solution contains xylitol, which may be toxic to dogs.	Gabapentin has been used for treating refractory epilepsy and as adjunct for analgesia (with other drugs).	100, 300, 400 mg capsules. 100, 300, 400, 600, 800 mg scored tablets. 50 mg/mL oral solution.	Anticonvulsant dose: 2.5–10 mg/kg q8–12h po. For analgesia: 10–15 mg/kg q8h po.

(continued)

Drug name (trade or other names)	Pharmacology and indications	Adverse effects and precautions	Dosing information and comments	Formulations	Dosage (unless otherwise indicated, dose is the same for dogs and cat)
Gentamicin sulfate (Gentocin)	Aminoglycoside antibiotic. Action is to inhibit bacteria protein synthesis via binding to 30S ribosome. Bactericidal. Broad spectrum of activity except streptococci and anaerobic bacteria.	Nephrotoxicity is the most dose-limiting toxicity. Ensure that patients have adequate fluid and electrolyte balance during therapy. Ototoxicity, vestibulotoxicity also are possible. *Drug interactions*: When used with anesthetic agents, neuromuscular blockade is possible. Do not mix in vial or syringe with other antibiotics.	Dosing regimens are based on sensitivity of organisms. Some studies have suggested that once-daily therapy (combining multiple doses into a single daily dose) is as efficacious as multiple treatments. Activity against some bacteria (e.g., *Pseudomonas*) is enhanced when combined with a β-lactam antibiotic. Nephrotoxicity is increased with persistently high trough concentrations.	50 and 100 mg/mL solution for injection.	Dog: 2–4 mg/kg q8h, or 9–14 mg/kg q24h IV, IM, SC. Cat: 3 mg/kg q8h, or 5–8 mg/kg q24h IV, IM, SC.
Gold sodium thiomalate (Myochrysine)	Gold therapy (for mechanism, see Aurothioglucose).	See Aurothioglucose.	Clinical studies have not been performed in animals. Efficacy and safety of this product are not available for animals. Aurothioglucose generally is used more often than Myochrysine.	10, 25 and 50 mg/mL injection.	1–5 mg IM on first week, then 2–10 mg IM on second week, then 1 mg/kg once/week IM maintenance.
Gold therapy	See Aurothioglucose, Gold sodium thiomalate, or Auranofin.				

Griseofulvin (microsize) (Fulvicin U/F)	Antifungal drug. Incorporates into skin layers and inhibits mitosis of fungi. Antifungal activity is limited to dermatophytes.	Adverse effects in animals include teratogenicity in cats; anemia and leukopenia in cats; anorexia, depression, vomiting, and diarrhea. Do not administer to pregnant cats.	A wide range of doses has been reported. Doses listed here represent the current consensus. Griseofulvin should be administered with food to enhance absorption.	125, 250, 500 mg tablets; 25 mg/mL oral suspension; 125 mg/mL oral syrup.	50 mg/kg q24h po (up to a maximum dose of 110–132 mg/kg/day in divided treatments).
Griseofulvin (ultramicrosize) (Fulvicin P/G, Gris-PEG)	Same as above.	Same as above.	Same as above. Ultramicrosize is absorbed to a greater extent, and doses should be less than microsize.	100, 125, 165, 250, 330 mg tablets.	30 mg/kg/day in divided treatments po.
Hydrocortisone (Cortef and generic)	Glucocorticoid antiinflammatory drug. Hydrocortisone has weaker antiinflammatory effects and greater mineralocorticoid effects compared with prednisolone or dexamethasone. Also used for replacement therapy.	Adverse effects are attributed to excessive glucocorticoid effects.	Dose requirements are related to severity of disease.	5, 10, 20 mg tablets.	Replacement therapy: 1–2 mg/kg q12h po. Antiinflammatory: 2.5–5 mg/kg q12h po.
Hydrocortisone sodium succinate (Solu-Cortef)	Same as hydrocortisone, except that this is a rapid-acting, injectable product.	Same as for hydrocortisone.	Same as for hydrocortisone. Prepare vials according to manufacturer's instructions.	Various size vials for injection.	Shock: 50–150 mg/kg IV q8h for two days. Antiinflammatory: 5 mg/kg q12h IV.

(continued)

Drug name (trade or other names)	Pharmacology and indications	Adverse effects and precautions	Dosing information and comments	Formulations	Dosage (unless otherwise indicated, dose is the same for dogs and cat)
Hydroxyurea (Hydrea)	Antineoplastic agent. Used in combination with other anticancer modalities for treatment of certain tumors. Has been used to treat polycythemia vera.	Only limited use in veterinary medicine. No adverse effects have been reported. In people, hydroxyurea causes leukopenia, anemia, thrombocytopenia.	Limited use in veterinary medicine.	500 mg capsules.	Dog: 50 mg/kg po q24h, 3 days/week. Cat: 25 mg/kg po q24h, 3 days/week.
Hydroxyzine (Atarax)	Antihistamine of the piperazine class. Used primarily to treat pruritus in animals.	Side effects of therapy are related primarily to antihistamine effects. Sedation occurs in some animals.	Clinical studies have shown hydroxyzine to be somewhat effective for treatment of pruritus in dogs.	10, 25, 50 mg tablets; 2 mg/mL oral solution.	Dog: 1–2 mg/kg q6–8h IM, po. Cat: safe dose not established.
Ibuprofen (Motrin, Advil, Nuprin)	NSAID. Produces antiinflammatory action via inhibition of prostaglandins.	Safe doses have not been established for dogs and cats. Vomiting and severe GI ulceration and hemorrhage have been reported in dogs.	Avoid use, especially in dogs.	200, 400, 600, 800 mg tablets.	Safe dose not established.
Imipenem (Primaxin)	β-lactam antibiotic with broad-spectrum activity. Action is similar to other β-lactams except that imipenem is the most active of all β-lactams. Used primarily for serious, multiple-resistant infections.	Allergic reactions may occur with β-lactam antibiotics. With rapid infusion or in patients with renal insufficiency, neurotoxicity may occur (seizures). Vomiting and nausea are possible. IM or SC injections may cause pain in dogs.	Reserve the use of this drug for only resistant, refractory infections. Observe manufacturer's instructions carefully for proper administration. For IV administration, add to IV fluids. For IM administration, add 2 mL lidocaine (1%); suspension is stable for only 1h.	250 or 500 mg vials for injection.	3–10 mg/kg q6–8h IV, SC or IM; usually 5 mg/kg q6–8h IV, IM, or SC.

Interferon (interferon-α, HuIFN-α) (Roferon)	Human interferon. Used to stimulate the immune system.	Adverse effects have not been reported in animals.	Doses and indications for animals have primarily been based on extrapolation of human recommendations or limited experimental studies. To prepare, add 3 million U to 1 L sterile saline and divide into aliquots and freeze. Thaw as needed for 30 U/mL solution.	5 and 10 million U/vial.	Dog: 2.5 million units/kg IV once daily for 3 days. Cat: 1 million units/kg IV once daily for 5 consecutive days on days 0, 14, and 60.
Isotretinoin (Accutane)	Keratinization stabilizing drug. Isotretinoin reduces sebaceous gland size and inhibits sebaceous gland activity, and decreases sebum secretion. In people, it is primarily used to treat acne. In animals, it has been used to treat sebaceous adenitis.	Absolutely contraindicated in pregnant animals. Adverse effects not reported for animals, although experimental studies have demonstrated that it can cause focal calcification (such as in myocardium and vessels).	Use in veterinary medicine is confined to limited clinical experience and extrapolation from human reports.	10, 20, 40 mg capsules.	Dog: 1–3 mg/kg/day (up to a maximum recommended dose of 3–4 mg/kg/day po). Cat: no dose established.
Itraconazole (Sporanox)	Azole (triazole) antifungal drug. Active against dermatophytes and systemic fungi, such as *Blastomyces*, *Histoplasma*, and *Coccidioides*. Also used for *Malassezia* dermatitis.	Itraconazole is better tolerated than ketoconazole. However, vomiting and hepatotoxicosis are possible, especially at high doses. In one study, hepatotoxicosis was more likely at high doses. 10–15% of dogs will develop high liver enzyme levels. High doses in cats caused vomiting and anorexia.	Doses in animals are based on studies in which itraconazole has been used to treat blastomycosis in dogs. In cats, lower doses have been effective for dermatophytes (see dosage section). Other uses or doses are based on empiricism or extrapolation from human literature.	100 mg capsules and 10 mg/mL oral liquid. Compounded formulations may not be absorbed as well as proprietary formulations.	Dog: 2.5 mg/kg q12h, or 5 mg/kg q24h po. For *Malassezia* dermatitis: 5 mg/kg q24h po for 2 days, repeated each week for 3 weeks. Dermatophytes: 3 mg/kg/day po for 15 days. Cat: 5 mg/kg q12h po. For dermatophyte infection in cat: 1.5–3.0 mg/kg (up to 5 mg/kg) q24h po for 15 days.

(continued)

Drug name (trade or other names)	Pharmacology and indications	Adverse effects and precautions	Dosing information and comments	Formulations	Dosage (unless otherwise indicated, dose is the same for dogs and cat)
Ivermectin (Heartgard, Ivomec, Eqvalan liquid)	Antiparasitic drug. Neurotoxic to parasites by potentiating effects of inhibitory neurotransmitter GABA.	Toxicity may occur at high doses and in breeds in which ivermectin crosses blood–brain barrier. Sensitive breeds include collies, Australian shepherd, sheltie, and old English sheepdog. Toxicity is neurotoxic, and signs include depression, ataxia, difficulty with vision, coma, and death. Ivermectin appears to be safe for pregnant animals. Do not administer to animals under 6 weeks of age. Animals with high microfilaremia may show adverse reactions to high doses.	Doses vary, depending on use. Heartworm prevention is lowest dose, other parasites require higher doses. Heartgard is only form approved for small animals; for other indications, large animal injectable products are often administered po, IM, or SC to small animals. For demodectic therapy, it is advised to start with 100 µg/kg/day and increase dose by 100 µg/kg/day to 600 µg/kg/day.	1% (10 mg/mL) injectable solution; 10 mg/mL oral solution; 18.7 mg/mL oral paste; 68, 136, and 272 µg tablets.	Heartworm preventative: 6 µg/kg every 30 days po in dogs and 24 µg/kg every 30 days po in cat. Microfilaricide: 50 µg/kg po 2 wk after adulticide therapy. Ectoparasite therapy (dog and cat): 200–300 µg/kg IM, SC, po. Endoparasites (dog and cat): 200–400 µg/kg weekly SC, po. *Demodex* therapy: start with 100 µg/kg/day and increase dose by 100 µg/kg/day to 600 µg/kg/day for 60–120 days po.
Kanamycin (Kantrim)	Aminoglycoside antibiotic with broad-spectrum activity.	Shares same properties with other aminoglycosides (see Amikacin, Gentamicin).	See Gentamicin.	200, 500 µg mg/mL injection.	10 µg/kg q12h or 20 µg/kg q24h IV IM, SC.

Ketamine (Ketalar, Ketavet, Vetalar)	Anesthetic agent. NMDA receptor antagonist. Exact mechanism of action is not known, but appears to act as dissociative agent. Rapidly metabolized and eliminated in most animals.	Causes pain with IM injection. Tremors, spasticity, and convulsive seizures have been reported. Increases cardiac output compared to other anesthetic agents. Do not use in animals with head injury because it may elevate CSF pressure.	Often used in combination with other anesthetics and anesthetic adjuncts, such as xylazine, acepromazine, or diazepam. IV doses generally less than IM doses.	100 mg/mL injection solution.	Dog: 5.5–22 mg/kg IV, IM (recommend adjunctive sedative or tranquilizer treatment). Cat: 2–25 mg/kg IV, IM (recommend adjunctive sedative or tranquilizer treatment). Dog and cat: Dose for constant rate infusion: 0.5 mg/kg IV followed by 10 µg/kg/min. May be used in combination with other analgesics.
Ketoconazole (Nizoral)	Azole (imidazole) antifungal drug. Similar mechanism of action as other azole antifungal agents. Inhibits ergosterol synthesis in fungal cell membrane. Fungistatic. Efficacious against dermatophytes and variety of systemic fungi, such as *Histoplasma*, *Blastomyces*, and *Coccidioides*. Also active against *Malassezia*.	Adverse effects in animals include dose-related vomiting, diarrhea, and hepatic injury. Enzyme elevations are common. Do not administer to pregnant animals. Ketoconazole causes endocrine abnormalities, most specifically inhibition of cortisol synthesis. *Drug interactions*: Ketoconazole will inhibit metabolism of other drugs (anticonvulsants, cyclosporine, cisapride).	Oral absorption depends on acidity in stomach. Do not administer with antisecretory drugs or antacids. Because of endocrine effects, ketoconazole has been used for short-term treatment of hyperadrenocorticism.	200 mg tablets; 100 mg/mL oral suspension (only available in Canada).	Dog: 10–15 mg/kg q8–12h po. For *Malassezia canis* infection: 5 mg/kg q24h po. For hyperadrenocorticism: 15 mg/kg q12h po. Cat: 5–10 mg/kg q8–12h po.

(continued)

Drug name (trade or other names)	Pharmacology and indications	Adverse effects and precautions	Dosing information and comments	Formulations	Dosage (unless otherwise indicated, dose is the same for dogs and cat)
Ketoprofen (Orudis KT [human OTC tablet]; Ketofen [veterinary injection])	NSAID. Antiinflammatory agent. Used to treat arthritis and other inflammatory disorders.	All NSAIDs share similar adverse effect of GI toxicity. Ketoprofen has been administered for 5 consecutive days in dogs without serious adverse effects. Most common side effect is vomiting. GI ulceration is possible in some animals.	Although not approved in the US, ketoprofen is approved for small animals in other countries. Doses listed are based on approved use in those countries. It is available as OTC drug for humans in the US.	12.5 mg tablet (OTC); 25, 50, 75 mg Rx human form; 100 mg/mL injection for horses.	1 mg/kg q24h po for up to 5 days. Initial dose can be given via injection at up to 2 mg/kg SC, IM, IV.
Ketorolac tromethamine (Toradol)	NSAID. Used for short-term relief of pain and inflammation. Acts by inhibiting cyclooxygenase enzyme (COX). Use of ketorolac has been evaluated clinically in dogs but not cats.	NSAIDs may cause GI ulceration. Ketorolac may cause GI lesions if administered more frequently than q8h. Do not administer more than 2 doses.	Available as 10 mg tablet and injection for IV or IM use. Clinical studies in dogs have shown safety and efficacy. Dosing q12h is recommended to avoid GI problems.	10 mg tablets; 15 and 30 mg/mL injection, in 10% alcohol.	Dog: 0.5 mg/kg q8–12h po, IM, IV. Cat: safe dose not established.
Levamisole hydrochloride (Levasole, Tramisol, Ergamisol)	Antiparasitic drug of the imidazothiazole class. Mechanism of action due to neuromuscular toxicity to parasites. Levamisole has been used for endoparasites in dogs and as microfilaricide. Levamisole has also been used as an immunostimulant; however, clinical reports of its efficacy are not available.	May produce cholinergic toxicity. May cause vomiting in some dogs.	In heartworm-positive dogs, it may sterilize female adult heartworms.	0.184 g bolus; 11.7 g per 13 g packet; 50 mg tablet (Ergamisol).	Dog: hookworms, 5–8 mg/kg once po (up to 10 mg/kg po for 2 days); microfilaricide, 10 mg/kg q24h po for 6–10 days; immunostimulant, 0.5–2 mg/kg 3 times/week po. Cat: endoparasites, 4.4 mg/kg once po; lungworms, 20–40 mg/kg q48h for 5 treatments po.

Levothyroxine sodium (Soloxine, Thyro-Tabs, Synthroid)	Replacement therapy for treating patients with hypothyroidism. Levothyroxine is T_4, which is converted in most patients to the active T_3.	High doses may produce thyrotoxicosis, which is uncommon (compared to people). *Drug interactions*: Patients receiving corticosteroids may have decreased ability to convert T_4 to T_3.	Thyroid supplementation should be guided by testing to confirm diagnosis and postmedication monitoring to adjust dose.	0.1–0.8 mg tablets (in 0.1 mg increments).	Dog: 18–22 µg/kg q12h po (adjust dose via monitoring). Cat: 10–20 µg/kg/day po (adjust dose via monitoring).
Lidocaine (Xylocaine and generic brands)	Local anesthetic. Lidocaine is also commonly used for acute treatment of cardiac arrhythmias. Class 1 antiarrhythmic. Decreases phase 0 depolarization without affecting conduction.	High doses cause CNS effects (tremors, twitches, and seizures). Lidocaine can produce cardiac arrhythmias but has greater effect on abnormal cardiac tissue than normal tissue. Cat are more susceptible to adverse effects, and lower doses should be used.	When used for local infiltration, many formulations contain epinephrine to prolong activity at injection site. Avoid epinephrine in patients with cardiac arrhythmias. Note that human formulations may contain epinephrine, but no veterinary formulations contain epinephrine. To increase pH, increase onset of action, and decrease pain from injection, one may add 1 mEq sodium bicarbonate to 10 mL lidocaine (use immediately after mixing).	5, 10, 15, 20 mg/mL injection.	Dog (antiarrhythmic): 2–4 mg/kg IV (to a maximum dose of 8 mg/kg over 10 min period); 25–75 µg/kg/min IV infusion; 6 mg/kg q1.5h IM. Cat (antiarrhythmic): 0.25–0.75 mg/kg IV slowly, or 10–40 µg/kg/min infusion. For epidural (dog and cat): 4.4 mg/kg of 2% solution.

(*continued*)

Drug name (trade or other names)	Pharmacology and indications	Adverse effects and precautions	Dosing information and comments	Formulations	Dosage (unless otherwise indicated, dose is the same for dogs and cat)
Lincomycin (Lincocin)	Lincosamide antibiotic, similar in mechanism to clindamycin and erythromycin. Spectrum includes primarily gram-positive bacteria. Used for pyoderma and other soft tissue infections.	Adverse effects uncommon. Lincomycin has caused vomiting and diarrhea in animals. Do *not* administer orally to rodents and rabbits.	Action of lincomycin and clindamycin is similar enough that clindamycin can be substituted for lincomycin.	100, 200, 500 mg tablets.	15–25 mg/kg q12h po. For pyoderma, doses as low as 10 mg/kg q12h have been used.
Linezolid (Zyvox)	Oxazolidinone antibiotic. Gram-positive spectrum that includes drug-resistant strains of *Enterococcus* and *Staphylococcus*. High expense limits routine use.	Adverse effects include diarrhea and nausea. Rarely in people, anemia and leukopenia have been observed. Use cautiously with monoamine oxidase inhibitors and serotonergic drugs.	Use in animals is reserved for only drug-resistant infections (e.g., MRSA) for which other drugs are ineffective.	400 and 600 mg tablets. 20 mg/mL oral suspension. 2 mg/ML injection.	10 mg/kg, q8–12h, po or IV.
Liothyronine (Cytomel)	Thyroid supplement. Liothyronine is equivalent to T_3.	Adverse effects have not been reported (see Levothyroxine sodium).	Doses of liothyronine should be adjusted on the basis of monitoring T_3 concentrations in patients.	60 µg tablets.	4.4 µg/kg q8h po. ForT_3 suppression test in cats: collect presample for T_4 and T_3, administer 25 µg q8h for 7 doses, then collect postsamples for T_3 and T_4 after last dose.
Lokivetmab (Cytopoint)	Caninized monoclonal antibody against IL-31. Reduces pruritus associated with allergic dermatitis.	Transient vomiting, diarrhea, lethargy. Treatment-induced immunogenicity may reduce efficacy.	Not for use in cats	10, 20, 30, and 40 mg single-use vials.	Dogs: 2 mg/kg subcutaneously repeated every 4–8 weeks.

Lomustine (CCNU) (CeeNU)	Anticancer drug – alkylating agent in the nitrosourea class. Chemotherapeutic agent. Highly lipid soluble and crosses blood–brain barrier. Used for lymphoma and brain tumors.	Myelosuppression, hepatotoxicosis, vomiting.	Administering on empty stomach decreases nausea. Monitor hemogram for evidence of myelosuppression.	10, 40, 100 mg capsules.	Dog: 70–90 mg/m^2 every 4 weeks po. For brain tumors 60–80 mg/m^2 q6–8 weeks po. Cat: 50–60 mg/m^2 po every 3–6 weeks or 10 mg per cat po every 3 weeks.
Lufenuron (Program)	Antiparasitic. Used for controlling fleas in animals. Inhibits development in hatching fleas. May be used for dermatophytes in dogs and cats, although efficacy has been questioned by some experts.	Adverse effects have not been reported. Appears to be relatively safe during pregnancy and in young animals.	Lufenuron may control flea development with administration once every 30 days in animals.	45, 90, 135, 204.9, 409.8 mg tablets; 135 and 270 mg suspension per unit pack.	Dog: 10 mg/kg po every 30 days. Cat: 30 mg/kg po every 30 days Cat injection: 10 mg/kg SC every 6 months. Antifungal dose – dog: 80 mg/kg; cat: 100 mg/kg. In endemic areas (e.g., catteries) treat cats once a month.
Lufenuron + milbemycin oxime (Sentinel tablets and Flavor Tabs)	Combination of two antiparasitic drugs. See Lufenuron or Milbemycin oxime. Used to protect against fleas, heartworms, roundworms, hookworms, and whipworms.	See Lufenuron or Milbemycin oxime.	See Lufenuron or Milbemycin oxime.	Milbemycin oxime/lufenuron ratio is as follows: 2.3/46 mg tablets; 5.75/115, 11.5/230, and 23/460 mg Flavor Tabs.	Dog: administer one tablet, every 30 days. Each tablet formulated for size of dog. Cat: This product is not registered for cats.

(*continued*)

Drug name (trade or other names)	Pharmacology and indications	Adverse effects and precautions	Dosing information and comments	Formulations	Dosage (unless otherwise indicated, dose is the same for dogs and cat)
L-Lysine (Enisyl-F)	Amino acid for treatment of herpes infections. Oral supplementation for cats with feline herpesvirus-1 (FHV-1) infection is associated with reduced viral shedding.	Well tolerated in cats.	Doses listed will reduce viral shedding. Powder can be mixed with food. Paste can be given directly.	250 mg/mL paste.	Cat: 400 mg po/day. Paste formulation 1–2 mL po to adult cats and 1 mL to kittens.
Marbofloxacin (Zeniquin)	Fluoroquinolone antimicrobial. Spectrum includes staphylococci, gram-negative bacilli, and some *Pseudomonas*.	May cause some nausea and vomiting at high doses. Avoid use in young animals. Safe for cats (ocular safety) at recommended dose.	Use susceptibility testing to guide therapy.	25, 50, 100, and 200 mg tablets.	2.75–5.55 mg/kg q24h po.
Maropitant (Cerenia)	Antiemetic. Neurokinin (NK) type-1 inhibitor. Maropitant acts to prevent vomiting caused by chemotherapy and motion sickness. It is also effective for inhibiting vomiting from both central and peripheral stimulation.	In clinical trials, there were few adverse effects in dogs. Salivation and muscle tremors occurred in some animals.	Studies have shown NK-1 inhibitors to be effective antiemetics for a variety of stimuli.	10 mg/mL injection; 16, 24, 60, or 160 mg tablets.	Dog: 1 mg/kg SC q24h for up to 5 days; 2 mg/kg po q24h for up to 5 days; for motion sickness, 8 mg/kg po q24h for up to 2 days. Cat: dose not established.

Meclizine (Antivert, generic)	Antiemetic and antihistamine. Used for treatment of motion sickness. Action may be caused by central anticholinergic actions. Also may suppress chemoreceptor trigger zone (CRTZ).	Adverse effects have not been reported in animals. Anticholinergic (atropine-like) effects may cause side effects.	Results of clinical studies in animals have not been reported. Use in animals is based on experience in people or anecdotal experiences in animals.	12.5, 25, 50 mg tablets.	Dog: 25 mg q24h po (for motion sickness, administer 1h prior to traveling). Cat: 12.5 mg q24h po.
Meclofenamate sodium (Arquel, Meclofen)	NSAID. Used for treatment of arthritis and other inflammatory disorders.	Adverse effects have not been reported in animals, but adverse effects common to other NSAIDs are possible.	Results of clinical studies in animals have not been reported. Use in animals is based on experience in people or anecdotal experiences in animals. Administer with food.	50, 100 mg capsules. Formulations for dogs are rarely available now.	Dog: 1 mg/kg po q24h for up to 5 days. Cat: not recommended.
Medetomidine (Domitor)	α_2-Adrenergic agonist. Used primarily as sedative, anesthetic adjunct, and analgesia.	α_2-Agonists decrease sympathetic output. Cardiovascular depression may occur. Medetomidine will cause an initial bradycardia and hypertension.	May be used for sedation, analgesia, and minor surgical procedures. Should be reversed with equal volume of atipamezole.	1.0 mg/mL injection.	750 μg/m^2 IV or 1000 μg/m^2 IM. Lower doses may be used for short-term sedation and analgesia.
Medroxyprogesterone acetate (Depo-Provera [injection]; Provera [tablets])	Progestin hormone. Derivative of acetoxyprogesterone. In animals, used as progesterone hormone treatment to control estrus cycle. Also used for management of some behavioral and dermatologic disorders (such as urine spraying in cats and alopecia).	Adverse effects include polyphagia, polydipsia, adrenal suppression (cat), increased risk of diabetes, pyometra, diarrhea, and increased risk of neoplasia.	Clinical studies in animals have studied primarily the reproductive use and effects on behavioral use. Medroxyprogesterone acetate may have fewer side effects than megestrol acetate.	150, 400 mg/mL suspension injection; 2.5, 5, 10 mg tablets.	1.1–2.2 mg/kg q7d IM. For behavioral use, 10–20 mg/kg is injected SC. For prostatic disease in dogs, use 3–5 mg/kg IM, SC.

(continued)

Drug name (trade or other names)	Pharmacology and indications	Adverse effects and precautions	Dosing information and comments	Formulations	Dosage (unless otherwise indicated, dose is the same for dogs and cat)
Megestrol acetate (Ovaban)	Progestin hormone.	Long-term use may produce adverse effects including increased risk of neoplasia and diabetes.	Avoid chronic use. Use for controlling behavior problems is discouraged.	5 mg tablets.	Dog – proestrus: 2 mg/kg q24h po for 8 days; anestrus: 0.5 mg/kg q24h po for 30 days; behavior: 2–4 mg/kg q24h for 8 days (reduce dose for maintenance). Cat – dermatologic therapy or urine spraying: 2.5–5 mg/cat q24h po for 1 week, then reduce to 5 mg once or twice/week; suppress estrus: 5 mg/cat/day for 3 days, then 2.5–5 mg once/week for 10 weeks.
Meloxicam (Mobic [human drug], Metacam [veterinary drug])	NSAID of the oxicam class. Meloxicam is relatively COX-1 sparing and has high COX-1:COX-2 ratio. It has been used in dogs and cats for pain and osteoarthritis.	Adverse effects are GI and include vomiting, diarrhea, and ulceration.	In studies in dogs, higher doses (up to 0.5 mg/kg) were more effective than lower doses but were associated with a higher incidence of GI adverse effects. Oral suspension is in a palatable flavor, which may be added to pet's food.	7.5 mg tablets (human). Veterinary forms: 1.5 mg/mL oral suspension, 5 mg/mL injection.	Dog: 0.2 mg/kg initial loading dose, then 0.1 mg/kg q24h po. Injection: 0.2 mg/kg IV or SC. Cat: single antipyretic dose, 0.3 mg/kg; long-term dose, 0.05 mg/kg q48–72h po. Injection: 0.2 mg/kg SC, one time.

Mepivacaine (Carbocaine-V)	Local anesthetic of the amide class. Medium potency and duration of action, compared to bupivacaine. Compared to lidocaine, longer acting, but equal potency.	Mepivacaine may cause less irritation to tissues than lidocaine.	For epidural use, do not exceed 8 mg/kg total dose. Duration of epidural is 2.5–3h.	2% (20 mg/mL) injection.	Variable dose for local infiltration. For epidural, 0.5 mL of 2% solution every 30 sec until reflexes are absent.
6-Mercaptopurine (Purinethol)	Anticancer agent. Antimetabolite agent that inhibits synthesis of purines in cancer cells.	Many side effects are possible that are common to anticancer therapy (many of which are unavoidable), including bone marrow suppression and anemia. Do not use in cats.	Used for various forms of cancer, including leukemia and lymphoma. Consult specific anticancer protocol for specific regimen.	50 mg tablets.	Dog: 50 mg/m2 q24h po. Cat: do not use.
Meropenem (Merrem IV)	Broad-spectrum carbapenem antibiotic; indicated primarily for resistant infections caused by bacteria resistant to other drugs. Bactericidal. More active than imipenem and ertapenem.	Risks similar to those of other β-lactam antibiotics. Meropenem does not cause seizures as frequently as imipenem. SC injections may cause slight hair loss at injection site.	Dosage guidelines have been extrapolated from pharmacokinetic studies in animals and not tested for efficacy in animals. Meropenem is more soluble than imipenem and can be injected via bolus rather than administered in fluid solutions.	500 mg/20 mL or 1 g/30 mL vial for injection.	8.5 mg/kg q12h SC up to 12 mg/kg q8h SC or 24 mg/kg IV q12h. For *Pseudomonas*: 12 mg/kg q8h SC or 25 mg/kg q8h IV.

(continued)

Drug name (trade or other names)	Pharmacology and indications	Adverse effects and precautions	Dosing information and comments	Formulations	Dosage (unless otherwise indicated, dose is the same for dogs and cat)
Methimazole (Tapazole)	Antithyroid drug. Used for treating hyperthyroidism, primarily in cats. Action is to serve as substrate for thyroid peroxidase and decrease incorporation of iodide into tyrosine molecules.	In people, it has caused agranulocytosis and leukopenia. In cats, lupus-like reactions are possible, such as vasculitis and bone marrow changes. Well tolerated in dogs.	Use in cats is based on experimental studies in hyperthyroid cats. Methimazole has, for the most part, replaced propylthiouracil for use in cats. Adjust maintenance dose by monitoring T_4 levels. Twice-daily dosing in cats shown to be more effective than once-daily dosing.	5 and 10 mg tablets.	Cat: 2.5 mg per cat q12h po × 7–14 days, then 5–10 mg per cat po q12h, and monitor T_4 concentrations.
Methocarbamol (Robaxin-V)	Skeletal muscle relaxant. Depresses polysynaptic reflexes. Used for treatment of skeletal muscle spasms.	Causes some depression and sedation of the CNS.	Results of clinical studies in animals have not been reported. Use in animals (and doses) based on experience in people or anecdotal experience in animals.	500, 750 mg tablets; 100 mg/mL injection.	44 mg/kg q8h po on the first day, then 22–44 mg/kg q8h po.

Methotrexate (MTX, Mexate, Folex, Rheumatrex, and generic)	Anticancer agent. Used for various carcinomas, leukemia, and lymphomas. Action is via antimetabolite action. Analogue of folic acid that binds dihydrofolate reductase. Inhibits DNA, RNA, and protein synthesis. In people, methotrexate is also commonly used for autoimmune diseases, such as rheumatoid arthritis.	Anticancer drugs cause predictable (and sometimes unavoidable) side effects that include bone marrow suppression, leukopenia, and immunosuppression. Hepatotoxicity has been reported in people from methotrexate therapy. *Drug interactions*: Concurrent use with NSAIDs may cause severe methotrexate toxicity. Do not administer with pyrimethamine, trimethoprim, or sulfonamides.	Use in animals has been based on experimental studies. There is only limited clinical information available. Consult specific anticancer protocols for precise dosage and regimen.	2.5 mg tablets; 2.5 or 25 mg/mL injection.	2.5–5 mg/m^2 q48h po (dose depends on specific protocol). Dog: 0.3–0.5 mg/kg once/week IV. Cat: 0.8 mg/kg IV every 2–3 weeks.
Methylprednisolone (Medrol)	Glucocorticoid antiinflammatory drug. Compared to prednisolone, methylprednisolone is 1.25 × more potent.	Same as for other glucocorticoids. Manufacturer suggests that methylprednisolone causes less PU/PD than prednisolone.	Use of methylprednisolone is similar to that of other corticosteroids. Dose adjustment should be made to account for difference in potency (see dose section.)	1, 2, 4, 8, 18, 32 mg tablets.	0.22–0.44 mg/kg q12–24h po.

(continued)

Drug name (trade or other names)	Pharmacology and indications	Adverse effects and precautions	Dosing information and comments	Formulations	Dosage (unless otherwise indicated, dose is the same for dogs and cat)
Methylprednisolone acetate (Depo-Medrol)	Depot form of methylprednisolone. Slowly absorbed from IM injection site, producing glucocorticoid effects for 3–4 weeks in some animals. Used for intralesional therapy, intraarticular therapy, and inflammatory conditions.	Many adverse effects are possible from use of corticosteroids. Cardiovascular problems (congestive heart failure) have been associated with use in cats. Chronic use of methylprednisolone acetate may cause long-term adverse effects.	Use of methylprednisolone acetate should be evaluated carefully because one injection will cause glucocorticoid effects that persist for several days to weeks.	20 or 40 mg/mL suspension for injection.	Dog: 1 mg/kg (or 20–40 mg/dog) IM every 1–3 weeks. Cat: 10–20 mg/cat IM every 1–3 weeks.
Methylprednisolone sodium succinate (Solu-Medrol)	Same as methylprednisolone, except that this is a water-soluble formulation intended for acute therapy when high IV doses are needed for rapid effect. Used for treatment of shock and CNS trauma.	Adverse effects are not expected from single administration; however, with repeated use, other side effects are possible.	Results of clinical studies in animals have not been reported. Use in animals (and doses) based on experience in people or anecdotal experience in animals.	1 and 2 g and 125 and 500 mg vials for injection.	For emergency use: 30 mg/kg IV and repeat at 15 mg/kg in 2–6h, IV.
Methyltestosterone (Android, generic)	Anabolic androgenic agent. Used for anabolic actions or testosterone hormone replacement therapy (androgenic deficiency). Testosterone has been used to stimulate erythropoiesis.	Adverse effects caused by excessive androgenic action of testosterone. Prostatic hyperplasia is possible in male dogs. Masculinization can occur in female dogs. Hepatopathy is more common with oral methylated testosterone formulations.	See also Testosterone cypionate, Testosterone propionate. Use of testosterone androgens has not been evaluated in clinical studies in animals. Use is based primarily on experimental evidence or experiences in people.	10, 25 mg tablets.	Dog: 5–25 mg/dog q24–48h po. Cat: 2.5–5 mg/cat q24–48h po.

Metoclopramide (Reglan, Maxolon)	Prokinetic drug. Centrally acting antiemetic. Stimulates motility of upper GI tract. Action is to inhibit dopamine receptors and enhance action of acetylcholine in GI tract. Used primarily for gastroparesis and treatment of vomiting. It is not effective for dogs with gastric dilation.	Adverse effects are primarily related to blockade of central dopaminergic receptors. Adverse effects similar to phenothiazines (e.g., acepromazine) have been reported, in addition to behavioral changes. Do not use in epileptic patients or with diseases caused by GI obstruction.	Results of clinical studies in animals have not been reported. Use in animals (and doses) based on experience in people or anecdotal experience in animals. Most use is for general antiemetic purposes, but doses as high as 2 mg/kg have been used to prevent vomiting during cancer chemotherapy.	10, 5 mg tablet; 1 mg/mL oral solution; 5 mg/mL injection.	0.2–0.5 mg/kg q6–8h IV, IM, po; CRI: loading dose of 0.4 mg/kg IV, followed by 0.3 mg/kg/h IV. In refractory patients, rates up to 1.0 mg/kg/h have been used.
Metronidazole (Flagyl and generic) and Metronidazole benzoate	Antibacterial and antiprotozoal drug. Disrupts DNA in organism via reaction with intracellular metabolite. Action is specific for anaerobic bacteria. Resistance is rare. Active against some protozoa, including *Giardia*; however, other drugs, such as fenbendazole, have been used for *Giardia*.	Most severe adverse effect is caused by toxicity to CNS. High doses have caused lethargy, CNS depression, ataxia, vomiting, and weakness. Metronidazole may be mutagenic. Fetal abnormalities have not been demonstrated in animals with recommended doses, but use cautiously during pregnancy. Cat may find broken tablets unpalatable.	Metronidazole is one of the most commonly used drugs for anaerobic infections. Although it is effective for giardiasis, other drugs used for giardiasis include albendazole, fenbendazole, and quinacrine. CNS toxicity is dose related. Maximum dose that should be administered is 50–65 mg/kg/day in any species. Although tablets have been broken or crushed for oral administration to cats, they find these unpalatable. When palatability is a problem in cats, consider metronidazole benzoate.	250, 500 mg tablet; 50 mg/mL suspension; 5 mg/mL injection; the benzoate form is not available commercially and must be obtained from compounding pharmacies. 20 mg of metronidazole benzoate = 12.4 mg metronidazole.	For anaerobes – dog: 15 mg/kg q12h, or 12 mg/kg q8h po; cat: 10–25 mg/kg q24h po. For *Giardia* – dog: 12–15 mg/kg q12h for 8 days po; cat: 17 mg/kg (1/3 tablet per cat) q24h for 8 days.

(continued)

Drug name (trade or other names)	Pharmacology and indications	Adverse effects and precautions	Dosing information and comments	Formulations	Dosage (unless otherwise indicated, dose is the same for dogs and cat)
Mibolerone (Cheque Drops)	Androgenic steroid. Used to suppress estrus.	Do not use in Bedlington terriers. Do not use with perianal adenoma or carcinoma. Many bitches show clitoral enlargement or discharge from treatment. Do not use in cats.	Treatment ordinarily is initiated 30 days prior to onset of estrus. It is not recommended to be used for more than 2 years.	55 μg/mL oral solution.	Dog: (2.6–5–μg/kg/day po) 0.45–11.3 kg, 30 μg; 11.8–22.7 kg, 60 μg; 23–45.3 kg, 120 μg; > 45.8 kg, 180 μg. Cat: safe dose not established.
Milbemycin oxime (Interceptor, Interceptor Flavor Tabs, and SafeHeart)	Antiparasitic drug. Action is similar to ivermectin. Acts as GABA agonist in nervous system of parasite. Used as heartworm preventative, miticide, and microfilaricide. Used to control infections of hookworm, roundworms, and whipworms. At high doses, it has been used to treat *Demodex* infections in dogs.	In susceptible dogs (collie breeds), milbemycin may cross the blood–brain barrier and produce CNS toxicosis (depression, lethargy, coma). At doses used for heartworm prevention, this effect is less likely.	Doses vary, depending on parasite treated. Consult dose column. Treatment of *Demodex* requires high dose administered daily. See also Lufenuron + milbemycin oxime.	2.3, 5.75, 11.5, and 23 mg tablet.	Dog: microfilaricide: 0.5 mg/kg; *Demodex*: 2 mg/kg q24h po for 60–120 days; heartworm prevention and control of endoparasites: 0.5 mg/kg every 30 days po. Cat: for heartworm and endoparasite control, 2.0 mg/kg every 30 days po.
Minocycline hydrochloride (Minocin Solodyn)	Tetracycline antibiotic. Similar to doxycycline.	Similar to other tetracyclines (doxycycline). Adverse effects have not been reported for minocycline. Oral absorption is not affected by calcium products as with other tetracyclines.	Minocycline has received little attention for clinical use in North America. Clinical use has not been reported, but properties are similar to doxycycline.	50, 75 and 100 mg tablets; or capsules 10 mg/mL oral suspension.	5–12.5 mg/kg q12h po.

Mitotane (*o,p*′-DDD) (Lysodren)	Adrenocortical cytotoxic agent. Causes suppression of adrenal cortex. Used to treat adrenal tumors and pituitary-dependent hyperadrenocorticism (PDH).	Adverse effects, especially during induction period, include lethargy, anorexia, ataxia, depression, vomiting. Corticosteroid supplementation (e.g., hydrocortisone or prednisolone) may be administered to minimize side effects.	Dose and frequency often are based on patient response. Adverse effects are common during initial therapy. Administration with food increases oral absorption. Maintenance dose should be adjusted on the basis of periodic cortisol measurements and ACTH stimulation tests. Cats usually have not responded to mitotane treatment.	500 mg tablets.	Dog – for PDH: 50 mg/kg/day (in divided doses) po for 5–10 days, then 50–70 mg/kg/week po; for adrenal tumor: 50–75 mg/kg/day for 10 days, then 75–100 mg/kg/week po.
Moxidectin (canine form: ProHeart; equine oral gel: Quest; cattle pour-on: Cydectin)	Antiparasitic drug. Neurotoxic to parasites by potentiating effects of inhibitory neurotransmitter GABA. Used for endo- and ectoparasites, as well as heartworm prevention.	Toxicity may occur at high doses and in species in which ivermectin crosses blood–brain barrier (collie breeds). Toxicity is neurotoxic, and signs include depression, ataxia, difficulty with vision, coma, and death.	Similar use as ivermectin. Extreme caution is recommended if equine formulation is considered for use in small animals. Toxic overdoses are likely because the equine formulation is highly concentrated.	30, 68, 136 μg tablets for dogs; 20 mg/mL equine oral gel; and 5 mg/mL cattle pour-on.	Dog – heartworm prevention: 3 μg/kg q30d po; endoparasites: 25–300 μg/kg. *Demodex*: 400 μg/kg/day po and up to 500 μg/kg/day for 21–22 weeks.
Moxifloxacin (Avelox)	Fluoroquinolone antibiotic of the new (4th) generation. Similar to other fluoroquinolones, except with greater activity against gram-positive and anaerobic bacteria.	Similar to those of other fluoroquinolones. Because of the increased spectrum of action on anaerobic bacteria, greater GI disturbance is expected from oral dose.	Doses and recommendations are based primarily on limited clinical experience and extrapolation from human studies.	400 mg tablet.	10 mg/kg q24h po.

(*continued*)

Drug name (trade or other names)	Pharmacology and indications	Adverse effects and precautions	Dosing information and comments	Formulations	Dosage (unless otherwise indicated, dose is the same for dogs and cat)
Mycophenolate (Cell Cept)	Mycophenolate is metabolized to mycophenolic acid. It is used to suppress immunity for transplantation and for treatment of immune-mediated diseases.	In dogs, gastrointestinal problems (diarrhea, vomiting) have been the most common effects reported. Use in veterinary medicine has been rare.	Mycophenolate is used in some patients that cannot tolerate other immunosuppressive drugs such as azathioprine or cyclophosphamide.	250 mg capsule.	Dog: 10 mg/kg q8h po. Cat: no dose established.
Naloxone (Narcan)	Opiate antagonist. Used to reverse effects from opiate agonists (such as morphine). Naloxone may be used to reverse sedation, anesthesia, and adverse effects caused by opiates.	Adverse effects are not reported. Tachycardia and hypertension have been reported in people.	Administration may have to be individualized based on response in each patient. Naloxone's duration of action is short in animals (60 min) and may have to be repeated.	20 or 400 μg/mL injection.	0.01–0.04 mg/kg IV, IM, SC, as needed, to reverse opiate.
Naltrexone (Trexan)	Opiate antagonist. Similar to naloxone, except that it is longer acting and administered orally. Used in people for treatment of opiate dependence. In animals, it has been used for treatment of some obsessive-compulsive behavioral disorders.	Adverse effects have not been reported in animals.	Treatment for obsessive-compulsive disorders in animals has been reported with naltrexone. Relapse rates may be high.	50 mg tablets.	Dog: for behavior problems: 2.2 mg/kg q12h po.

Naproxen (Naprosyn, Naxen, Aleve [naproxen sodium])	NSAID. Action is via inhibition of prostaglandins. Used for treatment of inflammatory disorders (e.g., arthritis).	Naproxen is a potent NSAID. Adverse effects attributed to GI toxicity are common to all NSAIDs. Naproxen has produced serious ulceration in dogs because elimination in dogs is many-fold slower than in people or horses.	Results of clinical studies in animals have not been reported. Use in animals (and doses) based on pharmacokinetic studies in experimental animals. Caution when using the OTC formulation designed for people because the tablet size is much larger than safe dose for dogs. 220 mg naproxen sodium is equivalent to 200 mg naproxen.	220 mg tablet (OTC); 25 mg/mL oral suspension; 250, 375, 500 mg tablets (Rx).	Dog: 5 mg initially, then 2 mg/kg q48h po. Cat: not recommended.
Neomycin (Biosol)	Aminoglycoside antibiotic. Neomycin differs from other aminoglycosides because it is administered only topically or orally. Systemic absorption is minimal from oral dose.	Although oral absorption is so small that systemic adverse effects are unlikely, some oral absorption has been demonstrated in young animals (calves). Alterations in intestinal bacterial flora from therapy may cause diarrhea.	Neomycin is primarily used for oral treatment of diarrhea. Efficacy for this indication (especially for nonspecific diarrhea) is questionable. Used also for treatment of hepatic encephalopathy.	500 mg bolus; 200 mg/mL oral liquid.	10–20 mg/kg q6–12h po.
Nilenpyram (Capstar)	Antiparasitic drug. It rapidly kills adult fleas.	No adverse reactions are reported. It was safe in studies in dogs and cats in which up to 10 × dose was administered.	Do not use in dogs or cats less than 1 kg (2 pounds) in weight. Do not use in cats or dogs less than 4 weeks of age.	Tablet: 11.4 or 57 mg.	1 mg/kg, po, daily as needed to kill fleas.

(continued)

Drug name (trade or other names)	Pharmacology and indications	Adverse effects and precautions	Dosing information and comments	Formulations	Dosage (unless otherwise indicated, dose is the same for dogs and cat)
Nitrofurantoin (Macrodantin, Furalan, Furatoin, Furadantin, and generic)	Antibacterial drug. Urinary antiseptic. Action is via reactive metabolites that damage DNA. Therapeutic concentrations are reached only in the urine. Not to be used for systemic infections.	Adverse effects include nausea, vomiting, and diarrhea. Turns urine color rust-yellow brown. Do not administer during pregnancy.	Two dosing forms exist. Microcrystalline is rapidly and completely absorbed. Macrocrystalline (Macrodantin) is more slowly absorbed and causes less GI irritation. Urine should be at acidic pH for maximum effect. Administer with food to increase absorption.	Macrodantin and generic: 25, 50, 100 mg capsules; Furalan, Furatoin, and generic: 50, 100 mg tablets; Furadantin: 5 mg/mL oral suspension.	10 mg/kg/day divided into four daily treatments, then 1 mg/kg at night po.
Nizatidine (Axid)	Histamine H2 blocking drug. Same as cimetidine, except up to 10 × more potent. Inhibits acid secretion in stomach. Used for ulcers and gastritis.	Side effects from nizatidine have not been reported in animals.	Results of clinical studies in animals have not been reported. Use in animals (and doses) based on experience in people or anecdotal experience in animals. Nizatidine and ranitidine have been shown to stimulate gastric emptying and colonic motility via anticholinesterase activity.	150, 300 mg capsules.	Dog: 2.5–5 mg/kg q24h po.
Norfloxacin (Noroxin)	Fluoroquinolone antibacterial drug. Same action as ciprofloxacin, except spectrum of activity is not as broad as with enrofloxacin or ciprofloxacin.	Adverse effects have not been reported in animals. Some effects are expected to be similar to cipro/enrofloxacin administration.	Use in animals (and doses) based on pharmacokinetic studies in experimental animals, experience in people, or anecdotal experience in animals.	400 mg tablets.	22 mg/kg q12h po.

Oclacitinib (Apoquel)	Janus kinase inhibitor. Reduces pruritus associated with allergic dermatitis in dogs.	Vomiting, diarrhea, increased risk of demodicosis, pneumonia, persistent infection.	Approved for dogs 1 year of age and older.	3.6, 5.4, and 16 mg tablets.	0.4–0.6 mg/kg q24h po.
Omeprazole (Prilosec)	Proton pump inhibitor. Omeprazole inhibits gastric acid secretion by inhibiting the K^+/H^+ pump. Omeprazole is more potent and longer acting than most available antisecretory drugs. Used for treatment and prevention of GI ulcers.	Side effects have not been reported in animals. *Drug interactions*: Do not administer with drugs that depend on stomach acid for absorption (e.g., ketoconazole).	Due to omeprazole's potency and accumulation in gastric cells, infrequent administration is possible.	20 mg capsules and equine paste.	Dog: 20 mg/dog q24h po (or 0.7 mg/kg q24h). Cat: 0.5–0.7 mg/kg q24h po.
o,p'-DDD	See Mitotane.				
Orbifloxacin (Orbax)	Fluoroquinolone antimicrobial. Same mechanism as enrofloxacin and ciprofloxacin. Spectrum includes staphylococci, gram-negative bacilli, and some *Pseudomonas*.	May cause some nausea and vomiting at high doses. Avoid use in young animals. Blindness in cats has not been reported with doses < 15 mg/kg/day.	Dose range is wide to account for susceptibility of bacteria. Dosing should be guided by susceptibility tests.	5.7, 22.7, and 68 mg tablets.	2.5–7.5 mg/kg q24h po.
Ormetoprim + sulfadimethoxine	Trimethoprim-like drug used in combination with sulfadimethoxine. (See Primor.)				

(continued)

Drug name (trade or other names)	Pharmacology and indications	Adverse effects and precautions	Dosing information and comments	Formulations	Dosage (unless otherwise indicated, dose is the same for dogs and cat)
Oxacillin (Prostaphlin and generic)	β-lactam antibiotic. Inhibits bacterial cell wall synthesis. Spectrum is limited to gram-positive bacteria, especially staphylococci.	Use cautiously in animals allergic to penicillin-like drugs.	Doses based on empiricism or extrapolation from human studies. No clinical efficacy studies available for dogs or cats. Administer on empty stomach, if possible.	250, 500 mg capsules; 50 mg/mL oral solution.	22–40 mg/kg q8h po.
Oxymorphone hydrochloride (Numorphan)	Opioid agonist. Action is similar to morphine, except that oxymorphone is more lipophilic than morphine and 10–15 × more potent than morphine.	Same adverse effects and precautions as morphine.	There is some evidence that oxymorphone may have fewer cardiovascular effects compared to morphine. Since oxymorphone is more lipophilic, it is readily absorbed from epidural injection.	1.5 and 1 mg/mL injection.	Analgesia: 0.1–0.2 mg/kg IV, SC, IM (as needed), redose with 0.05–0.1 mg/kg q1–2h. Preanesthetic: 0.025–0.05 mg/kg IM or SC. Sedation: 0.05–0.02 mg/kg (with or without acepromazine) IM, SC.
Oxytetracycline (Terramycin)	Tetracycline antibiotic. Same mechanism and spectrum as tetracycline. Oxytetracycline may be absorbed to higher extent.	Generally safe. Use cautiously in young animals. See precautions for tetracycline.	Oral dose forms are from large-animal use. Use of injectable long-acting forms has not been studied in small animals.	250 mg tablets; 100, 200 mg/mL injection.	7.5–10 mg/kg IV q12h; 20 mg/kg q12h po.

Paroxetine (Paxil)	Selective serotonin reuptake inhibitor (SSRI) much like fluoxetine (Prozac) in action. Used for obsessive-compulsive disorders, aggression, and other behavioral problems.	Some effects similar to fluoxetine, but in some animals, paroxetine is better tolerated.	Dosing recommendations are empirical.	10, 20, 30, 40 mg tablets.	Dog: 0.5 mg/kg q24h po. Cat: 1/8 to 1/4 of a 10 mg tablet q24h po.
Pentoxifylline (Trental)	Methylxanthine. Pentoxifylline is used primarily as a rheological agent in people (increases blood flow through narrow vessels). It may have anti-inflammatory action via inhibition of cytokine synthesis. Used in dogs for some dermatoses (dermatomyositis) and vasculitis.	May cause similar signs as other methylxanthines. Nausea and vomiting have been reported in people. When broken tablet is administered to cats, the taste is unpleasant.	Results of clinical studies in animals have not been reported. Use in animals (and doses) based on experience in people or anecdotal experience in animals.	400 mg tablets.	Dog – 10 mg/kg q12h and up to 15 mg/kg q8h po or 400 mg/dog for most animals. Cat: 1/4 of a 400 mg tablet (100 mg) q8–12h po.
Phenobarbital (Luminal and generic)	Long-acting barbiturate. Phenobarbital's major use is as an anticonvulsant, in which it potentiates inhibitory actions of GABA.	Adverse effects are dose related. Phenobarbital causes polyphagia, sedation, ataxia, and lethargy. Some tolerance develops to side effects after initial therapy. Hepatotoxicity has been reported in some dogs receiving high doses.	Phenobarbital doses should be carefully adjusted via monitoring serum/plasma concentrations. Optimum range for therapeutic effect is 15–40 μg/mL.	15, 30, 60, 100 mg tablets; 30, 60, 65, and 130 mg/mL injection; 4 mg/mL oral elixir solution.	Dog: 2–8 mg/kg q12h po. Cat: 2–4 mg/kg q12h po. Status epilepticus: administer in increments of 10–20 mg/kg IV (to effect).

(continued)

Drug name (trade or other names)	Pharmacology and indications	Adverse effects and precautions	Dosing information and comments	Formulations	Dosage (unless otherwise indicated, dose is the same for dogs and cat)
Phenylbutazone (Butazolidin and generic)	NSAID. Inhibits prostaglandin synthesis. Phenylbutazone is used primarily for arthritis and various forms of musculoskeletal pain and inflammation.	Phenylbutazone is generally well tolerated in dogs, but there is no data for cats. Adverse effects include GI toxicity. Do not administer injectable formulation IM. Phenylbutazone causes bone marrow depression in people, which also is possible in dogs.	Doses are based primarily on manufacturer's recommendations and clinical experience.	100, 200, 400 mg and 1 g tablets; 200 mg/mL injection.	Dog: 15–22 mg/kg q8–12h (44 mg/kg/day) po or IV (800 mg/dog maximum). Cat: 6–8 mg/kg q12h IV or po.
Phenylpropanolamine (PPA) (Proin PPA, Propalin syrup)	Adrenergic agonist. Used as decongestant, mild bronchodilator, and to increase tone of urinary sphincter.	Adverse effects are attributed to excess stimulation of adrenergic (α and β) receptors. Side effects: tachycardia, cardiac effects, CNS excitement, restlessness, and appetite suppression.	Phenylpropanolamine has been removed from human decongestant formulations. Only veterinary compounded formulations are available.	25, 50, 75 mg flavored tablet and 25 mg/mL vanilla-flavored oral solution.	Dog: 1 mg/kg, q12h, po. Increase to 1.5–2.0 mg/kg as needed, q8h po.
Piperacillin (Pipracil)	β-lactam antibiotic of the acylureidopenicillin class. Similar to other penicillins, except with high activity against *Pseudomonas aeruginosa*. Also good activity against streptococci.	Same precautions as for other injectable penicillins.	Reconstituted solution should be used within 24 hours (or 7 days if refrigerated). Piperacillin is combined with tazobactam (β-lactamase inhibitor) in Zosyn.	2, 3, 4, 40 g vials for injection.	40 mg/kg IV or IM q6h.

Piroxicam (Feldene and generic)	NSAID of the oxicam class. Prostaglandin synthesis inhibitor. Clinical effects are similar to other NSAIDs. Piroxicam has been used for treatment of transitional cell carcinoma in dogs.	Elimination of piroxicam is slow; use cautiously in dogs. Adverse effects are primarily GI toxicity (ulcers); see Flunixin meglumine.	Piroxicam is primarily used to treat arthritis and other musculoskeletal conditions, but there are reports of its activity for treating certain tumors (e.g., transitional cell carcinoma of bladder).	10 mg capsules.	Dog: 0.3 mg/kg q48h po. Cat: 0.3 mg/kg q24h po.
Polysulfated glycosaminoglycan (PSGAG) (Adequan Canine)	Large molecular weight compound similar to normal constituents of healthy joints. Chondroprotective. Inhibits enzymes that may degrade articular cartilage. Used primarily to treat or prevent degenerative joint disease.	Adverse effects are rare. Allergic reactions are possible. PSGAG has heparin-like effects and may potentiate bleeding problems in some animals.	Doses are derived from empirical evidence, experimental studies, and clinical studies in dogs. Although effective for acute arthritis, may not be as effective for chronic arthropathy.	100 mg/mL injection in 5 mL vial (for horses, vials are 250 mg/mL).	4.4 mg/kg IM, twice weekly for up to 4 weeks.
Praziquantel (Droncit)	Antiparasitic drug. Action on parasites related to neuromuscular toxicity and paralysis via altered permeability to calcium. Used primarily to treat infections caused by tapeworms.	Vomiting occurs at high doses. Anorexia and transient diarrhea have been reported. Safe in pregnant animals.	Dose recommendations based on label dose supplied by manufacturer.	23, 34 mg tablet; 56.8 mg/mL injection.	Dog (oral dose): < 6.8 kg: 7.5 mg/kg po, once; > 6.8 kg: 5 mg/kg po, once. Dog (injection): ≤ 2.3 kg: 7.5 mg/kg IM or SC, once; 2.7–4.5 kg: 6.3 mg/kg IM or SC, once; ≤ 5 kg: 5 mg/kg IM or SC, once. Cat (oral dosage): < 1.8 kg: 6.3 mg/kg po, once; > 1.8 kg: 5 mg/kg po, once; for *Paragonimus* infection use 25 mg/kg q8h po for 2–3 days. Cat (injection): 5 mg/kg IM or SC.

(continued)

Drug name (trade or other names)	Pharmacology and indications	Adverse effects and precautions	Dosing information and comments	Formulations	Dosage (unless otherwise indicated, dose is the same for dogs and cat)
Prednisolone (Delta-Cortef and many others)	Glucocorticoid antiinflammatory drug. Potency is approximately 4 × cortisol.	All glucocorticoids produce expected (and sometimes unavoidable) side effects. Chronic therapy may lead to several adverse effects.	Doses for prednisolone are based on severity of underlying condition.	5 and 20 mg tablets.	Dog (cats often require 2 × dog dose) – antiinflammatory: 0.5–1 mg/kg q12–24h IV, IM, po initially, then taper to q48h; immunosuppressive: 2.2–6.6 mg/kg/day IV, IM, po initially, then taper to 2–4 mg/kg q48h; replacement therapy: 0.2–0.3 mg/kg/day po.
Prednisolone sodium succinate (Solu-Delta-Cortef)	Same as for prednisolone, except that this is a water-soluble formulation intended for acute therapy when high IV doses are needed for rapid effect. Used for treatment of shock and CNS trauma.	Adverse effects are not expected from single administration; however, with repeated use, other side effects are possible.	Although shock doses are listed, efficacy for treatment of shock is questionable.	100, 200 mg vials for injection (10 and 50 mg/mL).	Shock: 15–30 mg/kg IV (repeat in 4–6h). CNS trauma: 15–30 mg/kg IV, taper to 1–2 mg/kg q12h.
Prednisone (Deltasone and generic; Meticorten for injection)	Same as for prednisolone, except that, after administration, prednisone is converted to prednisolone.	Adverse effects are same as for prednisolone.	Same as for prednisolone. In cats use prednisolone.	1, 2.5, 5, 10, 20, 25, and 50 mg tablets; 1 mg/mL syrup (Liquid Pred in 5% alcohol) and 1 mg/mL oral solution (in 5% alcohol).	Dogs convert prednisone to prednisolone, and doses are similar; in cats there is inadequate conversion of prednisone to prednisolone.

Primor (ormetoprim + sulfadimethoxine)	Antibacterial drug. Ormetoprim inhibits bacterial dihydrofolate reductase, sulfonamide competes with p-aminobenzoic acid (PABA) for synthesis of nucleic acids. Bactericidal/bacteriostatic. Broad antibacterial spectrum and active against some coccidia.	Several adverse effects have been reported from sulfonamides. Ormetoprim has been associated with CNS adverse effects.	Doses listed are based on manufacturer's recommendations. Controlled trials have demonstrated efficacy for treatment of pyoderma on once-daily schedule.	Combination tablet (ormetoprim + sulfadimethoxine).	27 mg/kg on first day, followed by 13.5 mg/kg q24h po.
Progesterone, repositol	See Medroxyprogesterone acetate.				
Propylthiouracil (PTU) (generic, Propyl-Thyracil)	Antithyroid drug. Compared to methimizole, PTU inhibits conversion of T_4 to T_3.	Adverse effects in cats include hemolytic anemia, thrombocytopenia, and other signs of immune-mediated disease.	Use of PTU in most cats has been replaced with methimazole.	50 and 100 mg tablets.	11 mg/kg q12h po.
Ranitidine hydrochloride (Zantac)	Histamine H2 antagonist. Same as cimetidine except 4–10 × more potent and longer acting.	Ranitidine may have fewer effects on endocrine function and drug interactions, compared to cimetidine.	Pharmacokinetic information in dogs suggests that ranitidine may be administered less often than cimetidine to achieve continuous suppression of stomach acid secretion. Ranitidine may stimulate stomach emptying and colon motility via anticholinesterase action.	75, 150, 300 mg tablets; 150, 300 mg capsules; 25 mg/mL injection.	Dog: 2 mg/kg q8h IV, po. Cat: 2.5 mg/kg q12h IV; 3.5 mg/kg q12h po.

(continued)

Drug name (trade or other names)	Pharmacology and indications	Adverse effects and precautions	Dosing information and comments	Formulations	Dosage (unless otherwise indicated, dose is the same for dogs and cat)
Retinoids	See Isotretinoin and Vitamin A				
Retinol	See Vitamin A.				
Rifampin (Rifadin)	Antibacterial. Action is to inhibit bacterial RNA synthesis. Spectrum of action includes staphylococci and mycobacteria. Other susceptible bacteria include streptococci. Used in people primarily for treatment of tuberculosis.	Adverse effects not reported in animals, but in people, hypersensitivity and flu-like symptoms are reported. *Drug interactions*: Multiple drug interactions are possible. Induces cytochrome P450 enzymes. Drugs affected include barbiturates, chloramphenicol, and corticosteroids.	Results of clinical studies in animals have not been reported. Use in animals (and doses) based on experience in people or anecdotal experience in animals. Rifampin is highly lipid soluble and has been used to treat intracellular infections.	150, 300 mg capsules; injection solution: 600 mg Rifadin IV.	5 mg/kg q12–24h po or 5–15 mg/kg q24h po.
Sarolaner	Antiparasitic drug. Isoxazoline: selective inhibitor of arthropod GABA and L-glutamate-gated chloride channels.	Vomiting, diarrhea, neurologic symptoms.	Labeled use: flea and tick preventative. Off-label efficacy against sarcoptid mites and demodicosis.	Dog: 5, 10, 20, 40, 80, and 120 mg.	Dog: 2 mg/kg every 4 weeks po.

Selamectin (Revolution)	Topical parasiticide and heartworm prevention.	Transient localized alopecia with or without inflammation at or near the site of application was observed in approximately 1% of 691 treated cats. Other signs observed rarely included GI signs, anorexia, lethargy, salivation, tachypnea, and muscle tremors.	Recommended for use in dogs 6 weeks of age or older and in cats 8 weeks of age or older.	Available in six separate dose strengths.	6–12 mg/kg topically every 30 days.
Selegiline (Anipryl [also known as deprenyl and L-deprenyl]; human dose form is Eldepryl)	Inhibits specific monoamine oxidase (MAO type B) to inhibit degradation of dopamine in CNS. In people, it is primarily used to treat Parkinson's disease and other neurodegenerative diseases (in combination with levodopa). In dogs, it is approved to control clinical signs of pituitary-dependent hyperadrenocorticism (Cushing's disease) and to treat cognitive dysfunction in geriatric dogs.	Adverse effects have not been reported in dogs. However, amphetamine-like signs can be produced in experimental animals. At high doses in dogs, hyperactivity has been observed (doses > 3 mg/kg). Do not use with other MAO inhibitors or drugs that inhibit serotonin reuptake.	In the multicenter trial performed by Deprenyl Animal Health, Inc., selegiline controlled the clinical signs of > 70% of dogs with hyperadrenocorticism. However, other investigators have reported efficacy rates as low as 20%.	2, 5, 10, 15, and 30 mg tablets.	Dog: begin with 1 mg/kg q24h po. If there is no response within 2 months, increase dose to maximum of 2 mg/kg q24h po. Cat: 0.25–0.5 mg/kg q12–24h po.

(continued)

Drug name (trade or other names)	Pharmacology and indications	Adverse effects and precautions	Dosing information and comments	Formulations	Dosage (unless otherwise indicated, dose is the same for dogs and cat)
Silymarin (Silybin, Marin, "milk thistle")	Contains silybin as the most active ingredient. It is also known as milk thistle, from which it is derived. Silymarin is a mixture of antihepatotoxic flavonolignans (derived from the plant *Silybum*).	No adverse reactions have been reported.	Silymarin is available in several dietary supplements. There may be variable content and absorption among products.	Silymarin tablets are widely available OTC. Commercial veterinary formulations (Marin) also contain zinc and vitamin E in a phosphatidylcholine complex in tablets for dogs and cats.	30 mg/kg/day po.
Stanozolol (Winstrol-V)	Anabolic steroid. Stanozolol has been used to decrease negative nitrogen balance in animals with chronic renal failure.	Stanozolol will produce anabolic effects with chronic use. There is increased risk of hepatic toxicity, with cats being at higher risk.	Monitor liver enzymes in treated animals.	50 mg/mL injection; 2 mg tablets.	Dog: 2 mg/dog (or range of 1–4 mg/dog) q12h po; 25–50 mg/dog/week IM. Cat: 1 mg/cat q12h po;2 5 mg/cat/week IM.
Sucralfate (Carafate, [Sulcrate in Canada])	Gastric mucosa protectant. Antiulcer agent. Binds to ulcerated tissue in GI tract to aid healing of ulcers. There is some evidence that sucralfate may act as a cytoprotectant (via prostaglandin synthesis).	Adverse effects have not been reported. Not absorbed systemically. *Drug interactions*: Sucralfate may decrease absorption of other orally administered drugs (e.g., fluoroquinolones and tetracyclines) via chelation with aluminum.	Dosing recommendations are based largely on empiricism. No clinical trials of efficacy in animals. Sucralfate may be administered concurrently with histamine type-2 inhibitors (e.g., cimetidine).	1 g tablets; 200 mg/mL oral suspension.	Dog: 0.5–1 g q8–12h po. Cat: 0.25 g q8–12h po.

Sulfadiazine (generic, combined with trimethoprim in Tribrissen)	Sulfonamides compete with PABA for enzyme that synthesizes dihydrofolic acid in bacteria. Synergistic with trimethoprim. Broad spectrum of activity, including some protozoa. Bacteriostatic.	Adverse effects associated with sulfonamides include allergic reactions, type II and III hypersensitivity, hypothyroidism (with prolonged therapy), keratoconjunctivitis sicca, and skin reactions.	Usually, sulfonamides are combined with trimethoprim or ormetoprim in 5:1 ratio to produce a synergistic effect.	500 mg tablets and trimethoprim + sulfadiazine available as 30, 120, 240, 480 and 960 mg tablets (although availability is limited).	100 mg/kg IV, po (loading dose), followed by 50 mg/kg q12h IV, po (see Trimethoprim + sulfadiazine section for additional dosing).
Sulfasalazine (sulfapyridine + mesalamine) (Azulfidine [Salazopyrin in Canada])	Sulfonamide + antiinflammatory drug. Used for treatment of colitis. Sulfonamide has little effect, salicylic acid (mesalamine) has antiinflammatory effects.	Adverse effects are all attributed to sulfonamide component. Keratoconjunctivitis sicca has been reported.	Usually used for treatment of idiopathic colitis, often in combination with dietary therapy.	500 mg tablets.	Dog: 10–30 mg/kg q8–12h po. Cat: 20 mg/kg q12h po.
Tepoxalin (Zubrin)	Analgesic drug and NSAID. Used to treat pain and inflammation in dogs, particularly osteoarthritis. Tepoxalin has lipoxygenase-inhibiting effects (decreases leukotrienes), and the active metabolite has cyclooxygenase-inhibiting effects (decreases prostaglandins), which is longer acting.	Most common adverse effects from the clinical trials have been GI related (nausea, vomiting, diarrhea).	When switching animals from another NSAID or corticosteroid to tepoxalin, allow 7-day washout. Long-term safety of tepoxalin has not been established in cats.	50, 100, and 200 mg tablets (Zydis freeze-dried tablet).	Dog: 10–20 mg/kg po initially, 10 mg/kg q24h po thereafter. Cat: safe dose not established.

(continued)

Drug name (trade or other names)	Pharmacology and indications	Adverse effects and precautions	Dosing information and comments	Formulations	Dosage (unless otherwise indicated, dose is the same for dogs and cat)
Terbinafine hydrochloride (Lamisil)	Antifungal drug effective against dermatophytes and *Malassezia*.	Vomiting and anorexia. Hepatotoxicity possible but not reported in animals.	Doses used in dogs and cats much higher than those used in humans.	250 mg tablets, 1% topical solution, 1% topical cream.	Dog: 30 mg/kg po (with food) q24h for 3 weeks. Cat: 30–40 mg/kg po q24h for at least 2 weeks.
Testosterone cypionate ester (Andro-Cyp, Andronate, Depo-Testosterone, and other forms) and Testosterone propionate ester (Testex [Malogen in Canada])	Testosterone ester. Similar effects as methyltestosterone. Testosterone esters are administered IM to avoid first-pass effects. Esters in oil are absorbed more slowly from IM injection. Esters are then hydrolyzed to free testosterone.	Adverse effects are attributed to androgenic and anabolic effects. Hepatic toxicity is also possible.	Clinical efficacy for chronic diseases has not been evaluated in small animals.	Testosterone cypionate 100, 200 mg/mL injection. Testosterone propionate 100 mg/mL injection.	Testosterone cypionate 1–2 mg/kg every 2–4 weeks IM (see also Methyltestosterone). Testosterone propionate 0.5–1 mg/kg 2–3 times/week IM.
Tetracycline (Panmycin)	Tetracycline antibiotic. Tetracyclines bind to 30S ribosomal subunit and inhibit protein synthesis. Usually bacteriostatic. Broad spectrum of activity, including bacteria, some protozoa, *Rickettsia*, *Ehrlichia*.	Tetracyclines in general may cause renal tubular necrosis at high doses. Tetracyclines can affect bone and teeth formation in young animals. Tetracyclines have been implicated in drug fever in cats. Hepatotoxicity may occur at high doses in susceptible individuals. *Drug interactions*: Tetracyclines bind to calcium-containing compounds, which decreases oral absorption.	Pharmacokinetic and experimental studies have been conducted in small animals, but no clinical studies. Do not use outdated solutions.	250, 500 mg capsules; 100 mg/mL suspension.	15–20 mg/kg q8h po; or 4.4–11 mg/kg q8h IV, IM.

Thyroid hormone	See Levothyroxine sodium and Liothyronine.				
Thyrotropin-releasing hormone (TRH)	Used to detect hyperthyroidism when T_4 is not elevated.	Adverse effects uncommon.	Used for diagnostic purposes.	Injection.	Collect baseline T_4, followed by 0.1 mg/kg IV. Collect post-TRH T_4 sample at 4h.
Thyrotropin, thyroid-stimulating hormone (TSH) (Thytropar, Thyrogen)	Thyroid-stimulating hormone is used for diagnostic testing. Stimulates normal secretion of thyroid hormone.	Adverse reactions rare. In people, allergic reactions have occurred.	For Thytropar: to prepare solution, add 2 mL NaCl to 10 U vial. Reconstituted solutions retain potency for 2 weeks at 2–8°C. Consult testing laboratory for specific guidelines for thyroid testing. For Thyrogen: reconstitute vial with 6 mL sterile water.	Old forms (Thytropar) are difficult to obtain. Human recombinant form (rh TSH) (Thyrogen) contains 1.1 mg/vial.	Dog: collect baseline sample, followed by 0.1 U/kg IV (maximum dose is 5 U); collect post-TSH sample at 6h. For human recombinant form: 50–100 μg per dog.
Ticarcillin + clavulanate (Timentin)	Same as ticarcillin, except clavulanic acid has been added to inhibit bacterial β-lactamase and increase spectrum. Clavulanate does not increase activity against *Pseudomonas*, however.	Same as for ticarcillin.	Same as for ticarcillin.	3 g per vial for injection.	Dose according to rate for ticarcillin.

(continued)

Drug name (trade or other names)	Pharmacology and indications	Adverse effects and precautions	Dosing information and comments	Formulations	Dosage (unless otherwise indicated, dose is the same for dogs and cat)
Ticarcillin disodium (Ticar, Ticillin)	β-lactam antibiotic. Action similar to ampicillin/amoxicillin. Spectrum similar to carbenicillin. Ticarcillin is primarily used for gram-negative infections, especially those caused by *Pseudomonas*.	Adverse effects are uncommon. However, allergic reactions are possible. High doses can produce seizures and decreased platelet function. *Drug interactions*: Do not combine in same syringe or in vial with aminoglycosides.	Ticarcillin is synergistic and often combined with aminoglycosides (e.g., amikacin, gentamicin). 1% lidocaine may be used for reconstitution to decrease pain from IM injection.	Vials containing 1, 3, 6, 20, and 30 g for injection.	33–50 mg/kg q4–6h IV, IM.
Tobramycin sulfate (Nebcin)	Aminoglycoside antibacterial drug. Similar mechanism of action and spectrum as amikacin, gentamicin.	Adverse effects similar to those of amikacin, gentamicin.	Dosing requirements vary depending on bacterial susceptibility. See dose schedules for gentamicin and amikacin.	40 mg/mL injection.	Dog: 2–4 mg/kg q8h IV, IM, SC or 9–14 mg/kg q24h IV, IM, SC. Cat: 3 mg/kg q8h IV, IM, SC or 5–8 mg/kg q24h, IV, IM, SC.
Tramadol hydrochloride (Ultram, and generic)	Analgesic drug. Tramadol has some μ-opioid receptor action, and it may also inhibit the reuptake of norepinephrine (NE) and serotonin (5 HT). The metabolite (desmethyltramadol) may have greater opiate effects than the parent drug.	Sedation may occur in some animals, especially at high doses. In cats, some vomiting, behavior changes, and mydriasis may be observed at high doses. At very high doses in dogs, seizures may occur.	Dosing information is based on experimental studies in dogs, and derived from clinical experience in dogs. Extended-release tablets are not equivalent.	Tramadol immediate-release tablets are available in 50 mg doses.	Dog: 5 mg/kg q6–8h po. Cat: safe dose not established.

Triamcinolone and Triamcinolone acetonide (Vetalog, Triamtabs, Aristocort, generic)	Glucocorticoid antiinflammatory drug. Triamcinolone has potency that is approximately equal to methylprednisolone (about 5 × cortisol and 1.25 × prednisolone), although some dermatologists suggest that potency is higher. Injectable suspension is slowly absorbed from IM or intralesional injection site. Used for intralesional therapy.	Adverse effects are similar to other corticosteroids. When used for ocular injections, there is some concern that granulomas may occur at injection site.	Note that cats may require higher doses than dogs (sometimes 2 ×).	Veterinary (Vetalog) 0.5 and 1.5 mg tablets; 2 or 6 mg/mL suspension injection. Human form: 1, 2, 4, 8, 16 mg tablets; 10 mg/mL injection.	Antiinflammatory: 0.5–1 mg/kg q12–24h po, then taper dose to 0.5–1 mg/kg q48h po. (However, manufacturer recommends doses of 0.11–0.22 mg/kg/day.) Triamcinolone acetonide injection: 0.1–0.2 mg/kg IM, SC, repeat in 7–10 days. Intralesional: 1.2–1.8 mg, or 1 mg for every cm diameter of tumor every 2 weeks.
Tribrissen	See Trimetho-prim + sulfadiazine.				
Triiodothyronine	See Liothyronine.				
Trilostane (Vetoryl)	Used for treatment of hypercortisolemia (Cushing's syndrome) in dogs. 3-β- hydroxysteroid dehydrogenase inhibitor, in dogs, for treatment of pituitary-dependent hyperadrenocorticism (PDH).	In one study, adverse effects consisted of 1 dog with transient lethargy and 1 dog with anorexia. Otherwise, it has been well tolerated. One should check electrolyte levels in treated patients because trilostane decreases aldosterone.	Trilostane is an efficacious and safe medication for treatment of dogs with PDH. It is registered in Europe for treatment of PDH but is not commercially available at this time in the US. It has been imported by veterinarians after obtaining permission from the Food and Drug Administration. Dose should be adjusted in individual patients based on cortisol measurements.	60 mg capsules. No formulations approved in the US.	Dog: median dose is 6.1 mg/kg/day but range is 3.9–9.2 mg/kg/day po, which is adjusted based on cortisol measurements. General dose is 30 mg q24h po for dogs that weigh < 5 kg, 60 mg q24h po for dogs that weigh = 5 kg, and 120 mg for dogs > 20 kg.

(continued)

Drug name (trade or other names)	Pharmacology and indications	Adverse effects and precautions	Dosing information and comments	Formulations	Dosage (unless otherwise indicated, dose is the same for dogs and cat)
Trimeprazine tartrate (Temaril [Panectyl in Canada])	Phenothiazine with antihistamine activity (similar to promethazine). Used for treating allergies and motion sickness.	Adverse effects similar to those of promethazine.	There is evidence that trimeprazine is more effective when combined with prednisone for treatment of pruritus. Combination product is Temaril-P.	2.5 mg/5 mL syrup; 2.5 mg tablet.	0.5 mg/kg q12h po.
Trimethoprim + sulfadiazine (Tribrissen, Tucoprim, and others)	Combines the antibacterial drug action of trimethoprim and a sulfonamide. Together, the combination is synergistic, with a broad spectrum of activity.	Adverse effects primarily caused by sulfonamide component.	Dosage recommendations vary. There is evidence that 30 mg/kg/day is efficacious for pyoderma; for other infections, 30 mg/kg twice daily has been recommended.	30, 120, 240, 480, 960 mg tablets (all formulations have ratio of 5:1 sulfa: trimethoprim). Some trimethoprim-sulfadiazine formulations are no longer available in US.	15 mg/kg q12h po, or 30 mg/kg q12–24h po (for *Toxoplasma*: 30 mg/kg q12h po).
Trimethoprim + sulfamethoxazole (Bactrim, Septra, and generic forms)	Combines the antibacterial drug action of trimethoprim and a sulfonamide. Together, the combination is synergistic, with a broad spectrum of activity.	Adverse effects primarily caused by sulfonamide component.	Dosage recommendations vary. There is evidence that 30 mg/kg/day is efficacious for pyoderma; for other infections, 30 mg/kg twice daily has been recommended.	480, 960 mg tablet; 240 mg/5 mL oral suspension (all formulations have ratio of 5:1 sulfa: trimethoprim).	15 mg/kg q12h po, or 30 mg/kg q12–24h po.
Tripelennamine citrate (Pelamine, PBZ)	Histamine (H) blocker. Similar in action to other antihistamines. Used to treat allergic disease.	Adverse effects similar to other antihistamines. Members of this class (ethanolamines) have greater antimuscarinic effects than other antihistamines.	There are no clinical reports of use in veterinary medicine. No evidence that it is more efficacious than other drugs in this class.	25, 50 mg tablets; 20 mg/mL injection.	1 mg/kg q12h po.

TSH (thyroid-stimulating hormone)	See Thyrotropin.				
Tylosin (Tylocine, Tylan, Tylosin tartrate)	Macrolide antibiotic. Tylosin is not used systemically, but has been administered to treat chronic diarrhea in dogs.	May cause diarrhea in some animals. Do not administer orally to rodents or rabbits.	Tylosin is rarely used in small animals. Powdered formulation (tylosin tartrate) has been administered on food for control of signs of colitis in dogs. Tablets are approved in Canada for treatment of colitis.	Available as soluble powder 3 g/tsp (tablets for dogs in Canada).	Dog and cat: 7–15 mg/kg q12–24h po. Dog (for colitis): 10–20 mg/kg q8h with food; if there is a response, increase the interval to q12–24h.
Vancomycin (Vancocin, Vancoled)	Antibacterial drug. Mechanism of action is to inhibit cell wall and cause bacterial cell lysis (via mechanism different from that of β - lactams). Spectrum includes staphylococci, streptococci, and enterococci (but not gram-negative bacteria). Used primarily for treatment of resistant staphylococci and enterococci.	Adverse effects have not been reported in animals. Administer IV; causes severe pain and tissue injury if administered IM or SC. Do not administer rapidly; use slow infusion, if possible (e.g., over 30 min). Adverse effects in people include renal injury (more common with older products that contained impurities) and histamine release.	Vancomycin use is not common in animals, but is valuable for treatment of enterococci or staphylococci that are resistant to other antibiotics. Doses are derived from pharmacokinetic studies in dogs. Monitoring of trough plasma concentrations is recommended to ensure proper dose. Maintain trough concentration above 5 μg/mL. Infusion solution can be prepared in 0.9% saline or 5% dextrose, but not alkalinizing solutions.	Vials for injection (0.5 to 10 g).	Dog: 15 mg/kg q6–8h IV infusion. Cat: 12–15 mg/kg q8h IV infusion.

(continued)

Drug name (trade or other names)	Pharmacology and indications	Adverse effects and precautions	Dosing information and comments	Formulations	Dosage (unless otherwise indicated, dose is the same for dogs and cat)
Vitamin A (retinoids) (Aquasol A)	Vitamin A supplement. See also Isotretinoin for analogues used for other conditions.	Excessive doses can cause bone or joint pain, dermatitis.	Dosing of vitamin is expressed as U or retinol equivalents (RE), or μg of retinol. 1 RE = 1 μg of retinol. 1 RE of vitamin A = 3.33 U of retinol.	Oral solution: 5000 U (1500 RE)/0.1 mL; 10 000, 25 000 and 50 000 U tablets.	625–800 U/kg q24h po (see dosing information section).
Vitamin D	See Ergocalciferol.				
Vitamin E (α-tocopherol) (Aquasol E and generic)	Vitamin considered as antioxidant. Used as supplement and as treatment of some immune-mediated dermatoses.	Side effects have not been reported.	Vitamin E has been proposed as treatment for a wide range of human illnesses, but evidence for efficacy in animals is lacking.	Wide variety of capsules, tablets, oral solution available (e.g., 1000 U/capsule).	100–400 U q12h po (or 400–600 U q12h po for immune-mediated skin disease).
Xylaxine hydrochloride (Rompun, and generic)	α_2-Adrenergic agonist. Used primarily for short-term anesthesia and analgesia.	Produces sedation and ataxia. Cardiac depression, heart block, and hypotension are possible with high doses. Produces emesis after IV injection, especially in cats.	Often used in combination with other drugs, e.g., ketamine.	20 and 100 mg/mL injection.	Dog: 1.1 mg/kg IV; 2.2 mg/kg IM. Cat: 1.1 mg/kg IM (emetic [cat only] dose is 0.4–0.5 mg/kg IV).

Yohimbine (Yobine)	α_2-Adrenergic antagonist. Used primarily to reverse actions of xylazine or detomidine. Atipamezole is more specific as a reversing agent.	High doses can cause tremors and seizures.	Reverses signs of sedation and anesthesia caused by α_2-agonists.	2 mg/mL injection.	0.11 mg/kg IV, or 0.25–0.5 mg/kg SC, IM.
Zidovudine (AZT) (Retrovir)	Antiviral drug. In people, used to treat AIDS. In animals, has been experimentally used for treatment of feline leukemia virus (FeLV) and feline immunodeficiency virus (FIV) viral infection in cats. AZT acts to inhibit the viral enzyme reverse transcriptase, which prevents conversion of viral RNA into DNA.	Anemia and leukopenia are adverse effects. Monitor the packed cell volume in treated cats and perform a complete blood count periodically.	At this time, experience with using AZT for treating viral disease in animals is largely experimental or anecdotal. Consult a more detailed reference for guidance. It may have helped some cats with FIV and may prevent persistent FeLV.	10 mg/mL syrup; 10 mg/mL injection.	Cat: 15 mg/kg q12h po to 20 mg/kg q8h po (doses as high as 30 mg/kg/day have been used).

Key to Table Abbreviations

ACE	angiotensin-converting enzyme
CHF	congestive heart failure
CNS	central nervous system
COX	cyclooxygenase
CSF	cerebrospinal fluid
g	gram
GABA	gamma amino butyric acid
GI	gastrointestinal
IM	intramuscular
INR	international normalization ratio
IV	intravenous
μg	microgram
mg	milligram
MIC	minimum inhibitory concentration
mL	milliliter
NSAID	nonsteroidal antiinflammatory drug
OTC	over the counter (without prescription)
po	per os (oral)
PU/PD	polyuria and polydipsia
q	every, as in q8h = every 8 hours
Rx	prescription only
SC	subcutaneous
U	units

Disclaimer for Dose Tables

Note: Doses listed are for dogs *and* cats, unless otherwise listed. Many of the doses listed are extra-label or are human drugs not approved for animals administered in an extra-label manner. Doses listed are based on best available information at the time of table editing. The author cannot ensure efficacy or absolute safety of drugs used according to recommendations in this table. Adverse effects may be possible from drugs listed in this table of which authors were not aware at the time of table preparation. Veterinarians using this table are encouraged to consult current literature, product labels and inserts, and the manufacturer's disclosure information for additional information on adverse effects, interactions, and efficacy that were not identified at the time these tables were prepared.

Modified from material provided for *Blackwell's Five-Minute Veterinary Consult: Canine and Feline* by Mark Papich.

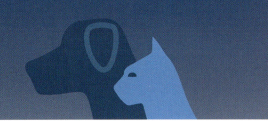

Index

Note: page numbers in *italics* refer to illustrations; those in **bold** to tables.

ABCB1 gene defect, 301, 551, 637
Abelcet *see* amphotericin B
ABLC *see* amphotericin B
abscess
  anal sac, 169, 170, *172*
  defined, 13
Abyssinian cat
  alopecia, 61, 228
  hypothyroidism, 417
  mycobacterial infections, 511, 512
acantholysis, **39**
  autoimmune blistering diseases, 188, 194, *210*
  dermatophytosis, 321, *331*
acanthosis, **39**
acanthosis nigricans, 433, *446*
Accutane *see* isotretinoin
acemannan, 715
acetate tape preparation, 47, *58*
acetic acid (vinegar) solutions, **485**, 548
acitretin, 369
acne, 62, 157–159
  canine, 157–159
  chin, 157, 158, 213
  feline, *105*, 157–159, *159–160*
acral lick dermatitis
  clinical features, 228–229, *235–236*
  diagnostics, 231–232
  differential diagnosis, 230
  secondary deep pyoderma, 213
  signalment/history, 228
  therapeutics, 233
acral mutilation syndrome, 65
acrodermatitis of bull terrier, 434–435
ACTH (corticotropin), **763**
  endogenous levels, 399, 411
  hypersecretion, 394
  stimulation tests, 340, 397–398, 403, 410–411
Acthar *see* ACTH
actinic comedones and furunculosis, 574, 575, 577, *580–581*
actinic dermatoses, 65, 574, 575–576, *580–582*
actinic keratosis (AK)
  clinical features, 62, *102*, 575–576, *582*, 618, 626
  diagnostics, 577, 622
  differential diagnosis, 577, 620, 621
  etiology/pathophysiology, 574, 615
  preneoplastic nature, 575, *585*, 619
  signalment/history, 616, 617
  therapeutics, 578, 623, 624
actinomycosis, 535–538, *540*
acute moist dermatitis (hot spot), 213, 214, *220*
  flea bite hypersensitivity, 241, *250*
adenitis, sebaceous *see* sebaceous adenitis
adenocarcinoma
  anal sac, 170–171
  cerumen gland, *560*
  pulmonary metastatic, *600, 688*
  sebaceous, 674, 676, 678, 680, *688*
S-adenosylmethionine, 668
Adequan Canine *see* polysulfated glycosaminoglycan
adnexal tumors *see* skin and adnexal tumors
adrenal dependent hyperadrenocorticism (ADH)
  canine, 394, 397, 399, 401, 403
  feline, 409
adrenalectomy, 400, 411
adrenal hyperplasia-like syndrome *see* alopecia X
adrenal neoplasia, 394, 397, 400, 403
adrenal sex hormone imbalance of plush-coated breeds *see* alopecia X
adrenocorticotropic hormone *see* ACTH
adverse drug reactions *see* drug reactions, cutaneous adverse
Advil *see* ibuprofen
affenpinscher, 731
Afghan hound, 674, 731
afoxolaner, 302, 638, **748**
Airedale terrier, 417, 673, 731
Akita, 731
  acral lick dermatitis, 228
  alopecia X, 338
  pemphigus foliaceus, 189
  sebaceous adenitis, 434, *450*, 648, 650, *651, 653*
  uveodermatologic syndrome, 65, 692, *695–697*
Alaskan malamute, 731
  alopecia X, 338
  lupus erythematosus, 468, 469

Blackwell's Five-Minute Veterinary Consult Clinical Companion: Small Animal Dermatology, Third Edition.
Karen Helton Rhodes and Alexander H. Werner.

Alaskan malamute (*Continued*)
  uveodermatologic syndrome, 692
  zinc-responsive dermatosis, 434
albinism, oculocutaneous, 66
alcohols, **149, 150**
aldehydes, **149, 150**
Aleve *see* naproxen
allergen-specific immunotherapy, 179–180
allergic contact dermatitis (ACD), 265–266, 267–268
allergic dermatitis, 64, *122*
  see also atopic disease
allergic miliary dermatitis, 351, 352, 353, 354, *362*
allergic (hypersensitivity) reactions
  atopic disease, 173–175
  contact dermatitis, 265
  drugs, 273, *281*
  eosinophilic plaque, 351
  flea bites *see* flea bite hypersensitivity
  food, 286–291
  hymenoptera stings, 241, 243
  insect bites and stings, 239–240, 351
  keratinization disorder, 435
  Malassezia dermatitis, 480
  miliary dermatitis, 351
  mosquito bites *see* mosquito bite hypersensitivity
  nodules and draining sinuses, 68
  otitis externa, 545, *558*
  tick bites *see* tick bite hypersensitivity
  vasculitis, 698
allergic threshold principle, 182
allergy testing, 178–179
  contact dermatitis, 267
  insect bite hypersensitivity, 245, *264*
allopurinol, 463
alopecia, 59–61
  adverse food reactions, 287, *292–293*
  atopic disease, 176, *184–185*
  canine flank, 60, *76–77*
  color dilution *see* color dilution alopecia
  congenital, 61
  estrous related, 60
  feline paraneoplastic *see* paraneoplastic alopecia, feline
  feline symmetric *see* feline symmetric alopecia
  foot, 591, *606*
  generalized/diffuse, 60–61, *81–94*
  patchy, 59, *69–74*
  pattern baldness in dogs, 60, *79–80*
  pinnal, 60
  postclipping, 60
  specific location, 60, *76–81*
  tail gland, 60, *81*
  traction, 60, *76*
alopecia areata, 59, *72*
alopecia mucinosa, 61
alopecia universalis, feline, 61
alopecia X
  clinical features, 60, *85*, 338, *343–344*
  therapeutics, 341
alpha 2-adrenergic antagonists, 303
alpha-hydroxy acids, 438
alpha toxins, staphylococcal, 145
Amblyomma maculatum, 243
American bulldog
  ichthyosis, 432, *441*
  mast cell tumors, 495, *504*
American bull terrier, 575, 616, 673
American cocker spaniel
  cryptococcosis, 522
  Malassezia dermatitis, 481
  primary seborrhea, 433, *443*
  superficial necrolytic dermatosis, 617, 666
  see also cocker spaniel
American foxhound, 731
American hairless terrier, 61
American Staffordshire terrier, 731
  demodicosis, 297
  ichthyosis, 432
  solar-induced dermatoses, 575, 616, 673
  see also Staffordshire bull terrier
American water spaniel, 60, *79*, 731
Amiglyde-V *see* amikacin
amikacin, **748**
  for mycobacterial infections, 516
  for nocardiosis, 538
  for otitis, 550
  for pyoderma, 151, **218**
Amikin *see* amikacin
amino acid infusions, 624, 668
amitraz, **748**
  for demodicosis, 300–301, 302
  for sarcoptid mites, 638
  toxicity, 303
amitraz-metaflumizone, 189
amitriptyline, 181, 234, **749**
ammonia, **149, 150**
amoxicillin, *124*, 538
amoxicillin + clavulanate, **749**
  for anal furunculosis/perianal fistula, 164
  cutaneous adverse reactions, *279*
  for eosinophilic granuloma complex, 354
  for otitis, 550
  for pyoderma, **218**
amphotericin B, **749–750**
  for deep mycoses, 524, 525–526
  for sporotrichosis, 661
ampicillin, 538, **750**
amyloid, defined, **39**
amyloidosis, cutaneous (primary nodular), 615, 617
  clinical features, 619, *627*
  diagnosis, 620, 622
  therapeutics, 623–624
Anafranil *see* clomipramine
anagen defluxion, 59
anagen hairs, 44, *51*
anal furunculosis/perianal fistula, 161–164, *165–168*
anal licking, 228, 230, 231, 232, *238*

anal sac
  adenocarcinoma, 170–171
  disorders, 169–171, *171–172*
  expression of contents, 170, 171
  impaction, 169, 170, *171–172*
  infection/abscessation, 169, 170, *172*
  neoplasia, 169
anal sacculitis, 169, 171
anaplastic carcinoma or sarcoma, 384
Ancef *see* cefazolin sodium
Ancobon *see* flucytosine
Andro-Cyp *see* testosterone
Android *see* methyltestosterone
Andronate *see* testosterone
angioedema, 243, *264,* 273
Angiostrongylus vasorum, 701
anonychia, 588
antibacterial soaps, 147
antibiotic resistance
  client education, 146–147
  emerging, 142–144
  etiology, 143–144
  historical background, 145–146
  systemic treatment options, 151–152
  transfer between species, 146, 727
antibiotics, 142–152
  for acne, 159
  for acral lick dermatitis, 233
  for anal furunculosis/perianal fistula, 164, *168*
  cutaneous adverse reactions, 272, *276–277, 279–280, 281*
  for eosinophilic granuloma complex, 354
  for methicillin-resistant staphylococci, 151–152
  for nocardiosis, 538
  for otitis, 549, 550
  for pemphigus/pemphigoid, 196
  for pyoderma, 217–220, **218–219**
  stewardship, 142, 143, 152
  topical therapy, 142, 151
  for vasculitis, 701
anti-cIL31 monoclonal antibody, 181
antifungal agents
  for deep mycoses, 524–526
  for dermatophytosis, 323–324
  for *Malassezia* dermatitis, 483
  for otitis, 549, 550
  for paronychia/onychomycosis, 594
  for sporotrichosis, 660–661
antihistamines
  for atopic disease, 181
  for cutaneous mastocytosis, 623
  for cutaneous mucinosis, 624
  for flea bites, 246
antimonial drugs, pentavalent, 462–463
Antirobe *see* clindamycin
Antisedan *see* atipamezole
antiseptics
  for ear cleaning, 549
  for *Malassezia* dermatitis, 483
  for vasculitis, 483
  see also chlorhexidine
antithyroglobulin antibodies, 417, 420
Antivert *see* meclizine
antiviral agents, 715
ant stings, 240–241, 243, *262–263*
apocrine cyst, *21*
apoptosis, **39**
Apoquel *see* oclacitinib
Aquasol A *see* vitamin A
Aquasol E *see* vitamin E
Aristocort *see* triamcinolone
armadillo protein, 188
Arquel *see* meclofenamate
L-asparaginase, 369
asthenia, cutaneous, 64
Atarax *see* hydroxyzine
atipamezole, 303, **750**
Atopica *see* cyclosporine
atopic disease (atopic dermatitis, AD), 173–182
  adverse food reactions and, 287
  clinical features, 176, *182–186*
  diagnostics, 177–179
  differential diagnosis, 177
  etiology/pathophysiology, 10, 173–175
  secondary pyoderma, 214, 220
  signalment/history, 175–176
  therapeutics, 179–181, 182
  T-lymphoma pathogenesis, 365
atopic-like dermatitis, 173, 174
atrophy, epidermal
  defined, **39**
  hyperadrenocorticism, 395, *406–407,* 410
atropine, **751**
auranofin, 196, **751**
aurothioglucose, **752**
aurotrichia, acquired, of miniature schnauzers, 66
Australian cattle dog, 228, 732
Australian kelpie, 732
Australian shepherd dog, 732
  cutaneous adverse drug reactions, 273
  ivermectin sensitivity, 301, 551, 637
  panniculitis, 563, *568*
  uveodermatologic syndrome, 692
Australian terrier, 432, 481, 732
autoimmune blistering diseases, 187–198
  clinical features, 190–192, *199–209*
  course and prognosis, 198
  diagnostics, 194–195
  differential diagnosis, 192–194
  etiology/pathophysiology, 187–189
  monitoring response to therapy, 197–198
  signalment/history, 189–190
  therapeutics, 195–197
autoimmune keratinization disorders, 435
autoimmune subepidermal blistering dermatoses (AISBD), 187
Avelox *see* moxifloxacin
Axid *see* nizatidine

azathioprine, **752**
  adverse effects, 197, 625
  for anal furunculosis/perianal fistula, 164
  for canine eosinophilic granuloma, 355
  for cutaneous adverse drug reactions, 275
  for epidermolysis bullosa acquisita, 197
  for lupus erythematosus, 472
  for panniculitis, 566
  for pemphigus complex, 196, 624
  for reactive systemic histiocytosis, 387
  for uveodermatologic syndrome, 693, 694
  for vasculitis, 702
azithromycin, **218**, 715, **752**
Azium *see* dexamethasone
AZT *see* zidovudine
Azulfidine *see* sulfasalazine

baby oil, 650
bacteria
  culture and identification, 28, 30–31, *34–35*
  cytology, **45**
  resident skin, 211–212
  transient skin, 212
bacterial dysbiosis, 211
bacterial infections
  acne, 158
  anal sac, 169, 170, *172*
  antibiotic resistance, 142–148
  categories, 213
  claw and clawfold, 66, *132*, 590
  client education, 146–147
  nodules and draining sinuses, 67–68
  otitis externa/media, 545, 547, 548
  surface, 213
  systemic therapy, 151–152
  topical therapy, 142, 151
  zoonotic potential, 146, 728
  see also folliculitis, bacterial; furunculosis; pyoderma, bacterial
bacterial overgrowth syndrome, 215, *225*
Bactrim *see* trimethoprim + sulfamethoxazole
ballooning degeneration, **39**
Banamine *see* flunixin meglumine
basal cell carcinoma, 676
basal cell tumors, 673
  clinical features, 676, *685*
  diagnostics, 677, 678
  differential diagnosis, 677
  prognosis, 679
  signalment/history, 673, 674, 675
  therapeutics, 678–679
basenji, 732
basset hound, 732
  congenital alopecia, 61
  Malassezia dermatitis, 481, *489*
  mast cell tumors, 495
  mycobacterial infections, 511
  nasodigital hyperkeratosis, 433–434
  primary seborrhea, 433, *443*, *444*
  solar-induced dermatoses, 575, 616, 673
  trichoepithelioma, 674
  uveodermatologic syndrome, 692
Baytril *see* enrofloxacin
beagle, 732
  amyloidosis, 617
  congenital alopecia, 61
  hyperadrenocorticism, 395
  hypothyroidism, 417
  juvenile polyarteritis syndrome, 63, 699
  mast cell tumors, 495
  nasodigital hyperkeratosis, 433–434
  photodermatoses, 575, 673
  sebaceous adenitis, 648, *657*
  skin tumors, 673
bearded collie, 732
Beauceron shepherd dog, 312, 732
Bedlington terrier, 732
bee stings, 240–241, 243, *264*
behavioral dermatoses, 227–234
  clinical features, 228–230, *235–238*
  comments, 234
  diagnostics, 231–232
  differential diagnosis, 230–231
  etiology/pathophysiology, 227–228
  secondary, 227
  signalment/history, 228
  therapeutics, 233–234
behavior modification therapy, 233, 234
Belgian sheepdog, 732
Belgian shepherd dog, 65
Belgian tervuren, 732
Benadryl *see* diphenhydramine
benzoyl peroxide, 151, 159, 437
Bernese mountain dog, 381, 732
betamethasone, 196, 197, 472, **753**
Biaxin *see* clarithromycin
bichon frise, 61, 732
biofilms, 144, 151
biological therapy, for atopic disease, 181
biopsy, 36–41
  atopic disease, 178–179
  contact dermatitis, 267
  dermatomyositis, 314
  dermatophytosis, 323, *336*
  indications, 36
  panniculitis, 565–566, *572–573*
  pathology report, 38, **38–41**, 41
  samples for bacterial culture, 30–31
  site selection, 36–37
  technique, 37–38, *41–42*
  touch imprints, 46, *54–55*
  vasculitis, 701
  see also histopathology
Biosol *see* neomycin
birman cat, 61
black flies (*Simulium* spp.), 240

cavalier King Charles spaniel, 734
  eosinophilic granuloma, 352
  ichthyosis, 62, 432
  Malassezia dermatitis, 481
  primary seborrhea, 433
  primary secretory otitis media, 543, 544, *554–555*
  sebaceous adenocarcinoma, 674
CCNU *see* lomustine
CeeNU *see* lomustine
Cefa-Drops *see* cefadroxil
cefadroxil, **218**, **755**
Cefa-Tabs *see* cefadroxil
cefazolin sodium, **755**
cefdinir, **756**
cefixime, **756**
Cefotan *see* cefotetan disodium
cefotaxime sodium, **756**
cefotetan disodium, **756**
cefovecin, **218**, *276–277*
cefoxitin sodium, **756**
cefpodoxime, **218**, **757**
ceftazidime, 550, **757**
ceftiofur, **757**
Celestone *see* betamethasone
CellCept *see* mycophenolate mofetil
cellulitis, canine juvenile, 63, *116*
cephalexin, **757**
  for acral lick dermatitis, 233
  for actinic dermatoses, 578, 623, 624
  for eosinophilic granuloma complex, 354
  induced pemphigus foliaceus, *109*
  for otitis, 550
  for pyoderma, **218**
  for sebaceous adenitis, 651
  for vasculitis, 701
cephalosporins, **218**, 272
Ceptaz *see* ceftazidime
ceramides, 438
Cerenia *see* maropitant
cerumen glands, 541
  adenocarcinoma, *560*
  hyperplasia, 544, 545, *553*
ceruminous cystomatosis, 545, *560*
cetirizine, 181, **758**
Chediak–Higashi syndrome, 66
chemotherapy
  for cutaneous lymphoma, 369–370, *378–379*
  for histiocytic sarcoma, 387
  for mast cell tumors, 498–499
  for skin and adnexal tumors, 679
Cheque Drops *see* mibolerone
Chesapeake Bay retriever, 734
Cheyletiella blakei, 634
Cheyletiella yasguri, 634, *641*
cheyletiellosis (*Cheyletiella* spp. infestation)
  clinical features, 62, *453*, 635, *645*
  diagnostics, 43, 47, 636, *646*
  etiology/pathophysiology, 634, *641*
  therapeutics, 637–638
  zoonotic potential, *729*
chihuahua, 60, 563, 673, 735
chin
  acne, 157, 158, 213
  swollen, eosinophilic granuloma, 158, *160*, 352, *359*
Chinese crested, 61, 617, 735
Chinese shar-pei, 735
  acral lick dermatitis, 228
  cutaneous amyloidosis, 617
  demodicosis, 297
  hypothyroidism, 417
  mast cell tumors, 495
  otitis, 543
  primary seborrhea, 433
  vasculitis, 698
  vitamin A-responsive dermatosis, 62
chipapillomavirus, 713
chlorambucil, **758**
  for cutaneous lymphocytosis, 625
  for cutaneous lymphoma, 369
  for eosinophilic granuloma, 355
  for lupus erythematosus, 472
  for mast cell tumors, 498
  for pemphigus complex, 196
  precautions, 625
  for vasculitis, 702
chloramphenicol, **759**
  for nocardiosis, 538
  for otitis, 550
  for pyoderma, 151, **218**
chlorhexidine, **149**, **150**
  for dermatophytosis, 324
  for keratinization disorders, 437
  for pyoderma, 151
Chloromycetin *see* chloramphenicol
chlorpheniramine, 181, 623, **759**
Chlor-Trimeton *see* chlorpheniramine
cholesterol clefts, **39**
CHOP chemotherapy, 369
chow chow, 735
  alopecia X, 338
  color dilution alopecia, 434
  hypothyroidism, 417
  lupus erythematosus, 468, 469
  melanocytic tumors, 673
  pemphigus foliaceus, 189
  uveodermatologic syndrome, 692
Chrysops spp. (deerflies), 240
chrysotherapy, 196, 198, **751–752**, **778**
cicalfate, 151
cimetidine, 499, 679, **759**
Cipro *see* ciprofloxacin
ciprofloxacin, **219**, 550, **760**
cisplatin, 679
civatte bodies, **39**
Claforan *see* cefotaxime sodium
clarithromycin, **760**

for mycobacterial infections, 515, 516
for nocardiosis, 538
Clavamox *see* amoxicillin + clavulanate
claw
anatomy, 588
dystrophy, 591, 594
claw and clawfold disorders, 588–594
asymmetrical claw disorders, 592
clinical features, *132–136*, 590–591, *595–614*
course and prognosis, 594
diagnostics, 593
differential diagnosis, 66, 591–593
etiology/pathophysiology, 589
signalment/history, 589–590
symmetrical claw disorders, 592–593
terminology, 588–589
therapeutics, 593–594
CLE *see* cutaneous lupus erythematosus
clefts, **39**
clemastine, **761**
Cleocin *see* clindamycin
Clinafarm EC *see* enilconazole
clindamycin, **761**
for anal furunculosis/perianal fistula, 164
for anal sacculitis, 171
for eosinophilic granuloma complex, 354
for otitis, 550
for pyoderma, 152, **218**
clofazimine, 515, 516, **761**
Clomicalm *see* clomipramine
clomipramine, 234, **762**
closed-patch testing, 267
cloxacillin sodium, **762**
Cloxapen *see* cloxacillin sodium
coagulase, 143, 144
Coccidioides immitis, 521, 523, 524, *534*
coccidioidomycosis, 522
course and prognosis, 526–527
diagnostics, 523, 524, *534*
therapeutics, 524–526
cocker spaniel, 743
atopic disease, 175
cutaneous amyloidosis, 617
cutaneous mastocytosis, 617
hypothyroidism, 417
idiopathic onychodystrophy, 589
keratinization disorder, 61, *91*, 433–434
leishmaniasis, 459
papillomavirus infections, 713
skin tumors, 673, 674
vitamin A-responsive dermatosis, 62, 433, *444*
see also American cocker spaniel
coconut oil, topical, **485**
colchicine, 197, 198, **762**
cold agglutinin disease, 63
collagen, 188
collagenolysis, **39**
collagenous nevi, multiple, 616, 617
clinical features, 619, *628–629*
diagnostics, 622
collie, 735
autoimmune blistering dermatoses, 189, 190
dermatomyositis, 65, 312, 589
gray collie syndrome, 66
ichthyosis, 432
ivermectin sensitivity, 301, 551, 637
lupus erythematosus, 468, 469
panniculitis, 563
testicular tumors, 339
ulcerative dermatosis, 64
see also border collie
colonization, vs infection, 212
color dilution alopecia
clinical features, 61, 65, *90*, 434
trichogram, 44, *52*, *449*
color dilution and cerebellar degeneration, Rhodesian ridgeback, 66
comedones, 13, *16*
acne, 158
actinic, 574, 575, 577, *580–581*
canine hyperadrenocorticism, 395
schnauzer comedo syndrome, 434, *452*
common brown spider (*Loxosceles unicolor*), 240, 242
compulsive disorders, 227
see also self-injurious dermatoses
computed tomography (CT scan)
for deep mycoses, 523
for hyperadrenocorticism, 397, 411
for otitis, 546
Contac 12 Hour Allergy *see* clemastine
contact dermatitis, 265–268
allergic (ACD), 265–266, 267–268
clinical features, 266, *268–271*
differential diagnosis, 177, 266–267
drug-induced, 266, *269*, 273, *276*
irritant (ICD), 265–266, 267–268, *268*, *271*
nasal planum, 67, *138*
coonhound, 522
corneocytes, 5, *5*, *7*
bundling of keratin, 5, *7*
envelope formation, 5, *7*
exfoliating (squames), *7*, *9*
corneodesmosomes, *9*
cornification, 5–6, *6–9*
cornification disorders *see* keratinization disorders
Cortef *see* hydrocortisone
corticosteroids
for acne, 159
for actinic dermatoses, 578, 623, 624
for anal furunculosis/perianal fistula, 164
for atopic disease, 179, 180
for contact dermatitis, 268
for cutaneous adverse drug reactions, 275
for cutaneous lymphocytosis, 623, 625
for cutaneous mastocytosis, 623
for cutaneous mucinosis, 624

corticosteroids (*Continued*)
for eosinophilic granuloma, 355, *364*
for epidermolysis bullosa acquisita, 197
for epitheliotropic lymphoma, 369
for histiocytic proliferative disorders, 386
for insect bites and stings, 246, 247
for keratinization disorders, 438, 439
for lupus erythematosus, 472
for mast cell tumors, 498
for otitis, 549, 550
for pemphigus complex, 195–196
precautions, 197, 625
for pyoderma, 217
for sarcoptid mites, 637, 638
for sterile nodular panniculitis, 566
for uveodermatologic syndrome, 693
see also dexamethasone; methylprednisolone; prednisolone
corticotropin *see* ACTH
cortisol-creatinine ratio, urine, 398–399, 410
Cortrosyn *see* cosyntropin
cosyntropin, **763**
cowpox virus infection, feline, 64, 712
COX-2, 365
COX-2 selective inhibitors, 578, 623, 679
crusting dermatoses, 63–65
crusts, 12, *15*
biopsy technique, 37
cytology, 46
histopathology, **39**
cryotherapy, for sporotrichosis, 661
cryptococcosis
clinical features, *118*, 521–522, *528–531*
course and prognosis, 526
diagnostics, 523, 524, *533*
therapeutics, 524–526
Cryptococcus gattii, 521
Cryptococcus neoformans, 521, *533*
Ctenocephalides felis felis, 239
CT scan *see* computed tomography
culture and identification, 28–31
bacteria, 28, 30–31, *34–35*
deep mycoses, 524, *534*
dermatophytes, 28–30, *33–34*, 322–323, *334–335*
Malassezia, 482, *493*
mycobacteria, 514
otitis, 547
culture media, dermatophyte, 28
curly-coated retriever, 735
Cushing's syndrome *see* hyperadrenocorticism
cutaneous adverse drug reactions *see* drug reactions, cutaneous adverse
cutaneous adverse food reactions *see* food reactions, cutaneous adverse
cutaneous and renal glomerular vasculopathy of greyhounds, 63, 699
cutaneous epitheliotropic lymphoma *see* epitheliotropic lymphoma, cutaneous
cutaneous lupus erythematosus (CLE), 467–472
clinical features, 469–470, *473–478*
course and prognosis, 472
diagnostics, 471
exfoliative *see* exfoliative cutaneous lupus erythematosus
mucous membrane (MCLE), 468, 469–470, 471, *476*
signalment/history, 468–469
therapeutics, 471–472
vesicular (VCLE), 468, 470, 471
see also discoid lupus erythematosus
cutaneous lymphocytosis *see* lymphocytosis, cutaneous
cutaneous mucinosis *see* mucinosis, cutaneous
cutaneous nonepitheliotropic lymphoma (CnEL), 365–370
clinical features, 366, *370–371*
diagnostics, 368
differential diagnosis, 367, 383
etiology/pathophysiology, 365
prognosis, 370
signalment/history, 366
therapeutics, 369
cutaneous T-cell lymphoma (CTCL), 365–370, *613*
see also cutaneous nonepitheliotropic lymphoma; epitheliotropic lymphoma
cyclic hematopoiesis, canine, 66
cyclic neutropenia, canine, 66
cyclooxygenase-2 *see* COX-2
cyclophosphamide, **763**
adverse effects, *73*, 198
for cutaneous lymphoma, 369
for mast cell tumors, 498, 499
cyclosporine, **764**
for anal furunculosis/perianal fistula, 163–164, *168*
for atopic disease, 180–181
for claw disorders, 594
for contact dermatitis, 268
for cutaneous adverse drug reactions, 275
for dermatomyositis, 315
for eosinophilic granuloma (complex), 355
for epidermolysis bullosa acquisita, 197
for keratinization disorders, 438
for lupus erythematosus, 472
for panniculitis, 566
for pemphigus complex, 196
for reactive histiocytosis, 386
for sebaceous adenitis, 650
side effects, 198
for uveodermatologic syndrome, 694
for vasculitis, 702
Cydectin *see* moxidectin
cyproheptadine, 234, **764**
cysts
cerumen, *562*
defined, 13, *21*
panniculitis vs, 564
cytokines, in atopic disease, 174–175

cytology, 43–48
  acetate tape preparation, 47, *58*
  for deep mycoses, 524, *533–534*
  direct impression smears, 46, *53–55*
  for epitheliotropic lymphoma, *55,* 368, *378*
  fine-needle aspiration, 46–47, *56–57*
  for leishmaniasis, 462, *465*
  for *Malassezia* dermatitis, 46, 47, *53–54,* 482, *492*
  for mast cell tumors, 496, *509*
  for mycobacterial infections, 514
  for nocardiosis, 538
  for otic disease, 45–46, *53,* 547–548
  skin scrapings, 43–44, *48–49*
  squeeze tape impressions, 44–45
  trichograms, 44, *50–52*
Cytomel *see* liothyronine
Cytopoint *see* lokivetmab
Cytoxan *see* cyclophosphamide

dacarbazine, 369
dachshund, 735–736
  acanthosis nigricans, 433, *446*
  allergic contact dermatitis, 266
  autoimmune blistering diseases, 189, 190
  claw disorders, 589
  color dilution alopecia, 434
  ear margin dermatosis/vasculitis, 62, *103,* 433, *445,* 699
  hyperadrenocorticism, 395
  hypothyroidism, 417
  idiopathic nodular panniculitis, 65, 563
  idiopathic sterile granuloma, 589, *598*
  Malassezia dermatitis, 481
  mast cell tumors, 495
  onychorrhexis, 66, *135,* 589, *595–596*
  primary seborrhea, 433
  sebaceous gland adenoma/hyperplasia, 673
  uveodermatologic syndrome, 692
dalmatian, 736
  acral lick dermatitis, 228
  actinic dermatoses, 575, 616
  atopic disease, 175
  cutaneous adverse drug reactions, 273
  panniculitis, 563
  pedal folliculitis and furunculosis, 214
  squamous cell carcinoma, 673
  vitamin A-responsive dermatosis, 62
danazol, **764**
Dandie Dinmont terrier, 736
Danocrine *see* danazol
Dantrium *see* dantrolene sodium
dantrolene sodium, **765**
dapsone, 702, **765**
Darier's sign, 495, *500–501*
o,p'-DDD *see* mitotane
Decadron *see* dexamethasone
Decaject SP *see* dexamethasone
deerflies (*Chrysops* spp.), 240
dell, **39**
Delta-Cortef *see* prednisolone
Deltasone *see* prednisone
d'emblee form of epitheliotropic lymphoma, 367
Demodex canis, 296, 300
  skin scrapings, 44, *49,* 299, *304*
  trichogram, *50, 311*
Demodex cati, 297
  identification, 44, 298, 299, *306*
Demodex cornei, 297
  identification, 43, 299, 300, *305*
Demodex felis, 297, 299, *306*
Demodex gatoi, 297, 298
  clinical features, 298, 299
  identification, 43, 299, 300, *306*
Demodex injai, 297
  clinical features, 298, *310*
  identification, 44, 299, *305*
demodicosis, 296–304
  canine hyperadrenocorticism, 395, *407*
  clinical features, 64, 298–299, *307–310*
    generalized alopecia, 60, *81,* 298, *307–308*
    localized alopecia, 59, *69–70,* 298–299, *307, 310*
    pododemodicosis, *132,* 298, *309, 599*
  course and prognosis, 303–304
  diagnostics, 299–300
    skin scrapings, 43–44, *49,* 299, *304*
    squeeze tape impressions, 44–45
    trichograms, 44, *50,* 299, *311*
  differential diagnosis, 177, 299
  juvenile-onset generalized (dog), 296, 297, *307–308*
  signalment/history, 297–298
  therapeutics, 300–303
dendritic cells (DC), 174
Depo-Estradiol Cypionate *see* estradiol cypionate
Depo-Medrol *see* methylprednisolone
Depo-Provera *see* medroxyprogesterone acetate
Depo-Testosterone *see* testosterone
L-deprenyl (selegiline), 402, 403, **809**
deracoxib, **765**
Deramaxx *see* deracoxib
Dermacenter andersoni, 243
Dermacenter occidentalis, 243
Dermacenter variabilis, 243
dermatofibrosis, nodular *see* nodular dermatofibrosis
dermatomyositis, canine familial, 312–316, 700
  associated conditions, 316
  clinical features, 313, *317–319, 707–708*
    alopecia, 60, *78*
    claw disorders, 589, *595*
    depigmentation, 65, *319*
    nasal planum, 67
  complications and prognosis, 315–316
  pregnancy, 316
  therapeutics, 314–315
dermatophytes, 28–30
  culture and identification, 28, 29, *33–34,* 322–323, *334–335*

dermatophytes (*Continued*)
  microscopic examination, 322, *333*
  polymerase chain reaction (PCR), 30
  sample collection, 28–29, *31–32, 334*
  trichograms, 44, *52*
dermatophyte test medium (DTM), 28, 29, 323
dermatophytosis, 320–326
  acantholytic, 321, *331*
  clinical features, 321, *326–331*
    alopecia, 59, 60, *82,* 321, *326–328*
    claw/foot, *330, 605, 606*
    exfoliative lesions, 62, *94*
    keratinization defects, 435, *454*
  diagnostics, 322–323, *332–336*
  differential diagnosis, 177, 322
  etiology/pathogenesis, 320
  granulomatous, 321, 323, *329*
  signalment/history, 321
  therapeutics, 323–325
  treatment goals (CCATS, Moriello), 325–326
  zoonotic, *330–331, 730*
dermoepidermal junction, **39**
dermonecrotoxin, 144
Dermoscent Essential-6 spot-on, 650
DES *see* diethylstilbestrol
deslorelin, 341
desmogleins (Dsg1 and Dsg3), 188, 195
desmoplasia, **39**
desmosomes, 187–188
desoxycorticosterone, **766**
desquamation, 5, *7, 9*
Devon rex cat
  hereditary hypotrichosis, 61
  Malassezia dermatitis, 481, 589
  squamous cell carcinoma, 673, 712
dexamethasone, **766**
  for autoimmune blistering diseases, 197
  for eosinophilic granuloma complex, 355
  for insect bites and stings, 247
  for otitis, 550
  for uveodermatologic syndrome, 693
dexamethasone suppression test
  high-dose (HDDST), 399, 411
  low-dose (LDDST), 398, 403, 411
Dexasone *see* dexamethasone
Dexavet *see* dexamethasone
diabetes mellitus
  clinical features, 338, *342*
  hyperadrenocorticism with, 409, 410, 412
  partial diffuse alopecia, 61, *90*
  superficial necrolytic dermatosis and, 665, 668
diapedesis, **39**
diascopy, 700, *710*
diazepam, **767**
dicloxacillin sodium, **767**
Dicural *see* difloxacin
diet
  for anal furunculosis/perianal fistula, 164
  for anal sac disorders, 171
  challenge and provocation trials, 289–290
  food elimination, 288–289
  for hypothyroidism, 421
  for *Malassezia* dermatitis, **485**
  for nocardiosis and actinomycosis, 537
  for pyoderma, 217
  raw, 288
  for superficial necrolytic dermatosis, 668
diethylstilbestrol (DES), **767**
  effects on hair coat, 339, *347*
  for sex hormone imbalances, 341
difloxacin, **219, 768**
Diflucan *see* fluconazole
dihydrostreptomycin, 515
dilated pore of Winer, 674, 675, 677, 678
dimenhydrinate, **768**
dimethyl sulfoxide (DMSO), 624
diphenhydramine, **768**
  for atopic disease, 181
  for cutaneous mucinosis, 624
  for mast cell tumors, 497
diphenoxylate, **769**
direct impression smears, 46, *53–55*
dirofilariasis, 701
dirty face syndrome (facial dermatitis) of Persian and Himalayan cats, 62, *104,* 435, *453*
discoid lupus erythematosus (DLE), 467–472
  clinical features, 67, 469, *473–475*
    crusting and erosive lesions, 63, *111*
    pigmentation changes, 65, *130*
  course and prognosis, 472
  diagnostics, 471
  facial-predominant, 468, 469, *473–475*
  generalized (GDLE), 468, 469, 471, *475–476*
  signalment/history, 468
  therapeutics, 471–472
  see also cutaneous lupus erythematosus
disinfectants, **149, 150,** 151
distemper, canine, 713
DLE *see* discoid lupus erythematosus
DMSO (dimethyl sulfoxide), 624
doberman pinscher, 736–737
  acne, 157
  color dilution alopecia, 61, *90,* 434
  cryptococcosis, 522
  cutaneous adverse drug reactions, 273
  deep mycoses, 522
  hypothyroidism, 417
  ichthyosis, 432
  leproid granuloma, 512
  melanocytic tumors, 673
  pemphigoid complex, 190
  primary seborrhea, 433
  self-injurious dermatoses, 228, *235*
  vitiligo, 65
DOCA pivalate *see* desoxycorticosterone
DOCP *see* desoxycorticosterone

dogue de Bordeaux, 432, 434, 737
Domitor *see* medetomidine
doramectin, 302, 637
doxepin, 181, 234
doxycycline, **769**
for autoimmune blistering diseases, 196
for claw disorders, 594
for eosinophilic granuloma complex, 355
for lupus erythematosus, 471–472
for mycobacterial infections, 515, 516
for nocardiosis, 538
for panniculitis, 566
for pyoderma, 152, **218**
for reactive cutaneous histiocytosis, 386
for sebaceous adenitis, 650
for vasculitis, 701
Dramamine *see* dimenhydrinate
Drisdol *see* ergocalciferol
Droncit *see* praziquantel
drug formulary, 747–820
drug reactions, cutaneous adverse (CADR), 272–275
clinical features, 273–274, *276–277*, *279–281*
contact dermatitis, 266, *269*, 273, *276*
crusted lesions, 64, *124*
nasal planum lesions, 67
pemphigus/pemphigoid, 188, 189, 273, *279–280*
pigmentation changes, 65
Dudley nose, 65
Duragesic *see* fentanyl
Dynapen *see* dicloxacillin sodium
dysbiosis, bacterial, 211
dyskeratosis, **39**
dystrophic mineralization, **39**, 396

ear
anatomy, 541–542
cleaning and flushing, 548–549
polyps, *558–559*
ear canal
biofilms, 144
cytology, **45**, 45–46
external, 541–542
middle, 542
sample collection, 31, 45, *53*, *562*
ticks, 240, 243
ear infections *see* otitis externa; otitis interna; otitis media
ear margin dermatosis/vasculitis, 62, *103*, 433, *445*, 699
ear mites, 544, *558*, 634
see also Otodectes cynotis
Echidnophaga gallinacea, 239, *248*
EGC *see* eosinophilic granuloma complex
eicosapentaenoic acid, 179
Elavil *see* amitriptyline
Eldepryl *see* selegiline
electrical shock injury, *611*
electromyography (EMG), 314
elimination diets, 288–289
Elizabethan collar, for dermatophytosis, 324
emollients, 438
endocrinopathies
atypical, 337–341, *342–350*
cutaneous xanthomatosis, *123*
keratinization disorders, 435, *455*
pyoderma secondary to, 216, 220, *223*
see also diabetes mellitus; hyperadrenocorticism; hyperthyroidism, feline; hypothyroidism
English bulldog
acne, 157
atopic disease, 175
demodicosis, 297
hypothyroidism, 417
idiopathic sterile granuloma, 589
mast cell tumors, 495, *506*
nasodigital hyperkeratosis, 433–434
pedal folliculitis and furunculosis, 214
pemphigus foliaceus, 189
primary seborrhea, 433
English bull terrier, 228, 673
English foxhound, 737
English pointer, 434, 740
English setter, 737
acral lick dermatitis, 228
atopic disease, 175
Malassezia dermatitis, 481
English springer spaniel, 433, 589, 743
see also springer spaniel
enilconazole, 324, **769**
Enisyl-F *see* L-lysine
enrofloxacin, **219**, 550, **770**
Enterocort *see* budesonide
eosinophilic granuloma
canine (CEG), 351–356
clinical features, 353, *363*
course and prognosis, 356
diagnostics, 353, 354
differential diagnosis, 353
signalment/history, 352
therapeutics, 354, 355
feline, 351, 352
clinical features, 352, *357–360*
diagnostics, 354
differential diagnosis, 158, *160*
footpad, 592, *610*
eosinophilic granuloma complex (EGC), feline, 351–356
clinical features, 64, *134*, 352–353, *356–362*
course and prognosis, 356
diagnostics, 353–354, *364*
differential diagnosis, 353
etiology/pathophysiology, 351
flea bite hypersensitivity, 242, *254*, 351
signalment/history, 352
therapeutics, 354–355
eosinophilic microabscess, **40**

eosinophilic nasal furunculosis, 63, *115*
eosinophilic plaque
  atopic disease, 176, *186*
  clinical features, *134*, 352, *356–357*
  diagnostics, 353, 354, *364*
  pathophysiology, 351
  signalment/history, 352
  therapeutics, 354–355
eosinophils, 351
epidermal collarettes, 13, *23*
  bacterial pyoderma, 215, *223, 226*
  sampling, 46
epidermal dysplasia, 433, *445*
epidermis, 3–10
  layers, *5*
  renewal time, 3
epidermolysis bullosa acquisita, 187
  clinical features, *25*, 64, *122*, 192, *209*
  course and prognosis, 198
  differential diagnosis, 193–194
  etiology/pathophysiology, 189
  pathologic findings, 195
  signalment/history, 190
  therapeutics, 197
epitheliotropic lymphoma, cutaneous (CEL), 365–370
  clinical features, *19*, 366–367, *372–377*
    alopecia, 61, *91–93*
    depigmentation, 65, *129*
    exfoliative lesions, 62, *100–101*, 366, *372–373*
    foot, *136*, 592, *612*
    nasal planum, 67, *129*
    ulcerative lesions, 64, *101*
  d'emblee form, 367
  diagnostics, *54–55*, 368–369, *378*
  differential diagnosis, 367
  etiology/pathophysiology, 365–366
  keratinization defects, 435, *457*
  prognosis, 370
  signalment/history, 366
  therapeutics, 369–370, *378–379*
Eqvalan liquid *see* ivermectin
Ergamisol *see* levamisole hydrochloride
ergocalciferol, **770**
erosion, 14, *25*
erosive dermatoses, 63–65
erythema ab igne, 65, *127*
erythema multiforme (EM), 63, *115*, 272–275
  clinical features, 274, *277–279, 281–283*
  feline herpes virus-associated, 712, *722*
  footpads, 592, *608*
  major, 274, *282–283*
  minor, 274, *282*
  "old dog" form, 274, 275, *282*
erythromycin, **219**, 538, **771**
Escherichia coli, 213
essential fatty acid supplements, 179, 438, 594, 650, 668
essential oils, **485**
estradiol, serum, 340
estradiol cypionate (ECP), **771**
estrogen imbalances, 60, 339, *345–349*
estrous related alopecia, 60
ethambutol, 515
ethyl alcohol, **149**
ethyl lactate, 151, 437
etodolac, **771**
EtoGesic *see* etodolac
Excenel *see* ceftiofur
excoriations, 13, *24*
  adverse food reactions, 287, *293, 295*
  atopic disease, 176, *183, 186*
exfoliative cutaneous lupus erythematosus (ECLE), 469, 471
  clinical features, 62, 63, *105*, 470, *477–478*
  prognosis, 472
exfoliative dermatoses, 62, *94–105*
  keratinization defects, 435, *457*
  leishmaniasis, 460, *463–464*
  thymoma-associated *see* thymoma-associated exfoliative dermatitis
exfoliative erythroderma
  adverse drug reactions, 272, 274
  differential diagnosis, 274
  epitheliotropic lymphoma, 366, 367, *372–373*
exfoliative staphylococcal toxin, 144
exocytosis, **39**
exotoxin, staphylococcal, 144

facial dermatitis (dirty face syndrome) of Persian and Himalayan cats, 62, *104*, 435, *453*
facial nerve (cranial nerve VII) deficits, 544, *557*
famcyclovir, *279*, 715, **772**
famotidine, **772**
fasciitis, nodular *see* nodular fasciitis
fatty acids
  dietary deficiency, *456*
  essential, supplements, 179, 438, 594, 650, 668
  topical therapy, 650
Feldene *see* piroxicam
feline calicivirus-associated dermatoses, 64, 712–713, *722*
feline coronavirus (FcoV), 712
feline cowpox virus infection, 64, 712
feline immunodeficiency virus (FIV)-associated dermatoses, 64, *120*, 712, *717–718*
  see also plasma cell pododermatitis, feline
feline infectious peritonitis, 712
feline leukemia virus (FeLV)-associated dermatoses, 64, 712, *716*
feline orofacial pain syndrome, 64, 713
feline papillomaviruses (FcaPV), 712
feline plasma cell pododermatitis *see* plasma cell pododermatitis, feline
feline rhinotracheitis, 712
feline sarcoma virus (FeSV), 712

feline symmetric alopecia
  clinical features, 229, *236–237*
  diagnostics, 232
  differential diagnosis, 61, 230
  signalment/history, 228
FeLV *see* feline leukemia virus
fentanyl, **772–773**
ferritin, serum, 384
fibroplasia, **39**
fibropruritic nodules, *19,* 241, *251*
fibrosis, **39**
fillagrin, *7,* 174
fine-needle aspiration, 46–47, *56–57*
Finnish spitz, 737
fipronil, 638
firocoxib, **773**
  for actinic keratosis, 578, 623, 679
fissures, 14, *26*
fistulae, 14
  panniculitis, 564, *569*
  perianal, *26,* 161–164, *165–168*
FIV *see* feline immunodeficiency virus
Flagyl *see* metronidazole
flame figures, **39**
flank alopecia, canine, 60, *76–77*
flank sucking, 228, 229, 230, 232
flat-coated retriever, 737
Flavor Tabs *see* lufenuron + milbemycin oxime
flea bite dermatitis (FBD), 239–240, 241
  clinical features, 241, *249*
  diagnostics, 245
  differential diagnosis, 243–244
  therapeutics, 246
flea bite hypersensitivity (FBH), 239–240, 241
  clinical features, 64, 241–242, *249–254*
  diagnostics, 245
  differential diagnosis, 177, 243–244
  eosinophilic granuloma complex, 242, *254,* 351
  therapeutics, 246
fleas, 239, 246, *248*
florfenicol, **773**
Florinef *see* fludrocortisone
fluconazole, **774**
  for deep mycoses, 525
  for dermatophytosis, 324
  for *Malassezia* dermatitis, 483
  for otitis, 550
  for paronychia, 594
  precautions, 484
Flucort *see* flumethasone
flucytosine, 526, **774**
fludrocortisone, **775**
flumethasone, **775**
flunixin meglumine, **776**
fluocinolone/fluocinolone-DMSO
  for acral lick dermatitis, 233
  for autoimmune blistering diseases, 196, 197
  for eosinophilic granuloma complex, 355
  for lupus erythematosus, 472
fluoroquinolones
  for methicillin-resistant staphylococci, 152
  for mycobacterial infections, 515, 516
  for nocardiosis, 538
  for pyoderma, **219**
5-fluorouracil, 679, 715, **776**
fluoxetine, 234, **777**
fluralaner, 302, 638, **777**
fly dermatitis, 240, 244, 246
  clinical features, 242, *255–257*
  diagnostics, 245
fly strike (myiasis), 240
Folex *see* methotrexate
follicular casts (keratin collaring), 13, *15*
  sebaceous adenitis, *98,* 434, *451,* 649, *654*
follicular dysplasias
  alopecia, 61, 62, *96*
  black hair, 60, *77*
follicular lipidosis, 61
folliculitis
  bacterial
    acne, 158
    canine hyperadrenocorticism, 396, *407, 408*
    crusted and ulcerative lesions, 63, *117*
    demodicosis, 298
    hypothyroidism, 419
    keratinization disorders, 433, 435, *445, 454*
    Malassezia dermatitis, 481
    patchy alopecia, 59, *70*
    sebaceous adenitis, 649, *655*
    superficial, 213
  dermatophytosis, 321, *329*
  feline lymphocytic mural, 61
  pyotraumatic, 213
food allergens, 286, 287, 288
food allergy, 286–291
  eosinophilic plaque, 351, *356*
  see also food reactions, cutaneous adverse
food challenge and provocation trials, 289–290
food elimination diet, 288–289
food intolerance, 286
food reactions, cutaneous adverse (CAFR), 286–291
  clinical features, 287–288, *291–295*
  diagnostics, 288–290
  otitis externa, 287, *291,* 545
footpads
  biopsy, 37
  crusted/hyperkeratotic/fissured, 592, *606–610*
  idiopathic (familial) hyperkeratosis, 434, *447,* 589, 592, *609*
  nodular lesions, 592, *612–614*
  sloughing/ulcerative, 592, *611*
foreign body reactions, 157, 214, 545
formaldehyde, **149**
formamidine, 300
formulary, drug, 747–820

Fortaz *see* ceftazidime
foxhound, 512
fox terrier, 737
  mast cell tumors, 495
  uveodermatologic syndrome, 692
  vitamin A-responsive dermatosis, 62
French bulldog, 737
  atopic disease, 175, *182*
  congenital alopecia, 61
  demodicosis, 297
  vitamin A-responsive dermatosis, 433
fulvestrant, 341
Fulvicin U/F *see* griseofulvin
fungal infections
  claw/clawfold, 66, 590, 591, 594, *601, 605*
  deep mycoses, 521–527
  nodules and draining sinuses, 68
  sporotrichosis, 658–661
  zoonotic, 728, *729*
  see also dermatophytosis; *Malassezia* dermatitis; onychomycosis
Fungizone *see* amphotericin B
Furadantin *see* nitrofurantoin
Furalan *see* nitrofurantoin
Furatoin *see* nitrofurantoin
furunculosis, 213
  acne, 158
  acral lick, 213
  actinic, 574, 575, 577, *580–581*
  anal, 161–164, *165–168*
  demodicosis, 298, *309*
  eosinophilic nasal, 63, *115*
  German shepherd dog, 213, 214
  interdigital, 213
  postgrooming, *225*
  pyotraumatic, 213
  see also pyoderma, bacterial
fusidic acid, 151

gabapentin, 234, 777
generic dog food dermatosis, 435
genodermatoses, canine, 731–745
gentamicin, 538, **778**
Gentocin *see* gentamicin
geriatric animals, keratinization disorders, 435
German shepherd dog, 737
  allergic contact dermatitis, 266
  anal furunculosis/perianal fistula, 161, *165*
  atopic disease, 175
  behavioral dermatoses, 228, *236*
  cryptococcosis, 522
  familial cutaneous vasculopathy, 63, 699
  folliculitis and furunculosis, 213, 214
  hypopituitary dwarfism, 338
  hypothyroidism, 417
  idiopathic onychomadesis, 589
  ivermectin sensitivity, 301, 637
  leishmaniasis, 459
  leproid granuloma, 512
  lichenoid psoriasiform dermatosis, 62
  lupus erythematosus, 467, 468, 469
  Malassezia dermatitis, 481
  nodular dermatofibrosis, 589, 592, 616
  paraneoplastic dermatoses, 617
  pemphigus, 189
  primary seborrhea, 433
  sebaceous adenitis, 434, 648, *653*
  symmetric lupoid onychodystrophy, 589, *597, 604*
  testicular tumors, 339
  trichoepithelioma, 674
  uveodermatologic syndrome, 692
  vitiligo, 65
German short-haired pointer, 740
  acne, 157
  exfoliative cutaneous lupus erythematosus, 62, 63, *105*
  hypothyroidism, 417
  lupus erythematosus, 469
  solar-induced dermatoses, 575, 616, 673
giant cell dermatosis, feline, 712
giant schnauzer, 738
  hypothyroidism, 417
  squamous cell carcinoma, 673
  symmetric lupoid onychodystrophy, 589
glucagon, plasma, 621, 667
glucagonoma, 616, 665
glutaraldehyde, **149**
golden retriever, 738
  acral lick dermatitis, 228
  allergic contact dermatitis, 266
  atopic disease, 175
  cutaneous lymphocytosis, 617
  flea bite hypersensitivity, 241, *251*
  footpad hyperkeratosis, 434, 589
  hypothyroidism, 417
  ichthyosis, 62, *99*, 432, *440*
  mast cell tumors, 495
  paraneoplastic dermatoses, 617
  pedal folliculitis and furunculosis, 214
  trichoepithelioma, 674
gold sodium thiomalate, **778**
gold therapy *see* chrysotherapy
Gordon setter, 433, 589, 738
gram-negative infections, 213
granuloma
  bacterial, 213
  canine leproid *see* leproid granuloma, canine
  eosinophilic *see* eosinophilic granuloma
  linear, 352, *357*
  sterile idiopathic interdigital, 589, *598*
granulomatous dermatitis, periadnexal multinodular, 384
granulomatous mycobacteriosis, feline multisystemic, 513
granulomatous sebaceous adenitis *see* sebaceous adenitis

Gravol *see* dimenhydrinate
gray collie syndrome, 66
Great Dane, 738
  acne, 157
  acral lick dermatitis, 228
  color dilution alopecia, 434
  cryptococcosis, 522
  epidermolysis bullosa acquisita, 64, 190
  hypothyroidism, 417
  idiopathic sterile granuloma, 589
  pedal folliculitis and furunculosis, 214
great Pyrenees, 738
Grenz zone, **39**
greyhound, 738
  cutaneous adverse drug reactions, 273
  cutaneous and renal glomerular vasculopathy, 63, 699
  ivermectin sensitivity, 301, 637
  pattern baldness, 60, *80*
  solar-induced dermatoses, 575, 616, 673
griseofulvin, 323–324, **779**
Gris-PEG *see* griseofulvin
growth hormone (GH)
  for alopecia X, 341
  responsive alopecia *see* alopecia X

hair coat, descriptive terms, 11
hair follicle tumors, 673
  clinical features, 676–677, *689–691*
  diagnostics, 677, 678
  differential diagnosis, 677
  prognosis, 680
  signalment/history, 674, 675
  therapeutics, 678–679
hair plucks, 28–29, 44, *50–52*
hand washing, 146–147
havanese, 434, 648, 738
head tilt, 544, *557*
Heartgard *see* ivermectin
hemangioma (HA), 574, 576, 577, *583*
hemangiosarcoma (HSA), 574, 576, 577, *584*
hemidesmosomes, 187–188
beta-hemolysin, 144
hemophagocytic syndrome, 384
hepatocutaneous syndrome *see* superficial necrolytic dermatosis
herpes virus-associated dermatoses
  canine, 713
  feline, *141*, 712, *721–722*
hidradenitis suppurativa, 161
high-dose dexamethasone suppression test (HDDST), 399, 411
Himalayan cat
  basal cell tumors, 673
  facial dermatitis (dirty face syndrome), 62, 435
  urticaria pigmentosa, 495
histiocytic proliferative disorders, 380–387
histiocytic sarcoma (malignant histiocytosis), 381
  clinical features, 383, *390–391, 392*
  diagnostics, 384, 385, 386
  therapeutics, 387
histiocytoma
  cutaneous, 380, 381
    clinical features, 382, *387–388*
    diagnostics, 384–385, *393*
    therapeutics, 386
  malignant fibrous, 382, 383, 385, 387
histiocytosis
  malignant *see* histiocytic sarcoma
  nasal planum, 67, *141*
  reactive cutaneous, 380
    clinical features, 63, *117*, 382, *389–390*
    diagnostics, 385, 386, *393*
    therapeutics, 386
  reactive systemic, 381
    clinical features, 382–383, *391–392*
    diagnostics, 385, 386
    therapeutics, 386–387
histopathology
  for cutaneous nonepitheliotropic lymphoma, 368
  for deep mycoses, 524
  for eosinophilic granuloma complex, 354
  for epitheliotropic lymphoma, 368–369
  for histiocytic proliferative disorders, 384–385
  for hypothyroidism, 420
  for leishmaniasis, 462, *466*
  for lupus erythematosus, 471
  for *Malassezia* dermatitis, 483
  for mycobacterial infections, 514
  for panniculitis, 565–566, *573*
  for paraneoplastic dermatoses, 621, 622, 623
  patterns, 41
  for photodermatoses, 577
  for preneoplastic dermatoses, 621, 622
  report, 38, **38**
  for skin and adnexal tumors, 677–678
  for superficial necrolytic dermatitis, 667
  terminology, **39–40**
  for viral dermatoses, 714–715
  see also biopsy
hookworm migration, 64
hormone replacement therapy, human topical *see* topical hormone replacement therapy, human
horn, cutaneous
  actinic keratosis, 575, 618
  canine papillomavirus infection, *602*, 713, *724*
Horner's syndrome, 544, *557*
hornet stings, 240–241, 243
horseflies (*Tabanus* spp.), 240
hot spot *see* acute moist dermatitis
hovawart, 648
HuIFN-α *see* interferon-alpha
humectants, 438
husky, 65, 674
  see also Siberian husky

hyaluronidase, 144
Hydrea *see* hydroxyurea
hydrocortisone, 472, **779**
hydrogen peroxide, 151
hydropic degeneration, **40**
hydroxyurea, **780**
hydroxyzine, **780**
  for atopic disease, 181
  for cutaneous mastocytosis, 623
  for cutaneous mucinosis, 624
hygiene hypothesis, 175
hymenoptera stings, 240–241
  clinical features, 243, *262–264*
  diagnostics, 246
  differential diagnosis, 245
  treatment, 247
hyperadrenocorticism (HAC)
  adrenal dependent *see* adrenal dependent hyperadrenocorticism
  canine, 394–403
    alopecia, 60, *83*, 395, *404*, *406*
    clinical features, 395–396, *404–408*
    course and prognosis, 403
    diagnostics, 397–399
    differential diagnosis, 396
    signalment/history, 395
    therapeutics, 400–402
    treatment monitoring, 403
  feline (skin fragility syndrome), 409–412
    clinical features, 60, *84*, 410, *412–415*
    therapeutics, 411–412
  iatrogenic, 394, 395, *408*, 409, *413–415*
  keratinization defects, 435, *455*
  pituitary dependent *see* pituitary dependent hyperadrenocorticism
  see also alopecia X
hyperandrogenism, 339, *350*
hyperestrogenism, 339, *348–349*
  alopecia, 60–61, *88–89*
hypergranulosis, **40**
hyperkeratosis, **40**
hyperlipidemia, 64, *123*, *613*
hyperpigmentation, 13, 65–66
  canine hyperadrenocorticism, 396, *407*
  postinflammatory, 65
hyperprogesteronemia, 339, *349*
hypersensitivity reactions *see* allergic reactions
hyperthyroidism, feline
  alopecia, 60, *87–88*
  clinical features, 338, *343*
hypoaminoacidemia, 665, 667
hypochlorite *see* bleach
hypogranulosis, **40**
hypomelanosis, **40**
hypophysectomy, 400
hypopigmentation, 13, 65–66, 67
hypopituitarism (pituitary dwarfism), 338, *344*
  alopecia, 60, *85*
  hypothyroidism with, 417, *423*
hypothalamic-pituitary-adrenal (HPA) axis abnormalities, 337
hypothyroidism, 416–422
  clinical features, 60, *86*, 418–419, *423–428*
  congenital, 417
  diagnostics, 419–421
  differential diagnosis, 419
  etiology/pathophysiology, 416–417
  keratinization defects, 435, *455*
  signalment/history, 417
  treatment, 421–422, *428–429*
hypotrichosis, feline hereditary, 61

Ibizan hound, 459
ibuprofen, **780**
ichthyosis, 62, *99*, 432
  epidermolytic, 432, *442*
  nonepidermolytic, 432, *440–441*
IgE (immunoglobulin E), 174, 178, 482
IIS-PAA (incomplete iron salt of polyacrylic acid), 151
IL-31, 175
Imaverol *see* enilconazole
imidacloprid, 302, 637
imipenem, 550, **780**
imiquimod, 369, 715
immune-mediated diseases
  claw and clawfold region, 66, *133–134*, 590, 591
  nasal planum, 67
  panniculitis, 563
  pigmentary abnormalities, 65
immunocompromised host
  cryptococcosis, 521
  dermatophytosis, 321
  mycobacterial infections, 510, 511
  nocardiosis, 535
immunohistochemistry
  for epitheliotropic lymphoma, 369
  for histiocytic proliferative disorders, 384, 385–386
  for viral dermatoses, 715
immunosuppressive therapy
  adverse effects, 197–198
  for anal furunculosis/perianal fistula, 163–164
  for atopic disease, 180–181
  for autoimmune blistering diseases, 195–196, 197
  for lupus erythematosus, 472
  for uveodermatologic syndrome, 693–694
  for vasculitis, 702
  see also azathioprine; chlorambucil; corticosteroids; cyclosporine; leflunomide; mycophenolate mofetil
impetigo, 213, 214, 220, *221–222*
impression smears, 46, *53–55*
Imuran *see* azathioprine
indolent ulcer (rodent ulcer), 351
  clinical features, *121*, 353, *361*
  diagnostics, 353, 354
  signalment/history, 352
  treatment, 355
infection, vs colonization, 212

infection control, 147–148, **149**, **150**
injection reactions, 59, *71*
insect bites and stings, 239–247
  clinical features, 241–243, *249–264*
  comments, 247
  diagnostics, 245–246
  differential diagnosis, 243–245
  etiology/pathophysiology, 239–241, *248*, 351
  signalment/history, 241
  therapeutics, 246–247
insecticide-induced dermatoses
  contact dermatitis, 266, *270*
  pemphigus foliaceus (PF), 189, *199*, 266
integrins, 188
Interceptor *see* milbemycin
interdigital furunculosis/nodules, 213, 214
interferon-alpha, 355, 715, **781**
intertrigo, 213, 214, *221*
intradermal skin testing (IDST)
  atopic disease, 178
  insect bite hypersensitivity, *264*
  Malassezia dermatitis, 482, 484
  mycobacterial infections, 513–514
intravenous immunoglobulin (IVIG), 275
iodism, 660
Irish setter, 738
  acral lick dermatitis, 228
  anal furunculosis/perianal fistula, 161
  atopic disease, 175
  color dilution alopecia, 434
  hypothyroidism, 417, 418
  ichthyosis, 432
  melanocytic tumors, 673
  primary seborrhea, 433
  psoriasiform-lichenoid dermatosis, 434
  sebaceous gland tumors, 674
  uveodermatologic syndrome, 692
Irish terrier, footpad hyperkeratosis, 434, 589, 738
Irish water spaniel, 61, 738
Irish wolfhound, 417
irritant contact dermatitis (ICD), 265–266, 267–268, *268*, *271*
ischemic dermatopathy, 700, *706*
  hereditary *see* dermatomyositis
  vaccine-induced, 700, *709*
isoniazid, 515
isopropyl alcohol, **149**
isotretinoin, **781**
  for acne, 159
  for actinic dermatoses, 578, 623
  for epitheliotropic lymphoma, 369
  precautions, 578, 625
  for primary seborrhea, 438
  for sebaceous adenitis, 650
Italian greyhound
  color dilution alopecia, 434, *448*
  pattern baldness, 60
  solar-induced dermatoses, 575, 616, 673
Italian spinone, 61
itraconazole, **781**
  for deep mycoses, 525
  for dermatophytosis, 323
  for *Malassezia* dermatitis, 483
  for onychomycosis, 594
  for otitis, 550
  precautions, 325, 484
  for sporotrichosis, 660
ivermectin, **782**
  for demodicosis, 301, 302–303
  for otitis, 550
  for sarcoptid mites, 637
  sensitivity testing, 301
  toxicity/precautions, 303, 551, 637
Ivomec *see* ivermectin
Ixodes dammini, 243
Ixodes ricini, 243
Ixodes scapularis, 243

Jack Russell terrier, 738
  cutaneous mastocytosis, 617
  ichthyosis, 62, 432
  neutrophilic leukocytoclastic vasculitis, 63, 699
  vasculitis, 698
JAK (Janus kinase) inhibitors, 181
JAK/STAT, 175
juvenile cellulitis, canine, 63, *116*
juvenile polyarteritis syndrome of beagles (JPS), 63, 699

kanamycin, **782**
Kantrim *see* kanamycin
keeshond, 338, *343*, 739
Keflex *see* cephalexin
Kefzol *see* cefazolin sodium
keratin
  bundling, 5, 7
  collaring *see* follicular casts
keratinization, 5–6, *6–9*, 430
keratinization disorders, 430–439
  clinical features, 436
  diagnostics, 436–437
  differential diagnosis, 436
  etiology/pathophysiology, 430–431
  exfoliative dermatosis, 62
  generalized/diffuse alopecia, 61, *91*
  primary, 431, 432–435
  secondary, 431, 435
  signalment/history, 431–435
  terminology, 431, 439
  therapeutics, 437–439
keratoacanthoma, subungual, *603*
keratoderma of dogue de Bordeaux, 432
keratohyalin granules, 48
kerion, 321, *329*
Kerry blue terrier, 739
  footpad hyperkeratosis, 434, 589
  papillomavirus infections, 713
  skin and adnexal tumors, 673, 674

Ketalar *see* ketamine
ketamine, **783**
Ketavet *see* ketamine
ketoconazole, **783**
  adverse effects/precautions, 65, 324–325, 402, 483–484
  for anal furunculosis/perianal fistula, 164
  for deep mycoses, 525–526
  for dermatophytosis, 324
  for hyperadrenocorticism, 402, 411
  for *Malassezia* dermatitis, 438, 483
  for otitis, 550
  for paronychia/onychomycosis, 594
  for sporotrichosis, 660
Ketofen *see* ketoprofen
ketoprofen, **784**
ketoroloc tromethamine, **784**
c-KIT mutations, 494
Kiupel grading system, mast cell tumors, 497
kuvasz, 739

labrador retriever, 739
  acral lick dermatitis, 228
  allergic contact dermatitis, 266
  color dilution alopecia, 61
  cutaneous mastocytosis, 617
  flea bite hypersensitivity, 241
  footpad hyperkeratosis, 434, 589
  ichthyosis, 432, *440*
  mast cell tumors, 495
  nasal parakeratosis, 62, 67, *103*, 432, *442*
  pedal folliculitis and furunculosis, 214
  primary seborrhea, 433
  vitamin A-responsive dermatosis, 62, 433
lactoferricin, 151
lactophenol cotton blue stain, 29, *33*
Lakeland terrier, 739
lamellar bodies, *7, 8*
laminin, 188
Lamisil *see* terbinafine
Lamprene *see* clofazimine
Latrodectus bishopi (red-legged widow spider), 240, 242
Latrodectus mactans (black widow spider), 240, 242
leflunomide, 196, 386–387, 472
Leishmania braziliensis, 458
Leishmania donovani complex, 458
Leishmania infantum, 458
leishmaniasis, 458–463
  cutaneous, 64, *120*, 460, 461, *463–465*
  diagnostics, 461–462, *465–466*
  pododermatitis, *600*
  therapeutics, 462–463, *466*
  visceral, 459–461
lentigo, 65, *130*
leproid granuloma, canine, 510
  clinical features, 513, *517–519*
  diagnostics, 514
  fly bites with, 242, *257*
  prognosis, 516
  signalment/history, 512
  treatment, 515, 516
leprosy syndrome, feline, 510
  client education and prognosis, 516
  clinical features, 512–513
  diagnostics, 514
  signalment/history, 511
  treatment, 515, 516
lesions, dermatologic
  under 1 cm in diameter, 13
  biopsy, 36–37
  description/terminology, 11–14, *14–27*
  distribution, 12
  over 1 cm in diameter, 13
  pattern, 12
  primary, 12–13
  sample collection, 30, *34–35*
  secondary, 13–14
  symptom checker, 59–69, *69–141*
Leukeran *see* chlorambucil
leukoderma, 13, *22*
  idiopathic *see* vitiligo
leukonychia, 588
leukotrichia, 13, *23*
  idiopathic *see* vitiligo
levamisole hydrochloride, **784**
Levasole *see* levamisole hydrochloride
levothyroxine (L-thyroxine), 421, 422, *428–429*, **785**
Lhasa apso, 739
  atopic disease, 175
  sebaceous adenitis, 648
  sebaceous gland tumors, 673
  superficial necrolytic dermatosis, 617, 666
lichenification, 13, *24*
  adverse food reactions, 287, *294*
  contact dermatitis, 266, *271*
lichenoid psoriasiform dermatosis, 62, *102*, 434, *452*
lidocaine, **785**
lime sulfur solutions, 302, 324, 325, 638
Lincocin *see* lincomycin
lincomycin, **786**
linear granuloma, 352, *357*
linezolid, 152, **786**
linoleic acid, 369
liothyronine, 422, **786**
lipid bilayer, 5, *8, 9*
lipoma, cutaneous, 565
Lodine *see* etodolac
lokivetmab, **786**
Lomotil *see* diphenoxylate
lomustine, **787**
  for cutaneous lymphocytosis, 625
  for epithelioid lymphoma, 369, *378–379*
  for mast cell tumors, 498, 499
  precautions, 625

low-dose dexamethasone suppression test (LDDST), 398, 403, 411
Loxosceles reclusa (brown recluse spider), 240, 242
Loxosceles unicolor (common brown spider), 240, 242
lufenuron, 325, **787**
lufenuron + milbemycin oxime, **787**
Luminal *see* phenobarbital
lung-digit syndrome, *136, 600, 688*
lupoid onychitis, symmetric, 589
lupoid onychodystrophy, symmetric, *133,* 589, 594, *596–597, 604*
lupus erythematosus (LE), 467–472
  cutaneous *see* cutaneous lupus erythematosus
  discoid *see* discoid lupus erythematosus
  keratinization disorder, 435, *456*
  systemic *see* systemic lupus erythematosus
lymphocytosis, cutaneous
  clinical features, 618, 619, *626*
  diagnostics, 622
  differential diagnosis, 620, 621
  etiology/pathophysiology, 615, 616
  signalment/history, 617
  therapeutics, 623, 625
lymphoma *see* cutaneous nonepitheliotropic lymphoma; epitheliotropic lymphoma
lymphomatoid granulomatosis, 383
lymphosarcoma, 565, *604*
L-lysine, 715, **788**
Lysodren *see* mitotane

MAB IBF9 antigen, 673
Macrodantin *see* nitrofurantoin
macromelanosome, 44, *52*
macronychia, 588
macular melanosis, 65
macules
  bacterial pyoderma, 215, *226*
  defined, 13, *17*
magnetic resonance imaging (MRI)
  for deep mycoses, 523
  for hyperadrenocorticism, 397, 411
  for otitis, 546
malamute, 417, 674
  see also Alaskan malamute
Malassezia dermatitis, 480–484
  adverse food reactions, 287, *291*
  atopic disease, 182, *183, 184*
  clinical features, 481, *486–492*
  diagnostics, 46, 47, *53–54,* 482–483, *492–493*
  differential diagnosis, 177, 482
  facts for pet owners, 484, **485**
  keratinization disorders, 432, 433, *444, 445, 448*
  paronychia, 589, *601*
  signalment/history, 481
  therapeutics, 438, 483–484
Malassezia pachydermatis, 480, 484
malignant fibrous histiocytoma, 381, 383, 385, 387
malnutrition, 435, *456*
Malogen *see* testosterone
Maltese, 699, 739
Manchester terrier, 60, 432, 739
marbofloxacin, **788**
  for mycobacterial infections, 515
  for otitis, 550
  for pyoderma, **219**
Marcaine *see* bupivacaine hydrochloride
Marin *see* silymarin
maropitant, **788**
mast cell tumors, 494–500
  canine grading systems, 497
  clinical features, 495–496, *500–509*
  course and prognosis, 499–500
  diagnostics, 496–497, *509*
  differential diagnosis, 496, 565
  signalment/history, 494–495
  therapeutics, 497–499
mastiff, 157, 214, 739
masitinib, 499
mastocytosis, cutaneous, 615, 617
  clinical features, *508,* 618
  diagnostics, 622
  differential diagnosis, 620
  therapeutics, 623
Maxolon *see* metoclopramide
mecA gene, 143
mechlorethamine, 369
meclizine, **789**
Meclofen *see* meclofenamate
meclofenamate, **789**
medetomidine, **789**
Medrol *see* methylprednisolone
medroxyprogesterone acetate, 341, **789**
Mefoxin *see* cefoxitin sodium
megestrol acetate, **790**
  adverse effects, 339, *349, 364, 414*
  for eosinophilic granuloma complex, 355
meglumine antimoniate, 463
melanin granules, 48
melanocytic tumors, 672–673
  clinical features, 676, *683–684*
  diagnostics, 677, 678
  differential diagnosis, 677
  malignant *see* melanoma, malignant
  prognosis, 679
  signalment/history, 673, 674, 675
  therapeutics, 678–679
melanoderma/alopecia of Yorkshire terriers, 60, 65
melanoma, malignant
  client education, 679
  clinical features, 66, *131, 614,* 676, *684*
  etiology/pathophysiology, 672–673
melanosis, **40**
melatonin, for alopecia X, 341
meloxicam, **790**
mepivacaine, **791**
6-mercaptopurine, **791**

meropenem, 550, **791**
Merrem IV *see* meropenem
mesenchymal stem cell injections, 164
metabolic epidermal necrosis *see* superficial necrolytic dermatosis
Metacam *see* meloxicam
methicillin resistance, 143–144, 145–146, 151–152
methicillin-resistant *Staphylococcus aureus* (MRSA), 143–144, 145–146
  community acquired (CA-MRSA), 145
  hospital acquired (HA-MRSA), 145
  infection control, 147
methicillin-resistant *Staphylococcus pseudintermedius* (MRSP), 142, 143–144, 145–146, *153–154*
methicillin-resistant *Staphylococcus schleiferi* (MRSS), 143–144, 145–146
methimazole, **792**
methocarbamol, **792**
methotrexate, **793**
methylprednisolone, **793–794**
  for atopic disease, 180
  for autoimmune blistering diseases, 197
  for eosinophilic granuloma (complex), 355
methyltestosterone, 341, **794**
Meticorten *see* prednisone
metoclopramide, **795**
metronidazole, 164, **795**
metyrapone, 411
Mexate *see* methotrexate
Mexican dog, 61
mibolerone, **796**
miconazole, 324
microabscesses, 40
microbiome, skin, 211–212
microneedling therapy, 341
micronychia, 588
Microsporum canis, 29, 320, 321
  clinical features, *326, 327–328, 330–331*
  culture and identification, *33, 34, 334–335*
  diagnostics, 322
  pododermatitis, *606*
  zoonotic potential, *331, 729–730*
Microsporum gypseum, 29, 320, 321
  clinical features, *326*
  culture and identification, *31, 33, 34, 334–335*
milbemycin, **796**
  for demodicosis, 301
  for sarcoptid mites, 637
  toxicity, 303
milia, 13, *16*
miliary dermatitis (cat)
  allergic, 351, 352, 353, 354, *362*
  bacterial pyoderma, 213, 215, *223*
  flea bite hypersensitivity, 241
milk thistle *see* silymarin
miltefosine, 463
miniature pinscher, 739
  hypopituitary dwarfism, 338
  pattern baldness, 60
  sebaceous adenitis, 648
miniature poodle, 741
  alopecia X, 338
  cutaneous adverse drug reactions, 273
  Malassezia dermatitis, 481
  panniculitis, 563
miniature schnauzer, 740
  acquired aurotrichia, 66
  atopic disease, 175
  cutaneous adverse drug reactions, 273, *279–280*
  hypothyroidism, 417
  mycobacterial infections, 511
  papillomavirus infections, 713
  primary seborrhea, 433
  schnauzer comedo syndrome, 434, *452*
  skin and adnexal tumors, 673, 674
  superficial suppurative necrolytic dermatitis, 274
  vitamin A-responsive dermatosis, 433
Minocin *see* minocycline
minocycline, **796**
  for claw disorders, 594
  for lupus erythematosus, 471–472
  for methicillin-resistant staphylococci, 152
  for nocardiosis, 538
  for panniculitis, 566
  for pemphigus/pemphigoid, 196
  for reactive cutaneous histiocytosis, 386
  for sebaceous adenitis, 650
  for vasculitis, 701–702
Mitaban *see* amitraz
mite infestations
  acetate tape preparation, 47
  exfoliative dermatosis, 62, *95*
  external ear canal, 544, *558*, 634
  skin scrapings, 43–44, *48–49*
  trichograms, 44, *50*
  see also cheyletiellosis; demodicosis; *Notoedres cati; Otodectes cynotis; Sarcoptes scabiei* var. *canis;* sarcoptid mites
mitotane, 341, 400–401, 411, **797**
mitoxantrone, 679
Mobic *see* meloxicam
moisturizers, 438
mosquito bite dermatitis, 240, 244, 247
  clinical features, 242, *257*
  diagnostics, 245
mosquito bite hypersensitivity, 240, 244
  clinical features, 64, 67, *121*, 242, *258–260*
  diagnostics, 245
  eosinophilic granuloma complex, 351
  therapeutics, 247
"moth-eaten" appearance, pyoderma, 214, 215, *223*
Motrin *see* ibuprofen
moxidectin, **797**
  for demodicosis, 302
  for otitis, 550
  for sarcoptid mites, 637

moxifloxacin, **797**
MRI *see* magnetic resonance imaging
MRSA *see* methicillin-resistant *Staphylococcus aureus*
MRSP *see* methicillin-resistant *Staphylococcus pseudintermedius*
MRSS *see* methicillin-resistant *Staphylococcus schleiferi*
MTX *see* methotrexate
mucinosis
  cutaneous (secondary), 615, 617, 619, 621, 622, 624, *627*
  defined, **40**
mucocutaneous pyoderma (MCP), 213, 214, *222*
  nasal planum, 67, *140*
mucous membrane cutaneous lupus erythematosus (MCLE), 468, 469–470, 471, *476*
mucous membrane pemphigoid
  clinical features, 63, 191, *208*
  etiology/pathophysiology, 189
  see also pemphigoid complex
Munro's microabscess, **40**
mupirocin ointment, 151, 159, 164, 550
muscle biopsy, 314
muzzle folliculitis/furunculosis, 157, 213
  see also acne
mycobacterial infections, 510–517
  clinical features, 512–513, *517–520*
  diagnostics, 513–514
  differential diagnosis, 513
  etiology/pathophysiology, 510–511
  signalment/history, 511–512
  therapeutics, 515–516
  zoonotic potential, 517
mycobacterial panniculitis, 511, 512, 513, *519–520*
mycobacteriosis
  feline multisystemic granulomatous, 513
  systemic nontuberculous (atypical), 511
    clinical features, 63, *119*, 513, *519–520*
    diagnostics, 514
    prognosis, 516
    signalment/history, 512
    treatment, 515, 516
Mycobacterium avium complex, 510, 511, 515
Mycobacterium bovis, 510, 511, 515
Mycobacterium lepraemurium, 511
Mycobacterium microti, 510, 511
Mycobacterium sp. strain Tarwin, 511
Mycobacterium tuberculosis, 510, 511, 515, 517
Mycobacterium visibile, 511
mycophenolate mofetil, **798**
  for epidermolysis bullosa acquisita, 197
  for lupus erythematosus, 472
  for pemphigus complex, 196
  side effects, 198
mycoses
  deep, 63, *118*, 521–527
  see also fungal infections; onychomycosis
mycosis fungoides *see* epitheliotropic lymphoma
myiasis, 240
Myochrysine *see* gold sodium thiomalate
myringotomy, *35*, 547, *562*
myxedema, 418, *425*, *426–427*
  see also hypothyroidism
myxedema coma, 422

N-acetyl-L-cysteine (NAC), 151, 548, 550
naloxone, **798**
naltrexone, **798**
Naprosyn *see* naproxen
naproxen, **799**
Narcan *see* naloxone
nasal arteritis, 67, *139*, 699, *706*
nasal furunculosis, eosinophilic, 63, *115*
nasal hypopigmentation, 65, 67
nasal parakeratosis, hereditary, of labradors, 62, 67, *103*, 432, *442*
nasal planum
  biopsy, 37
  dermatoses, 67, *137–141*
nasal pyoderma, 67, 213
nasal solar dermatitis, 67, *138*
nasodigital hyperkeratosis, idiopathic canine, 62, 67, *97*, 433–434, *446*
Naxcel *see* ceftiofur
Naxen *see* naproxen
Nebcin *see* tobramycin
necrolysis, **40**
necrolytic migratory erythema *see* superficial necrolytic dermatosis
neomycin, *269*, *276*, **799**
neoplasia
  claw/clawfold region, 66, *136*, 592, *603–604*, *605*
  cutaneous lymphoma *see* epitheliotropic lymphoma, cutaneous
  keratinization disorders, 435, *457*
  lymphoma *see* cutaneous nonepitheliotropic lymphoma
  mast cell tumors, 494–500
  nodular, 69
  onychomadesis, 591
  panniculitis, 565
  paraneoplastic syndromes *see* paraneoplastic dermatoses
  paronychia, 590
  pododermatitis, 590, *600*
  skin and adnexa *see* skin and adnexal tumors
  ultraviolet light induced, 575
  see also preneoplastic dermatoses; tumors
Neoral *see* cyclosporine
Neosar *see* cyclophosphamide
neuro-immuno-cutaneous-endocrine (NICE) model, 228
Neurontin *see* gabapentin
neutrophilic leukocytoclastic vasculitis of Jack Russell terriers, 63, 699
nevus/nevi, 66, *131*
  see also collagenous nevi, multiple

Newfoundland dog, 417, 617, 740
niacinamide
  for claw disorders, 594
  for lupus erythematosus, 472
  for panniculitis, 566
  for pemphigoid/pemphigus, 196
  for reactive cutaneous histiocytosis, 386
  for sebaceous adenitis, 650
  for vasculitis, 702
Nikolsky sign, 191
nilenpyram, **799**
nitrofurantoin, *279–280,* **800**
nitrogen mustard, 369
nizatidine, **800**
Nizoral *see* ketoconazole
nocardiosis, *119,* 535–538, *539–540*
nodular dermatofibrosis, 617
  clinical features, 619, *628–629*
  diagnostics, 622
  differential diagnosis, 621
  German shepherd dog, 589, 592, 616
  therapeutics, 624
nodular fasciitis, 615, 617, 618
  diagnostics, 622
  differential diagnosis, 620
nodules, 13, *19*
  etiology, 67–69
  fine-needle aspiration, 46–47
  foot, 592, *612–614*
  leishmaniasis, 460, *465*
  panniculitis, 564, *567–568*
norfloxacin, **800**
Norfolk terrier, 62, 432, 740
Noroxin *see* norfloxacin
Norwegian elkhound, 673, 740
Norwich terrier, 740
Notoedres cati (notoedric mange), 634, *640*
  clinical features, *95,* 635, *643–644*
  diagnostics, 43, 636
  therapeutics, 637–638
Novox *see* carprofen
Nuflor *see* florfenicol
Numorphan *see* oxymorphone
Nuprin *see* ibuprofen
nutrition *see* diet
nutritional disorders, 435, *456*

obsessive-compulsive disorder, 227
oclacitinib, 181, 275, **801**
octreotide, 624, 668
Old English sheepdog, 740
  cutaneous adverse drug reactions, 273
  hypothyroidism, 417
  ivermectin sensitivity, 301, 551, 637
  pilomatrixoma, 674
  pododemodicosis, 298
  uveodermatologic syndrome, 692
omeprazole, **801**
Omnicef *see* cefdinir
Omnipen *see* ampicillin
onychalgia, 588
onychatrophia, 588
onychauxis, 588
onychitis, 588
  symmetric lupoid, 589
onychoclasis, 588
onychocryptosis, 588
onychodystrophy, 588
  dermatomyositis, *595*
  dermatophytosis, *330, 605*
  idiopathic, 589
  symmetric lupoid, *133,* 589, 594, *596–597, 604*
  trauma-induced, 590, *599*
onychogryphosis, 589
onycholysis, 589, *596*
onychomadesis, 588, 590
  clinical features, 591, *596*
  idiopathic, 589
  treatment, 593, 594
onychomalacia, 588
onychomycosis, 588
  clinical features, 591, *605*
  treatment, 593, 594
onychopathy, 588
onychorrhexis, 588, 591
  in dachshunds, 66, *135,* 589, *595–596*
  demodicosis, *599*
  treatment, 593
onychoschizia, 588
o,p'-DDD *see* mitotane
Optimmune *see* cyclosporine
Orbax *see* orbifloxacin
orbifloxacin, **219**, 550, **801**
ormetoprim + sulfadimethoxine, **219**, 550, **801**, **807**
orofacial pain syndrome, feline, 64, 713
Ortoenin *see* cloxacillin sodium
Orudis KT *see* ketoprofen
osteomyelitis, petrous temporal bone and bulla, 548
osteosarcoma, *605*
otic cytology, **45**, 45–46, *53*
otitis externa, 541–551
  adverse food reactions, 287, *291,* 545
  clinical features, 543–544, *552–553*
  demodicosis, 298
  diagnostics, 546–548
  differential diagnosis, 544–545, *558–560*
  ear ticks, 240
  etiology/pathogenesis, 542
  sample collection, 31
  signalment/history, 543
  therapeutics, 548–551
otitis interna, 541–551
  clinical features, 544, *557*
  diagnostics, 546–548
  differential diagnosis, 545–546
  etiology/pathogenesis, 542
  signalment/history, 543
  therapeutics, 548–551

otitis media, 541–551
  clinical features, 544, *554–557*
  diagnostics, 546–548, *562*
  differential diagnosis, 544–545, *561*
  etiology/pathogenesis, 542
  primary secretory, 541, 543, 544, *554–555*
  sample collection, 31, *35*
  signalment/history, 543
  therapeutics, 151, 548–551
Otobius megnini, 243
Otodectes cynotis, *558*, 634, *641*
  clinical features, 635, *646*
  diagnostics, 43, 636
  therapeutics, 637–638
otoscopy, 546
ototoxicity, 541, 551
otter hound, 740
outside-inside-outside theory, atopic disease, 173–174
Ovaban *see* megestrol acetate
ovarian cysts/tumors, 339, 341, *345*
oxacillin, **802**
oxidizing agents, **149**, **150**
oxymorphone, **802**
oxytetracycline, **802**

p53 tumor suppressor gene, 494, 574, 615, 672, 711
pachyonychia, 588
paecilomycosis, 64
Pagetoid reticulosis, 366, 367, *377*
pancreatic/hepatic paraneoplastic alopecia, feline *see* paraneoplastic alopecia, feline
pancreatic tumors
  feline paraneoplastic alopecia, 616, 623
  panniculitis, 565
  superficial necrolytic dermatitis, 616, 665, 667, *671*
Panectyl *see* trimeprazine
panepidermal pustular pemphigus/pemphigus vegetans (PEP/Pveg)
  clinical features, 191, *206*
  course and prognosis, 198
  diagnostics, 194–195
  differential diagnosis, 193
  etiology/pathophysiology, 188
  signalment/history, 189
  therapeutics, 196
Panmycin *see* tetracycline
panniculitis, 563–566
  clinical features, *26*, 564, *567–570*
  diagnostics, 565–566, *571–573*
  mycobacterial, 511, 512, 513, *519–520*
  pancreatic, 565
  sterile (idiopathic) nodular (SNP), 65, *126*, 563, 564, 565, 566
papillomatosis, **40**
papillomaviruses, 711
  canine, *602*, 713, *723–726*
  feline, 712
papillon, 740
papule, 13, *17*
paraneoplastic alopecia, feline (pancreatic/hepatic), 616
  clinical features, 61, *93*, 619–620, *631–632*
  diagnostics, 623
  differential diagnosis, 621
  signalment/history, 617
  therapeutics, 625
paraneoplastic dermatoses, 615–625
  canine, 615–616
    clinical features, 619, *627–631*
    diagnostics, 621, 622
    differential diagnosis, 620–621
    signalment/history, 617
    therapeutics, 623–624
  feline, 616
    clinical features, 619–620, *631–633*
    diagnostics, 621, 623
    differential diagnosis, 621
    signalment/history, 617–618
    therapeutics, 625
paraneoplastic pemphigus (PP)
  clinical features, 191, *206–207*, 619, *629–630*
  course and prognosis, 198
  diagnostics, 194–195, 622
  differential diagnosis, 193, 621
  etiology/pathophysiology, 188, 616
  signalment/history, 189, 617
  therapeutics, 196, 624
parasitic diseases
  clawfold region, 66, *132*
  exfoliative dermatosis, 62, *95*
  keratinization defects, 435, *453*
  nodules and draining sinuses, 68
  zoonotic, 727–728, *729*
  see also mite infestations
paronychia, 588, 590
  bacterial, 66, *132*, 594, *601*
  clinical features, 590, *601–604*
  dermatophytosis, *330*
  direct impression smears, 46
  treatment, 593, 594
  yeast/*Malassezia*, 589, 594, *601*
paroxetine, 234, **803**
pars flaccida, 542, *551*
  swelling, 544, *554*
pars tensa, 542, *551–552*
Pasteurella multocida, 213
patches, 13, *19*
Patnaik grading system, mast cell tumors, 497
pattern baldness, 60, *79–80*
Pautrier's microabscess, **40**
Paxil *see* paroxetine
PBZ *see* tripelennamine citrate
PCR *see* polymerase chain reaction
pekingese, 339, 673, 740
Pelamine *see* tripelennamine citrate
pelodera, 64
Pembroke Welsh corgi, 740

pemphigoid complex, 187
  clinical features, 191, *208*
  course and prognosis, 198
  differential diagnosis, 193
  etiology/pathophysiology, 189
  pathologic findings, 195
  signalment/history, 190
  therapeutics, 196–197
pemphigus
  drug-induced, 188, 189, 273, *279–280*
  panepidermal pustular *see* panepidermal pustular pemphigus/pemphigus vegetans
  paraneoplastic *see* paraneoplastic pemphigus
pemphigus complex, 187
  clinical features, 61, 190–191, *199–207*
  course and prognosis, 198
  diagnostics, 194–195, *210*
  differential diagnosis, 192–193
  etiology/pathophysiology, 188
  keratinization disorder, 435
  nasal planum, 67, *137*
  signalment/history, 189
  therapeutics, 195–196
pemphigus erythematosus (PE)
  clinical features, *137,* 190, *204*
  course and prognosis, 198
  diagnostics, 194–195
  differential diagnosis, 192–193
  etiology/pathophysiology, 188
  signalment/history, 189
  therapeutics, 196
pemphigus foliaceus (PF)
  clinical features, *18,* 190, *199–203*
  course and prognosis, 198
  crusted/ulcerative lesions, 63, *106–109*
  diagnostics, *57,* 194–195, *210*
  differential diagnosis, 192
  drug-induced, *279–280*
  etiology/pathophysiology, 188
  foot, *133, 602–603, 606–607*
  insecticide-induced, 189, *199*
  signalment/history, 189
  therapeutics, 195–196
pemphigus vegetans *see* panepidermal pustular pemphigus/pemphigus vegetans
pemphigus vulgaris (PV)
  claw/clawfold region, 66, *134*
  clinical features, 63, *110, 137,* 190–191, *205*
  course and prognosis, 198
  diagnostics, 194–195
  differential diagnosis, 193
  etiology/pathophysiology, 188
  signalment/history, 189
  therapeutics, 195–196
penicillin-binding proteins (PBP), 143
penicillins, adverse reactions, 272
pentoxifylline, **803**
  for atopic disease, 181
  for claw disorders, 594
  for contact dermatitis, 268
  for cutaneous adverse drug reactions, 275
  for dermatomyositis, 315
  precautions, 702
  for sebaceous adenitis, 650
  for vasculitis, 701
Pepcid *see* famotidine
Percorten-V *see* desoxycorticosterone
Periactin *see* cyproheptadine
periadnexal multinodular granulomatous dermatitis, 384
perianal fistula, *26,* 161–164, *165–168*
peritonitis, feline infectious, 712
Persian cat
  Chediak–Higashi syndrome, 66
  facial dermatitis (dirty face syndrome), 62, *104,* 435, *453*
  oculocutaneous albinism, 66
  primary seborrhea in newborn, 435
  skin tumors, 673, 674
Phenetron *see* chlorpheniramine
phenobarbital, **803**
phenols, **149, 150**
phenylbutazone, **804**
phenylpropanolamine, **804**
phlebectasia, 395, *407*
photodermatoses, 574–578
phytosphingosines, 438
pigmentary incontinence, **40**
pigmentation abnormalities, 13, 65–66, *128–131*
  nasal planum, 67, *140–141*
  see also hyperpigmentation
pilomatrixoma, 674, 675, 678, *690*
pinnal alopecia, 60
pinnal-pedal reflex, 636
piperacillin (Pipracil), **804**
piroxicam, **805**
pit bull terrier, 157, 214, 266
pituitary dependent hyperadrenocorticism (PDH)
  canine, 394, 397, 399, 400, 403
  feline, 409
pituitary dwarfism *see* hypopituitarism
pituitary tumors, 394, 397, 400, 401
plakins, 188
plaques, 13, *20*
plasma cell chondritis, feline, 712
plasma cell pododermatitis, feline, 65, *126,* 592, *610,* 712
plasma cell stomatitis, feline, 712
plastic food bowl hypersensitivity, *138*
plectin, 188
pododemodicosis, *132,* 298, *309, 599*
pododermatitis, 588–594
  clinical features, *132,* 590–591, *595–614*
  course and prognosis, 594
  diagnostics, 593
  differential diagnosis, 591–593

etiology/pathophysiology, 589
feline plasma cell, 65, *126*, 592, *610*, 712
signalment/history, 589–590
therapeutics, 593–594
pointer, 522, 740
see also English pointer; German short-haired pointer
polyarteritis nodosa, 698, 699
polymerase chain reaction (PCR), 30, 462, 514
polyps
ear canal, 545, *558–559*
symmetric lupoid onychodystrophy, *604*
polysulfated glycosaminoglycan (PSGAG), **805**
pomeranian, 741
alopecia X, 338, *344*
panniculitis, 563
poodle, 741
allergic contact dermatitis, 266
anal licking, 228, *238*
color dilution alopecia, 434
hyperadrenocorticism, 395
hypothyroidism, 417
psoriasiform-lichenoid dermatosis, 434
skin and adnexal tumors, 673, 674
vaccination-associated vasculitis, 699
see also miniature poodle; standard poodle; toy poodle
Portuguese water dog, 60, 741
posaconazole, 525, 660
postgrooming pyoderma, 215, *225*
postinflammatory hyperpigmentation, 65
potassium iodide, supersaturated solution (SSKI), 660
pradofloxacin, 515, 516
praziquantel, **805**
prednisolone, **806**
for actinic dermatoses, 578, 623, 624
for atopic disease, 180
for contact dermatitis, 268
for cutaneous lymphocytosis, 625
for cutaneous mastocytosis, 623
for cutaneous mucinosis, 624
for dermatomyositis, 314
for eosinophilic granuloma (complex), 355
for epidermolysis bullosa acquisita, 197
for histiocytic proliferative disorders, 386
for insect bites and stings, 246, 247
for keratinization disorders, 438
for lupus erythematosus, 472
for mast cell tumors, 498
for otitis, 550
for pemphigus complex, 195–196, 624
for sarcoptid mites, 638
for sterile nodular panniculitis, 566
for superficial necrolytic dermatosis, 624, 668
for uveodermatologic syndrome, 693
for vasculitis, 701
prednisone, 400, **806**
preneoplastic dermatoses, 615–625
canine, 615
clinical features, 618, *626*
diagnostics, 621–622
differential diagnosis, 620
signalment/history, 616–617
therapeutics, 623
feline, 616
clinical features, 618
diagnostics, 621, 622
differential diagnosis, 621
signalment/history, 617
therapeutics, 624–625
solar-induced, 574, 575–576
preputial erythema, linear, *89*
Previcox *see* firocoxib
Prilosec *see* omeprazole
Primaxin *see* imipenem
Primor *see* ormetoprim + sulfadimethoxine
Principen *see* ampicillin
profillagrin, *7*
progesterone, elevated levels, 339, *349*
Program *see* lufenuron
ProHeart *see* moxidectin
Proin PPA *see* phenylpropanolamine
Propalin *see* phenylpropanolamine
Propionibacterium acnes, 715
propylene glycol, 438, 650
propylthiouracil (Propyl-Thyracil), **807**
Prostaphlin *see* oxacillin
protein A, staphylococcal, 144
Proteus spp., 213
protothecosis, 64
protozoan dermatitis, 458–463, *463–466*
zoonotic potential, 729
Provera *see* medroxyprogesterone acetate
Prozac *see* fluoxetine
pruritus
adverse food reactions, 288, 291, *295*
atopic disease, 176, 182, *186*
bacterial pyoderma and, 214
flea bite hypersensitivity, 241, *250*
interdigital erythema with, 591
sarcoptid mites, 634, 636, 638
pseudo-Cushing's syndrome *see* alopecia X
pseudohyperparathyroidism, 170
Pseudomonas aeruginosa
otitis externa/media, 544, 545, *553*
postgrooming furunculosis, 215, *225*
Pseudomonas spp. infections, *154*, 213
pseudo-Nikolsky sign, 274
pseudopelade, 61, *94*
pseudorabies, 713
psoriasiform lichenoid dermatosis, 62, *102*, 434, *452*
psychodermatoses *see* behavioral dermatoses
pug, 741
atopic disease, 175, *183*
mast cell tumors, 495
papillomavirus infections, 713

puli, 741
pulmonary carcinoma, metastatic (lung-digit syndrome), *136, 600, 688*
puppy impetigo, 213, 214, *221*
puppy strangles (canine juvenile cellulitis), 63, *116*
Purinethol *see* 6-mercaptopurine
pustular dermatitis
  contagious viral, 713
  leishmaniasis, 460
  superficial, 220
pustules, 13, *18*
  biopsy, 37
  fine-needle aspiration, 46–47
pyoderma, bacterial, 211–220
  antibiotic resistance, 142–144, 146
  canine exfoliative superficial, 213, 214, *223*
  clinical features, 214–215, *220–225*
  deep, 213, 214–215, *224*
    differential diagnosis, 564
    generalized, German shepherd dog, 213, 214
  diagnostics, 216
  differential diagnosis, 177, 215–216
  etiology/pathophysiology, 211–213
  hypothyroidism, 419
  idiopathic recurrent superficial, 214
  lesions, 215, *226*
  mucocutaneous *see* mucocutaneous pyoderma
  nasal, 67, 213
  pedal, 213
  postgrooming, 215, *225*
  signalment/history, 214
  skinfold *see* intertrigo
  superficial, 213, 214, *223, 226*
  superficial spreading, 213, 214, *223*
  therapeutics, 151–152, 217–220, **218–219**
  see also folliculitis; furunculosis
pyonychia, 588
pyotraumatic folliculitis and furunculosis, 213
  flea bite hypersensitivity, 241, *250–251*
pyrazinamide, 515
pythiosis, 64

quaternary ammonium compounds, **149, 150**
Quest *see* moxidectin
quorum sensing, 215

rabies vaccine, adverse reactions, 273, *280*
  ischemic dermopathy, 700, *709*
  patchy alopecia, 59, *71*
radiography
  for blastomycosis, 526
  for histiocytic proliferation disorders, 384
  for hyperadrenocorticism, 397
  for mycobacterial infections, 514
  for otitis media, 546
  for paraneoplastic dermatoses, 621
  for skin tumors, 677, 679
radiotherapy, 400, 498, 679
ranitidine, **807**
rapid sporulating medium (RSM), 28
rat tail appearance, 418, *426*, 649
raw diets, 288
Reconcile *see* fluoxetine
red-legged widow spider (*Latrodectus bishopi*), 240, 242
regional dermatoses, symptom checker, 59–69, *69–141*
Reglan *see* metoclopramide
renal cystadenocarcinoma, with nodular dermatofibrosis, 616
renal glomerular and cutaneous vasculopathy of greyhounds, 63, 699
retapamulin, 151
reticular degeneration, **40**
Retin-A *see* tretinoin
retinoids, **818**
  for acne, 159
  for epitheliotropic lymphoma, 369
  for photodermatoses, 578
  precautions, 439
  for primary seborrhea, 438
  see also isotretinoin; tretinoin; vitamin A
retinol *see* vitamin A
Retrovir *see* zidovudine
Revolution *see* selamectin
Rheumatrex *see* methotrexate
rhinotracheitis, feline, 712
Rhipicephalus sanguineus, 243
Rhodesian ridgeback, 741
  color dilution and cerebellar degeneration, 66
  ichthyosis, 432
  idiopathic onychodystrophy, 589
Ridaura *see* auranofin
Rifadin *see* rifampin
rifampin, **808**
  for methicillin-resistant staphylococci, 152
  for mycobacterial infections, 515, 516
  for pyoderma, **219**
Rimadyl *see* carprofen
ringworm *see* dermatophytosis
ringworm vaccine, 325
Robaxin-V *see* methocarbamol
rodent ulcer *see* indolent ulcer
Roferon *see* interferon-alpha
Rompun *see* xylaxine hydrochloride
rottweiler, 741–742
  acne, 157
  claw disorders, 589
  congenital alopecia, 61
  follicular lipidosis, 61
  leishmaniasis, 459
  vasculitis, 698
  vitiligo, 65

Sabouraud's dextrose agar, 28, 323
S-adenosylmethionine, 668
SafeHeart *see* milbemycin

St Bernard, 742
  flea bite hypersensitivity, 241
  nasal arteritis, 67, *139*, 699, *706*
  uveodermatologic syndrome, 692
Salazopyrin *see* sulfasalazine
saluki, 434, 742
samoyed, 742
  alopecia X, 338
  sebaceous adenitis, 434, 648
  uveodermatologic syndrome, 692
sample collection
  bacterial culture, 30–31, *34–35*
  cytology, 43–47
  dermatophytes, 28–29, *31–32*
  ear canal, 31, 45, *53*
  see also biopsy
sandflies, 458
Sarcoptes scabiei var. *canis* (sarcoptic mange, scabies), 634, *639*
  clinical features, 635, *642–643*
  diagnostics, 636
  differential diagnosis, 177
  therapeutics, 637–638
  zoonotic potential, *647*, *729*
sarcoptid mites, 634–638
  clinical features, 64, 635, *642–646*
  diagnostics, 636, *646*
  differential diagnosis, 636
  skin scrapings, 43, *49*
  therapeutics, 637–638
sarolaner, 302, 638, **808**
satellitosis, **40**
scabicides, 637–638
scabies *see Sarcoptes scabiei* var. *canis*
scaling, 12, *14*
  keratinization disorders, 430, 431, *440*
scar, 14, *27*
schipperke, 742
schnauzer comedo syndrome, 62, 434, *452*
scleroderma, localized, 59, *73*
sclerosis, **40**
Scottish deerhound, 417
Scottish terrier, 742
  allergic contact dermatitis, 266
  atopic disease, 175
  cutaneous adverse drug reactions, 273
  skin and adnexal tumors, 673, 674
  superficial necrolytic dermatosis, 617, 666
  vasculitis, 698
Sealyham terrier, 175, 742
sebaceous adenitis (granulomatous), 648–651, *652–657*
  diffuse alopecia, 60, *82*
  exfoliative dermatosis, 62, *97–98*
  keratinization defects, 434, *449–451*
  patchy alopecia, 59, *74*
  therapeutics, 650–651
sebaceous adenocarcinoma
  clinical features, 676, *688*
  histopathology, 678
  prognosis, 680
  signalment/history, 674
sebaceous adenoma
  clinical features, 676, *686–687*
  differential diagnosis, 677
  histopathology, 678
  predisposed breeds, 673
sebaceous epithelioma, 674, 678
sebaceous gland hyperplasia
  clinical features, 676, *686*
  histopathology, 678
  signalment/history, 433, 673
sebaceous gland tumors, 673
  clinical features, 676, *686–688*
  diagnostics, 677, 678
  prognosis, 680
  signalment/history, 673–674, 675
  therapeutics, 678–679
seborrhea, 430
  primary (idiopathic), 433, 435, 438, *443–444*
  terminology, 431
  see also keratinization disorders
seborrheic dermatitis, 338, 433, 481
selamectin, 550, 637, **809**
selective serotonin reuptake inhibitors (SSRIs), 234
selegiline (L-deprenyl), 402, 403, **809**
self-injurious dermatoses, 227–234
  adverse food reactions, 287, *292–294*
  atopic disease, 176, *183*, *185–186*
  clinical features, 228–230, *235–238*
  comments, 234
  diagnostics, 231–232
  differential diagnosis, 230–231
  etiology/pathophysiology, 227–228
  flea bite hypersensitivity, 241, *250*
  lesion types, 13, *24*
  signalment/history, 228
  therapeutics, 233–234
sensory dermatoses, cutaneous, 227
Sentinel tablets *see* lufenuron + milbemycin oxime
Septra *see* trimethoprim + sulfamethoxazole
serologic allergy tests, 178
serotonin syndrome, 234
Sertoli cell tumor, 61, *88*, *345–347*
sertraline, 234
sex hormone-related dermatoses, 337, 339, 341, *345–350*
Sézary cells, 368
Sézary syndrome (SS), 366, 367
shampoos
  for adverse food reactions, 290
  for atopic disease, 179
  for atypical endocrinopathies, 341
  for keratinization disorders, 437–438
  for pyoderma, 142, 151, 217, 219

shampoos (*Continued*)
  for sarcoptid mites, 638
  for sebaceous adenitis, 650
shar-pei *see* Chinese shar-pei
Shetland sheepdog (sheltie), 742
  autoimmune blistering dermatoses, 189, 190
  basal cell tumors, 673
  cutaneous adverse drug reactions, 273
  cutaneous lymphocytosis, 617
  dermatomyositis, 65, 312, 589
  ivermectin sensitivity, 301, 551, 637
  lupus erythematosus, 468, 469
  superficial necrolytic dermatosis, 617, 666
  testicular tumors, 339
  ulcerative dermatosis, 64
  uveodermatologic syndrome, 692
shiba inu, 692
shih tzu, 743
  Malassezia dermatitis, 481
  sebaceous gland tumors, 673, 674
  superficial necrolytic dermatosis, 617, 666
Siamese cat
  basal cell tumors, 673
  demodicosis, 297
  feline orofacial pain syndrome, 64, 713
  feline symmetric alopecia, 228, *237*
  hereditary hypotrichosis, 61
  mast cell tumors, 495, 496
  mycobacterial infections, 511
Siberian husky, 743
  alopecia X, 338
  eosinophilic granuloma, 352
  lupus erythematosus, 468, 469
  onychodystrophy, 589
  skin tumors, 673
  uveodermatologic syndrome, 692
  zinc-responsive dermatosis, 434, *447–448*
silken windhound, 301, 637
silky terrier, 481, 699, 743
silver preparations, topical, 151
silymarin (Silybin), 668, **810**
Simplicef *see* cefpodoxime
Simulium spp. (black flies), 240
sinuses, draining, 67–69
skin, 3–10
  functions, 3
  layers, *5*
  microbiome, 211–212
skin and adnexal tumors, 672–680
  client education/prognosis, 679–680
  clinical features, 675–677, *680–691*
  diagnostics, 677–678
  differential diagnosis, 677
  etiology/pathophysiology, 672–673
  signalment/history, 673–675
  therapeutics, 678–679
skin barrier, 3–10, 430
  "bricks and mortar" structure, 6, *9*
  formation process, 5–6, *6–9*
  impairment, 10
    atopic dermatitis, 10, 173–174
    keratinization disorders, 430, 431
  structure and function, 4, *4–5*
skinfold dermatitis/pyoderma (intertrigo), 213, 214, *221*
skin fragility syndrome, feline *see* hyperadrenocorticism (HAC), feline
skin scrapings
  deep, 44, *49*
  for demodicosis, 43–44, *49,* 299, *304*
  for sarcoptid mites, 43, *49,* 636
  superficial, 43, *48–49*
Skye terrier, 743
SLE *see* systemic lupus erythematosus
snow nose, 65
soap, 147
sodium stibogluconate, 463
soft-coated wheaten terrier, 432
solar dermatitis, 574
  clinical features, 575, *579–580*
  diagnostics, 577
  differential diagnosis, 576
  nasal, 67, *138*
solar elastosis, 577
solar-induced dermatoses, 574–578, 615, 672
solar vasculopathy, 699
Solenopsis spp. (fire ants), 243
Solganol *see* aurothioglucose
Solodyn *see* minocycline
Soloxine *see* levothyroxine
Solu-Cortef *see* hydrocortisone
Solu-Delta-Cortef *see* prednisolone
Solu-Medrol *see* methylprednisolone
Somali cat, 511
spaniel, 189, 674, 743
sphynx cat, 61, 481
spider bite dermatitis, 240
  clinical features, 242, *254–255*
  diagnostics, 245
  differential diagnosis, 244
  therapeutics, 246
spinone, 743
spitz, 338
spongiform microabscess, **40**
spongiosis, **40**
Sporanox *see* itraconazole
Sporothrix schenckii, 658
sporotrichosis, 658–661
  clinical features, 659, *662*
  diagnostics, 659, *663–664*
  therapeutics, 660–661
springer spaniel
  acral mutilation syndrome, 65
  lichenoid psoriasiform dermatosis, 62
  melanocytic tumors, 673

psoriasiform-lichenoid dermatosis, 434
see also English springer spaniel
squames (exfoliating corneocytes), *7, 9*
squamous cell carcinoma (SCC), cutaneous
client education/prognosis, 679
clinical features, 576, *585–587*, 675–676, *681–683*
diagnostics, 577, 677–678
differential diagnosis, 577, 677
etiology/pathophysiology, 672
premalignant lesions, 575
signalment/history, 673, 674–675
solar induced, 574, 672
therapeutics, 678–679
squamous cell carcinoma *in situ see* Bowen's disease
squeeze tape impressions, 44–45
stable flies (*Stomoxys calcitrans*), 240
Staffordshire bull terrier, 744
demodicosis, 297
leproid granuloma, 512
mast cell tumors, 495
tail biting or chasing, 228
see also American Staffordshire terrier
standard poodle, 741
sebaceous adenitis, *82, 98*, 434, *449–450*, 648, *651, 652*
trichoepithelioma, 674
standard schnauzer, 744
stanozolol, **810**
Staphage lysate, 217
staphoid A, 217
staph vaccine therapy, 217
staphylococcal scalded skin syndrome, 144
staphylococci, 143, 213
bacterial overgrowth syndrome, 215
biofilms, 144
coagulase-negative and -positive, 143
folliculitis *see* folliculitis, bacterial
methicillin resistance, 143–144
relationship with *Malassezia*, 484
virulence factors, 144–145
Staphylococcus aureus, 213
methicillin resistant *see* methicillin-resistant *Staphylococcus aureus*
zoonotic potential, 146
Staphylococcus pseudintermedius, 143, 144, 213
methicillin resistant *see* methicillin-resistant *Staphylococcus pseudintermedius*
resident vs transient strains, 212
zoonotic potential, 146
Staphylococcus schleiferi, 143, 213
methicillin resistant *see* methicillin-resistant *Staphylococcus schleiferi*
zoonotic potential, 146
sterile idiopathic interdigital granuloma, 589, *598*
sterile (idiopathic) nodular panniculitis (SNP), 65, *126*, 563, 564, 565, 566
Stevens–Johnson syndrome (SJS), 272–275
sticktight flea, 239, *248*
stratum basale, *5*
stratum corneum, 3, 4, *4, 5*
stratum granulosum, *5*
stratum spinosum, *5*
streptokinase, 144
streptolysin, 144
Sublimaze *see* fentanyl
sucralfate, 151, 499, **810**
Sulcrate *see* sucralfate
sulfadiazine, **811**
see also trimethoprim + sulfadiazine
sulfasalazine (sulfapyridine + mesalamine), 702, **811**
sulfonamides
adverse reactions, 272
potentiated, 151, **219**
sulfur/salicylic acid washes, 437
superantigens, 145, 215
superficial necrolytic dermatosis (SND), 665–668
clinical features, 62, 64, 619, *630–631*, 666, *669–670*
diagnostics, 622, 667, *671*
differential diagnosis, 621, 666–667
etiology/pathophysiology, 616, 665
footpads, *104, 135*, 592, *608*
signalment/history, 617, 666
therapeutics, 624, 668
supracaudal gland *see* tail gland
Suprax *see* cefixime
symptom checker, 59–69, *69–141*
Synthroid *see* levothyroxine
systemic lupus erythematosus (SLE), 63, *112*
clinical features, 470, *478–479, 705*
course and prognosis, 472
diagnostics, 471
nasal planum, 67
pigmentation abnormalities, 65
signalment/history, 469
therapeutics, 471–472

T_3 (triiodothyronine), 416, 420
T_4 (tetraiodothyronine), 416
free, 420
total, 419–420, 422
Tabanus spp. (horseflies), 240
tacrolimus ointment
for anal furunculosis/perianal fistula, 164
for cutaneous adverse drug reactions, 275
for lupus erythematosus, 472
for pemphigus complex, 196
Tagamet *see* cimetidine
tail biting/chasing
clinical features, 229–230, *237–238*
diagnostics, 232
differential diagnosis, 230–231
signalment/history, 228
tail gland
alopecia, 60, *81*
hyperplasia, 339, *350*
Tapazole *see* methimazole

target lesions, erythema multiforme, 274, *281*
Tavist *see* clemastine
tazarotene, 159
Tazicef *see* ceftazidime
T-cell lymphoma *see* cutaneous T-cell lymphoma
Tegopen *see* cloxacillin sodium
telogen defluxion, 61
telogen hairs, 44, *51*
Temaril *see* trimeprazine
tepoxalin, **811**
terbinafine, **812**
 for dermatophytosis, 324
 for *Malassezia* dermatitis, 483
 precautions, 484
 for sporotrichosis, 661
terminology, 11–14, *14–27*
 claw disorders, 588–589
 histopathology, **39–40**
Terramycin *see* oxytetracycline
Testex *see* testosterone
testicular tumors, 339, 341, *345–347*
testosterone, **812**
testosterone-responsive dermatoses, 61, 339
tetracycline, **812**
 for claw disorders, 594
 for lupus erythematosus, 471
 for nocardiosis, 538
 for panniculitis, 566
 for pemphigus/pemphigoid, 196
 for reactive cutaneous histiocytosis, 386
 for sebaceous adenitis, 650
 for vasculitis, 701
Th_1/Th_2/Th_{17} cells, 174–175
thrombovascular necrosis, proliferative, 699, *707*
thymoma-associated exfoliative dermatitis, feline, 616
 clinical features, 61, 62, *457*, 620, *632–633*
 diagnostics, 623
 differential diagnosis, 621
 footpads, 592, *609*
 therapeutics, 625
Thyrogen *see* thyrotropin
thyroid gland biopsy, 420
thyroid hormones, 416–417, 419–420
 supplementation, 420, 421–422, *428–429*
thyroiditis, lymphocytic, 417
thyroid-stimulating hormone (TSH) *see* thyrotropin
Thyro-Tabs *see* levothyroxine
thyrotoxicosis, 421
thyrotropin (TSH), 416, 417, **813**
 plasma levels, 420, 422
 stimulation test, 420–421
thyrotropin-releasing hormone (TRH), 416, **813**
 stimulation test, 421
L-thyroxine *see* levothyroxine
Thytropar *see* thyrotropin
Tibetan terrier, 744
Ticar *see* ticarcillin
ticarcillin, **814**
ticarcillin + clavulanate, 550, **813**
Ticillin *see* ticarcillin
tick bite dermatitis, 240, 244, 246
 clinical features, 242–243, *261*
 therapeutics, 247
tick bite hypersensitivity, 240, 244, 246
 clinical features, 242–243, *262*
 therapeutics, 247
tick paralysis, 243
ticks, 240, 243, *261*
Timentin *see* ticarcillin + clavulanate
tissue sampling *see* biopsy
tobramycin, **814**
toceranib phosphate, 499
α-tocopherol *see* vitamin E
toothbrush technique, sample collection, 29, *32, 334*
topical hormone replacement therapy, human
 clinical features, 61, *89*, 339, *348–349, 350*
 diagnostics, 340
topical therapy
 adverse reactions, 266, *269*, 273, *276*
 for atopic disease, 179
 for dermatophytosis, 324, 325, 326
 for epitheliotropic lymphoma, 369
 for keratinization disorders, 437–438
 for lupus erythematosus, 472
 for *Malassezia* dermatitis, 483
 for otitis, 549–550
 for pyoderma, 142, 151, 217, 220
 for sebaceous adenitis, 650
Toradol *see* ketoroloc tromethamine
touch imprints, 46, *54–55*
toxic epidermal necrolysis (TEN), 272–275
 clinical features, 63, *114*, 274, *283–285*
toxic shock syndrome toxins, 145
toy fox terrier, 417
toy poodle, 481, 741
traction alopecia, 60, *76*
tramadol, **814**
Tramisol *see* levamisole hydrochloride
transepidermal water loss (TEWL), 10, 431
trauma
 clawfold region, 66
 footpad sloughing/ulceration, 592, *611*
 see also self-injurious dermatoses
T_{reg} lymphocytes, 174, 175
Trental *see* pentoxifylline
tretinoin
 for acne, 159
 for actinic keratosis, 623, 624
 for photodermatoses, 578
Trexan *see* naltrexone
TRH *see* thyrotropin-releasing hormone
triamcinolone, **815**
 for autoimmune blistering diseases, 197
 for eosinophilic granuloma complex, 355
 for otitis, 550
Triamtabs *see* triamcinolone
Tribrissen *see* trimethoprim + sulfadiazine
trichoblastoma, 674, 675, 678, *691*

trichoepithelioma, 674, 675, 678, *689*
trichofolliculoma, 675, 677, 678, *691*
trichograms, 44, *50–52*
for demodicosis, 44, *50*, 299, *311*
tricholemmoma, 674, 675, *690*
Trichophyton mentagrophytes, 29, 320, 321
clinical features, *327, 328, 330*
culture and identification, *33, 34, 334–335*
onychomycosis, 591
trichorrhexis nodosa, 61
tricyclic antidepressants, 181, 234
triethylphosphine gold *see* auranofin
triiodothyronine *see* T_3
trilostane, **815**
for alopecia X, 341
for hyperadrenocorticism, 401–402, 411–412
trimeprazine, **816**
trimethoprim + sulfadiazine, **816**
for eosinophilic granuloma complex, 354
for nocardiosis, 538
for otitis, 550
trimethoprim + sulfamethoxazole, **219**, *281*, **816**
tripelennamine citrate, **816**
trizEDTA, 151
TSH *see* thyrotropin
tuberculosis, 510
client education and prognosis, 516
clinical features, 512
diagnostics, 513–514
signalment/history, 511
treatment, 515
zoonotic potential, 517
tumors, 13, *22*
fine-needle aspiration, 46–47
skin and adnexa *see* skin and adnexal tumors
see also neoplasia
Tylan *see* tylosin
Tylocine *see* tylosin
tylosin, **817**
tympanum, 542, *551–552*
assessing patency, 545, *561*
fluid accumulation behind, 544, *554–555*
rupture, 544, *556*
sample collection through, 31, *35*
tyrosine kinase inhibitors, 499
Tzanck preparation, 46

ulcer, 14, *25*
biopsy technique, 37
cytology, 46
indolent (rodent) *see* indolent ulcer
ulcerative dermatosis, 63–65
of collies and shelties, 64
leishmaniasis, 460, *464*
linear feline, 64
Ultram *see* tramadol
ultrasonography
for hyperadrenocorticism, 397, 399, 411
for hypothyroidism, 420
for paraneoplastic dermatoses, 621
for superficial necrolytic dermatitis, 667, *671*
ultraviolet light (UVL)-induced dermatoses, 574–578, 615, 672
urine cortisol-creatinine ratio, 398–399, 410
urticaria
adverse food reactions, 288, *294*
atopic disease, 176, *182*
drug-induced, 273, *281*
hymenoptera stings, 243
mast cell tumors, *500*
urticaria pigmentosa, 495, 496, *508*
uveodermatologic syndrome, canine, 692–694
clinical features, 692–693, *695–697*
depigmentation, 65, *129*
nasal planum, 67, *139*

vaccine reactions, cutaneous adverse, 273, *280*
ischemic dermatopathy, 699, 700, *709*
panniculitis, *570*
patchy alopecia, 59, *71*
vaccines, for pyoderma, 217
vacuolar degeneration, **40**
Valium *see* diazepam
Vancocin *see* vancomycin
Vancoled *see* vancomycin
vancomycin, 152, **817**
vasculitis, 698–702
clinical features, 63, *113*, 699–700, *703–709*
diagnostics, 700–701, *710*
differential diagnosis, 274, 700
drug-induced hypersensitivity, 274, 275
leukocytoclastic, 698
signalment/history, 698–699
therapeutics, 701–702
vasoproliferative plaque, 576, *583*
VDC-1101, 370
vesicles, 13, *18*, 37
vesicular cutaneous lupus erythematosus (VCLE), 468, 470, 471
vestibular (cranial nerve VIII) deficits, 544, 548, *557*
Vetalar *see* ketamine
Vetalog *see* triamcinolone
Vetergesic *see* buprenorphine hydrochloride
Vetoryl *see* trilostane
Vibramycin *see* doxycycline
vidarabine, 715
video-otoscopy, 546, *562*
vinblastine, 369, 498, 499
vincristine-cyclophosphamide-prednisolone (COP), 369
vinegar (acetic acid) solutions, **485**, 548
viral dermatoses, 711–715
clawfold region, 66, *602*
clinical features, 713
diagnostics, 714–715
differential diagnosis, 714
nasal planum, 67, *141*
signalment/history, 711–713

viral dermatoses (*Continued*)
therapeutics, 715
zoonotic, 728
vitamin A, **818**
for actinic keratosis, 623
for keratinization disorders, 438, 439
for photodermatoses, 578
for sebaceous adenitis, 651
see also retinoids
vitamin A-responsive dermatosis, 62, *95*, 433, *444*
vitamin C, 578, 623
vitamin D2, **770**
vitamin E, **818**
for actinic dermatoses, 578, 623
for dermatomyositis, 314
for lupus erythematosus, 472
for onychomadesis, 594
for panniculitis, 566
for pemphigus complex, 196
for skin and adnexal tumors, 679
for superficial necrolytic dermatitis, 668
for vasculitis, 701
vitiligo (idiopathic leukoderma/leukotrichia), *23*, 65, *128*
nasal planum, 67, *140*
vizsla, 744
sebaceous adenitis, 434, *451*, 648, *655–656*
Vogt Koyanagi Harada-like syndrome *see* uveodermatologic syndrome, canine
voriconazole, 324

walker hound, 522
walking dandruff, 634, 635
see also cheyletiellosis
wasp stings, 240–241, 243
weimaraner, 744
acne, 157
acral lick dermatitis, 228
allergic contact dermatitis, 266
blastomycosis, 522
mast cell tumors, 495
testicular tumors, 339
Welsh corgi, 617, 734, 740
Welsh terrier, 744
West Highland white terrier (westie), 744
allergic contact dermatitis, 266
atopic disease, 175
demodicosis, 297
epidermal dysplasia, 433
ichthyosis, 62, 432
Malassezia dermatitis, 481
primary seborrhea, 433
superficial necrolytic dermatosis, 617, 666
vitamin A-responsive dermatosis, 62
wheal, 13, *20*
wheaten terrier, 673, 744
whippet, 744
claw disorders, 589
color dilution alopecia, 434
long-haired, ivermectin sensitivity, 301, 637
pattern baldness, 60
solar-induced dermatoses, 575, 616, 673
squamous cell carcinoma, 673
Winer, dilated pore of, 674, 675, 677, 678
Winstrol-V *see* stanozolol
wire-haired fox terrier
allergic contact dermatitis, 266
atopic disease, 175
cutaneous adverse drug reactions, 273
demodicosis, 297
sebaceous gland hyperplasia, 433
Wood's lamp examination, *32*, 322, *332*

xanthomatosis, cutaneous, 64, *123*
feline diabetes mellitus, 338
footpads, 592, *613*
xylaxine hydrochloride, **818**
Xylocaine *see* lidocaine

yeast infections
atopic disease, 176, *183*
common misconceptions, **485**
diagnostics, **45**, 46, 47, *53–54*
ear, 547, 548
foot, 594, *601*
see also Malassezia dermatitis
yellow jackets, 240–241, 243
Yobine *see* yohimbine
yohimbine, 303, **819**
Yorkshire terrier, 744
color dilution alopecia, 61, 434
cutaneous adverse drug reactions, 273
ichthyosis, 62, 432
melanoderma/alopecia, 60, 65
vaccine-induced vasculitis, 699

Zantac *see* ranitidine
Zenecarp *see* carprofen
Zeniquin *see* marbofloxacin
zidovudine, 715, **819**
zinc-responsive dermatosis, 62, *96*, 434, *447–448*
zinc supplements, 668
Zithromax *see* azithromycin
zoonoses, 146–147, 727–728
blastomycosis, 527
coccidioidomycosis, 527
dermatophytosis, *330–331*, *729*
leishmaniasis, 458, 462
reverse, 146, 147
risk reduction, 147
sarcoptid mites, 634, 635, 638, *647*, *729*
sporotrichosis, 658–661
tuberculosis, 517
Zubrin *see* tepoxalin
Zyrtec *see* cetirizine
Zyvox *see* linezolid